Leffers

AF697014

FORENSIC MEDICINE

With a Foreword
from the point of view of Jurisprudence by

HARRY A. BLACKMUN

Associate Justice of the Supreme Court of the United States

and a Foreword
from the point of view of Forensic Science by

MILTON HELPERN

Late Chief Medical Examiner of the City of New York; Late Emeritus Professor of Forensic Medicine, New York University; Late Emeritus Professor of Pathology, Cornell University Medical College; Late President, American Academy of Compensation Medicine

FORENSIC MEDICINE

a study in trauma and environmental hazards

Volume I

MECHANICAL TRAUMA

edited by

C. G. TEDESCHI

Late Clinical Professor of Pathology, Boston University School of Medicine, and Late Director of Medical Education, Framingham Union Hospital, Framingham, Massachusetts

WILLIAM G. ECKERT

Editor of INFORM (International Reference Organization in Forensic Medicine and Science); Pathologist, St. Francis Hospital, Wichita, Kansas; Director, The Milton Helpern International Center for the Forensic Sciences, Wichita State University; Adjunct Professor of Forensic Medicine, Wichita State University

LUKE G. TEDESCHI

Director of Laboratories, Framingham Union Hospital, Framingham, Massachusetts; Associate Professor of Pathology, Boston University School of Medicine

associate editors:

HERBERT B. HECHTMAN
BERNARD KNIGHT
SHIELDS WARREN

1977 W. B. SAUNDERS COMPANY • Philadelphia • London • Toronto

W. B. Saunders Company: West Washington Square
Philadelphia, PA 19105

1 St. Anne's Road
Eastbourne, East Sussex BN21 3UN, England

1 Goldthorne Avenue
Toronto, Ontario M8Z 5T9, Canada

Forensic Medicine—Volume I, *Mechanical Trauma* Vol. I: ISBN 0-7216-8772-5
Volume II, *Physical Trauma* Vol. II: ISBN 0-7216-8773-3
Volume III, *Environmental Hazards* Vol. III: ISBN 0-7216-8774-1

© 1977 by W. B. Saunders Company. Copyright under the International Copyright Union. All rights reserved. This book is protected by copyright. No part of it may be reproduced, stored in a retrieval system, or transmitted in any form or by any means, electronic, mechanical, photocopying, recording, or otherwise, without written permission from the publisher. Made in the United States of America. Press of W. B. Saunders Company. Library of Congress catalog card number 74-4593.

Last digit is the print number: 9 8 7 6 5 4 3 2 1

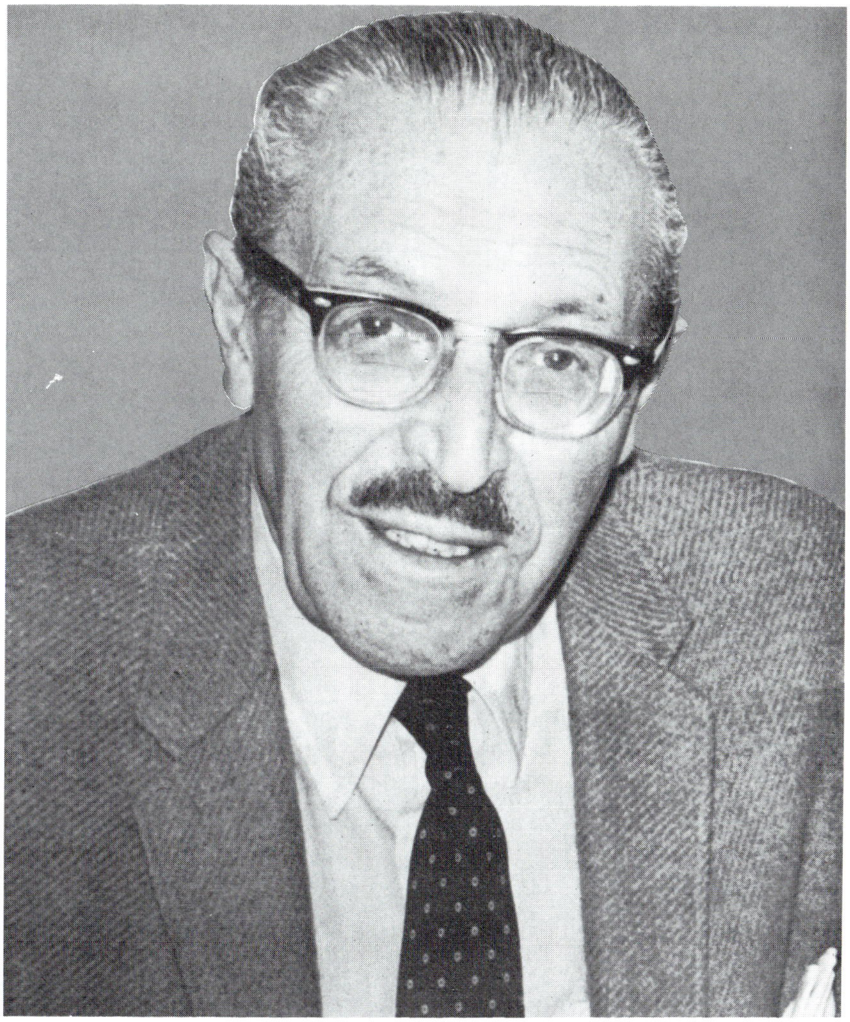

Dedicated to the memory of

C. G. TEDESCHI

by his associates in this work—
a lasting memorial to
his greatness as a person,
scientist, teacher, and writer

FOREWORD

Medicine and the Law long have been sister professions. Each serves the public. Neither dares or wants to be static. New learning constantly is sought, and as it is achieved, each profession adjusts happily and exultantly. What was almost absolute yesterday comes to be rejected today.

Despite this acknowledged fact of sisterhood and the further fact that each could learn much from the other, the paths of the two professions until comparatively recent years, it seems to me, have not been so close as one might expect and wish. Law and Medicine appear to have gone their respective ways, each engrossed in its own substantial problems and each concerned with its own development, except on those rare occasions of unavoidable intersection.

But it is encouraging that of late the two are drawing together, cognizant of their common problems and aware of their like responsibilities to the public each professes to serve. Their interests are not antagonistic and their concerns are not necessarily independent, although some lawyers and judges, and some physicians, act on occasion as though they were. My own happy personal experience with each profession has convinced me of the shortsightedness of assuming utter separateness.

Accordingly, it is gratifying that works, such as this one under the principal editorship of the Drs. Tedeschi and Eckert, and dealing with trauma of various kinds, with hazards to which man is exposed, and with the legal principles that are applicable to trauma and hazards, come to exposition and public print. *Forensic Medicine* should be of assistance to the physician who finds himself involved in the legal processes of his patient or examinee, to the forensic scientist who is positioned at the crossroads of the two professions, and to the attorney and the jurist who finds himself confronted with a medical feature of importance in a lawsuit or legal investigation.

May there be more of this type of endeavor as the future unfolds. After all, Mecicine and the Law are *service* professions—see *Virginia State Board of Pharmacy* v. *Virginia Citizens Consumer Council,* 425 U.S. 748, 773 n. 25, and 774 (1976)—and cooperation and understanding, rather than distance and isolation, should be their way of life.

HARRY A. BLACKMUN
Washington, D.C.

FOREWORD

Dr. Cesare George Tedeschi, a distinguished colleague for whom I had always had great admiration, honored me greatly when he invited me to write a Foreword to this monumental work on Forensic Medicine. He was then well along in assembling and editing it, and it is indeed very sad that his death on June 26, 1974, interrupted this great undertaking. Aware of his heritage and of the great contributions of the Italian Renaissance, especially of the versatile genius of that period, Leonardo da Vinci, Dr. Tedeschi has contributed much to our knowledge and understanding of the broad field of pathology and the interrelationships of its theoretic and practical subdivisions.

Forensic medicine is important not only as an offshoot of pathology but, in its own right, as an integral and essential part of that major discipline as well as of medicine in general and the public health. A perusal of the list of contributors to and the table of contents of this work indicates the breadth with which the subject is treated. Pathology is forensic medicine; forensic medicine is pathology.

The completion of the editing and assembling of this significant three-volume work was ably undertaken by Dr. Luke G. Tedeschi, his devoted son who, like his father before him, is Director of Laboratories at the Framingham Union Hospital in Massachusetts, and Dr. William Eckert, Pathologist at the St. Francis Hospital in Wichita, Kansas, Head of the medicolegal institute of the University of Wichita, Editor of INFORM, and President of the International Association of Forensic Sciences.

This three-volume contribution, *Forensic Medicine,* will be of great value to the legal profession, many of whose members must deal with its subject matter in their everyday work. They will find it informative and authoritative. By the same token, physicians involved in medicolegal responsibilities, who are required to understand the causation and mechanism of injuries and their complications, causal relationships in industrial medicine and workmen's compensation claims, who must attend those who sustain injury, and who must recognize and clarify medical issues that may come before the courts, will derive much help from this work not only in the area of direct trauma, but especially in that dealing with industrial and environmental hazards.

Milton Helpern

PREFACE

As we introduce this book to the reader, it is proper to ask what Forensic Medicine is. It may be defined as the application within jurisprudence of medical knowledge and the findings of its underlying sciences to the solution of questions of law. These questions concern the causes of death, identity of the living and dead, results of injuries of all kinds, effects of violent crimes and unnatural offenses, and the nature of toxic or lethal agents—those introduced by intent into the human structure, those ingested accidentally or in ignorance of their nature, and those more subtly introduced by environmental pollutants.

This work, then, brings together the professions of medicine and law, both having an ancient lineage, a tradition of respected practice, and a background of independent thought and investigation. Both have, too, an immediacy of function: To prevent, alleviate, and correct human ills by understanding the body of man and the regulation of society. Neither may disdain the right to be pragmatic, for pragmatism is the study of phenomena from the point of view of their discernible causes, antecedents, and effects.

The work may, hence, be seen as a bridge between two disciplines resting on the foundation of theoretical principles deduced from practice or observation and pursuing in parallel paths the same goal—the search for truth and the amendment of grievance, whether the wrong be of a physical or moral nature.

The custodian of the law has a more than perfunctory interest in what medicine has to offer. He wants to know how far medical science can go in answering with accuracy and reasonable certainty questions relevant to medicolegal problems. Similarly, the physician must be acquainted with the legal theories pertinent to trauma and hazards—in brief, with the concepts of negligence, malpractice, product liability, due cause, responsibility under the law, and the right to damages.

It is our hope that these volumes will be of value in the analysis and evaluation of problems related to both trauma and environmental hazard: problems that daily confront physicians, bioscientists—especially physiologists and toxicologists—attorneys, forensic scientists, and those charged with the enforcement of law, the examination of evidence, and the conduct of lawful inquiry.

This work has been the result of the expertness and unstinting cooperation of many individual writers who have been willing to set out and share their knowledge, and the result, too, of wise counsel and unfailing helpfulness from Associate Editors Herbert Hechtman, Bernard Knight, and Shields Warren.

Our appreciation is extended to John Dusseau, Vice President and Editor of the W. B. Saunders Company, whose insight into the need for this international effort facilitated our work. Our deepest gratitude also goes to Helen Clark for her valuable editorial and secretarial assistance, as well as for her steadfast patience and loyalty during many trying moments.

Above all, we are indebted to Cesare G. Tedeschi, who, despite failing health, originated the project and nurtured it through its early stages. We are sorry that he was not able to see his work brought to fruition.

THE EDITORS

CONTRIBUTORS

FREDERICK W. ACKROYD, M.D.
Associate Professor of Surgery, Harvard Medical School, Boston, Massachusetts. Chief of Surgical Services, Mount Auburn Hospital, Cambridge, Massachusetts.
Injuries of Liver, Pancreas, Spleen, and Gallbladder

GASPAR W. ANASTASI, M.D.
Associate Professor of Surgery (Plastic), Boston University Medical Center, Boston, Massachusetts. Chief of Plastic Surgery, University Hospital, Joseph P. Kennedy Memorial Hospital, Brighton Marine Hospital, Boston City Hospital, Boston, Massachusetts; Consultant in Plastic Surgery, Veterans Administration Hospital, Jamaica Plain, Massachusetts.
Facial Trauma

JAVIER ARIAS-STELLA, M.D., Ph.D., F.R.C. Path.
Universidad Peruana Cayetano Heredia, Lima, Peru. Chief Pathologist, Loayza Hospital, Lima, Peru.
High-Altitude Physiopathology

MARVIN E. ARONSON, M.D., F.A.A.F.S.
Medical Examiner, City of Philadelphia; Clinical Associate Professor of Forensic Pathology, Hahnemann Medical College; Visiting Lecturer in Forensic Pathology, Jefferson Medical College; Clinical Associate Professor of Forensic Pathology, Temple University; Adjunct Associate Professor of Pathology, University of Pennsylvania, Philadelphia, Pennsylvania. Chairman, Board of Consultants, International Association of Coroners and Medical Examiners; Regional Vice-President, Pennsylvania State Coroner's Association; Consultant, The Philadelphia County Medical Society Subcommittee on Mortality Survey, Philadelphia, Pennsylvania.
Forensic Roentgenology

ALBERT H. BANNER, Ph.D.
Professor of Zoology and Marine Biologist, Hawaii Institute of Marine Biology, University of Hawaii, Honolulu, Hawaii.
Hazardous Marine Animals

CHARLES J. BARR, LL.B.
Partner, Moore, Barr and Kerwin, Detroit, Michigan.
Drug and Device Litigation

STANTON O. BERG, LL.B.
Firearms Consultant, Minneapolis, Minnesota.
Ballistics Laboratory

ROBERT L. BERGER, M.D.
Professor of Surgery, Boston University School of Medicine, Director of Cardiothoracic Surgery, University Hospital and Boston City Hospital, Boston, Massachusetts.
Injuries of the Thorax

JOHN J. BYRNE, M.D.
Professor of Surgery, Boston University School of Medicine, Boston, Massachusetts. Director of Hand Surgery, Boston City Hospital and University Hospital, Boston, Massachusetts; Director of Surgery, Framingham Union Hospital, Framingham, Massachusetts.
Injuries of the Hand

GUIDO CALABRESI, LL.B.
John Thomas Smith Professor of Law, Yale University, New Haven, Connecticut.
Cost of Accidents

PIETRO CASTELNUOVO-TEDESCO, M.D.
James G. Blakemore Professor of Psychiatry, Vanderbilt University School of Medicine, Nashville, Tennessee.
Transplant, Body Image, Psychosis

JOHN S. CHAPMAN, M.D.
Professor of Internal Medicine, Southwestern Medical School, University of Texas Health Science Center, Dallas, Texas. Attending Physician, Parkland Memorial Hospital, Dallas, Texas; Consultant, Veterans Administration Hospital, East Texas Chest Hospital, and Baylor University Medical Center, Dallas, Texas, and Veterans Administration Hospital, Temple, Texas.
Fungal and Mycobacterial Infections

DAVID CHARLES, M.D.
Professor and Chairman of Obstetrics and Gynecology, Memorial University of Newfoundland, St. John's, Newfoundland.
Injuries of the Female Genital Tract

JOHN I. COE, M.D.
Professor, Department of Laboratory Medicine and Pathology, University of Minnesota Medical School, Minneapolis, Minnesota. Chief of Pathology, Hennepin County Medical Center, Minneapolis, Minnesota; Chief Medical Examiner, Hennepin County, Minneapolis, Minnesota.
Postmortem Chemistry

IRA A. COHEN, J.D.
Partner, Goldsmith, Cohen and Simon, New York, New York.
Law of Prenatal and Perinatal Injury

WARREN M. CROSBY, M.D.
Vice Chairman and Professor, Department of Gynecology and Obstetrics, University of Oklahoma College of Medicine, University of Oklahoma Health Sciences Center, Oklahoma City, Oklahoma.
Trauma and Pregnancy

JOANNE M. CUTTER, M.S.
Program Director, Medical Technology School, Framingham Union Hospital and Framingham State College, Framingham, Massachusetts.
Parasitic Diseases

ROBERT C. DAVIS, M.D.
Assistant Professor of Surgery, Boston University School of Medicine, Boston, Massachusetts. Visiting Surgeon, University Hospital; Attending Surgeon, Vascular Surgery,

Boston Veterans Administration Hospital; Consultant in Vascular Surgery, United States Public Health Hospital; Director, Vascular Surgery, Boston City Hospital, Boston, Massachusetts.
Vascular Injuries

DONALD J. DAWIDOFF, LL.B.
Member of the New York and District of Columbia Bars; Practicing Attorney, New York, New York.
Malpractice, Products Liability, Causation, Damages

BARRY C. DORN, M.D.
Major, United States Army Reserve, Fort Dix, New Jersey.
Injuries of the Musculoskeletal System

WILLIAM G. ECKERT, M.D.
Director, The Milton Helpern International Center for the Forensic Sciences, Wichita State University; Adjunct Professor of Forensic Medicine, Wichita State University, Wichita, Kansas. Editor of INFORM (International Reference Organization in Forensic Medicine and Science); Pathologist, St. Francis Hospital, Wichita, Kansas.
Self-Inflicted Wounds, Injuries Related to Atmospheric Pressure, Alcohol and Alcoholic Intoxication, Crash Injuries on the Road, Sex Crimes and Abnormal Sexual Behavior, Medicolegal Autopsy, Homicide and Suicide

THEODORE EHRENREICH, M.D.
Associate Clinical Professor of Community Medicine, Mt. Sinai School of Medicine of City University of New York; Assistant Professor of Forensic Medicine, New York University School of Medicine, New York, New York. Pathologist, Lutheran Medical Center, New York, New York.
Occupational and Environmental Disease

NILS-ÅKE EK
Head of Chemical Section, The National Laboratory of Forensic Science, Linköping, Sweden.
Arson Investigation

BERNARD J. FICARRA, M.D., Sc.D., Ph.D., LL.D., F.A.C.L.M., F.I.A. Law Sci.
Emeritus Professorial Research Associate in Physiology, Postgraduate School, Long Island University, Brooklyn, New York. Director of Medico-Legal Research, The Ficarra Foundation, Oyster Bay, New York.
Therapeutic Misadventures: Drugs

PIERRE A. FINCK, M.D.
Forensic Pathology Consultant, United States Army, Europe, and Seventh Army.
Carbon Monoxide Poisoning

CLAUDE ALBEE FRAZIER, M.D.
Consultant in Allergy, Memorial Mission Hospital and St. Joseph's Hospital, Asheville, North Carolina.
Insect Bites and Stings

MURRAY M. FREED, M.D.
Professor and Chairman, Department of Rehabilitation Medicine, Boston University School of Medicine, Boston, Massachusetts. Chief, Department of Rehabilitation

Medicine; Director, New England Regional Spinal Cord Injury Center in University Hospital, Boston, Massachusetts.
Disability from Spinal Cord Injury

PAUL SIGMUND FRIEDMAN, M.D., F.A.C.R., F.A.C.C.P., F.A.C.L.M., F.A.C. Nucl. Med.
Instructor in Radiology, Graduate School of the University of Pennsylvania, Philadelphia, Pennsylvania. Assistant Radiologist, Episcopal Hospital, Philadelphia, Pennsylvania; Consulting Radiologist, Malvern Institute for Psychiatric and Alcoholic Studies, Malvern, Pennsylvania.
Legal Problems Arising from Use of Radiation, Forensic Roentgenology

JOHAN CHRISTOPHER GIERTSEN, Dr. Med.
Professor of Forensic Medicine, University of Bergen, Bergen, Norway.
Drowning

LEE S. GOLDSMITH, M.D., LL.B., F.C.L.M.
Partner, Goldsmith, Cohen, and Simon, New York, New York.
Law of Prenatal and Perinatal Injury

RICHARD M. GOODMAN, J.D.
Attorney, Detroit, Michigan.
Drug and Device Litigation

JORDAN B. GREENFIELD, M.D.
Associate Clinical Professor of Radiology, Tufts University School of Medicine, Boston, Massachusetts. Director, Department of Ultrasound, Leonard Morse Hospital, Natick, Massachusetts; Radiologist, Leonard Morse Hospital, Natick, Massachusetts, and New England Medical Center, Boston, Massachusetts.
Medical Applications of Ultrasound

ROBERT ALAN HALL, O.B.E., C.Chem., M.R.I.C.
Principal Scientific Officer, Department of Commerce; Head of Explosives Section, The Northern Ireland Forensic Science Laboratory, Department of Commerce, Belfast, Northern Ireland.
Bomb and Explosives Investigation

JONATHAN P. HARVEY, J.D.
Attorney, Albany, New York.
Environmental Causes of Congenital Malformation, Informed Consent

HERBERT B. HECHTMAN, M.D.
Associate Professor of Surgery, Boston University School of Medicine, Boston, Massachusetts. Director of Surgical Intensive Care Unit, Trauma Center, and Emergency Room, University Hospital, Boston, Massachusetts.
Injuries of the Gastrointestinal Tract, Systemic Response to Trauma, Post Traumatic Embolism

MILTON HELPERN, M.D.
Late Emeritus Professor of Forensic Medicine, New York University; Late Emeritus Professor of Pathology, Cornell University Medical College, New York, New York. Late Chief Medical Examiner of the City of New York, New York; Late President, American Academy of Compensation Medicine.
The Pathologist in Compensation Cases

JORMA ILMARI HIRVONEN, M.D.
Professor of Forensic Medicine, University of Oulu, Oulu, Finland.
Hypothermic Injury

J. SUDLER HOOD, M.D.
Major, United States Army Reserve, Fort Dix, New Jersey.
Injuries of the Musculoskeletal System

THEODORE H. INGALLS, M.D.
Research Professor Emeritus of Preventive Medicine (Epidemiology), Boston University School of Medicine, Boston, Massachusetts. Senior Advisory Staff in Pathology, Research and Pediatrics, Framingham Union Hospital, Framingham, Massachusetts.
Café Coronary, Environmental Causes of Congenital Malformations

ROBERT J. JOLING, J.D.
Associate Professor of Medical Jurisprudence, University of Arizona College of Medicine, Tucson, Arizona.
Property of the Dead Body

E. STEWART JONES, JR., LL.D., J.D.
Attorney, Troy, New York.
Negligence

RONALD F. KAPLAN, M.D., F.A.C.S.
Clinical Instructor in Orthopedic Surgery, Boston University School of Medicine, Boston, Massachusetts. Associate Visiting Orthopedic Surgeon, University Hospital, Boston, Massachusetts.
Injuries of the Musculoskeletal System

ELLIS R. KERLEY, Ph.D.
Professor of Anthropology and Chairman, Department of Anthropology, University of Maryland, College Park, Maryland.
Forensic Anthropology

MOHANDAS M. KINI, M.D., Ph.D.
Assistant Professor of Ophthalmology, Boston University School of Medicine, Boston, Massachusetts. Associate Visiting Surgeon of Ophthalmology and Chief of the Retina Service, University Hospital, Boston, Massachusetts.
Injuries of the Eye

EDGAR W. KIVELA, Ph.D.
Chief, Division of Crime Detection, Bureau of Disease Control and Laboratory Services, Michigan Department of Public Health, Lansing, Michigan.
Toxicology Laboratory

BERNARD KNIGHT, M.D., B.Ch., F.R.C.Path., D.M.J., Barrister-at-Law
Reader in Forensic Pathology, Welsh National School of Medicine, Cardiff, Wales. Consultant Forensic Pathologist, The Royal Infirmary, Cardiff, Wales.
The Battered Child, Firearm Injuries, Blood Identification, Accidents in the Home and the Hospital, Industrial and Agricultural Hazards

ROBERT J. KRANE, M.D.
Assistant Professor of Urology, Boston University School of Medicine, Boston, Massachusetts. Associate Director, Urology Department, Boston City Hospital; Assistant Chief, Urology Department, University Hospital, Boston, Massachusetts.
Injuries of the Genitourinary System

HOWARD M. LEIBOWITZ, M.D.
Professor and Chairman, Department of Ophthalmology, Boston University School of Medicine, Boston, Massachusetts. Ophthalmologist-in-Chief, Boston University Medical Center, Boston, Massachusetts.
Injuries of the Eye

SIMMONS LESSELL, M.D.

Professor of Ophthalmology and Associate Professor of Neurology, Boston University School of Medicine, Boston, Massachusetts. Director, Department of Ophthalmology, Boston City Hospital; Visiting Surgeon of Ophthalmology, University Hospital, Boston, Massachusetts.

Injuries of the Eye

GERALD L. LOONEY, M.D.

Assistant Professor, University of Southern California School of Medicine, Los Angeles, California. Director of Research and Allied Health Training, Department of Emergency Medicine, Los Angeles County–University of California Medical Center, Los Angeles, California.

Emergency Care

ROBERT A. MacCREADY, M.D.

Retired Director, Diagnostic Laboratories of Massachusetts, Department of Public Health, Jamaica Plain, Massachusetts. Retired Lecturer on Microbiology, Harvard School of Public Health, Boston, Massachusetts.

Bacterial Food Poisoning

ANDREAS C. MAEHLY, Ph.D.

Professor, National Laboratory of Forensic Science, Linköping, Sweden.

Arson Investigation

ARTHUR KEITH MANT, M.D., F.R.C.Path.

Professor of Forensic Medicine, Guy's Hospital Medical School, London. Consultant in Forensic Medicine, King's College Hospital, London; Visiting Lecturer in Medical Jurisprudence, St. Mary's Hospital, Paddington, London.

Postmortem Injuries

THOMAS K. MARSHALL, M.D., F.R.C.Path.

Professor of Forensic Medicine, The Queen's University of Belfast, Northern Ireland. State Pathologist, Northern Ireland; Consultant in Pathology to the Northern Ireland Health and Social Services Boards, Belfast, Northern Ireland.

Explosion Injuries

JOHN R. McCORMICK, M.D.

Assistant Professor of Surgery, Boston University School of Medicine, Boston, Massachusetts. Assistant Visiting Surgeon, Cardiothoracic Surgery, University Hospital; Associate Visiting Surgeon and Assistant Director, Thoracic Surgery, Boston City Hospital, Boston, Massachusetts.

Injuries of the Thorax

PETER D. McGANN, M.D.

Resident in Orthopedic Surgery, University Hospital, Boston, Massachusetts.

Injuries of the Musculoskeletal System

DEREK McVITTY, O.B.E., A.I.W.Sc., F.I.Biol., F.L.S.F. Inst. F., A.I. Gas E.

Assistant Secretary, Department of Commerce, Government of Northern Ireland, Belfast, Northern Ireland.

Bomb and Explosives Investigation

JULIA FRANCES MORTON, D.Sc.

Research Associate Professor and Director of the Morton Collectanea, University of Miami, Coral Gables, Florida. Consultant, Poison Control Centers, Florida State Board of Health.

Poisonous Plants

MATTI K. MÖTTÖNEN, M.D.

Senior Lecturer of Forensic Medicine, University of Turku, Turku, Finland.
Postmortem Injury by Animals

PEKKA NUORTEVA, Ph.D.

Professor of Environmental Science, University of Helsinki, Department of Environmental Science, Helsinki, Finland. Former Custodian at the Zoological Museum, University of Helsinki, and Lecturer of Parasitology and Medical Entomology at the Veterinary Highschool, Helsinki, Finland.
Insects as Forensic Indicators

MATTI T. NUUTILA, M.D.

Department of Forensic Medicine, University of Turku, Finland.
Postmortem Injury by Animals

CARL A. OLSSON, M.D.

Professor and Chairman, Department of Urology, Boston University School of Medicine, Boston, Massachusetts. Urologist-in-Chief, University Hospital; Director of Urology, Boston City Hospital; Assistant Chief, Urology Section, Veteran's Administration Hospital, Boston, Massachusetts.
Injuries of the Genitourinary Tract

FRANK O. RAASCH, JR., M.D., Capt. (M.C.) U.S.N. (ret.)

Associate Professor of Pathology, University of California at San Diego, San Diego, California. Former Forensic Pathologist for the Navy (west coast); Consultant to the San Diego County Coroner, San Diego, California.
Drug Abuse

JYRKI RAEKALLIO, M.D.

Professor and Chairman, Department of Forensic Medicine, University of Turku, Turku, Finland.
Timing of the Wound

JOEL S. RANKIN, M.D.

Associate Professor of Obstetrics and Gynecology, Boston City Hospital, Boston, Massachusetts. Director of Obstetrics and Gynecology, Framingham Union Hospital, Framingham, Massachusetts.
Injuries of the Female Genital Tract

WILLIAM J. REALS, M.D.

Director of Laboratories and Vice-President for Medical Affairs, St. Joseph Medical Center, Wichita, Kansas.
Air Disaster Injuries

EVERETT R. RHOADES, M.D.

Professor of Medicine, University of Oklahoma College of Medicine, Oklahoma City, Oklahoma. Chief, Infectious Diseases Section, University of Oklahoma College of Medicine and Veterans Administration Hospital, Oklahoma City, Oklahoma.
Diseases Transmitted from Animals to Man

MARC RICHMAN, M.D.

Associate Clinical Professor of Ophthalmology, Boston University School of Medicine, Boston, Massachusetts. Visiting Surgeon of Ophthalmology, University Hospital, Boston, Massachusetts.
Injuries of the Eye

ABRAHAM ROSENTHAL, M.D., F.A.C.S., F.A.A.F.S.

Assistant Attending Surgeon, Maimonides Medical Center; Associate Attending Surgeon, Long Island College Hospital, Brooklyn, New York. Assistant Medical Examiner, Office of Chief Medical Examiner, City of New York, New York.

Complications of Surgical Procedures

ERIK A. RUDH

Electrical Engineer, Solna, Sweden.

Arson Investigation

FINDLAY E. RUSSELL, M.D., Ph.D.

Professor of Neurology, Physiology, and Biology, University of Southern California, Los Angeles, California. Attending Physician, Los Angeles County–University of Southern California Medical Center and White Memorial Hospital, Los Angeles, California, and Loma Linda University Medical Center, Loma Linda, California.

Venomous Snakes

ALFRED M. SADLER, JR., M.D.

Clinical Fellow in Medicine, Harvard Medical School, Boston, Massachusetts. Resident in Internal Medicine, Massachusetts General Hospital, Boston, Massachusetts.

Organ Transplantation and the Law

BLAIR L. SADLER, J.D.

Assistant Vice President, The Robert Wood Johnson Foundation, Princeton, New Jersey.

Organ Transplantation and the Law

ARTHUR FREDERICK SCHIFF, M.D.

Senior Attending Physician, Mercy Hospital, Miami; Attending Physician, Rape Treatment Center, Miami, Florida. Deputy Medical Examiner, Dade County, Florida.

Rape

PHILIP H. SECHZER, M.D.

Professor of Anesthesiology, Downstate Medical Center, State University of New York, Brooklyn, New York. Director of Anesthesiology, Maimonides Medical Center, Brooklyn, New York.

Complications of Anesthesia

IRVING J. SELIKOFF, M.D.

Professor of Community Medicine, Mount Sinai School of Medicine, City University of New York, New York, New York.

Occupational and Environmental Disease

MARK M. SHERMAN, M.D.

Chief Resident, Cardiothoracic Surgery, and Instructor in Surgery, University Hospital and Boston City Hospital, Boston, Massachusetts.

Injuries of the Thorax

ENDRE SOMOGYI, M.D., D.Sc.

Head and Professor of Forensic Medicine, Semmelweis Medical School Department of Forensic Medicine, Budapest, Hungary.

Injury by Electricity

M. STUART STRONG, M.D.

Professor of Otolaryngology, Boston University School of Medicine, Boston, Massa-

chusetts. Chief of Otolaryngology, University Hospital; Chief of Otolaryngology, Boston Veterans Administration Hospital, Boston, Massachusetts.
Injuries of the Auditory Apparatus

WILLIAM Q. STURNER, M.D., D.M.J., F.A.C.P.

Associate Professor, Department of Pathology and Laboratory Medicine; Director, Subsection of Forensic Medicine, Division of Biological and Medical Sciences, Brown University, Providence, Rhode Island. Consultant in Pathology, The Miriam Hospital and Rhode Island Hospital, Providence, Rhode Island.
Sudden Infant Death

CESARE G. TEDESCHI, M.D.

Late Clinical Professor of Pathology, Boston University School of Medicine, Boston, Massachusetts; Late Director of Medical Education, Framingham Union Hospital, Framingham, Massachusetts.
Injuries of Head and Spine, Injury by Electricity, Hyperthermic Injury

LUKE G. TEDESCHI, M.D.

Associate Professor of Pathology, Boston University School of Medicine, Boston, Massachusetts. Director of Laboratories, Framingham Union Hospital, Framingham, Massachusetts.
The Wound and Related Issues, Injuries to Adipose Tissue, Systemic Response to Trauma, Post-traumatic Embolism, Parasitic Diseases, Café Coronary

ABRAHAM TOWBIN, M.D.

Former Professor of Pathology, Chicago Medical School, Chicago, Illinois; Former Pathologist, Collaborative Perinatal Project, Department of Neuropathology, Harvard Medical School, Boston, Massachusetts. Pathologist, Massachusetts Department of Mental Health, Danvers State Hospital; Hathorne, Massachusetts; Associate in Pathology (Neonatology), Norwood Hospital, Norwood, Massachusetts.
Injury to the Fetus and Newborn

SOLCO W. TROMP, Ph.D.

Director, Biometeorological Research Center, Leiden, The Netherlands.
Environmental Effect on Accidents, Crime, Disease, and Suicide

CHARLES W. VAUGHAN, M.D.

Associate Professor of Otolaryngology, Boston University School of Medicine, Boston, Massachusetts. Associate Chief of Otolaryngology, University Hospital and Boston Veterans Administration Hospital, Boston, Massachusetts.
Injuries of the Auditory Apparatus

PAUL E. WALKER, J.D.

Member of the New York Bar; Practicing Attorney, New York, New York.
Products Liability

SHIELDS WARREN, M.D., LL.D. (Hon.), D.Sc. (Hon.)

Professor Emeritus of Pathology, Harvard Medical School at the New England Deaconess Hospital, Boston, Massachusetts. Consultant in Pathology, New England Deaconess Hospital, Boston, Massachusetts.
Occupational and Environmental Exposure to Ionizing Radiation

CHARLES L. WINEK, Ph.D.

Professor of Toxicology, School of Pharmacy, Duquesne University, Pittsburgh, Pennsylvania. Chief Toxicologist, Allegheny County Coroner's Office, Pittsburgh, Pennsylvania.
Chemical Injury

GERALD N. WOGAN, Ph.D.
Professor of Toxicology, Massachusetts Institute of Technology, Cambridge, Massachusetts.
Food-Borne Environmental Toxicants

EDWARD D. WOOLRIDGE, JR., D.D.S., LL.B., F.A.C.D.
Clinical Instructor, Department of Oral Health, Health Services, Tufts University School of Dental Medicine, Boston, Massachusetts. Chief of Dental Services, United States Coast Guard Academy Hospital, New London, Connecticut.
Oral Trauma, Forensic Odontology

JOHN P. WYSOCKI, M.D.
Assistant Professor of Surgery (Plastic), Boston University School of Medicine, Boston, Massachusetts. Assistant Surgeon, Boston City Hospital and University Hospital; Visiting Surgeon, Joseph P. Kennedy Memorial Hospital; Staff Surgeon, Veterans Administration Hospital, Boston, Massachusetts.
Facial Trauma

CONTENTS

VOLUME I

PART I TRAUMA BY PHYSICAL AGENTS........... 1

SECTION 1 MECHANICAL INJURY

CHAPTER 1

THE WOUND: AN INTRODUCTION TO RELATED ISSUES............. 3
Luke G. Tedeschi

CHAPTER 2

TIMING OF THE WOUND 22
Jyrki Raekallio

CHAPTER 3

THE WOUND: ASSESSMENT BY ORGAN SYSTEMS 29

I. Head and Spine 29
C. G. Tedeschi

II. Long-Term Disability from Spinal Cord Injury 76
Murray M. Freed

III. The Eye and Its Adnexa 88
Howard M. Leibowtiz, Mohandas M. Kini, Simmons Lessell, and Marc Richman

IV. Auditory Apparatus: The Cochlear-Vestibular System 132
Charles W. Vaughan and M. Stuart Strong

V. Facial Trauma 140
G. W. Anastasi and J. P. Wysocki

VI. Oral Trauma and Pathosis 147
Edward D. Woolridge, Jr.

VII. The Thorax 199
Mark M. Sherman, John R. McCormick, and Robert L. Berger

VIII. THE LIVER, PANCREAS, SPLEEN, AND GALLBLADDER 210
Frederick W. Ackroyd

IX. GASTROINTESTINAL TRACT 215
Herbert B. Hechtman

X. VASCULAR SYSTEM 221
Robert C. Davis

XI. GENITOURINARY TRACT 227
Carl A. Olsson and Robert J. Krane

XII. THE FEMALE GENITAL TRACT 243
David Charles and Joel Rankin

XIII. MUSCULOSKELETAL SYSTEM 259
Ronald F. Kaplan, Barry C. Dorn, J. Sudler Hood, and Peter D. McGann

XIV. ADIPOSE TISSUE 361
Luke G. Tedeschi

XV. THE HAND 365
John J. Byrne

CHAPTER 4

SYSTEMIC RESPONSE TO TRAUMA 386
Herbert B. Hechtman and Luke G. Tedeschi

CHAPTER 5

POSTTRAUMATIC EMBOLISM 406
Luke G. Tedeschi and Herbert B. Hechtman

CHAPTER 6

TRAUMA AND PREGNANCY 423
Warren M. Crosby

CHAPTER 7

TRAUMA IN PREGNANCY—INJURY TO THE FETUS AND NEWBORN 436
Abraham Towbin

CHAPTER 8

THE LAW OF PRENATAL AND PERINATAL INJURIES 487
Lee S. Goldsmith and Ira A. Cohen

CHAPTER 9

SELF-INFLICTED WOUNDS 496
William G. Eckert

CHAPTER 10

THE BATTERED CHILD 500

Bernard Knight

SECTION 2 INJURY BY FIREARMS, BOMBS, AND EXPLOSIVES

CHAPTER 11

FIREARM INJURIES 510

Bernard Knight

CHAPTER 12

THE FORENSIC BALLISTICS LABORATORY 527

Stanton O. Berg

CHAPTER 13

INVESTIGATION OF BOMBS AND EXPLOSIVES 570

Derek McVitty and Robert Alan Hall

CHAPTER 14

EXPLOSION INJURIES 612

T. K. Marshall

SECTION 3 BAROTRAUMA (DYSBARISM)

CHAPTER 15

INJURIES FROM INCREASED ATMOSPHERIC PRESSURE 636

William G. Eckert

CHAPTER 16

INJURIES RELATED TO LOW ATMOSPHERIC PRESSURE 641

William G. Eckert

SECTION 4

CHAPTER 17

INJURY BY ELECTRICAL FORCE 645

Endre Somogyi and C. G. Tedeschi

SECTION 5 INJURY BY IONIZING RADIATION

CHAPTER 18

EFFECTS OF OCCUPATIONAL AND ENVIRONMENTAL EXPOSURE TO IONIZING RADIATION 677

Shields Warren

CHAPTER 19

LEGAL PROBLEMS ARISING FROM THE UTILIZATION OF RADIATION 686

Paul S. Friedman

SECTION 6 THERMAL INJURY

CHAPTER 20

SYSTEMIC AND LOCALIZED HYPERTHERMIC INJURY 701

C. G. Tedeschi

CHAPTER 21

ARSON INVESTIGATION 730

Nils-Åke Ek, Andreas Maehly, and Erik Rudh

CHAPTER 22

SYSTEMIC AND LOCAL EFFECTS OF HYPOTHERMIA 758

Jorma Hirvonen

SECTION 7 ULTRASOUND INJURY

CHAPTER 23

APPLICATIONS OF ULTRASOUND IN MEDICINE 775

Jordan B. Greenfield

VOLUME II

PART II INJURY BY CHEMICAL AGENTS 785

CHAPTER 24

FOOD-BORNE ENVIRONMENTAL TOXICANTS 787

Gerald N. Wogan

CHAPTER 25

THE TOXICOLOGY LABORATORY 800

Edgar W. Kivela

CHAPTER 26

BLOOD IDENTIFICATION 810

Bernard Knight

CHAPTER 27

ALCOHOL AND ALCOHOLIC INTOXICATION 818

William G. Eckert

CHAPTER 28

DRUG ABUSE 826

Frank Raasch, Jr.

CHAPTER 29
EXPOSURE TO CARBON MONOXIDE 840
Pierre A. Finck

PART III CRASH INJURIES AND ACCIDENTS.................................. 851

CHAPTER 30
CRASH INJURIES ON THE ROAD 853
William G. Eckert

CHAPTER 31
THE EMERGENCY MEDICAL SYSTEM (PRE-HOSPITAL CARE) 865
Gerald L. Looney

CHAPTER 32
THE EMERGENCY MEDICAL SYSTEM (HOSPITAL CARE) 870
Gerald L. Looney

CHAPTER 33
AIR DISASTER TRAUMA 875
William J. Reals

CHAPTER 34
ACCIDENTS IN THE HOME 886
Bernard Knight

CHAPTER 35
ACCIDENTS IN THE HOSPITAL.. 901
Bernard Knight

CHAPTER 36
COST OF ACCIDENTS: A LEGAL AND ECONOMIC ANALYSIS.. 910
Guido Calabresi

PART IV SEX CRIMES.................................. 937

CHAPTER 37
RAPE 939
Arthur F. Schiff

CHAPTER 38
SEX CRIMES AND ABNORMAL SEXUAL BEHAVIOR 958
William G. Eckert

PART V DEATH 965

CHAPTER 39

PROPERTY OF THE DEAD BODY 967

Robert J. Joling

CHAPTER 40

ORGAN TRANSPLANTATION—THREE LEGAL ALTERNATIVES 978

Blair L. Sadler and Alfred M. Sadler, Jr.

CHAPTER 41

TRANSPLANT, BODY IMAGE, AND PSYCHOSIS 990

Pietro Castelnuovo-Tedesco

CHAPTER 42

THE MEDICOLEGAL AUTOPSY 995

William G. Eckert

CHAPTER 43

HOMICIDAL AND SUICIDAL DEATHS 1004

William G. Eckert

CHAPTER 44

SUDDEN, UNEXPECTED DEATH IN THE INFANT 1015

William Q. Sturner

CHAPTER 45

POSTMORTEM CHEMISTRY OF BLOOD, CEREBROSPINAL FLUID, AND VITREOUS HUMOR 1033

John I. Coe

CHAPTER 46

POSTMORTEM INJURIES 1061

A. Keith Mant

CHAPTER 47

SARCOSAPROPHAGOUS INSECTS AS FORENSIC INDICATORS 1072

Pekka Nuorteva

CHAPTER 48

POSTMORTEM INJURY CAUSED BY DOMESTIC ANIMALS, CRUSTACEANS, AND FISH 1096

M. Möttönen and M. Nuutila

PART VI EXAMINATION OF HUMAN REMAINS 1099

CHAPTER 49
FORENSIC ANTHROPOLOGY 1101
Ellis R. Kerley

CHAPTER 50
FORENSIC ODONTOLOGY 1116
Edward D. Woolridge, Jr.

CHAPTER 51
FORENSIC ROENTGENOLOGY 1154
Marvin E. Aronson and Paul S. Friedman

VOLUME III

PART I INDUSTRIAL AND AGRICULTURAL HAZARDS 1161

CHAPTER 52
AGRICULTURAL HAZARDS 1163
Bernard Knight

CHAPTER 53
HAZARDS OF THE FISHING INDUSTRY 1167
Bernard Knight

CHAPTER 54
HIGH-PRESSURE EQUIPMENT 1172
Bernard Knight

CHAPTER 55
LABORATORY HAZARDS 1175
Bernard Knight

CHAPTER 56
COAL MINING 1182
Bernard Knight

CHAPTER 57
RAILWAY HAZARDS 1186
Bernard Knight

PART II MEDICAL HAZARDS 1193

CHAPTER 58
THERAPEUTIC MISADVENTURES: DRUGS PRESCRIBED, TRIED, AND DECRIED 1195
Bernard J. Ficarra

CHAPTER 59
COMPLICATIONS OF MEDICOLEGAL IMPORTANCE ASSOCIATED WITH SURGICAL AND PARASURGICAL PROCEDURES 1226
Abraham Rosenthal

CHAPTER 60
COMPLICATIONS AND HAZARDS OF ANESTHESIA 1239
Philip H. Sechzer

CHAPTER 61
DRUG AND DEVICE LITIGATION 1261
Richard M. Goodman and Charles J. Barr

PART III ENVIRONMENTAL HAZARDS 1269

CHAPTER 62
MEDICOLEGAL ASPECTS OF OCCUPATIONAL AND ENVIRONMENTAL DISEASE 1271
Theodore Ehrenreich and Irving J. Selikoff

CHAPTER 63
PHYSIOPATHOLOGIC ASPECTS OF HIGH ALTITUDES 1293
Javier Arias-Stella

CHAPTER 64
DROWNING 1317
J. Chr. Giertsen

CHAPTER 65
FUNGAL AND MYCOBACTERIAL INFECTIONS 1334
John S. Chapman

CHAPTER 66
GEOGRAPHICALLY CONNECTED PARASITIC DISEASES 1343
Luke G. Tedeschi and Joanne M. Cutter

CHAPTER 67
INFECTIOUS DISEASES TRANSMITTED DIRECTLY OR INDIRECTLY FROM ANIMAL TO MAN 1369
Everett Rhoades

CHAPTER 68
HAZARDOUS MARINE ANIMALS 1378
Albert H. Banner

CHAPTER 69
TERRESTRIAL AND MARINE VENOMOUS SNAKES........................ 1437
Findlay Russell

CHAPTER 70
LOCAL AND SYSTEMIC EFFECTS FROM INSECT BITES AND STINGS 1445
Claude A. Frazier

CHAPTER 71
POISONOUS AND INJURIOUS HIGHER PLANTS AND FUNGI........ 1456
Julia F. Morton

CHAPTER 72
INJURY BY CHEMICAL AGENTS.. 1568
Charles L. Winek

CHAPTER 73
BACTERIAL FOOD POISONING.. 1588
Robert A. MacCready

CHAPTER 74
ASPHYXIATION BY FOOD (THE CAFÉ CORONARY)...................... 1614
Luke G. Tedeschi and Theodore H. Ingalls

CHAPTER 75
ENVIRONMENTAL FACTORS IN CAUSATION OF CONGENITAL MALFORMATIONS.. 1617
Theodore H. Ingalls and Jonathan P. Harvey

CHAPTER 76
INFLUENCE OF THE PHYSICAL ENVIRONMENT ON ACCIDENTS, CRIME, SUICIDE, AND DISEASE OF MAN................ 1627
S. W. Tromp

PART IV GENERAL LEGAL THEORIES PERTINENT TO TRAUMA AND HAZARDS 1643

CHAPTER 77
NEGLIGENCE... 1645
E. Stewart Jones, Jr.

CHAPTER 78
MALPRACTICE... 1651
Donald J. Dawidoff

CHAPTER 79
PRODUCTS LIABILITY 1656
Donald J. Dawidoff and Paul E. Walker

CHAPTER 80
CAUSATION 1661
Donald J. Dawidoff

CHAPTER 81
DAMAGES 1665
Donald J. Dawidoff

CHAPTER 82
THE DOCTRINE OF INFORMED CONSENT 1669
Jonathan P. Harvey

CHAPTER 83
THE RESPONSIBILITY OF THE PATHOLOGIST IN WORKMEN'S COMPENSATION CLAIMS 1675
Milton Helpern

INDEX i

Part I

TRAUMA BY PHYSICAL AGENTS

Section 1. MECHANICAL INJURY
Section 2. INJURY BY FIREARMS, BOMBS, AND EXPLOSIVES
Section 3. BAROTRAUMA (DYSBARISM)
Section 4. INJURY BY ELECTRICAL FORCE
Section 5. INJURY BY IONIZING RADIATION
Section 6. THERMAL INJURY
Section 7. ULTRASOUND INJURY

SECTION 1. MECHANICAL INJURY

chapter 1

THE WOUND: AN INTRODUCTION TO RELATED ISSUES

by Luke G. Tedeschi

The term *trauma*, as generally understood, means an injury (for instance, a wound) inflicted by a force upon a living tissue. It applies as well to emotional or mental stress resulting in a disordered psychic or behavioral state. Following trauma, a concurrence of effects, corporeal and psychic, is not uncommon, an association that obviously makes more complex the assessment of contingent forensic implications.

The history of trauma parallels the history of the evolution of man, with his aggressive instincts, creative ability, and endless ambition to conquer the environment without regard to the price he must pay to achieve his goals.

The first force used by man was of animal source—merely his own muscle strength. Additional force of the same nature was later drawn from stronger animals when horses, cattle, and elephants were subdued and brought under his dominion, to be employed in war and in peace as well for domestic purposes.

Instruments purposely designed for assault progressed rapidly with the advance of time from the primitive club to more refined weapons such as the axe, the dagger, the spear, the crossbow, and the catapult, to mention just a few. With the discovery of gunpowder came progressively more powerful firearms, and ultimately the splitting of the atom has brought the concept of injuring force to unforeseeable dimensions.

Pursuing a parallel course, the search for acceleration and speed led on one side to the discovery and exploitation of the chemical energy possessed by fossil fuels—coal and petroleum—and on the other to the development of high-velocity motorized vehicles, first a few, a mere curiosity, then more and more, no longer a curiosity but an integral part of a new system of life, congesting a grid of rails and roads that crisscross the planet in all directions. All this has become a source of injury far surpassing that of any weapon created for the purpose of assault. Finally, wings were added to equally motorized vehicles, and man learned how to travel in the skies and even to reach other planets. Expectedly, the toll of injury went higher.

CONCEPT OF FORCE AND LAWS OF MOTION

It took man several hundred thousand years to discover that force and its effects can be measured.

Galileo Galilei (1564–1642) opened the avenue to this gigantic undertaking by his enunciation of the principle of *inertia*. According to this principle, every object continues in its state of rest or uniform motion until that state is disrupted by an external force. This principle, applied to the field of mechanical trauma, finds support in the everyday observation that whether a wound occurs and, if it does, its basic characteristics are determined by the manner in which a moving object changes the state of rest of the tissue or by the manner in which the motion of the tissue is changed by meeting resistance.

Isaac Newton (1642–1727) pursued the avenue further. In the classic three laws that carry his name, he provided the methods by which force can be measured and quantitated. The first law is essentially a restatement of the Galilean principle of inertia. The second law supplies the equation that makes it possible to determine the change in velocity that takes place in a mass subjected to the influence of a given force.

$$F = \frac{d}{dt}(MV) = M\frac{dV}{dt} = Ma$$

Where

F is the applied force
$\frac{d}{dt}(MV)$ is the time rate of change of momentum of the object
M is the mass of the object
$\frac{dV}{dt}$ is the time rate of change of velocity of the object and
a is the acceleration of the object.

The third law states that for every action there is an equal reaction. This principle is exemplified by the case of a man sitting at a height. As he loses his balance, slips, and falls to the ground, his *potential energy* becomes converted in exactly the same amount to *kinetic energy*. On hitting the ground the body mass becomes decelerated and subjected to the effects of the equal, but opposite, reactionary force exercised by the ground. By equating the potential energy, expressed as *mgh*, to the kinetic energy, expressed as $\frac{1}{2}MV$, the velocity of the body mass at the time of impact with the ground can be determined by the equation

$$V = 2\ gh$$

where V is the velocity, g is the acceleration due to earth's gravity, and h is the height from which the fall took place. This equation is based on the principle of conservation of energy. According to the principles of conservation of momentum and energy, which are direct derivations of Newton's laws, the total momentum and energy of any system of elastically interacting bodies will remain constant as long as no external force or source of energy interferes with the system.

A direct application of these principles is found in the many problems that arise in coincidence with crashes on the road. When two vehicles collide, the parts that come into contact undergo compression at the moment of impact. At the instant of maximal compression, both vehicles have zero velocity. The kinetic energy that they possessed before the collision becomes stored in the form of elastic energy that is converted back to kinetic energy when the bodies of the vehicles rebound and fly apart. The speed of rebound is, in general, considerably less than the initial speed, which means that not all kinetic energy is restored. In this case, part of the kinetic energy is expended in causing distortion of the vehicles and part is transformed into thermic energy. In the case of collisions between objects in which all the kinetic energy is recovered, however, the rebound velocities of the objects are such that the total momentum is also conserved. Such a collision is called *elastic*.

The situation is entirely different when a moving vehicle hits a stationary or walking person crossing the path of the vehicle, because the collision is not elastic. In this case, at the moment of impact the vehicle undergoes deceleration, and the amount of kinetic energy lost by the vehicle is transferred to the victim of the accident. Part of the transferred energy is expended in producing body injury (primary impact) and the rest in setting the body in motion (kinetic energy). The body is thus accelerated on impact and consequently thrown to the ground, sustaining additional injuries (secondary impact). Ultimately when the body comes to rest, all the energy lost by the vehicle is absorbed by the person in the form of injuries.

The effects of a mechanical force on any given mass are determined by the elastic properties of the mass. This property is shared also by the human body. When an external force is applied to a part of the body, its constituent cellular components unavoidably are set in motion and become displaced from their original position. At this moment, elastic forces arise within the mass that tend to restore the composing particles to their original position and equilibrium. This restoring force is described in terms of a principle known as the *law of elasticity* (Hooke's law), which states that the force attempting to return the distorted mass to the original condition is proportional to the extent of the distortion. It is apparent that if the distortion exceeds the limits of elasticity of the mass, the mass will be torn apart. Hooke's law, applied to human tissues, well explains the formation of the wound. It leaves open, however, the unpredictability of its features, which are directly related on one side to the properties of the injuring force—its nature, velocity, weight, shape—and on the other to the peculiarities of the part struck—its degree of plasticity, tensile strength, and extent of relaxation at the moment of impact. This explains how wound patterns, although subject in some degree to the laws of mechanics, are so varied and unforeseeable in their characteristics.

TYPES OF WOUNDS

Mechanical trauma of adequate force, whatever the nature of the agent, usually leads to a wound. The latter may be limited to the tissues covering the outer and inner surfaces of the body, namely skin and mucous membranes, giving rise to a *superficial injury*, or may involve as well one or more of the deeper structures, such as the internal organs, causing a *penetrating* or *deep injury*. Any lesion, even the most insignificant from the medical standpoint, may constitute important legal evidence and lead to the disclosure of the agent or agents that were responsible for the injury (Figs. 1–1 through 1–6). Since only descriptive terms and not diagnoses should be used to record physical findings, accurate definition of terms is of primary importance.

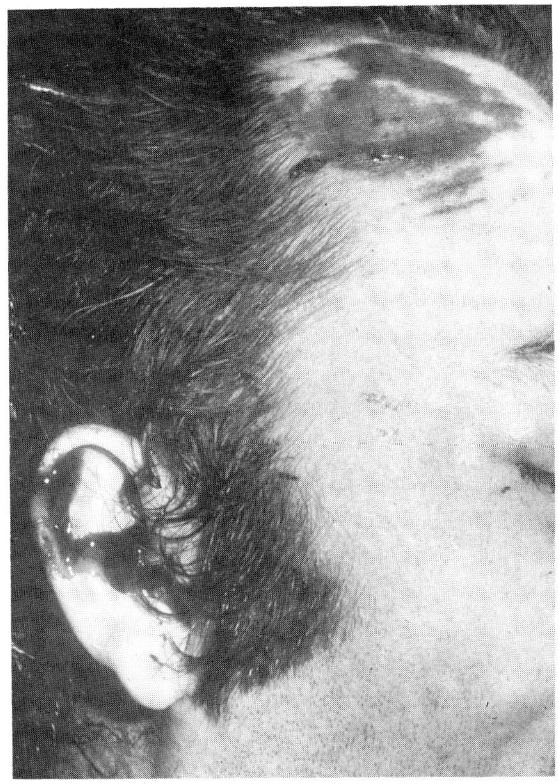

Figure 1–2. Multiple linear contusions in forehead. Head-on automobile crash. Notice the rivulet of blood escaping from the ear in conjunction with fracture of the buttress of the temporal bone.

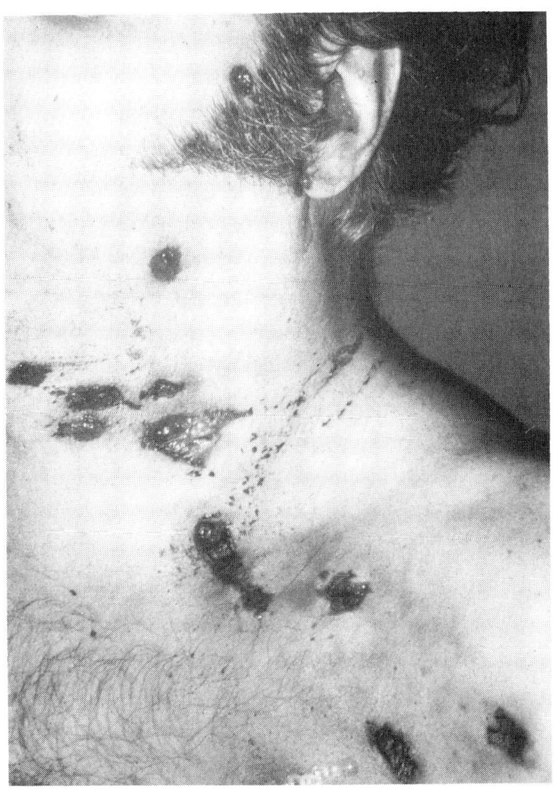

Figure 1–1. Multiple penetrating injuries from firearms. Gangland slaying. Immediate death.

Abrasion is the name given to a superficial wound. In the case of skin, the injury is limited to the epidermis; the mark left by a fingernail is an example.

Contusion means a hemorrhage, usually at the area where a blunt force was applied, as by an obtuse object without sharp edges. A contusion may or may not be associated with disruption of tissue continuity. The effused blood undergoes color changes, which to some extent reflect the rate of deterioration of the extravasated red blood cells. The significance of these changes is discussed in Chapter 2. A contusion should not be confused with *postmortem hypostasis*, which is usually limited to the dependent parts of the body. In postmortem hypostasis, the area of hemorrhagic discoloration blanches upon compression; in contrast, the area of discoloration related to a contusion does not change color upon compression because there is actual infiltration of blood into the tissue.

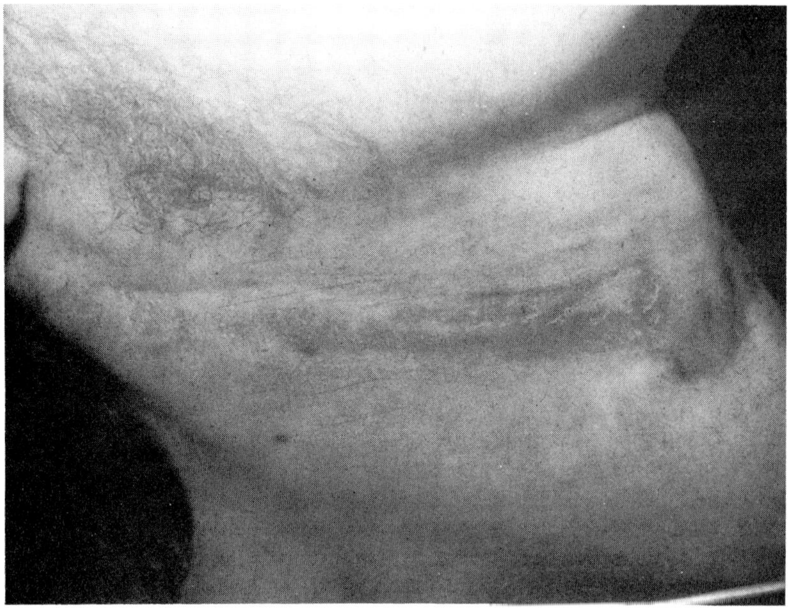

Figure 1–3. Patterned mark of cloth belt around the neck in suicidal hanging.

The same impact that gives rise to a superficial contusion may affect one or another of the deep bodily structures such as a viscus in the chest or abdomen, producing a visceral injury, or a bone, producing a fracture. Following the impact by a blunt object, a severe injury in a deep viscus or in the skeletal system may occur in the absence of visible change in the skin.

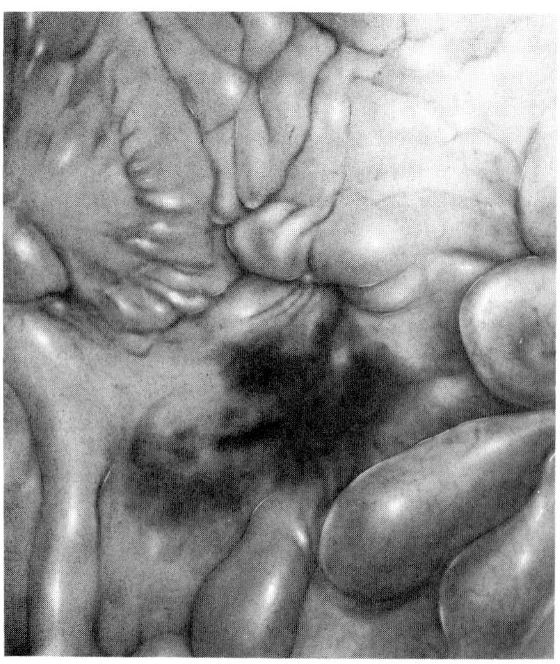

Figure 1–4. Retroperitoneal contusion from severe beating concurrent to assault.

An *incision wound* is produced by an object with a sharp edge, such as a knife or a piece of glass. The shape, direction, width, and depth of the wound, and eventually the presence of foreign particles (glass, soil) within it, can provide important clues to the accidental or suicidal or homicidal nature of the injury. Incised wounds can be further categorized as *therapeutic (surgical), accidental,* and *nonaccidental,* either *self-inflicted (suicidal)* or secondary to assault *(homicidal).* Incised wounds, within these different categories, frequently show distinguishing characteristics that allow reconstruction, with considerable accuracy, of the manner by which they have been produced.

A *laceration,* by definition, is irregular in shape—stellate, crescent-shaped, or Y-shaped; the shape itself can provide a clue to the reconstruction of the events. A laceration is usually the result of blunt impact and is more likely to occur where the integument is tightly stretched over bony structures such as the skull. Scalp lacerations resulting from a fall ordinarily occur on the posterior part of the head and are associated with skull fractures of the linear type; conversely, scalp lacerations at the top of the head are usually induced by moving objects striking the skull and are associated with depressed fractures. The term "laceration" is used most commonly to describe wounds affecting the skin and subcutaneous tissue, but it applies as well to the same type of injury in deep-seated internal structures. Following a blunt impact at the surface of the body, the oc-

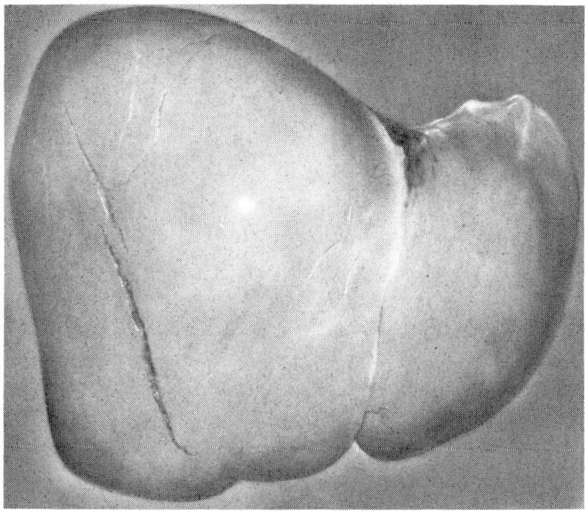

Figure 1–5. Traumatic laceration of liver concurrent to fractured ribs. Motorcycle crash.

currence of laceration and contusion in one or more of the internal organs, either by compression or displacement, is far from uncommon, and if the damage is extensive, the lesion is labeled a *crushing injury*. An injury of this type may be found beneath relatively intact skin.

Stab or *puncture wounds* are those induced by a rigid, slender object, and they may be so small as to be easily overlooked. As in the case of incised wounds, wounds resulting from the impact of a rigid, slender object can be accidental (from a fall on a pointed object), homicidal, or self-inflicted in a suicidal attempt. Careful assessment of the location and direction of the wound can provide objective evidence of whether the injury was self-inflicted or related to assault. Related to differences in the thrust of the force, disparities between the depth of the wound and the length of the weapon are not uncommon; for the same reason, wounds produced by the same object may display differences in size and shape. An incision wound or a stab or puncture wound can extend from the tegumental system into the deeper structures of the body, at varying depths, inducing a deeply seated injury; as such, it becomes a penetrating wound. When this is the case, important clues to the degree and direction of the force can be obtained by pursuing the track of the wound.

Patterned wound is the term suggested to denote tegumental lesions that by their pattern or location provide objective evidence of the type of injury incident to criminal assault, suicidal death, or accidental injury. The patterned bruise on the skin of the neck produced by a woven cord or band used in strangulation, the finger pressure marks on the neck in manual strangulation, the marks of the grid of a radiator or of a tire tread, the imprint of the muzzle produced by contact fire in a gunshot wound are all examples of patterned wounds.

The injurious effects of the striking force may take place at the point of impact or at some distance from it or may affect both local and distant areas; this is the case of the so-called *contralateral* or *contrecoup injury*.

Whatever the type of the wound, its location must be described in relation to a fixed anatomical landmark and its size must be recorded in units of measure, not by comparison to fruit or nuts, just because they vary in size.

Bullet wounds and injuries resulting from detonation of high explosives belong to a distinct category and they are considered in the section "Injuries by Firearms and Explosives."

Here it is enough to say that injuries produced by guns are affected by many variables. As a general rule, the wound of entrance is round and smaller than the wound of exit, which is irregular and stellate in shape. In the case of a *contact wound*, however, the gas blast effect may result in an entrance wound that is larger than the exit wound. Deposits of smoke

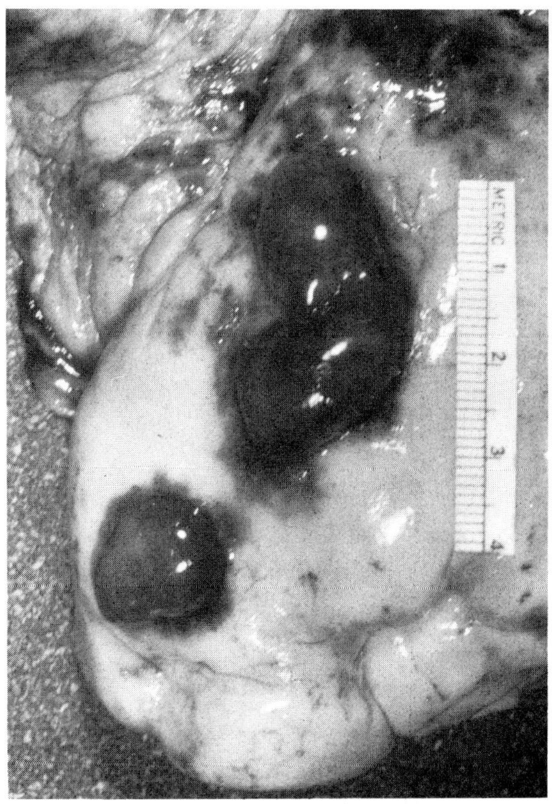

Figure 1–6. Multiple subpleural hematomas and pulmonary contusions secondary to fracture of chest wall (crushed chest syndrome). Automobile accident.

or unburned powder, and tattooing from unburned powder particles are valid indications of near-range firing. Whereas the pathologist forensically trained is fully aware of the importance of measuring exactly the extent of smoke-smudging or powder marks, the surgeon involved in a life-saving emergency procedure, in the course of debriding the skin wound, can fail to pay attention to the nature and distribution of this material and possibly neglect to submit the specimen for pathologic examination, inexorably affecting the course of the investigation.

The same is true of stab wounds. Information on the clean, ragged, sharp, or dull character of the incision and its exact size, depth, and direction is essential in any attempt to trace the weapon. By the same token, detection of associated bruising can provide useful information on the length of the knife, indicating that the haft of the weapon struck the skin. Proper recording of these data is vital. All these characteristics will be lost once the wound is surgically repaired.

The categorization of the wound at the site of the primary impact marks just the beginning of a series of events, the aftermath of which may have no consequential import, may be attended by immediate or delayed death, or may lead to sequelae the severity of which increases in direct proportion to the degree of trauma. Not infrequently the sequelae, rather than the primary injury, are responsible for the outcome of the morbid state initiated by the trauma.

Bleeding, either internal or external or both, frequently occurs in conjunction with severe mechanical trauma. This causes a reduction in circulating blood volume (hypovolemia), the magnitude of which varies with the nature and extent of the injury. *Hemorrhagic shock* is the term generally applied to this acute state of circulatory failure, which, unless promptly corrected, unavoidably leads to a progressively inadequate perfusion of tissues and organs.

The acute hypovolemia associated with the loss of blood as a rule is aggravated by the rapid shifting of extracellular fluid into the region of the injury, the deep tissues, and the body cavities as well. When the reduction in blood volume has reached a level of approximately 30 per cent, the arterial pressure begins to fall, and almost invariably this event is heralded by renal ischemia with consequent low urine output (oliguria) and by progressive upward cooling and pallor of the extremities.

In the attempt to compensate for the reduction in blood volume, the venous system contracts, maximally in the lower limbs, and this together with the oliguria and the coldness and pallor of the lower extremities establishes the presence of *compensated shock*. When the hypovolemia reaches a level above 30 per cent, the progressive decrease in blood pressure results in the classic manifestations of *decompensated shock*, which are primarily a reflection of cellular hypoxia secondary to deficient blood flow.

The decrease in cardiac output causes a decrease in cerebral blood flow and this in turn is responsible for the disarray in cellular structure and function that is mirrored by changes in mentation.

Although the brain constitutes only approximately 2 per cent of the body weight, it receives 15 per cent of the cardiac output and accounts for 20 per cent of the total basal oxygen consumption. As a rule, when the mean blood pressure reaches a level below 50 mm of mercury, the impairment in cerebral blood flow gives rise to a variety of alarming manifestations ranging from anxiety and restlessness to semicoma and coma.

Whereas in the young person organ failure associated with severe hemorrhagic shock primarily affects renal function, in the adult affected by the same condition, organ failure is inclined to affect, simultaneously or successively, practically all the vital organs of the body. The result is a broader spectrum of malefic disturbances. Respiratory difficulties and ventilatory failure are inherently associated with the state of acute systemic hypoxia. Cardiac disturbances also occur, affecting all major hemodynamic parameters (i.e., cardiac output, stroke volume, heart rate).

An important role in hemorrhagic shock has been attributed to factors other than hypoxia, primarily biochemical alterations that reflect changes in cellular metabolism.

Embolic phenomena also frequently occur. The embolus may consist of particles alien to the blood, such as fat globules (fat embolism), air bubbles (air embolism), foreign bodies (a bullet, for example), or, most commonly, a conglomerate of blood particles (a thrombus) that was turned loose from the intima of a blood vessel.

To the list of systemic disorders one can add the neurohormonal disorders concurrent to the stress of trauma, of which pulmonary edema, cardiac arrhythmias, and stress ulcers are the most common manifestations.

In the light of the nature of these sequelae, each one a life threatening event in itself, it is not surprising that mechanical trauma ranks third, immediately after heart disease and cancer, among the causes of death.

Deaths from trauma are listed in the vital statistics. There is no way to record the pain and anguish, the limitations of function, the aggravation of preexisting conditions that frequently attend the residual effects of injury. These are just the burdens that the victim of trauma must bear by himself.

In the same way that the physician tries to assess, heal, or correct to the best of his ability the physical wrongs attending the wound, the custodian of the law, pursuing a parallel path, looks into the causation of the injury, on the principle that the injured party is due amends.

As act one of the drama of the wound is brought to a close, act two begins and the custodian of the law steps onstage. Since he is not acquainted with the case, he asks to see the medical record. No effort should be spared by the physician in including in the record, accurately and in exact conformity to truth, the circumstances pertaining to the case. Maintenance of an exact record is one of the most important obligations of the physician to the victim of an injury. The custodian of the law has more than a perfunctory interest in what the medical record has to offer. From it he expects to learn how far the medical evidence can go in answering with accuracy and reasonable certainty questions relevant to the case.

As the drama of trauma unfolds in the court of law, it becomes apparent that there is no prototype case from which to draw information on matters of causation and effects. In every case of bodily or mental impairment in which trauma is the culprit, the theme of the drama varies. Diversified is the psychologic response of the individual and manifold are the manifestations of physical distress; the circumstances related to the injury are dissimilar, and the force that was responsible for the injury differs from case to case and often cannot be determined.

AGGRAVATING FACTORS

There are a few themes that are likely to recur periodically, however, that can be discussed theoretically. They include trauma and infection, trauma and heart disease, the mental reactions attending trauma, and trauma and tumor. These four situations deserve to be selected for another reason: they are best suited to illustrate the concept of aggravation.

Trauma and Infection

Upon disruption of the protective barrier provided by the normal continuity of the skin and mucosal membranes, bacteria that are normal inhabitants of the external environment may gain access to the injured tissue and set up a local infection. By the same token, bacteria are presumably present on any object that is capable of producing an injury.

Wounds associated with extensive crushing of tissue are more likely to become infected than simple incisional or puncture wounds. As a general rule, superficial wounds exposed to the air are less susceptible to bacterial contamination than penetrating wounds affecting deeper structures such as a joint space, a viscus, or any one of the serous cavities (pleural, peritoneal). A simple contusion, however, or even the irritation produced by friction of a contaminated object on the skin or on the mucosal lining of the internal passages may constitute a sufficient break through the protective barrier to allow the transfer of surface pathogens into the injured area.

This is what happens to hide porters, who not uncommonly develop the cutaneous lesions of anthrax in the weight-bearing areas, usually on the neck or on the upper surface of the shoulders. That relatively minor wounds may

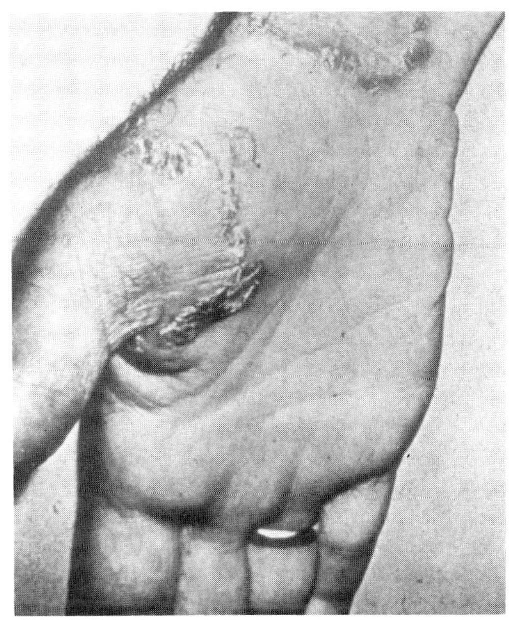

Figure 1–7. Malignant pustule of skin anthrax with vesiculation, formation of eschars, and central necrosis resulting in ragged black ulcers. Wool worker dying of septicemia and bronchopneumonia.

provide an adequate access to infection is further exemplified by the sequence of events that follow the accidental ingestion of a fishbone, a splinter, or a toothbrush bristle that leads to a small defect in the mucosa of the alimentary tract and ultimately to an apparently idiopathic mediastinal abscess, an empyema, or peritonitis.

The bacteria that are responsible for the primary infection of a wound are most commonly the normal inhabitants of the tissue involved in the trauma. For example, streptococci, staphylococci, *Escherichia coli, Proteus vulgaris,* usually present on normal skin, are also most frequently found in infected skin wounds. Pathogenic organisms kept in check under normal conditions by the general and local defenses of the host, suddenly become harmful upon loss or decrease of resistance brought about by the injury.

Soil is a frequent contaminant of superficial wounds. Most of the bacteria present in the soil derive from sewage disposal or from excrement of human or animal origin. They include *Clostridium tetani,* various organisms responsible for gas gangrene, and a large number of other pathogenic bacteria, fungi, spirochetes, protozoa, metazoa, and yeasts capable of contaminating a wound.

Pathogenic microorganisms not uncommonly are present in the blood of a normal individual *(benign bacteremia).* Usually these bacteria are quickly disposed of by the host's defenses and do not elicit signs or symptoms of disease. Concurrently to the stress of trauma and lowered resistance, however, these transient bacteria can easily migrate into the wound, setting up a localized infection. Dead cells, collections of blood or edema fluid, decreased blood supply coincidental to vascular thrombosis and rupture of blood channels, establish an ideal situation for bacterial growth.

Particular types of wound infections commonly arise among workers in trades involving the handling of animals, animal parts, leather, wool, or hair, and they can cause medicolegal conflicts on matters of compensation. This is primarily the case for the infections produced by *Pseudomonas mallei, Pasteurella tularensis,* and *Bacillus anthracis* that are usually transmitted directly from animal to man. Grooms, hostlers, and farmers are not infrequently exposed to *Pseudomonas mallei.* Infection from *Pasteurella tularensis* is relatively common in hunters and butchers who skin or dress game (woodchucks, muskrats, opossums, squirrels, skunks, and most frequently, wild rabbits). Anthrax infection in man is often derived from handling meat from sheep and cattle. Since anthrax bacilli are spore-forming organisms with long extracorporeal survival, leather or wool or hair workers are also likely to become infected (Fig. 1–7).

Tubercle bacilli, although widespread in the environment, rarely cause wound infection. Occasionally, however, they may become implanted in an accidental wound incurred in the handling of contaminated human or animal material. The ensuing lesion, not uncommon among pathologists and butchers, as a rule remains localized at the site of injury (so-called *local tuberculoma*) and it does not spread beyond the lymph nodes draining the area of infection (so-called *regional lymphadenitis*).

The general rule that microorganisms are incapable of gaining access to the tissues through an intact surface applies also to *Treponema pallidum,* the cause of syphilis. Both in genital and extragenital syphilis, it must be assumed that the agent of the disease has found its portal of entry through a preexisting abrasion, fissure, or ulcer.

The implant of bacteria in a wound is not necessarily followed by a wound infection. Whether an infection takes place depends on the dose of the inoculum, on the type of bacteria, on the degree of efficiency of the defensive mechanisms (both local and systemic) available to the host, and on other complex environmental factors—metabolic, immunologic, biochemical—that ultimately decide the fate of the bacterial implant.

The same factors also determine to a considerable extent the time lapse between the implant of the bacteria and the reaction of the host (so-called *incubation period*). In most wound infections, the incubation period is short, from a few hours to a few days. This is the case for the infections induced by staphylococci, streptococci, *C. welchii, E. coli;* other bacteria such as *B. anthracis, P. tularensis,* and *P. mallei* have a slightly longer incubation period, which may extend over a week. The manifest reaction to tubercle bacilli occurs within four to six weeks. The incubation period for *C. tetani* averages 5 to 14 days, but it can be much longer (even months), depending upon the time lapse required by the spores to develop into mature bacilli.

The bacterial contamination can remain localized, can spread by continuity, or can be carried to distant sites through the blood or lymph stream, giving rise to a systemic infection. It is apparent that the direct inoculation of the infective agent into the lumen of an injured blood vessel is more likely to produce a systemic infection than its passage through a simple superficial abrasion.

Since the time elapsing between the contamination of the wound and the reaction of the host is variable, the question may arise whether the infection occurred in coincidence with the original trauma *(primary infection)* or subsequent to it as the result of an accidental implant of bacteria, for instance, following application of contaminated dressings *(secondary infection).*

The concept of *aggravation* applies well to the situation by which trauma, in association with accident or assault, affects a preexisting infection, disturbing the local protective mechanisms and thus transforming a relatively innocuous process into a life-threatening condition. The invasion of the blood stream by bacteria that follows a blow to the mouth resulting in the loss or dislocation of infected teeth, the peritonitis that develops from the perforation of a gastric or duodenal ulcer subsequent to a blow to the abdomen, the activation or extension of a tuberculous lesion in the lungs in conjunction with a severe blow to the chest unavoidably bring up the question of *fortuitous circumstance* as against *causal relationship.*

The debilitated state attending any injury of some degree can enhance secondary fungal infection. When this occurs the problem of aggravation may arise and it may be difficult to apportion the responsibility between the fungus and the defective defense of the host—humoral or cellular or both—attending the injury.

It is unquestionable that certain types of therapy applied in the treatment of the traumatized patient may increase the circumstantial conversion of ordinarily innocent fungi into aggressive organisms capable of initiating a mycotic infection.

There is a growing awareness of the hazard of fungal infections following antibiotic and steroid treatment.

Antibiotics suppress sensitive bacteria, making available a surplus of nutrients to the fungus. Furthermore, they remove antifungal components produced by certain gram-negative bacteria and alter the supply of vitamins yielded by microbic organisms.

Adrenocorticosteroids and corticotropin also increase the susceptibility to fungal infection. The underlying factors are impairment of the reticuloendothelial system, depression of lymphoid tissue mass, and diminished antibody formation. Cortical steroid administration is, likewise, responsible for diminished leukocytic activity, clumping of leukocytes, and diminished blood flow that ultimately impair fixation and removal of bacteria and detoxification of their products (Figs. 1–8 and 1–9).

In a psychosomatic approach to infections, Bingham has proposed that stress can alter the cellular resistance to infection to the point at which an ordinarily harmless germ can gain a foothold in the functionally or structurally altered cells of the body, eliciting an infection.[1] Should this concept be accepted, every infectious process may be traced back to some preceding episode of physical or emotional stress. Stress as a factor predisposing to infection has

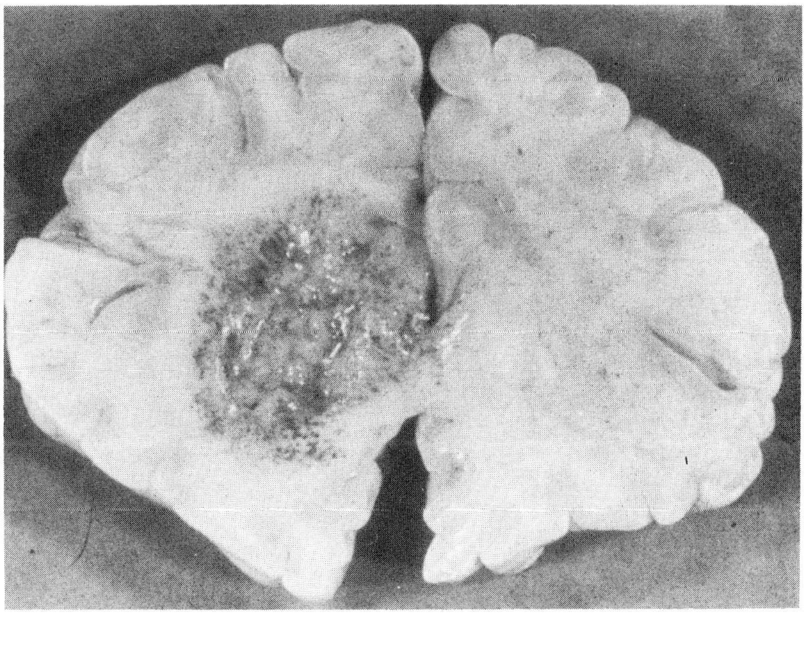

Figure 1–8. Mycotic abscess in the white matter of the right cerebral hemisphere *(Aspergillus fumigatus)* in a 37-year-old Caucasian woman with acute myelogenous leukemia treated by intense steroid and immunosuppressive therapy.

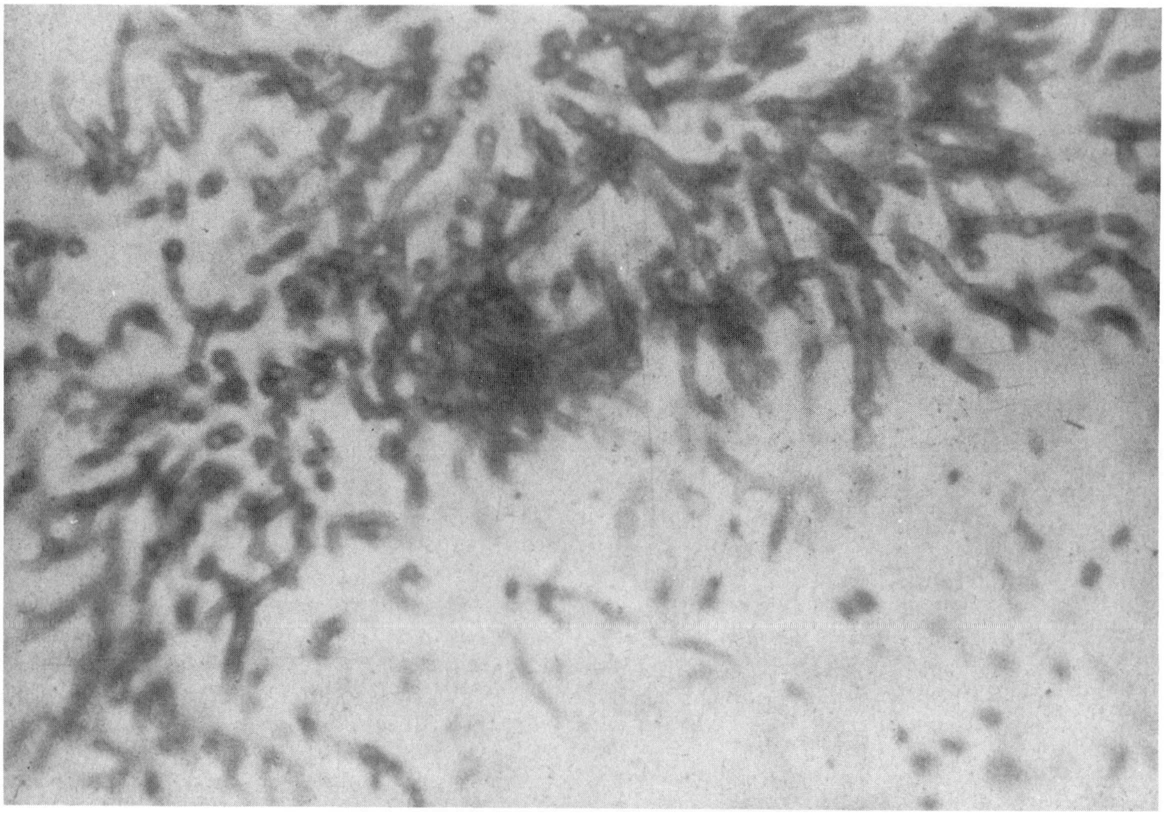

Figure 1–9. *Aspergillus fumigatus* organisms from brain abscess. Same case as Figure 1–8.

been demonstrated in the experimental animal but is difficult to prove in man. Nevertheless, in the light of day-to-day empirical observation, it is difficult to take a definite opposite stand.

Trauma and Heart Disease

The subject of trauma and stress as a cause of heart disease or of aggravation of preexisting heart disease deserves as much and possibily even more consideration than that of trauma and infection.

The mechanisms by which an injury induced by a mechanical force and the concurrent episode of stress may damage the heart or precipitate a crisis in an already diseased heart are multiple and complex. In most cases, causal relationships are drawn with difficulty, and controversy is likely to arise in matters of compensation. In abstract, two basic situations are most likely to find access to the courts of law: Direct injury to the heart, whether it be blunt or penetrating, and indirect injury, whenever the heart is damaged or a preexisting heart condition is aggravated by the systemic disturbances elicited by an injury to any part of the body and the attending stress.

Direct injury is given thorough consideration in Chapter 3–VII. In abstract, when the heart has been perforated or lacerated by a penetrating object (free missile or sharp object) or has been bruised or crushed by a violent impact against the chest, the ensuing death or disability can be reasonably attributed to the injury. Contusion of the heart is a common complication of steering wheel injuries in car collisions. As a general rule, the cause-and-effect relationship is substantiated by the absence of a symptom-free period, and if the victim dies, unmistakable evidence of cardiac damage is found at autopsy. It is also conceivable that blunt trauma to the chest can cause a broken rib to bruise the myocardium or one of the coronary arteries at the surface of the heart, causing a blood clot (thrombus) to form in the lumen of the damaged blood vessel (Figs. 1–10 and 1–11).[2]

In this situation, the causal relationship between the injury and the ensuing heart failure may remain a matter of speculation unless the sequence of events can be proved at postmortem examination.

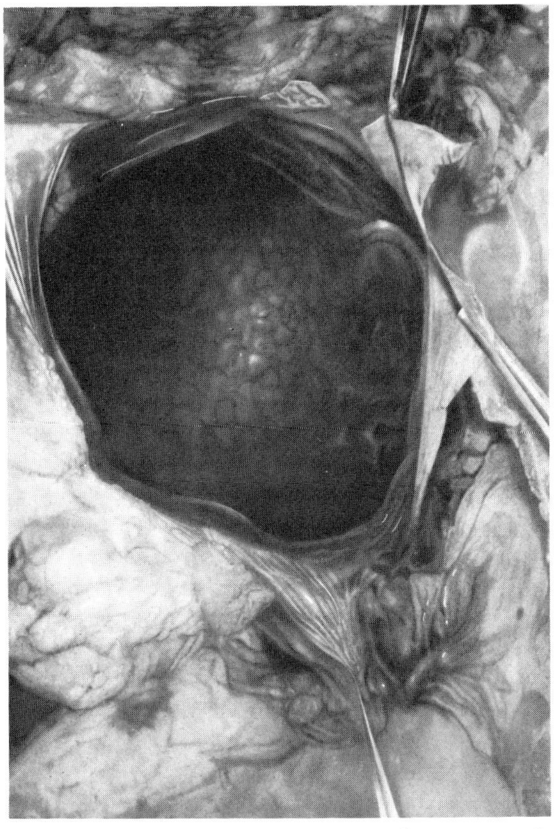

Figure 1–10. Direct heart injury: cardiac tamponade (hemopericardium) secondary to crash chest injury of sternum and ribs. Multiple ecchymosis and lacerations of the anterior wall of the heart, including partial transverse transection of ascending portion of aorta.

More difficult to prove is the concept of *indirect heart injury*. That disorders in rhythm and electrocardiographic changes frequently occur after trauma, particularly following head injuries, is common knowledge. Vagal overactivity, increased sympathetic tone, or excessive release of catecholamines, singly or in variable combinations, have been advocated to explain the occurrence of these cardiac disorders. It has recently been demonstrated that these disturbances can be underlain by lesions in the heart muscle visible under the light microscope (see Chapter 4).

A severe injury to any part of the body is usually associated with loss of blood and destruction of tissue. In concurrence with these events, there is the lowering of blood pressure, diminution of blood volume, and slowing of blood flow that are the characteristic hemodynamic alterations associated with shock. Shock predisposes to clotting of the blood (thrombus formation), and whenever the thrombus occurs in a coronary artery it can cause myocardial ischemia and death or, if this event is survived, a more or less permanent cardiac disability.[3-5]

Independently from shock, following a mechanical injury, the circulating blood may show a brief period of increased coagulability.[6, 7] In this case also a thrombus can develop in one of the coronary arteries, leading to death or cardiac disability.

A causal relationship between the trauma, the posttraumatic increase in the coagulability of the blood, and the occurrence of the coronary thrombosis may be accepted, provided laboratory evidence can be presented that following the trauma the blood coagulability was greater than normal, and that the manifestations of coronary thrombosis developed a few hours or, at most, a day or two after the injury.

More difficult to assess is the heart failure, or any other type of cardiac disorder, occurring in an individual with *anteceding history of heart disease* as an indirect effect of trauma (Fig. 1–13).

This introduces the concept of aggravation. The term *aggravation*, as generally understood, is applied to the injury that hastens death, leads to premature disability, or introduces features and complications that normally are not inclined to develop in the natural course of the disease process.

The most common conditions affecting the heart are coronary atherosclerosis, hypertensive heart disease, and valvular disease.

Severe injury and the attending anxiety, pain, anger, or fear associated with it may impose an extra load on an already diseased heart, ultimately leading to its failure.[8-10] Anxiety, in the broad sense, is a well-known cause of systemic physiologic changes, and the heart frequently acts as a focal point for anxiety. Measurable changes in pulse rate, cardiac output, stroke volume, peripheral resistance, and arterial blood pressure and increased oxygen consumption may well be expected to precipitate an episode of congestive heart failure in individuals with diminished cardiac reserve. Whenever the coronary circulation is impaired, the extra work imposed on the heart by the condition of anxiety may contribute to an anginal attack, as well as to a host of acute changes in heart rhythm, such as paroxysmal tachycardia, arrhythmia, flutter, and fibrillation, which are regarded as evidences of vasomotor instability or autonomic imbalance.

Since heart failure and death or a broad variety of arrhythmias are within the natural course of the illness of any patient affected by a heart condition, any attempt to recognize a causal relationship between the aggravation of

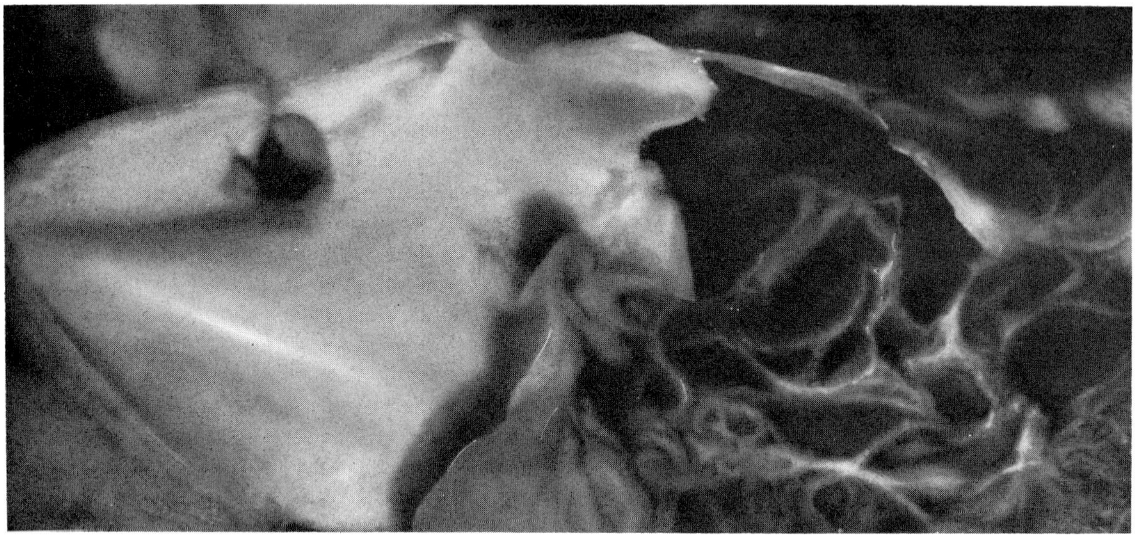

Figure 1–11. Partial transverse transection of ascending portion of aorta. Same case as Figure 1–10.

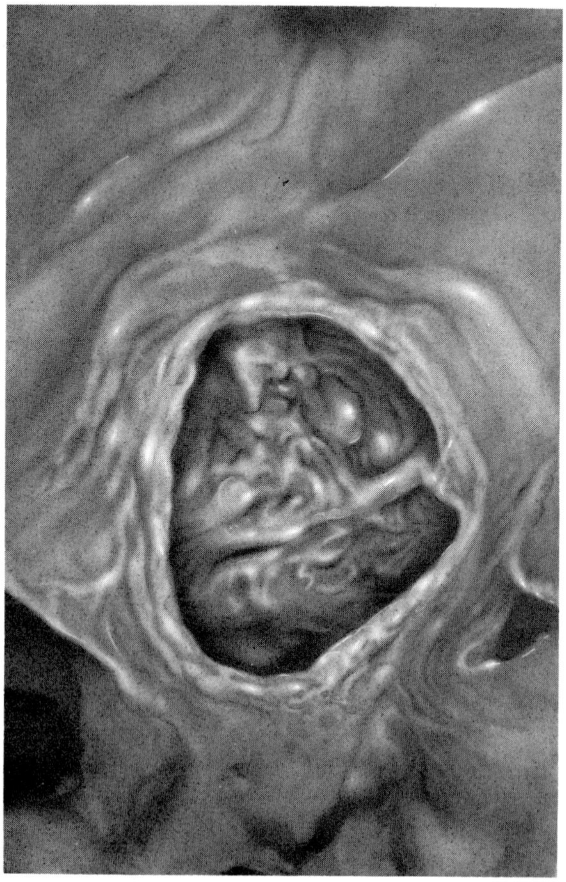

Figure 1–12. Sixty-four-year-old white woman found dead in the automobile she was driving following crash against telephone pole. Previous history of heart disease. Calcific aortic stenosis was found at postmortem examination.

the cardiac disorder and the trauma can reasonably lead to conflicts of opinion.

Criteria that have been advocated in support of the relationship include the concepts that the trauma must be of *some significance* and that the onset of symptoms must develop *shortly* after the event that precipitated the episode of cardiac distress.

The relative import of the concept of *some significance* is indicated by the disappointing but realistic observation that death does not always find a suitable explanation in detectable lesions at autopsy. This occurrence is particularly well documented in the case of blunt head trauma. Just to quote a single authoritative series, in 6 per cent of 1,367 cases of head injuries from blunt forces analyzed by Freytag, no morphologic changes could be detected in the vital centers of the brain.[11]

Equally nebulous and undependable is the concept that the symptoms must develop *shortly* after the event that precipitated the episode of cardiac distress. The weakness of the concept in this case rests in the fact that some time may elapse between the establishment of the disorder and the ability of the physician to demonstrate its existence by clinical and laboratory methods.

Whenever the circumstances of the case are indefinite, it is well to keep in mind that according to the laws of probability, a large proportion of the male population is expected to die or become disabled because of arteriosclerotic heart disease or one or another of its complications.

Since heart failure occurs in the natural course of events of any cardiac condition, and this may be sudden and unexpected, not infrequently the situation arises that the critical event occurs while the patient is standing or walking, or driving a vehicle. In the fall he can injure himself; even worse, if driving a car, he can lose control of the vehicle, injuring himself and causing physical and material damage to others.

Situations of this kind are far from uncommon. Injury concurrent to heart failure raises the question whether the fall and the ensuing injury precipitated the cardiac condition or whether the sudden failing of the heart was responsible for the loss of consciousness, the fall, and the injury.

As a general rule, if the injury was sufficiently severe to be considered incompatible with life, and if it can be shown that it occurred

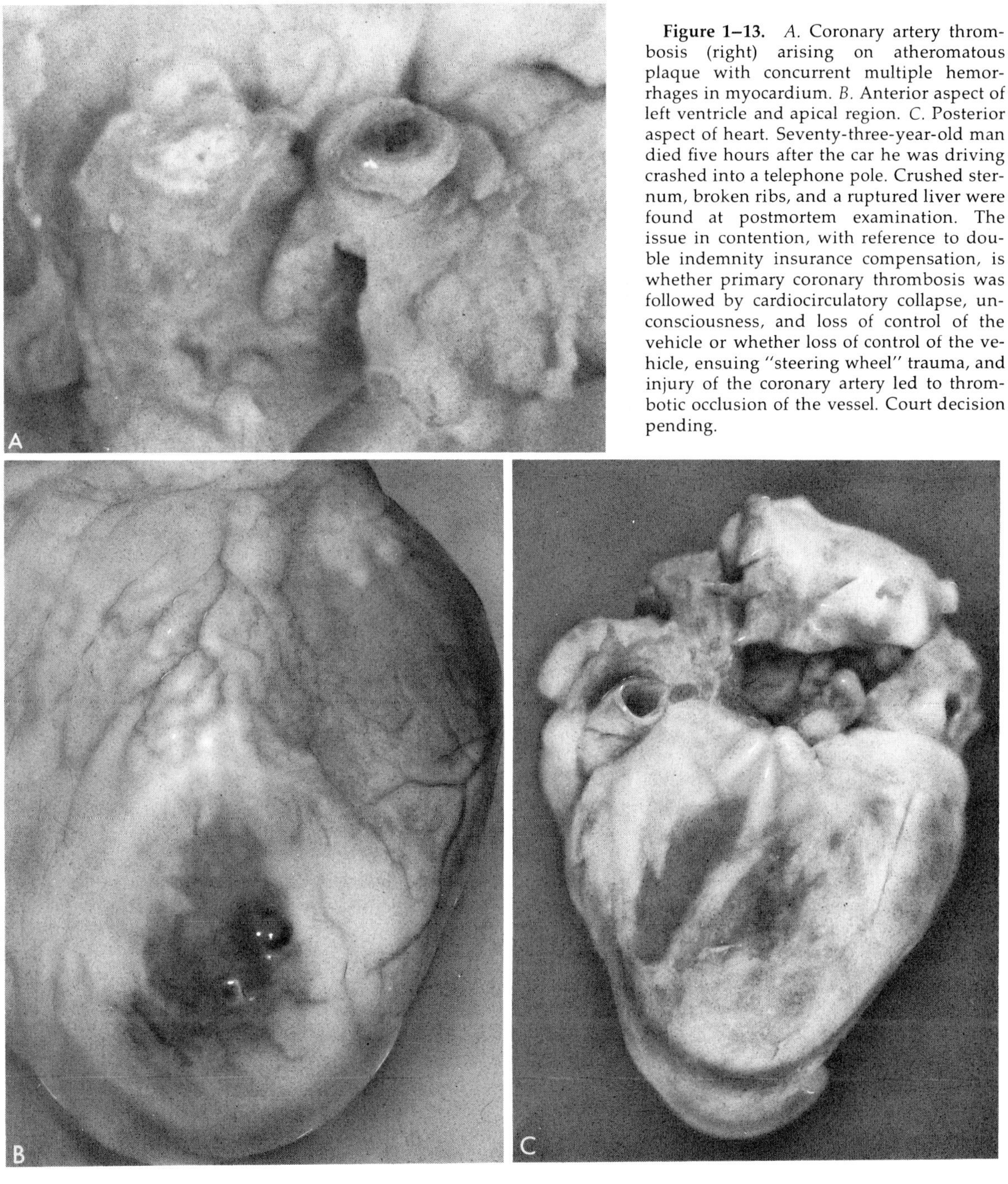

Figure 1–13. *A.* Coronary artery thrombosis (right) arising on atheromatous plaque with concurrent multiple hemorrhages in myocardium. *B.* Anterior aspect of left ventricle and apical region. *C.* Posterior aspect of heart. Seventy-three-year-old man died five hours after the car he was driving crashed into a telephone pole. Crushed sternum, broken ribs, and a ruptured liver were found at postmortem examination. The issue in contention, with reference to double indemnity insurance compensation, is whether primary coronary thrombosis was followed by cardiocirculatory collapse, unconsciousness, and loss of control of the vehicle or whether loss of control of the vehicle, ensuing "steering wheel" trauma, and injury of the coronary artery led to thrombotic occlusion of the vessel. Court decision pending.

before death, the death can be attributed to the injury. Conversely, if the injury per se was of a minor nature and, in contrast, the heart condition, as found at autopsy, provides an adequate explanation of death, the death can be attributed to the cardiac condition.

Following an injury, bacteria can gain access to the blood stream, lodge and grow in the heart valves, and give rise to an acute valvular infection *(acute bacterial endocarditis)*. This is attended by the formation of masses of fibrin, blood cells, and bacteria (so-called vegetations) at the surface of the heart valves (Fig. 1–14). Being friable, these vegetations can easily be detached by the blood flowing through the heart chambers, forming septic thromboemboli, which, as they are brought into the general circulation, can lodge in the brain, in the kidneys, or in other organs, causing septic infarcts.

The chance of an acute bacterial endocarditis is greatly increased in a person with preexisting valvular disease—in most cases, the end result of acute rheumatic fever. The links between injury, infection, bacteremia, preexisting valvular disease, and acute bacterial endocarditis are usually acknowledged and not debatable.

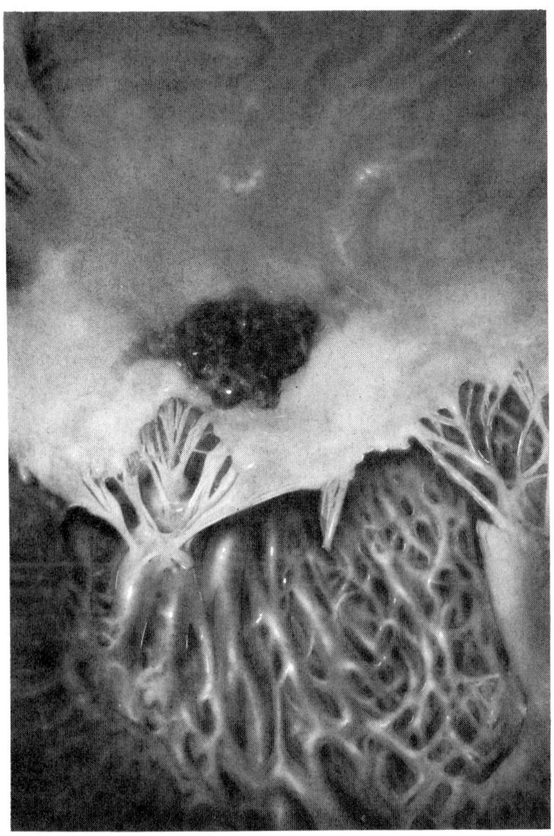

Figure 1–14. Acute vegetative bacterial endocarditis on normal mitral valve following osteomyelitis secondary to open fracture of tibia and fibula in a 28-year-old man. *E. coli* was obtained from blood and vegetation in mitral valve.

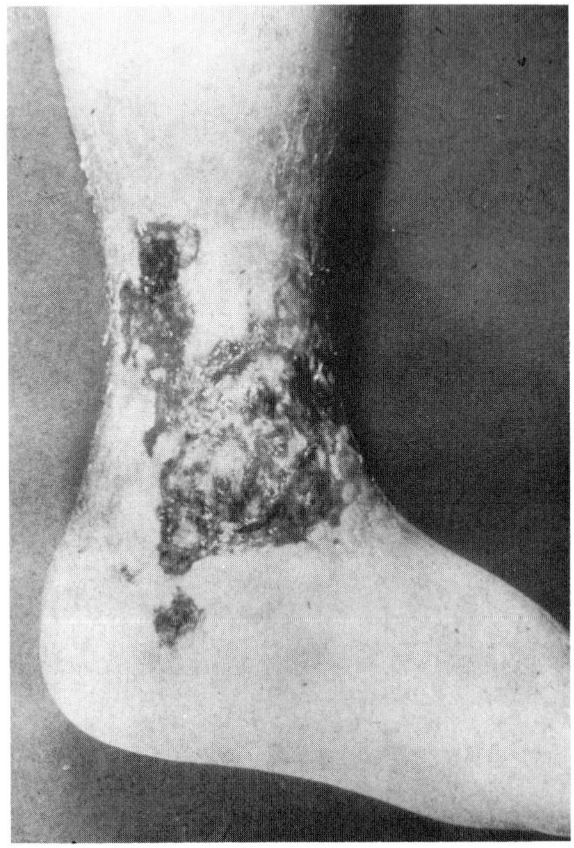

Figure 1–15. Dystrophic ulcer in lower limb of 68-year-old Caucasian man confined to bed for six months following multiple injuries sustained in a car accident. The lesion developed two months after the accident. There was no previous history of claudication.

The concept of trauma as an aggravating factor of preexisting coronary disease is duplicated in the issue of trauma and *peripheral arteriosclerosis.*

Gangrene, in the sense of death of tissue, usually in considerable mass, is a spontaneous event in the course of peripheral arteriosclerosis. It is well-acknowledged, however, that a severe contusion or a fracture, likely requiring confinement to bed, in a patient whose arteriosclerotic process was previously well compensated by collateral channels, can exhaust the collateral reserve and precipitate the development of gangrene in the injured extremity. Thrombotic occlusion in a previously diseased blood vessel may also be expected to occur, and this event may further accelerate the development of gangrene that otherwise might or might not have occurred spontaneously (Figs. 1–15 and 1–16).

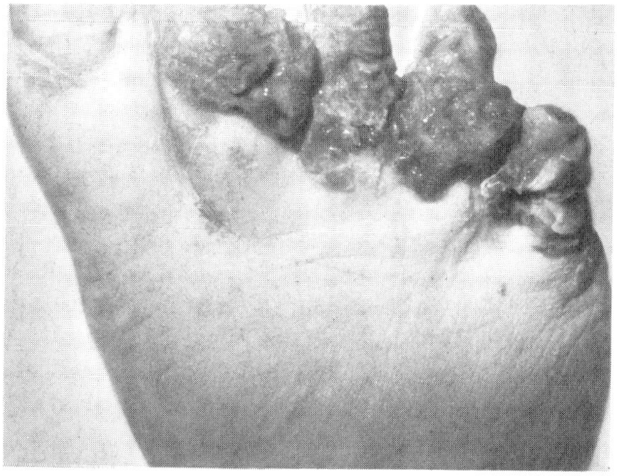

Figure 1–16. Dry gangrene of toes necessitating low leg amputation. Lumbosacral injury while at work, with fracture of vertebrae and spinal cord compression. The patient, a 64-year-old man, was bedridden for eight months. He had no previous history of claudication or any other evidence of lower limb vascular insufficiency. The question at issue is the possible role of immobilization in the development of the foot gangrene as against spontaneous occurrence.

It has been suggested that the concept of aggravation of preexisting disease must rest on the evidence that a nonhealing wound, gradually progressing to gangrene, developed not later than two weeks after the injury and that the preexisting arteriosclerotic process had been fairly well compensated, permitting the injured person to get around and walk for several blocks without pain.[12]

In the province of peripheral vascular disease, equally perplexing are the problems arising from the *rupture of a blood vessel* in concurrence with presumed physical exertion.

Increased intravascular pressure, either systemic or coincident to a strenuous physical effort, may cause a vessel to rupture.[13] The assumption in this case is that the walls of the vessel or the structures supporting it were weakened by preexisting disease or by a congenital structural disorder. Rupture of an aortic aneurysm or of a varicose vein exemplifies this situation. Generally acknowledged is the concept that any blood vessel, artery, or vein, weakened by preexisting disease, can rupture following exertion. Conversely, controversy may arise on the concept of whether a normal blood vessel (as far as it can be determined) can rupture in coincidence with muscular exertion.[14] Rupture of the inferior or deep epigastric artery, primarily in women who are or have been pregnant, under an episode of stress is well documented.[15] Similarly, many cases are on record of ruptured blood vessels following vigorous muscular effort in athletes and young males in military training.[16] Nevertheless against the contention that rupture of normal blood vessels may occur in connection with strenuous physical exertion are the results of direct tests showing the capacity of normal vessels to resist bursting tensions.

Trauma and Mental Reaction

Even relatively minor physical trauma, in the absence of organic brain damage may, in a mentally vulnerable personality, lead to a psychologic reaction that can delay return to functioning health.[17, 18] This is particularly common in the industrial setting in which the impact of compensation and claim settlements often tends to accentuate or prolong the disability, thereby interfering with rehabilitation. Thus, the ever-increasing present-day role of the psychiatrist in the area of medicine that deals with trauma. The range of mental disturbances that may follow injury includes a broad spectrum of effects. On one side are the deliberate malingering and the compensational neurosis *(attitudinal pathosis)* in which conscious mechanisms are primarily involved, and on the other, the *anxiety neurosis*, which is principally underlain by unconscious mechanisms.[19]

Unconscious and conscious motivation components probably exist in every case; ultimately, the personality of the individual and his potential for abnormal mental reactions are the major factors that determine whether a mental disturbance will occur, and, accordingly, its degree, type, and duration. The relative importance of the injury and the mental and emotional background of the individual provide the basic elements on which to assess any posttraumatic mental disorder.

In the absence of actual brain damage, nearly all posttraumatic mental disturbances represent either an aggravation of preexisting latent psychosis, primarily dementia praecox (schizophrenia) and manic-depressive states, or a tendency to psychosis. In a general sense, the injury comes to play the role of a precipitating factor.

Probably the same consideration applies to the chronic "war neurosis." A profuse literature indicates that the traumatic neurosis of war does not differ essentially from the traumatic neurosis of peacetime, both revealing a preexisting neurotic temperament or personality difficulties.[18]

It is generally accepted that the relation between injury and true posttraumatic psychosis rests on the demonstration that (1) the patient had been a mentally well-adjusted person prior to the injury; (2) the injury had produced organic damage to the central nervous system; (3) the injury, regardless of location, was of such magnitude as to reasonably threaten the very existence of the victim of the injury; (4) the injury was of a nature to affect the structure or the function of certain parts of the body to which emotional importance is attached (for example, genital organs, breasts, eyes, face, hands); (5) the victim was obsessed about the outcome from the time the injury was sustained; (6) the psychosis developed within a reasonable time after the occurrence of the injury; and (7) the psychotic thoughts had a positive relationship to the assault or accident that was responsible for the injury.

The differentiation between compensation neurosis and anxiety neurosis has practical implications. As a general rule, settlement tends to cure the former, whereas in the latter, the matter of compensation is of minor importance and indemnification has no effect on the mental disturbance.

Trauma and Subsequent Malignant Disease

Single Trauma

Since the cause of cancer is unknown, it can hardly be expected that a fair decision on the causal relationships between single, uncomplicated trauma and cancer be rendered by a court of law. A causal relationship between the two events, trauma and tumor, has not been established; nonetheless, cases of this sort continue to be filed in the courts, and occasional claims are being given favorable decisions.[20]

Against the assumption that a causal relation exists between single trauma and tumor are the 26,389 cases of injuries recorded by the New York State Industrial Compensation Bureau, among which 37 malignant tumors were found, an incidence parallel to that occurring in a similar group of uninjured persons.[21] This example, drawn from a very extensive literature, indicates that a causal relation between single trauma and cancer lacks statistical or scientific documentation.

The prerequisite to the assumption that any given case of cancer was caused by trauma rests in the fulfillment of the following postulates: (1) the part in which the tumor arose must be proved to have been normal before trauma; (2) the injury must have been of sufficient severity to produce tissue disruption; (3) the tumor must have originated in the part of the body that has sustained the injury; (4) it must be of the histologic type that could originate from the cells that have been disrupted by the trauma; and (5) it must develop within a certain period of time, between a minimum of three to four weeks and a maximum of three years, after receipt of the injury. Since it is well documented that a tumor can arise many years after exposure to a carcinogenic agent, some investigators have extended the upper limit of time to 10 to 20 years.

In fact, adequacy of the injury is difficult to establish. The term "adequacy" indeed has no meaning in the assessment of a condition the cause of which is not known. By the same token, tumors in all sites have a long silent period before revealing their presence; even the documentation of previous integrity of the tissues at roentgenologic examination cannot be considered as valid evidence inasmuch as a significant amount of tissue damage must occur before tissular distortion or destruction becomes obvious in x-ray films.

Very few case histories, when critically analyzed, fulfill the five classic postulates ruling the causative relation between single uncomplicated trauma and malignant change. It is more reasonable to say that trauma more frequently constitutes the event that reveals a tumor than the cause of its arising.

There is no organ in the human body in which the development of a cancer has not been attributed to prior trauma. The parts of the body most frequently implicated are the bones, testes, and breasts. Granted that traumatic cancer is difficult to prove on scientific terms, evidence to the contrary has been presented in individual cases, particularly in respect to tumors arising from the cerebral involucres; meningioma is an example.

Trauma as an Aggravating Factor

The role of trauma as an aggravating factor provides an equally complex challenge in compensation courts. Hemorrhage within a tumor, the perforation of the wall of a hollow viscus that results from the progressive infiltration of the growing tumor, the intensification of neurologic disorders associated with a tumor in the brain are natural features of neoplastic disease. Thus, the occurrence of any of these events following trauma can hardly be said to constitute aggravation. The concept of aggravation should be reserved for those situations in which the injury has introduced features detrimental to the patient that do not belong to the natural course of the tumor. On the other hand, this concept cannot be carried out with excessive inflexibility. For instance, although the occurrence of hemorrhage is within the natural course of neoplastic disease, it may be difficult to deny that an adequate blow in the region of a tumor may hasten the occurrence of a hemorrhage that, without the trauma, might or might not have occurred.

By the same token, the concepts of growth and rate of growth are implicitly inherent to the natural history of cancer. The term *acceleration* refers to an increase in the rate of growth. The idea that injury can accelerate the growth of a tumor lacks substantiation.

Another question related to trauma and tumor is whether a single injury can be responsible for the *conversion of a benign tumor into a malignant one.* Most investigators deny this possibility.

Equally debatable is whether trauma may aggravate the course of a tumor by hastening metastasis. The opinion generally held is that repeated rubbing or squeezing of a tumor can favor the development of metastasis, but that a single injury does not. It is also the prevailing opinion that a single trauma does not influence the localization of tumor particles circulating in the blood or lymph stream. In the light of occasional reports, however, in which substantial evidence is presented in support of a causal relation between trauma and localization of metastasis, in this situation also it is wise to keep an open mind.

Complicated Injury and Tumor

A single injury may initiate a chain of events that ultimately may become associated with a malignant tumor at the site of the original trauma *(complicated injury).* This is the case, for instance, for the skin cancer that originates in the proximity of a sinus tract draining a long-standing bone infection (osteomyelitis) that developed following a traumatic compound fracture. Two such cases are on record in our files (L.G.T., unpublished data). In a situation of this sort, medical science can support the concept of a causal connection between the original injury—bone fracture—and the ensuing

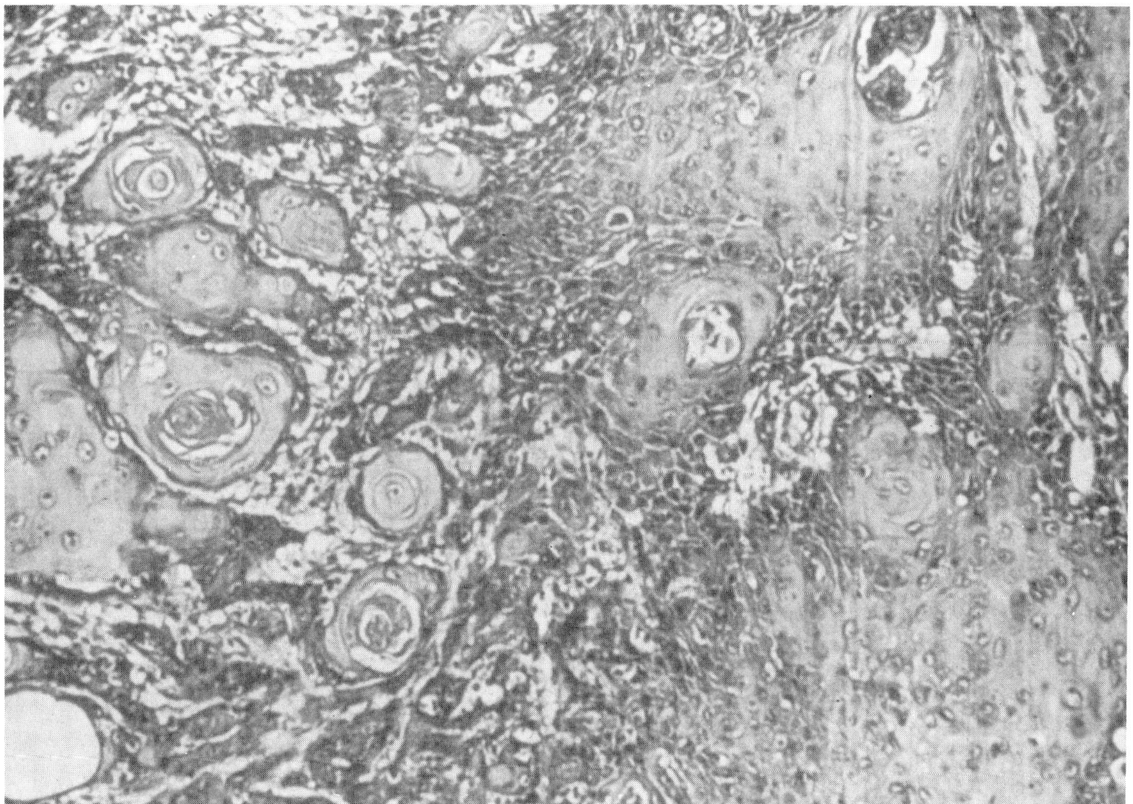

Figure 1–17. Epidermoid carcinoma at the site of a fistular tract in the left lower leg, the end result of chronic osteomyelitis in a 69-year-old man.

chronic irritation, which set up the environment best suited to tumor growth (Fig. 1–17). In the same category of complicated injury is the penetrating wound that introduces into the tissues foreign material with known carcinogenic properties. Thus, a cancer arising in the territory of imbedding of a bullet or shell splinter containing nickel or chromium, which are carcinogenic metals, may justifiably be considered related to the original trauma.

Repeated Trauma and Tumor

In the same way that the association of complicated injury and tumor usually provides favorable grounds for compensation, it is well accepted that *repeated* mechanical trauma over a period of years, to a limited surface of the body, can lead to the development of persistent abrasions or contusions and ultimately to a malignant growth, usually a skin cancer, at the site of continued irritation. This is not uncommon in certain trades, and whenever the chain of events can be established, the case falls into the category of industrial or occupational cancer.

Occupational Cancer

Industrial or *occupational cancer* is a field per se. It encompasses all the tumors that develop in concurrence with the repeated contact or exposure of the body to physical or chemical agents during certain phases of the individual's regular work. A tumor, to qualify as industrial or occupational, must arise in a given category of workmen more frequently than in a general population of comparable age and sex; it must occur in a particular portion of the body; and the incidence data must withstand critical statistical analysis. The assumption of a relation between occupation and tumor gains further strength if it can be proved that a tumor with the same general characteristics as that arising in the human following repeated contact with or exposure to the physical or chemical agent in question can be reproduced in experimental animals under comparable conditions of contact or exposure.

The correlation between exposure to arsenic among the workers in a broad spectrum of industries and the occurrence of cancer in body systems exposed to this metalloid is well supported by experiments in animals under conditions duplicating the exposure in man. Positive correlations are equally found among workers with asbestos, chrome, nickel and other metals, aromatic amines, azocompounds, and an endless list of other organic substances for which the ability to produce cancer is substantiated by controlled experiments.

The time interval between exposure to the carcinogenic agent and the arising of the cancer may extend over many years, and at the time the tumor has made its appearance, the individual may be engaged in a different occupation; thus, fact-finding is essential for accurate medical and legal opinion.

Industrial or occupational cancer rests on the concept that exposure to chronic irritants may provide in the targeted tissues a ground that is favorable to the development of a tumor. Mechanical trauma can provoke such a situation, but among the "irritants" it represents a statistically minor factor far surpassed by the chemical, physical, and biologic agents that crowd the environment.[22, 23] Because of the appreciation that pollutants can cause cancer, this aspect is receiving ever-growing consideration in relation to liability for cancer claims.

OUR PERMISSIVE KILLER

With at least 50 million injuries a year in the United States alone, resulting in 115,000 deaths and 400,000 permanent disabilities, the title of Ballinger and Drapanas's editorial "'Trauma' Our Permissive Killer" could not be more appropriate.[24, 25] Statistics indicate that more than one of every eight hospital beds in the United States is occupied by a victim of trauma and that trauma requires more hospital beds than heart disease and cancer.[24] Equally to the point is the subtitle of Seeley's monograph *Accidental Death and Disability: the Neglected Disease of Modern Society*.[26] Since trauma has become the most important health problem of our times, the approach to it is not different from that applied to any other disease: prevention and treatment are the base lines of the problem. Each provides a major challenge to the medical profession, to the law enforcement agencies, and to the public at large.

Along the line of prevention, the enforcing of rules and regulations that will produce a safer car is a step in the right direction. The same is true of the appeal for the manufacture of safer toys, household goods, and industrial machinery. The many "warnings" printed on the various containers and sprays that daily enter the American home are likewise aimed at protecting the consumer and the producer as well.

By the same token it is heartening to see that leading national agencies and institutions, such as the Highway Safety Bureau, the Consumer Testing Laboratories, the trauma committees of the American College of Surgeons, the National Academy of Sciences–National Research Council and the National Institute of Neurological Diseases and Strokes have established and are pursuing programs aimed at preventing injury and improving the methods of treatment. In both areas, emphasis is given to the role of research.

The first International Symposium on Trauma held in Washington, D.C., in May 1970, under the sponsorship of the National Institutes of Health, has awakened the public to the magnitude of the problem. It has also provided guidelines for improvement of the quality of and the distribution of care to the trauma victim. Improvement has already begun. The realization that rehabilitation begins with appropriate immediate care has led to the establishment of both trauma research units and community trauma centers. It has also led to the appreciation that even the most thoroughly capable general surgeon is not qualified to assume the overall responsibility for the management of the trauma victim. Adequate management requires proper monitoring of cardiac, renal, respiratory, and hepatic functions. Thus the need for detailed study of the patient and his responses by experts at all levels and from many disciplines. More and more it is being realized that emotional stress occasioned by the trauma is an integral part of the injury, that many biologic and biochemical disorders are part and parcel of the stress phenomenon, and that the psychologic aspects of trauma require as much attention as the medical and surgical aspects.

As Shires says "care and research combined in a single setting provide direct benefits to a given patient . . . [and] data gathered from many patients are of value in over-all improvement of knowledge for the care of every patient."[27]

REFERENCES

1. Bingham, C. T.: Psychosomatic approach to infections. Conn. State Med. J., *19*:731, 1955.
2. Tedeschi, L. G.: Fungal infections. In *Neuropathology: Methods and Diagnosis*. Edited by C. G. Tedeschi. Boston, Little, Brown and Company, 1970.
3. Blumgard, H. L., Schlesinger, M. J., and Zoil, P. W.: Multiple fresh coronary occlusions in patients with antecedent shock. Arch. Intern. Med., *68*:131, 1941.
4. Master, A. M., and Jaffie, H. L.: Factors in the onset of coronary occlusion and coronary insufficiency: effort, occupation, trauma, and emotion. J.A.M.A., *148*:794, 1952.
5. Moritz, A. R.: Trauma and heart disease. Western Reserve Univ. Law Rev., 5:133, 1954.
6. Schneider, R. A., and Zangari, V. M.: Variations in clotting time, relative viscosity, and other physiochemical properties of the blood accompanying physical and emotional stress in the normotensive and hypertensive subject. Psychosom. Med., *13*:289, 1951.
7. Biggs, R., and MacFarlane, R. G.: *Human Blood Coagulation*. 3rd Ed. Philadelphia, F. A. Davis Co., 1963.
8. Chambers, W. N., and Reiser, M. F.: Emotional stress in the precipitation of congestive heart failure. Psychosom. Med., *15*:38, 1953.
9. Weiss, E.: Emotional factors in cardiovascular disease. Pa. Med. J., *54*:319, 1951.
10. Weiss, E., Dlin, B., Rollin, H. R., Fischer, H. K., and Bepler, C. R.: Emotional factors in coronary occlusion. A.M.A. Arch. Intern. Med., *99*:628, 1957.
11. Freytag, E.: Autopsy findings in head injuries from blunt forces. Statistical evaluation of 1,367 cases. Arch. Pathol., *75*:402, 1963.
12. Fisher, M. M.: Trauma and peripheral vascular disease. Ind. Med. Surg., *21*:538, 1952.
13. Guy, C. C., and Wichowski, W. A.: Rupture of blood vessels by strenuous physical exertion. Am. J. Surg., *85*:418, 1953.
14. Longland, C. J.: Spontaneous rupture of pulmonary artery. J. Pathol. Bacteriol., *55*:103, 1943.
15. Payne, R. L.: Spontaneous rupture of superior and inferior epigastric arteries within rectus sheath. Ann. Surg., *108*:757, 1938.
16. St. John, F. B., Scudder, J., and Stevens, D. L.: Spontaneous rupture of axillary artery. Ann. Surg., *121*:882, 1945.
17. Brend, W. A.: *Traumatic Mental Disorders in Courts of Law, with a General Survey of Medical Evidence and Procedure in Civil Actions*. London, William Heinemann, Ltd., 1938.
18. Davidson, H. A.: *Forensic Psychiatry*. New York, The Ronald Press Co., 1952.
19. Kamman, G. R.: Traumatic neurosis, compensation neurosis or attitudinal pathosis? A.M.A. Arch. Neurol. Psychiatry, *65*:593, 1951.
20. Martin, W. F.: The relationship of a single act of trauma to subsequent malignancy—for the defense. American Bar Association Section of Insurance Law, 1955. In *Trauma and Disease*. Edited by A. R. Moritz and D. S. Helberg. New York, Central Book Co., Inc., 1959.
21. Stewart, F. W.: Occupational and post-traumatic cancer. Bull. N.Y. Acad. Med., *23*:145, 1947.
22. Seelig, M. G.: Compensation in one trauma cancer. J. Missouri Med. Assoc., *44*:27, 1947.
23. Moritz, A. R.: *Pathology of Trauma*. Philadelphia, Lea and Febiger, 1954.
24. Dunphy, J. E.: International trauma symposium: the challenge. Surgery, *69*:159, 1971.
25. Ballinger, W., and Drapanas, T.: Trauma: our permissive killer. Surgery, *69*:157, 1971.
26. Seeley, S.: *Accidental Death and Disability: the Neglected Disease of Modern Society*. National Academy of Sciences–National Research Council, 1966.
27. Shires, G. T.: The effect of trauma programs in the community. Surgery, *69*:162, 1971.

SECTION 1. MECHANICAL INJURY

chapter 2

TIMING OF THE WOUND

by Jyrki Raekallio

When examining a victim of violence no forensic pathologist is fulfilling his role when he confines his report to merely a numbered list of the wounds found. Of course, the nature, exact position, direction, and dimensions of every injury should be described, and it should, if possible, be photographed. Even the cause of death, however, is sometimes of less importance than the reconstruction of events, which may become possible with careful examination of the wounds and their proper timing. For example, a dead person may, after death, be run over by a car. If the examiner does not recognize that the injuries were caused after death, innocent people may be arrested and even found guilty. On the other hand, defective observations may lead to the acquittal of guilty persons. For example, the dead body of a murdered person may be put on a railroad track in order to simulate a suicide or an accident.

CLINICAL TIMING OF WOUNDS

Information concerning the age of wounds in *living persons* is often needed when examining an accused person or a complainant. It is not possible to determine exactly the age of a wound on the basis of its appearance to the naked eye. This is because the intensity of the local inflammatory reaction varies. Under average conditions, however, the edges of a wound are red and swollen after a lapse of about 12 hours.[1] A small wound may show scab formation after approximately 24 hours. Epithelium begins to grow at the edges of a wound after about 36 hours, and epithelialization of small clean wounds may be complete in four to five days.

Timing of bruises (contusions) must always be given with particular caution. After some 18 to 24 hours the blue or livid margins of the area become lighter, the whole area acquires a violet tint, and before its final disappearance, passes successively through shades of red-brown, green, yellow, and lemon color.[2]

When a wound has become infected, pus may be seen after a period of about 36 hours.[1] The wound's appearance to the naked eye depends to a large extent upon whether healing is proceeding with or without infection. Once infection has supervened, healing may be delayed, and it is often impossible to determine the age of the wound with any degree of accuracy.

VITAL REACTIONS: DISTINCTION BETWEEN ANTEMORTEM AND POSTMORTEM WOUNDS

In cases of *death by physical violence* there is always one major point to be determined by the forensic pathologist: whether the injuries were inflicted before death (intra vitam) or after it (post mortem). For the reconstruction of events, it is important to time the wound, i.e., to estimate the interval between trauma and death. The time of wounding is not necessarily that of death.

Ever since forensic medicine became an independent branch of science, the distinction between vital (antemortem, inflicted before death) and postmortem injuries has been one of its cardinal problems. As long ago as 1786 Plenk, in his *Elementa Medicinae et Chirurgiae Forensis*, emphasized the importance of recognizing vital reactions and differentiating them from postmortem phenomena.[3] Vital reactions in the forensic sense include all reactions of tissues and organs for which activities of living cells are necessary.[4] In earlier textbooks, such as that by Hofmann and Haberda in 1919, it was mainly the so-called systemic vital reactions that were discussed.[5] The word "systemic" refers to functioning circulatory and respiratory systems, which sustain life itself. The systemic vital reactions consist of hemorrhages, thrombi, emboli, and aspiration and swallowing of blood and foreign bodies and substances (for example, carbon monoxide).

It is interesting to note that classic systemic vital reactions have recently reattracted even greater interest because of modern advancement in medicine, including transplantation surgery. The recent technical advances in organ transplantation require that most organs be removed within a very short time of death so that the period of anoxia due to cessation of circulation can be kept to a minimum. This applies mainly to kidneys, heart, liver, and lungs at the present time, though this list is not complete. The determination of the moment of death has been discussed at length in medicolegal circles, but in most countries any statutory legal definition has been rejected. The World Medical Association (WHO) stated in 1968 (Chart of Sydney):

> This determination will be based on clinical judgement supplemented, if necessary, by a number of diagnostic aids, of which the electroencephalograph is currently most helpful. However, no single technological criterion is entirely satisfactory in the present state of medicine, nor can any one technological procedure be substituted by the overall judgement of the physician.

The legal requirements for obtaining tissues for transplantation are discussed in detail in Chapter 40. In connection with vital reactions it is sufficient to state that there is now great unanimity in medicolegal circles about the need for *several definitions of the moment of death.* The pronouncement of death in conventional cases, as for the purposes of *burial* and *autopsy*, may be based on the same criteria as previously, including cessation of respiration and circulation, and at least one of the classic secondary signs of death (for example, the lividity). For *organ transplantation*, numerous suggestions for determining the true moment of death have been put forward. This author suggests the following: an individual is dead when *infarction* of his brain tissue has advanced to such a degree that the essential cerebral functions have irreversibly been extinguished, irrespective of the presence or absence of cardiac function. The term "infarction" (which is very well accepted when it is applied to other organs than the brain) implies that the organ has "died," or ceased to function, owing to lack of blood supply. In most if not all cases of total brain infarction, the primary etiologic factor has been brain swelling with an increase in intracranial pressure and hence cessation of cerebral circulation.

The examination with the naked eye of wounds in corpses may be of some help when deciding whether the injuries are of antemortem origin. In the living body the extravasated blood is imbibed by the damaged tissues. The wound edges gape and become swollen after a lapse of about 12 hours. Later on, signs of inflammation and of healing dominate the picture. It may thus be possible to estimate that a wound is of antemortem origin if it shows evidence of a marked inflammatory reaction. This is not always the case, and a lapse of about 12 hours is far too long to satisfy the demands of a forensic examination. It is also customary to identify an antemortem wound by its profuse bleeding. Relatively recent investigations by Mueller and by Laiho, however, have shown that hemorrhages, even with abundant fibrin formation, are no longer reliable indicators of the antemortem origin of a wound.[6,7]

HISTOLOGIC EXAMINATION OF WOUNDS

Because of the uncertain and variable results of the naked-eye examination of wounds it is important to study the injuries microscopically. This is advisable both to distinguish between antemortem and postmortem wounds and to time wounds inflicted before death for the reconstruction of events. Walcher, Moritz, and many others have demonstrated that the leukocytic reaction is the earliest histologic sign of inflammation.[8,9] The exact time of the appearance of a distinct leukocytic infiltration is still a matter of debate. The discrepancy seems to be due to different opinions regarding the quantity of leukocytes to which the name leukocytic infiltration should be applied. The appearance of a few leukocytes in the wound periphery does not justify the diagnosis of a vital reaction, because these cells are a regular component of the connective tissue. According to Walcher and to Robertson and Hodge, perivascular cellular infiltration of polymorphonuclear leukocytes is clearly visible in cases with a survival period of about four hours or more.[8, 10] Dilatation of the capillaries and margination of leukocytes may be seen much earlier, even within a few minutes of the injury. It is important, however, to be aware that margination and a limited migration of leukocytes may occur in tissues in response to injury even after somatic death.[1] In subcutaneous adipose tissue the cellular reaction is demonstrable earlier (30 to 60 minutes in human material) than in the dermis.[11]

The first leukocytes to pass into the tissues are the polymorphonuclear neutrophils. Monocytes appear at a later stage and are seldom seen in the exudate before a lapse of about 12 hours.[1] In traumatic aseptic inflammation the exudation usually reaches its maximum intensity within 48 hours of the injury. Epithelial growth is clearly visible on the third day in most injuries.[10] The fibroblasts at the site of injury show reactive changes within a few hours, and these cells begin to undergo mitotic division about 15 hours after the injury. The rate of proliferation of the fibroblasts and the formation of new capillaries varies, but it usually takes at least three days for vascularized granulation tissue to develop. New collagen fibrils appear within four to five days of the injury. In small wounds a fibrous tissue scar may be apparent at the end of one week.[1] Usually at about 12 days, a definite stage of regression of cellular activity occurs in both epidermal and dermal tissue. Thereafter, the epithelium actually becomes atrophic, and reconstitution of normal rete pegs is not seen even after many weeks. The vascularity of the subepidermal tissue diminishes, and collagen fibers are restored. Even weeks after healing, elastic fibers are fewer in this new dermis than they are in adjoining undamaged skin.[10]

The histologic appearance of a wound depends to a large extent upon the presence or absence of *infection*. Infection delays healing to a variable extent; it is often impossible to time an infected wound with any degree of accuracy.

Histologic investigations have contributed substantially to the timing of wounds, and histologic examination is now—as in the past—absolutely indispensable. There still remains, however, a latent survival period of one to four (or even more) hours during which the distinction between antemortem and postmortem injuries is not possible by histologic methods.

HISTOCHEMICAL EXAMINATION OF WOUNDS

It is now known that morphologic changes are preceded by functional phenomena, and these, moreover, often correlate with the action of enzymes. *Enzymes* are proteins that possess the remarkable property of catalyzing biologic reactions. It is thus to be expected that the demonstration of enzymes, which cause many important phenomena, could reveal earlier reactions than could the visualization of the resulting morphologically demonstrable changes. This hypothesis has been proved true by applying the methods of enzyme histochemistry to the study of wound healing.[12-15] This is not surprising, since the importance of enzymes in the cells and tissues of healing wounds is readily recognized. It may even be appropriate to consider that the competence to heal is based on the enzyme functions in the participating cells and tissues. There can be no life without enzymes, and healing is an example of the enzymatically catalyzed processes in the organism on which its life depends.

Histochemical examination is based on the production of microscopically visible reactions by applying chemical tests to tissue sections prepared for microscopic study. For technical details the reader is referred to, for example, the textbook of histochemistry by Pearse.[16] The enzyme histochemical methods, applied to the timing of wounds, have been described and discussed in detail elsewhere.[13, 14] For histologic and histochemical examination, the wounds (or parts of them) are excised with their surroundings, about half an inch in each direction. One half of the tissue block is fixed overnight in neutral 10 per cent formalin at 4°C (refrigerator temperature) for the demonstration of esterase and phosphatase activity and for histologic examination. The other half is fresh frozen with isopentane chilled with dry ice, and the frozen specimen is subjected to the histochemical methods for detecting adenosine triphosphatases and aminopeptidases. The demonstration of enzymes in situ depends on their action on a specific substrate in the presence of other substances with which one of the decomposition products resulting from enzyme activity will form an insoluble deposit at the site of enzyme action. If this deposit is not already colored it is rendered visible by the use of suitable chemicals. To simplify, an increase in enzyme activity appears as an intensified color and a decrease in enzyme activity as a declining stainability. The forensic application of enzyme histochemical methods for the timing of wounds is

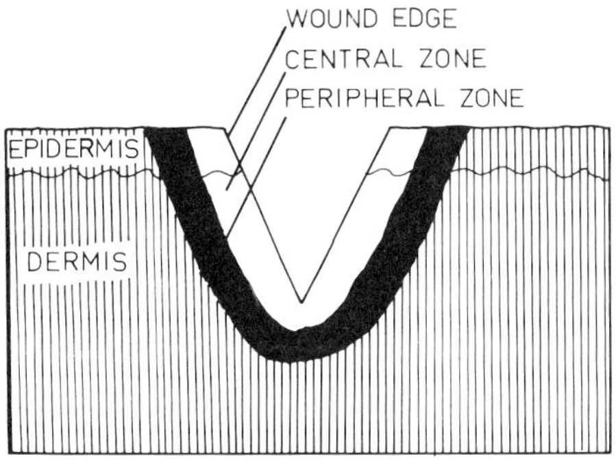

Figure 2–1. Schematic diagram of the zones, demonstrable by enzyme histochemistry, of an antemortem wound.

not possible without experience in enzyme histochemistry.

To summarize the results, two zones can be demonstrated around the antemortem wounds (Fig. 2–1).[12-15] In the immediate vicinity of the wound edge, a *central* (superficial) *zone*, 200 to 500 μ deep, shows decreasing enzyme activity. This should be considered as an early sign of imminent necrosis. The regressive phenomena in the central zone may be called *negative vital reactions*, since no such decrease in enzyme activity is observed in the wounds inflicted after death.[13]

Surrounding the central area, a *peripheral zone*, 100 to 300 μ deep, exhibits an increase in enzyme activity, which represents, among other things, an adaptive defense mechanism of the local connective tissue cells as an enzymatic response to injury.[13-15] This increase in enzyme activity in the peripheral zone may be called a *positive vital reaction* since there are no such changes in postmortem wounds.[13] Figure 2–2 is an example of this general pattern of enzyme activity in antemortem (vital) wounds. The activity of adenosine triphosphatases and esterases increases as early as about one hour after injury, the activity of aminopeptidases increases at about two hours, and those of acid phosphatases and of alkaline phosphatases at four and eight hours, respectively. The consecutive appearance of the positive vital reactions, demonstrable by the various methods of enzyme histochemistry, allows the construction of a biologic timetable that may be useful in the rough timing of antemortem wounds (Fig. 2–3).

It is important, in practice, that the histochemical vital reactions are recognizable several days after death. There are, however, certain exceptions in the biologic timetable when it is applied to human autopsy material. In material from 43 victims of traffic accidents there were five cases in which the enzyme appearances were exceptional.[17] For example, in one case (an 81-year-old man) alkaline phosphatase ac-

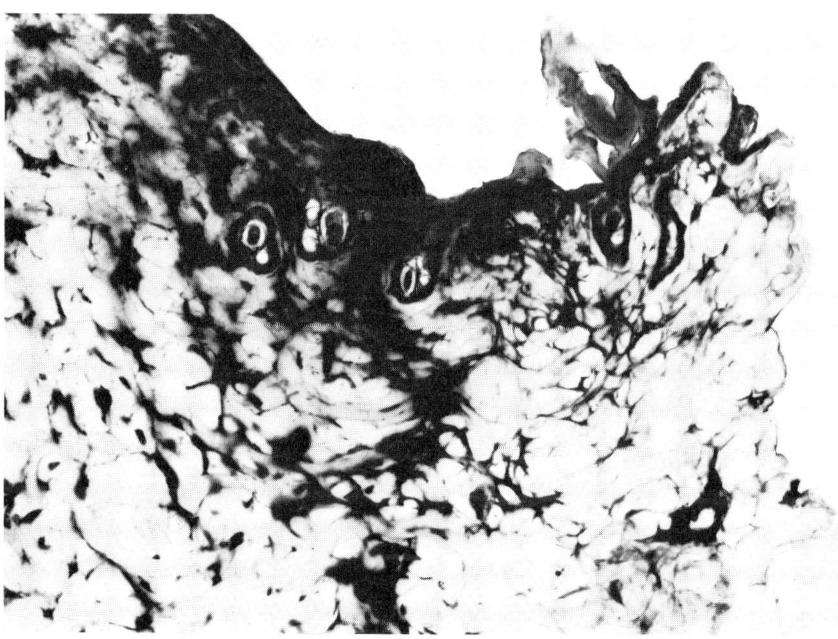

Figure 2–2. Adenosine triphosphatase activity in an incised wound. The victim survived for one and a half hours. The sample was removed at an autopsy performed two days after death. Histochemical determination was made by the method of Padykula and Herman. × 60.

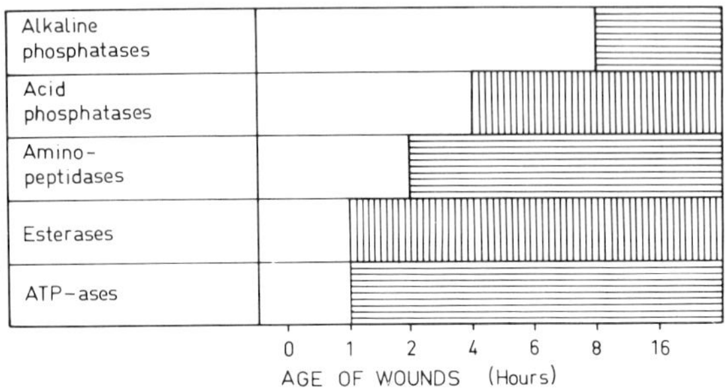

Figure 2–3. Schematic diagram of the histochemical timing of antemortem skin wounds.

tivity was not increased in the periphery of a lacerated wound inflicted 10 hours before death (from chest injury). This delay in the enzymatic response to injury may have been due to the senility of the victim. Conditions such as far-advanced senility, cachexia, and very severe and multiple injuries may impair the local reactivity of the skin.[8] On the other hand, Berg has shown that bleeding, a cold environment, and cranial fractures do not delay the inflammatory reaction.[18]

Histochemical findings are often of great, sometimes even decisive, help to the forensic pathologist when he is faced with the problem of timing of wounds. The following example illustrates this: A jealous young man believed that he had killed his fiancée when he hit her on the head with a stone. He placed the body on a railroad track in order to simulate an accident or a suicide. Four hours later a train arrived and caused fatal injuries to the body. A medicolegal autopsy was performed, and the wounds were studied with enzyme histochemical methods. According to the results, a laceration on her head was produced several hours before the fatal wounds caused by the train. The girl had obviously been unconscious after the blow to her head. The police were informed. The young man subsequently pleaded guilty when he realized that even the timetable of his crime was known.[15]

During recent years, studies by Fatteh, Lo Menzo, Lindner, Berg, and several other investigators have confirmed the presence of an early enzymatic response to injury in antemortem wounds and its absence in postmortem injuries.[18-21] The methods of enzyme histochemistry act, thus, as a guide to the estimation of the approximate age of wounds, especially those inflicted one to eight hours before death. Second, these methods reveal vital changes around skin wounds inflicted as little as one hour before death. This is about four to eight times earlier than was possible when only histologic techniques were available.

BIOCHEMICAL EXAMINATION OF WOUNDS

Although enzyme histochemical methods have considerably shortened the indeterminable period after wounding, there is still the very last hour before death, the study of which has presented a great challenge. The reaction to injury must be immediate, but the problem is: are we able to detect the very earliest reactions in a wound and thus to demonstrate its antemortem origin?

Histamine and serotonin (5-hydroxytryptamine) are vasoactive amines known to participate in the acute inflammatory process, especially in the earliest phase after injury. The first forensic application of the study of biogenic amines was published in 1965, when Fazekas and Virágos-Kis reported an increase in the free histamine content in an antemortem ligature mark due to hanging.[22] This observation prompted other investigators to study the histamine and serotonin content of skin wounds under controlled circumstances, i.e., initially in experimental animals.[23-26] The maximal increase in the free histamine content occurs within 20 to 30 minutes after wounding.[23] The increase in the serotonin content is demonstrable still earlier, the maximal increase occurring within 10 minutes after injury.[26]

In addition to experimental investigations, the serotonin and free histamine content of skin injuries have been studied in forensic autopsy materials.[24,27] In practice, a sample, about 2 g of the injured skin, is removed.[27] In addition, a control sample, equal in size, is taken from the neighboring intact skin of the same corpse. This is necessary since there are great individual and regional differences in the free histamine and serotonin content. The subcutaneous fat is removed from the samples before further processing, and the free histamine and serotonin in the wound samples are compared with those in the control samples. The modifications of the quantitative methods for the study of the biogenic amines, used in our laboratory in forensic practice, are as follows:

Extraction and Determination of Free Histamine

The extraction of free histamine from skin samples is performed as described by Fazekas and Virágos-Kis.[22] The free histamine content of the extract is measured spectrofluorometrically according to the method of Shore, Burkhalter, and Cohn.[28]

Reagents

Tyrode I solution: 200 g sodium chloride, 5 g potassium chloride, 5 g calcium chloride, 2.5 g magnesium chloride is dissolved with water to a final volume of 1000 ml. Tyrode II solution: 50 g sodium hydrogen carbonate and 5 g sodium dihydrogen phosphate is dissolved with water to a final volume of 1,000 ml. Eighty milliliters of Tyrode I solution and 40 ml of Tyrode II solution are mixed and diluted with water to 2,000 ml.
Sodium hydroxide, 5 N.
n-Butanol.
Sodium hydroxide, 0.1 N, saturated with sodium chloride.
Hydrochloric acid, 0.1 N.
n-Heptane.
Sodium hydroxide, 1 N.
o-Phthalaldehyde (OPT), 1 per cent in reagent grade absolute methanol.
Hydrochloric acid, 3 N.
Histamine standard solution: histamine hydrochloride in 0.1 N hydrochloric acid.

Procedure

The free histamine is extracted from the injured skin and from the control samples, which are cut with scissors into small pieces, with Tyrode solution (5 ml per gram) at 4°C for 12 to 15 hours. After incubation the solutions are filtered. An 0.8 ml aliquot of the filtrate is transferred to a shaking tube containing 0.1 ml of 5 N sodium hydroxide, 0.3 g of solid sodium chloride, and 2.0 ml of *n*-butanol. The tube is shaken for five minutes and then centrifuged. The aqueous phase is removed, and the organic phase is shaken for one minute with 1 ml of salt-saturated 0.1 N sodium hydroxide. After centrifugation, 1.8 ml of the butanol phase is transferred to a shaking tube containing 0.7 ml of 0.1 N hydrochloric acid and 3.0 ml of *n*-heptane. The mixture is shaken for one minute and centrifuged. To 0.5 ml of the aqueous phase, 0.1 ml of 1 N sodium hydroxide and 25 μl of *o*-phthalaldehyde reagent is added. After four minutes, 50 μl of 3 N hydrochloric acid is added. The contents of the tube is thoroughly mixed after each addition. The solution is activated at 360 mμ and the resultant fluorescence is measured at 450 mμ. To eliminate the fluorescence caused by the tissue itself or by the reagents, all the reagents are added to a separate aliquot of tissue extract, but reversing the order of addition of *o*-phthalaldehyde and 3 N hydrochloric acid.

Extraction and Determination of Serotonin

The method for the quantitative determination of serotonin is based on the spectrofluorometric method of Udenfriend, Weissbach, and Clark.[29]

Reagents

Borate buffer: to 94.2 g of boric acid, dissolved in 3 liters of water, 165 ml of 10 N sodium hydroxide is added. The buffer solution is then saturated with purified *n*-butanol and sodium chloride by adding these substances in excess and shaking. Excess *n*-butanol is removed by aspiration, and excess salt is permitted to settle. The final pH is approximately 10.
n-Butanol: reagent grade *n*-butanol is purified by shaking with an equal volume of 0.1 N sodium hydroxide, then with 0.1 N hydrochloric acid, and finally twice with distilled water.
Heptane: practical grade heptane is treated in the same manner as the *n*-butanol.
Serotonin standard solution: serotonin-creatininsulfate in 0.1 N hydrochloric acid.

Procedure

The serotonin is extracted from the skin samples that have been cut with scissors into small pieces with 0.1 N hydrochloric acid (5 ml per gram) at 4°C for 16 to 18 hours. After incubation the solutions are filtered. The pH of 1.5 ml of the filtrate is adjusted to approximately pH 10 by the addition of anhydrous sodium carbonate. To it 2.5 ml of borate buffer, 3.5 ml of water, 2.5 g of sodium chloride, and 7.5 ml of *n*-butanol are added and the mixture is shaken for 10 minutes. Centrifugation for 5 minutes follows. The aqueous layer is discarded. To 7 ml of the butanol phase, 7 ml of borate buffer is added and the mixture is again shaken and centrifuged as before. Five milliliters of the butanol phase is transferred to another bottle containing 10 ml of heptane and 1.5 ml of 0.1 N hydrochloric acid. The mixture is shaken for 10 minutes and centrifuged. The pH of 1.0 ml of the acid layer is adjusted to pH 2.5 with anhydrous sodium carbonate. The solution is activated at 295 mμ in the spectrophotofluorometer, and the resultant fluorescence is measured at 345 mμ.

On the basis of autopsy studies, a distinct increase in serotonin content indicates the antemortem origin of a wound even in man.[24, 27] According to our experience, the increase in the serotonin content of the injured tissue must be at least twofold, and that in histamine one and a half fold or more (as compared to a control sample of neighboring intact skin), in order to indicate with certainty that the wound was inflicted before death.

There is no increase in the histamine and serotonin content in postmortem wounds. The absence of the histamine reaction does not necessarily indicate that a wound was inflicted after death, but a positive histamine reaction, i.e., a distinct increase in the histamine content, does indicate the vital origin of an injury.[24, 25, 27] A distinct increase in the serotonin content also indicates a wound made before death, and the increase in serotonin seems to be more constant than that in histamine.[24, 27] The antemortem increase in both these amines remains well demonstrable during the first four to five days after death.[27] The changes in the serotonin and histamine content may thus be used in forensic practice.

Berg and Bonte have compared the results of biochemical determinations of serotonin and of histamine.[30] A great increase in the serotonin content with a simultaneous slight increase in histamine characterizes an agonal injury. In wounds inflicted 5 to 15 minutes before death there is a relatively greater increase in histamine than in serotonin. The case is just the reverse in injuries inflicted 15 to 60 minutes or more before death.

The biochemical serotonin and histamine determinations are most important in the timing of wound inflicted during the last hour before death and in the distinction between antemortem and postmortem injuries. Wounds inflicted more than one hour before death may be timed enzyme histochemically, and if the injuries were caused more than four to eight hours ante mortem, even histologically. Although the histochemical and biochemical methods have contributed substantially to the timing of wounds, the histologic examination is still absolutely indispensable in every case of forensic importance.

REFERENCES

1. Gordon, I., Turner, R., and Price, W.: *Medical Jurisprudence.* 2nd Ed. Edinburgh, E. & S. Livingstone, 1953.
2. Simpson, K.: *Taylor's Principles and Practice of Medical Jurisprudence.* 12th Ed. London, J. & A. Churchill Ltd., 1965.
3. Plenk 1786, cited by Orsós, F.: Die vitalen Reaktionen und ihre gerichtsmedizinische Bedeutung. Beitr. Pathol., *95*:163, 1935.
4. Gradwohl, R. B. H.: *Legal Medicine.* 1st Ed. St. Louis, C. V. Mosby Co., 1954.
5. Hofmann, E. R., and Haberda, A.: *Lehrbuch der gerichtlichen Medizin mit gleichmässiger Berücksichtigung der deutschen und österreichischen Gesetzgebung.* 10th Ed. Berlin, Urban & Schwarzenberg, 1919.
6. Mueller, B.: Zur Frage der Unterscheidung von vitalen beziehungsweise agonalen und postmortalen Blutungen. Acta Med. Leg. Soc., *17*:43, 1964.
7. Laiho, K.: Immunohistochemical studies on fibrin in vital and postmortem subcutaneous hemorrhages. Ann. Acad. Sci. Fenn. [Med.], *128*:1, 1967.
8. Walcher, K.: Über vitale Reaktionen. Dtsch. Z. Gesamte Gerichtl. Med., *15*:16, 1930.
9. Moritz, A. R.: *The Pathology of Trauma.* Philadelphia, Lea & Febiger, 1942.
10. Robertson, I., and Hodge, P. R.: Histopathology of healing abrasions. Forensic Sci., *1*:17, 1972.
11. Hirvonen, J.: Histochemical studies on vital reaction and traumatic fat necrosis in the interscapular adipose tissue of adult guinea pigs. Ann. Acad. Sci. Fenn. [Med.], *136*:1, 1968.
12. Raekallio, J.: Enzymes histochemically demonstrable in the earliest phase of wound healing. Nature (Lond.), *188*:234, 1960.
13. Raekallio, J.: Histochemical studies on vital and postmortem skin wounds. Experimental investigation on medicolegally significant vital reactions in an early phase of wound healing. Ann. Med. Exp. Fenn., *39*:Suppl. 6:1, 1961.
14. Raekallio, J.: *Enzyme Histochemistry of Wound Healing.* Stuttgart, Gustav Fischer Verlag, 1970.
15. Raekallio, J.: Determination of the age of wounds by histochemical and biochemical methods. Forensic Sci., *1*:3, 1972.
16. Pearse, A. G. E.: *Histochemistry, Theoretical and Applied.* London, J. & A. Churchill Ltd., Vol. 1, 1968, and Vol. 2, 1972.
17. Raekallio, J.: Application of histochemical methods to the study of traffic accidents. Acta Med. Leg. Soc. (Liege), *20*:171, 1967.
18. Berg, S.: Die Altersbestimmung von Hautverletzungen. Z. Rechtsmed., *70*:121, 1972.
19. Fatteh, A.: Histochemical distinction between antemortem and postmortem skin wounds. J. Forensic Sci., *11*:17, 1966.
20. Lo Menzo, G.: *Lesioni Vitali e Post-Mortali.* Catania, Edigraf, 1969.
21. Lindner, J.: Vitale Reaktionen. Acta Histochem. (Jena) Suppl., *9*:435, 1971.
22. Fazekas, I. G., and Virágos-Kis, E.: Der Gehalt der Erhängungsfurche an freiem Histamin als vitale Reaktion. Dtsch. Z. Gesamte Gerichtl. Med., *56*:250, 1965.
23. Raekallio, J., and Mäkinen, P.-L.: Histamine content as vital reaction. I. Experimental investigation. Zacchia, *41*:273, 1966.
24. Berg, S., Ditt, J., Friedrich, R., and Bonte, W.: Möglichkeiten der biochemischen Wundaltersbestimmung. Dtsch. Z. Gesamte Gerichtl. Med., *63*:183, 1968.
25. Merli, L. D., Gualdi, G., and Ronchi, G. U.: La diagnosi chronologica delle ferite cutanee. Zacchia, *44*:380, 1969.
26. Raekallio, J., and Mäkinen, P.-L.: Serotonin content as vital reaction. I. Experimental investigation. Zacchia, *44*:587, 1969.
27. Raekallio, J., and Mäkinen, P.-L.: Serotonin and histamine contents as vital reactions. II. Autopsy studies. Zacchia, *45*:403, 1970.
28. Shore, P. A., Burkhalter, A., and Cohn, V. H., Jr.: A method for the fluorometric assay of histamine in tissues. J. Pharmacol. Exp. Ther., *127*:182, 1959.
29. Udenfriend, S., Weissbach, H., Clark, C. T.: The estimation of 5-hydroxytryptamine (serotonin) in biological tissues. J. Biol. Chem., *215*:337, 1955.
30. Berg, S., and Bonte, W.: Praktische Erfahrungen mit der biochemischen Wundaltersbestimmung. Beitr. Gerichtl. Med., *28*:108, 1971.

SECTION 1. MECHANICAL INJURY

chapter 3

THE WOUND: ASSESSMENT BY ORGAN SYSTEMS

I. Head and Spine

by C. G. Tedeschi

"Head injury," as defined by the National Advisory Neurological Diseases and Stroke Council, "is a morbid state, resulting from gross or subtle structural changes in the scalp, skull, and/or the contents of the skull, produced by mechanical forces."[1] By the same definition the concept of "mechanical forces" is restricted to those forces applied externally to the head, thus excluding surgical ablations and internally acting forces such as increased intracranial pressure resulting from edema, hydrocephalus, or a mass-occupying lesion "*without* antecedent head trauma."[1]

This definition provides for a reasonably clear understanding of the problems directly concerned with the neurologic deficits that are likely to arise following an injury to the head. To be complete, however, it should take into account that the impact responsible for the injury need not be applied directly to the head.

According to the causative mechanisms, skull fractures and other injuries of the head may be classed as *direct* or *indirect* trauma. In the category of direct injuries are those resulting from a moving object striking a stationary head or a moving head striking a stationary object. Indirect injury is exemplified by a mechanical force applied to the chin and transmitted to the middle fossa by way of the mandible, or applied to the feet or buttocks and transmitted to the base of the cranium by way of the vertebral column.

The fatality rate from the epidemic of trauma on the highways increases steadily. Equally on the increase are sports-connected injuries and injuries from social upheaval and violence.

Although exact data are not available to determine the role played by head injury in the overall number of fatal or disabling accidents, presumably the toll is the highest. Estimates indicate that head trauma occurs in 71 per cent of persons injured in automobile accidents, in 50 per cent of persons injured in motorcycle accidents, in 70 per cent of persons injured in accidental falls in the home, and in 7 per cent of compensable work-related injuries.[2–5]

Lewin, in an analysis of mortality figures for nonmissile head injuries, quotes rates of 12 to 20 per cent and emphasizes that in 60 to 70 per cent of the fatal cases, death occurs within the first 24 hours.[6] Frequently these early deaths are due to the severity of the brain lesions, but this is not necessarily the case. Early fatalities can be caused by extracranial factors, primarily chest complications and systemic disorders that, if promptly recognized, may be amenable to effective treatment.

Trauma, as a general rule, carries medicolegal implications. Head injury adds complexity to the problem, for the reason that the full effects of the trauma cannot be completely evaluated until some time has elapsed after the alleged injury. The often ill-defined clinical manifestations, the impact of claim settlements, and deliberate malingering appose further difficulties to the problem of fair decision.

The remarkable capacity of the brain to recover from, or compensate for, the effects of injury has also to be kept in mind. As Lewin points out, aphasia and hemiplegia are commonly seen in the early days after injury, but they frequently resolve in the course of time and rather infrequently cause permanent disability.[6] Even in brain stem injury, which as a rule carries a high mortality rate, recovery is possible. Lewin mentions the case of a patient with clinical evidence of such a lesion who remained unconscious for six months following the injury and thereafter made a progressive recovery; 10 months after the accident she was talking and later was able to return home and look after her family.[6] Observations like this one stress the point that any final decision on claims for compensation for neurologic deficits and mental reactions following alleged head trauma should be deferred until after competent evaluation of the claimant's signs and symptoms at a distance of time from the original injury.

HISTORICAL BACKGROUND

Looking into the history of head trauma, we realize that it did not take long for man to appreciate that the head is one of the most vulnerable parts of the body. This is well attested by the creation of the protective helmet (iron hat) worn by warriors far back in antiquity and now as well, at war and at peace, while at work and in a variety of sport-connected activities.

We learn from the Egyptian papyrus of Edwin Smith and from the heroic poems of the Greek *(Iliad)* and Roman *(Aeneid)* literature that the cranial wounds of antiquity did not differ a great deal in their lethal or disabling effects from the cranial wounds of our times; what have changed through the ages are the methods of injury, both accidental and intentional assault, the basic reason for the change being a continuous upgrading of "force."

As Courville says, "the march of the conquerors has often been marked by the bones of their victims who dared dispute their way."[7] The head-hunters' hideouts in the Philippines, the skull houses of the South Sea Islanders, the military graveyards of ancient Peru, the ossuaries of Sedlec and Wisby, the skeletons of soldiers found in pharaohs' tombs, and ultimately, in our own times, the pits filled with the remains of the victims of war and persecution sadly bear witness to the violence and trauma in the evolution of mankind.[7-10] It becomes clear that the methods of injury have changed through the ages, but not their effects, nor man's nature.

Several studies are available on the characteristics of war wounds of the cranium in the Middle Ages, as disclosed by the analysis of human remains in the historical ossuaries. Courville's scrutiny of the skeletal material of 1,185 individuals interred in common graves on the battleground of Wisby* revealed that 44.9 per cent of the crania held the marks of injury, an indication not only of the frequency of wounds of the head but also of their lethal quality.[9]

Equally revealing is Courville's study of skulls found in Sedlec Ossuary, near Kuttenberg, Czechoslovakia, presumably from soldiers killed in the Thirty Years' War.[7] Findings ranged from surface irregularities or depressions with little loss of bone (contusions), probably resulting from edged weapons that failed to enter the cranial vault, to linear fractures, probably produced by heavier two-handed swords or battle-axes or pole arms. Depressed skull fractures and large and small irregular cranial defects involving the vault alone, or both vault and base, were also seen. Blade marks often betrayed the edged nature of the weapon that was responsible for the fatal blow; conversely, small, round cranial perforations left problematic the nature of the weapon. They might have been made by a pitchfork, since farm tools were used as instruments of war, or by the bolt of a crossbow, or by an arrow with a rounded metal point. Iron arrowheads mounted on wooden shafts were frequently used in the Middle Ages, and the sizes of the cranial defects indicate the considerable force with which such missiles could be fired from a crossbow. Not uncommonly, an arrowhead was found to rest deep within the cranial cavity, having produced a through-and-through wound.

An additional interesting point emerging from these studies was the remarkable degree of healing detected in old cranial defects and depressed fractures evidently sustained in previous conflicts or accidents. Equally remarkable was the absence of signs of past infections at the borders of these defects. This would suggest either a high degree of skill on the part of the military surgeons of the time or a benevolence on the part of mother nature far superior to that shown in our day.

The elegant woodcut of the "wound man," shown in Figure 3–I–1, carried with small modifications from one surgical treatise to another from the late fifteenth century for the following 250 years, disappoints the reader. One

*Battle of Wisby between the Danes and the Gotlanders fought on July 27, 1361.

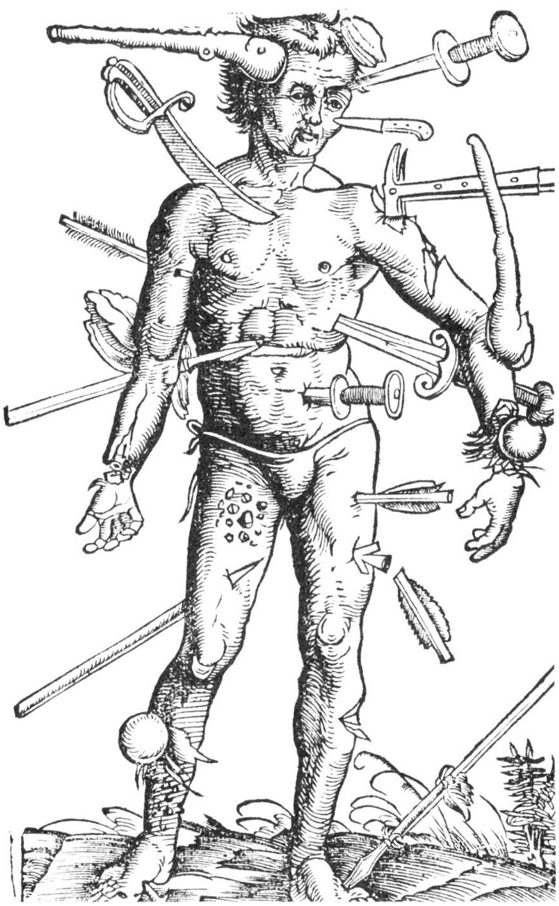

Figure 3–I–1. "Wound man."

would expect to find, beneath the well-drawn weapons and missiles striking the man's figure from head to toe, some information on how to treat the wounds inflicted by them, but this is not the case. Methods of treatment of cranial wounds throughout the Middle Ages still followed the tradition of the teaching of Hippocrates, carried on from generation to generation of surgeons for about 2,000 years, as exemplified in the commentary by Paaw in 1616.[11]

In spite of this deficiency, the "wound man," with his many injuries produced by still in situ flying stones, clubs, edged and penetrating weapons, knives, swords, arrows, and spears, gives a graphic impression of the weaponry of the times. Furthermore, the customary association of the "wound man" with other figures of astrological significance points to the superstition that attended medical and surgical practice in the Middle Ages. As Major elegantly says, "For a doctor (of that time) to doubt the validity of astrology was quite as unusual as for a priest to doubt the authority of the Church."[12]

When the "wound man" was first used in medical manuscripts is not exactly known. According to Courville, the figure is believed to date back to the early 1400's.[13] It is found also in a manuscript described by Sudhoff, variously dated from 1450 to 1485, and it appears again a few years later in the surgical treatises of Ketham (1491), Brunschwig (1497) and von Gersdorff (1517).[14-17] In the last-named, a distinction is drawn for the first time between head wounds "sine apertura volneris" (blunt or closed wounds), "apertura cranii" (open wounds), "incisu cerebri" (actual injury of the brain). The Brunschwig treatise *(Der Cirurgia. Hautwirckung der Wundarztny)* also deserves special recognition for giving the earliest consideration to gunshot wounds. Reproduced in almost every book dealing with the surgery of trauma throughout the Middle Ages, the "wound man" made his last appearance on the title page of the 1678 English edition of Paré's work.[13]

The state of knowledge of the treatment of head trauma at the time the "wound man" went into oblivion is well mirrored by an account of the subject presented by a distinguished Italian physician, Dr. Mattia Caterini, to the highly reputed Accademia dei Fisiocritici di Siena (13 December 1696).[18]

When to refer the victim of a head injury to the surgeon and when to apply conservative medical treatment are the main issues in the entire presentation. Although the benefits derived from draining the wound, curetting its edges, trephining the calvaria and removing bone fragments and foreign bodies are not denied, the learned physician points out the dangers associated with excessive surgery that often hastens the fatal course of events and adds to the discomfort of the already suffering patient. He also criticizes the common practice of pouring ink on the surface of open wounds, a fashionable procedure used by surgeons of that time to reveal fracture lines in the calvaria. The danger of this method, he says, rests in the ink's seeping between bone and dura mater or even deeper between dura and pial meninges, and not uncommonly into the brain itself, thus causing the entrance of undesirable foreign particles into the cranial cavity.

Obviously a physician, not a surgeon, Caterini maintains that results comparable to and often far better than those obtained by surgery can be attained by conservative medical treatment, including the application of ointments on the wound, repeated blood letting, and generous administration of laxatives and diuretics in order to drain through natural channels (veins) the humors that accumulate at the site of the wound.

The learned physician, in support of his arguments, profusely quotes and requotes the teachings of the old masters—Galenus, Aristotle, Hippocrates, Celsus. Other writings, closer to his time, are totally ignored except for a brief mention of the work of Fallopius. Literary omissions are, however, compensated for by good sense and evidently by considerable experience. He recommends that the patient be kept warm, and points out the poor prognosis associated with bloody discharge from the ears and mouth and nostrils, loss of consciousness, vomiting, vertigo, and delirium. In the system of examination of the patient with a cranial wound, he further stresses the value of inviting the patient to cough and blow his nose. The localized sharp pain elicited by these maneuvers may point out to the surgeon, he says, the exact area on the head on which to apply his iron implements.

It is apparent that the rational approach to the treatment of head trauma was still far away at the time of Caterini's presentation. It had to await, for more than 200 years, the advent of anesthesia and roentgenology, the introduction of sterile techniques, the discovery of antibiotic agents, and above all, the understanding that the effects of head trauma extend beyond the site of injury to disturb the function of practically all body systems. Stone by stone, however, the foundations to the rational approach to trauma were being built. It is significant that approximately one hundred years after the poor display of knowledge made by Dr. Caterini, the Royal Academy of Surgery of Paris (Académie Royale de Chirurgie) in 1776 announced a prize "to establish the theory of contrecoup lesions of the head and their effects *(établir la théorie des contrecoups dans les lésions de la tête et les conséquences qu'on peut en tirer).*"[19] The prize was not, to our knowledge, awarded and probably never will be, for the simple reason that no two head injuries are exactly alike; however, this announcement informs us that toward the end of the eighteenth century, empiric traumatology was being pushed aside by sound study of the mechanisms and theory of injury.

Of the same century, properly called the century of enlightenment, is the establishment, on the same soil of France, of military hospitals attended by military surgeons. Marie François Xavier Bichat (1771–1802), the founder of scientific histology and pathologic anatomy, was one of them, and this gives us an indication of the quality of the physicians recruited at that time by the Army Medical Corps. We learn from Peabodys that a *Journal de Médecine Militaire* was established in 1747 by an ordinance from Louis XV.[20] The journal, printed at the Crown's expense, was distributed at no cost to the health officers of the hospitals and regiments of the army of France. A perusal of the contents of the volume of 1782, kept in the rare book section of the Countway Library in Boston, gives us a clear perspective of how rapidly the study of trauma was progressing (Fig. 3–I–2). Wounds by firearms are discussed, and there are carefully described case reports on

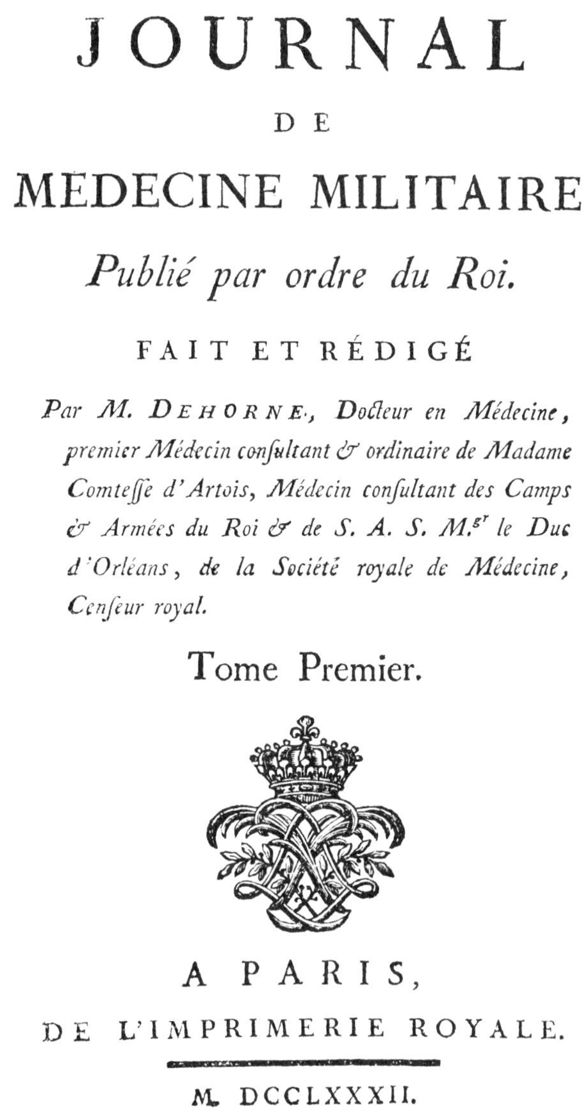
JOURNAL

DE

MEDECINE MILITAIRE.

Publié par ordre du Roi.

FAIT ET RÉDIGÉ

Par M. DEHORNE, Docteur en Médecine, premier Médecin consultant & ordinaire de Madame Comtesse d'Artois, Médecin consultant des Camps & Armées du Roi & de S. A. S. M.gr le Duc d'Orléans, de la Société royale de Médecine, Censeur royal.

Tome Premier.

A PARIS,

DE L'IMPRIMERIE ROYALE.

M. DCCLXXXII.

Figure 3–I–2. The title page of the *Journal de Médecine Militaire* of 1782. Established by order of King Louis XV, the journal was printed at the Crown's expense and distributed to the health officers of the hospitals and regiments of the army of France.

the severance of the Achilles tendon and on the fracture of the seventh cervical vertebra. The same volume also carries on page 137 what may be considered the first description of a case of diabetes insipidus ("Observations on an Extraordinary Thirst") by M. Roger, Surgeon Major of the Regiment of The Crown. Even more significant, as the Peabodys point out, is the leading article dealing with the care of patients in the military hospitals. It specifies that physicians will visit their patients twice a day, and whenever possible there shall be only one patient in each bed. Two reasons are given for this. The first is humanitarian, because it is distressing for a sick man to share a bed with a dying patient. The other is practical, because this policy diminishes the possibility of error in administering medications.

Obviously, the course of humanistic concern and that of medical knowledge were rapidly converging, preparing the ground for the explosion of scientific perception and social advancement that distinguishes our own century.

SYSTEM OF INVESTIGATION

The major objectives of the investigation are to establish the mechanisms of injury and the effects of trauma. The examiner must be aware that, in both civil and criminal cases, correct description of the findings may provide the only clue to how the injury was sustained.

The History

Obviously, the history is an important part of the investigation; in the case of head trauma, however, one must accept the fact that it is not always available, and even if available, it may not be entirely correct. Head injuries are frequently lethal, and as a result of the trauma, the victim may have died; he may be unconscious at the time of the investigation, or he may have lost consciousness momentarily when struck and may not have a clear recollection of the sequence of events. The examiner can also be misled by an incorrect history, either unintentionally given or deliberately constructed because claim settlements are foreseen. Equally equivocal and unreliable can be the histories obtained from eye witnesses.

Examination of the Body

Another important part of the investigation includes the general examination, first of the clothed and, subsequently, of the unclothed body. Since marks and trace evidence may be lost when the body is washed, this should not be allowed to take place prior to the examination.

Particularly in traffic accidents, glass particles, flakes of paint, or oil spots on the clothing of the victim may supply valuable information for reconstructing the modalities of the accident and identifying the responsible vehicle. Any evidence of this sort should be collected, placed in labeled jars, and made available to the police laboratory. Equally important is inspection of the scene of the accident and search for any kind of trace evidence that might aid in the reconstruction. The importance of documenting the findings photographically is never stressed enough. Photographs make it possible to reexamine the case at a later date; simple observations, such as that the victim was wearing a hearing apparatus or corrective eye lenses or had a wasted or deformed limb may have significant medicolegal implications, indicating that he was suffering from preexisting disabilities in hearing, vision, or locomotion.

Assessment of body build, skeletal deformities, and tegumental marks, and recording of the color of the eyes and the color and texture and distribution of the hair of the scalp are part of the identification of the body. This portion of the examination may also disclose hidden lesions in the chest, abdomen, or limbs that may have occurred concurrent to the head injury.

In the case of traffic accidents, the examination may likewise reveal which injuries resulted from the impact with the vehicle (injuries from primary impact) and which were caused by striking the ground or some other object (injuries by secondary impact).

Unidentified bodies require a special approach. Regardless of the presence or absence of visible lesions, photographs of the face should be taken and fingerprinting should be done. If the skin of the fingers is desiccated, the subcutaneous tissue of the terminal phalanges should be injected with water until rehydration is obtained. Scars must be properly described, teeth carefully examined, dentures noted, and if possible, x-rays of the mandible taken. Recording of prostheses, moles, and tattoos may provide additional means of identification.

An autopsy is usually performed on anyone who dies as a result of violence. In this case, ascertaining the state of death becomes an essential part of the examination. Cessation of cardiorespiratory function and loss of motion and consciousness are not absolute signs of death.

By the same token, drying of the exposed mucous membranes and epidermis due to evaporation of body fluids cannot be considered a valid sign, for an identical condition can be caused in the living by any disorder associated with severe loss of body fluids. The same is true for desiccation of the cornea.

As the heart weakens or ceases to function, the blood gravitates to the vessels in the dependent portions of the body, giving rise to the so-called *livor mortis.* It is well, however, to keep in mind that with exsanguinating hemorrhage, livor can be minimal or absent. Meaningful variations in color can also be found in carbon monoxide or cyanide poisoning, in which the livor is characteristically cherry red, or in methemoglobinemia, in which the discoloration is smoky gray to brown. With the onset of putrefaction and the ensuing production of hydrogen sulfide, the livor assumes a black-green tinge due to the formation of sulfmethemoglobin.

After death, the body undergoes a progressive decrease in temperature *(algor mortis),* and the skeletal muscle, myofibers, and smooth muscle acquire temporary stiffness *(rigor mortis),* which is thought to result from the breakdown of adenosine triphosphate (ATP) and its transformation to adenosine diphosphate (ADP); with the resynthesis of adenosine triphosphate, the rigor disappears. Thus, measurement of pupils after death is of little value inasmuch as they merely reflect the state of rigidity or flaccidity of the iris muscles.

Since both algor and rigor may take place in the living after the body has been exposed to freezing temperatures, these phenomena also, per se, do not constitute absolute signs of cessation of life. The earliest evidence of death is the absence of activity in the electroencephalogram; later there are the postmortem changes associated with autolysis and putrefaction.

Mechanisms of Injury

The goals of the examination in any injury by mechanical force include the study of the mechanisms by which the lesions have been produced. Unfortunately, in most of the cases that come under investigation, the magnitude and the direction of the force are not known, and this prevents exact reconstruction of the physical events responsible for the injury. The information available on the mechanisms of head injury is, for the most part, derived from skull-brain models and from experiments in animals or in human cadavers.[21-36] One of the major practical needs for such knowledge is to design a rationale of head protection.

The basic distinction between *compression concussion* and *acceleration concussion* is generally acknowledged. In compression concussion a moving force modifies the state of rest of the head. As a result, the skull, at the site of application of the force, either is fractured or locally deformed and generally distorted. The new curvatures of the distorted skull impinge upon the underlying brain, giving rise to increased pressure in some areas and diminished pressure in others. Thus, the nature and extent of injury depend not as much upon the violence of the impact between the external surface of the skull and the striking object as upon the impact between the inner surface of the skull and the subjacent intracranial structures.

The effects of the rebounding of the skull after the injuring force has ceased to impinge upon its external surface must also be considered. As this occurs, the sudden change in intracranial pressure causes the meningeal vessels to be pulled away from the brain, evulsed and torn, and the subjacent brain to undergo contusion of variable depth. This explains why an elastic skull, although less likely to be fractured than a rigid one, offers less protection to the underlying brain; it is more easily deformed or distorted when struck. This is the case in the skulls of children.

When forces of acceleration are operating, more severe effects are to be expected. As the brain is made to slide within its dural covering, entire anatomical units, and probably the individual neurons as well, are likely to be distorted and the connecting pathways to be bent, stretched, or torn in a direction determined by the direction of the accelerating force. The delicate vessels draining the cortical veins into the large venous sinuses and the small arteries that enter the base of the brain are also likely to be evulsed, which explains the frequency of subdural or subarachnoid hemorrhage. Contusions are likely to occur at the points where the accelerated brain is pushed forcibly against the highly irregular floor of the anterior fossa or the sharp edges of the wings of the sphenoid bone. In the space left vacant by the displaced brain, a zone of diminished pressure and the resulting suction will be responsible for additional brain damage.

It has been stated that if the head is prevented from moving at the moment of impact, no concussion occurs, whereas if even slight movements are allowed, concussion takes place.[28] Supporting this contention is the demonstration, by means of one of the earliest "skull-brain models," that to produce shear strains of the skull contents, a rotary acceleration is necessary.[26] Accordingly, it has been proposed that as a result of rotary acceleration, constituent particles of the brain are pulled apart, particularly around regions where it is locally fixed in relation to the skull, and if they do not join up properly when the immediate effect of the impact is over, nervous deficit is likely to follow. Thus, concussion has been related to minimal separation of constituent particles and contusion to maximal separation. Experiments on monkeys, in which the calvaria was replaced by a translucent plastic model, have shown that the acceleration following a blow to the head causes rotational gliding movements of the brain, the planes of which vary according to the site and direction of the blow.[23]

The smaller the area over which the energy of the impact is discharged in a fixed unit of time, the greater will be its intensity until a point is reached at which the injuring force penetrates the skull. This is exemplified by the gunshot wound. The penetration lessens the degree of acceleration to which the skull is subjected, and this explains why penetrating wounds, while causing severe local damage, often fail to produce concussion.

It has been suggested that in a hollow structure, such as the skull, the energy of impact is propagated by radiating waves of motion along meridional lines that diverge as they leave the site of impact and converge as they approach the opposite pole, giving rise, at the point of collision, to a *contralateral* or *contrecoup injury*.[37] In reality, cerebral lesions fitting the definition of contralateral injury, in the sense that a pole of the brain opposite the site of impact undergoes some damage, presumably can be caused by several different mechanisms. Converging of motion waves is one possibility. Another is that there are two impacts, the first at the site where the force is applied, the second where the advancing segments of the accelerated brain are brought suddenly to rest by the forces that resist its forward motion.[27]

A third concept is that contralateral injury results from traction as the brain is torn away from its coverings by the force of its own momentum.[38] Accordingly, application of a blow to the movable head is followed by a positive pressure in the area of brain underlying the zone of impact and by a negative pressure over the contralateral brain surface, where the brain pulls away from the skull.

A fourth concept, advanced by Saucerote in 1778 and revived in our time, is that a sound wave elicited by the impact is the most important physical factor responsible for the production of contrecoup lesions.[30,31] If the sound wave travels through the skull at a greater speed than through the skull contents, the negative pressure on the side contralateral to the impact will cause tearing of pia-arachnoidal membranes and brain contusion. If, instead, the opposite condition occurs, namely, that the sound wave travels at a greater speed through the cranial contents than through the skull, the initial contralateral pressure will be positive, and in this case, no contrecoup injury will take place.

A major objection to this view has been raised by Friede, who points out that if this is the mechanism responsible for contrecoup, any skull fracture should prevent the propagation of the sound wave and, therefore, of the injury, whereas, in actuality, the combination of skull fracture and contrecoup injury is far from uncommon.[33]

The cerebrospinal fluid plays an important role in protecting brain areas under mechanical stress. Whatever the thickness of the protective cushion of fluid under normal conditions, it should be understood that the fluid will shift during acceleration of the head, resulting in a thicker layer in the areas of negative pressure and a thinner layer in the areas of positive pressure.

EXAMINATION OF THE HEAD

In contrast to the clinical autopsy that follows well-established classic techniques, the evaluation of death by mechanical trauma involves problems so complex that the prosector is given a certain freedom of approach and allowed to choose the method best suited to the case under investigation.

There are, however, several advantages to examining the head first. Blood escapes from the circulatory system during excision of the organs of the chest and abdomen, and as a result, the blood content of brain and meninges necessarily loses its original pattern. There is the unavoidable contamination of the body associated with the autopsy, which prevents reliable culturing of microorganisms from the cranial contents. Finally, manipulation and severing of the neck vessels can result in air bubbles' being artificially drawn into the cerebral vessels, impairing fair evaluation of air embolism that might have occurred during life.

Even when a satisfactory cause of death has been established at the examination of the head, the operation should never be stopped, but should be extended to include all parts of the body. Every pathologist will recollect, at one time or another, examining the victim of a fall in whom, at the examination of the head, a skull fracture and some sort of presumably lethal intracranial injury was found and then, upon opening of the chest, a cardiac tamponade from a ruptured myocardial infarct was revealed that almost certainly antedated and caused the fall and the head trauma.

Scalp

The scalp is the portion of the soft tissues of the head that extends from the eyebrows anteriorly to the superior nuchal line posteriorly, and laterally from one temporal line to the other. Its primary function is to protect and insulate the skull. Without the protection given by the scalp, the human skull can be fractured by as little as 40 pounds per square inch (psi) of energy, whereas the skull of an intact cadaver head can withstand 425 to 900 psi.[39]

The scalp consists of five layers of tissue arranged in the following order: skin, dense connective tissue, galea aponeurotica, loose connective tissue, and periosteum (pericranium).

The skin is normally hair-bearing, a feature that adds protection and insulation. The layer of dense connective tissue between skin and galea can, in turn, be subdivided into two layers: a fatty layer, atrophy of which has been associated with baldness, and a deeper membranous layer that contains the major feeding vessels of the scalp. The latter derive from the superficial temporal, posterior auricular, supraorbital, supratrochlear, and occipital arteries, all branches of the external carotid artery. Knowledge of the course and direction of these vessels is particularly valuable to the neurosurgeon in planning the base of flaps. When severed, these vessels contract poorly and, because of this, give rise to severe hemorrhage.

The galea, a freely movable aponeurosis of dense fibrous tissue is structurally designed to absorb the force of external trauma, particularly glancing blows. It is pierced by numerous emissary veins that connect the veins of the scalp with the intracranial venous circulation. These communicating vessels provide an easy pathway for the propagation of infection from the scalp to the intracranial structures.

The layer of loose connective tissue between the galea and the periosteum has been properly called the "dangerous area of the scalp."[40] The loose composition of the connective tissue allows accumulation of blood or pus in conjunction with local hemorrhage or infection. The lack of anterior attachments of the superimposed aponeurotic layer explains the slow downward gravitation of blood, first in the upper and later in the lower eyelids, that is characteristically associated with laceration of the scalp extending into the subaponeurotic layer.

Any scalp lesion, even if per se insignificant, may constitute important medicolegal evidence. Careful exposure and examination of the cranium may confirm the impressions gained from a wound in the scalp. Not uncommonly at the area of application of a blunt force, the only visible alteration is a *contusion*, namely, a hemorrhage within the soft tissues of the scalp, with or without gross disruption of tissue continuity. The effused blood undergoes color changes, from dark red to dark blue, brown-yellow, and yellow-green, which reflect the rate of deterioration of the extravasated erythrocytes. Since this varies considerably from case to case, primarily in relation to environmental conditions, color changes fail to give any reliable indication of the age of the injury.

A contusion should be differentiated from *postmortem hypostasis*, which, as a rule, is limited to the dependent parts of the scalp, usually the occipital region. When the discoloration is due to postmortem hypostasis, the tissue blanches upon compression, and after incision blood can be readily obtained from the vessels; this in contrast to the discoloration produced by a contusion in which blood infiltrates the involved tissue.

Scalp lacerations are more likely to take place where the integument is tightly stretched over the calvaria. The shape of the laceration—stellate, linear, Y-shaped, penetrating, or crescent-shaped—may give a clue to how the wound occurred or was inflicted. Scalp lacerations at the vertex of the head are usually induced by moving objects striking the skull and are frequently associated with depressed fractures. Conversely, lacerations resulting from a fall ordinarily occur on the posterior part of the head and are associated with skull fractures of the linear type. It is well to remember that compound fractures of the skull may produce lacerations of the scalp that may be confused with those resulting from the impact that was responsible for the fracture. Extensive and boggy swelling under the scalp is an almost certain indication of subgaleal hemorrhage and skull fracture.

Sudden cardiovascular collapse while the individual is erect may lead to a fall to the ground, resulting in a scalp contusion, abrasion, or laceration, usually on the back of the head. This occurrence is particularly likely to take place in association with cerebral vascular accidents, convulsions, epileptic seizures, dizziness, or fainting spells. A concurrent intracranial hemorrhage, with or without skull fracture, is not uncommonly found under these circumstances, and the prosector is faced with the problem of deciding whether the fall was secondary to primary organic brain disease or vice versa, i.e., that the fall initiated the fatal course of events leading to the intracranial damage. This situation is illustrated by a case in which I was personally involved:[40]

...a known hypertensive died following a car accident. The autopsy revealed multiple contusions, a fractured skull, severe cerebral arteriosclerosis, and a massive unilateral intracerebral hematoma extending into both the corresponding lateral ventricle and the subarachnoidal space. Opinion was requested on the stand whether the deceased underwent cerebral hemorrhage, followed by loss of consciousness, which in turn, was responsible for the accident, or whether the accident was primarily responsible for the brain injury and demise.

The request for a positive opinion was met with much hesitation and lack of assurance.

Incised wounds produced by an object with a sharp edge differ from lacerations in the absence of denudation of hair at the edges of the wound and the presence of hair forced into the wound. Stab or puncture wounds made by a rigid slender object may be small enough to be easily overlooked. Usually they cause similar injuries to the underlying pericranium and bone.

Evaluation of homicidal or suicidal death by *bullet wounds* is dealt with in another chapter. Here it is sufficient to say that recognition of the entrance hole of the bullet is of primary importance. It is likely to be identified by the *contact ring*, so called because it represents the area with which the bullet first came in contact. Abrasion, bruising, tearing, and indentation of the surrounding skin are additional features. *Barrel impression* in contact shots is a distinctive feature of suicidal death. The hole subjacent to the contact ring is characteristically smaller than the exit wound and also smaller than the discharged bullet. No effort should be spared in recovering the missile, and much time can be saved by identifying its location with properly oriented roentgenograms. Since the prosector may be required, under oath, to recognize the missile, the bullet's base should be scratched with a recognition mark, avoiding alteration of the identifying characteristics on the bullet's side.

Although less dramatic than penetrating injuries, *tangential, grazing, glancing wounds* from high-velocity missiles and from metallic fragments of high-explosive shells present distinct clinical problems.[41] In this type of injury, an apparently innocent scalp laceration is frequently associated with considerable disturbance of function of the central nervous system that is related to localized damage of the brain directly beneath the scalp wound. Roentgenographic evidence of a depressed skull fracture, progressive focal neurologic symptoms or signs, evidence of increasing intracranial pressure, and seizures are the most common indications that an intracranial lesion has occurred in conjunction with the tangential scalp wound. The complicating factor of sepsis not infrequently makes it difficult to assess the relative importance of mechanical trauma and infection. Cortical contusion and laceration, subcortical hematoma, and epidural and subdural hematoma are the conditions most commonly found to explain the neurologic manifestations.

Total scalp avulsion also deserves distinct consideration. This unusual accident occurs almost exclusively in women whose hair has become entangled in the moving parts of a machine. The scalp first tents up from the skull, then tears at a point where the skin is thinner (usually at the supraorbital ridge), and then becomes separated from the skull along the loose subaponeurotic layer. Occasionally, some of the skin of the face and cheeks, and parts of the ears are torn away together with the scalp. Complications of this serious accident include meningitis, brain abscess, and tetanus. Accordingly, one of the major problems in treatment arises from the danger of infection. Another problem is how to cover the denuded skull. Replacement of the avulsed scalp has been attempted, but in most cases it has proved unsuccessful. Preferred treatment has been either application of tubed pedicle flaps from the neck or exposure of the diploë followed by immediate or delayed skin grafting.[42]

It is of interest that two cases have been recorded in which an epithelioma developed in the scar tissue subsequent to avulsion.[43, 44] The occurrence of keloid scars has also been described.[42]

Face

A few conceivable situations are worth mentioning. Diffuse subconjunctival hemorrhage and edema are almost certain indications of fracture of the anterior cranial fossa; in contrast, the limited, flame-shaped subconjunctival hemorrhage as a rule is caused by a contusion of the soft tissues of the eye. Swelling of the temporal muscle and retromastoid bruising are also reliable signs of fracture. On the other hand, bleeding from the nose or ears often comes from laceration of soft tissues. In this connection it is essential to make certain that the blood actually stems from the nose or ears rather than from a wound in the adjoining scalp or face. Occasionally, flow of blood from the ear is due to an isolated rupture of the drum membrane or a fracture of the bony external auditory canal. In the majority of cases, however, it is a sure sign of basal skull fracture of the longitudinal variety, involving the superior petrosal sinus, the sigmoid sinus, the jugular bulb, or the middle meningeal artery. When the internal carotid artery is injured, there is concurrent profuse bleeding from nose and mouth. Bilateral hemorrhage from the ear frequently signifies a bilateral longitudinal fracture of the temporal bones, occasionally combined with labyrinthine or transverse fracture.

Probing of the nose should not be omitted in the investigation of unexpected death in newborn infants. This simple procedure can lead to the disclosure of a posterior choanal atresia and thus to the explanation of a death that otherwise may escape recognition or mistakenly be attributed to foul play.

Swelling of the soft tissues of the face, associated with crepitation on palpation are certain indications of a broken nose. Splitting lacerations of the eyebrow, cheek, or lips are usually due to a localized impact, such as from a fist or boot. Impacts from hard objects used by an assailant, knuckle dusters for example, usually cause bone injuries that are far more serious than those produced by the bare fist. Face injuries similar to those inflicted by an assailant can be caused by a fall to the ground; however, in this case, the abrasions are likely to be limited to the protruding parts of the face: nose, cheeks, chin, and forehead.

The teeth are accessible to inspection, and description of their condition is an integral part of the examination, not only for identification of the body, but also for detection of evidence of trauma (bleeding gums, loose or broken teeth). Lacerations in the tongue and oral mucosa can also be related to assault.

SKULL AND SKULL FRACTURE

Skull

In discussing the different patterns of skull fractures, Bruns arrived at the conclusion that if all skulls were equally thick and equally elastic, the lines of fracture could be calculated on mathematical formulas.[45] In reality, the skull is not a homogeneous body, but is composed of panels of bone that differ in thickness and elasticity from individual to individual, and in the same individual in the different portions of the skull. The thickness of the calvaria ranges in the adult from 3 to 6 mm. It is thin in the squamous portion of the temporal bone and much thicker in the midfrontal, midoccipital, parietosphenoid, and parietopetrous buttresses. On the average, the bones are thicker in the Negro than in the Caucasian, but this is by no means an infallible rule. The skull is somewhat thinner in the female than in the male, and the outer table is always thicker than the brittle inner table. Bone density also varies. Areas of decreased density are frequently seen in the frontoparietal region, in the neighborhood of the coronal suture, above the roof of the orbit, and in a small segment above the internal occipital protuberance. In contrast, an arcuate area of increased density is usually present between the squamous portion of the temporal bone and the parietal bone.[46] This explains how skull fracture patterns, although subject to some extent to the laws of mechanics are so varied and unpredictable.

In the fetus, the skull consists of a fibrous membrane that becomes ossified through a process of cellular differentiation (intramembranous ossification). Ossification starts in well-individualized centers that make their appearance around the seventh week. In early infancy, the bones of the skull are thin and pliable, and the differentiation between inner and outer tables can hardly be seen. A distinct inner table does not become apparent until the age of two years. Fibrous septa pass through the open suture so that each bone becomes enveloped in a fibrous sheath. Patency of the fontanelles adds further protection from trauma to the infant skull. The posterior fontanelle is patent until about the sixth week and the anterior fontanelle until the ninth to the sixteenth month. The suture between the two frontal bones disappears during the third year of life.

This anatomical configuration and its relatively smaller size in proportion to the skull capacity permit the infant brain to withstand greater trauma than would be possible later in life. As Jackson says, "in an infant, a blow which would perhaps fracture an adult skull often produces only a dent, like that seen in a damaged Ping-Pong ball."[47]

With closure of the fontanelles and union of the sutures, the skull becomes a rigid cavity that gradually enlarges from a capacity of about 350 ml at birth to 1,400 or 1,500 ml at maturity. With advancing age, partial closure of the sutures takes place, and in the later decades of life, it is not uncommon to find complete bridging of at least some of the sutures. Partial closure begins during the second decade, and since this occurs when brain and skull have reached adult size, the closure has no pathologic implications. The considerable variations in the sequence with which obliteration of the sutures takes place, however, further prevent prediction of the effects of trauma.

In the adult, the rounded vault is composed of an inner table and an outer table of bone, between which lies a layer of cancellous bone—the diploë. This structural plan gives strength to the calvaria with economy in weight. The inner table of the vault of the skull is relatively smooth. The depressions produced by the impressions of the cerebral gyri (digital markings), the foramina of emissary veins, the erosions caused by the pacchionian granulations, and the grooves in which lie the anterior, middle, and posterior meningeal arteries are not the kind of deformities likely to damage the underlying brain when the calvaria is struck by a force.

Nevertheless, a fracture line running through one of the arterial grooves may tear the contained artery and give rise to an epidural hemorrhage. Since the grooves follow a tortuous course and as a rule are bilateral and symmetrical, their vascular origin is recognized at a glance; occasionally, however, they may appear straight, lack symmetrical configuration, and thus simulate fracture lines.

The diploic venous channels situated between the inner and the outer tables of the skull are variously distributed and in their course present areas of dilatation called venous lakes. These channels communicate with the meningeal veins and dural sinuses on one side and with the veins of the pericranial circulation on the other, thus establishing a pathway to the spread of infection from the outer to the inner structures of the head. A fracture crossing a venous channel or lake will produce an epidural hemorrhage.

In contrast to the vault, the base of the skull presents many jagged areas. In the anterior fossa, the almost razor-sharp lesser wings of the sphenoid, the cribriform plate of the ethmoid bone, and the crista galli represent as many threats to the integrity of the brain when it is pushed forward in accelerated motion. In the middle fossa, equal threats are provided by the clinoid processes, and in the posterior fossa by the foramen magnum, toward which the pressure wave caused by a blow descends along the brain stem to cause a shearing stress in that vital structure. Similarly, as a result of pressure from above, the uncus and tip of the temporal lobe can be forced beneath the sharp anterior edge of the tentorium. The ensuing pressure on the third cranial nerve, the posterior cerebral artery, and the cerebral peduncle explain the triad of neurologic manifestations associated with this occurrence, namely ipsilateral dilated pupil, contralateral hemiparesis, and not uncommonly, contralateral hemianopia.

The character of any lesion in the outer table of the skull may provide an important lead to the identification of the injuring agent. As a rule, the marks of the pericranial injury coincide with the marks of the scalp wound. These can be in the form of tangential or vertical cuts, as they might be made by a heavy knife, or in the form of indentations, as produced by a hammer, or of a tangential "egg top" lesion, such as may be caused by the impact of the head against an edge or an angular object.

Skull Fracture

It has been estimated, that in one of four fatal head injuries the skull escapes fracture. The practical implication is that roentgenologic evidence of absence of skull fracture should never be relied upon to determine whether the brain has been injured.[46]

Experimental observations indicate that the skull bends inward at the point of impact, and outward in the surrounding segments. Whenever the pressure at the point of impact surpasses the bending capacity of the calvaria, a fracture will take place in the outbent segments. (Fig. 3–I–3).[46, 48, 49]

Gurdjian and Webster, from strain gauge studies of deformations of the skull in human autopsy heads, have determined that the total time period of disturbance following the impact is in the neighborhood of 0.004 second.[50] During the first 0.0006 second, the scalp is compressed; the deformation of the skull resulting in fracture takes another 0.0006 second. At the moment of stress, the fracture line may open by several millimeters, to close again into a narrow line immediately afterward. Multiple linear fractures can be better tolerated than single ones, because they allow some degree of spontaneous decompression.

Courville's classification of skull fractures includes three major categories: depressed fractures, linear fractures, and fractures of specific

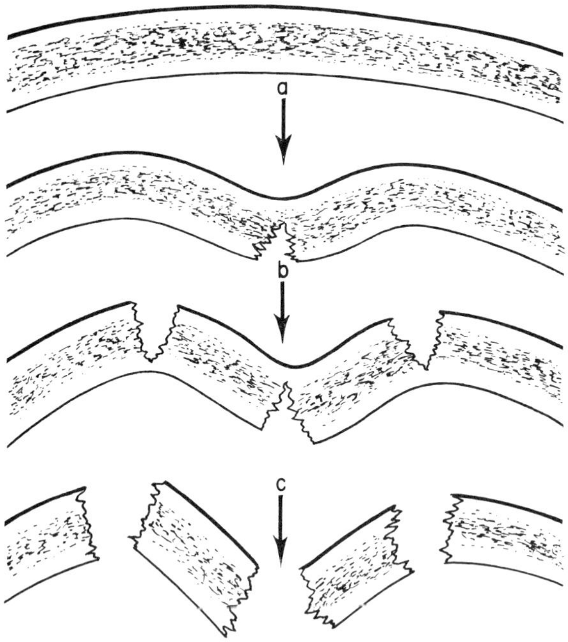

Figure 3–I–3. Effects of local deformity in the skull: *a*, bending of bone along the line of pressure; increase in longitudinal diameter and fracture of the inner table; *b*, multiple fractures along the longitudinal diameter in the outer table; *c*, fragmentation of bone at the site of impact and at a distance from the area of application of the force. (Redrawn from C. G. Tedeschi (Ed.): *Neuropathology: Methods and Diagnosis.* Boston, Little, Brown and Co., 1970.)

types.[51] Whether a depressed fracture or a linear fracture will occur depends upon the velocity, the kinetic energy, and to a lesser extent, the shape of the injuring object.[52]

Depressed Fractures

As a rule, depressed fractures result from the local impact of a moving object on the cranial vault. The area struck is driven along the same line of force into the subjacent structures, the depth varying according to the velocity of the injuring object (Fig. 3–I–4). Thus, an object moving at extremely high velocity, such as a high-powered rifle bullet, will not only perforate the skull, but will also cause fragments of bone to be driven into the substance of the brain. In contrast, the effects of a blunt object moving at a lower velocity, such as a hammer or brick, may be limited to a simple area of depression that absorbs most of the expended energy. Under these circumstances, there can be the association of a depressed fracture with one or more linear fractures that have resulted from distant outbending of the skull.

Linear Fractures

Linear fractures are usually caused by the impact of the moving head against a solid object, as in a fall to the ground. They can range from vertical to transverse or circumferential.

The middle meningeal artery frequently becomes torn in concurrence with a lateral fracture involving the parietal bone, thus causing an extradural hemorrhage. A fracture in the posterior or posterolateral aspect of the head often extends into the base of the skull, involving the hypoglossal foramen and the cranial nerves that transit through it. A linear fracture traversing the posterior aspect of the middle fossa frequently involves the petrous portion of the temporal bone. A manifestation of this is bloody discharge from the external auditory canal. It should, however, be kept in mind that bleeding from the ear can result from the simple rupture of the tympanic membrane.[53]

Fracture lines along the buttresses of the middle fossa may converge toward the region of the sella turcica; injury of the pituitary body has been recorded in concurrence with this event. In conjunction with fracture of the middle fossa, similarly, the formation of a carotid-cavernous fistula at the point where the internal carotid artery traverses the cavernous sinus is not uncommon.

Fractures of Specific Types

These include: *fractures by diastasis*, which extend into and separate suture lines, and the *meridional* and the closely related *bursting fractures;* both terms refer to the crushing of cranial bones at a distance from the point of impact. Usually these occur in falls from heights when the vertex undergoes sudden flattening.

In contrast to *simple fractures*, which are shallow and as a rule are not associated with brain damage, *complex fractures* are accompanied by fragmentation of the depressed part of the bone into several segments that are often driven into the subjacent dura and brain.

Indentation is the term applied to superficial abrasion of the outer table of the cranial vault; as a rule, this is not associated with intracranial damage.

Contrecoup fractures are uncommon and, as a rule, they occur in conjunction with a sudden increase in intracranial pressure. The thin bones of the orbital region are more likely to be affected. The extension of a fracture line from one lateral wall of the skull to the opposite one should not be misinterpreted as a contrecoup fracture.

Gutter fracture is the name used to indicate a

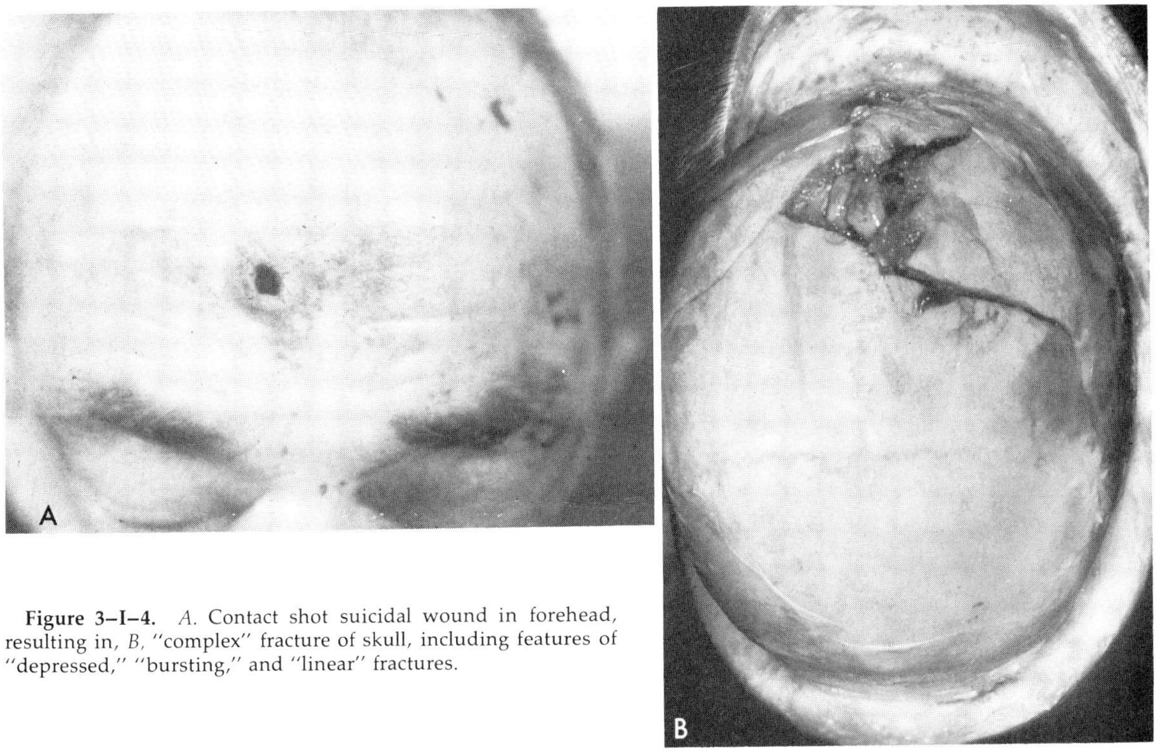

Figure 3–I–4. *A*. Contact shot suicidal wound in forehead, resulting in, *B*, "complex" fracture of skull, including features of "depressed," "bursting," and "linear" fractures.

furrow in the outer table of the skull, usually the result of a glancing blow from a rifled firearm missile. Externally these fractures present as gutters, but they are frequently accompanied by an irregular depressed fracture of the inner table of the skull.

Fracture-dislocation of the mandibular condyle into the middle cranial fossa is very rare and only a few cases are on record.[54] The mandibular joint is formed by the articulation of the condyle of the mandible with the articular fossa and the articular eminence of the temporal bone. The lateral aspect of the fossa is quite thick and is buttressed by the anterior and posterior roots of the zygomatic bone. This anatomical arrangement explains the infrequency of this type of injury. It is uncertain whether a congenital anomaly, either of the condyle or of the fossa, must exist for the dislocation of the mandibular condyle into the middle fossa to materialize. A congenitally small and ovoid condyle was present in the case reported by Whitacre.[54] It is also significant that all cases so far recorded in the medical literature were in teen-aged or young adult females.

Whenever evaluating the presence of skull fracture at autopsy, care should be taken against indiscreet use of chisel and hammer. The examination should not be considered complete until the dura is stripped away from the base of the skull. Linear basilar fractures can be missed unless this simple procedure is carried out. Tapping of the skull is a time-honored and still profitable method. The crack sound elicited in the presence of skull fracture provides almost definite evidence that there is a discontinuity within the skull.

Healing of Skull Fracture

Bony restoration may occur in infants through a process of cellular differentiation (intermembranous ossification). Conversely, in adults, the matrix of the skull is not conducive to satisfactory healing of a fracture; repair is usually brought about by proliferation of fibrous connective tissue, which eventually may become calcified. Absence of callus formation tends to protect the underlying brain from irritation that might result from the formation of an exuberant callus.

INTRACRANIAL LESIONS

Any force that deforms the skull locally or causes the position of the brain to be changed in relation to the skull may result in damage to the meninges, the cerebral vessels and the cranial nerves; may contuse or lacerate the brain substance; or may induce a neuronal injury of microscopic or submicroscopic dimensions. Actually, very many disorders of the central nervous system caused by mechanical trauma are due to injury of the accessory elements, namely, meninges and blood vessels, and the changes in the nervous tissue are of a secondary nature.

Injury of the Accessory Elements

Blood Vessels and Meninges

Following Penfield's demonstration of nerve fibers in the walls of intracerebral blood vessels, the concept that cerebral concussion is due to impairment of the regulating vasomotor functions of the brain has been given considerable attention.[55] It has been shown that mechanical stimulation of the pial arterial vessel will cause it to constrict. The stretching of the vessel itself appears to be an adequae stimulus to constriction.[56-58] A vascular response similar in nature, but on a much larger scale, may be suspected in blunt cerebral trauma when the new curvatures of the under surface of the distorted skull impinge upon the underlying brain, when the brain is pushed forcibly against the irregular surfaces of the inner skull, and when brain and meninges are pulled away from the skull by the negative pressure over the contralateral brain surface.

In a recent analysis of the vascular changes associated with cerebral concussion, Ectors has reached the conclusion that ischemia and anoxia can cause paralysis of the capillaries, precapillaries, and veins, accompanied by extreme dilatation and possibly hemorrhages.[59] This is followed by local edema, which causes a further decrease in circulatory flow.

The same mechanical forces that are responsible for the altered vasomotor response are also responsible for tearing of vessel walls, luminal occlusion by thrombus formation, and spilling of blood in the intracranial cavity. The hemorrhage may take place between skull and dura, resulting in an epidural hematoma, or between dura and meninges, giving rise to a subdural hematoma, or between pia and arachnoid, resulting in a subarachnoid hemorrhage (Fig. 3–I–5).

Epidural Hemorrhage. Epidural hemorrhage has been estimated to occur in 1 to 3.1 per cent of patients with cranial injury.[60, 61] As a rule, the hemorrhage is associated with a linear fracture that crosses the grooves of the meningeal vessels on the inner surface of the skull. Rupture of the middle meningeal artery or the accompanying veins or both is the most common cause of epidural hemorrhage, and this explains why the region most often affected is the temporoparietal area. The frontotemporal and parietooccipital regions are involved next in frequency, while frontal localization is rather uncommon.

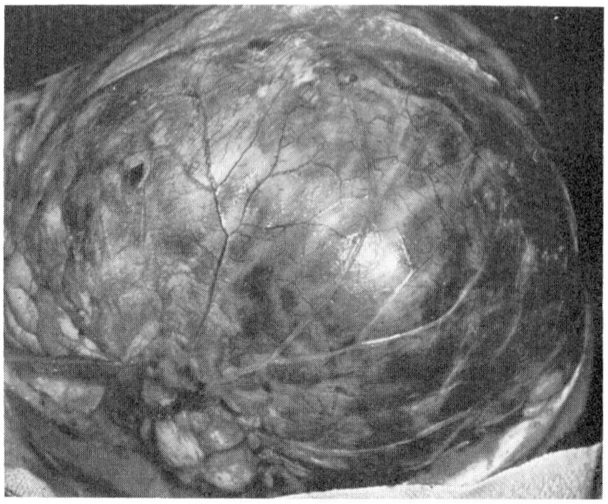

Figure 3–I–5. Subdural hematoma viewed through intact dura. Thirty-three-year-old woman was badly beaten on head. (From C. G. Tedeschi (Ed.): *Neuropathology: Methods and Diagnosis.* Boston, Little, Brown and Co., 1970. Reprinted by permission.)

Other sources of bleeding are the emissary veins and the dural sinuses, primarily the sagittal and lateral. The sagittal is more prone to involvement, in coincidence with midline depressed fractures of the crown of the skull.

Hemorrhage from diploic venous channels and lakes may also occur, but rarely does the blood clot become large enough to cause compression.

As the extravasated blood undergoes clotting, the resulting hematoma shows typical limitation due to the dural attachments at the suture lines.

Subdural Hemorrhage. Extravasated blood between dura and arachnoid constitutes a subdural hemorrhage. Tearing of the large veins entering the superior longitudinal sinus accounts for most of the cases of subdural bleeding. Less frequent causes include intracerebral hemorrhage with retrograde escape of blood through the wound track and tearing of dural sinuses or of arterial or venous channels in conjunction with contusion of the brain surface. Most of the subdural hemorrhages due to venous bleeding result from tears of veins that cross the zone between arachnoid and dura (communicating or bridging veins). The locations where these vessels are most frequently encountered include the lateral frontal region, the apex of the temporal lobe, and the subtentorial region (Fig. 3–I–6).[62, 63]

Lack of muscle fibers and thinness of fibrous walls and elastic lamina predispose these categories of veins to rupture as the brain slides within the skull. Cases in which the bleeding arises from a single small tear in a cortical artery are also being recognized with increasing frequency.[64]

The issue, whether or not a spontaneous nontraumatic subdural hemorrhage may occur, carries medicolegal implications. In this connection it is well to keep in mind that absence of a history of trauma does not preclude a hematoma of traumatic origin. Indeed, an apparently trivial head injury may precipitate bleeding from a blood vessel that is the site of a previous anatomical abnormality or a structural alteration induced by disease.[65]

Many explanations have been proposed to account for the latent interval between the injury and the onset of symptoms associated with the hematoma. There is one popular concept that recurrent hemorrhage causes progressive enlargement of the hematoma.[66] According to another view, the progressive disintegration of erythrocytes within the subdural space provides the osmotic impetus for enlargement of the hematoma.[67]

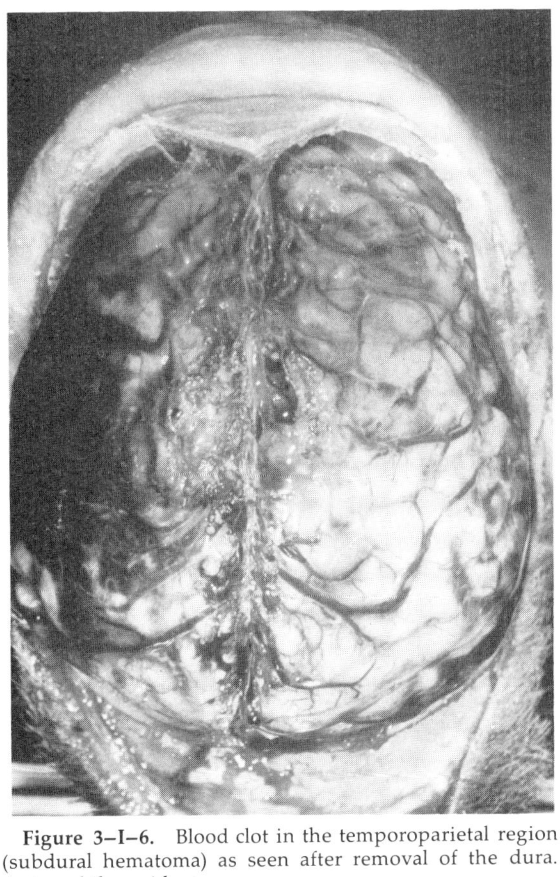

Figure 3–I–6. Blood clot in the temporoparietal region (subdural hematoma) as seen after removal of the dura. Automobile accident.

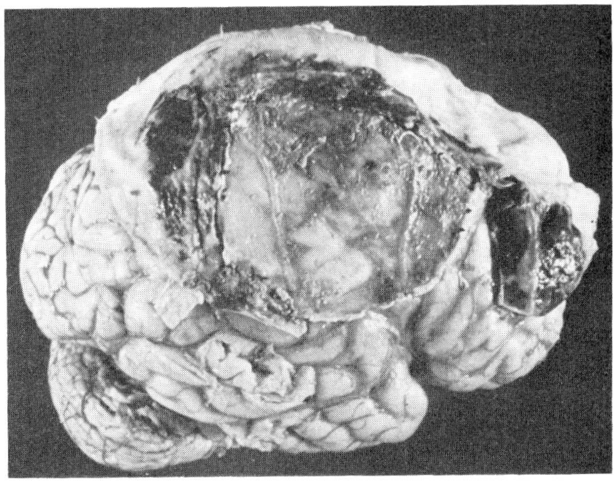

Figure 3–I–7. Chronic subdural hematoma in temporoparietal region in a 68-year-old white man with a history of accidental head injury sustained 44 days prior to death. Notice the area of hemorrhagic softening at the tip of the frontal lobe and the organizing subarachnoid hemorrhage on the dome of the cerebellum. (From C. G. Tedeschi (Ed.): *Neuropathology: Methods and Diagnosis.* Boston, Little, Brown and Co., 1970. Reprinted by permission.)

Since the subdural space has limited absorptive capacity, the blood clot undergoes organization rather than reabsorption (Fig. 3–I–7). The degree of thickening of the encapsulating membrane and its microscopic structure may provide information about the time of occurrence of the trauma. Adherence of the blood clot to the dura may take place as early as 24 hours after the beginning of the bleeding, and in two or three weeks the extravasated blood may become entirely encapsulated by a membrane of discrete thickness. A rusty discoloration of the inner aspect of the dura indicates an old subdural hemorrhage. In such cases, the presence of a subdural membrane can usually be demonstrated by scraping the inner aspect of the dura with a scalpel.[68] If this procedure fails to reveal a membrane, a cut is made through the thickness of the inner aspect of the dura, and an attempt is made to lift the subdural membrane. The normal dura consists of two apposed layers, and the inner layer should not be mistaken for a subdural membrane; whereas the latter can be lifted easily, the dural layers can be separated only with considerable difficulty.[68] The presence of hemosiderin deposits in the subdural membrane provides further evidence of previous subdural hemorrhage.

Difficulties in the timing of the injury may be

encountered upon rupture of newly formed blood channels attempting to organize a hematoma (chronic subdural hematoma). Under these circumstances, the contents of the hematoma consist of partially organized, roughly laminated blood clots intermingled with fresh blood. This is the condition that Virchow labeled *pachymeningitis interna chronica* or *pachymeningitis hemorrhagica*.

Calcification or ossification of the membrane enclosing the hematoma implies that the lesion is several months or even years old. Nevertheless, this criterion can be deceiving. In a case in our files, calcium deposits and osteoid plaques were found in the encapsulating membrane of a subdural hematoma that could be traced to head trauma sustained 62 days prior to death (Fig. 3–I–8).[69] Measurement of the protein content of the fluid portion of the hematoma has been suggested as a helpful procedure to estimate the age of the clot.[60] The protein content increases in the first 21 days and decreases thereafter. This is due to differences in osmotic pressure, which favor the diffusion of other fluids (possibly cerebrospinal fluid or blood serum) into the hematoma.

Relapsing juvenile chronic subdural hematoma refers to the sequence of events characterized by the occurrence of a traumatic subdural hematoma in infancy with relapse due to fresh bleeding and expansion of the old hematoma concurrent to a head injury later in life.[70] Actually, independently of new trauma, the same condition can be realized by the rupture of newly formed blood channels attempting to organize the hematoma, which results in bleeding into the sac of the old hematoma and onset of symptoms related to the expansion of the sac.

Hygroma and *hydroma* are equivalent terms used to indicate a saccular formation containing clear or yellow-tinged material—the end phase of a subdural hematoma. As the hematoma ages, the red blood cells disintegrate and are disposed of, and fluid, from various sources, is drawn into the sac. This condition must be differentiated from external hydrocephalus with brain agenesis, from postmeningitic subdural effusion, and from the loculated collection of cerebrospinal fluid in the subdural space caused by a laceration of the arachnoid membrane.

Subarachnoid Hemorrhage. In contrast to epidural and subdural hemorrhage, which are almost invariably associated with trauma, hemorrhage in the arachnoid space most frequently occurs in conjunction with the rupture of an aneurysm or a sclerosed blood vessel, vascular thrombosis, or occasionally one of the blood dyscrasias. Possibly the only conditions in which subarachnoid hemorrhage takes place in conjunction with head trauma alone are brain contusion with rupture of meningeal blood vessels and intracerebral hematoma extending into the subarachnoid space. Blood escaping into the subarachnoid space is likely to spread and give rise to a diffuse hemorrhage. An area of he-

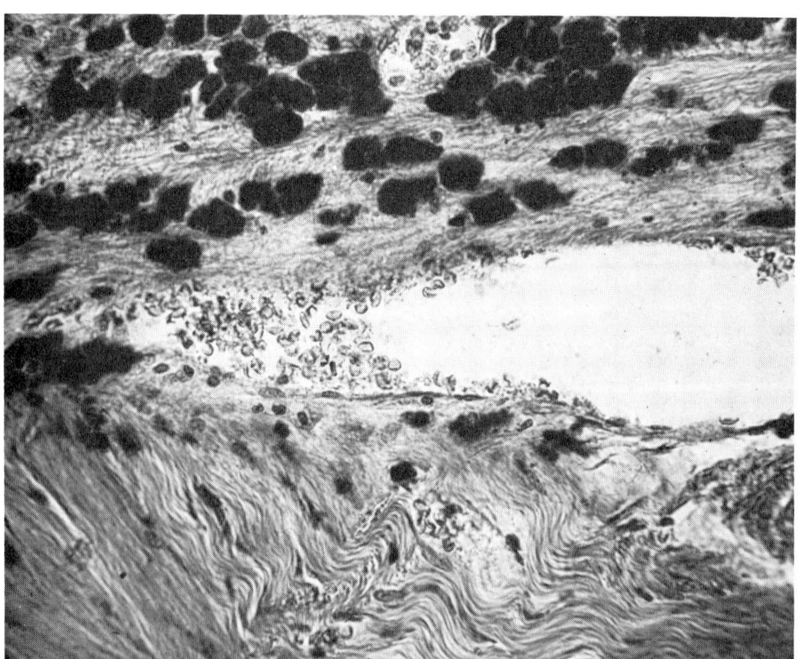

Figure 3–I–8. Microscopic view of wall of chronic subdural hematoma with prominent hemosiderin granules (prussian blue stain). Notice the newly formed blood channel. (From C. G. Tedeschi (Ed.): *Neuropathology: Methods and Diagnosis.* Boston, Little, Brown and Co., 1970. Reprinted by permission.)

morrhagic discoloration in the cerebral cortex often provides a clue to the source of the bleeding.

Superimposed Infection of Meningeal Membranes. Pus within the epidural or subdural space, or within the subarachnoid space is a clear indication that an infection has taken place.

Both *epidural* and *subdural abscesses* (empyema) usually arise in conjunction with open, penetrating wounds or by direct extension from neighboring foci of infection, most commonly osteomyelitis or thrombophlebitis. The bacteria most frequently responsible for the infection are streptococci, particularly of the anaerobic variety, and *Staphylococcus aureus*. The mortality rate is somewhat lower than in brain abscess because of the accessibility of the lesion to surgical drainage, but still approximates 30 per cent.[71]

The same sources of infection leading to a circumscribed empyema in the subdural or epidural space may give rise to leptomeningitis. In *traumatic leptomeningitis* the process is ordinarily confined to the convex surface of the brain adjacent to the source of infection; however, diffuse basal meningitis not infrequently follows a fracture of the oronasal region or a fracture involving the cranial sinuses. Recurrent bouts of meningitis may occur in conjunction with persistently opened fracture lines or with a fracture of the anterior fossa with subsequent invasion of bacteria from the nose or the accessory cranial sinuses.[72] On the average the infectious process manifests itself within two weeks of the injury, but it can become manifest from a few hours to several years after the trauma as well.[73]

Chronic traumatic cerebrospinal fluid rhinorrhea is a relatively frequent cause of recurrent meningitis when a dural defect establishes a fistulous tract between the subarachnoid space and the nasal cavity.

Cerebrospinal Fluid Rhinorrhea

The term refers to an escape of cerebrospinal fluid through the nose. The event is the result of a communication between the subarachnoid space and the nasal cavity, usually through the cribriform plate, the ethmoids, or the sphenoidal sinuses. Though most cases follow a fracture through the anterior fossa, the cerebrospinal fluid may escape through the nose from many other sites. Local injury is not invariable.

Although trauma is the most common cause of cerebrospinal fluid rhinorrhea, the same condition can be produced by several nontraumatic states such as hydrocephalus, congenital anomalies in the region of the cribriform plate, erosion of this area from osteomyelitis, and what Ommaya and his associates called focal atrophy.[74] Focal atrophy is a condition brought about later in life by reduction of the bulk of structures overlying the area of the cribriform plate or the sella turcica, with the result that arachnoid pouches may form and, through constant pulsation, erode the fragile bones in the anterior fossa.

Whereas nontraumatic cerebrospinal fluid rhinorrhea is insidious rather than sudden in onset and may last for years, in approximately 50 per cent of cases the traumatic type is of abrupt onset and not infrequently ceases spontaneously in between a week and six months. Concurrent anosmia is found in 78 per cent of cases. An equally frequent cause of traumatic leptomeningitis is *cerebrospinal fluid otorrhea*, when, as a result of trauma, a fistulous tract is established between the auricular canal and the leptomeninges.

Aerocele (Pneumatocele)

An intracranial inrush of air is likely to occur in both cerebrospinal fluid rhinorrhea and otorrhea, giving rise to an aerocele (pneumatocele).[75] The air may remain trapped in the subdural space, or enter further down in the subarachnoid space, or force its way into the lateral ventricles. It may also infiltrate the brain substance, forming an *air cyst*, which at a glance can simulate a postnecrotic cyst.

Brain Injury

From the mechanical standpoint, a relationship may be assumed to exist between the degree of shear strain induced by the trauma and the extent of the neuronal damage. Thus, a gradation of injuries can be expected, from frank, grossly noticeable cerebral lesions to ganglionic alterations of microscopic or submicroscopic dimensions.

Frank Cerebral Involvement

Hemorrhage. Hemorrhage, of variable dimensions, is one of the major features of traumatic brain lesions. It may range from irregularly scattered cortical and subcortical petechial hemorrhages to an intracerebral hematoma of such a large size as to constitute a space-occupying mass.

Duret probably was the first, in 1878, to call attention to the frequent localization of the petechial hemorrhages in the medulla oblongata and corpora restiformia, and he interpreted this occurrence as due to the convergence of wavelike forces elicited at the site of impact, toward the brain stem area, where they cause bursting of small blood vessels and bruising of the walls of the ventricles.[76] Petechial hemorrhages in the brain stem region are more frequently found in patients with a history of concussion and intact skull, but there is no general consensus on these points.

Contusional Patterns. *Cortical bruises* extending in a wedge shape into the subjacent white matter frequently attend vascular thrombosis. As the area of hemorrhagic necrosis undergoes absorption, a pseudocyst will develop in time. These pseudocysts contain fluid material of high protein content and are enclosed by a thin membrane of fibroglia; patchy areas of hemosiderin discoloration may give a hint to the origin of the lesion.

Equally frequent is the finding of short, linear, densely distributed bruises along the apices of several adjacent gyri.[77] The localization of the lesion at the *crest* of the gyri is highly characteristic of contusion; this in contrast to the same type of lesion in the *depths* of the gyri, which is usually associated with infarction.[68]

In conjunction with comminuted depressed fracture with in-driven bony fragments, a major hemorrhage can occur within the bulk of the cerebral hemispheres *(intracerebral hematoma)* (Fig. 3–I–9). This takes place in 1 to 1.7 per cent of cases of severe head injury.[78, 79] Accumulation of blood occurs by displacement rather than by destruction of tissue, and the blood tends to dissect along the bundles of myelinated nerve fibers. Intracerebral hematoma seldom reaches the pial surface because the U fibers prevent infiltration of blood into the cerebral cortex. Usually the blood finds its way into the ventricular system, and as this takes place there is a sudden increase in the intraventricular pressure.

In the early stages it is difficult to establish the age of the hemorrhage from the gross appearance of the lesion. With the passage of time, the clot gradually softens, and at two or three weeks a narrow rim of rusty color at the edge of the hemorrhage indicates that a local accumulation of hemosiderin-laden macrophages has taken place. Subsequently the color of the clot changes from brick red to rusty brown; the overall duration of the process of liquefaction and absorption depends upon the original size of the lesion.

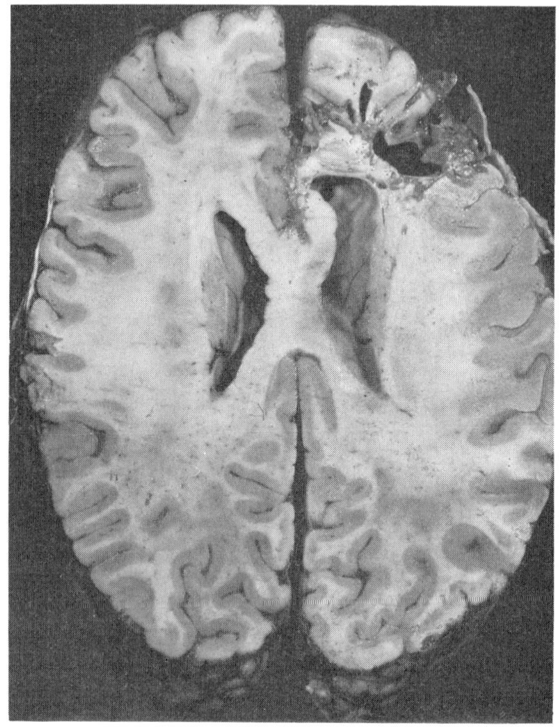

Figure 3–I–9. Laceration and hemorrhage in the right frontal temporal area resulting from in-driven fragments of the squamous portion of the temporal bone. Accidental head trauma involving a moving object and stationary head. (From C. G. Tedeschi (Ed.): *Neuropathology: Methods and Diagnosis.* Boston, Little, Brown and Co., 1970. Reprinted by permission.)

The expression *gutter cortical hemorrhage* is used to indicate a furrow of softened hemorrhagic cerebral tissue extending at variable depths from one pole of the brain to the opposite one. As a rule there is a concurrent gutter fracture in the calvaria, resulting from a glancing blow from a rifled firearm missile.

Contusions fitting the definition of *contralateral injury* are found most frequently at the points where the advancing surfaces of the sliding brain are suddenly brought to rest by the forces resisting forward motion (Fig. 3–I–10). The tips of the frontal and temporal lobes are most likely to be contused as they are pushed against the roof of the orbit, the lesser wing of the sphenoid, or the floor of the middle fossa.

Delayed intracranial hemorrhage (delayed traumatic apoplexy) refers to the condition described by Bollinger in 1891 and is characterized by the occurrence of a sudden intracranial hemorrhage some time after a mechanical brain injury.[80] Both *early* and *late* varieties are acknowledged.[81]

In the early variety, the hemorrhage takes place within a few weeks of the injury; in the late variety, the interval between the trauma

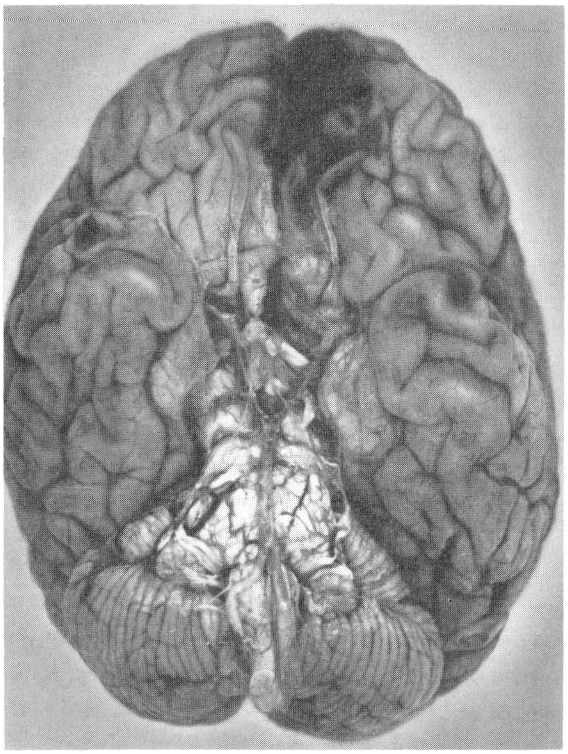

Figure 3–I–10. Hemorrhagic contusions at the tips of the temporal lobes and of the left frontal lobe, namely at the point where the advancing surfaces of the sliding brain were brought to sudden rest by the forces resisting forward motion. A 28-year-old white man was involved in a head-on automobile collision. (From C. G. Tedeschi (Ed.): *Neuropathology: Methods and Diagnosis.* Boston, Little, Brown and Co., 1970. Reprinted by permission.)

and the apoplexy may extend over a period of months or years.

Delayed hemorrhage has been variously explained as due to preexisting small vascular malformations *(cryptic hamartomas* or *microangiomas),* or as Bollinger originally suggested, to the rupture of an arterial wall weakened at the time of the trauma.[80, 82] Bollinger felt that the cortical damage resulting from closed head injury could lead to local necrosis of brain tissue, followed eventually by aneurysmal dilatation and ultimately by rupture of small arteries included in the area of softening.[80] Angiographic, surgical, and pathologic evidence of the traumatic aneurysms envisioned by Bollinger is now available.[83, 84] Despite the rarity of this condition, recognition of its occurrence is important. Once the aneurysm is identified, it is amenable to surgical treatment. The interval between the traumatic episode, the formation of the aneurysm, and its rupture may vary from a few hours to as long as 10 years.[83, 84] Whereas no controversy on matters of compensation is expected to arise when the trauma and the apoplexy occurred within a short time of each other, there could be difficulties in reaching an agreement when years have intervened between the two events.

Lindenberg's case of incarceration of a vertebral artery in a skull fracture and the report of Loop, White, and Shaw of entrapment of a basilar artery within a clivus fracture illustrate the mechanism by which a traumatic aneurysm may occur.[85, 86]

Ischemia. Ischemic brain damage, leading to frank infarction, has been paid relatively little attention; a recent study by Graham and Adams, however, indicates the incidence of ischemic brain damage in 55 per cent of 38 unselected brains from patients who had died as a result of blunt head injury.[87] Possible reasons why such a high rate of incidence has not been recorded in previous studies are that

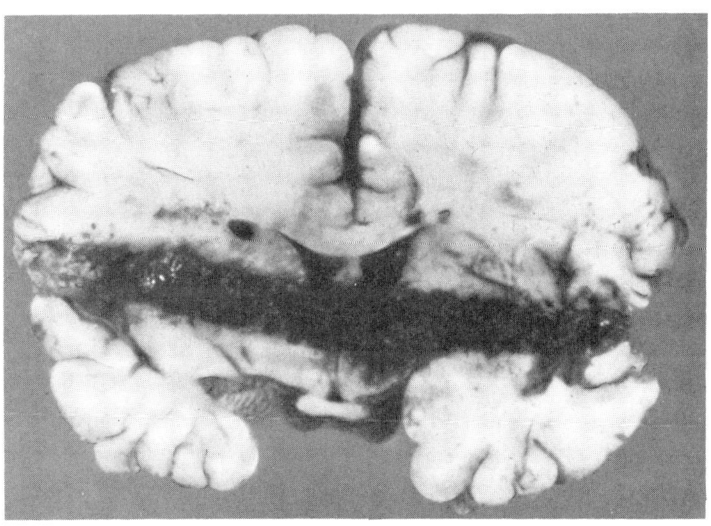

Figure 3–I–11. Complete transection of cerebral hemispheres from contact shot suicidal wound. Entrance hole in right temporal region, exit hole in left temporal region.

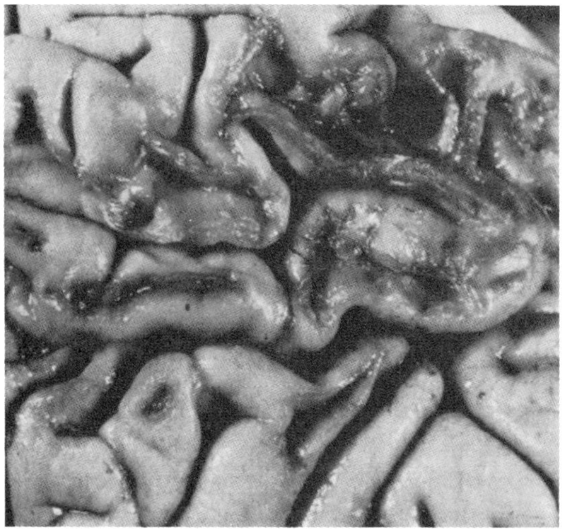

Figure 3–I–12. Contusion on the lateral aspect of cerebral hemisphere showing the characteristic longitudinal grooves along the crests of the convolutions. The 42-year-old construction worker died two months after an accidental fall from a height.

areas of recent necrosis can easily escape detection at the naked-eye examination of the brain. Ischemic brain damage can be found in any arterial territory, but particularly in boundary zones between major arteries.

The immediate alteration noticeable in the affected portion of brain is slight pallor or duskiness that is more pronounced in the gray matter. After two or three days, the ischemic area becomes swollen, moist, translucent; the microscopic counterpart is the total absence of staining of the affected white matter by the methods for myelin. As time advances, the ischemic area assumes progressive opacity, chalky white discoloration, and gradual increase in softening to the point of liquefaction.[68]

No generally applicable explanation of the pathogenesis of ischemic brain damage is available. A critical decrease in systolic blood pressure, however, and raised intracranial pressure are the two major factors most frequently found in the background of the lesion.

Cerebral Edema. The term "cerebral edema" refers to the excessive accumulation of fluid within the nervous tissue associated with volumetric enlargement of the brain. Not uncommonly the edema is the sole grossly noticeable change found in head injury. The brain is enlarged, the gyri are flattened, fissures and sulci are narrowed, and the ventricles are compressed. In some instances, the swelling of the brain is more severe in, or limited to, one cerebral hemisphere. This is often the case in unilateral subdural hematoma (Fig. 3–I–13). Since the subdural blood presses on both sides and crests of the convolutions, the compressed cerebral hemisphere is smaller and shows only slight evidence of gyral flattening.

There seems to be prevailing agreement that the white matter is the preferential site for edema. In the white matter the edema is characterized by swelling of the astrocytic processes and by widening of extracellular spaces. The myelinated nerve fibers are spread apart, especially around blood vessels, and hypertrophy, clasmatodendrosis, and Alzheimer's ameboid degeneration are characteristic astrocytic changes. The oligodendroglia are swollen and display nuclear homogenization and acidophilic change. Electron microscopy has brought forth evidence indicating that swelling of astroglial cytoplasm is due to changes in metabolism and uptake of extravasated serum proteins.[88-90] The remarkable preservation of the subcortical arcuate fibers has been pointed out by several investigators.[91]

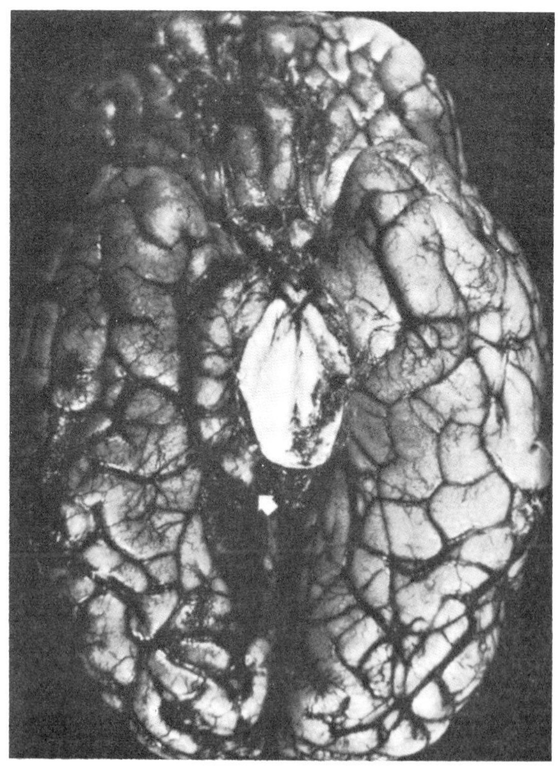

Figure 3–I–13. Transtentorial herniation due to right subdural hematoma. Notice the hemorrhagic necrosis of the right hippocampal gyrus at the point of compression against the edge of the tentorium. Hemorrhages are also present in the corpus callosum and left thalamus. (From C. G. Tedeschi (Ed.): *Neuropathology: Methods and Diagnosis.* Boston, Little, Brown and Co., 1970. Reprinted by permission.)

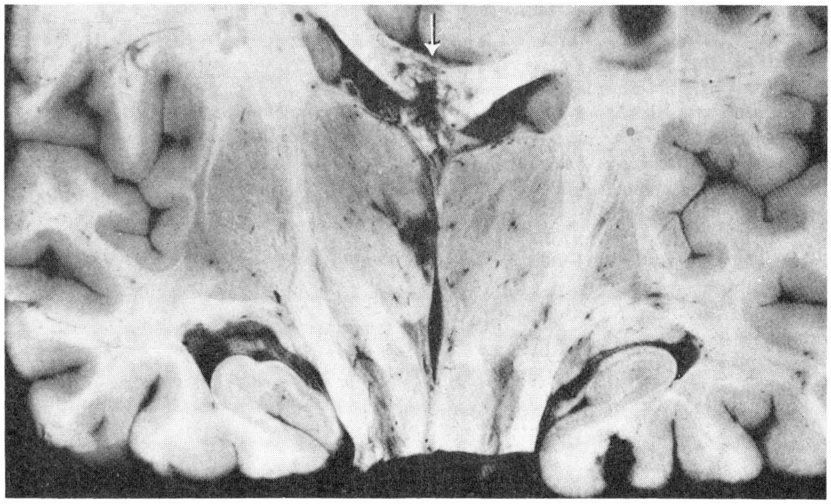

Figure 3–I–14. Herniation of the right temporal lobe caused by massive traumatic subdural hematoma. Notice the hemorrhagic infarction in the territory of the calcarine branch of the posterior cerebral artery, which was kinked against the tentorial edge (arrow). Contusions are visible around the anterior portion of the olfactory bulbs. (From C. G. Tedeschi, Ed.: *Neuropathology: Methods and Diagnosis.* Boston, Little, Brown and Co., 1970. Reprinted by permission.)

In the gray matter, the accumulation of fluid is confined to cells, primarily the astrocytes. Upon overdistention of the cell membranes and their rupture, however, outpouring of the cell contents may take place in the extracellular spaces.

Localization of enzymes at the ultrastructural level indicates that the histochemical changes in astrocytes are primarily related to dehydrogenases and phosphatases; it is debated whether this is due to actual activation of oxidative enzymes rather than to anoxic cellular damage.[90]

In spite of the great profusion of microscopic and ultramicroscopic changes described in association with cerebral edema, the prosector should be prepared to find a grossly swollen, wet brain but no substantiating microscopic evidence.

Suitable methods of investigation have shifted the interest of investigators from the static morphologic aspects of cerebral edema to the dynamics of underlying mechanisms (Fig. 3–I–14). This has led to the concept of two basically different types of cerebral edema, the *vasogenic* and the *cytotoxic*.[91] In the former, the edema is related to injury of the walls of the cerebral blood vessels, leading to escape of plasma components and water into the nervous tissue. In the latter, a toxic factor directly affects the metabolic functions of the cells in the parenchyma, causing cytoplasmic swelling. This concept has been favorably received; however, it must be assumed that in the vasogenic type of edema the fluid that escapes through the vessel walls must do some harm to some of the structural elements of the nervous tissue, and that in the cytotoxic type the swelling of the structural elements must adversely affect the permeability of the blood channels. It may also be expected that some injurious agent may act simultaneously on the walls of the blood vessels and on the cells of the parenchyma.

Distinctive ultrastructural features of the vasogenic type are enlargement of extracellular spaces in the white matter and cellular swelling affecting predominantly the astrocytes; in contrast, there is no enlargement of extracellular spaces in the cytotoxic type, and the swelling of the various cellular tissue components depends on the type of the cytotoxic agent. Differences have been equally noticed in the biochemical features of the edema fluid, basically consisting of plasma filtrate (including serum proteins) in the vasogenic type, and of plasma ultrafiltrate of a composition influenced by the nature of the noxious agent in the cytotoxic type.

The concept of two types of cerebral edema has mostly arisen from experimental studies. The same studies justify the contention that the cerebral edema associated with head trauma belongs to the vasogenic category.

It is to be hoped that this new classification may provide useful guidelines for a rational therapeutic approach.

Herniation of Anatomical Parts. Another threat connected with pronounced swelling of the brain is that brain parts located at the base of the cerebral hemispheres may become deformed, displaced, and ultimately pushed through the tentorial opening *(tentorial pressure cone of Jefferson)* or the occipital foramen *(cerebellar pressure cone of Cushing).*

Temporal lobe herniation may occur in conjunction with generalized brain swelling or in the presence of large blood clots situated close to the midsagittal plane. At the site of the imprint left by the tentorial edge on the hippocampal gyrus, the underlying tissue may show hemorrhagic pressure necrosis. Likewise, kinking of branches of the posterior cerebral artery against the tentorial edge may lead to sudden stagnation of circulation and hemorrhagic infarction of large portions of the temporal and occipital lobes.

Third ventricle downward shift can also occur and may constitute the predominant cause of hypothalamic dysfunction. When both temporal lobes herniate, the mesencephalon becomes compressed from the sides and elongated anteroposteriorly *(mesencephalon herniation).* Concurrently, the paramedian vessels may become stretched and eventually rupture causing the linear midline hemorrhages typical of herniation. The distortion of the diencephalon and midbrain are mainly responsible for the coma, the patient's decerebrate state, and the absence of reflex eye movements.[68] As the mesencephalon is pushed against the free edge of the tentorium, it may undergo pressure necrosis and cause damage to the contralateral cerebral peduncle, resulting in pyramidal tract signs. Downward displacement of the cerebral peduncles may also be responsible for pupillary abnormalities (dilatation of one pupil), which are probably related to damage of the parasympathetic fibers of the third cranial nerve.

Downward herniation through the foramen magnum is readily recognized at inspection of the inferior aspect of the cerebellum, which frequently shows necrosis of the extruded tissue due to compromised blood supply.

Upward displacement of cerebellar tissue is less common and in general occurs in concurrence with large accumulations of blood in the posterior fossa. When the herniation is very severe, the branches of the superior cerebellar arteries may become kinked against the edge of the tentorium, causing hemorrhagic infarction of the portion of cerebellum supplied by these vessels.

Hydrocephalus. The term "hydrocephalus" applies to an increased amount of cerebrospinal fluid in the subarachnoid spaces and in the cerebral ventricles. In conjunction with head trauma, the development of hydrocephalus from interference with absorption of cerebrospinal fluid secondary to blockage of arachnoidal granulations by extravasated blood is most unusual.[92] Equally uncertain is the role of increased secretion of cerebrospinal fluid due to abnormal activity of choroidal or ependymal cells.[93] Obstruction of the flow of fluid in the ventricular and subarachnoid pathways secondary to stricture of the aqueduct by bruising of its walls, periaqueductal edema, and obstruction of the third and fourth ventricles by torn-off brain tissue or blood clot are most frequently responsible for the occurrence of posttraumatic hydrocephalus.[94]

Cerebral Abscess. The avenues of infection most frequently leading to a brain abscess are epidural or subdural abscess, leptomeningitis, septic thrombophlebitis, a focus of osteomyelitis, or an ear infection.[95] In turn, cortical or subcortical abscesses can rupture and drain into the meninges, inducing a fulminating meningitis, or when deeply seated, can pierce through the walls of the ventricles. Unless of large size, a cerebral abscess can become entirely enveloped by a thick tissue of fibroglia and, so encapsulated, can remain silent until it is unexpectedly disclosed at postmortem examination. The virulence of the microorganism responsible for it probably plays an important role in determining the time required for an abscess to become manifest.

Among the unusual aspects of cerebral abscess is its occurrence after oral trauma and loss of teeth.[96] Among the 27 cases of fatal intracranial complications of tooth extractions reviewed by Haymaker, there are 8 brain abscesses and 11 cases of cavernous sinus thrombosis.[97] In an unpublished case in our files of head trauma coincident to assault, a brain abscess found at surgery one year later was presumably traced to a blow in the mouth that had resulted in the loss of several teeth. In the intervening time, the patient had complained of vague manifestations of a slowly progressing space-occupying lesion, which in retrospect were attributed to the expanding abscess.

Since it is well established that a state of transient bacteremia may occur after dental trauma, particularly when periodontal disease is present, it is not surprising that oral bacteria set free in circulation in concurrence with dental trauma may colonize at the site of a brain injury.[98, 99]

Nonstructural Neuronal Injury

Many cases are on record describing the occurrence of irreparable loss of cerebral functions following head trauma in which pathologic examination of the brain failed to offer any plausible explanation.[100] The concept of nonstructural neuronal injury has found, in our times, a suitable explanation in the theory of Denny-Brown and Russell that "excitation, excitation with reflex paralysis, excitation followed by complete paralysis, and complete paralysis alone" are the four degrees of nervous manifestations in which a head injury can be resolved.[101] Accordingly, it has been suggested that a generalized "molecular reaction," reversible in time and of a degree not likely to be noticed under the microscope, is responsible for the concussional state of short duration followed by recovery. Conversely, irreversible injury has been linked with failure of blood pressure, as in primary surgical shock.

Cerebral Injury of Microscopic Dimensions

The term *cerebral concussion* is generally used to indicate a purely functional disorder that is supposedly reversible and of a relatively minor nature. Profuse observations, however, indicate the occurrence of neuronal changes in the concussional state.[102] These changes attest to the fact that the line of demarcation between cerebral concussion and cerebral contusion is not as distinct as the definition of terms implies.

Since death seldom occurs in cerebral concussion, difficulties have always attended the investigation of its underlying mechanisms. Thus, most of the pathoanatomical observations on the brain during and after concussion have been largely based on animal experiments (Fig. 3–I–15). A further point that has held back the elucidation of the problem is the dif-

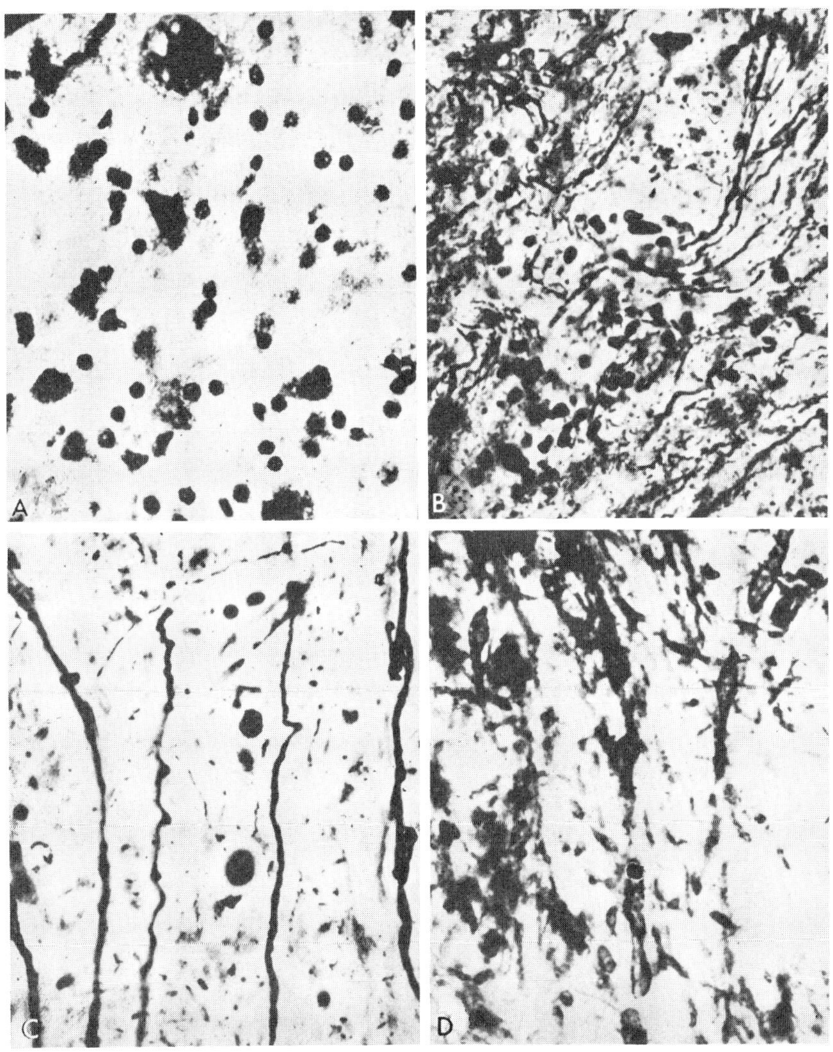

Figure 3–I–15. Moving object against stationary head in the experimental animal (rat). The animal received 11 subconcussive blows and at the last blow was unconscious for four minutes. It was killed three hours later. *A.*Tigrolysis and vacuolization of cortical nerve cell. *B.* Fragmentation of medullated axons, incipient granular disintegration and mobilization of microglia cells. *C.* Spreading apart of nerve fibers with bizarre loops and spirals. *D.* Varicose swelling and disintegration of myelin sheaths. (From C. G. Tedeschi: Cerebral injury by blunt mechanical trauma. Special reference to the effects of repeated impacts of minimal intensity; observations on experimental animals. Arch. Neurol. Psychiatry, *53*:333, 1945. Copyright 1945, American Medical Association. Reprinted by permission.)

ficulty in discriminating between the effects due to concussion and those caused by concurrent circulatory disorders, tissue edema, and eventually other associated alterations.

The duration of loss of consciousness is generally a fairly reliable yardstick for the degree of cerebral damage. The duration of the period in which memory of current events has not been stored is difficult to assess, however.[103] Furthermore, there are on record an endless number of cases of brain injuries associated with definite damage in which there was not even a recollection of a momentary dazed state.[104] For these reasons, retrograde amnesia has come to be considered a far more reliable index of the extent of intracranial damage than loss of consciousness.[105]

Electrophysiologic studies using superficial and deep recordings demonstrate that the period of unconsciousness correlates with the diminution of cortical electrical activity.[106, 107]

The brain stem, because of its location and mobility, is particularly likely to be involved in loss of consciousness incidental to the shearing effects of trauma or increase in intracranial pressure.[108] Changes in the brain stem reticular activating system and chromatolysis in large neurons of the midline reticular nuclei, red nuclei, and lateral vestibular nuclei have been shown in experimental animals submitted to acceleration concussion.[109, 110] Experimental evidence has also been presented that the chromatolysis of the brain stem neurons is due to interruption of ascending fibers in the mediocentral regions of the cervical spinal cord and that the axonal injury and attendant retrograde chromatolysis can be prevented by restricting the movements of the head at the time of the blow.[111, 112]

Equally well documented in the experimental animal is the occurrence of small foci of cortical ischemic necrosis, with concurrent disintegration of Nissl bodies, shrinkage, and chromatolysis of ganglion cells in conjunction with cerebral concussion.[102, 113] These findings suggest that microscopic neuronal injury may underlie the loss of function associated with cerebral concussion. Although one cannot be sure that these neuronal changes are of a secondary nature and caused by ischemia or other concurrent alterations, seemingly well-substantiated changes such as twisting and fragmentation of neuroaxons, fusiform swelling, and degeneration of myelin sheaths indicate the facility with which neuroaxons may be stretched, bent, or torn whenever the brain is subjected to shear strains that tend to alter its shape (Fig. 3–I–16).

Other common neuronal changes described in conjunction with cerebral concussion include *preservation necrosis*, an alteration characterized by an increased affinity for reduced silver of apparently morphologically intact cells. This alteration is likely to be found at the edges of necrotic areas and probably represents a manifestation of sudden ganglionic death associated with acute ischemia.

Nerve cells with several nuclei *(multinucleation)* can also be found; possibly they indicate barren attempts at cell regeneration.

Later in concussional injury, it is not uncommon to find nerve cells containing a yellow-

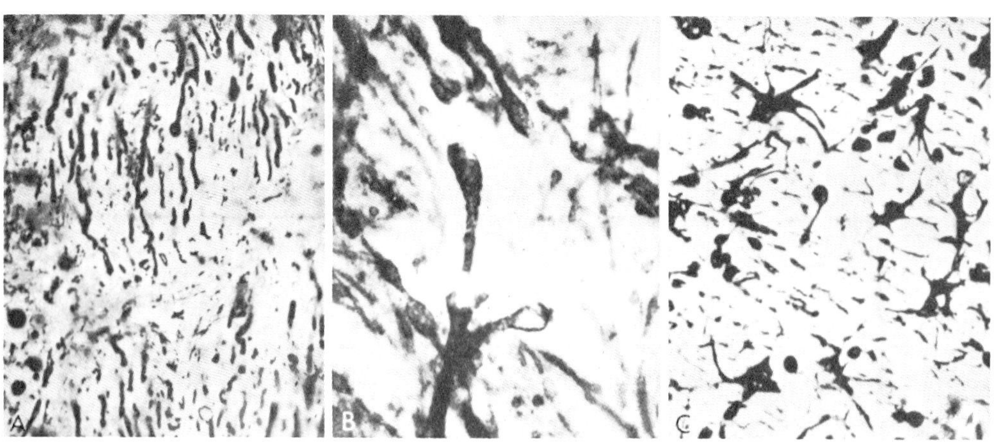

Figure 3–I–16. Experimental animal (rat) received 14 subconcussive blows in close succession on the stationary head; died 29 days later. Skull, brain, and meninges did not reveal abnormalities at gross inspection. *A* and *B*. Remnants of medullated axons, showing fusiform swelling, bulbs of retraction, and clublike formations at the end of fragmented fibers. *C*. Hyperplasia of astrocytes; a ball-like formation hanging at the end of a fragment of nerve fiber is noticeable at the center of the field. (From C. G. Tedeschi: Cerebral injury by blunt mechanical trauma. Special reference to the effects of repeated impacts of minimal intensity; observations on experimental animals. Arch. Neurol. Psychiatry, *53*:333, 1945. Copyright 1945, American Medical Association. Reprinted by permission.)

brown pigment *(pigmentary infiltration)* or showing calcium or iron depositions *(ferrugination)*. These changes lack specificity and can be found in other conditions not strictly related to trauma. More meaningful, in relation to trauma, is the detection of clublike formations *(balls of retraction)* at the ends of degenerated portions of fragmented fibers.

The value of the examination of frozen sections stained by a silver impregnation method for microglia (modified Weil-Davenport) has been stressed by Oppenheimer.[113] Under stimulation, such as may be provided by the neuronal damage resulting from the trauma, microglia cells become hypertrophic and multiply, giving rise to intensely argyrophilic aggregates that indirectly permit accurate assessment of the extent of neuronal destruction at various sites. This simple method has a particularly useful application in the identification of early neuronal lesions that otherwise could not be detected.

Ultrastructural and Biochemical Correlates

Among the early electron microscopic findings attending the neuronal chromatolysis associated with cerebral concussion, emphasis has been given to the dilation of Golgi's cisternae, dispersion of rough-surfaced endoplasmic reticulum, and detachment of ribonucleoprotein particles from the cell membranes.[114, 115]

Brown and his associates have shown alterations of axon terminals and presynaptic bulbs in the brain stem's reticular formation in animals in transient coma induced by controlled blows to the head, and later in the same experiment (7 to 10 days after the trauma), have noticed glycogen accumulation in dendrites, presynaptic boutons, and preterminal axons, seemingly associated with a decrease in synaptic vesicles from within the end bulb. Autophagic vacuoles, dilatation of membrane cisternae, and increased numbers of lysosome-like residual bodies were also found and can equally well be interpreted as evidence of degenerative changes and increased catabolic activity.[116]

The preferential accumulation of glycogen in astroglia and the nature of the changes in metabolic pathways that occur during the increased accumulation of glycogen remain poorly understood; a likely explanation, however, is that the glycogen accumulations are due to both an inhibition of anaerobic glycolysis and an increase in glycogenesis.

Concussion and the Blood-Brain Barrier

The concept of the blood-brain barrier originated with Ehrlich's demonstration that methylene blue injected into the vascular system of rabbits stained all tissues of the body except the central nervous system.[117] His explanation was that the capillary wall of the central nervous system had the ability to prevent inappropriate substances, such as dyes introduced in the general circulation, from reaching the nerve cells. The term "barrière hémato-encéphalique" (blood-brain barrier) was later introduced by Stern and Gautier in 1922 to in-

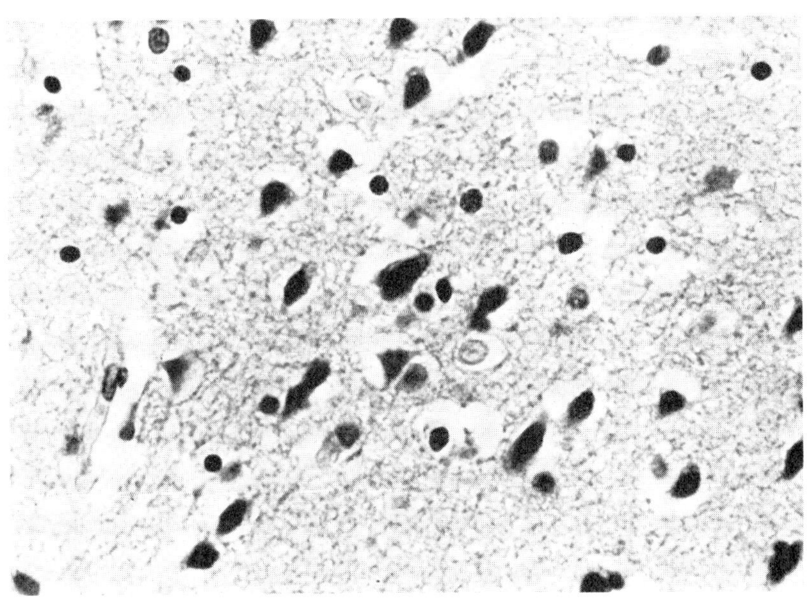

Figure 3–I–17. Ischemic changes in cerebral cortex. Hypovolemic shock following multiple injuries. (From C. G. Tedeschi (Ed.): *Neuropathology: Methods and Diagnosis.* Boston, Little, Brown and Co., 1970. Reprinted by permission.)

dicate the phenomenon that controls the passage of various substances into the brain.[118]

In spite of the general agreement on the existence of the barrier as a defense mechanism of the central nervous system, its anatomical site remains obscure. The vascular endothelium, the perivascular pia-glial membrane, the perivascular process of the astrocytes, have all been considered, at one time or another, as the sites of the barrier. Since electron microscopic studies have shown that the perivascular spaces represent an artificial separation, however, the perivascular foot plates of the astrocytes have come to be regarded as one of the probable sites of the barrier. Evidence has been presented that the capillary–glial basement membrane and the perivascular foot plates of the astrocytes may serve a regulatory and transport function in fluid and electrolyte homeostasis.

Blood-brain barrier mechanisms have also been shown in certain specialized cerebral adnexa, such as the pineal gland, adenohypophysis, hypothalamus, area postrema, and choroid plexus, whose difference from the conventional structures of the nervous tissue explain their patency to foreign proteins, anionic dyes, silver nitrate, and the like.

It is well documented that the blood-brain barrier is penetrated at the site of brain injury, including mechanical trauma.[119] The results of Fukui's experiments on the concussive effect of air pressure impacts on the exposed dura of rabbits receiving pre- and post-concussive administration of vital staining dyes suggest that functional impairment of the barrier may occur in the absence of visible neuronal changes.[120]

Enzyme Determinations in Evaluation of Acute Head Injury

Measurement of enzyme concentrations in body fluids has been widely applied to the assessment of tissue damage related to disease. Thus, glutamic oxaloacetic transaminase (GOT), commonly found in high concentrations in the heart, skeletal muscle, spleen, kidney, and liver, may show large increases in the blood serum in conjunction with disease, primarily that associated with heart and liver damage.

The blood-brain barrier prevents glutamic oxaloacetic transaminase from reaching the blood serum in coincidence with brain injury; abnormally increased concentrations have, however, been noted in the spinal fluid in a broad spectrum of diseases of the central nervous system.

An investigation by Smith and associates of the effects of craniocerebral trauma on its concentration in the spinal fluid has shown a significant relationship between the severity of the injury and the increase in glutamic oxaloacetic transaminase; the method was also found to be useful in prognosticating end results in the early phases of the injury.[121] Conversely blood serum determinations, of both the transaminase and the lactate dehydrogenase levels, have proved to be of no value in either the diagnosis or prognosis of cerebral lesions, including those induced by mechanical trauma.[122]

Creatine kinase (CK), because of its high concentration in brain tissue and relative scarcity in all other tissues (except bone and cardiac

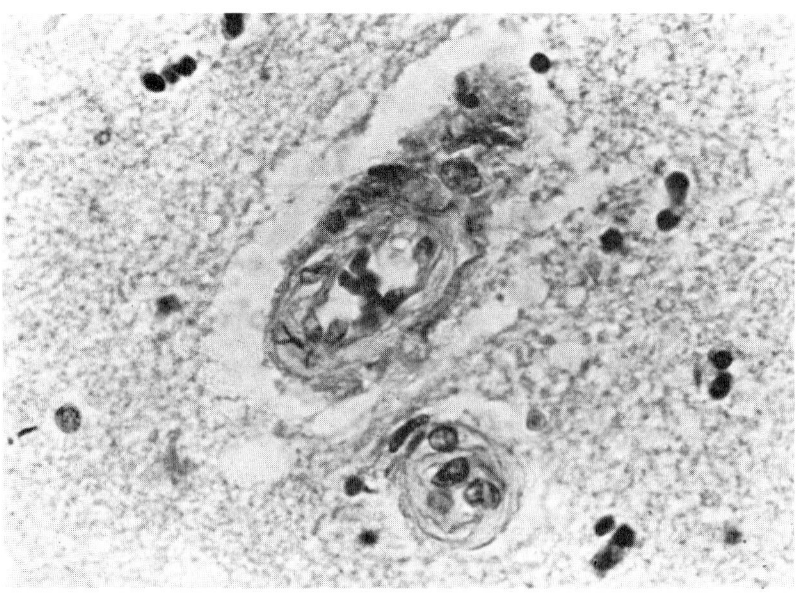

Figure 3–I–18. Intimal hyperplasia and acute ischemic changes in white matter. Hypovolemic shock following multiple injuries. Same case as Figure 3–I–10. (From C. G. Tedeschi (Ed.): *Neuropathology: Methods and Diagnosis*. Boston, Little, Brown and Co., 1970. Reprinted by permission.)

muscle) has received considerable attention. Kalbag, Park, and Pennington found a significant rise of serum creatine kinase levels in cases of acute head injury.[123] The isoenzyme pattern of the serum creatine kinase, however, for unexplained reasons, corresponded to that of muscle creatine kinase rather than to that of the brain enzyme.

In a similar assessment by Dubo and coworkers the degree of increase of creatine kinase activity in the blood serum did not correlate with the degree of severity of the posttraumatic neurologic deficit.[122] Thus, the results of the test were found to lack prognostic value.

Increased cerebrospinal fluid creatine kinase levels have been recorded by Herschkowitz and Cumings in various neurologic disorders.[124] No precise clinical correlation or prognostic inference could, however, be drawn in a similar study by Lisak and Craig.[125]

Timing of the Injury and Tissue Repair

Examination of a sample of cerebrospinal fluid obtained from the rachidian space may provide useful information on the time at which the injury occurred. When the fluid is bloody, the red blood cells are well preserved, and the supernatant of the centrifuged specimen is not blood-tinged, it can be assumed that the injury is only a few hours old. At least six hours have elapsed when the supernatant is hemoglobin-tinged, and frank xanthochromia can be taken as an indication that the injury occurred at least 12 to 24 hours before. As a rule, the color gradually fades away in two or three weeks. Of course, the observation loses its value in the presence of superseding bleeding.[126]

More reliable information on the time of the injury can be obtained from the histologic assessment of the process of tissue repair.[127, 131] The formation of intracellular cytoplasmic vacuoles in oligodendrocytes leading to cellular swelling is the earliest reactional change noticeable at the site of the injury. This is followed by swelling of microglia cells and by their streaming into the area of damage, an event that occurs at about the twelfth hour. Compound granular corpuscles can be seen 24 hours after the injury.

Whenever hemorrhage has taken place, hemosiderin-laden histiocytes make their appearance around the sixth day after the injury; they increase in number in the following days and reach their peak between the twelfth and fourteenth days, at which time hematoidin granules become noticeable. Subsequently, the histiocytes harboring the hemosiderin granules migrate into adjacent areas, primarily around the walls of the capillaries and smaller arteries.[132] Incrustation of blood vessel walls by iron salts, however, does not necessarily indicate previous hemorrhage. The same type of alteration is not uncommonly found in normal brains, primarily in the globus pallidus, a phenomenon that has been linked to a particular aspect of brain metabolism, possibly related to the respiration of the neuron.[133]

Following removal of the damaged nerve tissue, the final process of repair and healing of the wound is brought about by a proliferation of glia cells and mesodermal elements. The first evidence of glia mobilization—around the third day—is the hypertrophy of the cell body. Later, about the fourteenth day, the astrocytic processes begin to orient themselves toward the margins of the wound, and by the fourth week the damaged area is almost entirely replaced by a delicate web of glia cells and fibers. Not until the second month, however, does the glial network reach the degree of density to deserve the name of *protective scar*.[134] It must be realized that the formation of the scar may produce an amount of functional disturbance far greater than that induced by the primary injury.

Courville has made the distinction between *anisomorphic* and *isomorphic scars*.[135] In the former category, the glial elements are arranged in a netlike mesh; in the latter, they show a tendency to run parallel to the torn nerve fibers.

The extent of participation of fibroblasts and glia in the formation of the scar tissue may be linked to some extent to the nature of the wound. In missile wounds the scar is formed predominantly by fibroblasts springing from in-driven fragments of dura.[136] Continuity of the cerebral scar with the brain involucres may be responsible for the convulsive seizures that not uncommonly occur as a residual effect of missile wounds.[137] In contrast, the scar that ensues from blunt trauma is formed predominantly by glia cells and as a rule does not adhere to the brain coverings.

In time it may be difficult to differentiate the scar that follows a brain injury by mechanical force from the scar resulting from a brain injury from other causes. Common features of the brain injury healing process are meningeal thickening and adhesion, gyral shrinking and induration, and not uncommonly, hemosiderin staining and cortical cysts. Absolute evidence of remote trauma can, however, be provided by the disclosure, at microscopic examination of the scar, of fragments of twisted neuraxons, *end bulbs*, and *free balls* that appear early and maintain their identity for months and years after the accident.

Protracted Posttraumatic Encephalopathy

In spite of the restitution of vegetative functions, many victims of severe head trauma do not regain consciousness. This peculiar clinical state, variously referred to as "apallic syndrome," "akinetic mutism," or "coma vigile," is characterized by long-standing disorders of responsiveness ranging from varying degrees of coma to dementia.[138-140] Some of these patients will die within weeks or months from late complications or superseding disease; others may survive longer—for one or two years—and still others may eventually become responsive and show progressive improvement and adequate mental recovery.[141, 143]

According to Strich, the first recorded case of this condition is that of Rosenblath (1899), who examined the brain of a 17-year-old tightrope walker surviving for eight months in a "sleep-like state" after a head injury sustained in a fall.[144] Strich's dramatic description of this condition deserves verbatim transcription: The patient

> ... lies with his eyes open for much of the day and he appears to sleep for the rest of the time. He can easily be roused from sleep, though even when awake his reactions to the environment are very limited. He can cough, chew and swallow, and he follows sounds and moving objects with his eyes. Many are able to speak a few words and to obey commands. When first seen, he responds only to painful stimuli, often with generalized extensor spasms—the so-called "decerebrate" or "brainstem attacks."[144]

Cases fitting the label of protracted posttraumatic encephalopathy have been grouped by Jellinger and Seitelberger in the following five categories, each reflecting the degree of severity of the condition as judged by signs and symptoms:

- 4+ Category: Deep coma and/or fully developed acute mesencephalic syndrome;
- 3+ Category: Coma vigile, including all transitory stages from coma prolongatum, parasomnia, akinetic mutism to the fully developed "apallic" state. The latter is characterized by coma vigile, disturbed sleeping-waking rhythm, primitive reflex actions, lack of emotional response, vegetative and optomotor dysfunctions often associated with decerebrate posture, spastic tetraparesis, etc.;
- 2+ Category: Slight improvement of consciousness; normalization of the sleeping-waking rhythm, some interest in the environment, optic fixation, emotional responses, but no ability for verbal expression;
- 1+ Category: A state of partial recovery with normal regulation of sleep and wakefulness, beginning of purposive movements, some contact with the environment, differentiated recognition, ability to speak and write in the presence of severe mental and memory defects;
- 0 Category: A psycho-organic defect syndrome and post-traumatic dementia.[145]

In a pathologic condition characterized by such variability of clinical manifestations, ranging from deep posttraumatic coma to severe dementing syndrome, from partial mental recovery to full resocialization, it may be difficult to reach a reasonable decision with respect to degree of compensation and settlement of claims.

When the patient with protracted posttraumatic encephalopathy dies and the brain is examined, lesions visible to the naked eye often are few and inconspicuous; the results of the microscopic examination, however, are startling (Fig. 3–I–19). The prominent alteration is degeneration of myelin and nerve fibers in the white matter of the brain, with flow of axoplasm out of both cut ends, resulting in the formation of large blobs. The significance of these blobs, first described and named retraction balls or clubs by Ramón y Cajal in 1928, were subsequently stressed by others as direct evidence of tearing of nerve fibers by the shear stresses and strains set up during rotational acceleration of the head at the time of the trauma.[144, 146, 147]

Between the nerve fibers, large numbers of phagocytic cells containing the fatty products of myelin breakdown are usually present; in contrast, fibrous gliosis is absent or only slight.

In addition to these changes, which can be reasonably attributed to the direct mechanical effects of the trauma (primary lesions), Jellinger and Seitelberger have properly pointed out the role played by the "reactive" secondary lesions that arise from peripheral and cerebral circulatory disorders, from posttraumatic edema, and from increased intracranial pressure.[145] These secondary changes lack specificity; they are, however, equally important in determining the outcome of the encephalopathy.

The *punch-drunk syndrome* (dementia pugilistica) of professional fighters also belongs to the

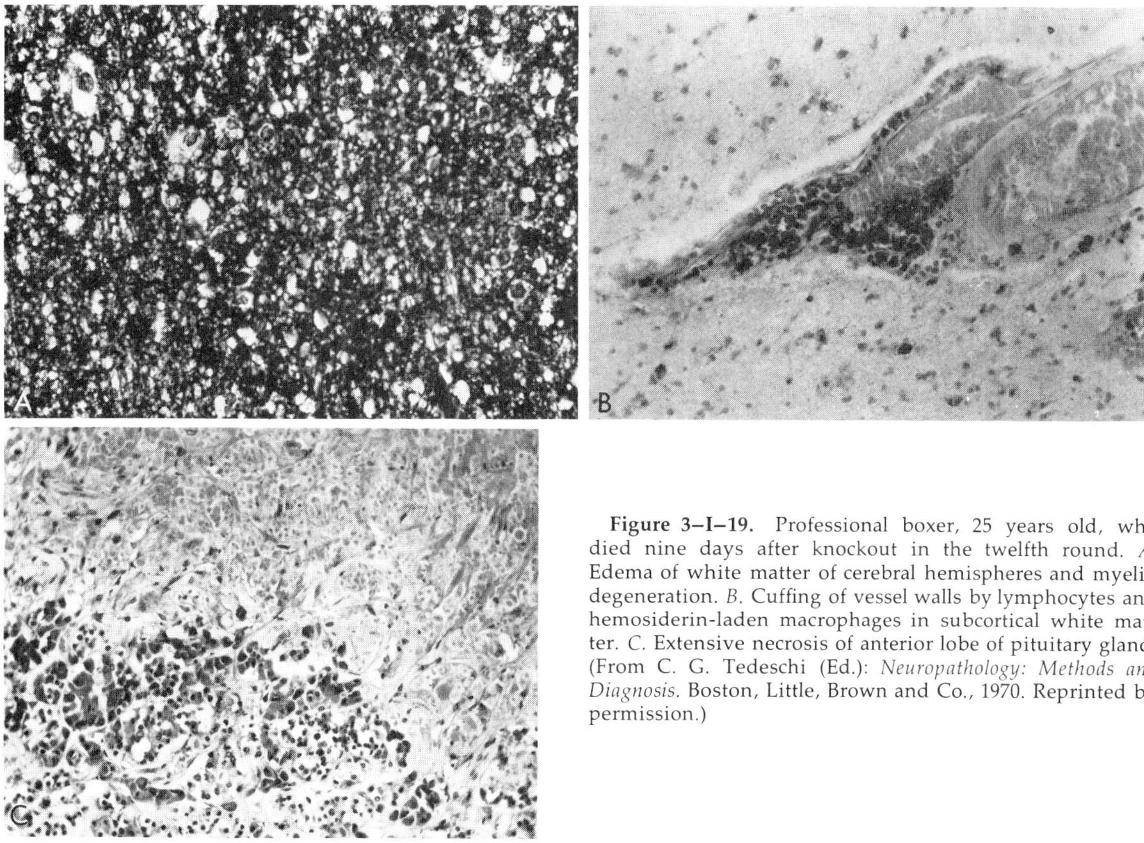

Figure 3–I–19. Professional boxer, 25 years old, who died nine days after knockout in the twelfth round. *A.* Edema of white matter of cerebral hemispheres and myelin degeneration. *B.* Cuffing of vessel walls by lymphocytes and hemosiderin-laden macrophages in subcortical white matter. *C.* Extensive necrosis of anterior lobe of pituitary gland. (From C. G. Tedeschi (Ed.): *Neuropathology: Methods and Diagnosis.* Boston, Little, Brown and Co., 1970. Reprinted by permission.)

posttraumatic encephalopathies. That the effects of cerebral trauma may be cumulative has been suspected since the demonstration by Koch and Filene in 1874 that experimental animals could be killed by repeated small blows on the head without showing any gross evidence of alterations in the brain.[150] Subsequently, Martland recognized in professional pugilists a distinct clinical syndrome characterized by fatigue, affective disorders, and hyperkinesis.[151] The occurrence of behavior disorders in prizefighters is now generally acknowledged, and several explanations have been offered to explain the phenomenon.[152-154]

According to Shaller and his associates, repeated blows to the head induce increased vulnerability of the cerebral vessels.[155] Denny-Brown and Russell have shown that paralysis of respiration of increasing duration and rise of blood pressure occur with successive blows.[156] A substrate of neuronal changes has been shown by Martland in patients with manifestations of this syndrome, and similar alterations have been described in experimental animals under conditions simulating the mechanisms of injury postulated in man.[147, 151]

Fatal injuries occur in boxing.[157] The prominent vascular thrombosis of pial veins and dural sinuses, the scattered perivascular hemosiderin deposits, and the numerous ischemic and hemorrhagic infarcts found at the examination of the brain point to the role of vascular changes among the factors primarily responsible for the progressive mental deterioration associated with dementia pugilistica (Fig. 3–I–20).

Psychoneurologic Sequelae of Head Injury

Although most patients who have sustained a head injury eventually recover in time, a certain number remain permanently incapacitated by the so-called *posttraumatic syndrome.* The most common symptoms of this condition are headache, dizziness, anxiety, irritability, insomnia, impairment of memory and concentration, and reduced tolerance to exertion and alcohol and heat.[158]

These symptoms signify a closely interlaced combination of organic and emotional proc-

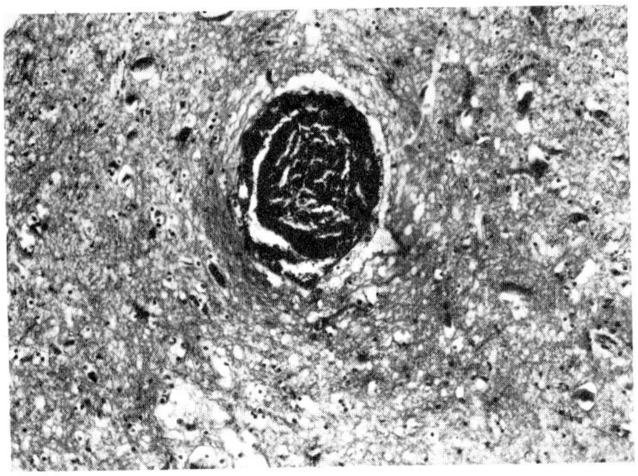

Figure 3–I–20. Amateur boxer, 20 years old, who died 55 hours after knockout in the second round. Recent thrombosis of pontine vein and ischemic necrosis and edema of surrounding nervous tissue. (From C. G. Tedeschi (Ed.): *Neuropathology: Methods and Diagnosis.* Boston, Little, Brown and Co., 1970. Reprinted by permission.)

esses. The former are related to damage to the brain and its involucres, such as vasomotor changes associated with brain stem damage, scarring in brain areas, and meningeal adhesions; the latter are of a more complex, unpredictable nature. The hope for compensation, when litigation is involved, often operates consciously or unconsciously to originate or prolong symptoms.

Well known is the importance of litigation as a determinant of exaggerated symptoms, false or distorted accounts, and perpetuation of neurologic disorders. Hyslop's analysis of 65 people who were claiming damages for posttraumatic epilepsy illustrates this point: 12 had never had a head injury, 7 had had seizures before the accident, and 28 had misrepresented the severity of the injury.[159] A similar trend is shown by Parker's survey indicating that 25 per cent of the individuals claiming damage for head injury had not been rendered unconscious at the time of the alleged trauma and that the nature of the accident was such that no damage to the head could possibly have taken place.[160]

Whereas in many cases the severity of the injury does not correlate with the severity of the psychoneurologic sequelae, a definite relation is frequently found between pretraumatic personality disorders and posttraumatic disturbances.[148]

The answer to the question of whether trauma can be regarded as capable of precipitating or aggravating a psychic or organic brain condition escapes generalization. It has been estimated that certain characteristics of intellectual impairment (mild dementia) became apparent only after removal of 90 to 120 g of cerebral hemisphere and that the excision of 30 to 60 g produced only slight departure from the preexcisional intellectual level.[160]

Much has been written on the relationship between trauma and paralysis agitans, general paresis, schizophrenia, manic depressive psychosis, encephalitis, and multiple sclerosis, but in the light of present knowledge, it seems that in the absence of organic changes related to the trauma, one cannot go much beyond the conclusion that head trauma can serve as a trigger mechanism and thus precipitate the manifestations of a preexisting latent disease.[161–166]

Trauma and Brain Tumor

Of the 313 patients with meningioma included in the classic monograph of Cushing and Eisenhardt, no fewer than 101 (93 intracranial and 8 spinal) had a history of trauma considered by the authors to be relevant to the tumor.[167] The nature of the trauma in this authoritative series varied; most commonly it consisted of a sharp blow on the vertex produced by contact with a hard object. Quite unique is the case of a child whose skull was fractured in the course of a high forceps delivery and who subsequently developed a meningioma in the injured falx.

In spite of the fact that in about 30 per cent of these cases there were medicolegal implications, the evidence presented in this study has not obtained the recognition that might have been expected.[168, 169]

As Sir Francis Walshe says, "in this litigious age the invoking of trauma as a factor in the genesis of any of the organic affections of the nervous system is not favored or it is met with profound skepticism."[170]

Whenever the issue of a causal relation between trauma and tumor is at stake, the possibility of chance association and fortuitous temporal relationship should be taken into account.

Life Expectancy in Head Injury

Lack of sufficient evidence prevents giving a clear-cut answer to the question of whether head injury shortens life expectancy; available information seems to suggest, however, that men with a history of head injury have a higher death rate than men in a normal population. A review of this subject by Walker and Erculei indicates that in the first 15 years after head injury, the death rate is three to four times as great as expected.[148] Similarly, on the basis of a study of Bavarian veterans of World War I made about 50 years after wounding, Walker and associates conclude that the life expectancy of men with head injuries, particularly those with posttraumatic epilepsy, is shorter than that of uninjured veterans and of the male German population within the same age group. Why epilepsy shortens the life span is not explained, and equally unanswered remains the question of why life expectancy is curtailed in both the epileptic and the nonepileptic with previous history of head trauma. Possibly "subtle functional changes related to the various cerebral impairments induced by the head injury render the general defense mechanisms of the body more vulnerable to the stresses of aging."[149]

BRAIN LESIONS FROM BLUNT TRAUMA IN EARLY INFANCY AND CHILDHOOD

The effects of blunt trauma to the head in an infant differ considerably from those occurring in a child, and under similar circumstances, the effects of the latter differ to some extent from those that are characteristic in the adult brain.

This is reasonably explained by the different tissular substrate. The infant skull lacks ossification of suture lines, the cranial bones are thinner, and it is not until two years of age that a recognizable inner table is laid down. Calcification is minimal, and as a result, the skull is more plastic. Furthermore, the intracranial fossae are shallower and the not yet myelinated brain has a much softer texture.

The marked pliability of the skull bones accounts for the infrequency of compound fractures. Conversely, quite unique to this age are the so-called "Ping-Pong ball fractures" that actually represent simple bony depressions or indentations mimicking a dent in a Ping-Pong ball. By the same token, the lack of ossification of the suture lines permits overriding of the bones and marked deformation of the skull without significant injury to the cranial contents.

Since the middle meningeal artery is not yet embedded in a groove, transection of this vessel in concurrence with temporal bone fracture does not occur as often as in the adult. *Extradural hemorrhage*, however, probably is as common, from tears in the tentorium or falx during the overriding of the skull bones.

Overriding of the bones of the skull may also cause tearing of the bridging veins extending from the cerebral cortex to the longitudinal sinus, giving rise to *subdural hemorrhage*.

It is well to keep in mind that in this age group the signs and symptoms of extradural or subdural hemorrhage can be imitated by an evanescent, acute focal cortical edema of the brain that, for reasons still poorly understood, is inclined to develop predominantly in children.[172]

In contrast to the hemorrhagic contusions of the mature brain, lesions in infants consist mainly of grossly visible, prominent *tears* in the cerebral white matter and smaller tears in the outermost layer of the cortex that extend parallel to the surface of the brain. Lindenberg and Freytag's authoritative study indicates that these characteristic tears are found only in young infants—five months or younger at the time of trauma.[173] Likewise, contrecoup injuries are uncommon before the age of three years and progressively increase in frequency thereafter.[174]

The tissue loss from tears of the infant brain is rather limited; nevertheless, neurologic deficit can be expected in surviving infants, as can epileptic attacks as well, as the result of precentral, central, and temporal lesions. Varying degrees of paraplegia may be produced by bilateral injury of the upper central convolutions, and speech development may be interfered with by a lesion in the posterior half of the temporal white matter. By the same token, destruction of residual matrix cells around the lateral ventricles may result in retarded or incomplete mental development, and whenever multiple tears occur at the time of injury, diffuse astrocytic fibrosis may interfere with myelination and lead to psychic or neurologic sequelae.[173]

Bleeding within the brain *(intracerebral hematoma)* may also occur. Frequently the hemorrhage dissects upward into the frontal lobe or downward into the temporal region. The clot expands, dissecting along the neural fibers rather than destroying nervous tissue, and this explains the not uncommon regression of symptoms.

Cerebral venous thromboses as a result of head trauma occur in the child almost as frequently as in the adult. Conversely, arterial thrombosis is much less common because of the absence of arteriosclerotic lesions that predispose to thrombus formation. Cerebral arterial occlusions in children have been recorded following trauma to head and neck, however, primarily in conjunction with open wounds and direct arterial wall lesions.[175]

There is no general agreement on the frequency with which children surviving a head injury develop manifestations of epilepsy, mental retardation, asocial behavior, and other symptoms of psychic insufficiency. Not infrequently the head injury has been viewed as a less important factor than the child's preexisting personality disorder or the unfavorable conditions in his environment.

Head banging is among the causes of intracranial injury in children. The range of behavior included under this heading varies from normal head rocking in infants to pathologic, violent striking of the head and face with fists and shoulders. This condition, which is considered a manifestation of a deprivation state, can lead to cerebral damage that basically does not differ from that in the punch-drunk syndrome of repeated trauma. Many childhood head bangers eventually develop cataracts during adolescence or adult life. It has been postulated that, as a result of repeated trauma to the head and eyes, the lens capsule undergoes an alteration in permeability, leading to exposure of the lens proteins to the fluid contents of the globe.[176]

PITUITARY INJURY IN CONJUNCTION WITH HEAD TRAUMA

Generally acknowledged is the discrepancy between the infrequency of pituitary disorders following craniocerebral trauma, as judged by manifestations of functional disturbances, and the frequency with which pituitary lesions are detected when the victim of the trauma dies and the gland is examined under the microscope. This is well attested by the meager 14 cases of posttraumatic hypopituitarism gathered from the world literature by Altman and Pruzanski, to which they added a case of their own.[177] By the same token, of the 595 cases of Simmond's disease reviewed by Escamilla and Lisser, only one could be presumably traced to previous head trauma.[178] Among the 2,000 cases of closed head injury investigated by Witter and Tascher, only 15 were found to display manifestations of anterior lobe insufficiency.[179]

Conversely, microscopic assessment of the pituitary gland in patients who die following head trauma points to a large incidence of pathologic changes: Boltz and Skala found evidence of lesions in 34 of 56 pituitary glands, Ceballos in 71 of 102, and Kornblum and Fisher in 62 of 100.[180-182] Individual case reports add further evidence that the pituitary gland, more commonly than previously thought, may undergo visible damage in conjunction with craniocerebral injury.[183, 184] The discrepancy between the relative rarity of clinical manifestations of pituitary dysfunction and the frequency with which pituitary lesions are detected under the microscope following head injury can be explained by the fact that large portions of the gland must be destroyed before manifestations of functional disorders become apparent.

The types of lesions most frequently found include capsular hemorrhage, stalk transection, swelling of the gland, and ischemic necrosis of the anterior lobe or the posterior lobe or both.

Capsular Hemorrhage

In over half the reported cases, the predominant pathologic change is capsular hemorrhage resulting either from seepage of blood from the subarachnoid cisterns at the base of the brain or from tearing of small arachnoid blood vessels situated between the diaphragma sellae and the dorsum of the gland. This occurrence, as a rule, is not associated with clinical manifestations.

Stalk Transection

Signs and symptoms of acute anterior lobe failure can be expected in conjunction with total transection of the pituitary stalk, an event that is unavoidably followed by infarct necrosis of the anterior lobe. This is due to the particular pattern of blood drainage of the anterior lobe, which is provided solely by the long and short hypothalamic-hypophyseal portal veins that arise from the capillary plexus within the stalk. Even when the disarrangement of the lobe is most extensive, it is not unusual to find that a few layers of peripheral subcapsular cells are still well preserved. These are the cells that are supplied and drained by the small capsular arteries and veins.

Transection of the stalk is generally associated with severe head injury and presumably results from shear stress at the time of impact. In conjunction with transection of the stalk, a fracture running through the body of the sphenoid bone is frequently found.

Swelling of the Gland

The pituitary gland is enclosed within the rigid bony structures of the sella turcica and is further protected and compartmentalized by the diaphragma sellae. A weak point in the overall anatomical structure is represented by the small circular opening in the diaphragma sellae that serves as a passage for the pituitary stalk. As a result of the shear stress incident to the trauma, the gland can swell considerably. As this occurs and the gland is pushed upward, the stalk is forced against the free edges of the diaphragm, and this may result in compression-occlusion of the hypothalamic-hypophyseal portal veins. The sudden suppression of blood flow may lead to a situation similar to that ensuing from the transection of the stalk, namely infarct necrosis of the anterior lobe.

Ischemic Necrosis of the Anterior Lobe

Whereas the lesion resulting from transection of the stalk and compression-occlusion of the hypothalamic-hypophyseal portal veins is essentially a venous infarct, an ischemic type of necrosis can arise in conjunction with systemic ischemia secondary to severe hemorrhage or shock. If damage to the gland is very extensive, the sudden withdrawal of pituitary control may precipitate fatal acute adrenal insufficiency. This situation is not different from that more familiarly associated with the postpartum Sheehan syndrome, and the pituitary lesion is also described in conjunction with increased intracranial pressure, shock, burns, brain edema, intracranial hemorrhage, hypertension, chronic renal disease, and other conditions.[181, 185–190]

Massive ischemic necrosis of the anterior lobe must be distinguished from the small focal infarcts that are not uncommonly found in the anterior lobe incident to head injury. These small lesions may presumably be attributed to partial interruption of blood flow. Since from two thirds to three fourths of the anterior lobe must be destroyed before evidence of anterior pituitary dysfunction becomes clinically manifest, confined small areas of damage are not significant as a cause of impaired glandular function.

Posterior Lobe Damage and Diabetes Insipidus

In coincidence with head trauma, hemorrhage and necrosis can be found with almost equal frequency in the anterior and posterior lobes of the gland. Lesions in the posterior lobe were noted by Kornblum and Fisher in 42 of the 100 pituitaries they examined.[182] The disproportion between the relatively frequent findings of posterior lobe damage and the rather uncommon occurrence of diabetes insipidus following head trauma, has been commented upon by several investigators. In the two cases of Kornblum and Fisher in which this condition was present, there was concurrent swelling of the brain and caudal shifting of hypothalamus and midbrain; thus, one remains in doubt whether the diabetes insipidus was related to the pituitary lesion or to the hypothalamic damage.[182]

Not much is known about the true incidence of diabetes insipidus in coincidence with head injury, and probably even less is known of the underlying relationships. In 6 of the 50 cases of diabetes insipidus analyzed by Blotner, there was a history of head trauma, but the same investigator cites patients with a history of concussion and diabetes insipidus who later were found to have a brain tumor.[192] Among the 2,500 patients with head injuries studied by Pickles, four developed diabetes insipidus, but in three of them the manifestations of this disorder were entirely gone four months after the head trauma.[193] In 5,000 cases of closed head injury, Porter and Miller found 13 cases of diabetes insipidus that they attributed to injury of' the pituitary stalk at the time of trauma.[194] In a case of posttraumatic diabetes insipidus reported by Henzi, scarring of the posterior lobe and tuber cinereum, extending into the region of the supraoptic nuclei, was the major finding at postmortem examination.[195] In another similar case reported by Goldman and Jacobs, the postmortem study revealed widespread sclerosis throughout the neurohypophysis and the hypothalamus.[196]

The histologic study of the hypothalamus by Treip, in 16 patients with fatal head injury, includes cases with manifestations of hypothalamic-pituitary dysfunction, such as electrolyte imbalance (hypernatremia), persistent hypothermia, and diabetes insipidus.[197] An attempt by this investigator to correlate lesions on one side and signs and symptoms on the other links the electrolyte imbalance to bilateral infarction of the ventromedial nuclei, persistent hypothermia to widespread damage to the periventricular gray matter, and the single case of diabetes insipidus to bilateral involvement of the supraoptic nucleus.

Although it is well established that the nervous system modulates the activities of the endocrine glands, understanding of the far-reaching extent of neurohormonal relations is still in the early stages of definition. The complexity of identifying central links is reflected in a recent report by Bartuska and associates, pointing to possible relationships between posttraumatic brain damage, hypertrichosis, and polycystic ovaries.[198]

INTRACRANIAL NERVE INJURY

Expectedly, the cranial nerves share with the brain and the other intracranial structures the effects of head trauma. The evidence of deficit of the affected nerve can become manifest immediately after the trauma or can appear some time later. Early manifestations presumably are caused by tearing of nerve fibers against the bony structures of the cranial cavity or by the shearing movement of the brain within the skull. Late effects can be due to a broad spectrum of factors, such as increased intracranial pressure or enveloping of the nerve trunk by an organizing blood clot or an inflammatory exudate.

Defects of smell following olfactory nerve injury are not uncommon in conjunction with frontal trauma and fracture of the cribriform plate of the ethmoid bones.[199] Disorders in vision can be caused by a lesion of the optic nerve itself or of the posterior parts of the visual pathway. The injury, in turn, can be due to an actual tear in the optic nerve, chiasma, or visual tracts, or to impairment in blood flow and ensuing ischemia. In the presence of blindness with retained reflexes for light, the cause must be sought in the visual pathways behind the lateral geniculate corpora; namely, in the optic radiation or in the visual cortex and underlying white matter.

Transient traumatic occipital blindness, also known as bilateral homonymous hemianopia, amaurosis corticalis, or cerebral (calcarine) blindness, is characterized by loss of vision with retention of the pupillary reactions to light and a normal ophthalmoscopic picture.[200, 201] The typical course is delayed complete blindness, of minutes to hours in duration, following a blunt injury to the skull. An interval with normal sight, from a few minutes to 24 hours, is highly characteristic of this condition. Although the symptoms are most frightening, the prognosis is favorable. To our knowledge, there are no published reports of autopsy findings in transitory cortical blindness. As such, the precise mechanism underlying this condition remains obscure. The transient nature of the disorder suggests some type of temporary cerebral dysfunction, presumably brought about by edema or a combination of edema and contusion of the occipital cortex and underlying white matter.

Bitemporal hemianopia is characteristic of the traumatic chiasm syndrome. This can be caused by a tear of the median portion of the chiasma in conjunction with fracture of the sphenoid bone, by avulsion in the absence of bony injury, or by impairment of blood flow. Cases are on record in which the hemianopia appeared several years after the head trauma.[202] The most frequently associated manifestations are hypothalamic disorders (polyuria), paralysis of the oculomotor nerve, and anosmia.[203]

About 3 per cent of surviving victims of a head injury show palsies of the third, fourth, and sixth cranial nerves, either singly or in combination. The sixth nerve is most frequently involved because of its long intracranial course.[204]

A variety of causes may be responsible for trigeminal nerve injury. In concurrence with a fracture of the upper margin of the orbit or even of a simple scalp wound in the same location, the supraorbital branch may become affected. Coincidentally with fracture of the maxillary bone, the infraorbital nerve may be involved. The upper division of the trigeminal nerve frequently is injured in conjunction with trauma that extends behind the eyeball.

Facial nerve paralysis occurs in 10 to 40 per cent of the patients with a longitudinal fracture of the temporal bone.[205] Longitudinal fracture is four times as frequent as transverse fracture and, as a rule, extends medially along the bony external canal to end either anteriorly in the region of the carotid canal or posteriorly in the mastoid region. A ruptured drum, bleeding into the middle ear and external canal, and when the dura overlying the tegmen is lacerated, cerebrospinal fluid otorrhea are the commonly associated manifestations. This type of fracture usually results from a force applied either to the condyle of the mandible or to the temporoparietal region. The less common transverse fracture is inclined to proceed through the labyrinthine capsule and to cross the facial canal. As in the case of the longitudinal fracture, blood or cerebrospinal fluid or both can leak through the fracture into the middle ear cavity, but since, as a rule, the eardrum is intact, there is no escape of fluid through the external canal. Transverse fracture most often occurs as a result of a blow to either the occipital or the occipitomastoid region. Although the facial nerve may be torn in conjunction with temporal bone fracture, the nerve palsy is usually due to pressure by blood extravasated in the bony canal.

Eighth nerve injury is not uncommon in fracture of the petrous portion of the temporal bone or retrolabyrinthine lesions in the auditory pathway (inferior colliculus, lateral lemniscus, superior olivary nucleus, cerebral cortex).[206]

Any fracture that involves the floor of the posterior fossa may affect the last four cranial nerves—glossopharyngeal, vagus, spinal accessory, and hypoglossal—and the cervical sympathetic trunk as well.

CRANIOCERVICAL AND SPINAL INJURY

In the Adult

It has been said that if a victim of an acute head injury should die instantaneously, he would be more likely to die of a twisted neck than a damaged brain.[207] The concept of head and neck as a single working unit is gaining acceptance. It is being realized more and more that any injuring force applied to either the head or neck must involve the craniospinal junction. Most impressive in this connection is Friede's demonstration that the chromatolysis of the brainstem neurons attending blunt trauma to the head is due to interruption of ascending fibers in the mediocentral regions of the cervical spinal cord.[208] From a study of the mechanisms of acceleration concussion in cats, this investigator has reached the conclusion that a blow accelerating the head produces an abrupt displacement of the craniocervical junction. This displacement affects the fibers located at the ventral circumference of the first segment of the cervical spinal cord, just opposite the odontoid process. Equally significant is Spicer and Strich's observation that hemorrhage in the posterior root ganglia can be found in patients who die from head injuries.[209]

Of the 22 bones that constitute the skull none are movable except the mandible. Conversely, the seven cervical vertebrae that form the neck have a multiplicity of movable joints. Mobility of the neck implies mobility of the head, and the end result of this unique dual arrangement is that a heavy immovable object (the head) is poised over a narrow stalk (the neck) capable of supplying a broad range of movements.

From the functional standpoint, the upper two cervical vertebrae provide rotational movement, and the lower five, flexion and extension. This explains why, as a general rule, rotational forces applied to the head are likely to injure the upper two vertebrae, and those causing extreme flexion and extension, the lower five.

The Brain

Brain lesion complicating whiplash injury is well documented.[210] Equally proved is the occurrence of electroencephalographic abnormalities, essentially of the same type as those occurring in closed head trauma, in almost one of two victims of whiplash injury.[211] The practical implication is that at least some of the psychoneurotic manifestations attending the sequelae of whiplash injury may be organically determined and due to injury of the brain.

The Spine

The usual history of a patient suffering from whiplash injury is that he was involved in an automobile accident, being struck from behind or from the side. When the striking force comes from behind, head and neck are subjected to hyperextension-flexion movements; when the force strikes from the side, head and neck are subjected to a sudden lateral to-and-fro motion.

Because the anterior longitudinal ligament does not provide sufficient protection to the cervical spine during the crash, it has been postulated, whiplash injury occurs, not during flexion of the neck, in which it is prevented by the contraction of the neck musculature, but rather, during overextension.

Injuries attending the whiplash injury range from tears and hemorrhages in the sternocleidomastoid muscle to rupture of the anterior longitudinal ligament and of the ventral part of the anulus fibrosus. Hemorrhages around the nerve roots, rupture of intervertebral disks, and fracture-dislocation of vertebrae are not uncommon in the most severe cases. Middle-aged and elderly people with preexisting cervical spondylosis are particularly vulnerable to this type of injury because hyperextension of the neck produces further narrowing of the spinal canal.

Atlantal fractures, atlantoaxial dislocation, and *displacement of the odontoid process* often follow a blow to the vertex, such as that resulting from the impact of the head against a cracking windshield in a head-on collision.

Fractures of the atlas constitute from 2 to 13 per cent of fractures of the cervical spine and about 1.3 per cent of fractures of the entire spinal column.[212, 213] For this type of injury to occur, certain conditions must be met. The cervical vertebrae must be vertically aligned beneath the atlas and rigidly held in position by the contracted muscles of the neck. Furthermore, the force transmitted through the skull must be driven in an axial direction. Thus the lesion is ultimately produced by the thrust of the neck musculature counter to the force transmitted from the skull to the atlas.[214]

The most common complaints attending fracture-dislocation of the atlas are suboccipital pain, headaches, stiffness of the neck, and frequently, difficulties in swallowing caused by hematoma formation in the parotid gland region and in the retropharyngeal area. Occipital neuralgia and painful paresthesias of the scalp are among the sequelae due to compression of the greater occipital nerve.[215]

The vertebral artery, because of its laxity, is rarely affected, but a few fatal cases of rupture of the artery are on record.[216] A number of cases have also been recorded of arteriovenous fistula formation.[217] Injury to the carotid artery is relatively more common owing to direct contusion, stretching, shearing effect, or arterial spasm. As a result of the injury, thrombosis may occur, but it is often difficult to determine whether the occlusion is antegrade, from a craniocervical lesion, or retrograde, from extension of an intracranial occlusion, which is often associated with basilar skull fracture.[218, 219]

Although the cervical region, because of its marked mobility, suffers the greatest incidence of spinal injuries, second and third in order of frequency are those of the lower thoracic and thoracolumbar vertebrae. As in the neck, injury to the lower vertebral segments is most commonly due to hyperflexion, vertical compression, and hyperextension.

In *hyperflexion*, laceration of the intervertebral ligaments drives the displaced portions of vertebrae posteriorly into the spinal canal. *Vertical strain* leads to compression fracture of the vertebral bodies, as a rule without change in their alignment. If the trauma is sufficiently severe to cause fracture of the vertebral bodies, there is almost invariably associated laceration of ligaments. Nevertheless, laceration of ligaments alone may allow sufficient dislocation of the vertebrae to compress the spinal cord or the nerve roots. In *hyperextension*, there is anterior displacement of the body and arch of the dislocated or fractured vertebrae, and this may reduce by half the sagittal diameter of the spinal canal.

Fractures may involve the vertebral body, the arches, and the spinous or transverse or articular processes, either singly or in unpredictable combinations. When bony fragments are driven into the spinal canal, the ensuing injury to the cord and nonnervous accessories does not differ from that induced by a simple dislocation.

Under a strain leading to hyperextension, compression of the spinal cord may be produced as well by the infolding of the ligamenta flava into the canal. It has been shown that any time the spine becomes extended, the ligamenta flava protrude into the canal.[220] Upon hyperextension, the protrusion, particularly at the level of the cervical enlargement, can reach a degree at which it occupies most of the available space and exerts pressure on the cord.

The Spinal Cord

As vertebrae or vertebral parts encroach upon the spinal canal, the spinal cord, its coverings, and its nerve roots may undergo varying degrees of compression and contusion. The pathologic change in the cord coverings in spinal trauma is basically the same as that arising in the intracranial coverings under comparable conditions. Blood extravasation may occur in the epidural, subdural, and subarachnoid spaces. Infection can also occur in any one of these areas in coincidence with septicemia originating from a distant focus of infection, from direct extension of an inflammatory process in the paraspinal tissues, or from a vertebra that is the site of osteomyelitis.

The occurrence of traumatic *subarachnoid-pleural fistula* is exceedingly rare but has been recorded.[221] This intriguing situation has been described following operations upon intrathoracic meningoceles, auto accidents with concurrent fracture of thoracic vertebrae, and gunshot injury.[221] Diagnosis is often delayed, largely because of the rarity or improbability of the condition and the subtle nature of the spinal injury that not uncommonly escapes radiologic demonstration.

As the result of a long-standing compression or a healed traumatic lesion or a localized infection that has subsided, the dura can become thickened and adhesions can develop between dura and arachnoid or between arachnoid and cord. Following fracture repair, exostosis at the vertebral margins may encroach upon the rachidian space or the intervertebral foramina.

Extending further the parallelism of lesions attending cranial and spinal mechanical injury, the distinction between *spinal concussion* and *spinal contusion* is equally poorly defined. By definition, the term "spinal concussion" is applied to a purely functional disorder that supposedly is reversible and of a minor nature. Sudden hydraulic changes in the cerebrospinal column, violent oscillations of the cord, momentary vertebral displacement, or evanescent edema have all been considered at one time or another in explanation of spinal concussion. As in head trauma, however, it is presumed that not infrequently the disorders in function are underlain by or associated with changes in nerve cells and fiber tracts, small hemorrhages, tissue edema, and microscopic areas of ischemic necrosis, which in turn may be responsible for crippling neurologic disorders.

In concurrence with interference with blood supply by hemorrhage or thrombosis, and in addition to spindle-shaped infarcts extending over several spinal segments, is the not uncommon finding, in the posterior horns and columns, of cylindrical cavities 1 or 2 mm in diameter, which probably represent the end results of colliquation necrosis.[222] The portion of the cord most vulnerable to defective blood supply is the fourth thoracic segment, which is the area of junction of the anterior and posterior spinal arteries (border zone).

Decrease in cardiac output or systemic hypotension usually affects the brain, leaving the cord intact. An infarct may, however, also take place in the spinal cord if the blood flow in the tributary vessels is compromised by arteriosclerosis or other processes.

Unequivocal alterations can be expected in *cord crush* injury and *contusion compression.* These terms expressively indicate the irreversible degeneration of nerve cells and fibers concurrent with fracture-dislocation of the spine and in-driven fragments of bone. Changes consist chiefly of swelling and fragmentation of myelin sheaths and axis cylinders, shrinkage, pyknosis of nerve cells, and disintegration of Nissl bodies. The nerve roots are frequently involved in the process.

Upon tearing of blood vessels, subarachnoidal or subdural hemorrhage may cause the bleeding to extend through the long axis of the cord *(hematorrhachis),* causing further compression and damage of fiber tracts. Tearing of dura and meninges is not common, but when it does occur, leakage of cerebrospinal fluid and superimposed infection are frequent complications.

Hematomyelia is the name given to a contusional lesion that is characterized by hemorrhage and softening in the gray matter at the point of impact. The end result of the lesion is gliosis and scarring enveloping a central fusiform cystic cavity.[223]

Penetrating injuries of the spine and cord by gunshot and stab wounds are entitled to special consideration (see Chapter 11). To round out the subject, here it is sufficient to say that high-velocity bullets characteristically have two major categories of effects: those related to the damage at the level of impact and those inherent in the jarring caused by the blast. The former include hemorrhage and necrosis in any of the structures in the track of the missile. The latter, in contrast, consist of minor lesions in an unpredictable distribution that may extend over several segments above and below the area of impact.

In the Infant and Young Child

The mechanisms underlying spinal injury in early infancy and childhood are the same as those operating later in life; the effects, however, are of a considerably different nature owing to the different characteristics of the tissular substrate.

A higher degree of plasticity, elasticity, and tensile strength of the spine texture affords to the very young a mobility that progressively declines during the process of aging. Great mobility, however, should not be interpreted as indicating greater protection from injury: in infancy and early childhood, muscular contraction is not as yet at its best to provide counterthrust at the site of impact. Although vertebral fracture and dislocation and transection injury of the cord are rare in infants, stretch injury by longitudinal traction and compression in coincidence with excessive flexion of the spinal axis may cause bleeding in the spinal canal and serious damage to the spinal cord and spinal nerve roots. Major injuries, particularly those involving the highly movable neck, may result in brain stem lesions with crippling of vital functions and sudden death—a sequence of events that in many ways duplicates the pathologic sequelae of spinal injury at birth.

An analysis of 2,000 persons with back pain or deformity has shown that 70 per cent of spinal lesions can be traced to problems caused by vertebral trauma or by vertebral trauma in association with degenerative changes of the spinal cord.[224] It is conceivable that not a few spinal disorders that appear later in life can be traced back to apparently insignificant trauma in infancy or childhood.

COMPLICATIONS OF SPINAL SURGERY

Possibly no other area of surgery is as likely to lead to failures, complications, disappointments, and litigations as that involving spinal operations. Tears of the dura may occur during laminectomy, and whenever they are not closed by adequate suture or by some other substance (absorbable gelatin foam) *arachnoid cysts* may develop. Since these cysts can be missed even by myelography, the possibility of their existence should be considered in the absence of any suitable explanation for recurrent pain.[225]

Complications due to *foreign bodies* left in the wound during the surgical procedure are quite inexcusable. Routine counting of sponges and cottonoid pads is common practice in all operating rooms. Failure to do so can be costly, both to the patient in terms of suffering and to the surgeon in terms of malpractice claims. A few such cases are recorded in Ford's article on local complications of lumbar disk surgery.[225] Before closure of the operative field, the wound should be carefully inspected and the surgeon in charge of the case should request a sponge and cottonoid pad count.

Other foreign bodies within the wound may result from broken instruments. Small set screws from a disk rongeur may become loose and drop into the wound. A replaceable blade may break and be lost in a disk space; search for it may considerably prolong the operation, increasing the risk to the patient; thus the indication to use a tenotomy knife, which is strong and in one piece.

Pyogenic infection of the intervertebral disk following a disk operation is another serious complication. The exact incidence of this occurrence is difficult to determine: the symptoms are bizarre, and not infrequently the physician is misled into a diagnosis of functional or psychoneurotic disorder; furthermore, roentgenographic evidence of the infection of the intervertebral space may not appear for 8 to 12 weeks after its onset.[226] Contamination of the surgical wound may occur from implantation of bacteria during the procedure or from circulating bacteria reaching the wound by way of blood vessels. In the case of lumbar spine infection, the possibility has also been entertained that bacteria can be drawn into the surgical field from septic foci in the genitourinary tract, reaching the vertebral bodies via the pelvic veins and the paravertebral plexus or, more likely, via the pelvic lymphatics and the general circulation. Once the bacteria reach the intervertebral space, they may remain confined to the disk or may progressively erode end plates and nucleus pulposus, ultimately leading to collapse of the interspace and interbody fusion. Paravertebral abscesses and epidural infection may occur, but rather infrequently. Fever and leukocytosis, the customary systemic manifestations of infection, as a rule are not prominent in sepsis of the intervertebral space. When they are present, extension of the process to adjacent tissues (paravertebral or epidural abscess) should be suspected.

Excruciating pain and elevated sedimentation rate are almost invariably present; since adequate treatment rests on the identification of the organism responsible for the infection and on application of the appropriate antibiotic treatment, exploratory needle aspiration should not be omitted. A positive result may establish the diagnosis several months before roentgenologic signs of erosion of the vertebral plates become manifest.

Although mostly localized in the lumbar region, pain can radiate to the testes, the groins, and the lower abdominal quadrants. Cases are on record of abdominal exploration before the exact diagnosis could be established.[226]

Of a different nature are some of the problems that may arise following cervical disk operation by the anterior approach. These complications have been analyzed by Cloward.[227] *Keloids* may occasionally form, particularly in dark-skinned people, and require removal. Obviously no fault can be attributed to the surgeon for this occurrence, which can develop for unexplained reasons following any operation wound affecting the skin.

During the surgical procedure the *cutaneous colli nerve* may be injured, and this may result in an area of numbness on the chin and side of the neck. As a rule, as the nerve regenerates, sensation returns within three to four weeks. Repair of the *recurrent laryngeal nerve* accidentally stretched or cut during the operation may take longer—from four to six months. This complication is promptly recognized by functional impairment or paralysis of the vocal cord and laryngeal muscles. It is conceivable that the *phrenic nerve* and the *sympathetic chain* can also be injured, the latter resulting in Horner's syndrome.

As a result of forceful retraction of the *larynx*, the patient may complain of mild hoarseness for a few days after the operation; by the same token forceful application of the retractor over the *esophagus* may lead to temporary difficulties in swallowing. Much more serious esophageal complications include *laceration of the esophagus,* followed by wound infection, osteomyelitis of the vertebra, and esophageal stricture, as in a case described by Cloward.[227] The same author mentions a case of displacement and migration through the esophagus of a displaced fragment of bone graft.

Retractor blades may also be responsible for accidental perforation of a high-lying dome of the *pleura*, a situation that, as a rule, can be promptly recognized and corrected. Puncture of the *vertebral artery*, with ensuing brisk hemorrhage, may follow probing through the intervertebral foramen with a sharp instrument. As Cloward says, this is an avoidable complication because sharp instruments should never be introduced into areas beyond the surgeon's vision.[227] Equally avoidable is *spinal cord* injury, a few instances of which have been recorded in coincidence with insertion of the bone graft under excessive pressure or plunging of the cervical drill into the spinal canal.

Paraplegia or *quadriplegia* following cervical disk operations is uncommon. When manifestations of these conditions become apparent, factors to be taken into account in addition to surgical trauma are mechanical compression of the cord by epidural abscess concurrent to spinal infection, or an alteration in the blood supply to the neural tissue caused by vascular thrombosis or pressure occlusion of epidural blood vessels.[228]

Postoperative hemorrhage at the site of the wound, graft displacement or fracture, collapse of the graft, and graft absorption are not always avoidable; they are just part and parcel of the risks inherent in a delicate operation.

Ford points out that even the useful myelogram carries some risks such as meningismus, arachnoiditis, and meningitis.[225] In the light of these not unlikely complications, the same investigator does not hesitate to advise restriction of myelography to only the cases in which surgery is contemplated.

Of all failures and adversities of disk surgery, the most feared is *unrelieved* or *recurrent pain*. Pain can be due to adjacent disks undergoing degenerative changes that progress, following the operation, to the symptomatic stage; or it can be caused by the formation of adhesions binding the nerve roots to the floor of the spinal canal and causing pressure on them.

The pain can be solely functional or psychogenic or due to the hope of gain from litigation.[229] It can also be real and excruciating. Any strain such as motion of the back or of the extremities, coughing or sneezing, even jarring of the bed, can initiate a painful spasm in the lumbar musculature. Ford mentions five patients with persistent discogenic pain who committed suicide.[225] Four did so after unsuccessful disk surgery, and the fifth one leaped from a tenth-floor window following myelography: "The day before contemplated surgery he told his roommates that he could not stand the pain any longer." Psychiatric evaluation of the patient whose pain has not been relieved by disk surgery can be indicated before deciding on further surgery, another type of therapy, or no therapy at all. In this connection, the following case in which the writer was actively involved, is worth reporting:

A 43-year-old veteran was transferred from a Veterans Administration Hospital in New York State to a Veterans Administration Hospital in the Boston area with the tentative diagnosis of a noncategorized malignant tumor of the lumbosacral spine. The history noted low back pain referred to an alleged fall on the back two months before. Diagnosis rested on the combined interpretation of a myelogram, roentgenologic studies, and the pathologic examination of a fragment of bone obtained at surgical exploration.

The slide accompanying the patient was reviewed by a panel of pathologists who all agreed that the lesion was consistent with the exuberant osteoblastic proliferation associated with callus formation. As the neurosurgeon in charge of the case conveyed the good news to the patient, he noticed a sudden change in mood, from rather indifferent to sad and worried. The following day the patient leaped to his death from an eighth-floor window.

In this particular case the low back pain was mild and presumably was not the cause of the successful suicide attempt. Why he did it remains a matter for speculation. A not unlikely interpretation is that the patient construed the news that no further surgery was contemplated as meaning that the malignant disease was so far advanced as to make useless any attempt at cure.

PERIPHERAL NERVE INJURY

Peripheral nerve injury may lead to three major categories of events: neurapraxia, axonotmesis, and neurotmesis.

Neurapraxia is characterized by a temporary loss of function in the absence of visible structural changes. In *axonotmesis* the axons are injured, but the enveloping connective tissue sheaths retain their continuity, allowing peripheral regeneration of nerve fibers without neuroma formation. In *neurotmesis* all or almost all of the nerve thickness is severed, and reinnervation is often prevented by the formation of a neuroma at the amputation stump.

The term *amputation neuroma* is applied to a disorganized mass of fibronervous tissue at the site of laceration of the nerve resulting from the piling up of regenerating axons, and Schwann cells that have been prevented from reaching their destination by an obstruction in their course. The obstruction can be interposed tissue or an organizing inflammatory exudate, a blood clot or a mass of fibroblastic cells.

The distal portion of the crushed or lacerated nerve becomes separated from the cell body and undergoes wallerian degeneration. The fibers of the proximal portion, still continuous with the cell bodies, also undergo wallerian degeneration, but for a very short distance. Regeneration of nerve fibers takes place through sprouting of new neurites from the severed axons at the proximal amputation stump as well as through the surviving Schwann cells. Maturation of the newly formed neurites gradually takes place with the formation of the myelin sheath, which is contributed in part by the axon and in part by the cell of Schwann.

In the human, the speed of growth has been estimated at between 2.5 and 3 mm a day.[230] Return to normal function is achieved when the motor neurites reach the old end-plates of the muscle fibers and the sensory neurites reenter the pacinian corpuscles.

Chemotactic influences, the syncytium of Schwann, and the direction of growth of the fibroblasts have been variously advocated to explain how the neurites can reach their destination.[230]

The three main causes of nerve injury are open wounds, traction, and fractures and dislocations.

Open wounds are by far the most common. In this category are the incised wounds, which are most frequently caused by glass. The injury can lead to complete or partial division of the involved nerve. Lacerated wounds are less common; like the incised wound, the laceration can lead to simple transection or to a substantial portion of nerve being torn away. The incidence rate of complete or partial division is so high (nearly 90 per cent) that surgical exploration is almost always necessary as soon as healing of the wound has taken place.[231]

The effects of the shock wave in a missile wound may vary considerably—from a fleeting paralysis, lasting a few minutes, to internal disruption of the nerve, ultimately causing moderate or severe intraneural fibrosis, the end effect of the pressure disturbance exercised by the missile traveling at high speed.

Traction injuries are less frequent. Peripheral nerves have great tensile strength, but limited elasticity; stretching can cause intraneural damage that may extend over a considerable length of the nerve. Experiments in animals indicate that the epineurium (the strongest neural structure) snaps first, and that thereafter the nerve fibers (the weakest structure) break anywhere at points remote from the site of epineurial rupture.[232] The vasa nervorum are damaged too, and the ensuing ischemia is responsible for additional alterations in the nerve fibers. Large effusions of blood (subepineurial hematoma) have also been recorded, in turn causing sustained pressure.[233] The end effects are reflected in interstitial fibrosis, segmental demyelination, and fragmentation of axons.

Sunderland and Bradley have determined the loads required to rupture four major nerves.[234] Their results are shown in Table 3–I–1.

In traction injury of severe degree, prognosis is poor. If recovery does not occur spontaneously, the longitudinal spread of the injury usually precludes surgical suture of the involved nerve. The most serious of the traction injuries is that affecting the brachial plexus, in which nerve roots can be torn away from the cord, an occurrence most commonly seen at birth (birth paralysis).

Fractures and dislocations may equally be responsible for traction injuries. Dislocation of the shoulder may injure the *axillary nerve*, and any nerve in the upper limb below the level of the clavicle may suffer traction injury in conjunction with a fracture of the shaft of the humerus or of both bones of the forearm. The *sciatic nerve* may be stretched in a posterior dislocation of the hip or a fracture of the acetabular rim. The *common peroneal nerve* is vulnerable to a knee dislocation, to a fracture of the tibia and fibula, and even to an inversion sprain of the ankle.

It is also possible for a nerve to be trapped between bony fragments or to be severed, particularly in connection with an open fracture.

Accidental stretching or severing of nerves may occur during the course of operations; not infrequently a retractor does the damage. In the light of medicolegal implications, this well-known surgical hazard is given further consideration in Chapter 59.

Nerve injury can arise, though less

TABLE 3–I–1. LOADS REQUIRED TO RUPTURE MAJOR NERVES*

Nerve	Load Required to Cause Rupture (kg)	Range of Loads (kg/mm² of cross-sectional area)
Median	7.3 to 22.3	1.0 to 3.1
Ulnar	6.5 to 15.5	1.0 to 2.2
Tibial	20.6 to 33.6	0.5 to 1.8
Common peroneal	11.8 to 21.4	0.8 to 1.9

*Modified from Sunderland, S., and Bradley, K. C.: Stress-strain phenomena in human peripheral nerve trunks. Brain, *84*:102, 1961.

frequently, as a result of a severe *percussive blow* or following undue pressure.[236, 237] The effects of pressure are directly proportional to the amount of force and the length of time it is applied; lesions in the compressed area may range from a momentary loss of function when the pressure is of short duration to fragmentation of axons and breakdown of myelin sheaths when the pressure is sustained over a considerable period of time. This is often the case with untreated prolapse of an intervertebral disk.

The nerve injury resulting from sustained pressure is probably due to a combination of direct mechanical trauma and ischemia. Not infrequently nerve function is reestablished on removal of the cause of the pressure; in these particular cases it must be assumed that nerves and spinal roots were not involved and that the injury was primarily extraneural.

The association of *nerve injury* and *vascular injury* is far from uncommon, and the combined effects can be most deleterious. Nerves and vessels (both arteries and veins) often lie close together; thus, in conjunction with an open wound they can be simultaneously affected at the same level. In this case the nerve is likely to undergo a local lesion at the site of the injury and a longitudinal one distal to it, the latter being caused by the ischemia resulting from the vascular injury. The same type of distal nerve damage may occur concurrently to an injury that affects the artery or the vein alone; this situation unavoidably generates ischemia that damages the nerve traversing the area of insufficient blood supply.

In the so-called *Volkmann's contracture* of the fingers and sometimes of the wrist, which develops rapidly after a severe injury in the region of the elbow joint or improper use of a tourniquet, the state of the muscle has attracted most attention. In reality, bone, tendon, and particularly nerves are affected, and the degree of nerve involvement is just a reflection of the severity of territorial ischemia.

Perhaps of all body injuries the most difficult to assess in their immediate and late effects are those related to peripheral nerves.

Among the consequences of nerve deficit, *muscle atrophy* is the most striking and the easiest to assess. Within the first few weeks after denervation the muscle fibers shrink rapidly and, when observed under the light microscope in a longitudinal section, present a wavy outline. The shrinkage is uneven, and some muscle fibers appear more wasted than others. Cross-striations are hardly seen, but not infrequently can still be shown under polarized light, quite a long time after denervation. With the passage of time, the muscle fibers finally disappear and are replaced by fat and fibrous tissue.

Spontaneous contraction of individual denervated muscle fibers characterizes the phenomenon generally known as *fibrillation*. This phenomenon becomes noticeable in very superficial muscles, those of the tongue primarily, within a week or less of denervation; it continues for months and gradually decreases with progressive atrophy of the muscle.

Wasting may be the first manifestation of *motor paralysis* to attract attention; however, *deformity* and *contractures* due to unbalanced muscle action are among the most devastating consequences of nerve injury. Clawing of the fingers and toes are familiar examples.

Well-demarcated areas of *anesthesia* and *analgesia* mirror the sensory paralysis resulting from loss of nerve function. Sensations of heat and cold, pressure sensibility, and postural and vibration sense are also lost. Yet the patient experiences spontaneous pain that he refers to the area of sensory loss; *phantom sensations*, indistinguishable from the phantom hallucinations after amputation, are also not uncommon.

The autonomic nerve fibers supplying the skin have about the same distribution as the sensory fibers. *Absence of sweating* (sudomotor paralysis) is one of the manifestations of involvement of the autonomic system, and the boundaries of anhidrosis match very closely those of analgesia and anesthesia. *Vasomotor* and *nutritional paralysis* are additional manifestations of autonomic disorders. Immediately after severance of the nerve, the skin of the affected area becomes hot, flushed, and dry (as after sympathectomy); then, after a variable period of time (weeks or months), the cold phase supervenes and persists until nerve regeneration has taken place. Absence of sweating makes the skin dry, thin, and scaly; alterations can also be noticed in the nails, such as increase in curvature, presence of prominent transverse ridges and retraction of the skin from the base of the nail.

Ulcers, *blisters*, and lesions that mimic *chilblains* occasionally occur. These are commonly due to accidental trauma, primarily burns or friction of the insensitive part against a hard object such as a nail in the sole of a shoe.

Disuse of the affected limb or part of the limb can lead to bone changes, and if the paralysis occurs early in life, arrested growth can cause shortening of the limb or deformity due to unbalanced muscular action.

Assessment of nerve deficit and overall loss of or reduction in function provides a real challenge in matters of compensation. As Sed-

TABLE 3–I–2. GRADING OF MOTOR AND SENSORY RECOVERY*

Motor (M) recovery		Sensory (S) recovery	
M0	No contraction	S0	Absence of sensibility in the autonomous area
M1	Return of perceptible contraction in the proximal muscles	S1	Recovery of deep cutaneous pain sensibility within the autonomous area of the nerve
M2	Return of perceptible contraction in both proximal and distal muscles	S2	Return of some degree of superficial cutaneous pain and tactile sensibility within the autonomous area of the nerve
M3	Return of function in both proximal and distal muscles of such degree that all *important* muscles are sufficiently powerful to act against resistance	S3	Return to superficial cutaneous pain and tactile sensibility throughout the autonomous area with disappearance of any previous overresponse
M4	Return of function as in Stage 3 with the addition that all synergic and independent movements are possible	S3+	Return of sensibility as in Stage 3 with the addition that there is some recovery of the two-point discrimination within the autonomous area
M5	Complete recovery	S4	Complete recovery

*From Seddon, H.: *Surgical Disorders of the Peripheral Nerves*. Edinburgh and London, Churchill Livingstone, 1972. Reprinted by permission.

don says, "For each nerve there is a particular value."[231] He further exemplifies this statement with the loss of sensibility associated with radial and ulnar nerve injury, an occurrence that has limited importance from the functional standpoint, as compared to injury of the median nerve that supplies two of the most important sensory areas in the body—the tips of the thumb and the index finger.

It must also be decided what *grade of recovery* can be expected, either by spontaneous nerve regeneration or after surgical repair. The system of grading introduced by the Nerve Injuries Committee of the British Medical Research Council (1954) and the American Veterans Administration monograph *Peripheral Nerve Regeneration* (1956), are both steps in the right direction.[231, 238] Grading of motor and sensory recovery according to the former report is given in Table 3–I–2.

The grading system has merits, but it is not always applicable, as for example, in injuries of the brachial plexus and to some extent of the sciatic nerve also; on the whole, it is more satisfactory to assess motor than sensory recovery.

The time taken for recovery to reach its final grade depends on several factors: the age of the patient, the level of the lesion, the time at which the lesion is repaired, and the extent of the gap.

As a general rule, it is well established that recovery in children is better than in adults. Conversely the higher (more proximal) the lesion the longer is the time required for final recovery. When surgery is indicated, the longer the interval between the injury and the surgical intervention, the poorer is the prognosis, and if the delay is excessive, the stage may be reached when the affected muscle has entered the irreversible phase of atrophy. Finally, the prognosis is worsened by the extent of the gap between the stumps of the severed nerve: the greater the gap, the less favorable the outlook for recovery.

REFERENCES

1. National Advisory Neurological Diseases and Stroke Council: A Survey of Current Head Injury Research, 1969. Bethesda, Md., U.S. Department of Health, Education and Welfare, 1969.
2. Poleck, D. G.: The body . . . what happens to it in a crash. Traffic Safety, April, 1967, p. 17.
3. Statistical Bulletin, Metropolitan Life Insurance Company: Motorcycle Accident Deaths Rising Rapidly. Vol. 49, October, 1968.
4. Statistical Bulletin, Metropolitan Life Insurance Company: Fatal and Non-fatal Accident Falls. Vol. 49, October, 1968.
5. National Safety Council: *Accident Facts*. 1968 Edition, p. 30.
6. Lewin, W.: Factors in the mortality of closed head injuries. Br. Med. J., *1*:1239, 1953.

HISTORICAL BACKGROUND

7. Courville, C. B.: War wounds of the cranium in the middle ages. II. As noted in the skulls of the Sedlec Ossuary near Kuttenberg, Czechoslovakia. Bull. Los Angeles Neurol. Soc., *30*:34, 1965.
8. Courville, C. B., and Abbott, K. H.: Cranial injuries of the pre-Columbian Incas. Bull. Los Angeles Neurol. Soc., *7*:107, 1942.
9. Courville, C. B.: War wounds of the cranium in the middle ages. I. As disclosed in the skeletal material from the Battle of Wisby (1361 A.D.). Bull. Los Angeles Neurol. Soc., *30*:27, 1965.
10. Winlock, H. E.: The Egyptian Expedition, 1925–1927, Section II. Bull. Metropolitan Museum of Art, New York, 1928, p. 3.
11. Paaw, P.: *Succenturiatus anatomicus, continens commentaria in Hippocratem, de capitis vulneribus*. . . . Lyons, Iodocum a Closter, 1616.
12. Major, R. H.: *A History of Medicine*. Vol. I. Springfield, Ill., Charles C Thomas, 1954, pp. 333–335.
13. Courville, C. B.: The "wound man" and craniocerebral injury. A transitional figure bridging the gap

between medieval astrological theories and scientific concepts of the Renaissance. Bull. Los Angeles Neurol. Soc., *26*:47, 1961.

14. Sudhoff, K.: *Studien zur Geschichte der Medizen. I. Tradition und Naturbeobachtung in den Illustrationen medizinischer Handschriften und Frühdrucke vornehmlich des 15 Jahrhunderts.* Leipzig, J. A. Barth, 1907.
15. Ketham, J.: *Fasciculus medicinae. Venice, De Gregorii, 1491. With an introduction . . . by Charles Singer.* Parts I and II. Florence, R. Lier & Co., 1925.
16. Brunschwig, H.: *Der Cirurgia. Hantwirckung der Wundarztny.* Strassburg, Johann Gruninger, 1497.
17. Gersdorff, H. von: *Feldtbuch der Wundtarztny.* Strassburg, Johannes Schotts, 1517.
18. Caterini, M.: Memorie Accademia Fisiocritici di Siena Codice L. III, Discorso LXXXIII, 13 Dicembre, 1696. From a study of Renato Marchi: Su alcuni pareri discordi in relatione al sistema di curare le ferite della testa (Dissenting opinions on the system to treat cranial wounds). Riv. Storia Med., *5*:214, 1961.
19. Lindenberg, R., and Freytag, E.: The mechanism of cerebral contusions. A pathologic-anatomic study. Arch. Pathol., *69*:440, 1960.
20. Peabody, C. N., and Peabody, C. N.: Le Journal De Médecine Militaire 1782. Massachusetts Physician, *31*:46, (Dec.) 1972.

SYSTEM OF INVESTIGATION

21. Ommaya, A. K., Hirsch, A. E., Flamm, E. S., and Mahone, R. H.: Cerebral concussion in the monkey: An experimental model. Science, *153*:211, 1966.
22. Lindenberg, R., and Freytag, E.: The mechanism of cerebral contusions. A pathologic-anatomic study. Arch. Pathol., *69*:440, 1960.
23. Pudenz, R. H., and Shelden, C. H.: The lucite calvarium—a method for direct observation of the brain: II. Cranial trauma and brain movement. J. Neurosurg., *3*:487, 1946.
24. Gurdjian, E. S., and Lissner, H. R.: Mechanism of head injury as studied by the cathode ray oscilloscope: preliminary report. J. Neurosurg., *1*:393, 1944.
25. Gross, A. G.: A new theory on the dynamics of brain concussion and brain injury. J. Neurosurg., *15*:548, 1958.
26. Holburn, A. H. S.: Mechanics of head injuries. Lancet, *2*:438, 1943.
27. Gurdjian, E. S., Lissner, H. R., Latimer, F. R., Haddad, B. F., and Webster, J. E.: Quantitative determination of acceleration and intracranial pressure in experimental head injury: preliminary report. Neurology (Minneap.), *3*:417, 1953.
28. Denny Brown, D., and Russell, W. R.: Experimental cerebral concussion. Brain, *64*:93, 1941.
29. Windle, W. F., Groat, R. A., and Fox, C. A.: Experimental structural alterations in the brain during and after concussion. Surg. Gynecol. Obstet., *79*:561, 1944
30. Saucerote: Mémoire sur les contre-coups dans les lésions de la tête. Mém. pour le prix Acad. roy. chir. *4*:368, 1778.
31. Sjövall, H.: The genesis of skull and brain injuries: an anatomical and physical study. Acta Pathol. Microbiol. Scand., Suppl. 48, 1943.
32. Gurdjian, E. S., Lissner, H. R., Evans, F. G., Patrick, L. M., and Hardy, W. G.: Intracranial pressure and acceleration accompanying head impacts in human cadavers. Surg. Gynecol. Obstet., *113*:185, 1961.
33. Friede, R. L.: Experimental concussion acceleration. Arch. Neurol. (Chicago), *4*:449, 1961.
34. Gosch, H. H., Gooding, E., and Schneider, R. C.: Distortion and displacement of the brain in experimental head injuries. Surg. Forum, *20*:425, 1969.
35. Evans, J. P., Mullan, S., Hekmatpanah, J., Moody, R. A., and Ishii, S.: A summary of current concepts of the dynamics of head injury. Trans. Am. Neurol. Assoc., *94*:256, 1969.
36. Tedeschi, C. G.: Cerebral injury by blunt mechanical trauma. Review of literature. Medicine (Baltimore), *24*:339, 1945.
37. Moritz, A. R.: *The Pathology of Trauma.* Philadelphia, Lea & Febiger, 1942.
38. Walker, A. E., Kollros, J. J., and Case, T.: The physiological basis of concussion. J. Neurosurg., *1*:103, 1944.

EXAMINATION OF THE HEAD

39. Jackson, F. E.: The pathophysiology of head injuries. Ciba Clinical Symposia, *18*:67, 1966.
40. Tedeschi, C. G. (Ed.): *Neuropathology: Methods and Diagnosis.* Boston, Little, Brown and Co., 1970.
41. Dodge, P. R., and Meirowsky, A. M.: Tangential wounds of scalp and skull. J. Neurosurg., *9*:472, 1951.
42. Hankins, E. A.: Total scalp avulsions. Ann. Surg., *158*:277, 1963.
43. Berard, M. E. M., and Henry, M.: Almost total cancerous degeneration of cranial vault due to noncicatrization following avulsion of scalp 20 years ago. Case. Lyon Chir., *32*:598, 1935.
44. Burns, E. L.: Epithelioma following avulsion. Case. Arch. Surg., *30*:266, 1935.

SKULL AND SKULL FRACTURE

45. Bruns, P. von: *Die Chirurgischen Krankheiten und Verletzungen des Gehirns und seiner Umhullungen. Undbuch der praktischen Chirurgie fur Arzte und Wundarzte.* Tubingen, 1854.
46. Tedeschi, C. G. (Ed.): *Neuropathology: Methods and Diagnosis.* Boston, Little, Brown and Company, 1970.
47. Jackson, F. E.: The pathophysiology of head injuries. Ciba Clinical Symposia, *18*:67, 1966.
48. LeCount, E. R., and Apfelback, C. W.: Pathologic anatomy of traumatic fractures of cranial bones and concomitant brain injuries. J.A.M.A., *74*:501, 1920.
49. Rowbotham, G. F.: *Acute Injuries of the Head. Their Diagnosis, Treatment, Complications and Sequels.* Baltimore, Williams & Wilkins Co., 1942.
50. Gurdjian, E. S., and Webster, J. E.: The mechanism and management of injuries of the head. J.A.M.A., *134*:1072, 1947.
51. Courville, C. B.: *Forensic Neuropathology: Lesions of the Brain and Spinal Cord of Medicolegal Importance.* Mundelein, Ill., Callaghan & Co., 1964.
52. Gurdjian, E. S., Webster, J. E., and Lissner, H. R.: The mechanism of skull fracture. J. Neurosurg., 7:106, 1970.
53. Browder, J.: Fracture of the skull. In *Injuries of the Brain and Spinal Cord and Their Coverings.* 4th. Ed. Edited by S. Brock. New York, Springer Publishing Co., 1960.
54. Whitacre, W. B. W.: Dislocation of the mandibular condyle into the middle cranial fossa: review of the literature and report of a case. Plast. Reconstr. Surg., *38*:23, 1966.

INTRACRANIAL LESIONS

55. Penfield, W.: Cerebral cortex in man; cerebral cortex and unconsciousness (Harvey Lecture). Arch. Neurol. Psychiatry, *40*:417, 1938.

56. Florey, H. W.: Microscopical observations on the circulation of the blood in the cerebral cortex. Brain, *48*:43, 1925.
57. Echlin, F. A.: Vasospasm and focal cerebral ischemia. Arch. Neurol. Psychiatry, *47*:77, 1942.
58. Riser, M., Meriel, P., and Planques: Les spasmes vasculaires en neurologie. Encéphale, *26*:510, 1931.
59. Ectors, L.: Paralysie vasculaire cérébrale. Acta Neurol. Belg., *69*:33, 1969.
60. Munro, D.: Cerebral subdural hematomas: a study of three hundred and ten verified cases. N. Engl. J. Med., *227*:87, 1942.
61. Voris, H. C.: The surgical treatment of extradural hematoma. J. Int. Coll. Surg., *10*:655, 1947.
62. Vance, B. M.: Ruptures of surface blood vessels on cerebral hemispheres as a cause of subdural hemorrhage. Arch. Surg., *61*:992, 1950.
63. Leary, T.: Subdural or intradural hemorrhages. Arch. Pathol., *28*:808, 1939.
64. Drake, C. G.: Subdural haematoma from arterial rupture. J. Neurosurg., *18*:597, 1961.
65. Scott, M.: Spontaneous nontraumatic subdural hematomas. J.A.M.A., *141*:596, 1949.
66. Putnam, T. J., and Cushing, H.: Chronic subdural hematoma; its pathology, its relation to pachymeningitis hemorrhagica and its surgical treatment. Arch. Surg., *11*:329, 1925.
67. Goodell, C. L., and Mealey, J.: Pathogenesis of chronic subdural hematoma. Arch. Neurol. (Chicago), *8*:429, 1963.
68. Romanul, F. C. A.: Examination of the brain and spinal cord. In *Neuropathology: Methods and Diagnosis.* Edited by C. G. Tedeschi. Boston, Little, Brown and Co., 1970.
69. Tedeschi, C. G. (Ed.): *Neuropathology: Methods and Diagnosis.* Boston, Little, Brown and Co., 1970, p. 278.
70. Davidoff, L. M., and Dyke, C. G.: Relapsing juvenile chronic subdural hematoma. Bull. Neurol. Inst., *7*:94, 1938.
71. Klein, J. O.: Bacterial infections. In *Neuropathology: Methods and Diagnosis.* Edited by C. G. Tedeschi. Boston, Little, Brown and Co., 1970.
72. Traut, E. F.: Recurrence of pneumococcic meningitis. J.A.M.A., *129*:273, 1945.
73. Appelbaum, E., and Abler, C.: Post-traumatic meningitis. In *Injuries of the Brain and Spinal Cord and Their Coverings.* Edited by S. Brock. New York, Springer Publishing Co., 1960.
74. Ommaya, A. K., Di Chiro, G., Baldwin, M., and Pennybacker, J. B.: Non-traumatic cerebrospinal fluid rhinorrhoea. J. Neurol. Neurosurg., Psychiatry, *31*:214, 1968.
75. Dandy, W. E.: Pneumocephalus, intracranial pneumatocele or aerocele. Arch. Surg., *12*:949, 1926.
76. Duret, H.: Etudes Experimentales et Cliniques sur les Traumatismes Cérébraux. Paris, A. Delahaye, 1878.
77. Lindenberg, R., and Freytag, E.: Morphology of cortical contusions. A.M.A. Arch. Pathol., *63*:23, 1957.
78. Echlin, F.: Traumatic subdural hematoma—acute, subacute and chronic; analysis of 70 operated cases. J. Neurosurg., *6*:294, 1949.
79. Gurdjian, E. S., and Webster, J. E.: *Head Injuries. Mechanisms, Diagnosis and Management.* Boston, Little, Brown and Co., 1958.
80. Bollinger, O.: Ueber Traumatische Spät-Apoplexie; ein Beitrag zur Lehre von der Hirnerschütterung. Internat. Beitr. Wissensch. Medicin Festschr. R. Virchow, *2*:457, 1891.
81. Symonds, C. P.: Delayed traumatic intracerebral hemorrhage. Br. Med. J., *1*:1048, 1940.
82. Krayenbühl, H., and Siebenmann, R.: Small vascular malformations as a cause of primary intracerebral hemorrhage. J. Neurosurg., *22*:7, 1965.
83. Burton, C., Velasco, F., and Dorman, J.: Traumatic aneurysm of a peripheral cerebral artery. Review and case report. J. Neurosurg., *28*:468, 1968.
84. Rumbaugh, C. L., Bergeron, T. B., Talalla, A., and Kurze, T.: Traumatic aneurysms of the cortical cerebral arteries. Radiographic aspects. Radiology, *96*:49, 1970.
85. Lindenberg, R.: Incarceration of a vertebral artery in the cleft of a longitudinal fracture of the skull. J. Neurosurg., *24*:908, 1966.
86. Loop, J. W., White, L. E., Jr., Shaw, C. M.: Traumatic occlusion of the basilar artery within a clivus fracture. Radiology, *83*:36, 1964.
87. Graham, D. J., and Adams, J. H.: Ischaemic brain damage in fatal head injuries. Lancet, *1*:265, (Feb. 6) 1971.
88. Miguel, J., and Otenasek, R.: The application of fluorescein labeled serum protein (FLSP) to the study of vascular permeability in the brain. Acta Neuropathol., *2*:144, 1962.
89. Luse, S. A., and Harris, B.: Electron microscopy of the brain in experimental edema. J. Neurosurg., *17*:439, 1960.
90. Rubinstein, L. J., Klatzo, I., and Miguel, J.: Histochemical observations on oxidative enzyme activity of glial cells in a local brain injury. J. Neuropathol. Exp. Neurol., *21*:116, 1962.
91. Klatzo, I.: Neuropathological aspects of brain edema. J. Neuropathol. Exp. Neurol., *26*:1, 1967.
92. Wortis, B. S., and McCullough, W. S.: Head injuries, an experimental study. Arch. Surg., *25*:529, 1932.
93. Rand, C. W., and Courville, C. B.: Histological studies of the brain in cases of fatal injury. II. Changes in the choroid plexus and ependyma. Arch. Surg., *23*:357, 1931.
94. Moritz, A. R., and Wortman, W. B.: Posttraumatic internal hydrocephalus. Am. J. Med. Sci., *195*:65, 1938.
95. King, L. E. J.: Brain abscess of traumatic origin. Am. J. Surg., *47*:348, 1940.
96. Javalet, A., Limbour, J., and Schilte, P.: Abcès cérébral d'origine dentaire. Rev. Otoneuroophthal., *34*:261, 1962.
97. Haymaker, W.: Fatal infections of the central nervous system and meninges after tooth extraction. Am. J. Orthod. (Oral Surg.), *31*:117, 1945.
98. Khairat, O.: The non-aerobes of post-extraction bacteremia. J. Dent. Res., *45*:1191, 1966.
99. Elliott, R. H., and Dunbar, J. M.: Streptococcal bacteraemia in children following dental extractions. Arch. Dis. Child., *43*:451, 1968.
100. Vance, M. B.: Fracture of skull: complications and causes of death. Review of 512 necropsies and of 61 cases studied clinically. Arch. Surg., *14*:1023, 1927.
101. Denny-Brown, D., and Russell, W. R.: Experimental cerebral concussion. Brain, *64*:93, 1941.
102. Tedeschi, C. G.: Cerebral injury by blunt mechanical trauma. Review of literature. Medicine (Baltimore), *24*:339, 1945.
103. Denny-Brown, D.: Brain trauma and concussion. Arch. Neurol. (Chicago), *5*:1, 1961.
104. Strauss, I., and Savitsky, N.: Head injury; neurologic and psychiatric aspects. Arch. Neurol. Psychhiatry, *31*:893, 1934.
105. Russell, W. R., and Smith, A.: Posttraumatic amnesia in closed head injury. Arch. Neurol. (Chicago), *5*:4, 1961.
106. Ward, J. W., and Clark, S. L.: Electroencephalogram

in experimental concussion and related conditions. J. Neurophysiol., *11*:59, 1948.
107. Williams, D., and Denny-Brown, D.: Cerebral electrical changes in experimental concussion. Brain, *64*:223, 1941.
108. Magoun, H. W.: *The Ascending Reticular System and Wakefulness in Brain Mechanism and Consciousness.* New York, Oxford University Press, 1954.
109. Chason, J. L., Hardy, W. G., Webster, J. E., and Gurdjian, E. S.: Alterations in cell structure of the brain associated with experimental concussion. J. Neurosurg., *15*:135, 1958.
110. Windle, W. F., and Groat, R. A.: Disappearance of nerve cells after concussion. Anat. Rec., *93*:201, 1945.
111. Friede, R. L.: Experimental concussion acceleration: pathology and mechanics. Arch. Neurol. (Chicago), *4*:449, 1961.
112. Friede, R. L.: Specific cord damage at the atlas level as a pathogenic mechanism in cerebral concussion. J. Neuropathol. Exp. Neurol., *19*:266, 1960.
113. Oppenheimer, D. R.: Microscopic lesions in the brain following head injury. J. Neurol. Neurosurg. Psychiatry, *31*:299, 1968.
114. Bodian, D.: An electron microscopic study of the monkey spinal cord. Bull. Johns Hopkins Hosp., *114*:13, 1964.
115. Kirkpatrick, J. B.: Chromatolysis in the hypoglossal nucleus of the rat (an electron microscopic analysis). J. Comp. Neurol., *132*:189, 1968.
116. Brown, W. J., Yoshida, N., Canty, T., and Verity, M. A.: Experimental concussion. Ultrastructural and biochemical correlates. Am. J. Pathol., *67*:41, 1972.
117. Ehrlich, P.: Ueber die Methylenblaureaktion der lebenden Nervensubstanz. Biol. Zbl., *6*:214, 1886.
118. Stern, L., and Gautier, R.: Recherches sur le liquide céphalo-rachidien. I. Les rapports entre le liquide céphalo-rachidien et la circulation sanguine. Arch. Int. Physiol., *17*:138, 1922.
119. Ommaya, A. K., Rockoff, S. D., and Baldwin, M.: Experimental concussion. A first report. J. Neurosurg., *21*:249, 1964.
120. Fukui, Y.: Morphological studies on experimental concussion with special reference to the vital staining of the nervous tissue. Jap. J. Leg. Med., *23*:1, 1969.
121. Smith, S. E., Cammack, K. V., Dodds, M. E., and Curry, G. J.: Glutamic oxalacetic transaminase in the evaluation of acute injury to the head. Am. J. Surg., *99*:713, 1960.
122. Dubo, H., Park, D. C., Pennington, R. J., Kalbag, R. M., and Walton, J. N.: Serum-creatine-kinase in cases of stroke, head injury and meningitis. Lancet, *2*:743, (Oct. 7) 1967.
123. Kalbag, R. M., Park, D. C., and Pennington, R. J.: Serum creatine kinase after head injuries and stroke. Proc. Assoc. Clin. Biochem., *4*:88, 1966.
124. Herschkowitz, N., and Cumings, J. N.: Creatine kinase in cerebrospinal fluid. J. Neurol. Neurosurg. Psychiatry, *27*:247, 1964.
125. Lisak, R. P., and Craig, F. A.: Lack of diagnostic value of creatine phosphokinase assay in spinal fluid. J.A.M.A., *199*:750, 1967.
126. Rezek, P. R., and Millard, M.: *Autopsy Pathology: A Guide for Pathologists and Clinicians.* Springfield, Charles C Thomas, 1963.
127. Alberca, R.: Intervention precox de la microglia en las heridas experimentales de la medulla del correjo. Bol. Soc. Espan. Biol., *11*:81, 1926.
128. Del Rio Hortega, P., and Penfield, W.: Cerebral cicatrix. The reaction of the neuroglia and microglia to brain wounds. Bull. Johns Hopkins Hosp., *41*:278, 1927.
129. Ferraro, A., and Davidoff, L. M.: The reaction of the oligodendroglia to injury of the brain. Arch. Pathol., *6*:1030, 1928.
130. Tedeschi, C. G.: Microscopic neuronal injury in rats submitted to concussive head trauma under different mechanisms. Proc. Soc. Exp. Biol. Med., *57*:266, 1944.
131. Rand, C. W., and Courville, C. B.: Histologic changes in brain in cases of fatal injury to head; reaction of microglia and oligodendroglia. Arch. Neurol. Psychiatry, *27*:605, 1932.
132. Strassmann, G.: Hemosiderin and tissue iron in the brain, its relationship, occurrence and importance. A study of ninety-three human brains. J. Neuropathol. Exp. Neurol., *4*:393, 1945.
133. Schmidt, M. B.: Die Stoerungen des Eisenstoffwechsels und ihre Folgen. Ergeb. Allg. Pathol., *35*:105, 1940.
134. Linnell, E. A.: The histology of neuroglial changes following cerebral trauma. Arch. Neurol. Psychiatry, *22*:926, 1929.
135. Courville, C. B.: *Forensic Neuropathology: Lesions of the Brain and Spinal Cord of Medicolegal Importance.* Mundelein, Ill., Callaghan & Co., 1964.
136. Penfield, W., and Buckley, R. C.: Punctures of the brain. The factors concerned in gliosis and cicatricial contraction. Arch. Neurol. Psychiatry, *20*:1, 1928.
137. Foerster, O., and Penfield, W.: Structural basis of traumatic epilepsy and results of radical operation. Brain, *53*:99, 1930.
138. Kretschmer, E.: Das apallische Syndrom. Z. Gesamte Neurol. Psychiatr., *169*:576, 1940.
139. Cairns, H., Oldfield, R., Pennybaker, J. B., and Whitteridge, D.: Akinetic mutism with an epidermoid cyst of the third ventricle (with report of an associated disturbance of brain potentials). Brain, *64*:273, 1941.
140. Alajouanine, Th.: Les altérations des états de conscience causées par les désordres neurologiques. 1er Congr. Int. Sci. Neurol., Brussels, 1957. Vol. 2. Brussels, Acta Medica Belgica, 1957, p. 19.
141. Carlsson, C.-A., von Essen, C., and Löfgren, J.: Factors affecting the clinical course of patients with severe head injuries. J. Neurosurg., *29*:242, 1968.
142. Frowein, R. A., Auf Der Haar, K., Terhaag, D., Kinzel, W., and Wieck, H. H.: Arbeitsfähigkeit und Abbausyndrome nach Hirntraumen mit langdauernder Bewusstlosigkeit. Monatsschr. Unfallheilkd., *71*:233, 1968.
143. Gerstenbrand, F.: *Das traumatische apallische Syndrom.* Vienna and New York, Springer, 1967.
144. Strich, S.: Shearing of nerve fibres as a cause of brain damage due to head injury. A pathological study of twenty cases. Lancet, *1*:443, 1961.
145. Jellinger, K., and Seitelberger, F.: Protracted posttraumatic encephalopathy. Pathology, pathogenesis and clinical implications. J. Neurol. Sci., *10*:51, 1970.
146. Ramón y Cajal, S. : *Degeneration and Regeneration of the Nervous System.* Vol. II. Translated by R. M. May. London, Oxford University Press, 1928.
147. Tedeschi, C. G.: Cerebral injury by blunt mechanical trauma. Special reference to the effects of repeated impacts of minimal intensity; observations on experimental animals. Arch. Neurol. Psychiatry, *53*:333, 1945.
148. Walker, A. E., and Erculei, F.: *Head Injured Men 15 Years Later.* Springfield, Ill., Charles C Thomas, 1968.

149. Walker, A. E., Leuchs, H. K., Lechtape-Grüter, H., Caveness, W. F., and Kretschman, C.: Life expectancy of head injured men with and without epilepsy. Arch. Neurol. (Chicago), *24*:95, 1971.
150. Koch, W., and Filene, W.: Beitrage zur experimentellen Chirurgie. Arch. Klin. Chir., *17*:190, 1874.
151. Martland, H. S.: Punch drunk. J.A.M.A., *91*:1103, 1928.
152. Carroll, E. J.: Punch-drunk. Am. J. Med. Sci., *191*: 706, 1936.
153. Millspaugh, J. A.: Dementia pugilistica. U.S. Nav. Med. Bull., *35*:297, 1937.
154. Winterstein, C. E.: Head injuries attributable to boxing. Lancet, *2*:719, 1937.
155. Shaller, W. F., Tamaki, K., and Newman, H.: Nature and significance of multiple petechial hemorrhages associated with trauma of the brain. Arch. Neurol. Psychiatry, *37*:1048, 1937.
156. Denny-Brown, D., and Russell, W. R.: Experimental cerebral concussion. Brain, *64*:93, 1941.
157. Strassmann, G. S., and Helpern, M.: Tödliche Hirn verletzungen im Boxkampf. Dtsch. Z. Gesamte Gerichtl. Med., *63*:70, 1968.
158. Auerbach, A. H., Scheflen, A. E., Reinhart, R. B., and Scholz, C. K.: The psychophysiologic sequelae of head injuries. Am. J. Psychiatry, *117*:499, 1960.
159. Hyslop, G. H.: Seizures, head injuries and litigants. Arch. Neurol. Psychiatry, *64*:736, 1950.
160. Parker, N.: Post-traumatic dementia. Proc. Aust. Assoc. Neurol., *6*:39, 1969.
161. Marburg, O.: Die traumatischen erkrankungen des Gehirns und Rückenmarks. In *Handbuch der Neurologie.* Edited by O. Bumke and O. Foerster. Berlin, Springer-Verlag, 1936. Vol. 11, pp. 1–77.
162. Klauder, J. V., and Solomon, H. C.: Trauma and general paresis. J.A.M.A., *96*:1, 1931.
163. Giaconia, A.: Sulle schizofrenie traumatiche. Schizofrenie, *4*:305, 1935.
164. Wechsler, I. S.: The relationship of brain injury to other organic diseases of the brain. In *Injuries of the Brain and Spinal Cord and Their Coverings.* 4th ed. Edited by S. Brock. New York, Springer Publishing Co., 1960.
165. Rabiner, A. M.: Influence of trauma in acute and chronic encephalitis. New York Med. J., *33*:796, 1933.
166. Harris, W.: The traumatic factor in organic nervous diseases. Br. Med. J., *2*:955, 1933.
167. Cushing, H., and Eisenhardt, L.: *Meningiomas. Their Classification, Regional Behaviour, Life History and Surgical End Results.* Springfield, Ill., Charles C Thomas, 1938.
168. Zülch, K. J.: *Brain Tumours. Their Biology and Pathology.* New York, Springer Publishing Co., 1957.
169. Editorial. Brain tumours and trauma. Br. Med. J., *3*:369, (Aug. 16)1969.
170. Walshe, F.: Head injuries as a factor in the aetiology of intracranial meningioma. Lancet, *2*:993, 1961.

BRAIN LESIONS FROM BLUNT TRAUMA IN EARLY INFANCY AND CHILDHOOD

171. Schneider, R. C.: Head injuries in infancy and childhood. Surg. Clin. North Am., *41*:1255, 1961.
172. Pickles, W.: Acute focal edema of the brain in children with head injuries. N. Engl. J. Med., *240*:92, 1949.
173. Lindenberg, R., and Freytag, E.: Morphology of brain lesions from blunt trauma in early infancy. Arch. Pathol., *87*:298, 1969.
174. Courville, C. B.: Contrecoup injuries of the brain in infancy. Remarks on the mechanism of fatal traumatic lesions in early life. Arch. Surg., *90*:157, 1965.
175. Frantzen, E., Jacobsen, H. H., and Therkelsen, J.: Cerebral artery occlusions in children due to trauma to the head and neck. A report of 6 cases verified by cerebral angiography. Neurology (Minneap.), *11*:695, 1961.
176. Spalter, H. F., Bemporad, J. R., and Sours, J. A.: Cataracts following chronic headbanging. Report of two cases. Arch. Ophthalmol., *83*:182, 1970.

PITUITARY INJURY IN CONJUNCTION WITH HEAD TRAUMA

177. Altman, R., and Pruzanski, W.: Post-traumatic hypopituitarism. Ann. Intern. Med., *55*:149, 1961.
178. Escamilla, R. F., and Lisser, H.: Simmonds disease. J. Clin. Endocrinol., *2*:65, (Feb.) 1942.
179. Witter, H., and Tascher, R.: Hypophysär-Hypothalamische Krankeitsbilder nach stumpfem Schadel Trauma. Fortschr. Neurol. Psychiatr., *25*:523, 1957.
180. Boltz, K., and Skala, O.: Zur Entstehung Traumatischer Hypophysenschäden. Acta Med. Leg. Soc. (Liege), *15*:45, 1962.
181. Ceballos, R.: Pituitary changes in head trauma. Ala. J. Med. Sci., *3*:185, (Apr.-June) 1966.
182. Kornblum, R. N., and Fisher, R. S.: Pituitary lesions in craniocerebral injuries. Arch. Pathol., *88*:242, (Sept.) 1969.
183. Adams, J. H., and Connor, R. C. R.: The shocked head injury. Lancet, *1*:263, (Jan. 29) 1966.
184. Tedeschi, C. G. (Ed.): *Neuropathology: Methods and Diagnosis.* Boston, Little, Brown and Co., 1970.
185. Sheehan, H. L., and Stanfield, J. P.: The pathogenesis of post-partum necrosis of the anterior lobe of the pituitary gland. Acta Endocrinol. (Kbh.), *37*:479, (Aug.) 1961.
186. Sheehan, H. L., and Murdoch, R.: Post-partum necrosis of the anterior pituitary: pathological and clinical aspects. J. Obstet. Gynaecol. Br. Commonw., *45*:456, (June) 1938.
187. Wolman, L.: Pituitary necrosis in raised intracranial pressure. J. Pathol. Bacteriol., *72*:575, 1956.
188. DeFaria, J. L., and DeOliveira, N. R.: Hypophysennekrose nach Schockzuständen. Beitr. Pathol. Anat., *127*:213, (Dec.) 1962.
189. Kerkhoven, cited by Fischer, H., and Spann, W.: *Pathologie des Trauma.* Munich, J. F. Bergman, 1967, p. 24.
190. Wanke, R., and Kricke, E.: Histologische Veränderungen der Hypophyse bei Traumatischen Hirnschaden und bei Hirntumoren. Beitr. Klin. Chir., *200*:165, 1960.
191. Plaut, A.: Pituitary necrosis in routine necropsies. Am. J. Pathol., *28*:883, (Sept.-Oct.) 1952.
192. Blotner, H.: *Diabetes Insipidus.* Edited by H. A. Christian. New York, Oxford University Press, 1951.
193. Pickles, W.: Disturbances of metabolism associated with head injuries. N. Engl. J. Med., *236*:858, 1947.
194. Porter, R. J., and Miller, R. A.: Diabetes insipidus following closed head injury. J. Neurol. Neurosurg. Psychiatry, *11*:258, 1948.
195. Henzi, H.: Zur pathologischen Anatomie des Diabetes insipidus. Monatsschr. Psychiatr. Neurol., *123*:292, 1952.
196. Goldman, K. P., and Jacobs, A.: Anterior and posterior pituitary failure after head injury. Br. Med. J., *5217*:1924, (Dec. 31) 1960.

197. Treip, C. S.: Hypothalamic lesions in head injury. Proc. Soc. Br. Neurol. Surgeons. J. Neurol. Neurosurg. Psychiatry, *33*:714, 1970.
198. Bartuska, D. G., Eskin, B. A., Smith, E. M., Dacou, C., and Dratman, M. B.: Brain damage, hypertrichosis and polycystic ovaries. Clinical evaluation of 7 cases. Am. J. Obstet. Gynecol., *99*:387, (Oct. 1) 1967.

INTRACRANIAL NERVE INJURY

199. Leigh, A. D.: Defects of smell after head injury. Lancet, *1*:438, 1943.
200. Griffith, J. F., and Dodge, P. R.: Transient blindness following head injury in children. N. Engl. J. Med., *278*:648, 1968.
201. Gjerris, F., and Mellemgaard, L.: Transitory cortical blindness in head injury. Acta Neurol. Scand., *45*:623, 1969.
202. Meyer, H. J.: Das chiasma Trauma. Klin. Monatsbl. Augenheilkd., *146*:833, 1965.
203. Francois, J., and Verriest, G.: Traumatic bitemporal hemianopsia. Ophtalmologica (Basel), Suppl.:332, 1969.
204. Tedeschi, C. G. (Ed.): *Neuropathology, Methods and Diagnosis.* Boston, Little, Brown and Co., 1970.
205. Kaseff, L. G.: Tomographic evaluation of trauma to the temporal bone. Radiology, *93*:321, 1969.
206. Kirikae, K., Eguchi, K., Okamoto, M., and Nakamura, K.: Histopathological changes in the auditory pathway in cases of fatal head injury. Acta Otolaryngol., *67*:341, 1969.

CRANIOCERVICAL AND SPINAL INJURY

207. Rao, D. B., Rao, K. S., Subrahmanyan, M. V., and Tirupathiah, K.: On the incidence of cranio-cervical injuries. Neurol. India, *17*:73, 1969.
208. Friede, R. L.: Specific cord damage at the atlas level as a pathogenic mechanism in cerebral concussion. J. Neuropathol. Exp. Neurol., *19*:266, 1960.
209. Spicer, E. J. F., and Strich, S. J.: Hemorrhages in posterior-root ganglia in patients dying from head injuries. Lancet, *2*:1389, 1967.
210. Shapiro, S. K., and Torres, F.: Brain injury complicating whiplash injuries. Minn. Med., *43*:473, 1960.
211. Torres, F., and Shapiro, S. K.: Electroencephalograms in whiplash injury. Arch. Neurol. (Chicago), *5*:28, 1961.
212. Cave, E. F. (Ed.): *Fractures and Other Injuries.* Chicago, Year Book Medical Publishers, Inc., 1958.
213. Putti, V.: *Le fratture vertebrali.* Bologna, Cappelli, 1942.
214. Sherk, H. H., and Nicholson, J. T.: Fractures of the atlas. J. Bone Joint Surg., *52A*:1017, 1970.
215. Delaire, J.: Swelling of the parotid region in conjunction with fracture of the atlas and external dislocation of one of its lateral masses. Rev. Stomatol., *67*:489, 1966.
216. Plant, H. F.: Injuries of the upper cervical spine and their x-ray findings. Ohio State Med. J., *34*:760, 1958.
217. Aronson, N. I.: Traumatic arteriovenous fistula of the vertebral vessels. Angiographic demonstration and rationale for treatment. Neurology (Minneap.), *11*:817, 1961.
218. Houck, W. S., Jackson, J. R., Odom, G. L., and Young, W. G.: Occlusion of the internal carotid artery in the neck secondary to closed trauma to the head and neck. Ann. Surg., *159*:219, 1964.
219. Murray, D. S.: Posttraumatic thrombosis of the internal carotid and vertebral arteries after non-penetrating injuries of the neck. Br. J. Surg., *44*:556, 1957.
220. Stoltmann, H. F., and Blackwood, W.: The role of the ligamenta flava in the pathogenesis of myelopathy in cervical spondylosis. Brain, *87*:45, 1964.
221. Saylor, M., Haine, R. A., and Dorner, R. A.: Traumatic subarachnoid-pleural fistula. J. Thorac. Cardiovasc. Surg., *59*:847, 1970.
222. Davison, C., and Keschner, M.: Myelitic and myelopathic lesions. IV. Traumatic lesions of the spinal cord. Arch. Neurol. Psychiatry, *30*:326, 1933.
223. Bailey, F. W.: Histological changes in the spinal cord of man in cases of fatal injury. IV. Alterations in the classical neuroglia. Bull. Los Angeles Neurol. Soc., *26*:32, 1961.
224. Nagel, D. A., Albright, J. A., Kristops, J. K., and Southwick, W. O.: Close look at spinal lesions. Open biopsy of vertebral lesions. J.A.M.A., *191*:975, 1965.

COMPLICATIONS OF SPINAL SURGERY

225. Ford, L. T.: Symposium: complications of lumbar disc surgery. Local complications. J. Bone Joint Surg., *50A*:418, 1968.
226. Sullivan, C. G.: Diagnosis and treatment of pyogenic infections of the intervertebral disc. Surg. Clin. North Am., *41*:1077, 1961.
227. Cloward, R. B.: Complications of anterior cervical disc operation and their treatment. Surgery, *69*:175, 1971.
228. Heusner, A. P.: Nontuberculous spinal epidural infection. N. Engl. J. Med., *239*:845, 1948.
229. Ford, L. T., and Lam, R. L.: Psychic aspect of low back pain, unpublished paper presented at the 1956 meeting of the American Academy of Orthopedic Surgeons.

PERIPHERAL NERVE INJURY

230. Speidel, C. C.: Studies of living nerves; phenomena of nerve irritation and recovery, degeneration and repair. J. Comp. Neurol., *61*:1, 1935.
231. Seddon, H.: *Surgical Disorders of the Peripheral Nerves.* Edinburgh and London, Churchill Livingstone, 1972.
232. Haftek, J.: Stretch injury of peripheral nerve. J. Bone Joint Surg., *52B*:354, 1970.
233. Nobel, W.: Peroneal palsy due to hematoma in the common peroneal nerve sheath after distal torsional fractures and inversion ankle sprains. J. Bone Joint Surg., *48A*:1484, 1966.
234. Sunderland, S., and Bradley, K. C.: Stress-strain phenomena in human peripheral nerve trunks. Brain, *84*:102, 1961.
235. Towbin, A.: Spinal cord and brain stem injury at birth. Arch. Pathol., *77*:620, 1964.
236. Denny-Brown, D., and Brenner, C.: Effect of percussion of nerve. J. Neurol. Psychiatry, *7*:76, 1944.
237. Denny-Brown, D., and Brenner, C.: Paralysis of nerve induced by direct pressure and by tourniquet. Arch. Neurol. Psychiatry, *51*:1, 1944.
238. Woodhall, B., and Beebee, G. W.: *Peripheral Nerve Regeneration.* Veterans Administration Monograph. Washington, D.C., U.S. Government Printing Office, 1956.

II. Long-Term Disability from Spinal Cord Injury

by Murray M. Freed

Since 1940 our understanding of the complications of and the care of individuals with spinal cord injury has developed more than it had during the previous 50 centuries. Yet it remains, because of its multisystem complications, one of the most demanding, not infrequently distressing, and always laborious experiences for all concerned—especially the patient. The earliest available documentary on spinal cord injury is found in the Edwin Smith surgical papyrus, estimated to have been written between 2500 and 3000 B.C. with certain commentaries added 1,000 years later.[1] Legend has it that the author was Imhotep, physician to the Pharoah. He described a man with a broken neck who was paralyzed in all his extremities, whose excretory function was characterized by constant dribbling, and whose muscles were wasting away. Under medical treatment was noted, "an ailment not to be treated." This dictum, because the injury's complications were poorly understood, was followed for millenia.

The century prior to World War I saw such advances in surgical procedures for spinal cord injury as laminectomy, nerve section, cordotomy, rhizotomy, and sympathectomy. During the Balkan wars of 1912–1913 there was a mortality rate of 95 per cent within a few weeks.[2] Thompson Walker, commenting in 1917, noted that of approximately 450 British soldiers with spinal cord injuries who had survived evacuation from World War I battlefields and been brought to the Star and Garter and King George hospitals, 179 died of urinary tract infection during a period of two years.[3] Among American troops during World War I, 80 per cent of the 2,324 men who had received injury to the spinal cord died before they could be returned from overseas.[4] Of the remainder, who were successfully evacuated to this country, 10 per cent survived the first year; in 1946 it was estimated that less than 1 per cent of those who survived the first year were still alive. Two decades after the end of World War I, Hinman wrote that most fatalities among patients with spinal cord injuries were still due to urinary tract infections and bedsores, and the failure to prevent or control these complications accounted for over 80 per cent of deaths.

Improved understanding of the management of the bladder dysfunction secondary to transverse myelopathy and improved nursing care for the prevention of bedsores accounted for significant changes in survival rates just prior to and during World War II. In the United States it was the work of the late Dr. Donald Munro, and in Great Britain of Sir Ludwig Guttmann, that made them prophets in the management of the spinal cord injury and the decrease in its complications.

In 1943 Munro reported a mortality rate of 0.575 in 40 patients during the previous nine-and-one-half-year period.[6] Sepsis of the genitourinary tract and bedsores accounted for 30.4 per cent of the deaths. In 1946, Kirk stated that there were at that time 1,400 paraplegic patients in service hospitals and that the results constituted a tribute to the professional competence of the Army doctors in the war.[7] In 1958, a Veterans Administration study of 5,743 patients with spinal cord injuries who survived the immediate handling and the potential early complications in service hospitals and who were subsequently treated, between 1946 and 1955, for their traumatic paraplegia or quadriplegia disclosed an overall mortality rate of 0.139.[8]

Because paralysis resulting from spinal cord injury is not a reportable medical condition, information on its incidence and prevalence has not been generally available. In the past decade information has begun to appear that is based on hospital admissions and to some extent on household surveys.

SCOPE OF THE PROBLEM

In 1957, Michaelis estimated, there were approximately 10 new cases of spinal injury per million of the population of a country.[9] In a study during the years 1960 to 1967 in Switzerland, Gehrig and Michaelis concluded that the annual incidence was 15 per million population with an annual increase of 1.7 per cent.[10] A 1967 Canadian estimate was 12 to 15 per million.[11] In 1969, Young reported estimates that the number of persons experiencing spinal injury in the United States ranged between 3,500 and 10,000 annually, an incidence of between 20 and 50 per million population.[12] Owens and Sharman found an incidence of 12.3 per million in New England in 1970 and predicted an annual increase to 15.6 by 1980 and 17.1 by 1990.[13] Brown gave an incidence of 20 to 30 per million population annually in the 14- to 50-year age group.[14]

Young noted that of the roughly 200 million population in the United States in 1969 it was estimated that the spinal cord injury population constituted approximately 500 per million or a total of 100,000 at that time.[12] Sharman and Owens estimated a prevalence of 46,700 in 1970 and predicted 75,200 by 1980 and 108,300 by 1990.[13] In the 14- to 50-year age group the prevalence was 161 per million for Hawaii in 1971, 121 per million for Nevada in 1970, and 119 per million for Maine and 121 per million for Massachusetts in 1972.[15, 16]

The Gehrig and Michaelis Swiss study disclosed that 36 per cent of spinal cord injuries occurred on the road and in traffic; 35 per cent occurred at work, and 29 per cent occurred at home and in sports. The Nevada study showed 52 per cent resulting from automobile accidents; in Maine the percentage was 51.6, while in Hawaii it was 21.[15, 16] A Canadian study of 1,737 cases in 1967–1968 revealed that 37 per cent were due to motor vehicle accidents, 37 per cent to industrial accidents, and 7 per cent to diving.[17]

THE TRAUMATIC EPISODE

Direct trauma of the spinal cord by compression resulting from a vertebral body fracture-dislocation is the most common cause of permanent spinal cord dysfunction resulting in paraplegia or quadriplegia. Less common are penetrating wounds due to gunshot and trauma from other missiles and fragments and on occasion stab wounds in the cervical spine region. Lipschitz, in his South African study of stab wounds, noted that since most stab wounds are inflicted haphazardly the chances are that a certain number will penetrate into the column and "destroy or damage the cord."[18]

Mechanisms of Injury

By definition, paraplegia is paralysis of the lower extremities and all or a portion of the trunk. When the arms are also involved, the term "quadriplegia" is used to describe the impairment.

Fracture-dislocation of the cervical spine is a consequence of sudden and violent flexion or, less frequently, of extension and rotational or horizontal forces. The vertebral fracture-dislocation may result from a direct blow or from acceleration injuries. Motor vehicle accidents are the leading cause of cervical cord trauma, with diving accidents the leading cause in sports injuries. Thoracic spine fractures may result from a direct blow such as occurs in a cave-in from violent flexion in the seated position or from a penetrating missile. Thoracolumbar fracture-dislocations are most common at the T12–L1 site and follow violent flexion such as occurs in a fall from a height. In such an occurrence the initial force may strike the calcanei, with the likelihood of fracturing these bony segments, following which the remaining force causes a sufficient degree of flexion at the thoracolumbar junction to produce a fracture-dislocation. The most common sites of fracture-dislocation injuries are the C5–6, C6–7, and T12–L1 junctions. Certain parts of the spine are relatively protected from injury, namely, the upper thoracic and lower lumbar regions.[19]

Those instances in which radiologic examination shows no fracture or dislocation but in which there is substantial cord damage prove to be hyperextension injuries to the cervical spine in persons with spondylosis.[20] The spinal cord, already compromised by a narrow canal, is compressed by the further narrowing caused by hyperextension of the cervical spine. In addition, Hughes points out, vertebral artery obstruction may occur in the absence of radiologic evidence of fracture and produce a central region of ischemia or infarction in the cervical cord.[20]

In the case of a fracture-dislocation with damage to the entire thickness of the cord, all function at and distal to the site of injury is lost. Thus, there is total sensorimotor loss in the area of the body supplied from the site of injury and below.

Following injury to the cord, vascular and biochemical changes lead to complete infarction and necrosis of the injured segment. The actual mechanism for reduction of spinal cord blood flow after trauma is poorly understood. According to Tator it may be a direct mechanical effect on the blood vessels or there may be a biochemical explanation.[21] There is not only a direct injury to the axons and blood vessels at the time of injury but also a secondary chain of events resulting in hypoxia, edema, and ultimate infarction. Osterholm and his co-workers were of the opinion that norepinephrine release at the site of injury causes severe vasoconstriction that leads to ischemia and hemorrhagic necrosis of the cord.[22]

For a clearer understanding of the signs and symptoms resulting from spinal cord damage, it is germane to describe the scheme of segmental distribution.[23] The surface regions of the body supplied by the sensory (dorsal) roots of a spinal cord segment through the spinal nerves are called dermatomes. These have been determined by clinical studies and documented (Fig. 3–II–1). The segmental innervation of voluntary muscles has also been recorded; most muscle groups are innervated from two or more spinal cord segments as shown in Table 3–II–1.

For better understanding of the complications of spinal cord injury and the prognosis, the description of the impairment is based on the functional level of motor and sensory loss rather than the anatomical location of the spinal column injury. Thus "a complete level below C5" or "a C5 sensorimotor quadriplegia" denotes that C5 is the last functioning segment of the spinal cord. This is the terminology in use at several of the leading spinal cord injury centers and is the one propounded by Michaelis.[9] For the pathologist additional information including the site of bony injury is described so that he may correlate the neurologic or orthopedic findings with the histologic findings, since the level of spinal cord involvement may be at variance with the bony injury.

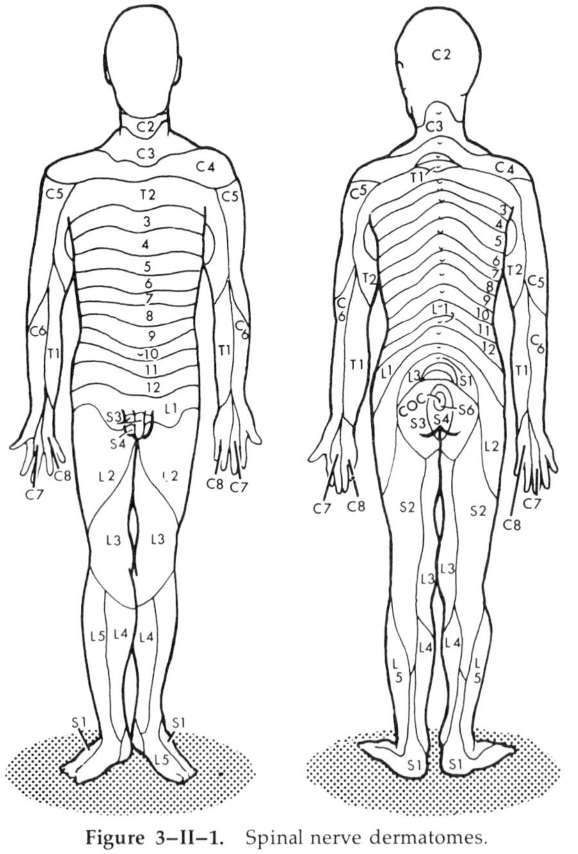

Figure 3–II–1. Spinal nerve dermatomes.

TABLE 3–II–1. SEGMENTAL INNERVATION OF MUSCLES

Neck	Flexion Extension Rotation	C1,2,3,4
Shoulder	Flexion Abduction Adduction Extension	C5,6 C5, 6 C5,6,7,8 C5,6,7,8
Elbow	Flexion Extension	C5,6 C7,8
Forearm	Pronation Supination	C6,7 C5,6,7
Wrist	Extension Flexion	C6,7 C6,7,T1
Hand	Gross extension of fingers Gross flexion of fingers Fine digital motion	C6,7,8 C7,8 T1 C8, T1
Back	Extension	C4 to L1
Chest muscles for breathing		T2 to T12
Diaphragm		C2,3,4
Abdominal muscles		T6 to L1
Hip	Flexion Abduction Adduction Extension Rotation	L2,3,4 L4,5, S1 L2,3,4 L4,5, S1 L4,5, S1,2
Knee	Extension Flexion	L2,3,4 L4,5, S1
Ankle		L4,5, S1,2
Foot		L5, S1,2
Bladder		S2,3,4
Bowel	Rectum and anal sphincter	S2,3,4
Generative system Erection Ejaculation	 Sacral cord Lumbar cord	 S2,3,4 L1,2,3,

Motor Loss

It is a rare individual who survives complete injury to the third or fourth cervical cord segments, since respiratory difficulties secondary to loss of function ensue. Damage below the fourth cervical segment spares the diaphragm for breathing; the only other significant musculoskeletal functions remaining are neck muscle function and the ability to shrug the shoulders.

Statistically there exist critical levels of spinal cord function (Table 3–II–2). The described levels of remaining musculoskeletal function are consistent with intact function at the specific spinal cord segment and all those proximal to it, with loss of function to a greater or lesser degree in all distal segments. From this it can be determined that the individual with a T1 level has complete innervation of all portions of the upper extremities, but lacks trunk and breathing musculature except for the diaphragm. The individual with a T12 level has normal upper extremities with a chain of strong fixators in the normal trunk to give virtually unlimited function of the upper extremities in the seated position.

The sensory sparing may be determined from the dermatome diagram (see Fig. 3–II–1).

Bladder Dysfunction

The bladder does not exist as an independent structure, but is part of a highly complex reflex mechanism. In normal micturition there is a balance between the expulsive and retentive forces so that after timely bladder emptying there is no postvoiding residual bladder urine. An understanding of this function clarifies the role of the reflex mechanisms in the neurogenic bladder.[24] Bors classified neurogenic bladders into two types on the basis of the neuronal involvement: upper motor neuron and lower motor neuron.[25] The presence of reflex activity in a neurogenic bladder is consistent with an upper motor neuron lesion, and the absence of reflex activity denotes lower motor neuron involvement. He suggested that the bulbocavernosus reflex be used to test the integrity of the spinal sacral reflex arc, thus ruling out trauma to the conus medullaris or cauda equina. Stimulation of the glans penis, of the vesical and urethral mucosa, or of the detrusor produces contraction of the pelvic floor musculature and the anal sphincter. Traction on an indwelling catheter also serves as a stimulus to this reflex. Bors and Comarr note that micturition starts as a purely spinal reflex in infancy and childhood, with the sacral segments of the cord as the only link for transmission of impulses to and from the target structures.[26] Thereafter this develops into a willed process; the spinal activity of smooth and striated muscle becoming integrated with brain function so that the sacral segments, later in life, are the sites for "transmission and modulation" of afferent and efferent impulses between the higher parts of the central nervous system and the so-called target organs.

The upper motor neuron reflex bladder functions without a catheter when there is reciprocation between action of the detrusor and the sphincter. Inability to empty occurs when there is lack of reciprocal action between these two or when voiding reflexes are aborted prior to completion of bladder emptying.

In the lower motor neuron bladder there is lack of reflex detrusor function, and the individual voids by vigorous abdominal straining.

TABLE 3–II–2. CRITICAL LEVELS OF SPINAL CORD FUNCTION

Level	Function
C5	Partial strength of all shoulder motions and elbow flexion.
C6	Normal power of all shoulder motions and elbow flexion; wrist extension, which indirectly permits gross grasping by the fingers
C7	Elbow extension, flexion, and extension of fingers
T1	Completely normal arms and hands
T6	Upper back extensors, upper intercostal muscles
T12	All muscles of thorax, abdomen, and back.
L4	Hip flexion, knee extension.
L5	Partial strength of all hip motions with normal flexion, partial strength of knee flexion, partial strength of ankle and foot motion

Bowel Dysfunction

The innervation for release of the anal sphincter tone is the same as that for bladder evacuation, the sensory innervation for appreciation of terminal bowel distention, the same as for bladder distention. The stimulus to bowel emptying is distention. Thus the individual with spinal cord injury prior to regulation training experiences alternating phases of constipation and uncontrolled defecation, since the voluntary muscle component inhibits bowel emptying.

Respiratory Dysfunction

Since the three major motors for breathing are the diaphragm innervated from C2 through C4, the intercostal muscles innervated from T2 through T12, and the abdominal muscles from T6 through L1, it becomes readily apparent that the individual with quadriplegia has been spared only the diaphragm. According to Bergofsky, this type of breathing is adequate at rest but requires abnormally large energy expenditure when large tidal volumes are needed to satisfy increased metabolic demands.[27] Thus the acute and chronic respiratory failure observed in quadriplegic patients arises from the inefficiency resulting from instability of the costal insertions of the diaphragm and the increased work of breathing due to increased intraabdominal pressure caused by unusually large excursions of the diaphragm.

Additionally, the lack of abdominal muscle also results in a cough that is feeble at best, with consequent difficulty in clearing secretions in respiratory infections. This same problem with cough is encountered in lower-level injuries down to the point at which there is significant intact function in the lower thoracic cord. Impaired respiratory function, including the inability to cough effectively, is especially hazardous in the patient with high-level spinal cord injury who develops respiratory tract infection; with pooling of secretions, airway obstruction leads to atelectasis.

LONG-TERM SEQUELAE

Sexual Dysfunction

Talbot points out that much of the misinformation that has "pervaded society and eventually the medical profession about spinal cord injury patients and their impotence is derived not from medical sources but from a literary source."[28] This source, *Lady Chatterly's Lover*, tells of a World War I paraplegic whom D. H. Lawrence deemed impotent. As Talbot notes, D. H. Lawrence, who was a considerable poet and novelist, was not a physiologist.

The sexual act in the male consists of erection, ejaculation, and orgasm. Erection may be induced by either of two stimuli, central or somesthetic and local tactile, and depends on the integrity of the second, third, and fourth spinal sacral segments for parasympathetic innervation and to a much lesser extent on the segments from T11 to L1 for sympathetic innervation.[29] Hyperemia results, through vasodilatation and patency of the arteriovenous shunts, from activity of the sacral innervation transmitted through the cauda equina and pelvic nerves (nervi erigentes).

In the spinally injured man, local tactile stimulation provides the mechanism for erection. The success in achieving erection by this method is dependent on the level of the spinal cord injury. In one collected series, the overall success rate has been stated to be 77 per cent.[29] In the Bors and Comarr study of 529 cases the success rate for erection in complete upper motor neuron lesions was 93 per cent while that in incomplete lesions was 99 per cent. Miller claims that erections occur in 80 per cent of patients with cervical cord lesions.[31] Much remains to be learned about this function in the man with spinal cord injury—certainly with understanding and communicating partners the success rate will be higher.

Ejaculation includes seminal emission and the ejaculation proper.[29] The first, dependent on the peristaltic action of the vasa deferentia, seminal vesicles, and prostate, is mediated through the sympathetic nervous system. The second results from contractions of the pelvic floor muscles and the bulbospongiosus and ischiocavernosus muscles.

Tarabulcy, in his collected series, stated that though 35 per cent had coitus, only 10 per cent achieved ejaculation.[29] The Bors and Comarr study described ejaculation in 5 per cent of those with complete lesions and 32 per cent of those with incomplete lesions.[30]

Orgasm has been described as a sensation resulting from contraction of the smooth muscles of the genitalia and the striated muscles of the pelvic floor coinciding with the ejaculation.[29] Because of the absence of peripheral sensory appreciation, the experience of orgasm is perforce altered in the man with spinal cord injury. Significant numbers of individuals, however, report pleasurable sensations in the genital region and also in an area of intact body surface innervation above the level of injury, particularly the nipple area (T5) when this is spared.

The estimates of the number of men with spinal cord injuries who have sired children has been on the order of 1 to 5 per cent.[29, 30] To date this has been ascribed to the lesser frequency of successful coitus (35 per cent), to loss of ejaculation and impaired spermatogenesis due to nutritional or hormonal or neurogenic causes or chronic urinary tract infection, and finally to occlusion of seminal passages due to infection.[29]

Recent studies have demonstrated that electric massage of the genitalia has tripled the overall incidence of ejaculation.[32] Use of intrathecal injections of prostigmin has produced specimens for study as well as for artificial insemination in individuals incapable of ejaculation.[32] These techniques are not without danger, since ejaculations may be accompanied by symptoms of severe autonomous dysreflexia, including hypertension and cardiac arrhythmia.[33]

The male with a cauda equina injury with consequent striated muscle paralysis has a dribbling ejaculation rather than the projectile type. Erection is achieved by some 25 per cent of such men, ejaculation by a lesser number, and progeny by 5 per cent.[30]

Less information is available concerning sexual function in the female because fewer women suffer spinal cord trauma. In our clinic the percentage has been under 10. The sequence of events in the sexual act corresponds to that in the male.[29] The tumescence of the clitoris and labia minora is the equivalent of erection. The seminal emission equivalent is contraction of the smooth muscle of the uterus, and the equivalent of ejaculation is the rhythmic contraction of the vaginal sphincter, the ischiocavernosus, and the pelvic floor musculature. Orgasm may be experienced as a pleasurable sensation at the level of demarcation between intact and lost sensation rather than vaginally; in some instances this sensation is vaginal in location.

Following injury, the woman with spinal cord injury may have an interval with loss of menstrual periods or irregularity with eventual return to regularity. The likelihood of pregnancy after spinal cord injury is unchanged, since fertility is unimpaired, and pregnancy and labor may proceed without complications. During labor in persons with a lesion at or above the T4–T5 level the manifestations of autonomic hyperreflexia may develop and should be distinguished from eclampsia.[34] It may be difficult to know when labor is beginning in patients with injuries above T10 because of lack of appreciation of uterine contractions.[35]

If the fetus has not been harmed in the accident in which the pregnant woman received the spinal cord injury and if the woman remains free of renal infection, there is all likelihood that a normal child will result.

> Pregnancy complicated by paraplegia is threatened more than in normal circumstances by the trauma itself, the immediate posttraumatic situation of the patient and by chronic infections and anemia in pregnancies, following cord injury.[36]

Orthostatic Hypotension

A not infrequent but dismaying problem encountered by patients with spinal cord injury, particularly those with quadriplegia, is the inability to tolerate the upright position because of orthostatic hypotension. This is characterized by nausea, lightheadedness, and even syncope. For most, this is of a temporary nature and passes with increasing periods in the upright position. For a small number, it persists and requires mechanical or pharmaceutical control. Deprived of the sympathetic response that prevents pooling of blood in dependent parts and with poor tissue turgor, which allows extravasation of fluid, orthostatic hypotension occurs.

Vallbona and his colleagues have suggested that in cases of complete transection of the cervical spinal cord and sympathetic denervation below the lesion, there is insufficient release of catecholamines in response to sudden positional changes.[37] Slow release of antidiuretic hormone, cortisol, and aldosterone may also play a role.

Temperature Adjustment

Maintenance of body temperature results from a balance of heat production and heat dissipation. Temperature-sensitive structures in the superficial and deep regions of the body act as a warning system to the central temperature-sensitive receptors in the anterior preoptic region of the hypothalamus.[38] A rise in central temperature results in vasodilatation and sweating in the periphery while central cooling results in vasoconstriction and shivering. Downey states that the central receptors probably play a dominant role in the thermoregulation, with skin responses functioning mainly in short-term regulation.[39]

According to Guttmann and his colleagues, T8 is the highest level at which a patient can maintain rectal temperature at 37°C in an environmental temperature from 18° to 40°C.[38] Patients with higher levels are poikilothermic in response to heating or cooling. In patients with spinal injury shivering occurs only in muscles innervated above the level of the lesion.[40] Miller comments on the presence of rudimentary thermoregulation at the cord level.[31]

Though the mechanism is not fully understood, the person with spinal cord injury does have difficulty adjusting to extremes of ambient temperature, and the higher the level the greater the difficulty.[41]

Metabolic Alterations

Bone

Prolonged bed rest is known to produce not only muscle atrophy but demineralization of bone as well. In the paralyzed individual this tendency is compounded, particularly in the bony structures below the level of the spinal cord lesion. The development of osteoporosis in the proximal femur makes the individual vulnerable to minimal trauma to the extent that even the ordinary activity of turning in bed may result in a hip fracture.

Serum Protein

In quadriplegics the median value of the total protein in both the immediate and late postinjury states is at the lower limits of normal.[42] In the later stages there is a gradual increase in the gamma globulin fraction. Once the serum protein changes have occurred, there is rarely return to normal.[43]

Cooper and Hoen described temporary elevation of urinary 17-ketosteroid levels during the first 48 hours after spinal injury.[44] Thereafter 50 per cent of paraplegic males showed a decrease for a period of 10 weeks to 7 years. Kaplan and his co-workers noted that, in their study of 60 patients, 63.3 per cent showed little or no 17-ketosteroid response to ACTH and 58.3 per cent showed little or no 17-hydroxysteroid response.[45]

Gynecomastia

Breast enlargement, either unilateral or bilateral, is not uncommon in the patient with spinal cord injury. In our own experience the incidence has been up to 5 per cent. The enlargement has been ascribed to an increase of circulatory estrogens resulting from hepatic dysfunction. Cooper and his colleagues commented that the liver impairment resolves within 8 to 10 weeks.[46]

Autonomic Dysreflexia

Autonomic dysreflexia is characterized by elevation of blood pressure on the order of 100 to 200 mm of mercury systolic and 50 to 100 mm of mercury diastolic, headache, slowing of the pulse, flushing and sweating of the face, and nasal congestion. The possibility of convulsions and cerebral hemorrhage with death exists.[47]

The phenomenon may occur in individuals with injuries above T7 and is not infrequent in those with high thoracic or cervical levels of injury when reflex function is retained in segments of the spinal cord below the level of injury. Young comments that the autonomic systems (sympathetic and sacral parasympathetic) remain without control from higher regulatory centers. Thus the reflex mechanisms function in "unrestricted reflex revelry with disastrous consequences to the patient."[48]

Elicited by noxious stimuli to the body parts below the level of injury, the reflex most frequently occurs in response to distention of bladder and bowel. Rossier and his co-workers note that during labor in patients with high thoracic or cervical levels of injury the manifestations of autonomic dysreflexia should not be confused with preeclampsia.[49]

Based on reflex activity, either viscerovascular or somatovascular, the syndrome occurs because of impaired vascular segmental activity resulting from spinal cord damage above the splanchnic outflow, that is above levels between T4 and T6. Bors and Comarr note that autonomic dysreflexia may reach a peak after a lapse of time following the spinal cord injury and then subside, but may recur after many years of quiescence.[26]

POTENTIAL COMPLICATIONS

Infection and Calculus Formation

The normal urinary tract is bacteria-free except adjacent to the distal portion of the urethra, and ordinarily the urine is sterile. The neurogenic bladder with large postvoiding residual urine volumes due to obstructive uropathy or impaired expulsive force provides the milieu for bacteria growth. Further, the indwelling catheter, when this is required, provides an entrance mechanism for bacteria from the external environment into the bladder.

The normal bladder mucosa is ordinarily resistant to bacterial entrance; the neurogenic bladder mucosa does not have this protective mechanism.

The person with spinal cord injury is also prone to kidney bacterial infection since obstruction to urine flow makes the kidney more liable to infection; the neurogenic bladder dysfunction results in bladder infection, which in turn results in kidney infection. The spread of infection is, in a significant number of instances, fostered by the presence of vesicoureteral reflux due to involvement of the intramural portion of the ureters and of the ureteral orifice that is sufficient to interfere with normal function. In the absence of reflux, however, bacteria can reach the kidney by the ascending route.

Urinary stasis favors precipitation of salts

resulting in calculus formation. Also, the presence of infection as well as a foreign body in the bladder sets the stage for formation of stones in the bladder and kidney and less commonly in the prostate and seminal vesicles. The presence of calculus also concurrently fosters the infection. The incidence of urinary tract calculi has been stated to be from 22.5 to 42 per cent.

Ischemic Ulceration

Decubitus ulcers or ischemic ulcerations are one of the major problems confronting any patient who remains in one position, either sitting or recumbent, for prolonged periods of time.[50] The most frequently involved areas are the sacrum, the trochanters of the hip, the ischial rami, and the malleoli and heels. These are sites with relatively little tissue interposed between the skin and bony prominences. Thus, the person with spinal cord injury, who may be unable to move or turn himself frequently and who has no sensation of pressure, is especially prone to ulceration because he lacks perception of pressure and because circulation to denervated areas is inadequate.

Munro wrote that the propensity for development of ulcers was based on interruption of the autonomic reflex arcs that controlled circulation to the skin; therefore, there was no response to pressure in the normal protective manner.[50] Later Kosiak demonstrated that decubitus ulcers were ischemic in nature and resulted from prolonged tissue ischemia when pressure applied exceeded capillary pressure at sites overlying bony prominences.[51, 52]

> Because hydrostatic pressures in capillaries are low and because cessation of flow occurs even in the presence of positive arterial pressure it seems logical that complete tissue ischemia may be present when pressures on the order of capillary pressure are applied.[53]

Thus an ischemic destructive process occurs with application of high pressure of short duration or prolonged low pressure. According to Kosiak these are localized areas of cellular necrosis; the microscopic changes are characterized by edema, loss of cross-striations and myofibrils, hyalinization of fibers, neutrophilic infiltration, and phagocytosis by neutrophils and macrophages.[52, 53] In animal studies these changes were produced by pressure of 50 mm of mercury for one hour in animals with a ligated femoral artery, but did not occur with pressure of 100 mm of mercury for two hours in the normal animal.

Thrombophlebitis and Phlebothrombosis

Among the complications to which the patient with spinal cord injury is subject are phlebothrombosis and thrombophlebitis.[54, 55] Bors, in a study of 99 paraplegic patients, described a 58 per cent incidence of deep vein occlusion detected by venography.[56] The occlusion was more significant in those with spastic than in those with flaccid paraplegia. Philipps studied 25 paraplegic patients both clinically and radiologically; 7 of the 50 limbs showed evidence of deep venous thrombosis.[57] Watson reported an overall incidence of 12.5 per cent in 431 patients, and Walsh described thrombosis in 13.2 per cent of 500 patients.[58, 59]

The etiologic basis proposed has been sluggish venous return due to the faulty muscle pump and the action of gravity against venous return.[57] A consequent complication is pulmonary embolization. Shull and Rose note that subclinical episodes of pulmonary embolization may occur more frequently than is commonly recognized.

Dietrick and Russi found pulmonary infarction in 2 of 55 paraplegic patients in whom they reviewed the necropsy findings.[60] Freed and co-workers' study of 243 patients, of whom 54 died during a 25-year period ending in 1955, revealed that five deaths were due to pulmonary embolization.[55] Walsh and Tribe cited a 3 per cent mortality rate, and Watson described an incidence rate of pulmonary embolism of 5 per cent and a mortality rate of 1.5 per cent.[58, 59]

Ectopic Bone Formation

Ectopic bone formation, extraosseous bone formation or paraosteoarthropathy, is said to occur in up to 49 per cent of individuals with spinal cord injury.[61] Forming below the body level involved by the spinal cord lesion, it is most often found adjacent to the hips, knees, shoulders, and elbows. In the vast majority of instances it is noted as an incidental finding in radiographic studies made for other reasons. In rare instances the process is so extensive that joint range of motion is impaired. The phenomenon is the result of metaplastic osteogenesis of apparently rapid onset, associated with some chrondrogenesis, forming corticospongiosal bone of lamellar structure; after 30 months, mineralization approaches that of normal young adult bone.[62] X-ray evidence and alkaline phosphatase determinations are no indicators of maturation.[61, 62] When uptake ratios determined from serial bone scans show a progressive decrease, however, it may be concluded that the process has reached maturity, and when surgical intervention is necessary the risk of postoperative recurrence is minimal.[62]

Malignant Disease

Melzak noted that since infection of the urinary tract is still very common in the patient with spinal cord injury it would be appropriate to study the incidence of bladder cancer in these individuals.[63] In Great Britain's National Spinal Injuries Centre his 20-year study beginning in 1944 of 3,800 persons with spinal cord injury resulted in the finding of 11 cases of bladder cancer, an incidence of 0.28 per cent. The earliest was diagnosed after 13 years, the latest after 42 years. The youngest patient was 37 years old. Because the vast majority of his patients smoked he hesitated to accuse smoking as the cause; it is, however, recognized that smokers have a greater incidence of bladder carcinoma. The only common factors proved to be long-standing chronic urinary infection and cystitis, and long-standing catheter drainage. Bors and Comarr found malignant genitourinary tract disease in 0.64 per cent of 2,322 patients.[30] The diagnosis was made 10 to 22 years following injury.

Hypertension

In his postmortem study of 122 paraplegics between 1945 and 1962 Tribe found a surprisingly large incidence of hypertension. "Critical assessment of both clinical and pathologic evidence revealed 41 cases of definite hypertension amongst the 122 paraplegics."[64] He concluded that the hypertension was associated with chronic pyelonephritis. Hypertension was an infrequent finding in other studies.[55, 65–68]

Amyloid Disease

Chronic suppurative infection in the urinary tract, in bedsores, and in underlying bone resulting in disturbance of protein metabolism may be responsible for amyloid disease of the secondary type in patients with spinal cord injury. The amyloidosis is widespread, with the most serious involvement in the kidney.

Gastrointestinal Function

The transport of products of digestion through the intestine results from peristaltic action that arises from the autonomic plexuses within the bowel wall. Quadriplegic individuals are known to have a high rate of incidence of peptic ulcer that may well be of the stress type.[69] Miller points out that this ulcer phenomenon may be due to unopposed vagal action, as are the ileus and hypermotility.[31]

Pain

> Many patients with injuries to the spinal cord or cauda equina experience pain at some time in early or late course of their illness.[70]

Persistent intractable pain is a problem in a limited number of individuals with spinal cord injury. Gooddy suggests that the pain experienced below the level of the spinal cord lesion may be transmitted through the sympathetic nervous system.[71]

Krueger believed that in most instances the pain originates from lesions of the intraspinal contents, either from intact or partially intact nerve roots or from neuroma formation in severed roots or at the proximal stump of the severed spinal cord, or in the transitional zone immediately above the lesion in cases of nontransecting spinal cord injuries.[70]

Another type of pain has been labeled "visceral pain" and follows distention by enemas or distention of the urinary bladder.[72] This discomfort is abdominal in nature. Visceral abnormality such as peptic ulcer or cholecystitis may also produce vague nonlocalizing abdominal discomfort.

Spasticity

The altered reflex activity of the spinal cord below the level of injury may produce an incapacitating situation for the injured person. Limitations are imposed on his physical functioning in activities of daily living and thus his rehabilitation. This occurs because of the resultant rigid posture or forceful, uncontrollable motions of the limbs innervated below the level of spinal cord injury.

Better understanding of the causes of this phenomenon (which may include stimuli such as infection, decubitus ulceration, bowel or bladder distention, and emotional tension) and availability of conservative and surgical measures have done much to minimize this complication.

SPECIALIZED HOSPITAL UNITS FOR CARE OF THE PATIENT WITH SPINAL CORD INJURY

The great advantage of using a categorically oriented system of care for the patient with spinal cord injury was first proved by Dr. Donald Munro in the 1930's in his unit in the Boston City Hospital. That a significant number of such patients could not only survive but could also return to a productive and functional life status was later confirmed by Guttmann in England, Weiss in Poland, Cheshire in Australia, Michaelis and Rossier in Switzerland, Bors and Talbot in the United States Veterans Administration, Gregg in Ireland, Meinecke in Germany, and Young and Freed in the United States.[73-83]

The complex nature of the manifestations of spinal cord injury and the potential for life-threatening complications, as well as for complications whose avoidance could decrease the hospital stay and minimize the psychologic trauma, makes mandatory the provision of care in a facility especially organized for providing holistic care for this injury. The Department of Health, Education, and Welfare is currently funding a regional system of spinal cord injury centers across the United States as a demonstration project.

A lifetime of care begins after discharge from the hospital. The ongoing goals include refinement of physical gains already achieved, maintenance of achieved functional ability and adjustment, and identification of potential or already developed problems. This care includes regular outpatient reevaluation as well as periodic inpatient study at intervals of 6 to 18 months.

Upon departure from the hospital, the person with spinal cord injury will, when possible, be discharged to his home, which will have been physically altered. His family will have become familiar with his total needs, and ideally his schooling, retraining, and vocational placement will have been arranged.

SPECIAL CONSIDERATIONS

Provided with adapted devices to exploit the full potential of his physical functioning and with removal of architectural barriers in the home and community, the individual with spinal cord injury, no matter what the level, can leave his home, make his way by wheelchair (the most essential equipment for mobility) and hand-control-operated motor vehicle, and participate in educational, vocational, recreational, and even social welfare pursuits in behalf of others.

These accomplishments require doors sufficiently wide to permit wheelchair entrance and egress; replacement of entrance stairs by ramps with grades of no greater than 8 per cent; widening of corridors to allow maneuverability of wheelchairs; construction of bathrooms both in public buildings and at home to allow maneuverability in the chair and transfer from the chair onto the toilet and return; and adjustment of public telephones, electric light switches, plugs, elevator operating buttons, and door latches to the height of the person seated in the wheelchair. Internal environmental temperature adjustment is also important in view of the intolerance of the person with spinal cord injury to extremes of heat and cold. Elevator accessibility in multistoried school buildings will permit him to attend regular classroom instruction with his peers.

Prejudice by potential employers and real estate managers remains a problem, as does that of transportation companies. The potential of the person with spinal cord injury, in the absence of medical and psychologic complications but even in the presence of multiple physical impairment, is unmeasurable.

Rusk avers:

> You don't get fine china by putting clay in the sun. You have to put the clay through the white heat of the kiln if you want to make porcelain. Heat breaks some pieces. Disability breaks some people. But once the clay goes through the white-hot fire and comes out whole, it can never be clay again; once a person overcomes a disability through his own courage, determination and hard work, he has a depth of spirit you and I know little about.[84]

In conclusion we quote Sir Ludwig Guttmann:

> One could only wish that the community at large would also recognize the new talents exhibited by paraplegics and other severely disabled in the field of training and employment. The old prejudice towards a person in a wheelchair dies hard. Indeed, there is still a great need for educating the public as a whole to give their disabled fellow men, women and children fair chances for their social reintegration by providing more and better facilities both in places of employment and in particular in ordinary schools and universities, to give wheelchair users the opportunity to be educated in company with their able-bodied fellows.[72]

REFERENCES

1. Elsberg, C. A.: The Edwin Smith surgical papyrus and the diagnosis and treatment of injuries to the skull and spine 5000 years ago. Ann. Med. Hist., *3*:271, 1931.
2. Poer, D. H.: Newer concepts in the treatment of the paralyzed patient due to war-time injuries of the spinal cord. Ann. Surg., *123*:510, 1946.
3. Thompson Walker, J. W.: Hunterian Lecture on the bladder in gunshot and other injuries of the spinal cord. Lancet, *1*:173, 1917.
4. Kuhn, W. G.: The care and rehabilitation of patients with injuries of the spinal cord. J. Neurosurg., *4*:40, 1947.
5. Hinman, F.: The treatment of paralytic bladder in cases of spinal cord injury. Surgery, *4*:649, 1938.
6. Munro, D.: Thoracic and lumbosacral cord injuries. J.A.M.A., *122*:1055, 1943.
7. Kirk, N. T.: Wartime activities of the Army Medical Department. N. Engl. J. Med., *235*:182, 1946.
8. Controller, Department of Medicine and Surgery: Mortality Report on Spinal Cord Injury. Reports and Statistics Service, Veterans Administration, (Nov. 13) 1958.
9. Michaelis, L. S.: Discussion of papers read at the 1967 Scientific Meeting of the International Medical Society of Paraplegia. Paraplegia, *5*:180, 1967.
10. Gehrig, R., and Michaelis, L. S.: Statistics of acute paraplegia and tetraplegia on a national scale. Paraplegia, *6*:93, 1968.
11. Canadian Neurosurgical Society: Report of a Sub-Committee. Paraplegic Care in Canada. 1969.
12. Young, J. S.: The Southwest Regional System for Treatment of Spinal Injury. Proposal to U.S. Department of Health, Education, and Welfare, April 25, 1969.
13. Sharman, G. J., and Owens, K. A., Jr.: Spinal Cord Injury. Report to the National Paraplegia Foundation, Boston, September 1970.
14. Brown, L. M.: Maine's Spinal Cord Injured. Study Report to Bureau of Rehabilitation, Department of Health and Welfare, Augusta, Maine, August 1972.
15. Wilcox, E., Kuwamoto, H., and Shauffer, E. S.: Statewide census of spinal cord injured persons. Hawaii. December 1971. (Cited in 12.)
16. Wilcox, E.: Statewide census of spinal injured persons. Nevada, 1970. (Cited in 13.)
17. Canadian Paraplegic Association: Paraplegic Survey, 1967–68.
18. Lipschitz, R.: Associated injuries and complications of stab wounds of the spinal cord. Paraplegia, 5:75, 1967.
19. Griffiths, H. J.: The radiology of spinal cord injury; a review article. Proceedings 18th U.S. Veterans Administration Spinal Cord Injury Conference, October 1971. Washington, U.S. Government Printing Office, 1972, p. 43.
20. Hughes, J. T.: Vertebral artery insufficiency in acute cervical spine trauma. Paraplegia, *3*:2, 1964.
21. Tator, C. H.: Acute spinal cord injury. A review of recent studies of treatment and pathophysiology. Can. Med. Assoc. J., *107*:142, 1972.
22. Osterholm, J. L., Mathews, G. J., Irvin, J. D., and Evangelakos, E. T.: A review of altered norepinephrine metabolism attending severe spinal injury. Proceedings: 18th U.S. Veterans Administration Spinal Cord Injury Conference, October 1971. Washington, U.S. Government Printing Office, 1972, p. 17.
23. Freed, M. M.: Teaching Syllabus; Rehabilitation Medicine. Boston University School of Medicine, 1972.
24. Abramson, A. S.: The neurogenic bladder. Arch. Phys. Med. Rehabil., *48*:480, 1967.
25. Bors, E.: Neurogenic bladder. Urol. Survey, *7*:177, 1957.
26. Bors, E., and Comarr, A. E.: Neurologic Urology. Baltimore, University Park Press, 1971.
27. Bergofsky, E. J.: Quantitation of function of respiratory muscles in normal individuals and quadriplegic patients. Arch. Phys. Med. Rehabil., *45*:575, 1964.
28. Talbot, H.: Discussion of papers read at the meeting of the International Medical Society of Paraplegia. Paraplegia, *9*:63, 1971.
29. Tarabulcy, E.: Sexual function in the normal and in paraplegia. Paraplegia, *10*:201, 1972.
30. Bors, E., and Comarr, A. E.: Neurological disturbances of sexual function with special reference to 529 patients with spinal cord injury. Urol. Survey, *10*:191, 1960.
31. Miller, J. M., III: Autonomic function in the isolated spinal cord. In *Physiological Basis of Rehabilitation Medicine.* Edited by J. A. Downey and R. C. Darling. Philadelphia, W. B. Saunders Co., 1971.
32. Guttmann, L., and Walsh, J. J.: Prostigmin assessment test of fertility in spinal man. Paraplegia, *9*:39, 1971.
33. Rossier, A. B., Ziegler, W. H., Duchosal, P. W., and Meylan, J.: Sexual function and dysreflexia. Paraplegia, *9*:51, 1971.
34. Rossier, A. B., Ruffieux, M., and Ziegler, W. H.: Pregnancy and labour in high traumatic spinal cord lesions. Paraplegia, *7*:210, 1970.
35. Robertson, D. N. S.: Pregnancy and labour in the paraplegic. Paraplegia, *10*:209, 1972.
36. Guller, H., and Paeslack, V.: Pregnancy damage and birth complications in the children of paraplegic women. Paraplegia, *10*:213, 1972.
37. Vallbona, C., Lipscomb, H. S., and Carter, R. E.: Endocrine response to orthostatic hypotension in quadriplegia. Arch. Phys. Med. Rehabil., *47*:412, 1966.
38. Guttmann, L., Silva, J., and Wyndham, C. H.: Thermoregulation in spinal man. J. Physiol. (Lond.), *142*:406, 1958.
39. Downey, J. A.: Physiology of temperature regulation in man. In *Physiological Basis of Rehabilitation Medicine.* Edited by J. A. Downey and R. C. Darling. Philadelphia, W. B. Saunders Co., 1971.
40. Sherrington, C. S.: Notes on temperature after spinal transection, with some observations on shivering. J. Physiol. (Lond.), *58*:405, 1924.
41. Johnson, R. H.: Temperature regulation in paraplegia. Paraplegia, *9*:137, 1971.
42. Arieff, A. J., Pyzik, S. W., Tigay, E. L., and Bersohn, J.: Some metabolic studies in quadriplegia following spinal cord injury. Ill. Med. J., *117*:219, 1960.
43. Robinson, R.: Serum protein changes following spinal cord injuries. Proc. R. Soc. Med., *47*:1109, 1954.
44. Cooper, I. S., and Hoen, T. T.: Metabolic disorders in paraplegics. Neurology (Minneap.), *2*:332, 1952.
45. Kaplan, L., Powell, B. R., Grynbaum, B. B., and Rusk, H. A.: *Comprehensive Follow-up Study of Spinal Cord Dysfunction and its Resultant Disabilities.* Chap. V., New York, Institution of Rehabilitation Medicine, 1966.
46. Cooper, I. S., Rynearson, E. H., MacCarty, C. S., and Power, M. H.: Metabolic consequences in spinal cord injury. J. Clin. Endocrinol., *10*:858, 1950.
47. Thompson, C. E., and Witham, A.: Paroxysmal hypertension in spinal cord injuries. N. Engl. J. Med., *239*:291, 1948.
48. Young, J. S.: Use of guanethidine in control of sympathetic hyperreflexia in persons with cervical and thoracic cord lesions. Arch. Phys. Med. Rehabil., *44*:204, 1963.
49. Rossier, A. B., Ruffieux, M., and Ziegler, W. H.: Preg-

nancy and labour in high traumatic spinal cord lesions. Paraplegia, *7*:210, 1970.
50. Munro, D.: Care of the back following spinal cord injuries. N. Engl. J. Med., *233*:391, 1940.
51. Kosiak, M.: Etiology of decubitus ulcers. Arch. Phys. Med. Rehabil., *42*:19, 1961.
52. Kosiak, M.: An effective method of preventing decubitus ulcers. Arch. Phys. Med. Rehabil., *47*:724, 1966.
53. Kosiak, M.: Etiology and pathology of ischemic ulcerations. Arch. Phys. Med. Rehabil., *40*:62, 1959.
54. Shull, J. B., and Rose, D. L.: Pulmonary embolism in patients with spinal cord injuries. Arch. Phys. Med. Rehabil., *47*:444, 1966.
55. Freed, M. M., Bakst, H. J., and Barrie, D. L.: Life expectancy, survival rates and causes of death in civilian patients with spinal cord trauma. Arch. Phys. Med. Rehabil., *47*:457, 1966.
56. Bors, E., Conrad, C. A., and Massell, T. B.: Venous occlusion of lower extremities in paraplegic patients. Surg. Gynecol. Obstet., *99*:451, 1954.
57. Philipps, R. S.: The incidence of deep venous thrombosis in paraplegics. Paraplegia, *1*:116, 1963.
58. Watson, N.: Venous thrombosis and pulmonary embolism in spinal cord injury. Paraplegia, *6*:113, 1968.
59. Walsh, J. J., and Tribe, C.: Phlebothrombosis and pulmonary embolism in paraplegia. Paraplegia, *3*:209, 1965.
60. Dietrick, R. B., and Russi, S.: Tabulation and review of autopsy findings in 55 paraplegics. J.A.M.A., *166*:41, 1958.
61. Nicholas, J. J.: Ectopic bone formation in patients with spinal cord injury. Arch. Phys. Med. Rehabil., *54*:8, 1973.
62. Rossier, A. B., Bussat, P., Infante, F., Zender, R., et al.: Current facts on para-osteo-arthropathy. Paraplegia, *11*:36, 1973.
63. Melzak, J.: The incidence of bladder cancer in paraplegia. Paraplegia, *4*:85, 1966.
64. Tribe, C. R.: Causes of death in early and late stages of paraplegia. Paraplegia, *1*:19, 1963.
65. Ebel, A.: Discussion of the pathology in selected cases of spinal cord injury. Proceedings: 9th Annual Clinical Spinal Cord Injury Conference, October 1960. Washington, U.S. Government Printing Office, 1961.
66. Finkle, J. R.: Discussion of the pathology in selected cases of spinal cord injury. Proceedings: 9th Annual Clinical Spinal Cord Injury Conference, October 1960. Washington, U.S. Government Printing Office, 1961.
67. Halladay, L. W.: Discussion of the pathology in selected cases of spinal cord injury. Proceedings: 9th Annual Clinical Spinal Cord Injury Conference, October 1960. Washington, U.S. Government Printing Office, 1961.
68. Lowry, R.: Discussion of the pathology in selected cases of spinal cord injury. Proceedings: 9th Annual Clinical Spinal Cord Injury Conference, October 1960. Washington, U.S. Government Printing Office, 1961.
69. Freed, M. M., and Corcoran, P. J.: Unpublished data.
70. Krueger, E. G.: Management of painful states in injuries of the spinal cord and cauda equina. Am. J. Phys. Med., *39*:103, 1960.
71. Gooddy, Y.: On the nature of pain. Brain, *80*:118, 1957.
72. Guttmann, L.: *Spinal Cord Injuries.* Oxford, Blackwell Scientific Publications, 1973.
73. Guttmann, L.: History of the National Spinal Injuries Centre, Stoke Mandeville Hospital, Aylesbury. Paraplegia, *5*:115, 1967.
74. Weiss, M.: Fifteen years' experience on rehabilitation of paraplegics at the Rehabilitation Institute of Warsaw University. Paraplegia, *5*:158, 1967.
75. Chesire, D. J. E.: The complete and centralised treatment of paraplegia. Paraplegia, *6*:59, 1969.
76. Michaelis, L.: Opening of the Swiss Paraplegic Centre in Basle. Paraplegia, *5*:158, 1967.
77. Rossier, A. B.: Organization and function of the French Swiss Paraplegic Centre. Paraplegia, *5*:166, 1968.
78. Bors, E.: The Spinal Cord Injury Center of the Veterans Administration Hospital, Long Beach, California. Paraplegia, *5*:126, 1967.
79. Talbot, H. S.: Rehabilitation in a changing world. Paraplegia, *7*:146, 1969.
80. Gregg, T. M.: Organization of a Spinal Injury Unit within a Rehabilitation Centre. Paraplegia, *5*:163, 1967.
81. Meinecke, F. W.: Opening of the Centre For Spinal Injuries and other severely disabled persons at the Orthopaedic Clinic of Heidelberg University. Paraplegia, *5*:104, 1967.
82. Young, J. S.: Development of systems of spinal injury management with a correlation to the development of other esoteric health care systems. Ariz. Med., *27*:1, 1970.
83. Freed, M. M.: The Spinal Cord Injury Center, Scope. B.U.M.C., *1*:16, (Nov.–Dec.) 1968.
84. Rusk, H. A.: *A World to Care For.* New York, Random House, 1972.

III. The Eye and Its Adnexa

by Howard M. Leibowitz, Mohandas M. Kini, Simmons Lessell, and Marc Richman

Nature appears to have recognized the susceptibility of the eye to trauma and has afforded it protection accordingly. Situated deep within the bony orbital cavity, it is cushioned by generous amounts of soft fatty tissue. Superiorly, the globe obtains further protection from a thick overhanging projection of bone, the orbital rim. Medially, it is similarly protected by the nose. Objects that threaten the eye and can be seen induce a rapid reflex closure of the eyelids and a reflex turning of the head. Intrusion of foreign material into the conjunctival cul-de-sac or its contact with the anterior surface of the eye produces a copious flow of tears that washes away or dilutes the offending material.

Despite this anatomical and physiologic protection, ocular injuries are common. The structural delicacy of the eye and its functional significance make all such injuries potentially major ones. Trauma of a magnitude that would cause little concern elsewhere produces disastrous consequences in the eye. The resultant disability, economic loss, and human misery are strikingly disproportionate to the extent of the injury.

Ocular injuries are extremely difficult to classify according to etiology since the list of causal factors is almost endless. They can, however, be separated into mechanical and nonmechanical categories. The former includes concussions and contusions of the globe, wounds and perforating injuries, and the effects of foreign body retention. The latter embraces such diverse causal entities as thermal, ultrasonic, electrical, radiational, chemical, stress, and toxicologic injuries. For purposes of organization, mechanical ocular injuries are discussed according to their location at the following sites: lids and lacrimal apparatus, conjunctiva, cornea, sclera, anterior chamber, iris and ciliary body, lens, vitreous humor, choroid and retina, optic nerve, extraocular muscles, and orbit (Fig. 3–III–1).

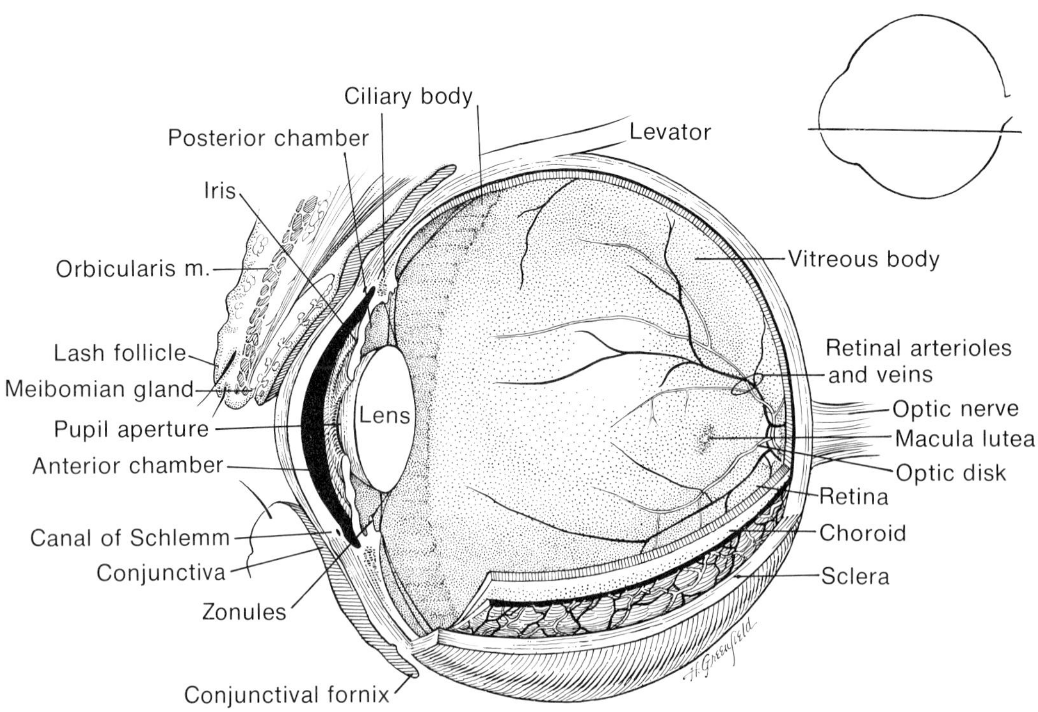

Figure 3–III–1. Anatomy of the eye and eyelids.

MECHANICAL INJURIES

Lids and Lacrimal Apparatus

The eyelids are movable structures lying anterior to the globe, protecting it from injury, excessive light, and dehydration. The upper eyelid is demarcated superiorly by the eyebrow, while the lower eyelid merges, usually without specific demarcation, into the skin of the cheek. The upper lid contains a special elevator muscle, the levator palpebrae superioris, which makes it much more mobile than the lower. In the open position, the lid margins meet at the inner and outer canthi and form an elliptical space, the palpebral fissure.

Eyelid Structure

Structurally, the eyelids consist of a series of layers. From anterior to posterior they are: the skin, a layer of subcutaneous areolar tissue, a layer of striated muscle, submuscular areolar tissue, a fibrous layer (including the tarsal plates), a layer of smooth muscle, and the mucous membrane or conjunctiva.

The skin of the eyelids is among the thinnest in the body. In youth, it is very elastic and recovers rapidly after being distended. The subcutaneous areolar layer consists of loose connective tissue containing no fat, permitting the skin to be easily lifted off the underlying muscle. The layer of striated muscle is formed by fibers of the palpebral portion of the orbicularis oculi, arranged concentrically around the palpebral fissure and innervated by branches of the seventh cranial nerve.

Between the orbicularis muscle and the underlying tarsal plate is the submuscular areolar tissue, which resembles the subcutaneous layer and communicates superiorly with the subaponeurotic layer of the scalp. Via this plane, blood or pus from a scalp injury may gain entrance into the upper lid. The main nerves to the eyelids lie in this layer.

The fibrous layer consists of two parts: a thickened central portion, the tarsal plates, and a thinner peripheral portion, the septum orbitale. The tarsal plates are constructed of dense fibrous tissue and are shaped like the letter D lying on its side. They give the lids their shape and support, molding themselves to the shape of the eye. The extremities of the tarsal plates are attached to the orbital margin by strong fibrous structures called the medial and lateral palpebral ligaments. The concave posterior surface of each tarsal plate is covered by mucous membrane, the conjunctiva. In addition to lining the posterior surface of the lids, the conjunctiva is reflected onto the globe, covering the anterior sclera and becoming continuous with the corneal epithelium at the limbus. The conjunctiva thus forms a continuous circular cul-de-sac, the fornix conjunctivae, connecting the lids to the eye.

Lacrimal Apparatus

The lacrimal gland consists of two portions, a large orbital portion above and a small palpebral portion below. The orbital portion lies in a bony fossa in the anterior and outer part of the orbital roof. The palpebral portion is located in the outer part of the upper fornix, where it lies, for the most part, on the palpebral conjunctiva and may be seen through the conjunctiva when the upper lid is everted.

The glands of Krause are accessory lacrimal glands located under the palpebral conjunctiva from the fornix to the convex border of the tarsus. Fine ducts running from both portions of the lacrimal gland open by approximately a dozen small orifices into the lateral portion of the superior fornix.

The puncta is a small aperture situated on a tiny elevation, the papilla lacrimalis, at the medial portion of each lid margin.

The canaliculi, an upper and a lower tubular structure, run initially in a vertical direction but then turn at right angles, course horizontally and medially along the lid border, and join to form a common canaliculus that enters the lacrimal sac, which is a membranous structure located in the lacrimal fossa in the anterior part of the medial wall of the orbit.

The nasolacrimal duct, an inferior extension of the lacrimal sac, forms the final portion of the lacrimal drainage system and terminates in the inferior meatus of the nose.

Injuries of the Eyelids

Blunt force striking the eyelids is a common occurrence, producing the classic "black eye." Injuries of this type are frequently documented at birth, the result of trauma during passage through the birth canal or by the instruments used to assist delivery. With increasing age, the causes of similar injury are legion—the blow from a fist, the impact of a ball, the collision with a door, the encounter with an adversary in a contact sport, the crash into a part of the vehicle during an automobile accident. All such applications of blunt force to the lids produce almost instantaneous swelling because of the looseness of the tissue and the paucity of subcutaneous tissue. The swelling is a manifestation of edema and hemorrhage. Not infrequently, it completely closes the eye and renders the tissues of the lid extremely taut, making it extremely difficult if not impossible to separate the lids to examine the globe. Extravasation of blood into the subcutaneous tissues of the lid is responsible for the "black eye." The blood and edema fluid may diffuse through the loose subcutaneous tissue of the lid across the bridge of the nose into the lids of the opposite eye. The skin over the bridge of the nose, however, is thick and firmly bound down to the underlying tissue so that it neither swells nor readily permits subcutaneous blood to be seen. Consequently, the continuity of lid ecchymosis is not apparent, which may lead to the mistaken interpretation that a second independent hemorrhage has occurred on the opposite side. In any event, anchorage of the fascia prevents the hemorrhage from spreading above the eyebrow, into the cheek, or inferiorly into the upper lip unless these areas are injured. Generally, the hemorrhage and edema resorb without complication or permanent residua in two to three weeks.

A blunt force may also rupture or tear the lids and surrounding soft tissues by compressing them between the offending object and the underlying bone. The resultant wound can resemble one inflicted by a sharp instrument. A wound of this type, however, has certain features that help to differentiate it from an incision produced by a sharp edge. The lacerated wound always extends down to the bone and is more extensive at its deepest portion than superficially It does not gape and is frequently bridged by attenuated strands of tissue.

If the blunt force is severe enough, one or both of the canthal ligaments may be ruptured or disinserted from their bony attachments. Force of this degree generally produces concomitant bony fractures and often considerable damage to the globe. Injury to the canthal ligaments is manifested by distortion of the lids and deformity of the palpebral fissure. The latter is generally shortened and is usually pulled downward by scarring. Involvement of the inner canthus is often associated with injury to the lacrimal passages and generally interferes with the apposition of the lower lid to the globe; both conditions result in tearing. Similarly, traumatic ptosis (drooping upper lid) may follow a concussive injury of the orbital rim. This results from damage either to the tendon of the levator palpebrae superioris or to the palpebral branch of the oculomotor nerve, which innervates the muscle.

Penetrating wounds of the lid are common and may be produced by a large variety of sharp instruments. A lesion of this type may be superficial and involve only an abrasion of the skin. Even such superficial injuries often are accompanied by much edema and hemorrhage that make them appear serious. Generally, however, they are relatively unimportant and heal rapidly without sequelae.

Incised wounds of the lid vary in clinical significance, depending largely on their direction, depth, and location. Horizontal cuts in the lid usually do not gape, while vertical incisions, which sever the orbicularis muscle fibers transversely, gape widely and bleed profusely. Division of the tendon of the levator palpebrae superioris produces complete ptosis. Involvement of the lid margin may be followed by its distortion, causing entropion and trichiasis, or by the formation of a coloboma. The latter is disfiguring and is of particular concern in the more severe injuries of this type when a portion of the lid is amputated. Subsequent exposure of the cornea then becomes the paramount problem.

Puncture or stab wounds are usually of far less importance to the lids and their function. The major concern here must be the involvement of deeper structures, including the cranial contents. Lacerated wounds are of considerably greater significance. As already noted, this type of injury may follow a severe contusion in which the tissues are ruptured when they are suddenly compressed between the causal agent and the underlying bone. The same type of ragged wound may be produced when a blunt object is driven into the tissues with sufficient force to perforate them. There is extensive tearing of tissues, and because of the magnitude of the forces involved, there is often major injury to the globe or the orbital tissues.

All forms of penetrating injuries of the lid may be complicated by infection. This may delay healing, produce extensive cicatricial deformities of the lid, and progress to produce orbital cellulitis or even intracranial involvement. Fortunately, the rich vascular supply of the area offers considerable protection and accounts for the relative infrequency of serious infection and its favorable response to therapy.

Lacrimal Gland and Duct Injuries

Damage to the lacrimal gland itself following blunt trauma to the orbital area is rare. Most such injuries occur in children in whom the superior and lateral portions of the orbital rim are not fully developed. Among such injuries, the most common presentation is dislocation of the gland with prolapse into the tissues of the upper lid. The palpable mass is freely movable in the superior and lateral direction from which it originated and generally may be repositioned without difficulty.

Disturbance of the lacrimal passages is a much more common occurrence and may follow blunt trauma. Avulsion of the medial palpebral ligament with deformation of the lids at the inner canthus may result in sufficient displacement of the punctum to interfere with the drainage of tears through the canalicular system. In more severe injuries in which the lids themselves are torn or avulsed, the lacrimal drainage apparatus, particularly the canaliculi, may be torn or severed. This is encountered most frequently in incisional types of injuries involving the medial portion of the lower lid (Fig. 3–III–2). The lacrimal passages are transected, the ends remain separated in the ensuing scar tissue, and the continuity of the tubular channel is permanently interrupted. The result is excessive tearing, at times accompanied by chronic infective dacryocystitis.

Conjunctiva

The conjunctiva is a thin, transparent mucous membrane that forms a continuous layer lining the posterior surface of the lids and covering the anterior scleral portion of the globe. Although all parts of the conjunctiva are continuous, the portion that lines the lids is called the palpebral conjunctiva, while the portion covering the anterior sclera is called the bulbar conjunctiva. The intermediate portion, which forms the limit of the conjunctival sac

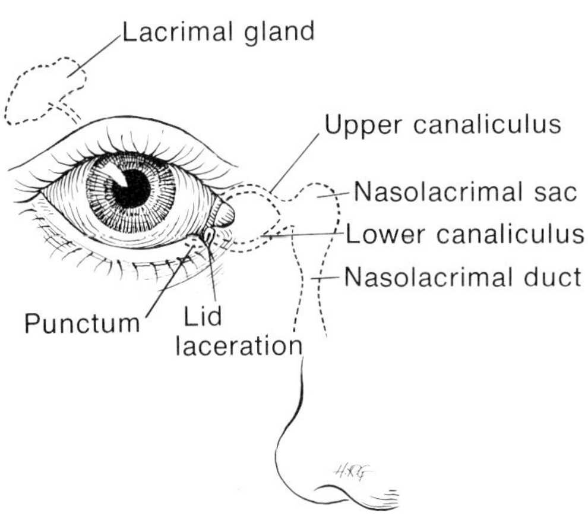

Figure 3–III–2. Incisional injury of the medial portion of the lower lid transecting the lower canaliculus.

where the tissue is reflected from the lids onto the globe, is referred to as the fornix. The conjunctiva overlying the tarsal plates is thin, transparent, and very vascular, the latter characteristic imparting the normal reddish color to the area. This conjunctiva is firmly adherent to the tarsus; it is almost impossible to separate the two by dissection. Therefore, gaps in the palpebral conjunctiva produced by injury cannot be repaired simply by dissecting neighboring flaps and drawing them over the bare area. The bulbar conjunctiva is also very thin and is so transparent that the white sclera readily shows through it, giving rise to the term "the white of the eye." In contrast to the conjunctiva lining the tarsal plates, it is very loosely connected to the underlying tissues.

Goblet cells, true unicellular mucous glands, are present in all portions of the conjunctiva but are most numerous in the fornix.They are of major importance for proper moistening and protection of the conjunctiva and cornea; their destruction through injury or disease leads to desiccation of both tissues. The conjunctiva also contains accessory lacrimal glands responsible for much of basal tear production.

The effect of blunt trauma upon the conjunctiva is highly predictable from the structure of the tissue. Since it is thin, loosely attached to the underlying globe, and very fragile (particularly its vascular component), hemorrhages are common after contusions. These hemorrhages vary in size from small petechiae to relatively large extravasations. The great majority involve the bulbar conjunctiva, because the connective tissue loosely attaching it to the globe provides adequate space for the blood. The more secure attachment of the palpebral conjunctiva to the tarsus of the lid provides significant resistance to dissection by blood.

Regardless of its location beneath the bulbar conjunctiva, the blood tends to migrate toward the limbus. Following local trauma, the blood is initially bright red in color but gradually changes to orange and yellow with the metabolic breakdown of hemoglobin. A subconjunctival hemorrhage often causes the patient considerable apprehension because of the disfigurement it produces, but it almost invariably resorbs in a centripetal direction over approximately a two-week period, leaving no sequelae.

Blood may also seep under the bulbar conjunctiva following a fracture of one of the bones of the orbit or a fracture of the base of the skull. This can often be distinguished from a subconjunctival hemorrhage of local origin because it does not appear until 12 to 24 hours after injury and it is purple from the outset. Moreover, when the hemorrhage is due to a fracture, it is densest and most extensive posteriorly and no posterior edge is clinically discernible; anteriorly, it may not reach the limbus. In all but the most extensive hemorrhages of conjunctival origin, the densest area lies next to the limbus and the color tends to fade or disappear posteriorly.

Blunt trauma may produce hyperemia and translucent swelling of the conjunctiva. In the bulbar portion, the laxity of the subconjunctival tissue permits the accumulation of serum transudate. The tissue may bulge considerably, overriding the peripheral cornea, and in the more severe cases may protrude between the lids. This condition is called chemosis. If the traumatic event produces an abnormal communication between the nasal cavity or the accessory sinuses and the orbit, the subconjunctival tissue and the subcutaneous tissues of the lid become distended by air (emphysema). The bulbar conjunctiva then may balloon out in a manner resembling chemosis, but its emphysematous nature may be distinguished by crepitus on pressure. Finally, the conjunctiva may be bruised and even lacerated by direct blunt impact, but the thinness and mobility of the tissue prevent most such injuries from being extensive.

Perforating wounds of the conjunctiva tend to bleed freely because the tissue is heavily vascularized. This invariably causes a degree of alarm well out of proportion to the volume of blood involved. Despite their frightening appearance, wounds of the conjunctiva are in themselves generally trivial. They are relatively asymptomatic and usually heal rapidly without complication. Abrasions of the conjunctiva are quite rare, since the tissue is loosely attached to the underlying sclera and moves away from a minor impact. Most injuries are therefore caused by sharp objects and are incisional in nature. They are generally associated with a considerable amount of ecchymosis and either sub- or intraconjunctival edema as described for contusions. When the wound edges are relatively close, the lesion tends to heal rapidly, but large, ragged, and irregular conjunctival wounds may be followed by a significant degree of cicatricial tissue or by cyst formation if they are neglected.

Cornea

The cornea is an avascular and transparent structure that functions as the major optical element of the eye. It consists largely of connective tissue and forms approximately the anterior one fifth of the eye.

Structure of the Cornea

Microscopically, the cornea is composed of five layers (Fig. 3–III–3). From anterior to posterior they are: the epithelium, Bowman's membrane, the substantia propria or stroma, Descemet's membrane, and the endothelium.

The epithelium lines the corneal surface. It is only 100 μ or less in thickness and consists of about five layers of stratified, nonkeratinized epithelium. It is heavily innervated by the ophthalmic branch of the fifth cranial nerve, contains many free nerve endings, and is exquisitely sensitive to pain. The corneal epithelium regenerates rapidly and replaces itself without scar formation following injury.

Bowman's membrane lies beneath the epithelium and consists of modified substantia propria. It is thin (about 12 μ) and appears structureless under the light microscope. There are no firm attachments between it and the epithelium, and the two layers may be mechanically separated without difficulty. The anterior surface of Bowman's membrane is parallel to the corneal surface, accounting for the frequent difficulty in visualizing epithelial defects without the aid of a diagnostic stain. Destruction of Bowman's membrane is not followed by regeneration of the structure; the epithelium fills in the defect directly.

Approximately 90 per cent of the cornea is made up by the substantia propria. This layer is composed of transparent, modified connective tissue, arranged in lamellae, and contains cellular elements that lie between the lamellae. Each of the roughly 60 lamellae, in turn, consists of a broad band of fibrils that runs the entire length of the cornea parallel to its surface.

Descemet's membrane is a strong, thin (approximately 6 μ), structureless membrane lying posterior to the substantia propria. Unlike Bowman's membrane, it is sharply defined from the corneal stroma, and if destroyed, can be re-formed, presumably by the corneal endothelium. Though not composed of true elastic tissue, if wounded, it tends to gape, and the cut edges tend to curl up.

The endothelium is a monolayer of hexagonal cells arranged along the inner surface of Descemet's membrane. These cells are fragile, very susceptible to injury, and have limited regenerative capacity. The highly critical physiologic control of corneal hydration is largely situated in this layer. Normally, the cornea tends to imbibe water and swell, the result of a negative

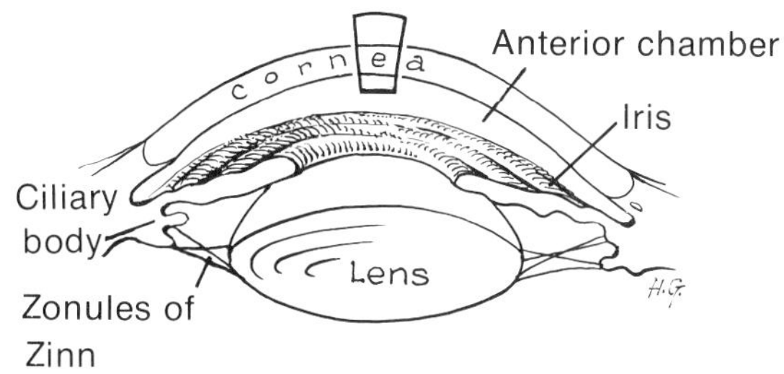

A

Figure 3–III–3. *A*. Anatomy of the anterior segment of the eye. Microscopic anatomy of the cornea.

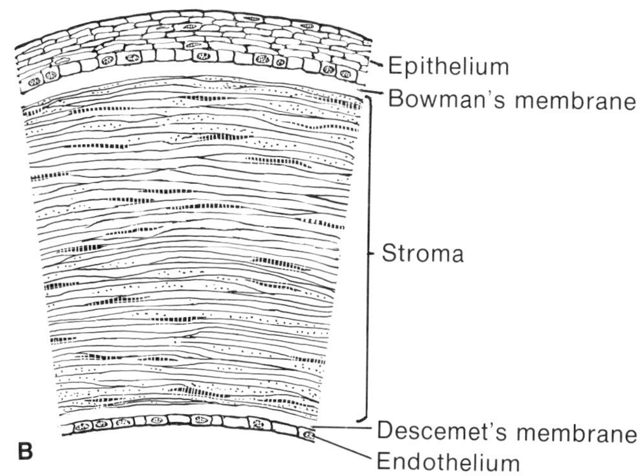

B

pressure present within the stroma and referred to as the swelling pressure. Excess fluid in the stroma disrupts the spatial correlation between fibrils, causing a dispersion of light, which in turn produces a loss in the transparency of the tissue. Similarly, edema of the corneal epithelium causes a significant degree of light scattering, which also interferes greatly with image formation. In the normal situation, the swelling pressure of the cornea is counteracted by the endothelium, where fluid is actively transported out of the tissue. This process requires metabolic energy to produce the state of relative deturgescence necessary for corneal transparency. Loss of endothelial cell function through injury or disease therefore results in edema of the corneal epithelium and stroma, a decrease in corneal transparency, and a visual deficit. In addition, the endothelium appears to act as a partial physical barrier preventing aqueous humor from entering the cornea. Disruption of this layer decreases the effectiveness of the barrier, contributes to the degree of corneal edema and clouding, and so adds to the severity of visual loss.

Blunt Injury of the Cornea

Blunt force may injure the superficial cornea directly, producing an abrasion of the corneal epithelium and edema of the underlying anterior stroma. Disruption of the anterior corneal surface produces a temporary decrease in visual acuity. The rapidly regenerating epithelium generally heals within a day or two, however, and the edema clears shortly thereafter, leaving no permanent residua.

More frequently, blunt force distorts the cornea and produces adverse effects deep in the tissue. This type of compression trauma may injure the cornea at birth. It presents as a diffuse, steamy opacity of the corneal stroma, the result of edema, and generally clears in approximately one week. More severe compression injuries of this type produce ruptures in Descemet's membrane. This again may result in opacification of the cornea at birth, but ultimately the tissue regains its transparency; multiple gray, translucent opacities are then discernible deep in the cornea. The opacities are generally linear and variable in number.

Each one is associated with a tear in Descemet's membrane, which is seen with the slit-lamp biomicroscope as a double contoured linear streak made up of two bright lines with a dark space between them. Often bright reflexes are noted at the sides of each linear opacity, indicating that the torn edge of Descemet's membrane has curled up in a spiral form, a reflection of the membrane's elasticity. Alternatively, if the break in Descemet's membrane is extensive enough, a portion of the torn edge may float freely in the anterior chamber. The membrane's tendency to curl generally precludes healing. Nonetheless, when the injury occurs at birth, the endothelium tends to cover the area devoid of Descemet's membrane. Often it secretes a hyalinelike material, producing a new Descemet's membrane and in some areas a reduplication of Descemet's membrane. A retrocorneal membrane has also been reported after this type of birth trauma.

In the adult, all corneal layers usually remain structurally intact following blunt trauma, and no morphologic damage is evident with the biomicroscope. Nonetheless, edematous changes are evident within the stroma, typically as a disk-shaped gray opacity. Though the cause has not been fully substantiated, the lesion appears to be due to a temporary disturbance of the corneal endothelial cells by the concussion and subsequent distortion of the cornea. It is not clear whether the physical barrier presented by the endothelial layer is disrupted so that aqueous humor is more freely able to percolate into the cornea or whether the endothelial cells are less able to pump water from the stroma. In any event, the edema generally clears without specific therapy in a variable period of time.

If the blunt force causing the injury is of sufficient magnitude, it produces a more severe injury, again manifested by tears in Descemet's membrane and interruption in the continuity of the endothelial layer in the involved area. This, in turn, is associated with more extensive edema of the corneal stroma, the lesion being larger and denser. Here again, the corneal opacity tends to clear without specific therapy after the residual endothelial cells enlarge to cover those areas devoid of endothelium and effect resorption of the edema fluid. In the most severe injuries of this type, however, the degree of structural damage is beyond the reparative capability of the endothelium. Permanent edema, scarring, and opacification of the cornea ensue.

Multiple tiny, golden-brown deposits may, with the aid of the biomicroscope, be seen to lie on the endothelium after blunt trauma. These deposits are derived from the pigmented epithelium of the iris. The pigment is dislodged from the iris in the traumatic episode and carried by the circulating aqueous humor into the anterior chamber where it is deposited diffusely and irregularly over the posterior corneal surface. It generally produces no corneal injury or visual loss in and of itself and may diminish with time.

When a considerable blunt force is applied directly to the cornea itself, the indentation of the cornea may be so great that the tissue may be lacerated. The laceration may involve the stroma, Descemet's membrane, and the endothelium while the epithelium and Bowman's

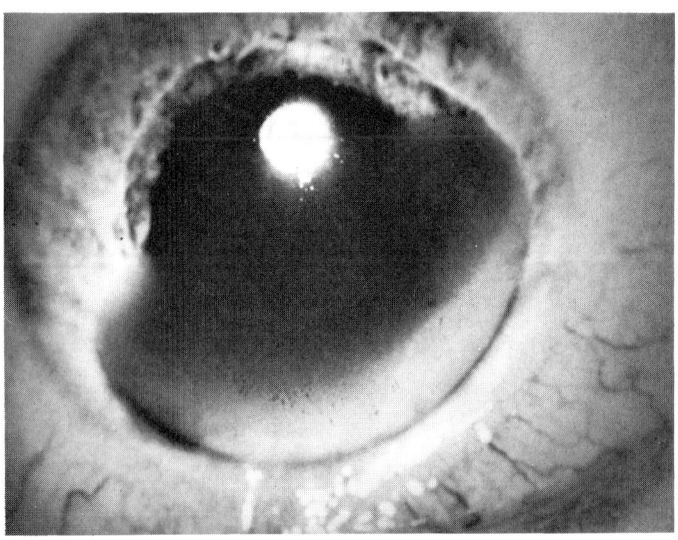

Figure 3–III–4. Bloodstaining of the cornea.

membrane remain intact, or complete rupture of the cornea may occur. In the latter instance, the force involved and the extreme elevation in intraocular pressure that it generates make prolapse of intraocular tissue an invariable occurrence. Fortunately, such injuries are rare.

A most dramatic result of blunt ocular trauma is bloodstaining of the cornea (Fig. 3–III–4). This occurs when the contusion has produced bleeding into the anterior chamber (hyphema) as described subsequently. The anterior chamber must be largely or wholly filled with blood, and concomitant elevation of the intraocular pressure seems to be a prerequisite. The metabolic breakdown products of hemoglobin appear to be driven through a compromised endothelium by the increased intraocular pressure. The opacity tends to involve most of the corneal area. It is initially a rusty brown, but with time it changes to greenish yellow. Over an extended period of time, minimally several months but most often on the order of several years, it tends to resorb, often leaving a clear cornea. Histologically, the staining material has been shown to vary. Large amorphous masses of pigmented granules as well as minute round, oval, or rod-shaped highly refractile bodies have been observed between the stromal lamellae. The latter form has also been noted between the basal epithelial cells and Bowman's membrane, while pigmented granules have been reported within the keratocytes. The full thickness of the corneal stroma appears to be involved. Good visual acuity may eventually be recovered if the original injury has not produced intractable glaucoma or seriously damaged other parts of the eye. Poor vision for a period of years while the corneal opacity is clearing may produce strabismus, and if the injury occurs in a child before the age of five or six, it may cause irreversible amblyopia.

Wounds of the Cornea

Incisional wounds of the cornea may be nonperforating or perforating. Nonperforating incisional wounds may in turn be superficial or deep. Several types of causal factors are capable of causing incisional corneal injuries, each producing a characteristic type of wound. A sharp edge or object will produce a clean, well-defined cut. A small foreign body traveling with great speed may cause a minute perforation. A blunt object striking the area with great force will produce a contused and jagged laceration, while a relatively large projectile traveling at high velocity may produce a shattering wound.

Nonperforating Wounds. It is important to divide nonperforating corneal wounds into superficial and deep types. This separation is important because corneal epithelium regenerates rapidly without the formation of scar tissue. A wound involving the epithelium only, therefore, heals with no permanent disruption of the optical transparency of the cornea. A wound of the corneal stroma, on the other hand, forms scar tissue, which is translucent and interferes with the ability of the cornea to form an optical image upon the retina (Fig. 3–III–5). A wound of the corneal stroma therefore produces a permanent deficit in visual acuity if it is central in location.

A superficial wound of the cornea, termed a corneal abrasion, is essentially a traumatic scraping of the epithelial layer from the underlying Bowman's membrane. That membrane and the remainder of the cornea are intact and uninjured. Many types of minor trauma are capable of producing a corneal abrasion. These include injury from a fingernail, from the edge of a piece of paper, from a small foreign body under the upper eyelid, and from improper manipulation or wear of contact lenses.

The cornea has very extensive sensory innervation, accounting for the extreme severity of clinical symptoms produced by a relatively minor injury. A corneal abrasion results in exposure of the sensory nerve endings, causing acute pain, photophobia, lacrimation, and blepharospasm, all of which begin promptly after the injury. Examination reveals injection of the deep perilimbal vessels, bilateral tearing, and

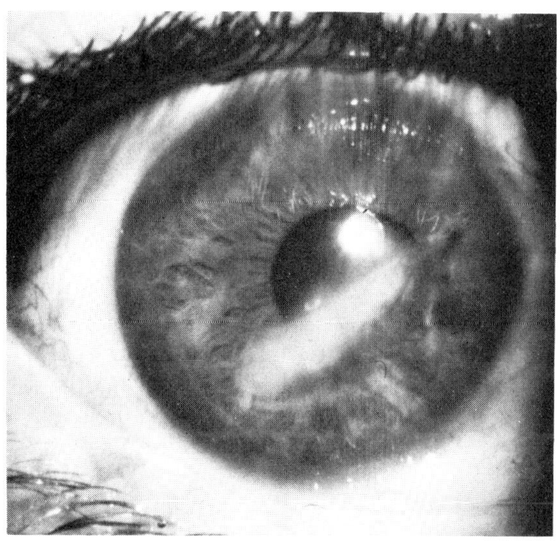

Figure 3–III–5. Corneal scar following a perforating wound of the cornea.

often reflex miosis in the involved eye. The transparency of the tissue and the superficial nature of the lesion often combine to make the abrasion difficult to discern, but it may be delineated by the topical application of fluorescein. The dye does not adhere to the normal corneal surface but stains any area devoid of epithelial cells a brilliant green color, particularly if the eye is examined with cobalt blue light, which causes the dye to fluoresce. The epithelium regenerates rapidly, and a small abrasion may be completely healed within 12 hours; a cornea completely denuded of epithelium will generally reepithelialize completely in approximately three days.

The corneal epithelium acts as a very effective barrier against invasion by microorganisms; an abrasion, however, provides a ready portal of entry for microorganisms that may be introduced by the traumatic agent or that are already present in the conjunctival sac. Therefore, although the injury itself is relatively minor, it offers a great potential for secondary corneal infection (Fig. 3–III–6).

A traumatic corneal abrasion may be followed by an entity called recurrent erosion of the cornea. The original abrasion is generally fairly minor and heals without complication. Sometime thereafter, generally on the order of weeks to months, the patient suddenly experiences the acute onset of pain, photophobia, lacrimation, and blepharospasm, the same symptoms that characterized the original abrasion. The same eye is invariably involved, and the symptoms characteristically occur immediately upon awakening. These may disappear spontaneously within an hour or persist up to 24 to 36 hours. In those cases in which the symptoms rapidly terminate, the eye may be free from abnormality by the time the patient is examined by his ophthalmologist. In those patients whose symptoms persist, examination may reveal injection of the deep perilimbal vessels and either an area of the cornea in which the epithelium is raised and gray or an area devoid of epithelium. The site of the recurrent lesion is generally but not invariably the same as that of the original injury.

The entity is presumably due to an injury of the basement membrane of the corneal epithelium at the time of the original injury. As a result, although the epithelium regenerates rapidly and appears to heal, it adheres very poorly to the underlying tissue. During sleep, tear flow is normally diminished and the relative drying of the conjunctiva allows the palpebral conjunctiva of the closed lid to adhere to the underlying corneal epithelium. This degree of adherence normally causes no difficulty, but when the attachment of the corneal epithelium to the underlying structure is abnormal, the epithelium may be torn from the cornea, accounting for the characteristic onset of symptoms immediately upon awakening. Intermittent recurrences may continue to take place at varying intervals for years, usually at the same site but, again, by no means invariably.

Because of the extreme thinness of the cornea (it is approximately 0.5 mm thick at its center and approximately 1.0 mm thick at its extreme periphery), nonperforating corneal wounds involving the deep stroma are relatively rare. When they occur, they may be caused by a sharp instrument producing a clean in-

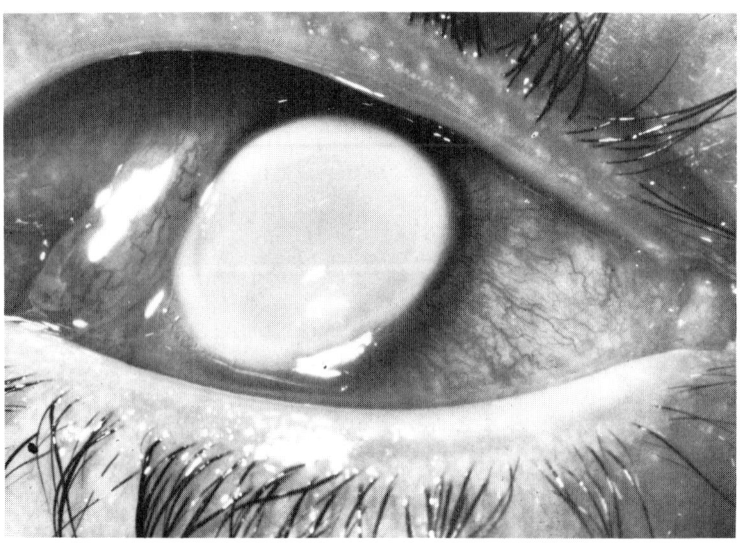

Figure 3–III–6. Fungal (aspergillus) infection involving the entire cornea following a minor abrasion of the corneal epithelium by a mascara brush.

cision, or by a pointed object producing a nonperforating puncture. Flying foreign bodies, such as glass from broken spectacles, have been known to cause this type of injury. A significant proportion of these injuries result from an object striking the cornea tangentially, producing a flat type of wound or actually excising part of the thickness of a portion of the cornea. Clinically, the symptoms of this type of injury generally are the same as those described for an abrasion, namely pain, photophobia, lacrimation, and blepharospasm. Examination reveals a break in the epithelium, which may be limited to the site of entry of the wound or may be more extensive. The corneal stroma bordering the incisional wound is swollen and gray, having lost its transparency because of imbibition of fluid. If it is a clean, vertical incision, the edema may cause the wound margins to be tightly apposed, in which case the epithelium will regenerate and the wound will tend to heal relatively rapidly. With healing, the edema and opacification tend to decrease. In a flap type of wound, the degree of apposition will depend upon the mobility of the flap, but the injured tissue will invariably demonstrate edema and loss of transparency. All such shearing wounds involving the corneal stroma produce some permanent scarring. The effect of the translucent scar tissue upon vision will depend upon the density of the scar and upon its location. A relatively lucent scar in the center of the cornea may produce profound visual loss, while a much more dense and severe scar in the corneal periphery may have no effect at all upon vision.

Significant complications following this type of injury include infection and irregular astigmatism. In the former, microorganisms gain entry, via the wound, deep into the corneal stroma where they can devastate the tissue. The latter problem, even if the wound heals without incident, is capable of deforming the tissue, permanently interfering with its optical performance.

Perforating Wounds. Perforating wounds of the cornea are relatively common. Because such injuries have numerous causes, the types of wounds encountered are varied. Incisional and puncture wounds are the most common and show great variability in size. Regardless of size, however, any such wound represents an emergency; prompt restoration of the integrity of the globe must be accomplished if further disorganization of intraocular contents and introduction of infecting agents are to be avoided.

Perforating corneal wounds may be simple, that is, their edges may be well apposed without intraocular contents interposed between them, or they may be complicated. In the case of the simple wound, fluid is imbibed through the cut surfaces, causing the wound edges to swell. This, coupled with an outpouring of fibrinous exudative material, tends to maintain the wound edges in apposition and may permit partial re-formation of the anterior chamber even before the appropriate therapeutic measures are initiated. If the traumatic incident has not injured intraocular structures, the situation is compatible with a favorable visual outcome.

More frequently, the perforating corneal wound is a complicated one. The edges of the wound are in faulty apposition; they overlap considerably or they gape widely. One or more of the intraocular tissues are incarcerated between the lips of the wound, carried there at the time of perforation by the rush of escaping aqueous humor. Left to its own devices, the incarcerated tissue consolidates with the fibrovascular mass generated by the healing processes to form a dense, opaque mass, an adherent leukoma. This will produce mechanical closure of the wound but may lead to secondary glaucoma and chronic irritability of the injured eye.

Incarceration of the iris is most commonly encountered. The tissue either may be caught in the posterior part of the wound to form an anterior synechia or may protrude through the wound as a prolapse of the iris (Fig. 3–III–7). Less commonly, portions of the crystalline lens may be incarcerated in the wound, an event that is invariably associated with prolapse of the iris. Cataract formation results, and the lenticular material may initiate a violent inflammatory

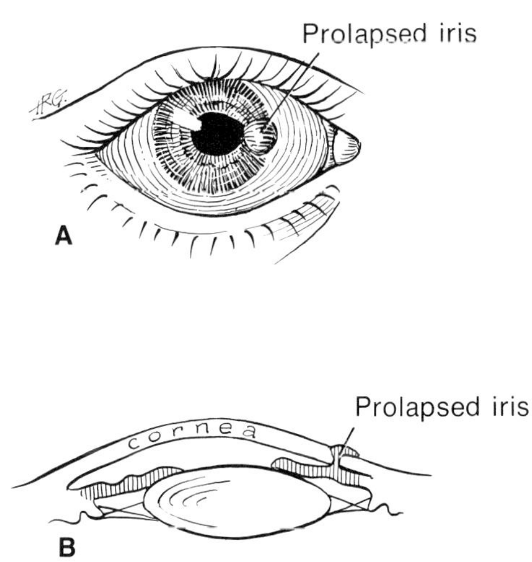

Figure 3–III–7. Prolapse of iris tissue through perforating wound in cornea.

reaction. Similarly, the vitreous humor may be incarcerated in the wound and contribute to an inflammatory response similar to that caused by lens material. Finally, in the most extensive injuries, the ciliary body, the choroid, and the retina may become incarcerated in the wound or prolapse out of the globe.

Incarceration or prolapse of intraocular structures leads to further complications. When wound apposition or healing is delayed, corneal or conjunctival epithelium may proliferate through the wound into the anterior chamber, a condition called epithelialization of the anterior chamber. These cells actively multiply on the posterior corneal surface, and the process may continue so that a sheet of epithelial cells lines the angle of the anterior chamber and the anterior and posterior surfaces of the iris as well as the surface of the ciliary body and lens. Uveitis and secondary glaucoma result, and most such eyes are irretrievable. If the posterior portions of the corneal wound are malapposed, particularly if endothelial damage at the borders of the wound has been extensive, an overgrowth of regenerating fibrous tissue into the anterior chamber may ensue, producing a retrocorneal membrane.

In an extensive wound with gaping edges, complicated by incarceration of uveal tissue, an ectatic scar called a staphyloma may result. Initially, the staphyloma is composed merely of prolapsed iris covered by epithelium. The epithelium thickens, and inflammation of the iris results in the formation of granulation tissue on its surface. This gradually develops into scar tissue, merging with similar tissue derived from the cornea and remnants of lens. With time the iris stroma gradually atrophies and is replaced by fibrous tissue. The thickness of the staphyloma and therefore the degree of ectasia vary with the amount of scar tissue formed.

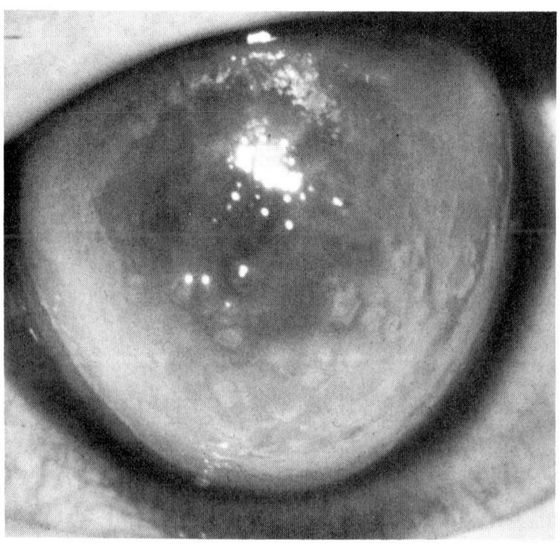

Figure 3–III–8. Bullous keratopathy—edema of the corneal epithelium and stroma with blister-like structures (bullae) in the corneal epithelium.

These complications may irreversibly injure the corneal endothelium. This is especially true of anterior synechiae, prolapse of the lens or vitreous, epithelialization of the anterior chamber, and formation of a retrocorneal membrane; all mechanically destroy endothelial cells and produce edema of the corneal epithelium and stroma. In the more severe cases, the intact edematous epithelium is lifted up from Bowman's membrane, forming blister-like structures called bullae. From time to time, bullae rupture, exposing free nerve endings; the entity, called bullous keratopathy, is therefore quite painful (Fig. 3–III–8).

Sclera

The sclera forms approximately 80 per cent of the eye's outer coat. It is a relatively avascular, white, fibrous material composed of interdigitating fibers of collagen, interspersed by a ground substance containing mucopolysaccharides, which supports and protects the vital inner structures of the eye. Scleral thickness varies considerably in different eyes and in different parts of the same eye. From the corneoscleral junction to the insertion of the rectus muscles, its thickness is approximately 0.6 mm. Posterior to the insertion of the recti, it thins to 0.3 mm and gradually increases to a thickness of 1 mm posteriorly.

Ruptures of the sclera may be divided into two types: contusion ruptures due to direct impingement of a slowly moving blunt force upon the globe; and concussion ruptures due to passage of a high-velocity missile through the orbit, producing concussion waves with sufficient energy to burst the globe. These ruptures are almost always accompanied by severe injury and disorganization of internal ocular structures. While a direct rupture of the sclera may occur, with the tissue giving way at the point of impact, such injuries are rare. They are caused only by blunt objects small enough to enter the bony orbit and strike the globe directly. In such intances the globe is forced backward in the orbit, where it is cushioned by the orbital fat. The force of the blow is largely dissipated by the soft tissue mass, which accounts for the rarity of the lesion.

In contrast, an indirect scleral rupture occurs relatively commonly following severe contusions of the globe. Usually it is caused by a large blunt object traveling obliquely so that, at least in part, it is driven between the globe and the orbital wall. The globe is therefore forced sideways against the orbital wall. The most common site of impact is the inferotemporal part of the globe where it is least protected by the orbital rim. The typical rupture is concentric to the limbus and, within the globe, begins at the extreme periphery of the anterior chamber. It travels posteriorly through the sclera and surfaces 2 to 4 mm behind the limbus. This is due to the greater strength of the sclera anteriorly and the support provided by the insertion of the extraocular muscles posteriorly. In the great majority of cases, it occurs opposite the point of impact and is therefore located in the upper nasal quadrant.

Clinically, scleral ruptures are accompanied by bruised and edematous lids, subconjunctival and intraocular hemorrhage, and disruption of intraocular structures. The latter may also prolapse through the break in the sclera. Injuries of this type are more apt to occur in older patients with less resilient sclerae, in patients with uncontrolled glaucoma, and in patients with collagen diseases, such as rheumatoid arthritis, which produce scleral thinning and ectasia. The prognosis for the ruptured globe is poor. Intraocular infection is of immediate concern, and secondary glaucoma, traumatic uveitis, retinal detachment, and sympathetic ophthalmia are among the complications that may be encountered. Proliferation of fibrous tissue in the posterior segment of the globe and phthisis bulbi due to failure of normal aqueous humor production may ultimately destroy the eye.

Perforating scleral injuries produced by a sharp object may be followed by rapid and uncomplicated healing if the wound is clean and has well-apposed edges. If uveal and retinal tissues are incarcerated in it, however, complications often occur. Even if the wound is surgically repaired, the uvea may be infiltrated by inflammatory cells and fibroblasts. A mass of granulation tissue fills the wound, and the retina frequently is incorporated into the scar tissue. Retinal detachment can occur, particularly if vitreous humor prolapses and is lost through the wound. The vitreous humor subsequently contracts and produces sufficient traction on the retina to detach it. Finally, neovascularization can occur at the site of injury, with proliferation of new vessels anteriorly to the ciliary body and posteriorly to the optic disk. Massive retinal detachment and phthisis bulbi follow.

Anterior Chamber

The anterior chamber is a fluid-filled space bounded anteriorly by the cornea and at its extreme periphery by sclera, and posteriorly by the iris, by a part of the ciliary body, and by that portion of the anterior lens surface that presents at the pupillary aperture. The extreme periphery of the anterior chamber is called the angle and contains the trabecular meshwork and the canal of Schlemm. The trabecular meshwork is composed of fenestrated collagen bundles whose pores permit the intraocular fluid, the aqueous humor, to flow from the anterior chamber into the canal of Schlemm, a circular channel lying in the fibrous tissue of the corneoscleral junction (Fig. 3–III–9). From here the aqueous humor gains access to the general circulation via the aqueous and anterior ciliary veins.

It is generally agreed that the aqueous humor is a dialysate of plasma that is produced by the epithelium of the ciliary body and enters the eye in the posterior chamber. The latter is a triangular-shaped space, of which the apex is formed by the pupillary portion of the iris resting on the anterior lens, and the base by the ciliary processes and the valleys between them. It is limited anteriorly by the iris and posteriorly by the lens and its suspensory ligament. Like the anterior chamber, it is filled with aqueous humor, which normally flows between the posterior iris border and the lens, through the pupillary opening, and into the anterior chamber.

Secondary Glaucoma

Trauma to the anterior chamber per se produces ocular morbidity and loss of function primarily as a result of secondary glaucoma. Glaucoma is an entity wherein the intraocular pressure is abnormally elevated. This results in ischemia and atrophy of the optic nerve, with progressive irreversible loss of visual field. As noted, the aqueous humor circulates from the posterior chamber where it originates, through the pupil, and into the anterior chamber, it percolates through the trabecular meshwork into the canal of Schlemm to leave the eye as shown in Figure 3–III–9. Since the eye is a closed system, the level of intraocular pressure is a function of two variables, the rate of production of aqueous humor and its rate of egress from the eye.

Elevations in intraocular pressure (normal range, up to 23 mm of mercury) occur as the result of a variety of mechanisms. Regardless of

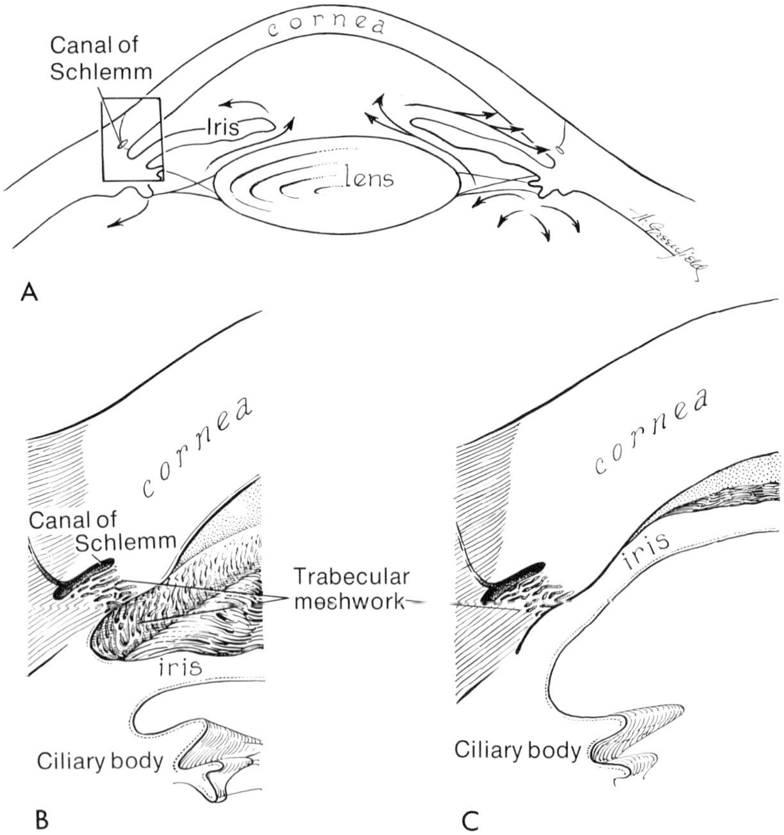

Figure 3–III–9. *A.* Diagram of the normal circulation of the aqueous humor. *B.* Anatomy of the angle of the anterior chamber. *C.* Obstruction of aqueous outflow caused by apposition of the peripheral iris to the trabecular meshwork.

the specific mechanism involved, all types of traumatic glaucoma have as their common denominator an obstruction to aqueous outflow. A continued secretion of aqueous humor into the posterior chamber coupled with a blocked outflow facility results in increased intraocular pressure. This outflow block can occur in one of the following three ways or a combination thereof: (1) Direct trauma to the angle structures and subsequent fibrosis interfere with aqueous flow into the canal of Schlemm. (2) Traumatic debris of any nature (e.g., lens material, pigment, inflammatory cells) blocks the trabecular pores, impairing aqueous outflow. (3) Pupillary block can occur. The pupillary margin of the iris lies adjacent to or in contact with the anterior lens capsule. In the latter instance only a potential space exists between the two structures. Nonetheless, under normal circumstances, aqueous humor is able to pass from the posterior to the anterior chamber. Any condition producing a greater approximation or adherence of the iris to the lens causes an increased resistance to aqueous flow between the two chambers. This, in turn, creates a pressure differential between the posterior and anterior chambers; aqueous humor continues to be produced in the posterior chamber, and since it is unable to escape, it increases the pressure there. The resultant force moves the peripheral iris against the trabecular meshwork, creating a direct block to aqueous outflow, and the "closed" angle causes a precipitous rise in intraocular pressure (see Fig. 3–III–9*C*). This is a surgical emergency, and appropriate therapy permits the iris to fall back to its former position. The angle "opens," normal aqueous outflow ensues, and the intraocular pressure drops to a normal level. If pupillary block is not broken within a reasonable period, the peripheral iris permanently adheres to the trabecular meshwork. This is called a peripheral anterior synechia, and functionally the involved part of the angle is permanently destroyed.

Severe blunt ocular trauma may be followed by a period of elevated intraocular pressure. This may occur in the absence of blood in the anterior chamber, but pigment or cells are almost invariably present in the aqueous humor. If the situation is not complicated by secondary hemorrhage or damage to the structures in the

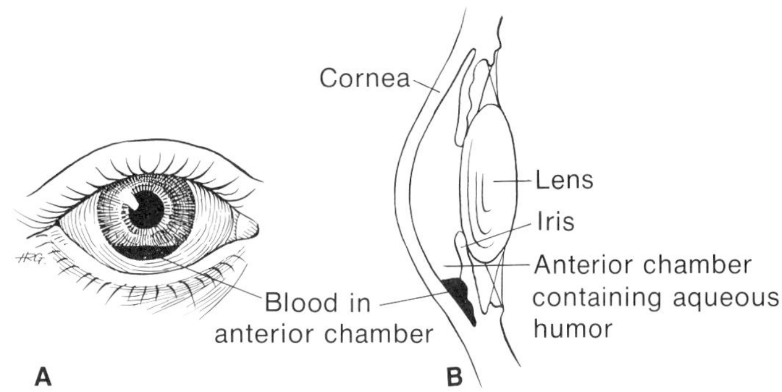

Figure 3–III–10. Hyphema—blood in the anterior chamber. In this instance the blood only partially fills the anterior chamber, producing a grossly discernible fluid level interface with the aqueous humor.

angle of the anterior chamber, then glaucoma of this type can be expected to resolve in one to two weeks.

Hemorrhage

Unfortunately, contusion injuries are frequently complicated by hemorrhage into the anterior chamber (hyphema). Severe bleeding of this type may occur immediately after injury, or its onset may be delayed for as long as a week. Children are more frequently affected than adults. The hemorrhage apparently originates from a ruptured iris vessel, most commonly located in the root of the iris. If the blood does not fill the anterior chamber, it tends to remain a relatively bright red and settles inferiorly, producing a grossly discernible fluid level interface with the aqueous humor (Fig. 3–III–10). The great majority of such hyphemata resorb rapidly, generally in less than one week, without permanent residua. In approximately 20 per cent of cases, however, a secondary hyphema occurs spontaneously, characteristically on the second to fourth day after the original hemorrhage. Frequently, the secondary hyphema is more profuse than the primary one and may fill the entire anterior chamber. It tends to clot and take on a darker hue, appearing almost black and giving rise to the term "eight ball hemorrhage" (Fig. 3–III–11). The large clot in the anterior chamber and the breakdown products of blood and inflammatory debris may combine to obstruct the passage of aqueous humor through the trabecular meshwork, giving rise to severe secondary glaucoma. The situation may be further complicated by bloodstaining of the cornea as described earlier (see Fig. 3–III–4).

A severe contusion of the globe may also damage the angle of the anterior chamber directly, producing a tear in the root of the iris that extends into the ciliary body proper and separates the ciliary muscle from its attachment to the scleral spur. The structural changes may be seen by gonioscopy. There is a retrodisplace-

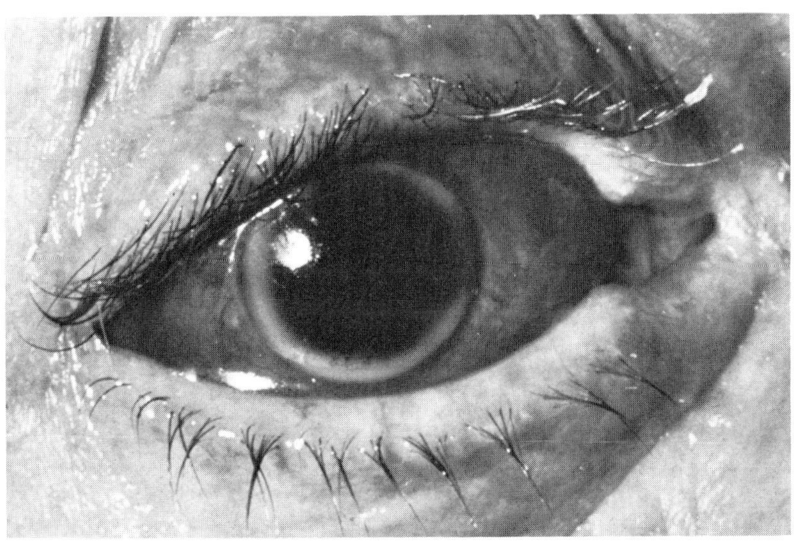

Figure 3–III–11. "Eight ball hemorrhage"—blood fills the entire anterior chamber. The clot appears almost black.

ment of the iris root (angle recession), and often the anterior chamber of the involved eye appears deeper than that of the fellow eye, although this difference is frequently subtle. Angle recession may occur in a small area, or it may be present throughout the entire ocular circumference. The initial appearance of glaucoma following the injury varies, as does its severity, but once established, it tends to be permanent. Two types of glaucoma related to damage of the angle structures are recognized, differentiated by the length of the interval between injury and intraocular pressure elevation. The earlier, more common variety usually develops within days or weeks of the injury; the later, more rare variety has its onset years after the original trauma. The severity of the glaucoma in the early-onset type tends to be directly proportional to the extent of damage to the angle. This relationship does not appear to hold for the late-onset disease. The injury causes the filtration portion of the trabecular meshwork to lose some of its permeability to aqueous humor, largely because of scarring and fibrosis of the structure or the development of a cuticular, avascular membrane covering it, accounting for the rise in intraocular pressure.

As noted previously, perforating wounds of the cornea and sclera are often accompanied by iris prolapse, by incarceration of iris in the wound, or by damage to the lens. Direct injury to these structures is discussed in the following sections. It should, however, be emphasized here that following repair, the iris may remain adherent to the back of the peripheral cornea (peripheral anterior synechia), closing the angle and preventing normal outflow of aqueous humor from the eye (see Fig. 3–III–9). If a sufficient portion of the total circumference is involved, glaucoma results.

Infection and Inflammation

When the integrity of the anterior chamber is lost through perforating trauma, a major concern is intraocular infection. The contents of the globe act as an excellent culture medium, and useful vision is rarely recovered after a bacterial or fungal endophthalmitis. This tragic complication usually becomes manifest during the first 24 or 48 hours after injury. Thereafter, its likelihood of occurring decreases significantly, but sporadic cases with onset several months after injury are on record. Clinically, such eyes are intensely inflamed and painful. They exhibit marked conjunctival injection and chemosis, corneal edema with keratic precipitates, hypopyon, and an increased protein and cellular content of the aqueous humor. Frank pus may drain from the wound.

A severe inflammatory reaction is evident with a marked outpouring of polymorphonuclear leukocytes from the blood vessels of the iris and ciliary processes. Many of the white cells gravitate and settle in the inferior portion of the anterior chamber, forming a grossly visible collection of pus (hypopyon) (Fig. 3–III–12). Necrosis of the inflamed uveal tissue produces a scattering of pigment and cellular debris that floats in the aqueous humor and is eventually phagocytosed by macrophages. Even if the replicating infecting organism is promptly brought under control by antibiotic therapy, the inflammatory response elicited by foreign particles and toxins is capable of irreversibly damaging the delicate ocular structures.

The acute cellular phase of inflammation is often followed by organization of the inflammatory exudate into vascularized connective tissue. Membranes form on the anterior surface of the iris, covering the pupil and frequently binding it to the lens. Cyclitic membranes form along the plane of the anterior vitreous face, their extremities being connected to the ciliary processes. These membranes are tenacious and usually cause total destruction and functional loss of all structures involved.

Other problems complicating penetrating injuries of the anterior chamber are sympathetic ophthalmia and epithelialization of the anterior chamber. These are discussed in other sections of this chapter.

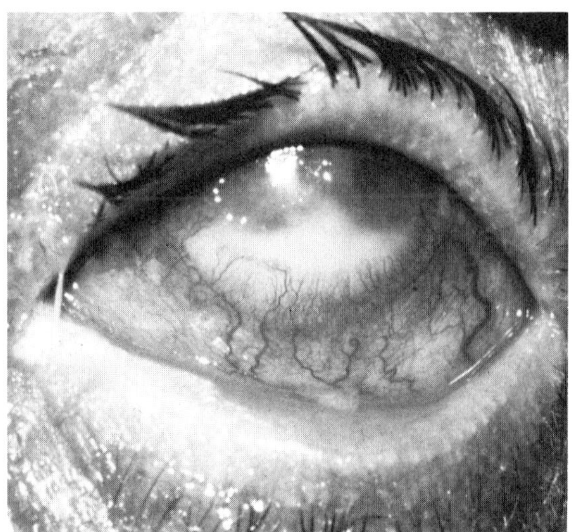

Figure 3–III–12. Hypopyon—pus in the anterior chamber.

Iris and Ciliary Body

Beneath the outer fibrous protective coat of the eye (consisting of the cornea and sclera) lies a highly vascularized layer called the uvea or uveal tract. It consists of three continuous structures, which from posterior to anterior are known as the choroid, ciliary body, and iris. This discussion deals with the anterior portion of the uveal tract, the iris and the ciliary body.

Iris

The iris is a thin circular disk of tissue lying more or less in a frontal plane. It is attached at its periphery or root to the middle of the anterior surface of the ciliary body and is perforated near its center by a circular aperture called the pupil. The size of the pupil varies with the level of light; it constricts in bright light and dilates widely in dim light, thus regulating the amount of light reaching the retina.

The anterior iris surface is characterized by a series of radiating ridges that indicate the position of blood vessels. These lie in the loose connective tissue stroma and form the bulk of the iris. Their course is sinuous to allow for the movements of the iris. At the root of the iris (actually in the anterior ciliary body) and 1 to 2 mm from the pupillary margin, there are circular vascular anastomoses known as the major and the minor arterial circles of the iris respectively. The former is indeed arterial, but the latter contains both arterial and venous elements. These structures are connected by the radial arteries, while the veins unite to form trunks that, along with those of the ciliary body, feed into the venae vorticosae.

In addition to the blood vessels, the vascular iris stroma contains pigment cells, nerves, and a muscle, the sphincter pupillae. The latter is a predominantly circular band of smooth muscle that surrounds the pupil. It receives parasympathetic innervation via the third cranial nerve and the short ciliary nerves, and causes the pupil to constrict. Immediately posterior to the vascular iris stroma is a second sheet of smooth muscle, the dilator pupillae, which is innervated by the sympathetic nervous system via the ciliary nerves, and as its name implies, produces dilatation of the pupil. Finally, the posterior surface of the iris is lined by two layers of heavily pigmented epithelial cells. The anterior of these two layers consists of flat spindle cells; the dilator fibers are processes of these spindle cells that have only partially developed into muscle. The posterior layer consists of large polyhedral or cubical cells that tend to lose their dark brown pigment granules following trauma. The pigment epithelium curls around the pupillary margin of the iris and is grossly evident as a black fringe.

The iris is responsible for the color of the eye. Most newborn Caucasians have blue eyes, because the iris stroma contains little pigment at birth and the darkly pigmented epithelium on the posterior iris surface appears blue through the translucent stroma (in much the same manner that the superficial veins containing dark red blood appear blue through the skin). With time, pigment is deposited in the anterior stroma, and the amount of pigment deposition determines the subsequent color of the eye. If little pigment is deposited, the eye remains blue or gray, while if much pigment is deposited it becomes brown.

Ciliary Body

The ciliary body, the middle portion of the vascular layer, is continuous with the iris periphery anteriorly and the choroid posteriorly. Externally it lies adjacent to the sclera, the potential suprachoroidal space between them, while its internal surface is covered by the pigmented epithelial extension of the retina. Structurally, the ciliary body has three basic parts: the ciliary muscle, the corona ciliaris, and the pars planum. The ciliary muscle lies anteriorly and consists of outer longitudinal fibers, which essentially run in an anterior-posterior direction, and inner circular fibers, which essentially are parallel to the limbus. Both portions are smooth muscle, innervated by the ciliary nerves, and both function to slacken the suspensory ligament of the lens during the process of accommodation. The longitudinal fibers presumably also are involved in control of the pore size of the trabecular meshwork.

The corona ciliaris contains the ciliary processes, about 70 in number, located on the inner surface of the ciliary body. They are irregular folds, approximately 2 mm in length and 0.5 to 1 mm high. The valleys between the ciliary processes give rise to the zonules of Zinn, the suspensory ligaments of the lens. Each process consists essentially of blood vessels embedded in connective tissue. The pars plana of the ciliary body contains a vascular layer much like that of the choroid. It contains no choriocapillaris, however, and with the exception of the cornea, it is the least vascular area of the eye. The internal surface of the ciliary body is lined by two layers of epithelial cells, the outer of which is pigmented and the inner (i.e., that next to the vitreous humor) nonpigmented.

Injuries of Iris and Ciliary Body

Most concussion injuries of the iris result largely from the sudden impact of a pressure wave of aqueous humor being driven backward by the traumatized cornea, thus forcing the iris against the relatively unyielding lens. This affects the various structures of the iris in a detrimental manner, and each responds with a highly individual reaction. The adverse effect of the concussion on the nerves and muscles produces dilatation of the pupil associated with paralysis of accommodation. The functions of the iris and the ciliary muscle are usually simultaneously affected, but occasionally iridoplegia may occur alone. The pupil is moderately dilated, often eccentric, and usually exhibits diminished reactions to light.

The vascular reaction in the anterior uvea following a concussion injury is characterized initially by an ischemic spasm followed by prolonged reactive vasodilatation. Clinically, this presents as circumcorneal injection with hyperemia and edema of the iris and ciliary body. Increased vascular permeability may be documented with the slit-lamp biomicroscope by the presence of a Tyndall effect, white cells, and in the more severe cases, collections of fibrin in the aqueous humor. Clumps of white cells and fibrin collect on the corneal endothelium to form keratic precipitates. Small hemorrhages may be visible deep in the interstitial tissue of the iris but are of no consequence and resorb spontaneously. Hyphema and secondary glaucoma may ensue, as discussed earlier.

The vascular reaction accounts for the almost invariable presence of an inflammatory response in the anterior uveal tract after trauma. Known as iridocyclitis, it may be transient and of little consequence, or it may be of considerable severity and quite resistant to therapy. In the latter instance, it may produce a lowered intraocular pressure because the inflammatory response in the ciliary body interferes with aqueous humor production, or it may produce glaucoma because the inflammatory cells and fibrin block the pores of the trabecular meshwork and interfere with aqueous humor outflow. Moreover, the outpouring of protein and leukocytes from the congested uveal tissues into the aqueous humor promotes fibrinous adhesion between the anterior lens capsule and the pigment epithelium of the iris. If the lens is absent, the adhesion can develop between the iris and the anterior vitreous face. When the adhesions involve the entire pupillary circumference, pupillary block may develop with the consequences already described.

Lacerations and tears of the anterior uveal tissue may also follow severe contusions. There is some controversy over the exact forces producing these lesions, but among those implicated are: (1) lateral dilatation of the corneoscleral ring, compensating for the anterior-posterior compression of the globe; (2) contraction of the iris sphincter, occurring immediately after blunt trauma to the cornea and preceding the onset of traumatic mydriasis; (3) the impact of the iris onto the lens and the lateral displacement of aqueous humor, both produced by the compression wave; and possibly (4) rebound of the lens against the posterior iris.

Injuries in this group include interstitial tears of the sphincter, lacerations at the pupillary border, tears in the iris stroma, dehiscences of the pigment epithelium, and iridodialysis, in which the iris is torn from its insertion on the ciliary body (Fig. 3–III–13). Recession of the anterior chamber angle has been discussed. All such injuries may be accompanied by gross hemorrhage, producing a hyphema, and all are permanent, since the iris shows no tendency to heal when cut. Many injuries of this type are followed by atrophy of the injured iris stroma.

Perforating wounds of the globe have been discussed, and their effects upon the iris per se are not of major significance. As noted, wounds of the iris are characterized by the absence of healing. They also bleed minimally, presum-

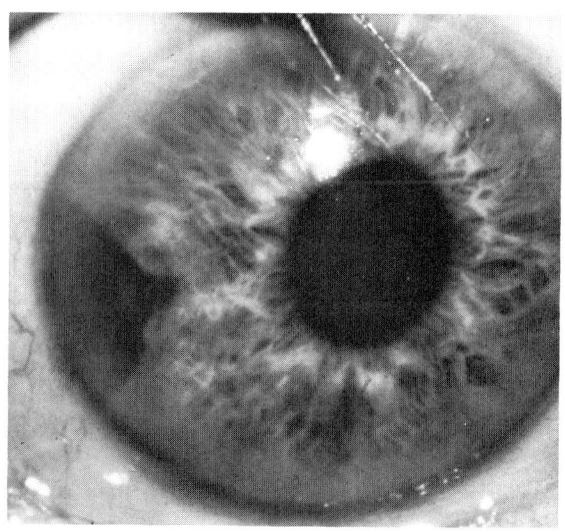

Figure 3–III–13. Iridodialysis—the iris is torn from its insertion on the ciliary body.

ably because of active retraction of their thick-walled vessels. If an extensive portion of the iris is wounded or if it must be excised during repair of the perforating injury, the patient may thenceforth suffer from the effects of glare in bright light because of the loss of pupillary function. Penetrating wounds affecting the ciliary body, on the other hand, are characterized by considerable hemorrhage, an intense leukocytic infiltrative response, and the formation of large amounts of granulation tissue. Healing is accomplished by consolidation of the fibrous tissue with scar formation and loss of function. Chronic uveitis may also follow such an injury, with disastrous results.

Lens

The crystalline lens of the eye is a transparent biconvex structure whose anterior surface lies in contact with the pupillary margin of the iris and whose posterior surface occupies the hyaloid fossa of the anterior vitreous body. It is the second of the major optical elements of the eye (the first being the cornea), and in youth it is capable of changing its shape to permit clear near vision, a process called accommodation. With age, the lens becomes more sclerotic, the ability to accommodate is lost (presbyopia), and near vision becomes blurred unless aided by spectacles.

The lens is entirely ensheathed within a transparent, amorphous, highly elastic envelope, the lens capsule. Beneath the anterior lens capsule lies a single layer of cuboidal cells, the anterior epithelium. Toward the equator, the rounded margin at which the anterior and posterior lens surfaces meet, the epithelial cells gradually become columnar and are converted into lens fibers. The great bulk of the lens is composed of these lens fibers, which are long, prismatic, six-sided bands that are laid down in two zones, an outer, softer, more fluid cortex and a central, harder, less fluid nucleus. The lens is maintained in its normal location by a delicate, membrane-like suspensory apparatus, the zonules of Zinn, which are attached to the lens capsule around its entire circumference and connect it to the ciliary processes.

Concussion injuries to the lens are common; the forces involved injure the lens capsule and interfere with its ability to regulate the interchange of fluid between the aqueous humor and the lens. As a result, the lens imbibes water from the aqueous humor that bathes it, and swells. The individual lens fibers have a high protein content, and the traumatic episode causes the protein to precipitate. This sequence of events results in loss of lenticular transparency, producing an opacified lens or cataract. The nature of the opacity, that is, its size, shape, and location within the lens as well as its course of progression, is quite variable and depends largely on the type and severity of the traumatic event and upon the age of the patient.

In addition, the relatively exposed position of the lens accounts for its frequent involvement in penetrating wounds of the globe wherein the lens capsule is injured and cataract formation results. Here too, the extent of the opacity varies; it may be small and localized, caused by a tiny puncture of the capsule that

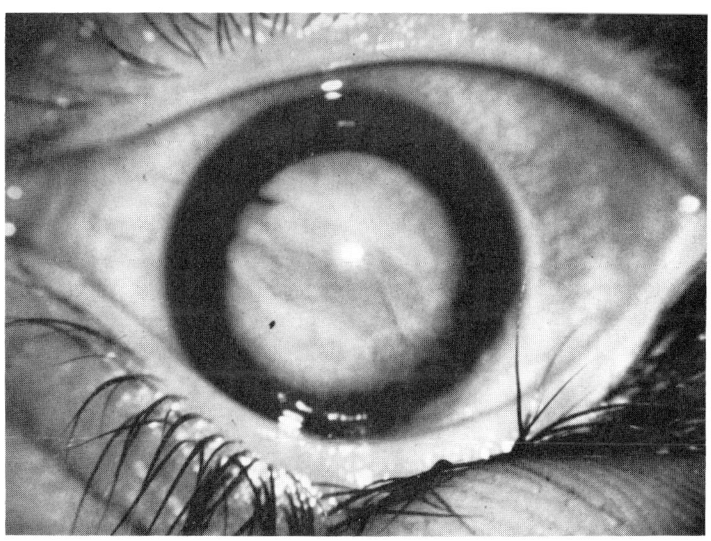

Figure 3–III–14. Traumatic cataract following a penetrating wound of the globe.

subsequently seals, or it may affect the entire lens, causing it to become swollen and white rapidly if the capsule is widely lacerated (Fig. 3–III–14).

A cataract interferes with the ability of the eye to focus light upon the retina and consequently interferes with vision. When the cataract is of traumatic origin, it may produce additional secondary complications. The lens may swell sufficiently to occlude the pupil totally, causing pupillary block and angle-closure glaucoma. As the lens imbibes water, liquefaction of the protein in the lens cortex occurs. Occasionally, the liquefied protein may leak through a break in the lens capsule and initiate a severe inflammatory response histologically characterized by macrophage invasion. The protein-laden macrophages mechanically plug the pores of the trabecular meshwork, decrease the outflow of aqueous humor, and cause secondary glaucoma. In this situation, the eye is red and painful as it is in angle-closure glaucoma resulting from pupillary block. It can, however, be differentiated from angle closure by the deep anterior chamber containing aqueous humor with high levels of protein and inflammatory cells. The intraocular inflammatory reaction may, at times, be so pronounced that hypopyon is present.

Blunt trauma may injure the zonular attachments between the lens and ciliary processes with or without simultaneous injury to the lens itself. Rupture of these zonules allows the lens to sink as a result of gravity (subluxation) or to leave its usual position immediately posterior to the iris and to move forward into the anterior chamber or backward into the vitreous cavity (dislocation) (Figs. 3–III–15 and 3–III–16). Abnormalities in the position of the lens result in a tremulous movement of the iris (iridodenesis) when the eyes move. Other diagnostic signs of an abnormality in lens position include direct observation of the curved edge of the lens in the pupillary space and the presence of the entire lens in the anterior chamber following its anterior dislocation.

The direction in which the lens moves following injury to the zonules is in part dependent upon the extent of zonular involvement. If only a portion of the zonules are ruptured, the lens will tend to travel in the direction of the remaining attached zonules. Displacement of the lens from its normal position produces significant optical distortions that may reduce visual acuity. Complete dislocation of the lens requires rupture of all the zonules. If the dislocation is posterior, the lens generally falls to the bottom of the vitreous cavity where it may move about freely or gradually become fibrosed to the ciliary body or retina or both. If the former condition occurs, the lens may pass in and out of the visual axis, producing significant visual symptoms. A lens dislocated posteriorly in the inferior vitreous cavity, however, often causes no problems other than the requirement for spectacles or a contact lens to correct optically the traumatic aphakia. If, on the other hand, the lens capsule is simultaneously injured, the lens protein leaking into and mixing with the vitreous humor may incite a severe inflammatory reaction. Complete dislocation of the lens in a forward direction so that it comes to lie entirely in the anterior chamber generally constitutes an ocular

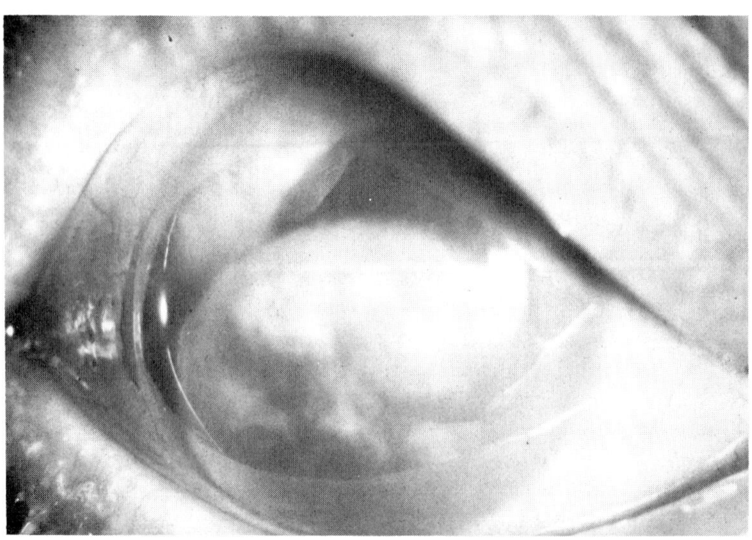

Figure 3–III–15. Anterior dislocation of the lens into the anterior chamber.

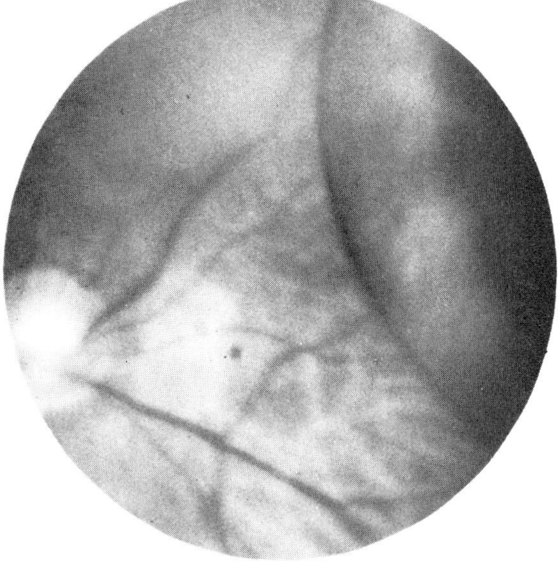

Figure 3–III–16. Posterior dislocation of the lens into the vitreous cavity. The edge of the lens is visible immediately anterior to the retina. The optic disk is seen at left.

emergency. Aqueous outflow is substantially blocked, resulting in a marked elevation of intraocular pressure, while apposition of the lens to the posterior corneal surface mechanically injures the endothelium, causing corneal edema and opacification.

Vitreous Humor

The vitreous humor or vitreous body is a colorless and highly transparent gellike mass that occupies approximately 80 per cent of the interior volume of the eye. It is formed by a network of collagen fibrils interacting with molecules of hyaluronic acid, and in the normal eye, it contains no blood vessels and only a small number of cells. The vitreous body fills the space bounded by the lens and its zonules anteriorly and by the ciliary body, retina, and optic disk posteriorly. It is anchored to the latter three structures, but this attachment is strongest at the peripheral retina and the pars plana of the ciliary body, where it is referred to as the vitreous base. The anterior extension of the vitreous base may lie as much as 1.5 mm in front of the ora serrata. The vitreous body may also adhere to the posterior lens capsule, forming the so-called hyaloideocapsular ligament.

Concussion injuries of the eye almost invariably produce reactive vasodilatation in the posterior segment of the globe. The resultant increased vascular permeability permits the extravasation of protein-rich, plasmoid material into the vitreous humor. Formed cellular elements and pigment granules may also be observed, and in the more severe forms of violence there may be an associated disruption of the fibrillar vitreous framework and liquefaction of the gel (syneresis). The vitreous body may be torn from its attachment at the ora serrata (anterior detachment) or at the optic disk (posterior detachment). Hemorrhage into the vitreous is a not-uncommon sequel to this type of injury and most often is due to a retinal tear, although blood from the ciliary region may seep into the anterior vitreous. A traumatic vitreous hemorrhage is slow to absorb, and although vision may return to normal, residual debris and fibrous membranes often persist and may subsequently lead to retinal detachment. Traumatic episodes causing zonular injury (with subluxation or dislocation of the lens) or iridodialysis are frequently characterized by prolapse of the vitreous humor into the anterior chamber. If the vitreous persists as a gel, the herniation has a well-demarcated border. If, however, it becomes more fluid it may fill the entire anterior chamber, at times interfering with aqueous humor outflow and causing secondary glaucoma.

Perforating wounds of the eye generally disrupt the vitreous body more extensively than concussion injuries. Every such wound must be considered as potentially infected, particularly if the vitreous body is involved, since it is an excellent culture medium for microorganisms. Introduced inside the eye, they can produce a devastating endophthalmitis capable of permanently destroying ocular function. Staphylococcus, streptococcus, pneumococcus, and pseudomonas are most frequently implicated, but even the usually nonpathogenic organisms that constitute the normal flora of the conjunctival sac are equally capable of destruction if they gain entrance into the eye. The virulence of the infection is greater if the lens has been injured simultaneously. Lens cortex also is an excellent culture medium, and when it mixes with vitreous it initiates an inflammatory response that augments the reaction to the replicating organism. The suppurative process in the vitreous body spreads to and involves the retina, resulting in its disorganization. Finally, the vitreous exudate itself becomes transformed into fibrous tissue, which degenerates and contracts, pulls upon and detaches the retina, and ultimately produces phthisis bulbi.

Even if the injured eye escapes infection and the destructive processes just described, its long-term prognosis for vision must remain guarded. Fibrosis, a normal and desirable healing process in most injured tissues, may be too gross a means of repair for the delicate architecture and physiologic processes of the eye and may actually compromise ocular function. Aside from inflammation at the actual perforation site, hemorrhage into and direct injury of the vitreous body can incite excessive fibrosis (Fig. 3–III–17). Similarly, injury of the lens and ciliary epithelium may be followed by metaplasia of these structures that extends into the vitreous cavity and contributes to the organization of the vitreous humor. This may lead to retinal detachment and interfere with essential physiologic mechanisms of the eye.

Choroid and Retina

The choroid is the posterior segment of the uveal tract, the vascular layer of the eye. It lies between the outer sclera and inner retina, and anterior to the ora serrata of the retina it is continuous with the ciliary body. The choroid is a thin membranelike structure made up almost entirely of blood vessels of various sizes. These give rise to a large bed of capillaries, the choriocapillaris, which is in direct contact with the retinal pigment epithelium through an elastic membrane called Bruch's membrane.

The retina is the inner, neural layer of the eye. It surrounds much of the vitreous cavity and, in turn, is enveloped by the choroid. Structurally, it is a gossamer-thin, translucent tissue composed largely of a highly complex arrangement of nerve fibers that function as the light-sensitive apparatus of the eye. The retina contains two types of photoreceptors, the rods and the cones, which function to convert optical images into neural impulses for transmission to the brain in order to produce what we know as vision. The rods function most effectively at lower levels of illumination, the cones in bright light. Both are arranged in a single cell layer supported by protoplasmic processes of the outermost retinal layer, the pigment epithelium, which is the major nutritive source for the photoreceptors.

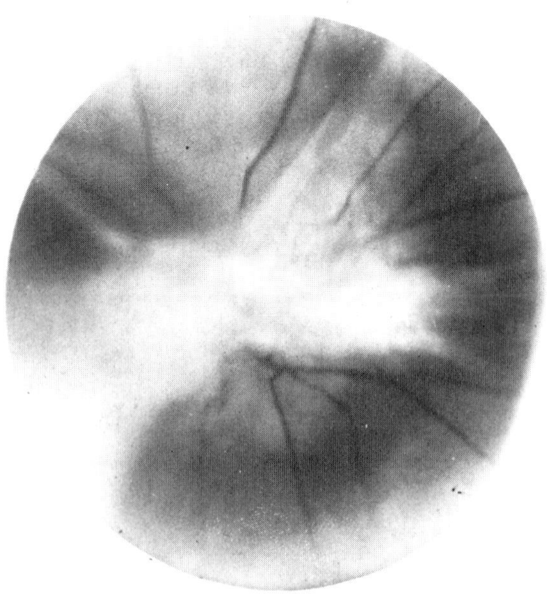

Figure 3–III–17. Fibrous membrane in the vitreous humor following removal of an intraocular foreign body from the vitreous cavity.

The rods and cones form only one of three retinal neuronal layer . Each photoreceptor is connected to an intermediate neuron in the biopolar cell layer, which in turn is linked to a third neuron in the ganglion cell layer. The latter continues as a long axon through the optic nerve to the visual centers of the brain. The neuronal elements are supported by a scaffolding that consists of two membranes, the internal and external limiting membranes, and an intricate network of glial cells that provide important metabolic support for the retinal neurons.

The functional center of the retina is the macula lutea, an area approximately 3 mm in diameter located slightly temporal to the optic disk. The area is responsible for the sharpest levels of visual acuity and is able to subserve this function because the photoreceptors are more densely packed here. The very center of the macula, the fovea centralis, is characterized by tall slender cones and the absence of rods. It subserves the best vision of all. The retina ends anteriorly at the ora serrata, located 7.5 to 8.5 mm posterior to the limbus. The degree of functional and structural differentiation of the retina decreases as one proceeds from the macula anteriorly to the ora serrata.

Choroidal Responses to Injury

The response of the choroid to contusion injury, like that of the anterior uveal tract, is characterized by vasodilatation, edema, and hemorrhage. The hemorrhage can seep into the vitreous body, or it can detach the choroid and collect in the suprachoroidal space between the choroid and sclera. Detachment of the choroid can also occur after blunt injury as a result of a serous exudation from the choroidal blood vessels. This carries a more favorable prognosis than hemorrhagic detachment.

Choroidal ruptures are often seen after concussion injuries to the choroid (Fig. 3–III–18).

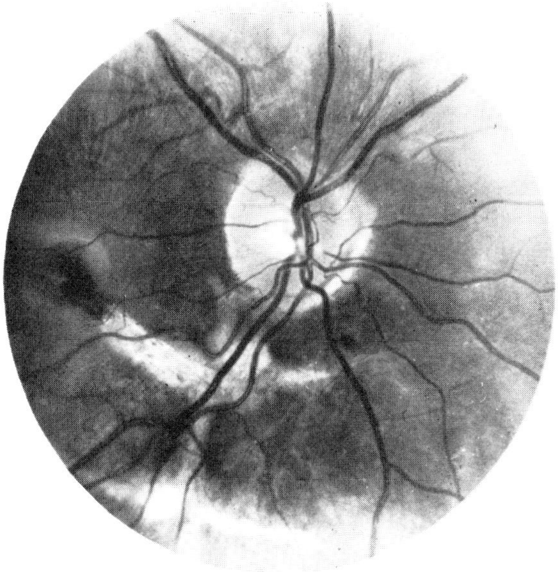

Figure 3–III–18. Choroidal rupture.

Classically, this lesion is a crescentic white patch, 3 to 4 mm from the optic disk, with the concavity of the crescent turned toward the disk. The white patch is the exposed sclera viewed without any overlying retinal pigment epithelium or choroid. Several ruptures can arise from the same injury. The choroidal scar and the proliferation of pigment at its borders can produce traction folds that extend into the macula. Histologically, there is a tear in Bruch's membrane and the choriocapillaris. The function of the overlying retina is usually lost with a corresponding nerve fiber bundle defect in the visual field. Less commonly, rupture of the choroid is due to injury causing interruption of the posterior ciliary vessels. The optic nerve is often involved in these cases and becomes atrophic.

Retinal Response to Injury

Concussion and Contusion. The retina's response to concussion or contusion is similar to that of the choroid. The vascular changes consist of ischemia followed by reactive hyperemia, increased permeability, and escape of blood or serous exudate into the surrounding tissues. Whether the initiating trauma is a contusion or a concussion, the clinical picture consists of commotio retinae, retinal hemorrhage, retinal tear or detachment, and macular cyst or hole formation.

Commotio retinae (Berlin's edema) is the most frequent retinal effect of concussion. Within 24 hours after injury, edema imparts a milky white appearance to the retina, most commonly in the periphery or at the posterior pole of the fundus. The macula stands out as a cherry red spot, and the affected area may have tiny hemorrhages. The posterior pole of the fundus is frequently affected because its rich vascular supply provides a source for the extravasation of copious amounts of edema fluid. The edema clears within a few days, although in some cases, it is followed by concussion necrosis, which leads to the formation of clumps of fibrous tissue.

Concussion hemorrhages of the retina may be intraretinal, subretinal, preretinal, or within the vitreous (Fig. 3–III–19). Retinal hemorrhages are very common at birth, potential traumatic factors being prolonged labor, use of forceps, and abnormal presentation. Usually these hemorrhages clear rapidly with no obvious disturbance of retinal structure or function.

Retinal tears produced in a healthy eye by a concussion injury are infrequent and are generally limited to the macula and ora serrata. If, however, the involved eye contains degenerative retinal changes associated with myopia, age, or healed peripheral inflammation, even a slight injury can produce a retinal tear. The presumed causal mechanism for these peripheral tears is a thrust and recoil of the vitreous to which the retina is adherent. At the ora serrata, the vitreous framework has the firmest anchorage, whereas the retina in this region is

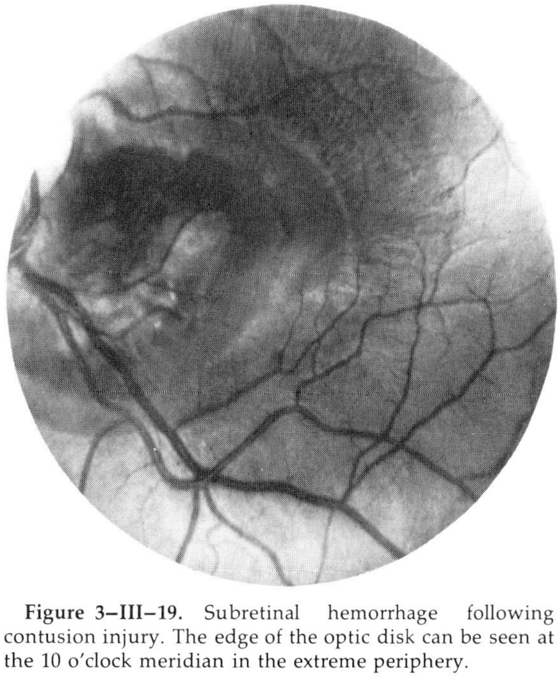

Figure 3–III–19. Subretinal hemorrhage following contusion injury. The edge of the optic disk can be seen at the 10 o'clock meridian in the extreme periphery.

thinnest, least supported by blood vessels, and most prone to degenerative changes.

Retinal tears may predispose to detachment of the retina. The time interval between injury and the onset of retinal detachment is variable. Only a small percentage of such retinal detachments occur immediately after injury and a long latent period (up to several years) is perfectly consistent with a retinal detachment caused by ocular contusion. In this instance, the retina is undoubtedly torn at the time of the injury. Nonetheless, a detachment need not occur at this time or it may be localized to a small area if the eye is healthy and the vitreous gel is solid. If, on the other hand, the vitreous humor is fluid, it will tend to flow through the retinal tear and lift the neural retina from the pigment epithelium, which remains attached to the choroid (Fig. 3–III–20). The vitreous often becomes fluid as part of the normal aging process, in myopic eyes, and in eyes in which there is an intraocular inflammatory process. Thus, in these instances and in eyes with peripheral retinal degenerative changes, even relatively minor trauma can initiate a chain of events that lead to retinal detachment.

A macular cyst or hole may result from the edema produced by blunt trauma or may occur as a direct sequela of the concussion forces (Fig. 3–III–21). A limited retinal detachment may follow the formation of a macular hole, and on occasion, the detachment may be extensive. When the lesion is a true cyst with retinal tissue present on its inner wall, some degree of central vision may be retained. If the lesion is a true macular hole, total and permanent loss of central vision invariably results.

Head injuries, compression injuries of the chest and abdomen, and fractures of the long bones may cause a traumatic retinopathy

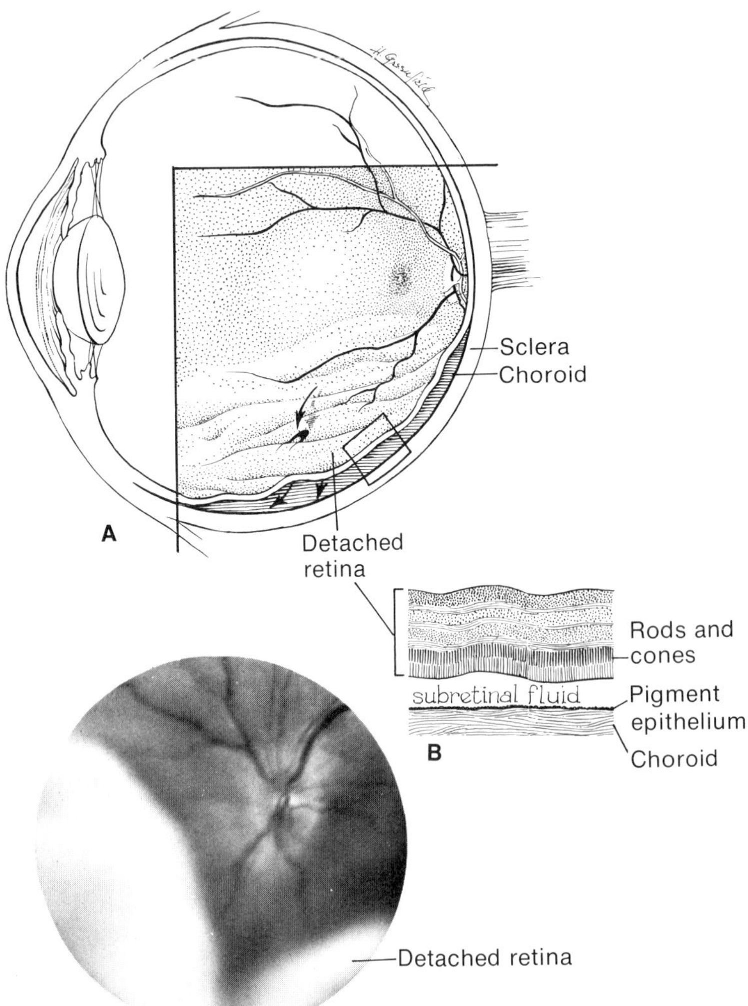

Figure 3–III–20. Mechanism of retinal detachment. *A.* Horseshoe-shaped tear in retina. Arrows indicate fluid from vitreous humor flowing through retinal tear and lifting retina from its normal position. *B.* Histological cross-section of retinal detachment demonstrating that the subretinal fluid separates the neuroepithelial retinal structures (including the rods and cones) from the retinal pigment epithelium. *C.* Clinical photograph illustrating balloonlike folds of detached retina.

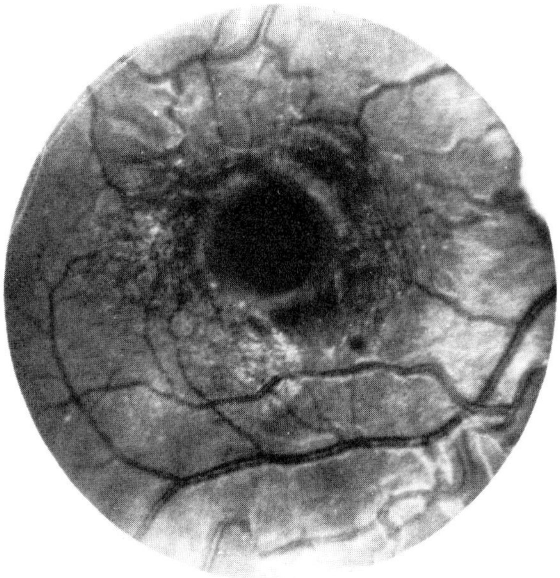

Figure 3–III–21. Macular hole following blunt ocular trauma.

(Purtscher's retinopathy) (Fig. 3–III–22). This entity is characterized by superficial white round exudative patches in a perivenous location and associated retinal hemorrhages. The condition appears within a few days after the injury and tends to disappear within a period of several weeks. Visual impairment depends upon the extent of macular involvement. The etiology of this retinal disturbance following remote injury is not entirely clear. It has been suggested that the multiple hemorrhages are due to a sudden venous reflux from a compression phenomenon. It is also probable that multiple fat emboli released from the marrow of long bones may lead to a vascular spasm causing the retinal exudates and hemorrhages.

The ocular manifestations of the battered baby syndrome primarily involve the retina and choroid. Intraocular hemorrhage is the most common ocular finding, with retinal, preretinal, and vitreous hemorrhage predominating. An associated subdural hematoma may be found. Although a majority of the intraocular hemorrhages clear, a substantial number progress to vitreous organization or macular scarring. A peculiar type of chorioretinal atrophy, with multiple atrophic areas each characterized by a gray center surrounded by black pigmentation, has been observed in the periphery of the retina. The commonest cause of severe permanent loss of vision in these battered babies, however, is irreversible injury to the visual pathways in the brain. Just as in other forms of blunt trauma, periorbital hematomas, subluxation of the lens, traumatic cataract, and retinal detachment also frequently occur.

Perforating Injuries. Perforating injuries involving the choroid and retina are among those least likely to enjoy a successful visual outcome despite early surgical restoration of the integrity of the globe. Both structures are apt to be torn. The choroidal tear is generally accompanied by copious hemorrhage, while the retinal tear may initiate a retinal detachment. Fibroblastic proliferation may occur during absorption of vitreous hemorrhage, and subsequent traction upon the retina by these bands may also produce retinal detachment. Direct damage to retinal tissue results in irreversible loss of function of the involved area. The potential for serious intraocular infection is great, while incarceration of uveal tissue in the wound can produce an equally serious sterile uveitis; both processes can endanger the functional survival of the eye.

A perforating wound involving uveal tissue may give rise to an entity called sympathetic ophthalmitis. This is a specific inflammation of unknown etiology involving the entire uveal tract of *both* eyes following ocular trauma to only *one* eye. It is more apt to occur if the prolapsed uveal tissue is iris or ciliary body. Sympathetic ophthalmitis is characterized by a severe chronic bilateral uveitis that appears in the injured eye at a variable time after the injury and in the second eye some time thereaf-

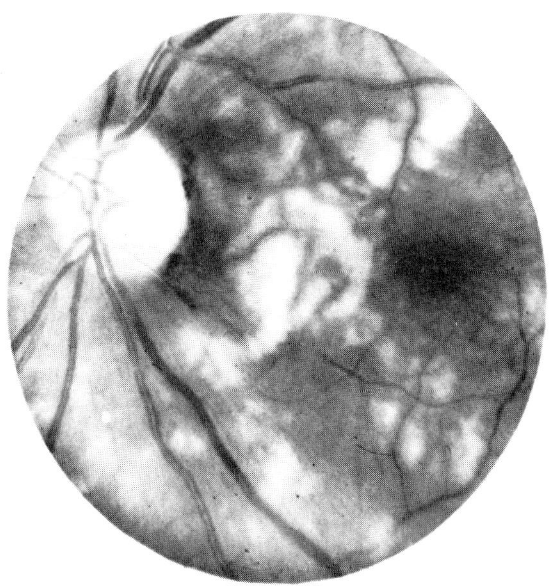

Figure 3–III–22. Purtscher's retinopathy—traumatic retinopathy following compression injury of chest and abdomen.

ter. Both the clinical and pathologic findings in the two eyes are basically identical. An incubation period of approximately 10 days appears to be necessary for the development of the disease. Enucleation of the injured eye within 10 days of the traumatic episode seems to virtually preclude involvement of the second eye. There appear to be no known cases of sympathetic ophthalmitis among casualties of the Korean and Vietnam wars despite a large number of perforating eye injuries. This is attributed to the prompt initiation of surgical therapy with excision of the prolapsed uveal tissue and closure of the ocular wound.

Clinically, sympathetic ophthalmitis consists of an extensive granulomatous uveitis with coarse deposits of inflammatory cells on the corneal endothelium, in the angle of the anterior chamber, on the iris, and in the pupil. The aqueous humor is very turbid because of a high protein level and contains many inflammatory cells and fibrin. Other objective findings include conjunctival and ciliary injection, corneal edema, edema and inflammation of the iris (often with large nodules on its surface), posterior synechiae, lens opacity, turbidity of the vitreous because of the large number of inflammatory cells it harbors, edema of the retina and optic disk, and elevated intraocular pressure. The predominant finding on histologic examination is a massive infiltration by mononuclear cells of the entire uveal tract but particularly of the choroid. Masses of epithelioid cells are also present, and in the more chronic cases these coalesce to form multinucleated giant cells. There is a definite tendency of these inflammatory cellular elements to form nodular aggregates. Symptoms include photophobia, lacrimation, and loss of vision. The entity tends to be chronic and progressive. As already noted, early enucleation of the injured eye appears to be effective prophylaxis against involvement of the uninjured eye but loses much of that effectiveness subsequent to the tenth day after injury. Once active inflammation appears in the second eye, enucleation of the injured eye no longer exerts any effect upon the course of the disease in the second eye. Treatment with corticosteroids has improved the visual prognosis of these eyes, but in many cases the functional outcome nonetheless remains guarded.

Foreign Bodies. One additional mode of ocular trauma, the intraocular foreign body, deserves mention here. It may involve the choroid and retina, but of course, may also affect other parts of the eye. Indeed, a whole spectrum of direct injuries and complications may be seen. The majority of such injuries result from the use of a hammer and chisel (or other combination in which steel strikes steel) or the use of machine tools. Military injuries are an exception. Multiple foreign bodies, often not metallic and often contaminated by dirt and stone, are the most common causal agents here. These eyes are also generally subjected to more simultaneous contusion than is incurred in civilian life. All these factors contribute to the poorer prognosis of the military injury. In civilian industrial accidents, approximately 90 per cent of intraocular foreign bodies are magnetic. Brass and copper are the most commonly encountered nonmagnetic metallic materials. Others are aluminum, nickel, and zinc. Wood, glass, stone, and organic materials such as eyelashes also contribute their quota.

The diagnosis of an intraocular foreign body can often be made from the history, and frequently the offending particle can be directly visualized with the slit-lamp biomicroscope or the ophthalmoscope. When it is not visible, localization of the foreign body may be aided by radiologic or ultrasonic examination. Demonstration by x-ray depends upon the density of the foreign body; metallic particles can be easily seen, whereas glass cannot, in the conventional radiograph. Ultrasonic probes, used with a magnet, can distinguish between a magnetic and a nonmagnetic foreign body. The differentiation is important since the presence or absence of this property determines the manner and degree of trauma required to remove the foreign body from the eye and often gives information about its relative toxicity to ocular structures. Ultrasonic energy beamed into the eye is reflected by each surface within the eye; the reflected beam is monitored by a probe placed over the eye. The axial length of the globe and the location of the foreign body can be determined simultaneously, indicating whether the foreign body lies inside or outside the eye.

Initially, an intraocular foreign body produces a perforating wound in cornea or sclera, and uveal tissue may become incarcerated in or prolapse through the wound. The final position of the foreign body and the amount of damage it causes depend upon its site of entry, its velocity, its direction, its size, and whether or not it is sterile. High-velocity foreign bodies are often sterilized by the heat they generate, but this is not invariable and intraocular infection may supervene.

The foreign body may come to rest in the anterior chamber, rub against and mechanically injure the corneal endothelium, and cause corneal edema (Fig. 3–III–23). It may pass into or

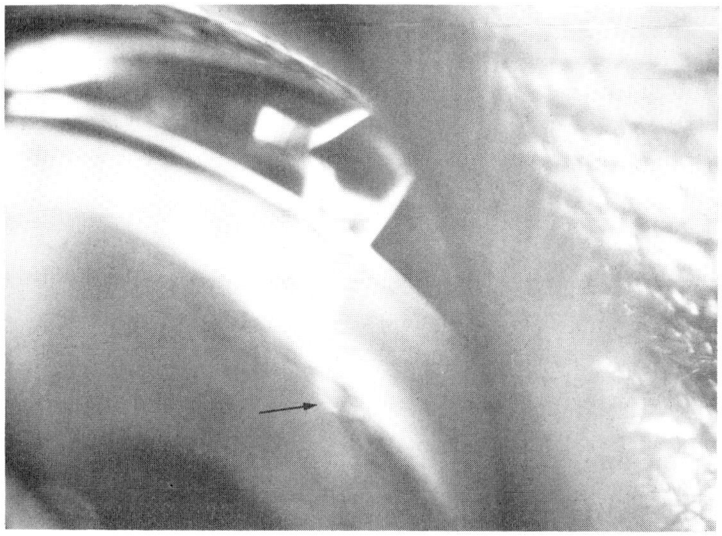

Figure 3–III–23. Glass foreign body wedged in the angle of the anterior chamber, causing edema of the overlying cornea.

through the lens, producing a cataract (Fig. 3–III–24). If it passes through the lens, the lenticular cortical material may mix with the vitreous humor and incite an intense inflammatory reaction. The injured, swollen lens may cause anterior or posterior synechiae or pupillary block, any of which may lead to glaucoma. Most intraocular foreign bodies come to lie in the vitreous cavity, however, since it occupies most of the volume of the globe, and they often gravitate to the surface of the retina at the equator (Fig. 3–III–25). Those traveling with a great deal of momentum may ricochet off the wall of the globe or incarcerate themselves in the retina, choroid, or sclera, producing chorioretinal tears and hemorrhage or retinal detachment or both. A few may produce a double perforation, passing entirely through the globe and becoming lodged in the orbit.

The composition of the intraocular foreign body profoundly influences its effect upon the eye. Vegetable material tends to provoke a marked inflammatory reaction and is commonly associated with fungal endophthalmitis.

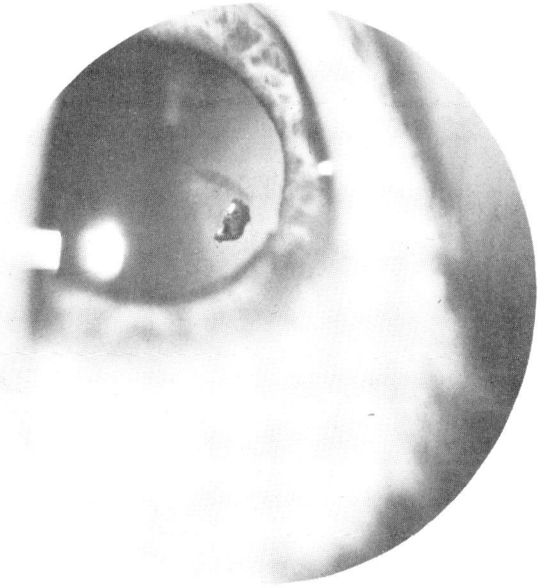

Figure 3–III–24. Steel fragment in the crystalline lens of the eye. The lens subsequently became cataractous.

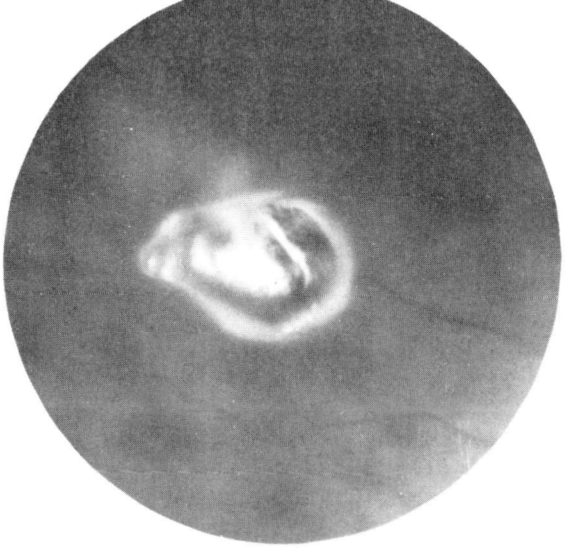

Figure 3–III–25. Metallic foreign body in the retina.

Inert foreign bodies such as glass, stone, or heavy metals usually incite very little inflammation, often because they become encapsulated by fibrous tissue, and frequently are better left alone because the intraocular manipulations involved in their removal may be more harmful to the globe. In contrast, other metallic foreign bodies, such as iron and copper, can cause late complications that make their early removal advisable.

Siderosis is the term applied to the effects produced by the absorption of iron pigment in various ocular tissues. An iron foreign body may oxidize within the eye, and the ionized forms of the metal precipitate as insoluble salts in several intraocular locations. The degree of oxidation depends largely upon the composition of the foreign body, its size, the number of particles, its location within the eye, whether or not it is encapsulated by fibrous tissue or organizing hemorrhages, and the length of time it has been retained within the eye. The process is generally an insidious one, but the delayed effects of the absorption of iron can be disastrous to the ultimate visual capacity of the involved eye. The severity of the pathologic effects is directly proportional to the ferrous content of the foreign particle.

Siderosis occurs between two months and two years after the injury. Definite signs of the disease are decreased vision, night-blindness, increased dark adaptation time, and concentric contraction of the visual field. Clinical examination reveals a rusty appearance of the cornea and iris, sluggish pupillary reaction, mild iritis, progressive cataractous changes in the lens, and pigmentary degeneration of the retina with glial proliferation. Glaucoma frequently occurs. The electroretinogram is extinguished early. The iron pigment is deposited primarily in the region of the foreign body itself, but it diffuses throughout the globe with preferential deposition in epithelial structures. Thus, dense deposition is seen in the trabeculae of the chamber angle, the iris musculature, and in the epithelial layers of the lens, ciliary body, and retina. It is believed that removal of the foreign body after siderosis has become established does not improve the prognosis of the eye. The retinal damage is inexorable and progressive.

Chalcosis is a disease similar to siderosis but induced by copper, which, in pure form, causes severe intraocular inflammation. The commonest source of copper foreign bodies is an exploding cartridge case or other copper alloy broken in an industrial accident. Increased use of copper alloys has resulted in a marked decrease in the intensity of the usual intraocular reaction, and foreign particles containing some copper have been observed for years within the eye without apparent damage.

Clinically the disease is characterized by a blue-green ring (Kayser-Fleischer ring) deposited on Descemet's membrane in the peripheral cornea (similar to that seen in Wilson's hepatolenticular degeneration), a sunflower cataract under the anterior capsule of the lens, metallic particles in the aqueous, greenish color of the iris, and deposition of copper particles in the vitreous and zonules and retina. In the retina the color has been described as resembling tiny pieces of gold leaf arranged along the main trunks of the blood vessels. The electroretinogram shows responses similar to those in siderosis. Copper particles seem to be preferentially deposited in or on the limiting membranes of the eye rather than intracellularly like the iron pigment in siderosis.

Optic Nerve

The optic nerve is a bundle of myelinated nerve fibers that extends from the back of the eye to the optic chiasm of the brain. Anatomically it may be divided into four segments: an ocular segment that passes through the lamina cribrosa of the sclera; an orbital segment, about 30 mm in length, which is longer than the distance between the posterior globe and the optic canal (this segment therefore has a sinuous course and lies lax in the orbit); an intracanalicular segment that passes through the optic foramen and lies within the optic canal of the sphenoid bone; and an intracranial segment that extends from the optic canal to the optic chiasm. The optic nerve is covered by three concentric layers of sheaths, called meninges, which are continuous with identical structures covering the brain. Outermost of these three layers is the dura, composed of dense connective tissue. Within the dura is the arachnoid, and most centrally lies the pia, which clothes the optic nerve and sends fibers into it to form septa within the nerve. The space between the arachnoid and pia contains cerebrospinal fluid and is continuous with the corresponding intracranial space. The optic nerve itself consists of nerve fibers that are the axons of the retinal ganglion cells, and more closely resembles a tract of the brain than a peripheral nerve. It contains fibers that subserve vision and others that control the pupil.

The anatomical location within the orbit of most of the optic nerve makes it illogical and artificial to divide a discussion of the effects of mechanical trauma on the two structures. The results of such injury to the optic nerve therefore are covered in the section on the orbit.

Extraocular Muscles

Each eye has six extraocular muscles, the medial, lateral, superior, and inferior rectus muscles, and the superior and inferior oblique muscles (Fig. 3–III–26). The medial and lateral recti control the motion of the eye in a horizontal plane in the direction indicated by their names. Similarly, the superior and inferior recti are primarily responsible for elevation and depression of the eye but also have secondary torsional actions around the anterior-posterior axis of the globe. The superior and inferior obliques are responsible for torsional eye movements in the primary position of gaze; they also have depressor and elevator actions respectively when the eyes are adducted.

The four rectus muscles and the superior oblique all originate near the apex of the orbit. They lie in the most peripheral portion of the orbit, and as they fan out anteriorly to their insertions they form a muscle cone that contains the remainder of the orbital structures with the exception of the sensory nerves responsible for sensation in the forehead and cheek. The muscle bellies of the four recti run directly forward to insert anterior to the equator around the globe at approximately 90-degree intervals. The superior oblique also runs directly forward, but has a functional origin at the trochlea, a pulleylike structure on the nasal orbital wall. The tendon of the superior oblique passes through the trochlea, then runs backward and laterally to insert underneath the superior rectus posterior to the equator of the globe. The sixth extraocular muscle, the inferior oblique, originates anteriorly at the inferior portion of the nasal orbital wall, whence it runs obliquely (laterally and backward) to insert in the sclera posterior to the equator.

As with the optic nerve, the location of the extraocular muscles totally within the orbit renders mechanical trauma to these structures virtually inseparable from orbital injury. Therefore, direct injury to the extraocular muscles is discussed in the succeeding section.

Orbit

The orbits are pear-shaped bony cavities within the skull that contain the eye and related structures, including the extraocular muscles, the optic nerve, the lacrimal gland, fibers of the autonomic nervous system, and blood vessels responsible for nourishment of the orbital tissues. The orbits are separated from each other by the nasal and sinus cavities. The medial orbital walls are parallel, but the lateral walls diverge. Anteriorly, a bony rim overhangs the edge so that the widest point lies behind the orbital opening. Each orbit is about 40 mm deep and has a volume of 30 cc, about one fifth of which is occupied by the globe.

All the walls of the orbit are formed by bones of the skull. The lateral orbital wall is the strongest, but as noted earlier, the globe is most exposed laterally. The superior orbital wall is also the floor of the anterior cranial fossa; it is thin in children but usually strong in adults, accounting for the greater incidence of perforating wounds of the orbital roof in children. The floor of the orbit forms the roof of the subjacent maxillary sinus or antrum and is relatively weak. The medial orbital wall includes the ethmoid bone, which in part is so thin that it is referred to as the "paper plate." These an-

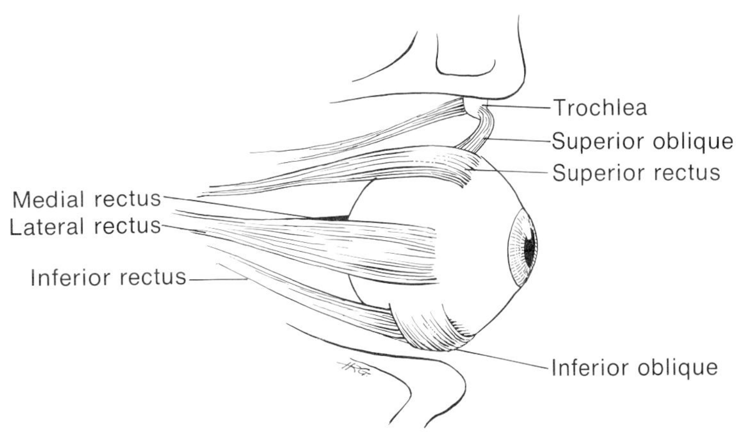

Figure 3–III–26. The extraocular muscles.

atomical peculiarities explain why the majority of orbital fractures involve the floor and medial wall.

There are important communications between the orbit and other cranial cavities. The superior orbital fissure is a pork chop–shaped opening near the apex of the orbit through which pass the nerves that innervate the extraocular muscles (cranial nerves III, IV, and VI), the sensory nerves that supply the eye and forehead (the first division of cranial nerve V), and the veins that return blood from the eye to the venous sinuses located in the cranial cavity. The optic nerve and the ophthalmic artery (the primary vascular source of the eye and orbital contents) pass through a narrow canal adjacent to the superior orbital fissure called the optic canal. It is directed down and out and lies in proximity to the sphenoid sinus. The inferior orbital fissure, located in the lateral portion of the orbital floor, communicates with the pterygopalatine fossa and transmits the second division of cranial nerve V. This branch is responsible for sensation in the skin of the cheek and the gums of the upper teeth. Injury involving the orbital floor may thus affect the perception of sensations in these areas.

The important anatomical relationships of the orbit are as follows. Above is the anterior fossa of the cranial cavity. It contains the frontal lobes of the brain and the olfactory apparatus, as well as the coverings of the brain (the meninges). Behind the apex of the orbit lies the middle cranial fossa, with the tip of the temporal lobe abutting the posterior wall of the orbit. The carotid artery, the optic chiasm, the cavernous sinus, and the pituitary gland are in the medial portion of the cranial cavity behind the orbital apex. Medially the orbit is related to the sphenoid and ethmoid sinuses. Inferiorly lies the maxillary sinus.

The close relationship between the eye and its related structures, on the one hand, and the central nervous system on the other, is reflected in the observation that mechanical trauma to the orbit not only may damage the orbital contents but also may damage the cranial contents. The converse is also true. Traumatic lesions of the brain, its blood vessels, and its meningeal coverings can also produce ocular and orbital symptoms and signs.

Intraorbital Hemorrhage

A blow to the eye or to the orbital wall may cause intraorbital bleeding. The hemorrhage generally stops spontaneously, largely as a result of the increased intraorbital pressure it produces, but nonetheless may result in striking symptoms and signs. The eye protrudes (exophthalmos or proptosis) because the blood occupies the orbital space behind the globe and pushes it forward. Pain may be present, and the pressure on the extraocular muscles may restrict the movement of the involved eye. As a result, the eyes become misaligned, and double vision (diplopia) occurs. Compression of the branches of the trigeminal nerve may cause numbness over the forehead. The blood can dissect into the lids and under the conjunctiva, producing cosmetic disfigurement but no functional problems. In the absence of associated injuries, complete resolution usually occurs within a period of weeks or (rarely) months. Patients with bleeding disorders (either endogenous or the result of anticoagulant therapy) may develop orbital hemorrhages after seemingly insignificant trauma.

The occurrence of visual loss in association with orbital hemorrhage always raises the possibility of compression of the optic nerve by the hemorrhage. This is probably an exceedingly rare mechanism. In actuality, visual impairment in the presence of orbital hemorrhage is usually due to some other direct effect of the initiating trauma upon the optic nerve or the eye itself. Even in cases of extreme proptosis, visual failure cannot be blamed on compromise of the optic nerve by the hemorrhage or stretching of the nerve. The extreme resistance of the optic nerve to damage by stretching is perhaps best illustrated by the retention of good visual function after displacement of the globe into the anterior cranial fossa.

Because of its anterior location, the trochlea is readily accessible to either blunt or penetrating orbital trauma. This structure is easily palpable if one inserts a finger between the globe and the orbital rim in the upper inner corner. A properly directed blow can separate the pulley from the orbital wall, producing an apparent paralysis of the superior oblique muscle. The effective loss of function of this muscle results in a deviation of the visual axis of the eye, clinically manifest as paralytic strabismus with diplopia. Since the primary function of the superior oblique is internal torsion of the globe, this injury is followed by an external rotation of the eye around an anterior-posterior axis. The patient characteristically turns or tilts his head to the side opposite the injury in an attempt to compensate for the abnormal ocular position and to eliminate the diplopia.

Fractures

An object large enough to compress the globe without rupturing it, yet big enough to be stopped by the orbital rim, may strike the eye. The resultant forces are displaced equatorially throughout the orbit. If powerful enough, these forces fracture the weakest of the orbital walls. Anatomically, these are the floor, as shown in Figure 3–III–27, and the medial wall at the level of the ethmoid sinus. If the floor fracture is large enough, the orbital contents immediately above it, i.e., fat and the inferior oblique and rectus muscles, drop through the hole into the maxillary antrum. This results in enophthalmos, an apparent recession of the eyeball in the orbit. Plain x-rays and tomograms of the orbit can generally outline the fracture, and the maxillary antrum may show a hemorrhagic fluid level. In the acute phase, the lids are swollen and ecchymotic. The skin below the orbital rim may be insensitive because of involvement of the infraorbital nerve. If the eye is enophthalmic this ocular displacement may cause diplopia in the primary position. The most noteworthy finding is an inability to elevate the affected eye; the restricted motion results from entrapment of the inferior rectus muscle and its surrounding structures in the fracture site. If uncorrected, healing and fibrosis follow, permanently preventing upward motion of the eye. This, in turn, causes a marked increase in diplopia during attempted upward gaze. The anesthesia of the infraorbital nerve is usually temporary, and normal sensation returns with time. Associated fractures of the medial wall of the orbit, the "paper plate" of the ethmoid, probably occur with the same frequency as fractures of the orbital floor. They usually remain clinically silent because the medial rectus is rarely trapped in the fracture. If this occurs, the patient is unable to turn his eye laterally in the normal manner. He will experience diplopia in the primary position of gaze if the trapped medial rectus muscle pulls the eye inward, and the degree of diplopia will increase during attempted lateral gaze with the involved eye.

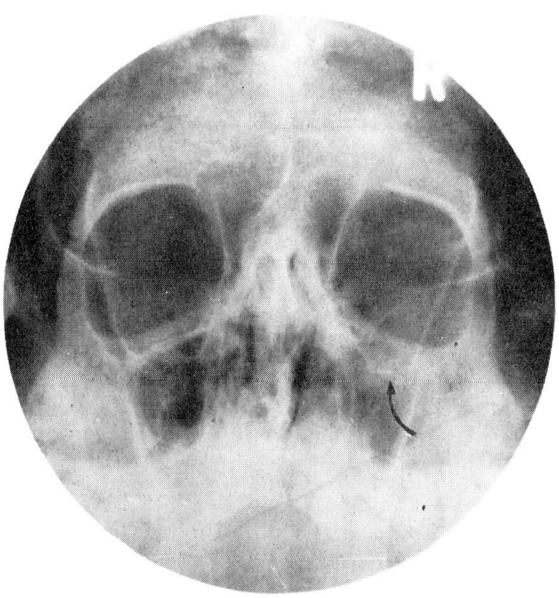

Figure 3–III–27. X-ray illustrating an orbital floor fracture on the right with blood and soft tissue in the right maxillary sinus.

Orbital roof fractures occur either because of direct penetration of the roof by a missile, or indirectly, as a result of a blow directed toward the cranial vault or orbital rim. Some orbital roof fractures produce no ocular signs or symptoms. Others may cause proptosis, in which case one of several mechanisms may be at fault. A blood clot overlying the roof of the orbit may be interfering with venous return from the orbit with resultant congestion, or it may be causing remolding of the orbital roof with a resultant decrease in orbital volume. Alternatively, the bony defect produced by the fracture may be so large that the brain and its meninges herniate through it into the orbit and push the globe anteriorly. In this instance, the exophthalmos may be pulsating, a posttraumatic finding that much more commonly indicates an abnormal communication between the carotid artery and the large venous sinuses at the base of the brain.

Orbital roof fractures are most apt to affect those orbital structures closest to the roof. The most important of these are the levator palpebrae superioris muscle, which elevates the lid, and the superior rectus muscle, which contributes to the elevation of the globe. Injury to these structures will therefore cause the upper lid to droop (ptosis), and the involved eye will be directed lower than its fellow eye (hypotropia). If the ptotic lid does not interfere with vision, diplopia in which the images are separated vertically will be present and be most pronounced on upward gaze. Damage to the branch of the trigeminal nerve that subserves sensory function over the forehead can also occur. Numbness and impaired sensation on the involved side, extending from the upper lid back to the level of the ear, result.

Missiles and foreign objects produce orbital roof fractures. The wound of entry, most commonly in the upper lid, may be surprisingly small and appear innocuous. Initially, few clinical signs and symptoms are manifest, and the fracture may be unsuspected. Children are particularly susceptible to this type of wound, probably because of the thinness of the orbital roof. The potential neurologic consequences are significant. Objects as large as plastic knobs from the dashboard of an automobile have been recovered from the frontal lobe after their transorbital passage.

Orbital Syndromes

The term orbital apex syndrome is used to refer to the concurrence of signs that indicate involvement of all the structures in the apex of the orbit. These include impaired vision, abnormality of extraocular muscle function, and impaired sensation over the forehead. The simultaneous occurrence of these signs helps localize the site of injury to the apex of the orbit but provides no information about etiology. Orbital apex syndromes attributable to mechanical trauma generally indicate a "sharp" injury. This could be produced either by penetration of the orbit by a foreign object (such as a knife) or by an extensive fracture of the orbital roof that "guillotined" the structures in question.

A lesion that specifically involves the structures passing through the superior orbital fissure produces impaired mobility of the globe in all directions, a drooping upper lid, and impaired sensation over the forehead, but no defect in vision. The pupil may be enlarged owing to compromise of the branches of the autonomic nervous system responsible for maintaining pupillary constriction. Thus the superior orbital fissure syndrome also serves to identify the location of the abnormality, but again fails to indicate the cause. The syndrome is likely to be due to a sharp object that penetrates the orbit and transfixes structures in the superior orbital fissure. It may also occur as the result of a fracture of the posterior portion of the roof of the orbit. Blood clots that abut the intracranial side of the superior orbital fissure may produce the same set of symptoms. In evaluating the mechanisms of injury one must be constantly aware of the seemingly circuitous, but actually very direct, means by which objects can penetrate to such remote areas as the superior orbital fissure. For example, the superior orbital fissure syndrome can occur after injections designed to produce anesthesia of the upper teeth. The long needle may enter the lateral portion of the orbit through the inferior orbital fissure and then be directed into the superior orbital fissure.

The optic nerve is susceptible to injury in its intracanalicular segment as well as in the adjacent intraorbital and intracranial segments. A variety of mechanisms may be implicated. Direct injuries to the optic nerve may occur in the course of surgical procedures in the cranial cavity or in the orbit. The nerve can be impaled by hypodermic needles inserted into the orbit intentionally during the induction of local anesthesia for ophthalmic surgery, or accidentally, most commonly during induction of local anesthesia for dental surgery. Penetration with damage to the optic nerve may, of course, also occur in the course of nonmedical accidental trauma. Fractures of the bones surrounding the optic canal may lacerate the nerve, while bone fragments may literally "skewer" it. These fractures may not be demonstrable by x-ray.

Injury to the intracanalicular segment of the optic nerve may also occur indirectly. There may be bleeding around the nerve, causing compression and visual loss, or necrosis due to swelling and impairment of its blood supply. At times, there may be a delay between the occurrence of the injury and the onset of visual loss, but commonly the patient notes impaired vision from the outset. The external evidence of trauma may often be insignificant and inconsistent with the tragic irreversible visual loss that ensues.

Air can find its way into the orbital soft tissues if a communication develops between one of the paranasal sinuses and the orbit. As elsewhere in the body, the presence of air within tissues that do not normally contain air is called emphysema, and this specific type is known as orbital emphysema. Most commonly, it is caused by a fracture of the medial orbital wall producing a communication between the ethmoid sinus and the orbit, The air may dissect forward and appear in the lids and under the conjunctiva. It may first appear or suddenly increase in amount after the patient blows his nose. Palpation of the tissue produces a crackling sensation (crepitus). The conjunctiva may balloon markedly, and the globe may become exophthalmic, giving the patient a rather grotesque appearance. While the signs are sometimes striking, orbital emphysema is, however, self-limited and unlikely to produce any harmful residua. Nonetheless, there is a potential for infection of the orbit because of its communication with the sinus.

Foreign Bodies

A similar potential for infection exists when a foreign body pentrates into the orbit and is retained within the orbital cavity. Depending on its physical properties (e.g., size, composition), the foreign body may or may not be visible on x-ray. Metallic objects of sufficient size are usually demonstrable, while those of plastic, glass, or wood are generally not visible by x-ray examination. An orbital foreign body may produce symptoms if it causes sufficient damage at the time of penetration or if it leads to subsequent abscess formation. Otherwise these foreign bodies tend to be asymptomatic.

Most infections of the orbit are due to low-velocity, nonmetallic foreign bodies, since fast-moving foreign bodies, particularly those of metal, generate sufficient heat en route to sterilize themselves. Infection is particularly apt to follow the introduction of vegetable matter into the orbit, in which case the infection may be fungal rather than bacterial. The resulting abscess may be more dramatic than the initiating trauma. The infection is likely to become chronic and drain through a communication between the orbit and the point of entry in the skin. Thus, in a typical case, the patient may experience a penetrating wound that initially produces few symptoms and leaves him with little or no deficit. Subsequently, however, the eye begins to protrude, and limitation of motion and ocular pain appear, indicating the presence of an orbital abscess.

NONMECHANICAL INJURIES

Although initial emphasis has been given to mechanical injury, other types of trauma may injure the eye. Their discussion is organized around the source of the injury rather than about its location within the eye.

Thermal Injuries

Thermal injuries can be divided into two broad categories, burns due to flame, and contact burns due to hot bodies or fluids (scalds). Flame burns commonly involve the face, but the eyes are rarely affected. The lashes and brows may be scorched, the skin of the lids may be burned, and the face may be extensively injured, but reflex closure of the lids is generally sufficiently rapid to protect the eye. Despite the delicacy of the skin of the lids, the tarsal plates usually remain intact to preserve the integrity of the globe. Only when the flames spread with explosive force and rapidity is the cornea damaged. Even then, the damage often is superficial, limited to only the corneal epithelium. In such cases, regeneration of the epithelium occurs within 48 hours, leaving no residua. In rare instances, when the heat is intense and prolonged, the eyes may be permanently damaged, but in such cases survival is rare. Indeed, the worst ocular damage usually is encountered secondarily as a result of destruction or cicatricial distortion of the eyelids. The absence of functional lid tissue or the presence of cicatricial ectropion may cause exposure keratopathy with ulceration, secondary infection, and ultimately perforation of the cornea. Entropion of the lid after a flame burn of the face may cause trichiasis, traumatizing the cornea and similarly producing ulceration, infection, and perforation.

Contact burns are encountered in industry, for instance, when flying fragments of glowing metal enter the fornix before the blink reflex can act to prevent it. Both the conjunctiva and the cornea may be involved, and the burn may be severe enough to produce permanent scarring of both structures. The conjunctival burn results in loss of goblet cells and the accessory lacrimal glands. This, in turn, causes severe keratoconjunctivitis sicca (dry eye), keratinization of the corneal epithelium, neovascularization and opacification of the cornea, and permanent visual loss. The more severe forms of corneal involvement cause the tissue to become gray and opaque, its appearance very much resembling ground glass. Often the involved tissue becomes necrotic and sloughs, leaving an ulcer. Contact burns incurred in the home frequently are caused by hot fluids. Tragically, these accidents often involve young children whose inquisitiveness leads them to overturn boiling liquid from the kitchen range upon themselves. The same hazard may, however, be encountered in industry as a result of a bursting boiler or steam pipe. Large areas of the face including the eyelids may be burned, but generally not as severely as by flames; the skin loss is more commonly of partial thickness rather than full thickness. The blink reflex often protects the eyes or at least decreases the severity of the injury. As with flame burns, the most significant ocular defects may result from cicatricial deformities of the lids, rather than directly from the thermal contact.

Exposure to extreme cold may produce lesions remarkably similar to those due to heat in both their clinical and their histologic characteristics. They occur more rarely, however, and invariably are encountered as the result of exposure in survivors of mountain climbing expeditions, high altitude flying, shipwrecks, airplane crashes, and the like. The pathologic processes are considerably accelerated by the presence of a high wind, icy seas, or contact of the skin with metal such as spectacle frames. The unclothed parts of the body, including the face, tend to be preferentially affected. Down to a critical temperature (approximately −5°C) the cold has no gross effect upon individual cells; the pathologic effect is upon small blood vessels. The exposed skin, including that of the lids, is primarily involved and becomes necrotic and sloughs. The avascular cornea is initially spared but may be involved secondarily by exposure if the eyelids are lost.

Ultrasonic Injuries

Sound waves at frequencies audible to the human ear are not known to produce ocular injury, but ultrasonic vibrations (above 20,000 cps) have the demonstrated ability to damage the eye. Exposure of the eyelids to ultrasonic energy may be followed by epilation, ulceration of the skin, and edema. High intensities of radiation will destroy the corneal epithelium and produce necrosis of the stroma. Ultrasonic irradiation can also irreversibly liquefy the vitreous humor, cause cataracts, and produce an adhesive chorioretinal lesion. The precise mechanisms by which ultrasonic waves create these pathologic changes in the eye are not fully understood. Fortunately, however, these effects have been documented in experimental animals, and at present, are largely of theoretical interest only. This form of energy is not a common source of industrial or domestic injury.

Electrical Injuries

Electrical injuries are caused by the passage of an electric current through the body. With the exception of nerves, tissues are generally poor conductors of electricity, and their high resistance undoubtedly accounts for the thermal effects of electrical injuries. When a current passes through the orbital region, the hair of the head, the brows, and the eyelashes may be singed, and there may be accompanying superficial burns of the lids. Following more severe, deeper electrical burns, the substance of the lids including the tarsal plates may be lost. Histologically, these electrothermal burns are indistinguishable from other hyperthermal injuries.

The anterior segment of the eye may be damaged considerably as the result of lightning or a high-voltage electrical burn. Pathologic findings include conjunctival hyperemia and chemosis, ciliary injection, and subconjunctival hemorrhage. Usually these abnormalities are transient and subside within two weeks. Corneal stromal opacities may be demonstrable beneath an intact epithelium. These often are largely a manifestation of edema and clear spontaneously. Alternatively, a more destructive electric burn may cause the corneal epithelium to become necrotic and slough. Corneal sensation is diminished, and stromal ulceration and secondary infection may ensue. Iridocyclitis of varying degrees of severity invariably occurs, generally accompanied by pupillary miosis and sometimes by the formation of synechiae. Changes in the retina and choroid are infrequent but do occur. They include retinal edema, particularly at the posterior pole of the fundus (including the macula), punctate pigmentary degeneration, retinal hemorrhages, swelling of the optic disk, and patches of chorioretinitis that progress to patches of chorioretinal atrophy.

The most common ocular sequel of electrical injury, however, is cataract. These generally appear as a delayed effect some time after the accident and may occur in the absence of any other ocular damage. Current as low as 200 volts has been reported to be cataractogenic, and the degree of lens change has not been considered to be directly proportional to the strength of the current. It is possible, however, that the severity of the cataract is in fact a function of current strength but that the relationship has been obscured by such factors as variations in the duration of action of the current, the distance of the points of contact from the eye, the direction taken by the current in the body, and the dryness of the skin. Both direct and alternating current can produce cataracts. Those produced by lightning are usually bilateral, while unilateral cataracts are more common after industrial accidents. In the unilateral injury, the lens on the side of electrical contact is involved as a rule. When the point of contact is on one side and the lens changes are bilateral, the proximal eye usually demonstrates cataractous involvement first. The latent period between injury and the appearance of lens opacities varies considerably; the cataract may appear almost instantaneously or be delayed for years.

The cataract has characteristic form and structure, the changes occurring predominantly in the lens epithelium and in the subcapsular cortex beneath it. Both the anterior and posterior surfaces may be affected, but the former is more commonly involved after an industrial accident. Typically, a number of vacuoles of varying sizes appear immediately beneath the capsule. Multiple gray opacities, sometimes in the capsule itself but more characteristically in the subcapsular layers of the cortex, follow; these differ widely in size, shape, distribution, density, and rate of progression. Some eventually mature so that the lens becomes completely milky and occasionally causes acute glaucoma as it swells. The precise mechanisms by which electric current induces cataract formation are not known.

Radiational Injuries

A wide range of wavelengths of the electromagnetic spectrum are capable of injuring ocular tissues. Each type of radiant energy can do so, but only insofar as it is absorbed by the ocular tissues. A latent period generally lapses between the absorption of the energy and the appearance of its biologic effects. This varies with the wavelength of the energy and the tissue in which it is absorbed; the longest wavelengths have the shortest latent period. Thus, the latent period following infrared radiation is negligible so that an "instantaneous" burn results, while the latent period following ultraviolet irradiation is on the order of hours, and that after ionizing radiation is weeks to months. For any particular wavelength the latent period varies with the intensity of the exposure. With increasing energy levels, the pathologic changes increase until a maximum level is reached, and thereafter the changes are constant. The vulnerability of the tissue to radiational injuries varies with its ability to repair itself. For example, the lens, with its sluggish metabolism and limited reparative capacity, is more likely to sustain cumulative damage following repetitive insults than the richly vascularized tissues of the eye. Repeated dosage of any radiation tends to have a cumulative effect, provided the interval between radiational exposures does not exceed the period during which physiologic repair occurs.

Short-Wave Diathermy

Thermal lesions have been produced experimentally in a number of locations in the eye and its adnexa by short-wave diathermy. The current traverses the tissues directly, tending to concentrate along the path of least resistance, so that deep heating is produced much more effectively than by the local application of surface heat. The lesion produced is nonspecific in nature, initially characterized by vasodilatation, cellular proliferation, and acceleration of vital activities. When a critical temperature is reached, tissue death occurs because of coagulation of protein and inflammation. This type of thermal lesion is rarely encountered clinically, however, because diathermy for salutary purposes is not widely used by ophthalmologists, and when it is used, the limits of tolerance are rarely exceeded. On the other hand, ophthalmic surgeons do make use of the destructive properties of this energy form to achieve therapeutic benefit. In the operation of cyclodiathermy, it is used to destroy a portion of the ciliary body in order to decrease formation of aqueous humor and thereby lower the intraocular pressure in glaucoma. Similarly, in certain surgical procedures used to repair retinal detachment, diathermy is used to damage tissue and incite inflammation so that the repair processes will cause the detached retina to adhere to the choroid.

Microwaves

Microwaves produce similar thermal lesions. Experimental pathologic changes can be produced in the eye and are comparable to those seen after exposure to short-wave diathermy. The cataractogenic action of microwaves has received some notoriety in the ophthalmic literature, and indeed there is considerable experimental evidence to support the potential of microwaves to cause cataracts. To date, only a few reports of such lesions occurring in man as a result of occupational exposure have appeared. In each instance, the patient had had many direct ocular exposures to very high levels of microwave radiation over a considerable period of time. The authors are unaware of any documented case of cataract formation attributable to the conventional domestic type of microwave oven.

Infrared Radiation

Radiation in the near infrared portion of the electromagnetic spectrum is readily absorbed in the posterior pigmented epithelial layer of the iris. Thermal energy is generated, and the resultant temperature rise at the anterior surface of the lens is of sufficient magnitude to cause a cataract. Clinically, this type of heat cataract is rare, but its occurrence has been well documented in glassblowers and in workers exposed to the radiation of industrial furnaces. Its clinical appearance is highly characteristic. It starts as a well-defined opacity in the outer layers of the posterior cortex and develops into a sharply circumscribed, dense, axial, disk-shaped or flower petal–shaped posterior cortical cataract. It tends to progress inexorably, and as opacification of the lens proceeds, the cataract ultimately becomes indistinguishable from the common senile variety. Associated with the posterior cortical opacity is a splitting of the zonular lamella of the anterior capsule within the pupillary aperture. Considerable sheets of this capsular layer may be stripped from the underlying lens; the peripheral portion of the sheet curls inward and axially, and floats freely in the anterior chamber.

Most of the visible and paravisible (near infrared) electromagnetic energy incident upon the eye is absorbed by the pigmented epithelial layer of the retina and by the choroidal pigment. Heat is generated, and the resultant lesions are thermally induced. The lesion is therefore not related to any particular wavelength but depends only on the concentration of energy in the tissue. All radiation of this type is subject to optical refraction and is brought to a focus, usually on the macula. The density of energy incident upon this small region of the retina can be quite high, and a destructive chorioretinal lesion may therefore be produced by levels of radiation that cause no damage to other ocular structures.

Clinically, chorioretinal burns of this type are produced by looking at the sun. Ordinarily, the extreme brightness of the sun prevents prolonged fixation and thereby keeps such injuries to a minimum. During an eclipse, however, prolonged gazing at the sun is possible, and the inapparent but intense solar radiation is focused upon the macula, causing a chorioretinal burn. The effects vary in degree from the prolonged persistence of a negative afterimage of the sun or the appearance of scotomata to the permanent loss of central vision with the objective signs of a retinal burn. The ophthalmoscopic signs are fairly typical. Initially, the macula may appear somewhat darker than usual; in the more severe cases, it may be raised and edematous with some minute hemorrhages or a dark central spot surrounded by an edematous retinal detachment. At the fovea, one or more yellowish-white spots rapidly develop, surrounded by an irregular zone of mottled pigmentation. In the worst cases, a typical macular hole may develop.

Laser Burns

The destructive processes encountered in the chorioretinal lesions of solar eclipse burns are put to therapeutic use in the method of photocoagulation. High-intensity visible light is delivered in a controlled manner through either a direct ophthalmoscope or a slit-lamp biomicroscope. Most commonly, the source of radiant energy is a xenon arc or a ruby or argon laser. The energy is absorbed in the retinal pigment epithelium and choroidal pigment, where it produces coagulation necrosis of all retinal layers. It is used to treat holes in the retina while this structure is still in contact with the choroid. The area of retina surrounding the hole is soldered to the choroid by a thermal scar, preventing subsequent retinal detachment. Photocoagulation also seems to be of value for obliterating abnormal blood vessels in retinal vasculopathies, particularly diabetic retinopathy.

Lasers emit high-power, monochromatic, highly directional radiation. Most lasers available at present operate in the visible and near-infrared portions of the spectrum, but they are not limited to this range. The carbon dioxide laser, for example, emits an invisible beam in the mid-infrared region of the spectrum. The light produced by these instruments is of great intensity and capable of causing severe chorioretinal burns. As just indicated, they provide the power source for several types of photocoagulators. If the beam strikes the iris, visible laser radiation is absorbed in the pigment epithelium of that structure, and the heat generated can produce cataracts, iris atrophy, and anterior uveitis. If power levels are sufficiently high, secondary corneal damage may occur. The damage resulting from ocular exposure to the radiation emitted by the carbon dioxide laser differs from that produced by visible laser radiation. Whereas the absorption of visible light is dependent upon the degree of tissue pigmentation, the infrared radiation emitted by the carbon dioxide laser is largely absorbed by water. Its absorption by tissues is therefore dependent upon the water content of the tissue. Since the cornea is more than 75 per cent water, radiation emitted by the carbon dioxide laser, if directed at the eye, is predominantly absorbed in the cornea, and heat is generated there. If the intensity of the incident beam and the duration of exposure to the beam are adequate, the resultant temperature rise within the cornea is sufficient to produce thermal denaturation and coagulation of proteins, and gross corneal opacification instantaneously ensues. At higher levels of radiation, stromal ulceration and even immediate corneal perforation may occur. Ocular injury from laser radiation is most apt to occur in patients undergoing laser photocoagulation for ocular disease and in the operators of laser systems used for industrial, military, research, or clinical purposes. Both types of accidents have been reported.

Ultraviolet Radiation

Ultraviolet radiation may adversely affect the skin (including the skin of the eyelids) and the eye. Skin injury is manifest as a diffuse, homogenous erythema appearing six to eight hours after irradiation. If the dose is sufficiently large, blistering, small hemorrhages, and edema may be observed. As the acute reaction subsides, the superficial layers of the epidermis are exfoliated, and the pigmentation characteristic of sunburn develops in the deeper layers.

Similarly, ultraviolet light can induce an acute inflammatory reaction in the conjunctiva and cornea (photophthalmia). This condition may occur under natural conditions or, more commonly, as an accident among those who either work with ultraviolet rays or otherwise are exposed to a source rich in short wavelengths. Experimental data indicate that the most effective wavelength for producing keratitis is 288 mμ, but the action spectrum capable of inciting a photophthalmic reaction is approximately 305 mμ to 250 mμ. Ordinarily, sunlight, even when reinforced by the light of a sky free from atmospheric contamination of moisture or dust (which absorb ultraviolet radiation), does not cause photophthalmia. When these sources are reinforced by a dazzling reflection from an extensive surface such as the sea, the desert, or particularly a snow or ice field with its high reflection factor, however, and an exposure of several hours to this combined radiational source is experienced, then the critical threshold of abiotic damage by ultraviolet rays may be exceeded and photophthalmia results. Under conditions of nature, this problem is most commonly encountered after exposure to bright sunlight on a snow field and is usually called snowblindness, a most inaccurate term since the symptoms are caused not by the snow but by the solar energy reflected in part by the snow, and since actual blindness rarely occurs. It is of interest that given the appropriate environmental conditions, animals do not escape this affliction; indeed, it has been described in the polar bear. Unlike the skin, in which the pigmentation that follows the initial exposure produces tolerance, the cornea acquires no such tolerance to repeated exposure.

Industrial photophthalmia (flash eye) is apt to occur in any occupation in which insufficiently screened sources of light rich in ultraviolet radiation are used. This includes the medical employment of ultraviolet radiation. The most acute symptoms, however, are encountered among workers with inadequate ocular protection engaged in oxyacetylene or arc welding. Short exposures are additive within a period of up to 24 hours and therefore are cumulatively dangerous.

Regardless of the source of the ultraviolet radiation, the clinical picture is the same and is characteristic. There is always a latent period between exposure and the onset of symptoms. Its length varies directly with the intensity and the duration of the exposure, but most commonly it is about 6 to 10 hours. The first symptom generally is a sensation like that caused by a foreign body, ranging in degree from a slight pricking to considerable discomfort likened to an eye full of sand. If the patient has been exposed to moderately intense radiation, as is often the case, frank ocular pain occurs accompanied by marked photophobia, profuse lacrimation, and striking blepharospasm. In most instances, the objective signs are surprisingly mild in view of the patient's particularly miserable and helpless state. The conjunctiva is red and occasionally chemotic, and the pupil tends to be constricted (miosis). The surface of the cornea has lost its luster and appears gray and irregular, but usually the epithelial layer is intact. Application of fluorescein stain gives it a stippled appearance. The entity usually is self-limited, with most of the discomfort subsiding within 48 hours.

Ionizing Radiation

As it traverses a tissue, ionizing radiation (x- and γ-rays) dissipates its energy by the liberation of ions. There seems to be no essential qualitative difference in the biologic action of various types of ionizing radiation. They appear to differ only quantitatively in relation to such factors as their penetrability, the density of the ionization to which they give rise, and the amount of energy they have available for dissipation. The vast majority of injuries to the eye and adnexa caused by this form of radiation result from therapeutic irradiation of the eye or neighboring structures. Generally, the irradiation is used to treat malignant disease and a considerable dose is required. Most such injuries consequently are a side effect that is rendered acceptable by the fatal nature of the primary disease under treatment. The ocular sequelae of ionizing radiation are widely appreciated, and careful protection of the eye is routinely practiced. As a result, the incidence of this type of injury has decreased considerably.

In the skin, the acute reaction may either heal completely or become chronic. Exposure to any type of ionizing radiation is invariably followed by a mild and transient edema within

24 hours. After a variable latent period, measured in days to weeks depending on the dose employed, a sustained hyperemia reappears, followed by a dry and then a moist desquamation of the superficial layer of epidermis. Reepithelialization is followed by fading of the erythema and ultimately of the edema. Epilation frequently occurs but is of cosmetic consequence only. The involved area may break down subsequent to minor trauma, and occasionally a squamous cell carcinoma will develop years after exposure. This has been exceptionally rare on the lids and has occurred only when excessive irradiation has previously caused considerable skin damage. With modern therapeutic techniques, even shrinkage of tissues of the lids due to vascular changes that lead to fibrosis and contracture in the dermis is rare, but ectropion or entropion may occasionally develop.

The immediate conjunctival reaction to ionizing radiation is characterized by hyperemia, edema, and chemosis, and is accompanied by a watery discharge that may become mucopurulent. Conjunctival injection may persist for months and even years. Some months after irradiation, scarring ensues, and the atrophic, scarred tissue becomes adherent to the underlying sclera. After diffuse irradiation, the entire conjunctival sac may be involved. Extensive areas of radionecrosis appear, the fornices become obliterated, symblepharon develops, and ocular motility is impaired. The reaction of the conjunctival vessels is typical, with alternate dilatations and constrictions, and large telangiectases. More severe effects include deformities of the lid, with ectropion or entropion and obliteration of the puncta (due to associated scarring and contracture of the lid and conjunctiva), and the localized loss of conjunctival glandular tissue, metaplasia of the irradiated conjunctiva, and keratosis. These more extreme sequelae are rarely seen now.

Punctate erosions of the corneal epithelium that heal rapidly and spontaneously are almost invariably seen after ocular exposure to ionizing radiation. Apart from this, the corneal complications of radiotherapy are delayed in onset. They may occur either as a direct effect of the radiation or indirectly in response to decreased or abnormal lacrimal secretions. After a latent period of weeks to months, it may be noted that corneal sensation is reduced or absent. Subsequently, the cornea loses its normal surface luster, there is loss of epithelium with superficial ulceration, and the stroma is invaded by inflammatory cells causing loss of transparency. The corneal ulcer may be central or peripheral in location and is characteristically indolent and slow to heal. Interstitial keratitis with neovascular invasion of the corneal stroma may occur, even in those cases that heal; in the worst instances, necrosis of corneal tissue progressing to perforation and extrusion of intraocular contents may be encountered. Hypesthesia generally ensures that the process is relatively painless and may give rise to a false sense of security, leading the patient to delay in seeking help.

Scleral complications following exposure to ionizing radiation are very uncommon. Those reported, primarily necrosis of the sclera, are produced only by very high radiation dosages. Similarly, large doses of ionizing radiation may cause vascular changes in the iris and ciliary body, while the tissues of the retina and optic nerve, particularly after they are fully developed, are even less sensitive. Clinical lesions have rarely been reported and have invariably been associated with very high dosage of radiation. With modern techniques of radiotherapy they have been largely eliminated.

The ocular lesion in this group that has perhaps been the object of the most intense investigation is radiation cataract. The subcapsular epithelium of the lens is unusually sensitive to ionizing radiation; indeed, it is the most radiosensitive part of the adult eye and may be damaged at radiation levels that do not adversely affect other parts of the eye. The injury produced in the germinal zone of the epithelium, located at the equator of the lens, is manifest by opacification in the posterior cortex. A considerable latent period elapses, however, between exposure to the ionizing radiation and the clinical appearance of the cataract and onset of visual symptoms. Its length varies a great deal. In general, the younger the patient and the greater the dose of radiation, the shorter is the interval before the lens opacities become evident. In most instances, the latent period is on the order of years. With x-radiation of the usual therapeutic type (100 to 250 kv), the minimal cataractogenic dose after a single exposure is usually considered to be 500 to 600 R. Cases have been reported, however, in which cataracts have appeared after a single exposure of as little as 200 R. The susceptibility of the lens epithelium is an inverse function of the patient's age. Fractionation of a given total radiation dose results in a longer latent period and fewer dense opacities.

The clinical appearance of radiation cataract is remarkably characteristic. Dotlike opacities are noted in the axial portion of the posterior capsule, imparting to it a granular appearance that ultimately assumes a ring shape. Vacuoles form in the posterior cortex anterior to the posterior capsule. Additional granular spots appear in the central portion of the posterior cortex, and this part of the lens gradually clouds. Thereafter, a hard central plaque, denser at its margins than at its center, develops at the posterior pole of the lens. Meanwhile, a gray haze and vacuoles appear in the pupillary region of the anterior subcapsular segment of the lens. Opacification seems to spread from the posterior pole, and in many cases, the lens finally becomes completely opaque.

No attempt has been made in the foregoing discussion to separate out the effects of an atomic blast. Visible and infrared radiation are emitted and cause the chorioretinal burns and other damage just detailed. Ionizing radiation in the form of gamma rays and fast neutrons is also emitted and is capable of producing radiation cataracts and the like. In those receiving sufficient total body exposure to induce radiation sickness, ocular damage may be secondary to injury of more radiosensitive tissues, particularly the hematopoietic system. Findings in the eye are predominantly hemorrhagic and include subconjunctival, retinal, vitreous, and anterior chamber bleeding. Fluffy retinal exudates and multiple foci of septic choroiditis may also be encountered.

Chemical Injuries

Chemical injuries of the eye are relatively common, and a markedly heterogeneous collection of causal agents may be at fault. As a result, the damage encountered may vary in severity from transient conjunctival hyperemia, which clears rapidly with little or no therapy, to disastrous tissue necrosis with rapid and irreversible loss of vision in one or both eyes. A number of prevalent activities and routine situations provide ample opportunity for the occurrence of this type of injury. Industry is undoubtedly responsible for the majority of chemical hazards and appears to have a virtually unlimited capability for producing new compounds capable of damaging the eye. Agriculture and its related activities present significant chemical dangers from toxic materials of animal and vegetable origin and from a wide variety of caustic fertilizers and insecticides. Laboratory accidents still contribute a considerable quota of these injuries, as do domestic accidents. The policeman seeking to disperse a rioting mob or to subdue those engaged in criminal activity and the jealous or angered person intent on revenge are still other sources. This discussion is limited to injury caused by external contact of the chemical with the eye. Those substances that exert a damaging effect on the eyes and their connections with the central nervous system through systemic absorption are covered in the section on toxicologic injuries.

Several factors determine the type and severity of the injury a chemical causes. The most important of these factors are the duration of contact of the chemical with the eye, its ability to penetrate into ocular tissues, and its reactivity with those tissues. The duration of contact of the offending agent with the eye is dependent, in turn, on its concentration, its ability to produce immediate discomfort, and the ease with which the chemical can be diluted or removed from the ocular surface. Pain may stimulate lacrimation, diluting the chemical, and also stimulates the victim to irrigate his eyes promptly. Unfortunately, it may also induce uncontrollable blepharospasm, which impedes attempts at immediate lavage. Agents that instantly injure corneal nerves and produce analgesia, such as ammonia or sulfur dioxide, are even more dangerous, however. The absence of discomfort may lull the patient into a false sense of security about the extent of the damage inflicted and cause him to delay remedial measures.

The concentration of a noxious agent coming into contact with the eye depends in part on its physical state. A gas arrives in less concentration than does a splash of liquid. A solid particle may act as a reservoir of toxic material that is progressively dissolved rather than being diluted by tears. This is particularly true if removal of the particle is delayed or is mechanically difficult, a situation encountered in its most devastating form with particles of lime, which cling tenaciously to the ocular tissues despite copious irrigation. The aqueous solubility of the offending agent is, of course, most important, since chemicals tend to react on conjunctiva and cornea only when they come into solution.

Although the specific mechanisms by which various chemicals injure ocular tissues are extremely diverse, they cannot be differentiated by either clinical or histologic appearances. ✓ Both acids and alkalis cause a rapid and drastic coagulation of proteins with cellular death. The essential difference between them is that alkalis penetrate the cornea readily by saponification of the cellular barriers and denaturation of the mucopolysaccharides, and thus cause more damage. Except for minor differences in the intensity of their reaction and the degree to which the effects spread, other substances of widely diverse action show no generic differences in their clinical pathologic effects. The various cellular changes produced by most substances, regardless of the chemical group to which they belong, show few distinctive characteristics.

Ocular Responses to Chemical Injury

The reaction of the conjunctiva is characterized by hyperemia, edema, and lacrimation. Leukocytes may migrate in quantity from the blood vessels and combine with cellular debris to form a mucoid discharge. After more severe injury, the edema may lead to considerable chemosis and the vascular injury to local hemorrhage. Ultimately coagulation necrosis results. If the process is acute, the damaged mucous membrane is treated as a foreign body and is sloughed or cleared away by phagocytic action. If it is chronic and cell death occurs gradually, the damaged mucosa may be retained and may remain pale, translucent, and permanently ischemic, or may eventually become revascularized. Damage at the limbus involving the limbal vessels may have a deleterious effect on corneal nutrition and therefore assumes added significance. Healing occurs by the formation of new connective tissue and regeneration of epithelium. The latter is effected by a sliding of epithelial cells adjacent to the injured region over the raw area and by the mitotic division of neighboring cells. In more destructive injuries the damaged mucosa is replaced by fibrous tissue that may become too exuberant in its proliferation. This leads to the formation of fibrous bands between the lids and the globe (anterior symblepharon), obliteration of the conjunctival fornix (posterior symblepharon), or the fusion of all conjunctival surfaces (total symblepharon).

As might be expected, the earliest changes in the cornea appear in the epithelium that has been in direct contact with the causal agent. Initially, this may present as edema of the epithelial cells, clinically visible with the slit-lamp biomicroscope. If the traumatic event interferes with cohesion between cells or between the epithelium and the underlying Bowman's membrane, fluid accumulates with the formation of vesicular blebs or bullae that may give rise to a considerable degree of irritation, lacrimation, and photophobia. These vesicles may increase in size and burst, leaving areas of Bowman's membrane devoid of epithelial covering, a phenomenon that is often accompanied by a marked increase in the severity of the subjective symptoms. Following more severe lesions, areas of the epithelium (or even the entire layer) suffer coagulation, lose their transparency, rapidly become necrotic, and are sloughed. If the damage is confined to the epithelium, healing will take place by epithelial sliding and mitosis of the surrounding cells.

Penetration of chemical agents into the stroma leads to denaturation and coagulation of proteins there and a consequent loss of transparency. An inflammatory response is initiated, and a chemotactic stimulus attracts large numbers of polymorphonuclear leukocytes to the area. Degranulation of these infiltrating cells causes significant amounts of hydrolytic enzymes to be released within the corneal stroma with resulting tissue necrosis and ulceration. Many noxious chemical agents are capable of penetrating completely through the stroma to damage the endothelial cells. Since the endothelium bears primary responsibility for maintaining the delicate water balance necessary for transparency of the cornea, its injury is followed by edema and opacification.

Vascularization of the cornea is often a prominent feature of chemical injuries (Fig. 3–III–28). The ingrowth of new vessels may occur at either a superficial or a deep level of the cornea, and not infrequently both types of vessels appear. The mechanism that stimulates corneal neovascularization has not been entirely elucidated, but it appears certain that

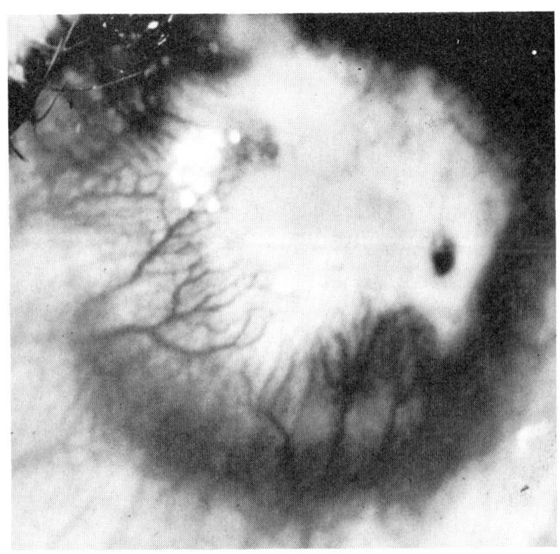

Figure 3–III–28. Chemical (sulfur dioxide) injury of the eye, characterized by dense scarring and neovascularization. The black oval spot is a perforating ulcer.

stromal edema plays a role. The new vessels invade the cornea from the limbus and may ultimately involve the entire cornea. As the acute inflammatory phase subsides, many of the newly formed vessels cease to transport blood. Most, however, persist indefinitely as patent channels and may be seen on retroillumination with the slit-lamp biomicroscope as fine empty tubes known as ghost vessels. If the corneal stroma has been severely damaged at the limbus, subconjunctival connective tissue as well as blood vessels and epithelial cells may migrate into the injured area, forming a fibrovascular mass referred to clinically as a pseudopterygium.

A violent iritis results if the caustic chemical gains access to the anterior chamber in quantity. The aqueous humor becomes plasmoid, containing a high concentration of protein, large numbers of inflammatory cells, and copious amounts of fibrin. The contents of the anterior chamber may become grossly gelatinous. Secondary glaucoma may follow, either because of mechanical blockage of the trabecular meshwork by this material, because of the formation of anterior and posterior synechiae, or because the anterior ciliary vessels and the drainage system from the canal of Schlemm have become necrotic and been obliterated by the direct action of the chemical. Other disastrous consequences include cataract, atrophy of the ciliary body, phthisis bulbi, and perforation of the globe.

Strong acids produce denaturation and coagulation of all the proteins with which they come into contact to form insoluble acid proteinates. The protein denaturation is irreversible; recovery does not follow neutralization of the acid, and tissue destruction is permanent. Further tissue penetration by the acid is prevented by the barrier created by the dense layer of precipitated protein, and continued activity is neutralized by the buffering action of the tissues themselves. The lesion therefore tends to be sharply delimited to the area of initial contact and tends to be nonprogressive.

Alkali burns usually cause even greater violence to the eye than do acid burns. Strong alkalis produce a shift of the hydrogen ion concentration beyond the limits of stability of tissue proteins, resulting in their degradation. Moreover, alkali dissociates and saponifies fatty acids, thereby specifically destroying lipoid cellular membranes; this enables it to penetrate rapidly into the involved tissue. Because they are hygroscopic, various alkalis also extract water from cells, another factor that contributes to necrosis. The combination of alkali with lipids to form soluble compounds causes the tissue to soften and become gelatinous, just the opposite of the hard dry coagulation necrosis caused by acids. As a result, alkali burns spread more widely and may remain active for several days.

Thus, the general clinical pictures of an acid and an alkali burn of the eye differ markedly. The acid burn produces a sharply defined coagulative injury whose maximum damage occurs almost instantly and is followed by rapid healing. In contrast, the alkali burn produces damage that is widespread, uncontrolled, and progressive. In the conjunctiva, it is manifested by rapidly developing edema and chemosis, extensive necrosis, and a purulent-appearing dis-

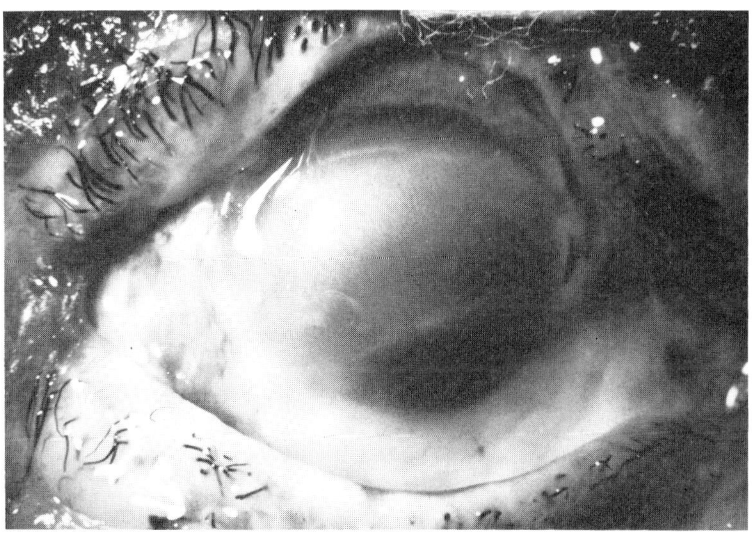

Figure 3–III–29. Chemical (sodium hydroxide) injury of the eye, characterized by an ischemic, necrotic conjunctiva, complete opacification of the cornea, and perforating ulceration of the inferior cornea with prolapse of the iris.

charge, with attempts at repair of the destruction leading to prolific fibroblastic proliferation and symblepharon. In the cornea, there are epithelial disintegration and sloughing, pronounced stromal edema, cellular infiltration, neovascularization, fibrosis, opacification, and a marked tendency toward ulceration and staphyloma formation. Severe iritis is a frequent accompaniment, damaging surrounding structures and causing glaucoma. The processes all tend to be progressive, and perforating ulceration may occur some time after the traumatic insult (Fig. 3–III–29). The ultimate outcome must remain in doubt for a relatively prolonged period.

As noted earlier, the number and types of chemicals capable of exerting an adverse effect upon the eye are extremely large. The range of severity and the specific effects of each are correspondingly large and diverse and beyond the scope of this work. Reference works in which pathologic changes created by individual compounds are discussed in detail are cited at the end of Chapter 3–III.

Stress Injuries

Ocular abnormality may be encountered as a result of three types of stress: abnormal barometric pressure and particularly a sudden variation in barometric pressure, vibration, and acceleration.

A sudden relative diminution of the atmospheric pressure permits air held in solution in the blood and tissue fluids at the higher pressure to be released. If this occurs rapidly, the released air forms bubbles in the tissues, in the blood, and in the lungs. Decompression sickness results and is seen when workers in compressed air are too rapidly decompressed (caisson disease), when deep sea divers surface too rapidly (divers' paralysis), and when aviators ascend too rapidly (aviators' aeroembolism). The general symptoms of decompression sickness are extremely varied, since virtually every organ in the body may be affected. Ocular effects occur and may be dramatic, but they are not common. These changes include subconjunctival, retinal, and choroidal hemorrhages; bubbles of gas may be visible in the retinal blood vessels. The retina may present a picture of central retinal artery occlusion with gray-white retinal edema and a cherry-red spot at the macula. The inert nitrogen in the liberated air not only represents a mechanical danger but also, because of its great fat solubility, is responsible for the tendency toward accumulation of bubbles in central nervous tissue. Thus, while blockage of the circulation by nitrogen emboli may produce ischemic infarction of tissues, the gas may also damage neuronal cells directly. Both types of damage may affect the intracranial visual pathways and are manifested by nystagmus, paresis of the extraocular muscles, visual field defects, pupillary abnormalities, partial optic atrophy, and papilledema.

Ocular signs and symptoms occur at low barometric pressure such as is encountered in mountain climbing and in flying without compression of the cabin atmosphere. The critical altitude seems to be about 12,000 feet above sea level, and abnormalities increase, both in severity and in incidence, with increasingly higher altitudes. The essential defect in the atmosphere at high altitudes that is responsible for the ocular difficulties is lack of oxygen. Objective signs include conjunctival hemorrhages, retinal vasodilatation, pupillary dilatation, strabismus, retinal hemorrhages, and edema of the optic nerve. Functional changes in vision are more common. They include decreased visual acuity, peripheral constriction of the visual fields, impaired dark adaptation, depressed stereopsis, diplopia, and the appearance of visual illusions. All appear attributable to depressed function of the central nervous system, not of the eye, and are rapidly reversed by the inhalation of oxygen.

Vibrational stresses may also have a detrimental effect upon vision. Visual acuity is reduced by a factor of about 25 per cent by rapid vibrations even though their amplitude may be very small, that is, on the order of a few millimeters. The degree of reduction in vision appears to be determined by the effective vibration of the head, particularly in the vertical direction. At higher frequencies or greater amplitudes of vibration, vision rapidly becomes impossible.

Similarly, sudden changes of motion, either in magnitude or direction, of acceleration or deceleration, may affect visual performance. Gravitational forces are primarily responsible for these effects. When the force acts from the head to the feet (as when a pilot pulls out of a power dive), the acceleration is called positive ($+g$); when the force acts from feet to head (as in an outside loop), the acceleration is called negative. The symptoms of positive acceleration are primarily visual. Initially there is blanching of the face, sagging of the soft tissues and ptosis, slumping of the trunk in the seat, venous distention in the lower extremities, and tachycardia. Associated with this is a "graying" or dimming of vision, followed by loss of the peripheral visual field that leaves the central area intact, and finally a sudden and complete "black-out" followed by loss of consciousness. Visual impairment is not accompanied by loss of hearing or smell, nor by nausea, giddiness, or pain. The symptoms of negative acceleration are a flushed feeling of the face, a throbbing sensation in the head as if the skull were about to burst and the eyes to be forced out of their sockets, mental confusion, muscular incoordination, and occasionally a "red-out" of vision. Consciousness is not lost. Conjunctival and retinal hemorrhages may occur. The visual symptoms of positive acceleration result from exsanguination of the eyes due to lack of carotid arterial circulation; those of negative acceleration are the result of vascular congestion. No residual abnormalities have been noted.

Toxicologic Injuries

The ingenuity of man in devising an increasing number of useful chemical compounds and drugs was commented upon earlier. Virtually all these compounds are toxic if ingested, and even those that exhibit salutary pharmacologic effects are usually toxic if taken in excess. Most of the structures of the visual apparatus may be damaged by the systemic absorption of a toxic chemical or drug. The number of compounds with toxic ocular effects is large, and the amount of available data describing these effects is enormous. A comprehensive discussion of ocular toxicology is therefore beyond the scope of this text, and the reader is referred to the references at the end of the chapter for more detailed information. This section attempts only to highlight the subject.

Inorganic Poisons

Inorganic poisons affecting the eye are mainly metallic salts. Characteristically they cause keratoconjunctivitis, oculomotor disturbances, optic neuropathy, or papilledema. Lead causes kidney dysfunction, which in turn can produce a retinopathy. It has also been documented to produce optic neuropathy, pupillary paresis, papilledema, ocular motor palsies, and amaurosis associated with encephalopathy. Arsenic produces eczema of the lids and conjunctivitis that in the most severe cases may be exfoliative. Keratitis frequently occurs that may be characterized by a massive loss of the epithelium, edema, neovascularization, necrosis, and ulceration of the stroma. Optic neuropathy and optic atrophy also have been documented. Silver may be deposited in the conjunctiva and cornea, imparting to it a slate gray discoloration. Prolonged absorption of mercury may lead to impregnation of the lens (mercurialentis), producing a brownish discoloration in the anterior pupillary portion. Gold may cause an exfoliative dermatitis resembling that due to arsenic and also may be associated with conjunctivitis and keratitis, the latter involving marginal ulceration or interstitial stromal opacities.

Organic Poisons

Conjunctival and lacrimal reactions have been attributed to a number of substances; most are of minor importance. Sulfadiazine, however, has produced a severe ulcerative conjunctivitis that resembles the lesions of erythema multiforme or pemphigus and is followed by extensive enough scarring to cause symblepharon. Although not due to systemic absorption, topical administration of epinephrine for the treatment of glaucoma has resulted in permanent black pigmentation of the conjunctiva and cornea and persistent epiphora due to obstruction of the lacrimal passages by the accumulated decomposition products of the drug.

Quinacrine, an antimalarial drug, may occasionally give rise to reversible edema of the epithelium and anterior stroma of the cornea. Corneal deposits have been documented to occur as a result of systemic ingestion of chlorpromazine, indomethacin, and chloroquine. Phenolphthalein has produced toxic necrosis of the cornea with destruction of the epithelium and stromal ulceration severe enough to cause perforation.

Several organic compounds exert toxic effects on the uveal tract and retina. Chronic benzene poisoning among rotogravure workers and among workers in the rubber, linoleum, and paint industries has demonstrated that benzene causes hemorrhages in the lids and conjunctiva as well as in the iris, choroid, and retina. It also causes optic neuropathy, optic atrophy, and papilledema. Two groups of drugs, however, the synthetic antimalarials, such as chloroquine, and the phenothiazines, used primarily as tranquilizers, have perhaps received the greatest attention because of their retinotoxicity. The discovery of the therapeutic effectiveness of chloroquine and related compounds in rheumatoid arthritis and other connective tissue disorders led to its administration in higher dosage and over more prolonged periods than had been used for antimalarial purposes. This, in turn, caused an increase in ocular side effects, most distressing of which was a delayed toxic retinopathy with specific predilection for the macula. Typically, the macular areas of both retinas contain a pigmented lesion that resembles the bull's eye of a target and results in a permanent and often profound decrease in visual acuity. It has been suggested that this toxic effect is produced by damage to the retinal pigment epithelium where chloroquine accumulates in association with melanin. Similar findings can, however, be produced experimentally in the albino rat, and it is therefore probable that binding of the drug to intracellular nucleoproteins is a more important factor in its toxic action. Among the phenothiazines, thioridazine has most often been found to cause a pigmentary retinopathy in humans.

Also of interest is the retinotoxic effect of epinephrine, which is not seen after systemic administration but rather following topical instillation. It occurs only in aphakic eyes and is characterized by macular edema associated with small hemorrhages or cystic changes in the perimacular region. A marked loss of vision with a central or paracentral scotoma in the visual field results. Termination of the medication is generally followed by complete visual recovery within approximately a six-month period, but its resumption is followed by a recurrence of visual symptoms and abnormal retinal findings.

Although it is not an organic chemical compound, oxygen must be mentioned in any discussion of retinal toxicity. Oxygen has a toxic action on the immature retina and exerts its adverse effect upon the immature retinal blood vessels rather than upon the neural tissue. When administered to newborn premature infants, oxygen causes obliteration of the developing immature retinal vessels. Prolific neovascularization results, accompanied by a profuse proliferation of fibrous tissue. This extends into the vitreous humor, and the entire process leads to the formation of a retrolental fibrovascular membrane, which, because of the traction it places on the retina, may cause retinal detachment. The entity is known as retrolental fibroplasia (Fig. 3–III–30).

A number of organic agents, given systemically, are followed by the appearance of lens opacities and the development of a frank cataract. Naphthalene is a potent cataractogenic agent that has produced documented lens changes in man that closely resemble those seen in senile cataract. Dinitrophenol, a chemical that increases oxidative metabolism and has been used in the past as a weight-reducing agent, produces anterior and posterior subcapsular lens opacities that usually proceed rapidly

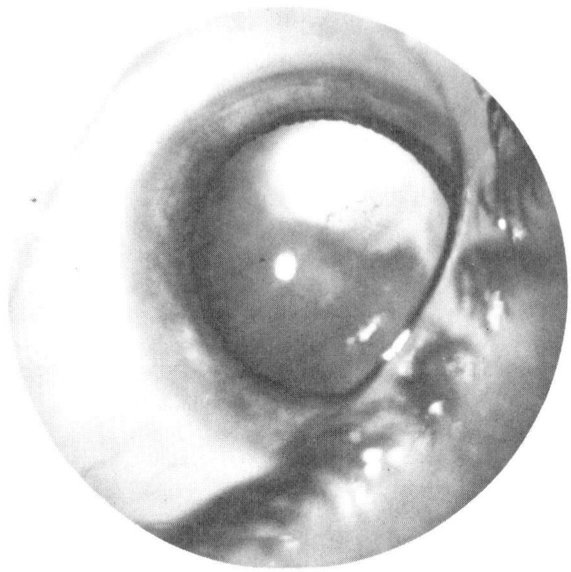

Figure 3–III–30. Retrolental fibroplasia.

to involve the cortex and nucleus of the lens with advanced cataractous changes. Among the drugs that cause cataracts are the morphine group, the corticosteroids, the phenothiazines, chloroquine, the sulfonamides, and the cholinesterase inhibitors. Perhaps because of the prevalence of corticosteroid use as well as the large doses prescribed and the prolonged periods of administration, the cataracts that follow its administration have attracted the greatest attention. They generally are seen in patients who have received the drug for periods longer than a year, and their incidence is directly correlated with drug dosage and duration of therapy. Characteristically, the cataract induced by corticosteroids is initially located in the posterior subcapsular area, directly in front of the posterior pole of the lens, and tends to progress. Cataracts have also been reported after the topical administration of corticosteroids, but many of these occurred in eyes with intraocular inflammatory disease capable of producing similar lens changes. The pathogenetic mechanisms by which corticosteroids produce lens opacities are not known.

Topical application of corticosteroids is also well documented as a cause of glaucoma in a substantial portion of the population. The drug produces an increased resistance to the outflow of aqueous humor from the anterior chamber, presumably as a result of structural changes it creates in the trabecular meshwork. Systemically administered corticosteroids, on the other hand, have comparatively little tendency to induce glaucoma. Most such eyes alleged to have glaucoma as a result of systemically administered corticosteroids have also been affected with intraocular inflammatory processes that are themselves capable of causing secondary glaucoma. Anticholinergic (atropine, scopolamine) and adrenergic (epinephrine, phenylephrine) drugs may induce angle-closure glaucoma after systemic administration but only if they produce pupillary dilatation in anatomically predisposed eyes. The systemically administered anticholinergic drugs may also aggravate existing open-angle glaucoma if it causes paralysis of accommodation.

A host of agents, largely drugs, have been implicated in the etiology of toxic optic neuropathies, but a definite cause and effect relationship is often difficult to establish. It may be impossible to distinguish between the effects on the optic nerve of an illness itself and of the drugs used to treat the illness. In many instances, there is exposure to a variety of agents, and it is difficult to be certain which (if any) is responsible for the optic neuropathy that developed in the course of treatment. Indeed, the diagnosis of toxic optic neuropathy presents major difficulties. The characteristics of this entity may be summarized as follows: (1) Blurred vision is the predominant symptom. (2) Symptoms are usually bilateral. Initially only one eye may be involved, but with time the second eye becomes symptomatic. (3) The disorder develops slowly over a period of weeks or months. (4) The disease is painless. (5) The disease does not produce total blindness. (6) There is usually some impairment of color perception as revealed by the standard test plates designed to detect congenital color blindness. (7) On visual field testing, there is a scotoma (non-seeing area) involving the point of fixation (central scotoma) or one extending from the point of fixation to include the physiologic blind spot (centrocecal scotoma). (8) Fundus examination may be normal early in the course of the illness. With time, the optic disk may become pale or swollen and congested, and there may be accompanying hemorrhages. (9) There is often potential for visual recovery if the offending chemical is discontinued.

Among the drugs most recently incriminated as a cause of optic neuropathy are the oral contraceptives, generally a mixture of estrogen and progesterone-like compounds. They are alleged to produce vascular occlusions in the blood supply of the optic nerve, which in turn cause the neuropathy. Interestingly, this mechanism permits them to violate two of the foregoing general rules. The entity they cause may be unilateral, and it may be rapid or sudden in onset. Among the clinical findings observed in association with "the pill" are papilledema, retinal edema, occlusion of the central retinal artery, venous congestion with hemorrhages, and retrobulbar neuritis. In several instances, the symptoms and signs disappeared on withdrawal of the drug, but the causal relationship is as yet not definitely established. Other hormones, notably the corticosteroids, may cause pseudotumor cerebri and papilledema.

The group of entities known as toxic amblyopias must be included here. The term is generally used to designate those conditions wherein visual loss results from the absorption of external poisons that affect the subchiasmal portion of the visual pathway, the ganglion cells of the retina, or their continuation, the fibers of the optic nerve. They tend to have a selective affinity for the papillomacular bundle, which explains the central or centrocecal scotoma already alluded to. Compounds included in this group are ethyl alcohol, methyl alcohol, carbon disulfide, isoniazid, ethambutol, and the aniline dyes. Tobacco has also been implicated as an etiologic agent in this condition, but as in the case of ethyl alcohol, there are many authorities who take exception to this. They believe that the toxic amblyopia seen in patients who smoke and drink heavily is due neither to the tobacco nor to the alcohol but rather to a nutritional deficiency caused by the poor dietary habits of these individuals. There is also a second, less prevalent group of toxic amblyopias in which the visual field defect takes the form of a concentric peripheral contraction, advancing to a general depression of the visual field. The reason for this difference is not known, but the compounds that cause it include quinine, carbon tetrachloride, ergot, salicylic acid, and organic arsenic.

SELECTED READINGS

1. Chandler, P. A., and Grant, W. M.: *Lectures on Glaucoma.* Philadelphia, Lea & Febiger, 1965.
2. Duke-Elder, W. S., and MacFaul, P. A.: *System of Ophthalmology XIV, Injuries, Part 1—Mechanical Injuries.* St. Louis, C. V. Mosby Co., 1972.
3. Duke-Elder, W. S., and MacFaul, P. A.: *System of Ophthalmology XIV, Injuries, Part 2—Non-Mechanical Injuries.* St. Louis, C. V. Mosby Co., 1972.
4. Grant, W. M.: *Toxicology of the Eye.* 2nd Ed. Springfield, Ill., Charles C Thomas, 1972.
5. Hogan, M. J., and Zimmerman, L. E.: *Ophthalmic Pathology.* 2nd Ed. Philadelphia, W. B. Saunders Co., 1962.
6. Lindenberg, R., Walsh, F. B., and Sacks, J. G.: *Neuropathology of Vision: An Atlas.* Philadelphia, Lea & Febiger, 1973.
7. Walsh, F. B., and Hoyt, W. F.: *Clinical Neuro-ophthalmology.* Baltimore, Williams & Wilkins Co., 1969.

IV. Auditory Apparatus: The Cochlear-Vestibular System

by Charles W. Vaughan and M. Stuart Strong

The ear is a sensory organ with a dual function. It is concerned with the perception of sound and with the perception of movement and of position of the head, i.e., it contributes to the sense of balance. It is conveniently divided into three parts: the external ear, the middle ear, and the inner ear.

The external ear includes the pinna and the ear canal. The pinna consists of a pliable cartilage intimately covered with thin skin that contains the normal skin appendages of hair, secretory glands, and sensory nerve endings. It is slightly cup-shaped to aid in its modest function of collecting sound waves and directing them into the ear canal. Some animals have well-developed muscles that can change the direction of the pinna, but in man these are rudimentary and ineffective. The external ear canal is approximately 25 to 30 mm in length and is lined with skin that in its outer half contains hair follicles, seborrheic glands, and special glands for the production of cerumen. The inner half of the canal is supported by bone of the skull. The eardrum (tympanic membrane) closes off the depth of the ear canal. It is a thin, cone-shaped, flexible membrane that serves to collect sound energy.

The middle ear is an air-filled space. Anteriorly the eustachian tube connects the middle ear space with the nasopharynx. This tube is normally closed so that sounds, fluids, foods, and the like in the respiratory and digestive tracts cannot enter into the middle ear space. Contraction of the palate muscles opens the tube so that there can be equilibration of air pressure between the middle ear and the external environment. Posteriorly the middle ear space connects to the mastoid air system. The mastoid process serves as the attachment for a large, head-supporting muscle, the sternocleidomastoid muscle, and it is probable that the function of the mastoid air cell system is to "lighten the head" by pneumatizing an otherwise unnecessarily heavy bone.

The middle ear space is crossed by three ossicles (ear bones), which serve to transmit the sound energy from the tympanic membrane to the inner ear. The malleus attaches to the tympanic membrane. The incus is interposed between it and the stapes. The foot plate of the stapes fits within the oval window of the inner ear wherein it acts like a piston to transmit sound energy to the fluid-filled space of the inner ear. This somewhat complicated system amplifies the incoming sound energy, thereby preventing the 99.9 per cent loss of sound energy that would otherwise occur at the air-fluid interface of the external environment and the inner ear fluids.

Two muscles attach to the ossicular chain by means of tendons. The stapedius muscle attaches to the neck of the stapes and the tensor tympani attaches to the handle of the malleus. They react to the stimulus of loud sounds and probably serve to protect the internal ear by damping excess movement of the ossicular chain.

The *inner ear* (labyrinth) is contained in the petrous portion of the temporal bone and is composed of the interconnecting sensory organs for hearing (the cochlea) and for equilibrium (the vestibular system). These structures float in a fluid system, the perilymph, and are themselves filled with fluid, the endolymph.

The *cochlea* is coiled upon itself like a snail's shell with its largest coil, the basal turn, forming the medial wall of the middle ear. The cochlea contains the organ of Corti, the sensory end-organ for hearing. It extends along the entire length of the cochlea and contains approximately 24,000 hair cells that are spatially arranged so that those in the basal regions are stimulated by high-pitched sounds and those in the apical end by low-pitched sounds. Ganglion cells receive impulses from the organ of Corti hair cells and transmit these impulses along their axons, which form the auditory portion of the eighth cranial nerve. The eighth nerve exits through the internal auditory canal in the posterior portion of the temporal bone and almost immediately enters the brain stem. The auditory cortex is in the superior and transverse gyrus of the temporal lobe.

The *vestibular (equilibrium) portion* of the inner ear is composed of the utricle and the three semicircular canals. These contain the cristae, which are the end-organs for equilibrium. The utricular end-organ is stimulated by gravity, centrifugal force, and linear movements and is concerned with the sense of position in space. The semicircular canals are stimulated by acceleration or rotation, and regulate the sense of movement in space. Axons from these sense organs make up the remainder of the eighth cranial nerve. They terminate in the vestibular nuclei in the brain stem, which in turn connect with the oculomotor nuclei and with nuclei of the vagus nerve.

The *facial (seventh cranial) nerve* also traverses the temporal bone. It enters the internal auditory canal with the eighth nerve, passes to the medial wall of the middle ear, where it continues posteriorly in a bony canal (the fallopian canal), and then turns around the oval window to run inferiorly to its exit at the stylomastoid foramen at the base of the skull—the longest pathway through bone of any nerve in the body. It innervates the facial muscles of expression to show joy, sorrow, surprise, and the like.

The nervus intermedius is also associated with the seventh nerve, following its path and giving off the greater superficial petrosal nerve, which is parasympathetic, i.e., secretory, to the nose and the eye. It finally becomes the chorda tympani, which contains sensory taste fibers from the anterior two thirds of the tongue. It also sends parasympathetic secretory fibers to the submaxillary salivary gland.

The sensory innervation of the ear (pain, touch) is complex in that it involves fibers from five different cranial nerve groups, including cranial nerves five, seven, nine, and ten, and also upper cervical sensory fibers. Therefore, pain may be referred to the ear from areas as distant as the teeth, palate, larynx, cervical spine, or esophagus.

MEASUREMENTS OF THE COCHLEAR-VESTIBULAR SYSTEM

Tests of Auditory Function

Tests of hearing are usually subjective in nature, i.e., are based upon the patient's interpretation and response to an auditory stimulus. The use of whispered voice, tuning forks, or watch ticks is readily available but is almost entirely qualitative. Quantitative evaluation is provided by the audiometric examination, but it should be remembered that this is still subjective in nature. A large variety of audiometric assessments is available to help determine the anatomical site of the hearing loss and whether it is conductive, cochlear, retrocochlear, or functional. These include, but are by no means limited to, the following:

Pure-tone audiometry: The lowest sound pressure level at which the patient reports hearing a tone of a single frequency is determined, commonly 250, 500, 1,000, 2,000, 4,000, and 8,000 cycles per second (Hz).

Air conduction: Sound is presented into the air of the ear canal.

Bone conduction: Sound is applied to the bone of the skull.

Speech reception threshold (SRT): The lowest sound pressure level at which the patient correctly identifies 50 per cent of a list of two-syllable words.

Speech discrimination (discrimination): Determined by the percentage of monosyllabic words that the patient correctly repeats when they are presented to him at a comfortable level of loudness.

Alternate binaural loudness balance (ABLB): Varying sound pressures are alternately applied to the ears until the patient reports that the sound intensity appears to be the same in each ear. An ear that "recruits" will be unusually sensitive to increasing sound pressures, so while a diseased ear may not hear soft sounds very well, a slightly louder sound may be perceived as uncomfortably loud.

Short increment sensitivity index (SISI): Tests the patient's ability to recognize very slight increases in sound intensity superimposed upon a steady tone. An ear that "recruits" is better able to detect these slight changes of intensity and, therefore, will score higher than will the normal ear.

Tone decay: A pure tone is presented to the ear at a sound pressure level that is just barely perceivable. The normal ear will fatigue slightly, so that the intensity may have to be increased by 10 to 15 db over a 60-second time period. A decay of more than 30 db over a 60-second time period is considered pathologic.

Békésy audiometry: This is a semiautomatic measuring system that tends to summarize the various forms of pure-tone audiometric testing.

Objective methods of evaluating hearing are available. In the past these included psychogalvanic skin resistance testing and evoked response audiometry employing computer measurements of the electroencephalographic patterns. Both are expensive, time consuming, and unfortunately, not consistent or reliable. Impedance audiometry provides the only practical clinical method of objective evaluation; it measures the reflex activity of the stapedius muscle in response to sounds and, therefore, requires no interpretation by the patient. The Stenger test is a subjective test that can nevertheless rule in or out a complaint of significant *unilateral* hearing loss.

Hearing loss is commonly described as conductive or sensorineural. Sensorineural loss is further described as cochlear or retrocochlear. A conductive hearing loss shows on audiometric testing as a loss of pure-tone perception by air conduction. All other test results are normal. A cochlear hearing loss shows as a decrease in the pure-tone response to both air and bone conduction, a moderate loss in discrimination, evidence of recruitment on the alternate binaural loudness balance test, and a positive (high score) short increment sensitivity index. A retrocochlear hearing loss shows as a decrease in pure-tone perception by air and bone testing, a marked decrease in discrimination, an abnormal tone-decay perception, and frequently an early loss of the stapedius reflex.

The Decibel

Hearing loss is described in terms of decibels. The decibel is a ratio, not an absolute value, comparing the relationship between two sound intensities. Since the range of hearing is remarkable, extending from an almost infinitesimally low intensity to a trillionfold increase in energy, a logarithmic system is used to deal conveniently with such large numbers. In this case the log 10 is used. Thus, 10 decibels is 10 times the threshold of hearing of zero decibels. Twenty decibels is a hundredfold increase in power, 30 decibels is a thousandfold increase, and so on. A soft whisper is 30 db; average speech, about 60 db; a loud shout at 1 foot, 120 db; and sound is painfully loud at about 140 db.

Measurements of Equilibrium

Many objective tests are available, such as observation of the patient's ability to stand, walk, or point. It should be remembered, however, that these may nevertheless be under the patient's control.

Nystagmus is a reflex activity not directly under the patient's control. It consists of eye movements that are rhythmic, with a fast and a slow component; if present, it usually indicates pathologic change. Electronystagmographic (ENG) recordings provide a permanent and quantitative record of nystagmus and other eye movements, and they can further provide evidence of whether the symptoms of vertigo have a basis in fact and whether they are central or peripheral in origin. In the tests the patient is first examined for nystagmus.

Gaze nystagmus is seen when the patient has his eyes open and fixed upon an object that is displaced, either horizontally or vertically, from his normal line of vision. When present, gaze nystagmus always indicates disease. *Spontaneous nystagmus* occurs while the patient is in a "neutral" or normal position with the eyes closed or, if with the eyes open, unable to fixate, as when in the dark. *Positional nystagmus* also occurs with the eyes closed or unable to fixate, but with the patient in one or more nonneutral positions, e.g., prone, supine, lateral, head down.

Spontaneous and positional nystagmus occur normally in a small percentage of patients, but usually they indicate pathologic change, especially if they are persistent and intense.

The ear is then further tested by subjecting it to abnormal labyrinthine stimuli, such as caloric (hot and cold) testing, rotational testing, or fistula testing. Special tests of occulomotor function (pendulum, optokinetic) may also be employed to test the smooth tracking and saccadic eye movements mediated by the central nervous system.

Radiographs of the Temporal Bone

Standard x-ray projections, the Laws (lateral) and the Towne (frontooccipital), may be supplemented by other views normally included in a skull film series, namely an anteroposterior and a Stenvers. None of these, however, will demonstrate fractures of the temporal bone with any reliability. It is essential that polytomography of the temporal bone be carried out and that the films be examined by a radiologist who is skilled in their evaluation and who has been advised to look for a fracture in a specific region, as may be suggested by the physical examination and by special testing, such as audiometry.

TYPES OF INJURY

Mechanical Injury

The simplest form of injury is caused by the external ear scraping or rubbing against an object. The resultant abrasion can be expected to heal well and leave no significant sequelae, unless tattooing by some foreign object, such as gravel, has occurred.

If the ear is cut, torn, or lacerated by a sharp object, the pinna can be expected to heal well, provided the wound is closed within a reasonable time, i.e., several hours. It is rare that the resultant scar is cosmetically important. The normal folds and convolutions of the pinna tend to disguise minor disfigurement, and since there are no stress lines in the ear, the resultant scar is not prone to enlargement unless the patient has a tendency to form keloids.

It is uncommon that cuts or lacerations produce any damage to the middle or inner ear structures because these are protected by the bony skull. There are, however, two exceptions to this. In the first, a thin instrument such as a stick, nail, hairpin, or ice pick may penetrate the depths of the ear canal and tympanic membrane, and thus enter the middle ear and possibly even the inner ear spaces. The signs and symptoms are immediate and dramatic, and depend upon the depth of penetration. If only the middle ear space is entered, there will be bleeding, pain, and usually a conductive hearing loss. If the laceration is promptly repaired and if any ossicular chain discontinuity is reconstructed, the disability may not be permanent. If the inner ear is injured there will also be an immediate sensorineural hearing loss with associated vertigo. These changes are often permanent. The vertigo usually subsides over a 2- to 6-week period, however, as the central nervous system produces a gradual inhibition of the impulses from the uninvolved vestibular system. The facial nerve, passing as it does along the medial wall of the ear space, may also be affected, which results in facial paralysis and loss, on the involved side, both of taste on the anterior two thirds of the tongue and of submaxillary gland secretions. Surgical exploration and repair of the nerve injury may promote a return of function.

Second, lacerations in the postaural (mastoid) region in the infant, before the development of the mastoid tip (usually before six months of age), may injure the seventh (facial) nerve and produce facial paralysis on the involved side. Unless the ends of the nerve are reapproximated, the deformity will be permanent.

A more severe sharp injury to the ear (e.g., a tearing, biting, or cutting) may result in loss of a part or all of the external ear. Brisk bleeding ensues, since the blood supply to this region is generous. The bleeding, however, is not a threat and is easily controlled with pressure. Since the pinna is largely composed of cartilage, its metabolic demands are minimal. If the parts can be recovered, they may be sutured into place with a reasonable expectancy of success. Infection must be guarded against by careful regard to asepsis. Cartilage infection is rare, but catastrophic if it occurs, resulting in loss of cartilage and a shrunken "prunelike" pinna. Partial or total loss of the pinna is cosmetically important, but it has no functional significance.

Blows to the ear by blunt instruments may produce a variety of injuries. The simplest is that seen when the ear is "boxed," as by a closed fist. This produces a contusion or bruise. The resultant bleeding commonly occurs below the perichondrium, since there is little or no soft tissue between the skin and the perichondrium to absorb the force of the energy. Bleeding in this area is poorly absorbed, and unless evacuated by aspiration or by incision, the clot may become organized and subsequently replaced by scar tissue to give the pinna the thickened appearance commonly known as "cauliflower ear."

Flat trauma delivered to the ear canal, such as a slap to the side of the head, may so compress (more than 25 psi) the column of air in the ear canal that it ruptures the tympanic membrane.[1] This will produce bleeding, pain, and a hearing loss that is primarily conductive. If the force has been great enough to violently thrust the stapes foot plate into the vestibule, then there may be some cochlear-vestibular symptoms as well. These are usually temporary. The conductive hearing loss will remain until either the drum heals spontaneously or injury to the tympanic membrane or the ossicular chain or both is surgically repaired.

Blunt trauma to the head insufficient to cause loss of consciousness or to cause fractures of the skull or temporal bone may, nevertheless, still produce significant injury to the cochlear-vestibular system.[2] Symptoms of vertigo or hearing loss or both may ensue on one or both sides. Such injuries may occur in falls or in beatings about the head, in which it has been demonstrated that closed head, coup, and contrecoup injuries may occur. These may be of two types. First, there may be damage to the sound conducting system, most commonly a disruption of the ossicular chain.[3] With surgical repair the prognosis in this type is usually quite good. Second, there may be sensorineural injury.[4-8] Any concussion may cause permanent damage to the neural portions of the cochlear-vestibular system. In experimental animals it has been shown that hemorrhages and edema may occur in the central nervous system or in the cochlear-vestibular system. These findings have also been noted in autopsy specimens.[9-11] These patients will complain of hearing loss, tinnitus, or both. The most common audiologic finding is a bilateral high-frequency hearing loss. Frequently the auditory discrimination is also reduced. The slope of the curve is similar to that associated with noise-induced hearing loss, with a characteristic notch at 4,000 cycles. Therefore, the relation of hearing loss to trauma is frequently difficult to prove except on a historical basis. Without a prior audiometric examination, a history of hearing loss or of normalcy, even from a reliable and honest patient, is remarkably unreliable.

Dizziness may be an even more common complaint.[12-15] It is historically more reliable. Most people know quite well when they are dizzy and an adequate examination (which includes neurologic evaluation, electroencephalography, electronystagmography, and x-rays of the skull and cervical spine) will usually verify the presence of a pathologic condition although the exact nature of the injury may still be open to speculation.

The imbalance caused by peripheral labyrinthine injury is self-limiting and usually resolves in two to six weeks if it is unilateral. If bilateral, it may be severely disturbing, with slow and tedious resolution or even permanent disability. Damage to the neural reflexes emanating from the neck is also usually limited in duration. If the vertigo is related to central nervous system injury, it may be more prolonged, and the prognosis is especially poor if there is electroencephalographic evidence of damage.[16]

Fistulization of the sealing membranes of the round or oval windows may also occur, possibly by the shear force of stapes foot plate impaction or by sudden increase in intracranial fluid pressure.[17-19] This fistula produces a variable reduction in perilymphatic fluid pressure and a resultant "hydrops" of the cochlear-vestibular system on the involved side. Auditory complaints of fluctuating hearing loss, tinnitus, and poor discrimination are confirmed by audiometric examination and show a pattern consistent with cochlear disease. Episodic vertigo is usually positional in nature and especially likely to occur when the involved ear is lowermost. The "fistula" test may be positive and the electronystagmogram may show a decreased response to caloric stimulus. These injuries may be self-limiting as spontaneous repair occurs or they may require surgical repair of the leak or leaks. The prognosis depends upon the extent of the neural damage prior to the repair.

"*Whiplash*" involving rapid changes in acceleration, as commonly occurs in moving vehicle accidents, and *barotrauma* such as occurs in a blast injury, or even in the rapid atmospheric changes of an *aircraft decompression* or the changes involved in *skin diving* have produced similar cochlear-vestibular injuries.[4, 12, 21]

Temporal Bone Fracture

A blunt force, sufficient to fracture the temporal bone, is usually associated with brain concussion and at least a short period of unconsciousness. This is not always true, however. Temporal bone fractures are usually associated with evidence of skull fracture elsewhere, but again, this is not always true. They almost invariably produce some permanent damage. The signs and symptoms thereof depend upon the type of fracture.

Transverse Fracture

This occurs in about 20 per cent of temporal bone fractures and usually results from blows to the frontal or occipital areas.[6] The fracture line runs across or perpendicular to the long axis of the temporal bone and may cross the contents of the internal auditory canal, namely the seventh and eighth nerves, the nervus intermedius, and the blood supply to the inner ear. More commonly, it may pass through the labyrinthine capsule. The fracture line is frequently difficult to detect, even with polytomography, and the diagnosis may rest upon the demonstration of other skull fracture lines, plus the clinical evidence of injury, namely hemotympanum, nystagmus and vertigo, sensorineural deafness, and in 50 per cent of cases, facial paralysis.[3, 7, 22] Permanent damage is the usual sequela.

Longitudinal Fracture

This occurs in 70 to 80 per cent of temporal bone fractures and usually results from blows to the temporal or parietal areas.[6] The fracture line extends along the length (parallel with the long axis) of the temporal bone, and the resultant injuries depend upon its exact path through the temporal bone.[3, 7] Invariably there is bleeding into the middle ear space, and if the tympanic membrane or canal wall is lacerated, there will be bleeding from the external ear canal. If the fracture has torn the dura there may be leakage of cerebrospinal fluid as well. With fluid in the middle ear space there is a conductive hearing loss. Frequently this hearing loss may be further compounded by traumatic dislocation of the ossicles. If the fracture has crossed the fallopian canal and seventh nerve, facial paralysis will ensue (in 20 per cent of longitudinal fractures), and if it has injured the vestibule, cochlea, or semicircular canals, the patient will have sensorineural deafness in the involved ear and be vertiginous as well.[22]

Mixed fractures, both transverse and longitudinal, may occur and both ears can be involved.[3]

These injuries are not uncommonly overlooked since they usually occur in association with other major trauma and the attention of the physician is, therefore, attracted to the more life-threatening injuries. But it should be remembered that in closed head injuries the ear is the most commonly involved sense organ. If the damage to the ear has severely injured the sensorineural portion, there is no therapy that will significantly improve it. It should also be remembered, however, that injury to the conductive system can be surgically repaired, a fistula can be closed, and injury to the seventh nerve should not be overlooked, since significant recovery may be expected if the nerve is surgically repaired as soon as the patient is capable of undergoing the necessary surgical exploration.[23] Some nerves may be capable of recovery up to 6 to 12 months following injury. Symptomatic fistulas have been closed many years after their onset, and improvement has followed. Conductive system damage can be repaired at any time the patient's general health permits.

Thermal Injury

The external ear, projecting as it does from the side of the head, is highly exposed and easily injured by thermal extremes. Compared to, say the fingers, it is also relatively free of sensory nerve endings, and extreme cold may produce freezing (frostbite) before the individual is aware of it. Nevertheless, the ear tolerates freezing quite well and, if gently warmed, often will recover without serious sequelae. Burns behave much as burns elsewhere; the ultimate outcome, in loss of tissue, depends upon the extent of damage.

The middle and internal ears are basically protected from most extremes of temperature except those that are therapeutically induced. Freezing techniques (cryotherapy) are currently employed for treatment in such disorders as Ménière' disease and glomus tumor. These are generally well controlled and well tolerated, although occasionally the freezing may produce a seventh nerve paresis that, fortunately, is usually only temporary. Sparks from a welder's torch are an exception to the rule; they not infrequently enter the ear canal, reach the tympanic membrane, and burn their way through it. This produces a perforation of the eardrum that is particularly difficult to heal, and the ear subsequently is prone to recurrent otitis media.

Chemical Injury

Chemical injury to the ear is surprisingly not uncommon. Almost all the medications employed in otitis externa contain antibiotics. When topically applied, these drugs are likely to produce an allergic skin reaction; medications containing neomycin are most notorious for this effect.

Many chemicals and medications are also toxic to the cochlear-vestibular system.[24, 25] The toxicity is related to the concentration of the medication in the blood serum, and therefore, elimination (output) is as important as dosage (input). Salicylates (aspirin) will produce tinnitus and sensory hearing loss, the decibel level of which corresponds roughly to the blood level of the drug.[26] Fortunately, this effect is completely reversible. Most ototoxic drugs, however, produce permanent and frequently progressive damage to the cochlear-vestibular system. A partial list of these substances includes:

- Streptomycin
- Neomycin
- Gentamicin
- Viomycin
- Polymyxin B
- Ethacrynic acid
- Carbon monoxide
- Heavy metals
- Dihydrostreptomycin
- Kanamycin
- Vancomycin
- Chloramphenicol
- Ristocetin
- Furosemide
- Analine dyes
- Quinine

Streptomycin and gentamicin are unique in this group in that the vestibular (balance) system is more sensitive to them than the cochlear (auditory), and therefore, often ataxia will develop before hearing loss is noted. This distinction is used therapeutically on occasion.

Radiation Injury

Ionizing radiation produces no significant injury to the inner ear until fairly high exposure levels are reached. Neural tissue is rather resistant to x-radiation. Even with the biologic effect of 5,000 to 6,000 R, delivered over a six-week period, it is uncommon to find a significant cochlear or vestibular injury related to it.[27] On occasion, however, one can document audiometric evidence of a hearing loss resembling presbycusis. Mucositis of the membranes of the middle ear space and eustachian tube is a common complication of therapeutic levels of x-radiation to this area. If severe and protracted it may go on to produce a permanent eustachian tube obstruction and a subsequent chronic accumulation of fluid in the middle ear spaces with a resultant conductive hearing loss.

Noise-Induced Trauma

Exposure to noise can produce a hearing loss. This usually begins in the 4,000 Hz area, but for practical purposes "loss" is defined as an average loss of 25 db or more (ISO) at 500, 1,000, and 2,000 Hz.[28] Although there is still much to learn about the relationship of noise exposure and hearing loss, the following generalities are more or less accepted.

The important parameters of noise exposure are: the overall noise level, the spectral composition of the noise, the duration and distribution of exposure, and the total lifetime exposure.[29-32]

Noise levels below about 80 dbA ("A" indicates measurement with "A" network of the sound level meter) are considered quite safe.[33] At this level there may be some slight auditory fatigue, but it leaves no permanent effects. At the opposite extreme, very high levels of sound pressure, 190 to 200 db, may produce a force sufficient to rupture the tympanic membrane and to destroy the organ of Corti. Total deafness has resulted from a single on-deck exposure to the blast of a 16-inch cannon.

The spectral composition of noise is highly variable. Sounds are usually made up of many frequencies at different intensities. Different sound frequencies have greater or lesser importance to hearing. While the normal ear can hear from roughly 64 to perhaps 20,000 Hz, the most important frequencies are those necessary for the comprehension of speech, largely in the 250- to 2,000-Hz range. Excess sound energy of very low frequency produces no significant harm unless it is presented at "blast" intensity. Ultrasonic frequencies, those above 20,000 Hz, have the capacity to produce cellular disruption, but only above fairly high sound pressure levels (110 db or more), and such levels are quite rare.[34]

Frequencies in the 2,000- to 3,000-Hz region have the potential to produce the greatest amount of damage to the organ of Corti, other factors being equal.[35] Even so, hearing loss can occur from overstimulation by a specific frequency above or below these middle ranges. The organ of Corti is spatially arranged so that specific frequencies will stimulate specific areas of it; overstimulation by specific frequencies will produce specific areas of damage. The basal portion is primarily affected by high-frequency energy, the apical end by low.[36]

The duration and distribution of the noise exposure appear to have equal importance to the actual level of intensity. While it is true that a single intense impulse, such as a cannon blast, may permanently damage the organ of Corti, this is an unusual occurrence. The ear apparently has a great capacity to recover from noise-induced damage, and if it is allowed frequent or prolonged periods of quiet, full recovery may be expected even from a noise of high intensity.[37] Sound pressure levels exceeding 80 dbA, however, if continued over an eight-hour period, five days a week, will usually produce a permanent hearing loss.[33] Further, the extent of the loss will increase in a somewhat linear fashion, with an increase in sound pressure levels, so that 83 dbA will produce twice the loss of 80 dbA (each 3-db increment equaling a doubling of sound pressure).

The combination of impulse noise superimposed on a steady noise produces effects that have not been documented in man, although common experience in groups such as tank corps personnel suggests that these combinations are especially damaging. Recent animal experiments substantiate this.[38]

It has been commonly assumed that total energy exposure determines the amount of damage, i.e., two hours of exposure to specific sound level will produce twice the damage that one hour of exposure at the same level will produce, and that the total lifetime damage is related to the total lifetime exposure. Our previous discussion of the ear's capacity to recover, however, makes obvious that this is an imperfect generality.

Noise-induced loss of hearing is the result of mechanical and biochemical disturbances of the organ of Corti, recognized primarily as damage to the hair cells.[39] This occurs initially where the sound wave activity is at its maximum, specifically at a point about 10 mm from the end of the basal turn.[35] Here are the hair cell receptors for the 4,000-Hz sounds. Audiometric examination, therefore, will initially show a hearing loss in this region, commonly referred to as a "4,000-Hz dip" or "a C-5 dip." Since this frequency is not important in the comprehension of speech, the affected individual does not usually recognize the presence of a hearing loss. With continued noise exposure a wider band of hair cells is injured, and the audiometric dip becomes deeper and wider. Eventually frequencies important for speech comprehension become involved, and the individual recognizes that he is having difficulty. He can hear but he does not understand.

There is considerable individual variation in susceptibility to noise-induced hearing loss. This may result from individual anatomical and metabolic variations. Further, if there is a degree of conductive loss, such as the presence of a tympanic membrane perforation or otosclerosis, this will tend to protect the ear from abnormal sound pressures. Ototoxic chemicals and drugs, on the other hand, greatly potentiate the damage of auditory trauma.[40] Susceptibility has not been shown to be related to age or sex. Nor has it been proved that a hearing loss from auditory trauma indicates that the ear is unduly sensitive to such trauma (largely because of the difficulty in experimentally demonstrating this). Common sense, however, would imply that a person with hearing loss from acoustic trauma should avoid future similar exposure if at all possible.

Effective treatment of noise-induced hearing loss is unknown. If the hair cells are not severely damaged, they will recover, if allowed a period of rest. If the hair cells have been destroyed, however, they will not replace themselves. The loss is permanent. Hearing aids are sometimes useful, but they are never an adequate substitute for normal hearing. If a hair cell has been destroyed, no amount of energy applied to it can make it respond.

Prophylaxis by reduction of the sound pressure levels reaching the organ of Corti is the only rational course. An excellent short discussion of this is contained in the "Guide for Conservation of Hearing in Noise," a supplement to the *Transactions of the American Academy of Ophthalmology and Otolaryngology*, revised in 1969.

REFERENCES

1. Keller, D. A., Jr.: A study of the relationship of air pressure to myringo puncture. Laryngoscope, *68*:2015, 1958.
2. Bandini, A.: Cochlear and vestibular function in 227 cases of skull injury J. Neurol. Neurosurg. Psychiatry *8*:79, 1945.
3. Hough, J. V. D., and Stuart, W. D.: Middle ear injuries in skull trauma. Laryngoscope, *78*:899, 1969.
4. Barber, H. O.: Head injury audiological and vestibular findings. Ann. Otol. Rhinol. Laryngol., *78*:239, 1969.
5. Fox, M. S.,: Auditory and vestibular disorders in head trauma—medicolegal aspects. Ann. Otol. Rhinol. Laryngol., *78*:180, 1969.
6. Proctor, B., Gurdjian, E. S., and Webster, J. E.: The ear in head trauma. Laryngoscope, *66*:16, 1956.
7. Grove, W. E.: Hearing impairment due to craniocerebral trauma. Ann. Otol. Rhinol. Laryngol., *56*:264, 1947.
8. Guerrier, Y., DeJean, Y., and Galy, G.: Les surdités de transmission dans les traumatismes fermés du crâne. Cahiers O. R. L., *1*:11, 1965–66.
9. Ward, P. H.: The histopathology of auditory and vestibular disorders in head trauma. Ann. Otol. Rhinol. Laryngol., *78*:227, 1969.
10. Schuknecht, H. F., Neff, W., and Perlman, H.: An experimental study of auditory damage following blows to the head. Ann. Otol. Rhinol. Laryngol., *60*:274, 1951.
11. Schuknecht, H. F.: Mechanism of inner ear injury from blows to the head. Ann. Otol. Rhinol. Laryngol., *78*:253, 1969.
12. Toglia, J. U., Rosenberg, R. E., and Ronis, M. L.: Post traumatic dizziness. Arch. Otolaryngol., *92*:485, 1970.
13. Pearson, B. W., and Barber, H. O.: Head injury. Some otoneurologic sequelae. Arch. Otolaryngol., *97*:81, 1973.
14. Ishikura, T.: Clinical studies on post-traumatic vertigo. In *Proceedings of the VIII International Congress of Otorhinolaryngology* Tokyo, Excepta Medica, 1965.
15. Phillips, D. G.: Investigations of vestibular function after head injury without fracture of the petrosal bone: comments on clinical and legal aspects. Inform Med., *18*:15, 226, 1963.
16. Greiner, G., Rohmer, F., Collard, M., et al.: Corrélations électroencéphalographiques et électronystagmographiques dans le syndrome postcommotionnel (à propos de cent cas). Rev. Neurol. (Paris), *115*:188, 1966.
17. Stroud, M. H., and Calcaterra, T. C.: Spontaneous perilymph fistulas. Laryngoscope, *80*:479, 1970.
18. Goodhill, V., Brockman, S. J., Harris, I., et al.: Sudden deafness and labyrinthine window ruptures. Ann. Otol. Rhinol. Laryngol., *82*:2, 1973.
19. Healy, G. B., Strong, M. S., and Sampogna, D.: Ataxia, vertigo and hearing loss. Arch. Otolaryngol., *100*: 130, 1974.
20. Rubin, W.: Whiplash with vestibular involvement, Arch. Otolaryngol., *97*:85, 1973.
21. Henry. G. H.: Blast injuries. Laryngoscope, *55*:663, 1945.
22. Kettel, K.: Peripheral facial palsy in fractures of temporal bone. Arch. Otolaryngol., *51*:25, 1950.
23. Alford, B. R., Weber, S. C., and Session, R. B.: Neurodiagnostic studies in facial paralysis. Ann. Otol. Rhinol. Laryngol., *79*:227, 1970.
24. Kohonen, A.: Effect of some ototoxic drugs upon the pattern and innervation of cochlear sensory cells in the guinea pig. II. Review of literature concerning ototoxic antibiotics. Acta Otolaryngol. (Stockh.), Suppl. 208, 19, 1965.
25. Mathog, R. H., Thomas, W. G., and Hudson, W. R.: The ototoxicity of new and potent diuretics. A preliminary study Arch. Otolaryngol., *92*:7, 1970.
26. Myers, E. N., and Bernstein, J. M.: Salicylate ototoxicity A clinical experimental study. Arch. Otolaryngol., *82*:5, 483, 1965.
27. Borsani, S. J., and Blanchard, C. L.: Ionizing radiation and the ears. J.A.M.A., *181*:958, 1962.
28. Davis, H., and Kranz, F. W.: The internal standard ref-

erence zero for pure-tone audiometers, and its relation to the evaluation of impairment of hearing. J. Speech Hear. Res., 7:1964.
29. Burns, W.: *Noise and Man* London, John Murray, Ltd., 1968.
30. Eldredge, D. H., and Miller, J. D.: Acceptable noise exposures–damage risk criteria. In Ward, W. D., and Fricke, J. E. (Eds.): Noise as a Public Health Hazard. A.S.H.A. Rep., *4*:110, 1969.
31. Glorig, A., Ward, W. D., and Nixon, J.: Damage risk criteria and noise induced hearing loss. Arch. Otolaryngol., *74*:413, 1961.
32 Ward, W. D.: The identification and treatment of noise induced hearing loss. Otolaryngol. Clin. North Am., *2*:89, 1969.
33. Baughan, W. L.: Noise control—percent of population protected. Int. Audiol., 5:331, 1966.
34. Davis, H., Parrack, H. O., and Eldredge, D. H.: Hazards of intense sound and ultrasound. Ann. Otol. Rhinol. Laryngol., *58*:732, 1949.
35. Lehnhardt, E.: Die Berufsschäden des Ohres. Arch. Ohren. Nsen. Kehlkopfheilkd., *185*:11, 1965.
36. Wittmaack, D.: Über Schädigung des Gehörs durch Schalleinwirkung. Z. Ohrenheilkd., *54*:37, 1907.
37. Ward, W. D.: Hearing of naval aircraft maintenance personnel. J. Acoust. Soc. Am., *29*:1289, 1957.
38. Henderson, D., Hamernik, R. P., and Crossley, J.: New data for noise standards. Laryngoscope, *84*:714, 1974.
39. Davis, H., et al.: Acoustic trauma in the guinea pig. J. Acoust. Soc. Am., *25*:1180, 1953.
40. Sato, T. A.: A study on experimental acoustic trauma in animals treated with specific poisons for auditory organ. J. Otorhinolaryngol. Soc. Jap., *60*:31, 1957.

SELECTED READING

Paparella, M. M., and Shumrick, D. A.: *Otolaryngology*, Vol. I. Basic Sciences and Related Disciplines. Philadelphia, W. B. Saunders Company, 1973.

V. Facial Trauma

by G. W. Anastasi and J. P. Wysocki

At any time in his career a plastic surgeon may be called upon to care for a patient who has suffered facial injury. These injuries may result from automobile accidents, knife wounds, and gunshot wounds. They may also result from industrial mishaps and athletic injuries in which both bony and soft-tissue structures of the face are damaged. The force that can cause massive soft-tissue injury may also cause fractures of the facial bones and damage to the salivary glands and ducts and the facial nerve. Injuries to the eyes and their adnexa can be caused by any such force and are also frequently associated with soft-tissue injuries of the face. Thorough knowledge, therefore, of the anatomy and function of the structures of the maxillofacial area is essential if we are to provide optimal care of the patient with facial injuries.

Avoidance of permanent facial disfigurement and serious functional disturbance often depends upon proper primary management of the maxillofacial injury.

EMERGENCY TREATMENT

Airway Obstruction

A major consideration in all maxillofacial injuries is the problem of airway. Injuries about the mouth, nose, and cheeks as well as lacerations of the tongue and palate are often associated with profuse bleeding into the oral cavity. These can obstruct the airway, resulting in the need for emergency procedures such as tracheostomy or endotracheal intubation. Removing clots and debris from the mouth will improve airway problems, but emergency endotracheal intubation or tracheostomy may be necessary in those cases in which the obstruction cannot be removed easily. Prophylactic endotracheal intubation or tracheostomy is justifiable whenever it is the opinion of the physician that the airway is obstructed or will be obstructed by swelling at a later date. In view of this it is essential that all emergency triage areas be prepared to perform tracheostomies or intubation when the need arises.

For the emergency tracheostomy the patient is placed in the recumbent position with the neck hyperextended. A midline incision is made through the skin and subcutaneous tissue. The tracheal rings are then palpated, and a vertical incision is made in the midline of the trachea. Preferably the incision should be at the level of the third and fourth tracheal rings. At this point a cannula is inserted and stabilized about the patient's neck to maintain the airway opening.

Hemorrhage

Hemorrhagic shock is not a frequent problem in injuries of the face. It is imperative, however, that active bleeding be controlled immediately. Pressure dressings, while not always effective, should be applied when possible to prevent excessive loss of blood. By placing the patient in a moderate sitting position and applying pressure over the wound, one can control most bleeding in the maxillofacial area. In those cases in which extensive lacerations have occurred and larger vessels have been cut, clamping the bleeding vessel with hemostats may be the only means of controlling bleeding. The clamping should be done carefully and accurately under good light; blind clamping in this area must be condemned because of the danger of injuring important nerves and their branches. Pressure alone will usually suffice until a surgeon familiar with this area is available.

Clinical Examination

Once the patient's respiration, blood pressure, and pulse are stable and there are no active bleeding or airway problems, it is appropriate to begin the clinical examination. This involves an accurate and thorough examination of both soft-tissue injuries and skeletal injuries. A thorough neurologic examination should also be performed to rule out injury to the central nervous system. Examination may reveal only minor injuries such as superficial lacerations, abrasions, or contusions, or one may find more serious injuries such as fractures, injury to the facial nerve, or injury to the parotid duct. Of significance is the frequent association of facial injuries with injuries to the head (with concomitant neurologic disorders) and wounds of the chest, abdomen, spine, or extremities, as well as blunt injuries to the abdomen with lacerations of the liver or spleen. The treatment of soft-tissue facial trauma is seldom, if ever, a life-saving one. Satisfactory repair of soft-tissue defects may be obtained immediately or may be postponed for up to 24 to 48 hours. Of far more importance is the treatment of the associated injuries; these may be life-threatening. It is therefore essential to rule out any concomitant injury. Appropriate consultation with neurosurgeons, general surgeons, ophthalmologists, and chest surgeons is recommended. Only after the physician has established that the patient's vital signs are stable should soft-tissue repairs be started. In life-threatening situations, wound closure of the face and repair of facial fractures become secondary. Wet dressings applied to open wounds maintain the viability of soft tissue for 24 to 48 hours and permit primary closure later. Careful and coordinated planning among the specialists involved in treating maxillofacial trauma is desirable if an optimal result is to be obtained.

Facial Injury Associated with Head Injury

Craniofacial injury should be suspected in a patient with any facial injury who has been unconscious or who demonstrates hemiplegia or paraplegia, abnormal reflexes, convulsions, or delirium. Appropriate neurologic or neurosurgical consultation is mandatory in all cases of suspected head injuries.

SOFT-TISSUE WOUNDS OF THE FACE

Wound cleansing is essential as a first step in the repair of soft-tissue wounds of the face. This should be done in an unhurried and careful manner. No attempt should be made to perform extensive debridement. The cleansing should be done meticulously and carefully under local anesthesia. All foreign bodies should be removed gently, and the wound should be irrigated with saline solution. Clots and foreign material can be removed by copious irrigation. Mechanical scrubbing with brushes, which in many cases may not only lead to bleeding but also cause irritation to the patient, is usually unnecessary. Once the wound cleaning has been completed, exploration of the wound should be done. The physician should record all findings pertaining to soft-tissue damage, fractures, injuries to the facial nerve, and severed submaxillary or parotid ducts. Debridement of the facial area, because of the excellent blood supply, should be very conservative; when any doubt exists about the viability of tissue, that tissue should not be removed.

Abrasions

Abrasions and contusions of the face usually require no suturing. They are handled by good wound cleansing and conservative debridement. They are then dressed with a lubricated gauze such as Xeroform or Adaptic, and a dry dressing is applied over this. Usually abrasions and contusions of the face heal within 10 days.

Lacerations

If one is dealing with a *simple laceration* with no injury to any vital structure of the face, skillful, unhurried suturing will result most often in a very satisfactory repair. The wound should be closed anatomically: muscular layer, subcutaneous tissue, and skin. Absorbable sutures are used beneath the skin. The skin may be closed with interrupted or continuous sutures of fine silk or nylon. Sutures in this area may be removed safely in five days and as late as seven days after the wound has been closed. The ultimate aim in suturing any wound is to have a primary union of the wound with minimal scarring.

Treatment of more complicated *extensive lacerations* of the face requires thorough knowledge of facial anatomy and landmarks. Extensive lacerations in which flaps of tissue are elevated are commonly seen in automobile accidents. The edges of these flaps are usually beveled, making closure extremely difficult. They should be debrided by cutting back on the flap at right angles in order to obtain a better closure of the wound. One must keep in mind the rich vascularization of the face, which permits survival of flaps maintained by small narrow pedicles. If tissue does not survive, it will be appropriate at a later date to perform a secondary repair; many of the flaps that are questionable when seen at the time of initial injury do survive, and therefore again the plea for conservatism.

Lacerations associated with soft-tissue loss are problematic at times. If the loss is small a primary closure usually can be obtained by undermining the tissue and closing the wound without tension. In those cases in which a significant loss of soft tissue has occurred it is best to treat the wound with saline dressings. Skin grafting can be done when the wound is covered with healthy granulation tissue. This usually takes 7 to 10 days. Skin grafting and construction of flaps are usually not considered emergency room procedures. Patients with extensive soft-tissue wounds of the face should be admitted to the hospital, and the surgery for resurfacing should be done in the operating room when the wound appears free of infection and necrotic tissue.

Lips and Oral Cavity

Repair of lacerations of the lips and adjacent areas also requires an anatomical closure. This includes mucosa, muscle, and skin. Mucosal lacerations within the oral cavity should be repaired, and an absorbable suture is suitable for these closures. The vermillion borders of the lips serve as convenient landmarks for the repair.

Submaxillary and Parotid Glands and Ducts

When leakage of clear fluid is noted in a deep wound of the cheek region, one should suspect a laceration of the parotid duct (Stensen's duct). Lacerations that injure the parotid gland itself often result in localized collections of salivary juice, but these will eventually be resolved and do not need any definitive work other than drainage, perhaps. If the main parotid duct has been divided, however, and the ends can be seen through the wound, a polyethylene catheter may be placed inside the mouth, into the duct, and threaded through the cut ends of the duct as visualized through the wound. The duct is then repaired around the catheter, which is left in place for 7 to 10 days; it can then be removed and the duct will have healed satisfactorily. Any and all reconstruction of the parotid duct or the submaxillary duct should be done in the operating theater under optimal conditions. Exploration of Stensen's duct, with its proximity to the facial nerve, in an emergency room is to be condemned. In those cases in which the severed ends of the parotid duct cannot be repaired it is recommended that the proximal end be sutured to the oral mucosa to permit intraoral drainage. Failure to ligate or reroute the proximal duct will lead to fistula formation.

The Facial Nerve

It is essential that a thorough peripheral neurologic examination, particularly of the facial nerve, be performed on all patients who have sustained facial injury. The facial nerve is responsible for facial expression, and its function is evaluated by testing the muscles of expression. In those cases in which facial nerve injury is suspected, exploration and identification of the nerve must be done within 72 hours of the injury, preferably through existing wounds. After this period of time the nerve apparently loses its ability to conduct electrical impulses. Exploration and repair are best performed using microsurgical technique. Suturing of the nerve is done with very fine (7-0 to 10-0) sutures, depending upon the location of the injury. Primary repair of the nerve should be the aim of the surgeon. In cases in which this is impossible, grafting procedures utilizing the greater auricular nerve or spinal accessory nerve are advised. When the fine peripheral branches of the facial nerve have been divided, repairs are not necessary, since restoration of function can occur spontaneously because cross-innervation is present. Repairs are necessary, however, in all major branches of the facial nerve as well as in its main trunk.

Eyelids and Adnexa

Eyelid lacerations demand meticulous approximation. Closure on all eyelid injuries should involve conjunctiva, tarsal plate, muscle, and skin. Injuries to the lacrimal duct should be suspected whenever there are lacerations of the lower lid near the medial canthus. Consultation with an ophthalmologist is mandatory in all cases of trauma to the eye and orbit. Preservation of tissue and protection of the eye are paramount in reconstructing eyelid injuries. Exploration and repair of the lacrimal apparatus are best performed using microsurgical technique. (See also Chapter 3–III, The Eye and Its Adnexa.)

FRACTURES OF FACIAL BONES

In the United States, the majority of facial bone fractures result from automobile accidents. Not unusually, however, they result from violent forces exerted on the face by assault with either a fist or a heavy object. In dealing with facial bone fractures, the reconstructive surgeon should aim to achieve a pleasing aesthetic result and also to restore function. The presence of concomitant injuries to other parts of the body should, however, always be considered, particularly with fractures incurred in automobile accidents. Facial bone fractures should never be considered emergencies. Of prime importance in all patients with fractured facial bones is maintenance of adequate airway and prevention of hemorrhagic shock. Optimal reduction of the fractures may be carried out within 7 to 10 days of the injury.

Early Management

An adequate airway is of extreme importance in all patients with facial fractures. When examining a patient with facial injuries, the examiner should be alert for foreign bodies such as broken teeth, blood clots, pieces of glass, debris, dislodged and broken dentures, and bits of clothing that may have been forced into the oral cavity, nose, and pharynx. These must be removed and an adequate airway maintained. If any doubt about the airway exists, an immediate tracheostomy or endotracheal intubation should be done. Tracheostomy, as described earlier, is a surgical procedure whereby an artificial opening into the trachea is made for the purpose of permitting proper exchange of air for the patient.

Hemorrhagic shock due to blood loss from concomitant injuries such as ruptured spleen, torn liver, or fractured hip, as well as blood loss from extensive soft-tissue injury, should be controlled by immediately establishing an intravenous line and utilizing blood and plasma expanders to correct the hypovolemia. Airway obstruction and hemorrhagic shock represent the two major problems in the early management of the patient with facial bone fractures. It is only when these two conditions are under satisfactory control that the physician should undertake a diagnostic work-up.

History and Examination

An adequate history of the cause of the injury, be it an automobile accident or assault with a fist or a foreign object, is essential.

Once the vital signs have been stabilized and an airway established, the patient should be thoroughly examined. One must first attempt to rule out the existence of any injuries to the brain, spinal cord, and intrathoracic and intraabdominal viscera, and any major fractures of the extremities or hips before undertaking a thorough facial examination. Treatment of maxillofacial injuries should be deferred until it is established that no major concomitant injuries exist.

Signs of Facial Bone Fractures

About 80 per cent of facial fractures can be diagnosed by physical examination. A common sign of facial bone fracture is malocclusion of the teeth. This occurs with fractures of the mandible or the maxilla or both. In fractures of the zygoma, a depression of the cheek bone is noted on the side of the fracture. Facial fractures may often be palpable, and in certain of them, movement of the fracture fragments may be detected. Trismus, the inability to open the mouth, should be regarded with suspicion in the diagnosis of facial bone fractures. Anesthesia over the cheek, upper lip, and gums usually indicates zygomatic fractures.

Radiologic Examination

After the physical examination the next most important step in the diagnosis is the radiologic examination. Probably the single most important view is the Waters projection; in this the maxilla, maxillary sinus floors, rims of the orbit, and zygomatic bones are visualized. The submental vertex projection, which demonstrates the mandible, should also be ordered, as well as x-rays of the zygomatic arches. These views will most aid the physician in making a diagnosis of a facial fracture. In patients with possible injuries of the cervical spine, x-rays should be deferred until the patient has been cleared by a neurosurgeon.

Fractures of the Mandible

The mandible is probably the strongest of all the facial bones. In spite of this, however, mandibular fractures represent two thirds of all the facial fractures that occur. Fractures of the mandible are typically classified as either closed fractures, i.e., no break in the skin, or open or compound fractures in which skin and mucosa have been lacerated.

The symptoms associated with fractures of the mandible include pain, malocclusion, and trismus. The signs most commonly noted by the physician are swelling, crepitation, and sometimes distortion of the chin. Respiratory distress due to displacement of the tongue into the throat may result from fractures of the symphysis.

Fractures of the mandible may be multiple or single.

Treatment of Mandibular Fractures

The goal in treatment of mandibular fractures is to restore dental occlusion and facial symmetry. Intermaxillary fixation is necessary for all fractures of the mandible. Simple, noncompound fractures occurring in the body of the mandible in patients with sufficient healthy teeth are usually managed by closed reduction and intermaxillary fixation (wiring of the jaws). Symphysis fractures, certain ramus fractures, and compound fractures are best treated by open reduction followed by intermaxillary fixation. The subcondylar fracture can also be treated by closed reduction.

Fractures of the mandible in edentulous patients are reduced and most commonly treated by using the patient's own dentures or specially constructed splints fixed to the maxilla, to the mandible, or to both with circumferential wiring to assure proper occlusal relationships.

Intermaxillary fixation, in all cases, is usually maintained for four to five weeks or until fracture stability is achieved. In the closed reduction technique the teeth are wired to arch bars made of stainless steel, which are bent to conform to the contours of the upper and lower jaws. The arch bar is wired to the teeth with No. 25 stainless steel wire. The upper and lower jaws are then placed in occlusion by fixing the upper arch bar to the lower one with small rubber bands or wire.

For open reduction, skin or intraoral incisions must be made near the fracture area. The stabilization usually necessitates drilling several holes on either side of the margin of the fracture and then threading stainless steel wire through these holes to obtain interosseous fixation of the fracture. In open reduction one uses not only interosseous wiring but also intermaxillary fixation utilizing the arch bars just described. In both the closed and open methods of reduction, the jaw usually remains wired until clinical evidence of stability rather than x-ray evidence determines healing. This usually occurs in six to eight weeks.

Fractures of the Maxilla

The violent force exerted in an automobile accident in which the driver or passenger is thrown up against the dashboard or steering wheel, or through the windshield, is the most frequent cause of fractures of the maxilla. The magnitude of maxillary fractures and the frequent concomitant skull or orbital injuries associated with them make thorough understanding of these fractures imperative.

LeFort Classification

Fractures of the maxilla have historically been classified according to the LeFort system. The three standard classic types of maxillary fractures have therefore been categorized as LeFort I, LeFort II, and LeFort III. The first, the LeFort I, requires the least amount of force to produce, and the last, the LeFort III, requires the most force to produce.

A *LeFort I fracture* is classically a transverse fracture through the maxilla just above the level of the teeth. If one were to place a ruler horizontally just beneath the nose, the line drawn at this point would represent the level of the LeFort I fracture. The fracture usually includes the lower portion of the wall of the maxilla, the palatine bone, the pterygoid process of the sphenoid bone, and the alveolar process. If improperly treated, this fracture will result in occlusal abnormalities.

The *LeFort II fracture* is referred to as the pyramidal fracture or fracture of the middle third of the face. The force required to cause this fracture is greater than that required to cause the LeFort I fracture, and the fracture is more complex and severe than the LeFort I. In this fracture the middle third of the face is telescoped backward. There is often disruption of the lacrimal system. The fracture may pass through the floor of the skull (cribriform plate), resulting in a spinal fluid leak caused by tears in the dura mater (brain covering). The bones involved in the LeFort II fracture are the nasal, lacrimal, orbital, and ethmoid bones, the zygoma, the maxillary sinus, the pterygoid and cribriform plates, and possibly the frontal sinus. If one were to place the left and right index fingers on either side of the nose with the tips of the fingers overlying the root of the nose to form a triangle the base of which would be the upper lip, one would be demarcating the classic lines of the LeFort II fracture.

The *LeFort III fracture* is the most severe facial fracture. It involves complete separation of the bones of the face from the cranial vault. The force required to produce such a fracture is much greater than the force needed to cause the LeFort II fracture. It would seem unlikely that there would not be concomitant injuries elsewhere in the patient who has sustained a LeFort III fracture. Therefore, the complexities of this fracture are not only in the severity of facial fracture but also in the danger of its association with life-threatening injuries elsewhere in the body. Neurologic as well as intrathoracic and intraabdominal problems (i.e., ruptured spleen, torn liver) are commonly seen with LeFort III fractures. The traumatic force of this fracture is so great that the facial bones are actually detached from the cranium. The line of fracture can be visualized by placing a ruler in a horizontal position across the level of the eyes from one temporal area to another. The skull is separated from the facial bones, giving the face an elongated "mule-like" appearance.

The symptoms of fractures of the maxilla are those that are commonly seen with any of the facial bone fractures. They include pain, malocclusion, excessive salivation, difficulty in swallowing, double vision, and epistaxis. A cerebrospinal fluid leak through the nose is common with both LeFort II and LeFort III fractures, but it is not seen with the LeFort I fracture. The pushed-in appearance of the LeFort II fracture and the elongation of the face in the LeFort III fracture make it possible on occasion to diagnose these injuries on the basis of these findings.

Treatment of Maxillary Fractures

Several important principles must be stated that apply to the management and treatment of all maxillary fractures. A high index of suspicion of associated injuries, particularly in LeFort II and III fractures, must be maintained. The fractures themselves are never emergencies. They should be considered secondary in importance to establishment of an airway and prevention of shock. Tracheostomies are commonly necessary in LeFort III fractures and are not infrequently used in LeFort II fractures to insure a proper airway. LeFort I fractures can be managed without tracheostomy. Whenever there is any question of airway obstruction, however, tracheostomy or endotracheal intubation must be done. Restoration of facial symmetry and occlusion as well as ocular and nasal function is the basis of treatment of all fractures. The LeFort II and III fractures require intermaxillary fixation and wire suspension to a stable point above the fracture line to maintain the reduction and immobilization of the fractured bones. Frequently, open reduction and direct interosseous wiring are required in these LeFort fractures.

LeFort I Fracture. In the LeFort I fracture the previously described intermaxillary fixation utilizing arch bars is most commonly done. This fixation is usually maintained for four to six weeks. It is important that the fracture be maintained in fixation until stability of the bone has been demonstrated by physical examination, not by radiologic examination alone. If after a four- to six-week period there is still movement across the fracture line, fixation must be maintained for an additional two to three weeks.

LeFort II Fracture. In this fracture one needs not only intermaxillary fixation but also wire suspension either from the zygomatic arch or from a stable point in the skull above the fracture line. The combination of intermaxillary fixation and suspension wiring guarantees the stability and immobilization necessary to correct this fracture. As stated earlier, in LeFort II fractures there is danger of tears of the dura (brain cover) caused by fractures of the cribriform plate. Leakage of fluid from the nose in these cases should be looked upon with great suspicion. A simple test, utilizing a glucose-sensitive tape, of the drainage from the nose will differentiate between mucus and cerebrospinal fluid. Positive results in tests for sugar or in other more sophisticated tests indicate the existence of a cerebrospinal fluid leak. A negative result usually indicates that the drainage from the nose is normal mucus. A neurologic or neurosurgical consultation should be obtained in all cases of suspected LeFort II fractures with cerebrospinal fluid leaks. It is felt by some physicians that when there is spinal fluid leakage, reduction of the fracture should be deferred until the leakage has ceased. Today, however, many feel that under antibiotic coverage, even in the face of spinal fluid leakage, it is safe and probably advisable to reduce these fractures. The spinal fluid leakage usually will cease spontaneously after the fracture has been reduced. There have been cases reported in which leakage has persisted for months and occasionally as long as a year. It is fair to say, however, that in the majority of the cases, it does cease spontaneously.

LeFort III Fractures. Principles governing the management of LeFort II fractures also apply to the LeFort III fractures. As stated earlier, a high index of suspicion for the presence of life-threatening injuries must be maintained in the LeFort III fracture. Elective tracheostomy is commonly employed in these patients.

Fractures of the Zygoma

Fractures of the zygoma (cheek bone), unlike the previously described maxillary fractures, usually occur as a result of a violent blow to the face from a fist or heavy object. These fractures are most commonly seen in assaults or athletic injuries. Symptoms of fracture of the zygoma include paresthesia (numbness) of the cheek due to contusion of the infraorbital nerve. Paresthesia will also involve the upper lip and gingiva on the affected side. There is usually a depression of the cheek bone on the side of the fracture and difficulty in opening the mouth (trismus) due to impingement of the coronoid process of the mandible. A step deformity in the infraorbital rim and fracture of the floor of the orbit are also seen in zygoma fractures. Owing to the thickness and heaviness of the body of the bone, blows to the zygoma usually result in the fracture of three weak areas about its periphery. These are the frontozygomatic suture, the zygomaticomaxillary suture, and the zygomaticotemporal suture. Because the fracture affects these three areas, the zygomatic fracture is often referred to as a tripod fracture. Of great importance in the zygomatic fracture is the associated fracture of the orbital floor with the possibility of herniation of orbital contents into the maxillary sinus and eye muscle imbalance. This can cause diplopia (double vision), particularly noted on upward gaze. A high index of suspicion for the fracture of the orbital floor should always be maintained in zygomatic fractures.

The diagnosis of the zygomatic fracture can be made most commonly by observation of the signs and symptoms previously mentioned and by radiologic examination. The most helpful x-rays are the Waters view, the submental vertex view, and the zygomatic arch view. Occasionally special views of the orbit and sinus, including tomograms, are needed.

Treatment of Zygomatic Fractures

As in the case of all facial bone fractures, fractures of the zygoma are never considered emergencies and their treatment may be delayed 10 days to two weeks. It is imperative that before any treatment be undertaken a thorough review of the patient be made to rule out the presence of any life-threatening concomitant injuries that should be managed before treatment of the zygomatic fracture. Once the patient's condition is stable, treatment of the fracture may be undertaken. It is advisable to allow four or five days before reducing a zygomatic fracture. This permits the edema to subside; the reduced fracture may then be compared with the unaffected side of the face. In cases in which extensive swelling and edema are present, it becomes extremely difficult to know when the reduction has been satisfactorily accomplished because comparison of the two cheek bones is impossible.

Reduction of zygomatic fractures can be done by any one of three classic methods. An eyebrow incision (Dingman technique) permits reduction to be done with an exposure of the fracture of the frontozygomatic suture. In severely depressed, unstable fractures, the zygoma can then be wired to the frontal bone. Other possibilities are approaches through the temporal hair-bearing area (Gillie's technique) and intraoral approaches.

Fractures of the Orbit

Diagnosis of these fractures has been discussed with that of zygomatic fractures. Findings of the enophthalmos and diplopia along with positive x-ray evidence of fracture of the orbital floor should be viewed with suspicion.

The orbital fracture is often called a "blow-out" fracture. If the rim and floor are fractured it is called an "impure" blow-out fracture. If only the floor is involved it is called a "pure blow-out." The pure blow-out fracture is not associated with a zygomatic fracture and is caused by a direct blow to the orbit.

Treatment of Orbital Fractures

Exploration of the orbital floor should be done in all cases in which there is entrapment of the inferior rectus muscle in an orbital floor fracture. Entrapment can be diagnosed by applying traction on the inferior rectus muscle (forced duction) to determine limitation of eye motion. Elevation of the orbital contents and reconstruction of the floor by either a prosthetic implant (Silastic) or autogenous cartilage or bone should be done at the time of exploration.

SELECTED READINGS

1. Ballinger, W. F., Rutherford, R. B., and Zuidema, G. D.: *The Management of Trauma.* Philadelphia, W. B. Saunders Co., 1973.
2. Barsky, A. J.: *Principles and Practice of Plastic Surgery.* Baltimore, Williams & Wilkins Co., 1950.
3. Converse, J. M.: *Reconstructive Plastic Surgery.* Philadelphia, W. B. Saunders Co., 1964.
4. Converse, J. M., and Smith, B.: Reconstruction of the floor of the orbit by bone grafts. Arch. Ophthalmol. (Chicago), *44*:1, 1950.
5. Converse, J. M., and Smith, B.: Naso-orbital fractures and traumatic deformities of the medial canthus. Plast. Reconstr. Surg., *38*:147, 1966.
6. Dingman, R. O., and Natvig, P.: *Surgery of Facial Fractures.* Philadelphia, W. B. Saunders Co., 1964.
7. Erich, J. B.: Fractures of the facial bones. Milit. Surg., *88*:637, 1941.
8. Hayward, J. R.: Treatment methods for jaw fractures. J. Oral Surg., *20*:273, 1962.
9. Kazanjian, V. H., and Converse, J. M.: *The Surgical Treatment of Facial Injuries.* 3rd Ed. Baltimore, Williams & Wilkins Co., 1963.
10. McCoy, F. J., Chandler, R. A., Magnan, C. G., Jr., Moore, J. R., and Siemsen, G.: An analysis of facial fractures and their complications. Plast. Reconstr. Surg., *29*:381, 1962.
11. Peacock, E. E., Jr.: Management of facial fractures in unconscious patients. Am. Surg., *24*:639, 1958.
12. Rowe, N. L., and Killey, H. C.: *Fractures of the Facial Skeleton.* Baltimore, Williams & Wilkins Co., 1955.

VI. ORAL TRAUMA AND PATHOSIS

by Edward D. Woolridge, Jr.

The term "oral trauma" refers to an injury to the structures of mastication. These structures comprise the teeth, their supporting periodontium, the maxilla and mandible with their various muscle and ligament attachments, the temporomandibular joints, the lips and tongue, and the nervous and vascular systems that supply these tissues.

ETIOLOGY AND PREVALENCE OF ORAL TRAUMA

A review of the literature concerning the incidence of oral trauma reveals a disparity between the 4 per cent reported by Kessler in 1953 and the 14 per cent reported by Akpata in 1969.[1, 2] It has been noted, however, that in a subsequent study, Kessler reported figures closer to the fourteenth percentile.[3] Other investigators, Grundy, Ellis, Wallentin, Buttner, Beck, Schutzmannsky, and McEwen and coworkers, have reported various percentages between 4 and 14 per cent.[4-10] These studies were conducted from 1922 through 1969 at various locations throughout the world.

The etiology and prevalence of oral trauma vary significantly according to the age of the individual. It has been the author's observation that there is a drastic increase in the incidence of injury when the young child begins learning to walk and run. According to Andreasen and Schutzmannsky, most dental injuries occur shortly before school age and are primarily due to falls.[9, 11] The incidence of child abuse has increased significantly since these investigations were conducted by Andreasen and Schutzmannsky, and with it, unfortunately, the oral manifestations of the battered child syndrome.[12] (This subject is discussed in Chapter 50, Forensic Odontology.)

Playground injuries are quite common after the child is of school age.[13] These injuries result in fractured and luxated anterior teeth, lacerations of the lip and gingiva, and chin abrasions. Many of them are due to the misuse of playground equipment or to falls caused by the child's carelessness or, in some cases, lack of coordination. Another common type of injury in this age group occurs at drinking fountains; the incisal angles of anterior teeth are fractured in situations in which the child falls or his head is pushed while he is using the fountain. Also prevalent in this young school-age group are bicycle accidents resulting in fractured teeth and injuries to the lips and chin.[11]

In the teenage group, oral trauma is frequently associated with athletic participation and automobile accidents.[14, 15] The incidence of these injuries has, however, declined in the past few years. This is primarily due to the dental consciousness of our society at present and the wearing of mouth guards by those engaged in sports activities. Many youth organizations now make the wearing of such guards a mandatory requirement for participation in sports.

Heretofore, many of the dental injuries that occurred in automobile accidents were due to the driver or passenger hitting the steering wheel or dashboard. It is believed that, with the advent of seat belts and cushioned dashboards, the incidence of these injuries may decline in the future.

Injuries sustained during fights are common in older age groups. Complete avulsion and luxation of teeth, fractures of roots and supporting bone, and mandibular fractures are characteristic of this type of trauma.[11] Trauma of this nature is frequently encountered in military and penal clinical dentistry.

Recently the incidence of drug abuse has increased, and with the increase, drastic oral manifestations such as fractured posterior teeth have appeared in many narcotic addicts. Frequently, owing to a hypoglycemic condition and a physiologic craving for refined carbohydrates, the addict has more dental disease than is found in a more normal population.[16, 17] The problem is worsened in these unhealthy dentitions because opiate derivatives apparently produce tooth grinding.[18] Greater anxiety is exhibited by bruxistic patients, and worry and nervousness are common findings in bruxism.[19, 20] Therefore, it is believed that bruxism frequently is a contributing factor in the relatively large incidence of fractured posterior teeth noted in narcotic addicts. (This subject is further discussed in Chapter 50, Forensic Odontology.)

APPEARANCE OF NORMAL TISSUES

For the sake of comparison, a review of the appearance of normal oral structures should prove beneficial.

The normal gingiva in the adult is pinkish gray in color, firm, and stippled, and has a thin marginal contour around the necks of the teeth and a pointed papillary contour between the teeth (Fig. 3–VI–1*A*).

There is a similar appearance in the deciduous (primary) dentition of the young child, except the teeth are narrower and shorter and frequently have wider spacing between them in the anterior area (Fig. 3–VI–1*B*).

Microscopically, the normal gingiva appears as a thick, cornified epithelium that has prickle cells and a granular layer. The lamina propria, a dense connective tissue, has a papillary area that extends with fingerlike projections into the epithelium.

The microscopic appearance of the tongue consists of papillae that are cone-shaped, making the section appear velvety. Hairlike tufts are formed by cornified epithelium, and skeletal muscle fibers are also apparent.

The mucous membranes of the hard palate consist of dense, fibrous connective tissue that is similar to that of the gingiva. There is a stratum granulosum and a keratinized layer, giving the epithelium a thicker, more cornified appearance than that of the normal gingivae.

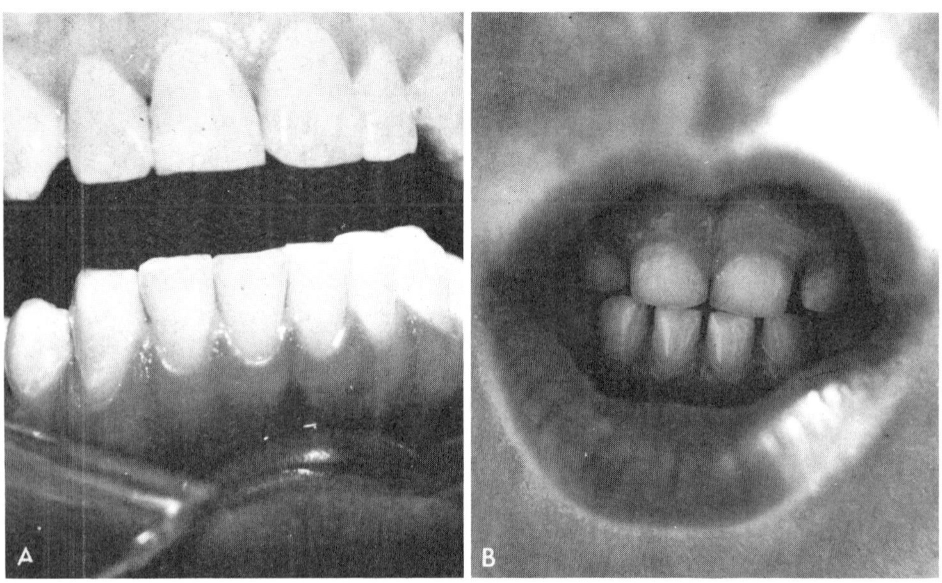

Figure 3–VI–1. *A*. Normal adult dentition. *B*. Normal deciduous dentition.

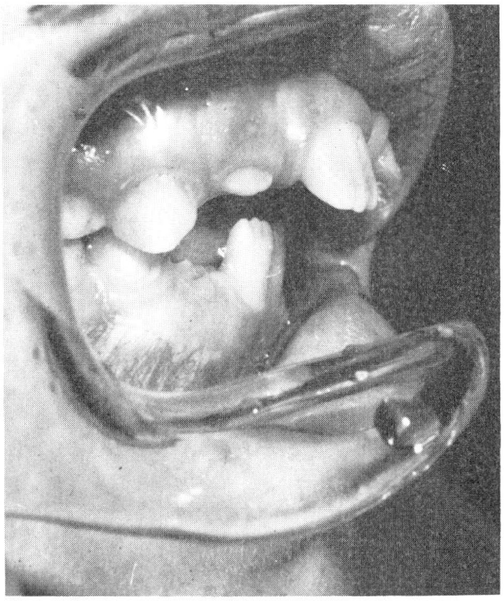

Figure 3–VI–2. Protruding teeth with fracture.

Microscopically, the mucous membrane that lines the soft palate, the ventral surface of the tongue, the lips, and the cheeks is noncornified, stratified squamous epithelium. A stratum of dense interlacing tissue forms the lamina propria, which does not extend as deeply into the epithelium as it does in the normal gingiva.

MODIFYING FACTORS IN ORAL TRAUMA

Obviously, there is a relationship between protruding anterior teeth and the incidence of oral trauma (Fig. 3–VI–2). It has been reported that children with this condition are much more prone to tooth injuries than those with more normal dentitions.[21]

Incomplete lip coverage is closely associated with protrusion of anterior teeth. Conditions of this nature, in which the soft tissues do not provide sufficient protection for the teeth, are significant factors predisposing the teeth to injury.[10, 21, 22]

It has been noted that *large existing dental restorations* influence the effects and incidence of oral trauma. The author has observed numerous fractures of these teeth after relatively minor trauma that would have been insignificant to a normal tooth.

Existing disease is a significant predisposing factor in oral trauma. Teeth with large carious lesions are weaker and therefore more susceptible to fracture.

External and internal root resorption weakens the tooth and renders it more susceptible to fracture (Fig. 3–VI–3). This entity is described later in the section on acute mechanical trauma to developed dental tissues.

Endodontically treated teeth appear more brittle than normal teeth and fractures in them are not infrequent. This characteristic is believed to be due to a loss in moisture content within the tooth that results from the removal of vital pulpal tissues. This is a controversial issue in the field of endodontics; more research in this area is necessary to prove or disprove the belief. Most endodontically treated teeth also have large lingual restorations, which tend to weaken the tooth and lower its resistance to excessive force.

Bone cysts are of great clinical importance because of their frequency of occurrence and

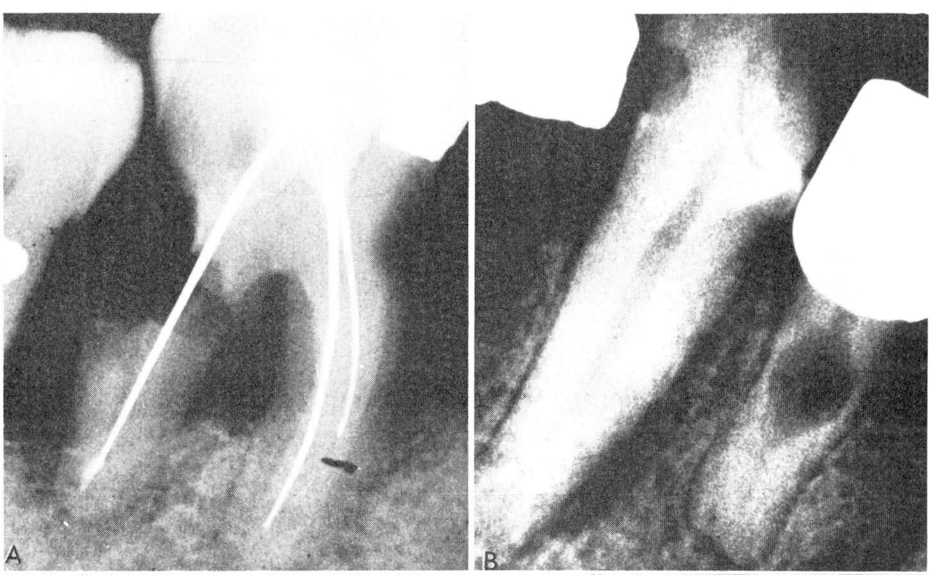

Figure 3–VI–3. *A,* External root resorption. *B,* Internal root resorption.

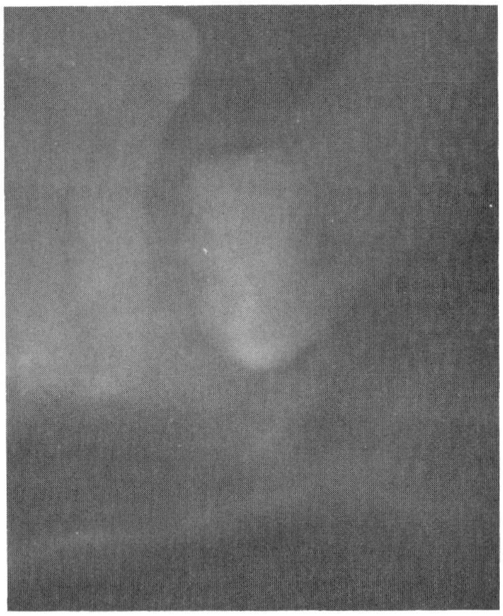

Figure 3–VI–4. Follicular cyst in third molar area.

their predisposition to fracture.[29] They exert a great influence on the incidence and effects of oral trauma. Lesions such as the cystic formation shown in Figure 3–VI–4 in the area of the unerupted third molar tend to weaken the mandible, thereby making it very fragile and more susceptible to fracture.

General Conditions Predisposing to Trauma

Systemic conditions that render a person irresponsible for his actions are predisposing factors in oral trauma. Some of the more common of these are encephalitis, diabetes, fatigue, epilepsy, brain lesions, and cerebral hemorrhage. According to Andreasen, 107 epileptic patients were examined to determine the incidence of oral trauma.[23] This study showed that 38 per cent of such injuries were probably due to falls during convulsive seizures. Tongue biting is also common in this disease (Fig. 3–VI–5). To my knowledge, however, there are no similar studies of significance concerning this subject.

Systemic Diseases and Oral Trauma

A disturbance of the endocrine glands may weaken bone, which greatly influences the effects of oral trauma. A significant condition of this nature is hyperparathyroidism.

Hyperparathyroidism. Hyperparathyroidism is a disorder in which abnormally increased activity of the parathyroid glands causes loss of calcium from the bones. It is marked by tenderness in the bones, spontaneous fractures, and osteitis fibrosa.[24]

A common cause of the disease is a tumor of the parathyroid gland.[25] The resulting increase in the amount of parathormone secreted acts on the kidney to increase urinary excretion of phosphorus. This is followed by a decrease in serum phosphorus, in the serum being less saturated with calcium phosphate, and more calcium phosphate entering the serum from the skeleton, which yields calcium when necessary to complete the change in chemical equilibrium.[26]

Clinically, there is a localized gingival enlargement, firm in consistency, with a smooth surface and dark red color (Fig. 3–VI–6*A*).

The first manifestations of the disease often appear in the oral cavity. They are seen radiographically as clear-cut or diffuse radiolucent areas with loss of the lamina dura (Fig. 3–VI–6*B*).

A bone biopsy appears vascular, and there are many fibroblasts and giant cells that are osteoclastic in nature. Obviously, the bone is weakened and mandibular fracture from relatively minor trauma is not uncommon.

Other conditions that make oral structures more susceptible to trauma are: Paget's disease (osteitis deformans), eosinophilic granuloma, Gaucher's disease, Hand-Schüller-Christian disease, Letterer-Siwe disease, osteogenesis imperfecta, congenital anemia (Cooley's), osteopetrosis, (marble bones, osteosclerosis fragilis generalisata) and osteomyelitis.

Paget's Disease. Paget's disease (osteitis deformans) is a rarefying osteitis leading to bow-

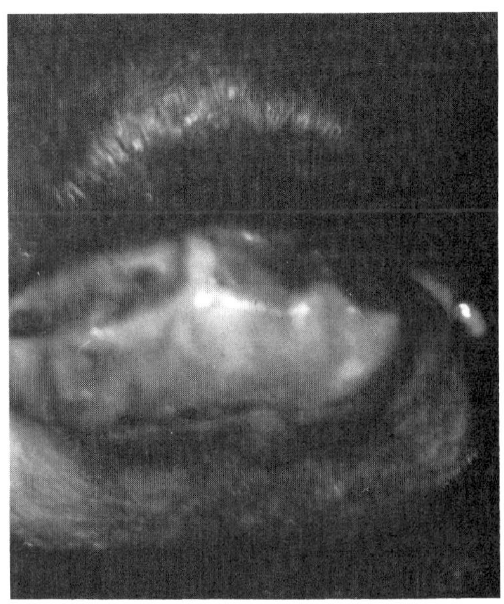

Figure 3–VI–5. Tongue bite during epileptic seizure.

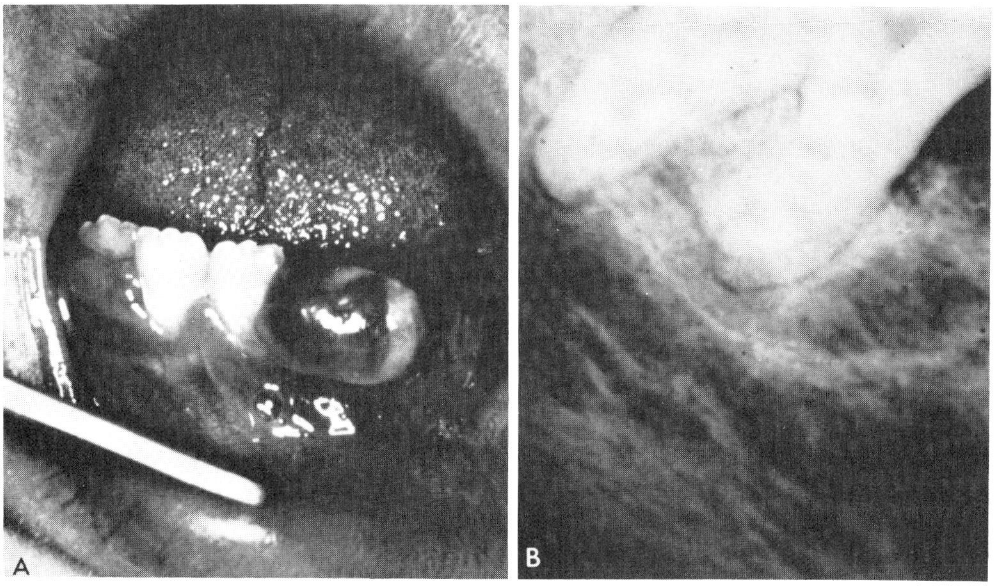

Figure 3–VI–6. Hyperparathyroidism. *A*. Clinical appearance. *B*. Radiographic appearance.

ing of the long bones and deformation of flat bones.[24] It is of unknown etiology, and in early stages it renders the bone very soft and susceptible to fracture. Frequently it is manifested clinically by an enlargement of the skull, the maxilla, and to a lesser extent, the mandible (Fig. 3–VI–7*A*). The radiographic appearance depends upon the stage of the disease (Fig. 3–VI–7*B*). Resorptive changes with an increase of radiolucency and an alteration of the trabecular pattern appear early. Later, when the resorbed bone is being replaced by fibrous tissue and poorly calcified bone trabeculae, the radiographs have the appearance of ground glass. When the disease is of long standing there is a cotton-wool appearance due to sclerosis, which is demonstrated radiographically as more irregular radiopaque areas.

Microscopically, the tissue shows evidence of excessive lacunar resorption that is osteoclastic in nature, plus the apposition of bone that is of inferior quality and quite porous.

Eosinophilic Granuloma. A benign destructive process, eosinophilic granuloma is neoplastic in nature and may appear first in the oral cavity. When this occurs it is characterized by an infiltration of granulation tissue from the marrow space into the oral epithelium.[27] This results in excessive bone loss and greater susceptibility to fracture.

The etiology of this disease is not completely agreed upon by all authorities; most of them appear to view it as an inflammatory reaction in which trauma may play an aggravating role.[27]

Clinically, there are ulceration of the mucosa and drifting of loose teeth owing to bone loss, which in turn weakens the bones affected.

The lesions appear radiographically as osteo-

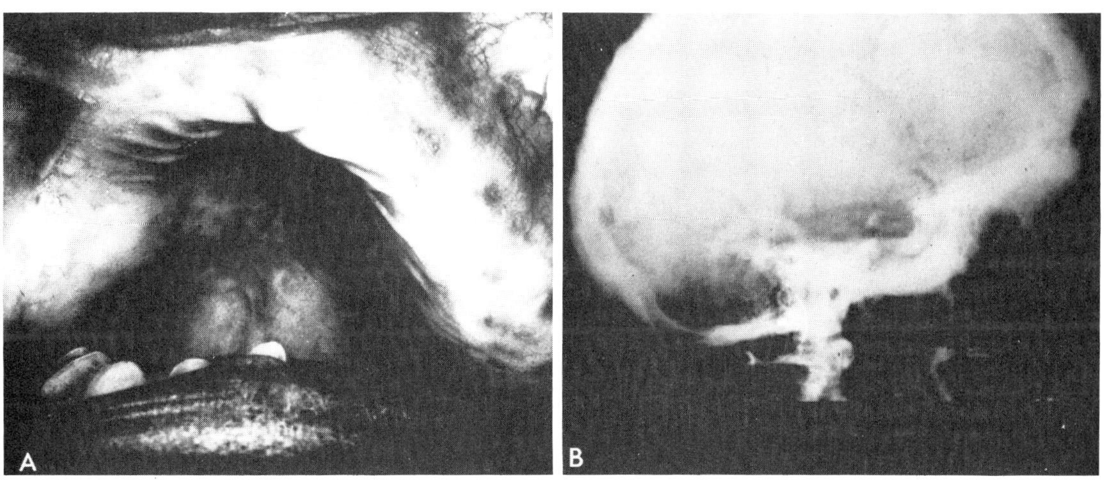

Figure 3–VI–7. Paget's disease. *A*. Clinical appearance. *B*. Radiographic appearance.

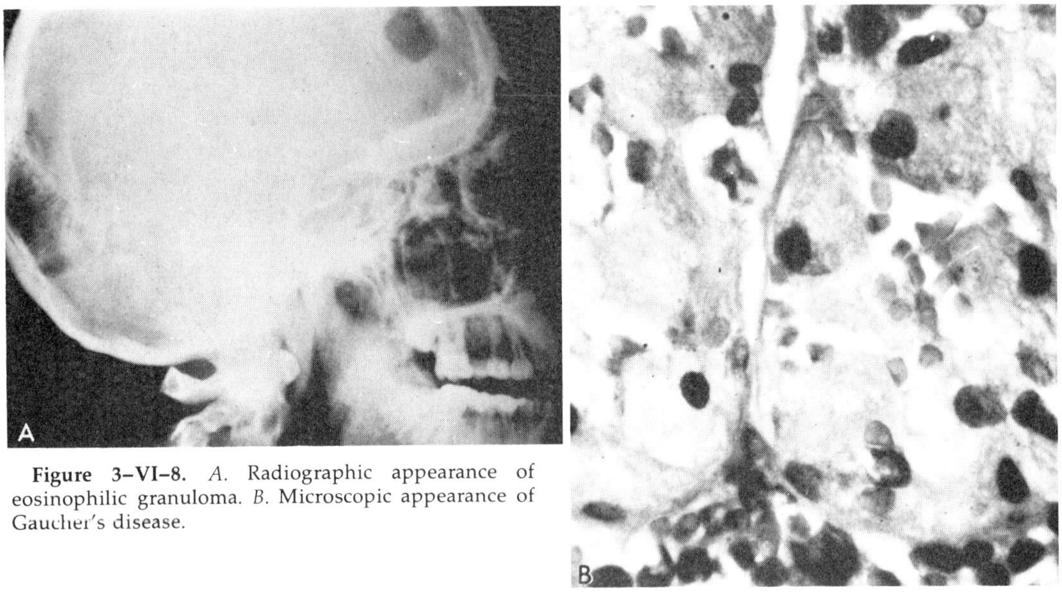

Figure 3–VI–8. *A.* Radiographic appearance of eosinophilic granuloma. *B.* Microscopic appearance of Gaucher's disease.

porotic areas that are sharply demarcated and resemble cyst formations (Fig. 3–VI–8*A*).

Microscopically, a large number of histiocytes with large, pale, oval nuclei are revealed. The eosinophils spread between the histiocytes and give a picture similar to that in an allergic reaction. The cytoplasm appears pale in color and foamy in texture.

Gaucher's Disease. In this disease, which affects the reticuloendothelial system, kerasin is deposited in the reticular cells of the liver, spleen, lymph nodes, and bone marrow.[28] It is of unknown etiology.

The radiographic appearance is one of extreme porosity, and large cystlike radiolucent areas appear in the weakened cancellous bone. Microscopic examination reveals large foamy cells occurring in bundles (Fig. 3–VI–8*B*). They are elongated and have striations and are commonly known as Gaucher cells.

Hand-Schüller-Christian Disease. This is a type of cholesterol lipoidosis. Clinically, it is manifested by a triad of defects in the membranous bones, exophthalmos, and diabetes insipidus.[24]

Thought to be congenital, it occurs predominantly in the Jewish race and generally in the male.[29] The disease involves the bones primarily, with the maxilla and mandible frequently affected. It manifests itself by re-

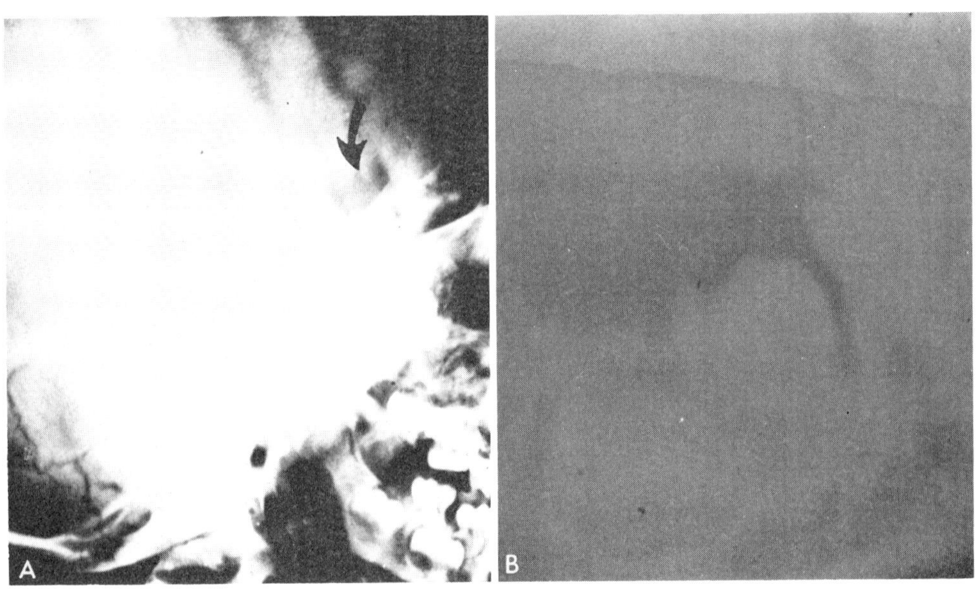

Figure 3–VI–9. *A,* Radiographic appearance of Hand-Schüller-Christian disease. *Arrow,* bone defect. *B,* Radiographic appearance of Letterer-Siwe disease.

placement of normal bone marrow by proliferating macrophages, weakening the bones and making them more susceptible to fracture.

Radiographically, the bone defects vary from round to ovoid in appearance, with well-defined margins (Fig. 3–VI–9*A*).

Letterer-Siwe Disease. This disorder is a nonfamilial, nonlipid reticuloendotheliosis that frequently occurs in early childhood and is considered fatal. It involves the jaws in a manner similar to that of Hand-Schüller-Christian disease and closely resembles it radiographically (Fig. 3–VI–9*B*). A microscopic examination reveals a proliferation of histiocytes that are nonlipidized.

Osteogenesis Imperfecta. Osteogenesis imperfecta is an inherited condition in which the bones are usually brittle and subject to fracture.[24] Its radiographic appearance in the jaw is one of generalized osteoporosis, showing a thinning with very little radiopacity.

Microscopic findings include imperfect calcification and a fibrous, vascular marrow, with only a few osteoblasts.

Cooley's Anemia. Cooley's anemia (thalassemia) is a genetically determined hemolytic anemia that occurs primarily in families of Mediterranean stock.[24] Clinically, the person has large, protruding upper incisors and a prominent premaxilla that give him mongoloid features.

Microscopic findings show that the fatty marrow of the spongiosa is replaced by red blood cells.

Radiographically, there appears to be a widening in the trabecular bone pattern with a marked increase in radiolucency and osteoporosis (Fig. 3–VI–10*A*). This picture explains why these persons are more susceptible to fractures than normal individuals.

Osteopetrosis. Osteopetrosis (marble bones) is the name of a condition in which there are bandlike areas of condensed bone at the epiphyseal lines of long bones and condensation of the edges of smaller bones.[24]

This disease is of unknown etiology, but is generally thought to be hereditary in nature. It is manifested by a marked increase in osteoblastic activity that causes closing of the red marrow, and the bones of the jaws become very brittle. Fractures from trivial causes occur frequently, owing to the decreased elasticity and greater fragility of the tissues.[29]

Radiographs show areas of dense opacity that may be general or localized.

Microscopically, there is a great increase in the number of bone trabeculae, causing marrow spaces to be narrow or obliterating them. The osteoblasts appear in irregular lines and only a few are present.

Osteomyelitis. Osteomyelitis is an inflammation of bone that is caused by a pyogenic organism.[24] This condition may be localized or it may be general throughout the bone involved. It may be the result of dental infection, trauma, or hematogenous transportation of bacteria.[29] The bone marrow is affected through inflammatory lesions that produce pus. The disease is clinically manifested by pain, swelling and pus in the area, lymphadenopathy, elevated temperature, and "bad breath."

Radiographic findings depend upon the stage of the disease. In the chronic condition there appear to be canals in the bone. The

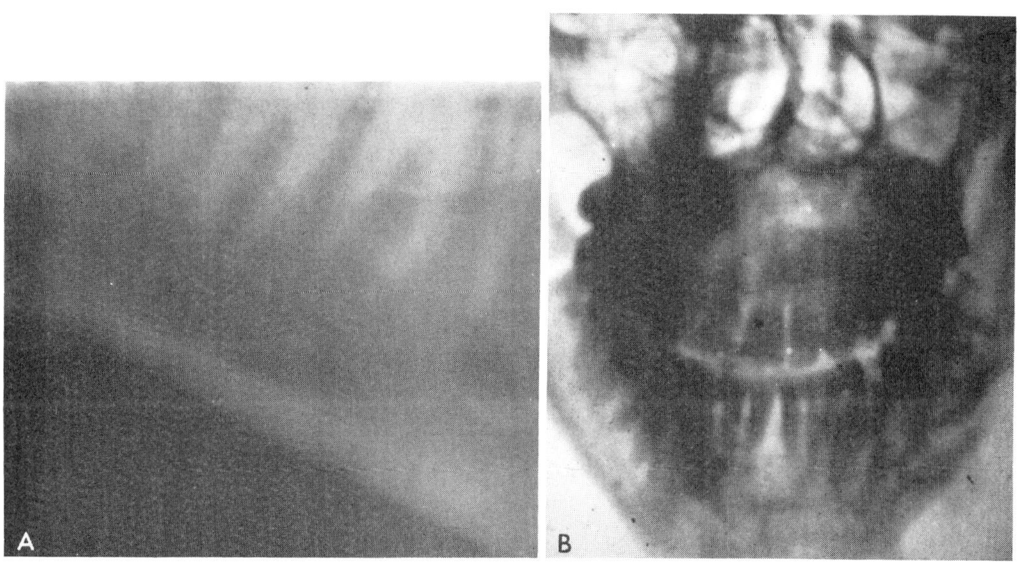

Figure 3–VI–10. *A.* Radiographic appearance of Cooley's anemia. *B.* Radiographic appearance of osteomyelitis with pathologic fracture.

sequestra appear extremely radiopaque and stand out in distinct contrast to normal bone trabeculae. A pathologic fracture at the angle of the mandible is noted in the case illustrated in (Figure 3–VI–10*B*).

Microscopic examination reveals an inflammatory infiltration of the marrow spaces of the spongiosa. This infiltration is primarily by lymphocytes, neutrophils, polymorphonuclear leukocytes, and plasma cells.

Leukemia. *Blood dyscrasias* are predisposing factors that influence the extent of dental injury in that they weaken the oral tissues, therefore making them more susceptible to trauma. Some of these are hemophilia, purpura, anemia, agranulocytosis, and leukemia. The influence of all of them on injury to the oral cavity is similar to that observed in acute leukemia.

Leukemia is a fatal disease involving the blood forming organs that is characterized by a marked increase in the number of leukocytes and their precursors in the blood.[24] It is of unknown etiology and, in the oral cavity, manifests itself clinically by gingivitis and stomatitis. The gingiva is hyperplastic; there is spontaneous hemorrhage; gingival ulceration occurs in later stages. The gingival biopsy shows marked proliferation of histiocytic elements.

Habits such as bruxism, bobby pin biting, and cheek biting render the oral tissues more susceptible and thereby influence the extent of injury in case of trauma. (This is discussed further in the section on trauma related to abnormal habits.)

Minimizing Factors in Oral Trauma

Morphologic variations play a vital role in minimizing the extent of injury in oral trauma. One variation is the "shovel-shaped" incisor, which is manifested by prominent mesial and distal ridges (Fig. 3–VI–11). The presence of this morphologic variation on the lingual surfaces of incisors is commonly noted by anthropologists and odontologists.[30] It has been observed that shovel-shaped incisors are found with great frequency in mongoloid peoples such as the Orientals, American Indians, and Eskimos.[31, 32]

Apparently, the typical structure of these teeth reinforces the incisal edges; it is reported that of over 1,000 teeth treated for fracture, none have been shovel-shaped incisors.[33]

Another important factor in resistance to trauma is the variation in *bone density* among different races. It has been reported that compact bone is more dense in the Negroid group than in the Caucasoid.[92] It is believed that this difference makes persons of the Negroid race less susceptible to fracture than others, when subjected to similar traumatic forces.

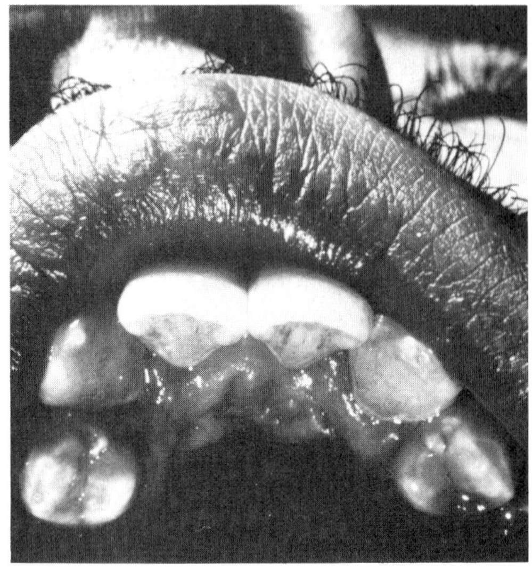

Figure 3–VI–11. Clinical appearance of the "shovel-shaped" incisor.

PRINCIPLES OF ORAL TRAUMA

There are two types of forces that cause injury to oral structures: *direct impact,* in which there is impact on the individual structure (e.g., fracture of an anterior tooth due to a fall against a drinking fountain), and *indirect impact* in which the force is applied to the mandibular arch, closing it forcefully against the maxillary arch. Fractured posterior teeth are a common result of the latter type of impact, and fractured anterior teeth are more frequently found in direct impact trauma.

Naturally, research in the actual mechanics involved in oral trauma is very difficult to conduct. Therefore, the following discussion of this subject is based on clinical observations of the author.

The *stability of the victim* plays a vital role in the type of trauma inflicted by a given force. For example, if one's reflexes permit him to move away from the impacting force, a minor abrasion may result from the blow that would otherwise have resulted in fractured teeth or even bone if one remained stable or moved toward it.

The type of tooth fracture frequently depends upon the *direction of the impact.* For instance, the impact usually hits the tooth on the labial surface at approximately a 90-degree angle to the long axis of the root. It has been

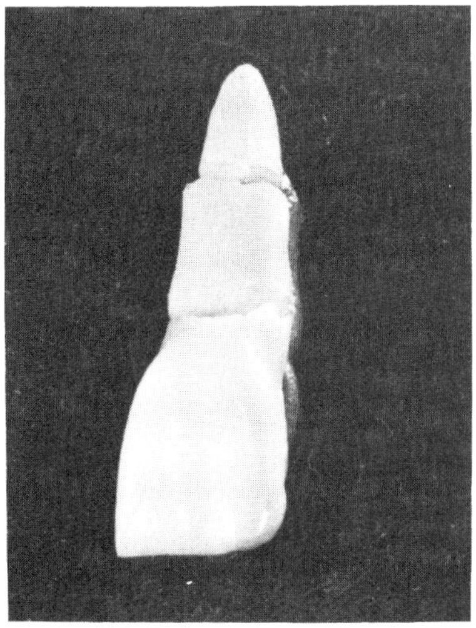

Figure 3–VI–12. Typical fracture lines from direct frontal impact.

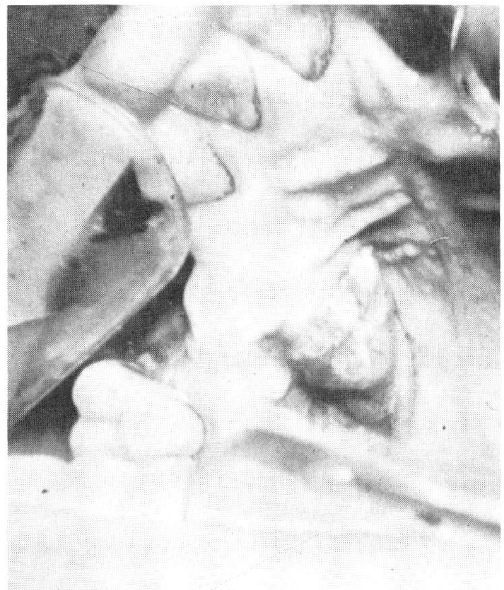

Figure 3–VI–13. Crown fractures due to bullet impact.

noted that injury from such impact frequently results in fractures involving both the crown and the root. Usually these fractures are parallel to each other and perpendicular to the direction of the original force (Fig. 3–VI–12).

The *velocity of the force* plays an interesting role in this type of injury. From observations it appears that tooth injury from high-velocity impact results in crown fractures alone, and injury to the supporting structures is insignificant (Fig. 3–VI–13). On the other hand, the opposite manifestations appear in cases of injury from low-velocity impact.

The *size of the impacting object* influences the type of trauma sustained. Large objects frequently injure the supporting structures, and crown fractures are infrequent in these instances (Fig. 3–VI–14).

The *shape of the offending object* exerts a great influence on the type of trauma. Generally speaking, crown fractures alone are common when the impacting object contacts a small area of the dentition; the supporting periodontal structures are more often affected when the object is larger and more blunt.

The *jaw relationship* at the time of impact is important: if the mandible is in a protruded position, the type of trauma caused by direct impact is often noted in the area of the lower anterior teeth (Fig. 3–VI–15*A*). The type of

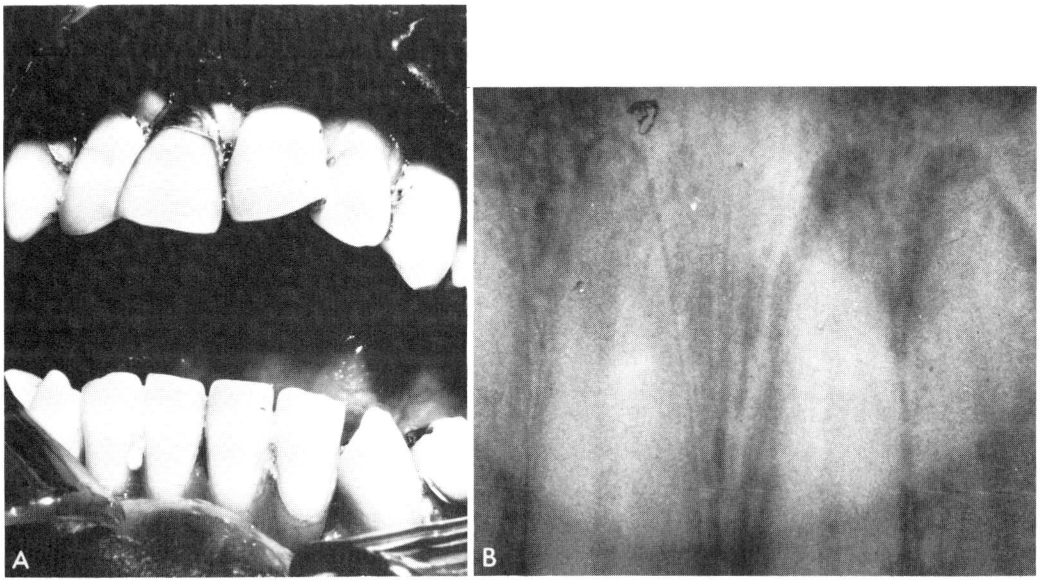

Figure 3–VI–14. *A*. Clinical appearance of tooth luxation from impact of a fist. *B*. Radiographic appearance of tooth luxation.

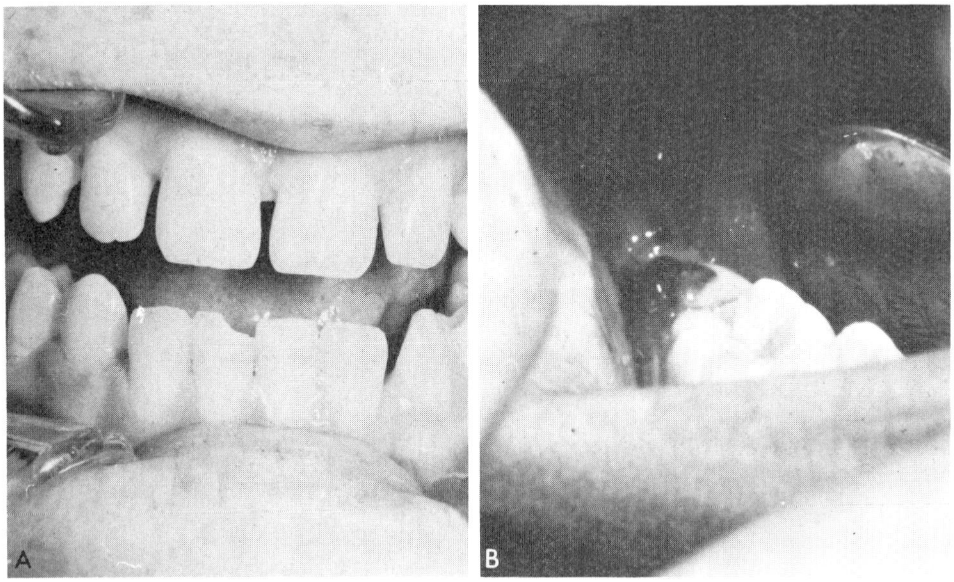

Figure 3–VI–15. *A.* Fractured incisor with mandible in protrusive position. *B.* Gingival injury in second molar area.

trauma caused by indirect impact in this situation is noted in the posterior area because the soft tissue of the mandible closes forcefully against the upper molars (Fig. 3–VI–15*B*).

The *character of the force* affects the type of trauma in that the risk of crown fracture appears minimized when the force is of softer, more elastic nature. In contrast, the supporting periodontal strúctures are more often affected by forces of this nature.

The *age of the victim* influences the type of trauma he may experience. In a young person, when the impact is large and blunt, the incidence of crown fracture is slight. This is probably because the supporting periodontal structures, in this age group, are very elastic, and these structures absorb the forces more readily than those of an older person.

CLASSIFICATION OF ORAL TRAUMA

It is appropriate to utilize the classification system adopted by the World Health Organization in its *International Classification of Diseases, Application to Dentistry and Stomatology, 1969,* since it has been adopted in America and non-English speaking nationalities can use this English version by recourse to the *Dental Lexicon.*[35-37] Another feature of this system is that it can

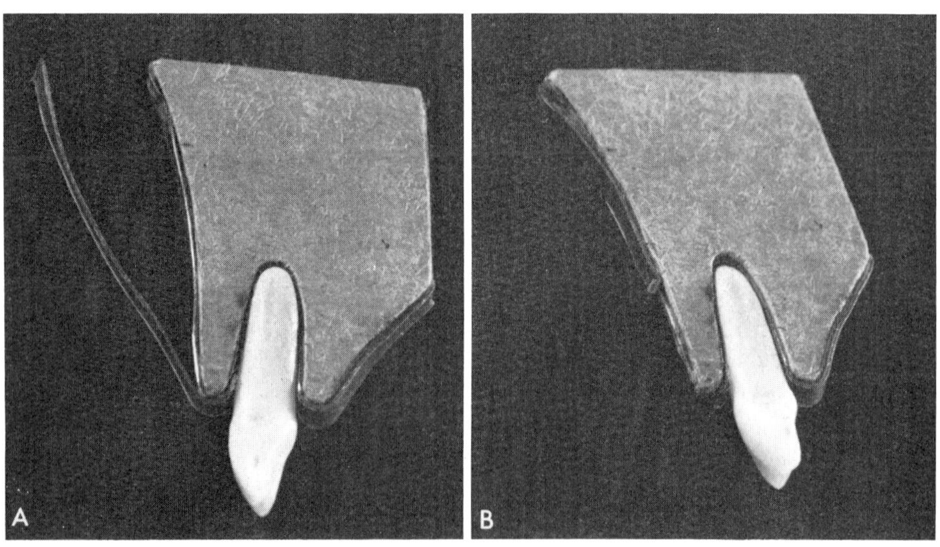

Figure 3–VI–16. *A.* Gingival or oral mucosal contusion N920.X1. *B.* Abrasion N920.X1. (Courtesy of G. T. Ward, D.D.S.)

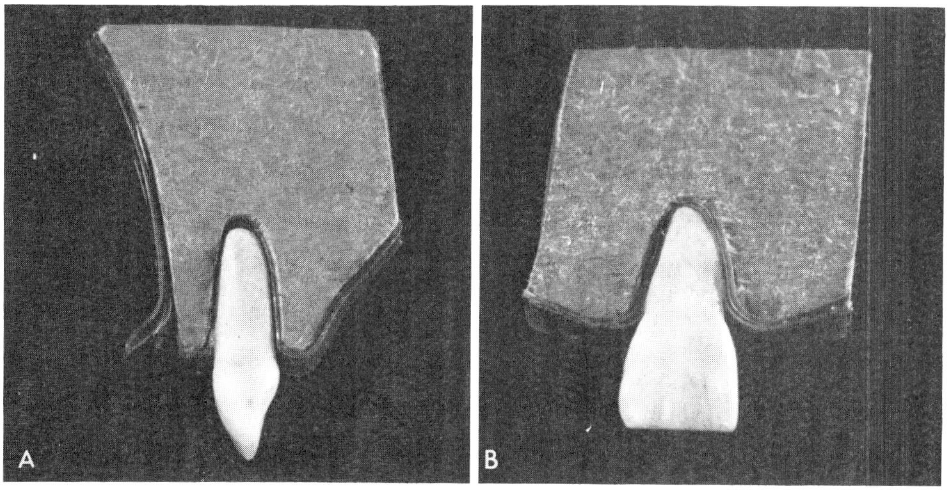

Figure 3–VI–17. *A.* Gingival or oral mucosal laceration N873.7. *B.* Fracture of enamel N873.70. (Courtesy of G. T. Ward, D.D.S.)

be utilized for both deciduous (primary) and succedaneous (permanent) dentitions.

The pertinent entities are classified as follows:

Gingival or Oral Mucosal Injury

N920.X1 Gingival or oral mucosal contusion (Fig. 3–VI–16*A*). This is a bruise and frequently associated with injury from a blunt object.

N920.X1 Gingival or oral mucosal abrasion (Fig. 3–VI–16*B*). An area is denuded of skin; this is frequently associated with mechanical trauma from a rough object.

N873.7 Gingival or oral mucosal laceration (Fig. 3–VI–17*A*). This is a tearing or cutting of the tissues and is frequently associated with trauma from a sharp object.

Hard and Pulpal Tissue Injury

N873.70 Fracture of enamel (Fig. 3–VI–17*B*).

N873.71 Fracture of enamel and dentin with no pulpal exposure (Fig. 3–VI–18*A*).

N873.72 Fracture of enamel and dentin with pulpal exposure (Fig. 3–VI–18*B*).

N873.73 Fracture of root (Fig. 3–VI–19*A*).

N873.74 Fracture of crown and root (Fig. 3–VI–19*B*).

Supporting Periodontal Injury

N873.75 Tooth luxation. This is dislocation and loosening of a tooth (Fig. 3–VI–20*A*).

N873.76 Tooth intrusion. The tooth is luxated inward into the alveolar socket (Fig. 3–VI–20*B*).

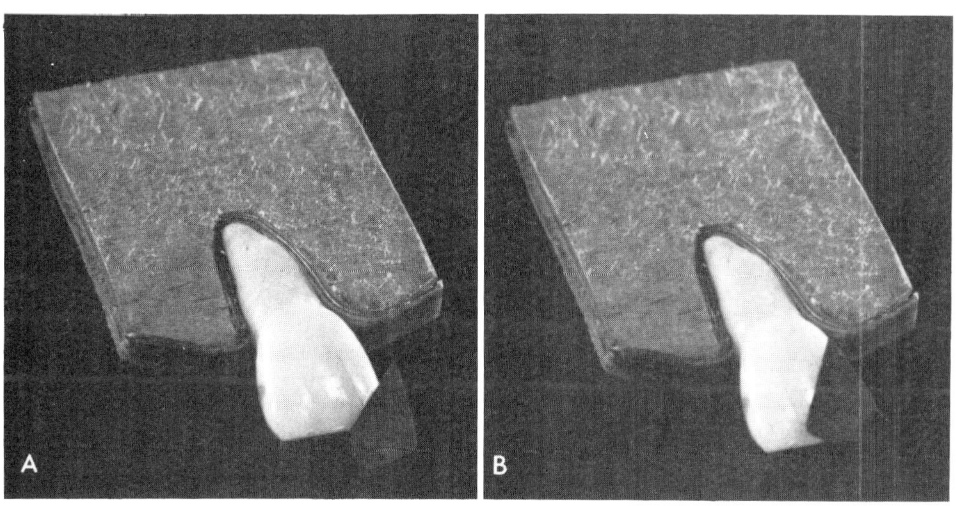

Figure 3–VI–18. *A.* Fracture of enamel and dentin with no pulpal exposure N873.71. *B.* Pulpal exposure N873.72. (Courtesy of G. T. Ward, D.D.S.)

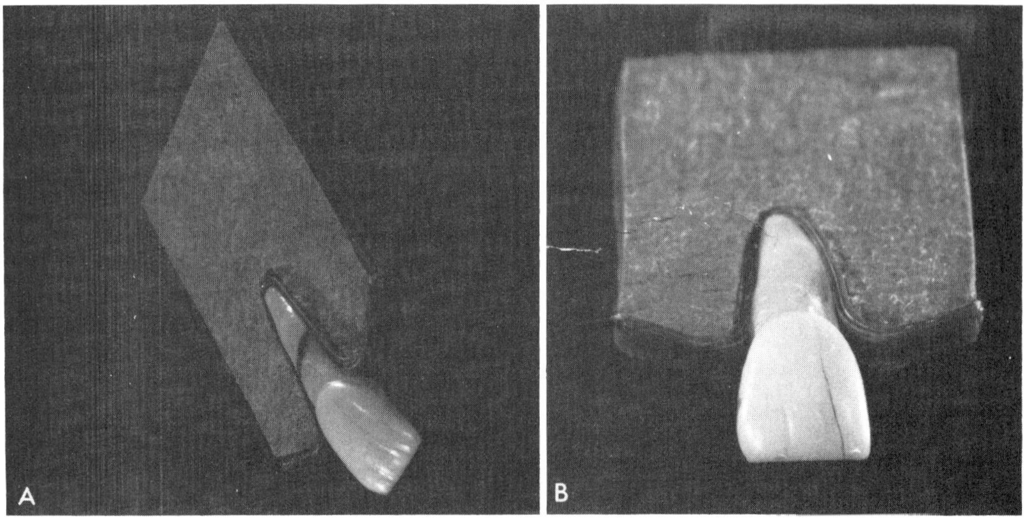

Figure 3–VI–19. *A*. Fracture of root N873.73. *B*. Fracture of crown and root N873.74. (Courtesy of G. T. Ward, D.D.S.)

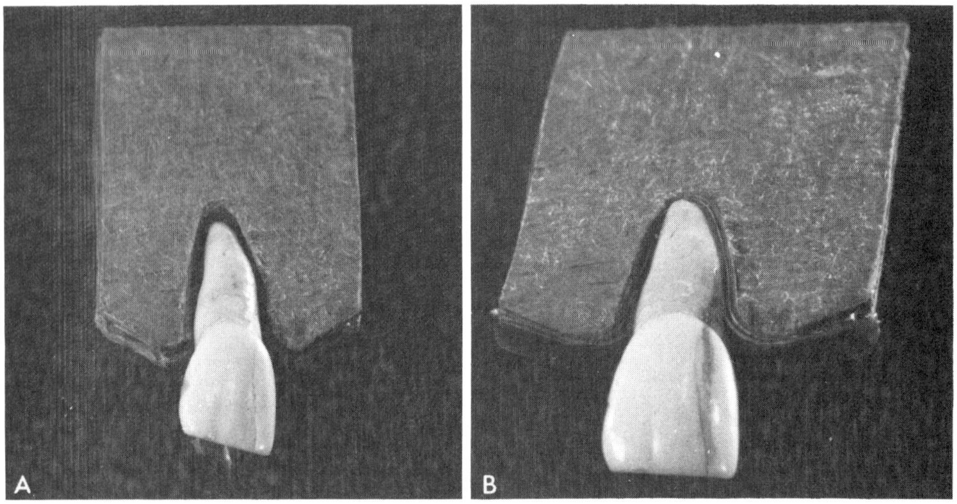

Figure 3–VI–20. *A*. Tooth luxation N873.75. *B*. Tooth intrusion N873.76. (Courtesy of G. T. Ward, D.D.S.)

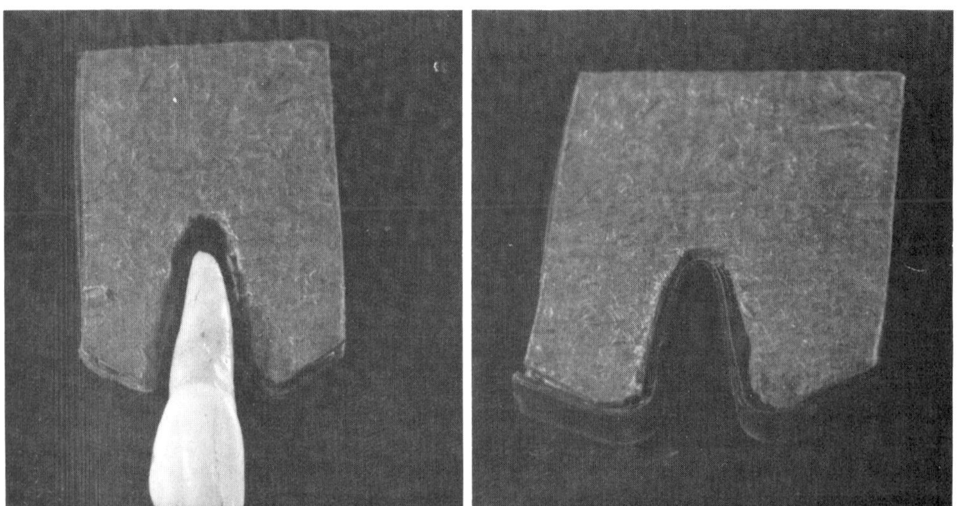

Figure 3–VI–21. *A*. Tooth extrusion N873.77. *B*. Tooth avulsion N873.78. (Courtesy of G. T. Ward, D.D.S.)

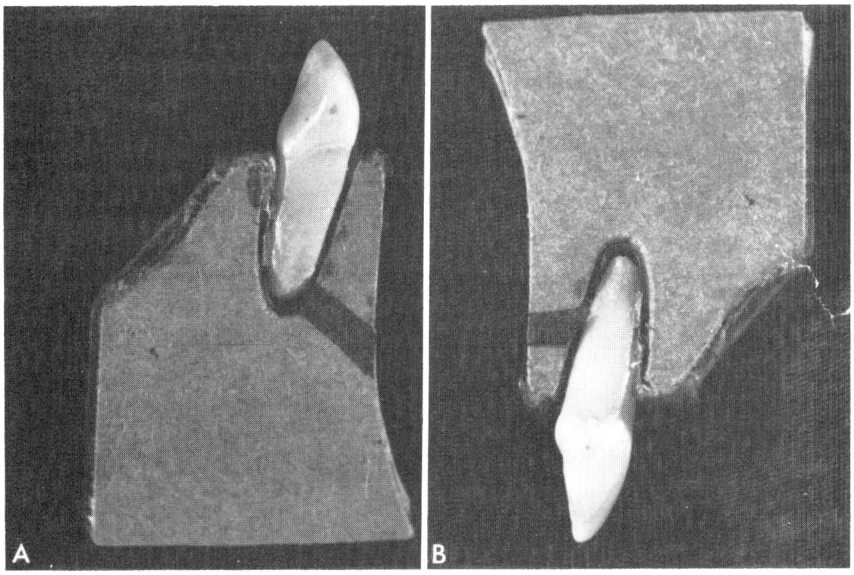

Figure 3–VI–22. *A.* Mandibular alveolus fracture N802.20. *B.* Maxillary alveolus fracture N802.40. (Courtesy of G. T. Ward, D.D.S.)

N873.77 Tooth extrusion. The tooth is displaced from the socket in an occlusal direction (Fig. 3–VI–21*A*).

N873.78 Tooth avulsion. The tooth is completely out of the alveolar socket (Fig. 3–VI–21*B*).

Supporting Bone Injury

N802.20 Fracture of mandibular buccal or lingual alveolus (Fig. 3–VI–22*A*).

N802.40 Fracture of maxillary buccal or lingual alveolus (Fig. 3–VI–22*B*).

N802.20 Fracture of mandibular alveolar process (Fig. 3–VI–23*A*).

N802.40 Fracture of maxillary alveolar process (Fig. 3–VI–23*B*).

N802.21 Fracture of mandible (Fig. 3–VI–24*A*).

N802.42 Fracture of maxilla (Fig. 3–VI–24*B*).

EXTRINSIC FACTORS IN ORAL TRAUMA

Acute Mechanical Trauma to Developing Hard Tissues

Calcification Defects. Defects due to trauma to the developing primary tooth germ appear

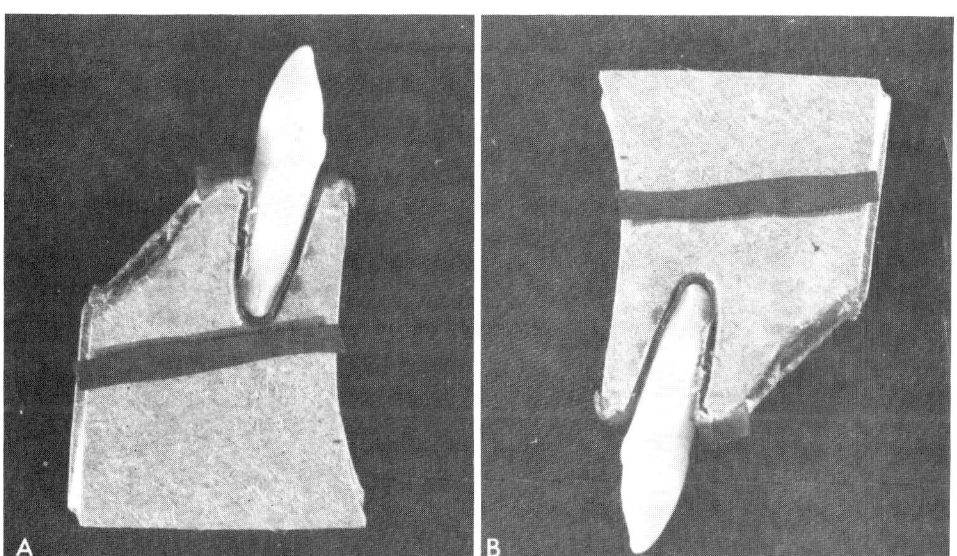

Figure 3–VI–23. *A.* Mandibular alveolar process fracture N802.20. *B.* Maxillary alveolar process fracture N802.40. (Courtesy of G. T. Ward, D.D.S.)

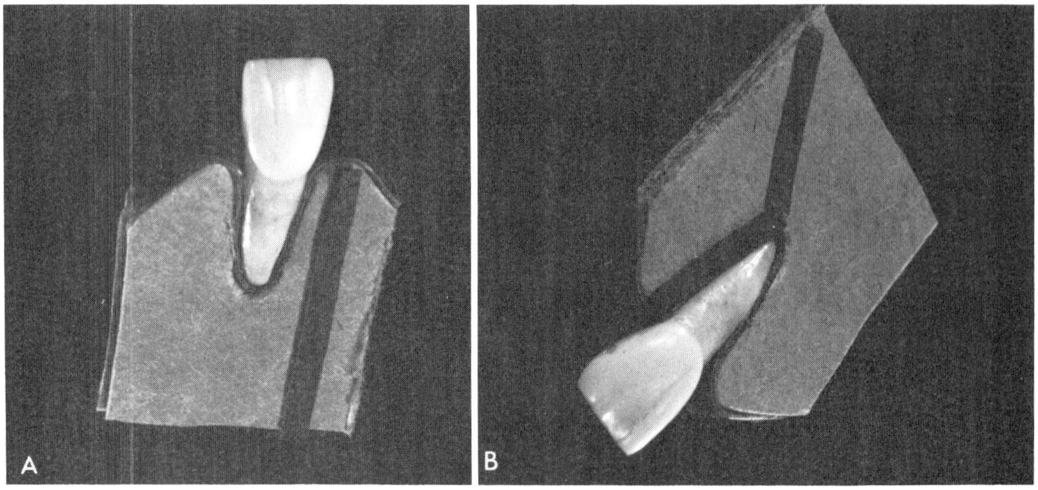

Figure 3–VI–24. *A.* Jaw fracture (mandible) N802.21. *B.* Jaw fracture (maxilla) N802.42. (Courtesy of G. T. Ward, D.D.S.)

clinically as white or yellowish brown areas (Fig. 3–VI–25). These usually occur on the labial surface of the crown in the permanent dentition. It has been reported that these changes occur in 23 per cent of cases in which there has been injury to the primary dentition.[38] Apparently, these color changes are due to interference with the maturation stage of mineralization.[39]

The pathogenesis of these color changes is not completely understood, but apparently the displaced primary tooth may traumatize tissue adjacent to the permanent tooth germ and even the odontogenic epithelium. This in turn may interfere with the final mineralization of enamel.[39]

Circular Enamel Hypoplasia. Another manifestation of trauma experienced during the formative stages of the permanent tooth germ is circular enamel hypoplasia (Fig. 3–VI–26).[40] This is probably due to localized damage to the ameloblasts. Such damage could be from traumatic displacement of already formed hard tissue adjacent to developing soft tissues.[23]

Radiographically, there is a transverse radiolucent line appearing at the place of enamel indentation. Frequently, this can be seen before tooth eruption.

Malformations Resembling Odontomas. These are sequelae to trauma experienced by the primary dentition. Cases that have been reported have occurred primarily in the upper incisor area.[39, 41-43] Apparently, the type of trauma affecting the primary dentition between

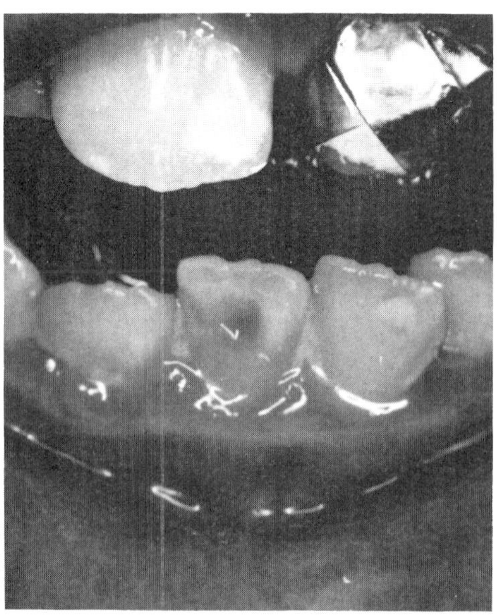

Figure 3–VI–25. White defect on upper central incisor and brown defect on lower central incisor. Also note the brownish white defect on adjacent lower central incisor.

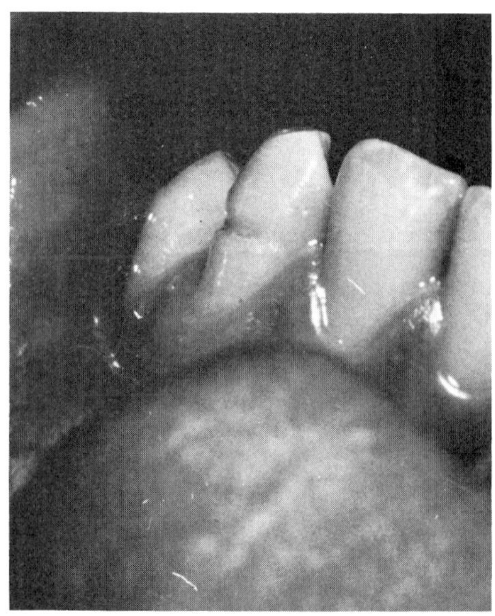

Figure 3–VI–26. Circular enamel hypoplasia of lower cuspid.

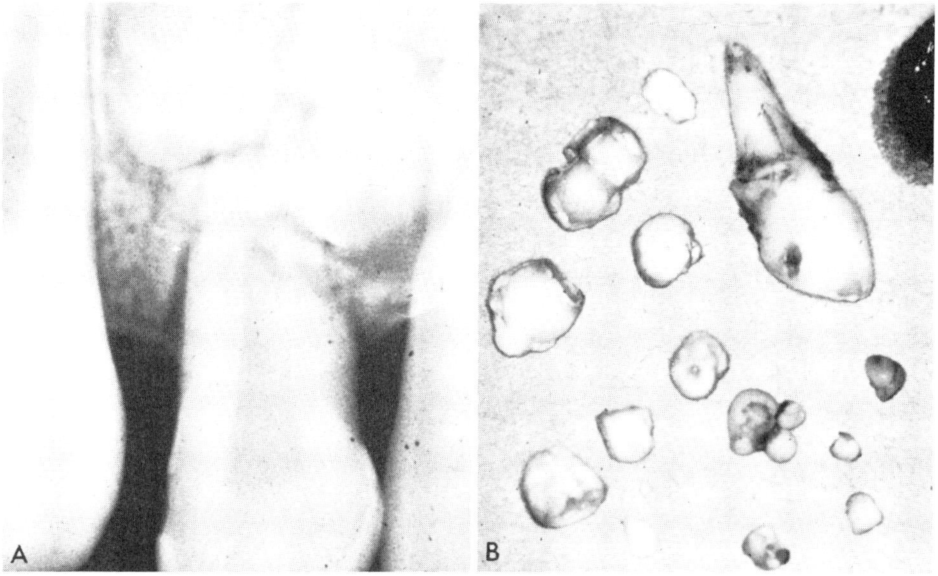

Figure 3–VI–27. *A.* Radiographic appearance of malformations. *B.* Postoperative appearance of malformations.

the ages of one and three years is prone to cause intrusive luxation or avulsion.[39]

Radiographically, there are many radiopaque areas of hard tissue that resemble normal types of tooth structure (Fig. 3–VI–27*A*). When the lesions are removed these are frequently found to be cementum, enamel, and dentin, and are part of a separate tooth formation (Fig. 3–VI–27*B*).

Root or Crown Dilacerations. Distortion of the root or crown occurs when there is traumatic displacement (avulsive or intrusive in nature) to the primary dentition at the approximate age of two to three years (Fig. 3–VI–28*A*). These distortions may appear on the labial, lingual, mesial, or distal portion of root surface. It is noted that the frequency of occurrence of this condition is 3 per cent after injuries to the primary dentition.[38]

Theoretically, this entity is due to displacement of a mineralized tooth portion together with enamel epithelium in relation to the dental papilla and cervical loops.[44, 45]

Arrest of Root Formation. Partial or complete arrest of root formation is an uncommon complication of trauma to the primary dentition. The frequency of occurrence in permanent teeth is approximately 2 per cent.[46-48] This en-

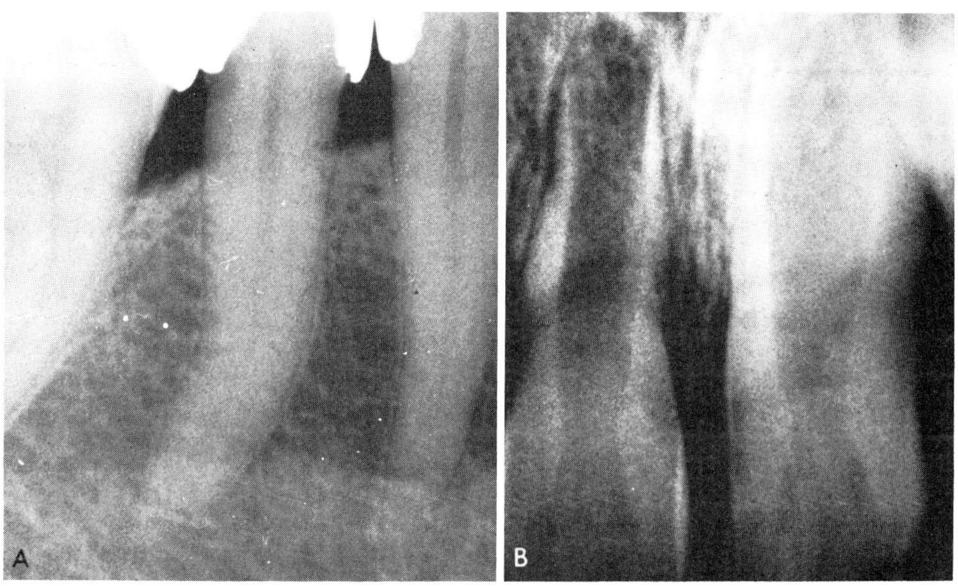

Figure 3–VI–28. *A.* Root dilaceration. *B.* Arrest of root formation.

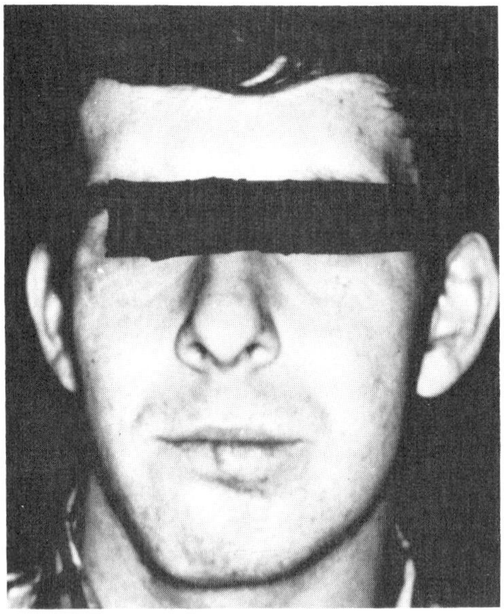

Figure 3–VI–29. Facial asymmetry.

tity is most often seen in the maxillary dentition and is due to trauma (usually of avulsive nature) to the primary dentition between the ages of five and seven.[39]

Apparently the pathogenesis of this malformation varies. Some cases show diminution of root formation even though there is no evidence of acute injury in the hard tissue.[48] There are, however, cases that demonstrate the typical calcio-traumatic line, indicating a separation of hard tissue formed before and after injury.[47, 49]

Radiographically, these teeth show the typical shortening of the root (Fig. 3–VI–28*B*). Root resorption has also been noted with this entity.[49, 50]

Trauma Affecting Growth and Development

The author has observed a considerable number of cases in which trauma has influenced the growth and development of the jaws. These sequelae are manifested by facial asymmetry, shown in Figure 3–VI–29, and micrognathism (underdevelopment of the jaws). On the basis of the patients' history it is believed that *facial asymmetry* is frequently related to a lateral traumatic force to the side of the mandible, whereas, in *micromandible* the associated injury is to the symphyseal area (Fig. 3–VI–30*A*).

Micromaxilla is often a hereditary trait; it has, however, been noted that this entity could possibly be due to the absence of the anterior nasal spine resulting from trauma (Fig. 3–VI–30*B*).[96]

The time of the traumatic experience in all three entities appears to be at a young age when the growth centers are affected.

Abnormal Tooth Eruption Due to Trauma

It has been noted that trauma is the most likely cause of *tooth eruption in an abnormal pattern.*[82] Clinically, these cases vary greatly and are very unpredictable.

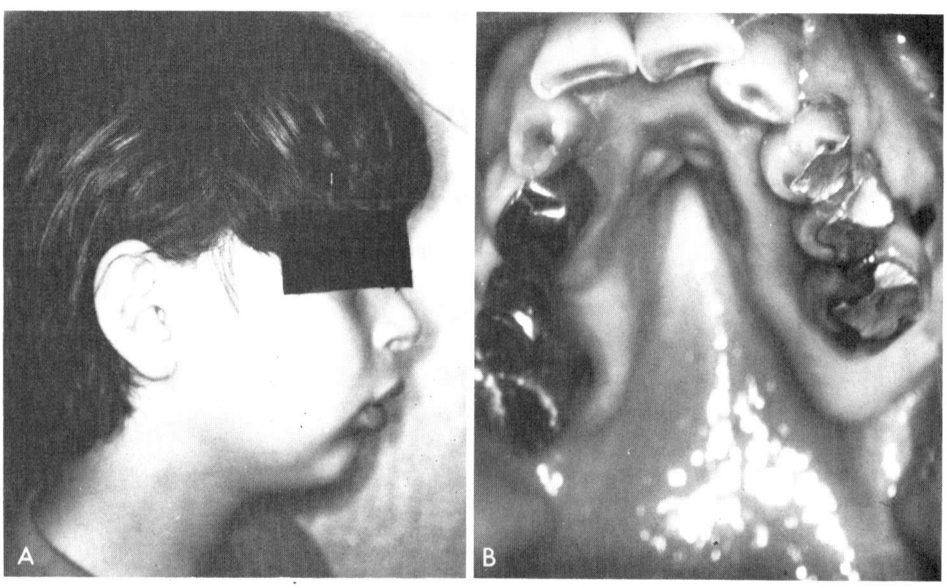

Figure 3–VI–30. *A.* Micromandible. *B.* Micromaxilla.

Trauma Resulting from Childbirth

A review of the literature reveals that oral trauma in childbirth is infrequent and is not well documented in suspected cases, so therefore, it appears insignificant.

One important point is discussed, however; the possibility of deformation of the maxilla from the obstetrician's inserting his fingers into the baby's mouth to facilitate passage through the birth canal. This practice is unacceptable from a dental standpoint because of the plasticity of the areas receiving the force. Temporary deformation is probable, and permanent damage to the maxilla could possibly result.[82]

Acute Mechanical Trauma to Developed Hard Tissue

Tooth Injuries

Trauma without Fracture. When a tooth is traumatized to a minor degree and the force is not of sufficient magnitude to cause inflammation, the capillaries will dilate and fill to their capacity with red blood cells. This condition is referred to as *pulpal hyperemia.* When the injury is more severe this hyperemia is followed by an inflammatory condition manifested by exudation due to the dilation of the blood vessels. Their walls appear more permeable nearest the site of injury. Fluid is extravasated from these vessels and enters into the connective tissue, causing an elevation of intrapulpal pressure.[51] At this time there is a migration of odontoblast nuclei into the dentinal tubules that is referred

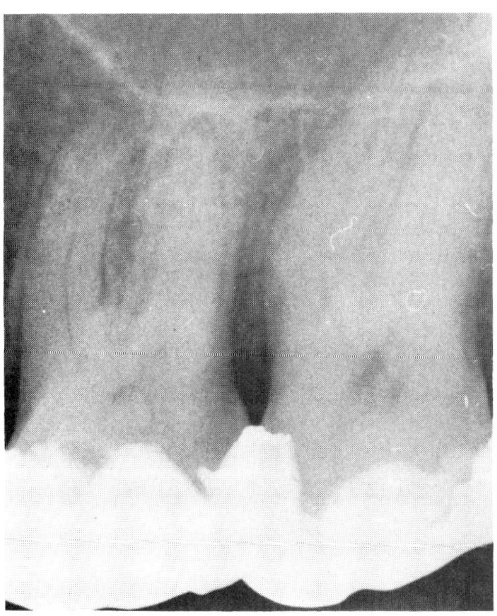

Figure 3–VI–31. Radiographic appearance of a pulp stone.

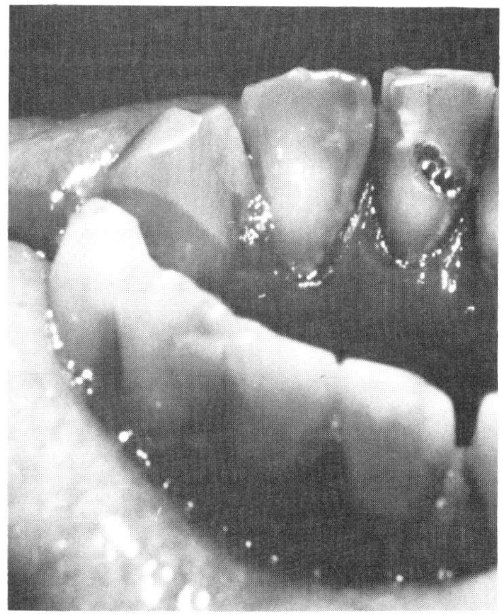

Figure 3–VI–32. Clinical appearance of a pulp polyp.

to as the initial pulpal reaction to injury.[52] It is easily demonstrated microscopically. These odontoblast cells are believed to break down, giving off by-products that act as further irritants to this inflammatory process.[52] This condition is referred to as *pulpitis.*

Calcific degeneration is a form of pulpal deterioration and is exemplified by pulp stones or denticles, which are made up of calcific substances in necrotic degenerated tissue (Fig. 3–VI–31). Frequently, these calcium deposits are developed as a reaction to oral trauma. They appear to occur in the pulpal tissue and are usually not attached to the dentinal wall.

It has been suggested that the rods of calcium fuse and may obliterate the pulp.[56] These teeth are usually asymptomatic, but the deposits are very significant in cases in which endodontic therapy is attempted.

Pulpitis may exist in an acute or chronic stage. In the chronic hyperplastic stage it is referred to as a *pulp polyp.*[53] This lesion appears very vascular, is relatively asymptomatic, and frequently occurs on the occlusal surface of posterior teeth. The one shown in Figure 3–VI–32 was on the lingual surface of a lower incisor; it was opened and left untreated for a long period of time.

Microscopically, this entity appears as though there were a well-defined layer of epithelium covering the hypertrophic part of the pulp. There is also an infiltration of mononuclear cells that extends apically.

Dental granuloma is a mass of granulation tissue that is usually surrounded by a fibrous sac that is continuous with the periodontal membrane and attached to the tooth's root.[24]

Microscopically, the relatively dense connective tissue is infiltrated with polymorphonuclear and endothelial leukocytes, fibroblasts and fibrous tissue, and islands of epithelial cells.

Radiographically, the root of the tooth appears roughened from the irregular absorption of the cementum. There are relatively well-defined areas of radiolucency that vary in size.

Necrosis refers to the death of tissue, sometimes of groups of cells in localized areas but usually of individual cells.[24]

Its incidence in trauma to the permanent dentition has been found to vary from 24 to 59 per cent.[71, 72] It has also been noted that there is a high rate of occurrence associated with trauma that is intrusive in nature and a lower rate following subluxations. [60, 61]

This occurs equally frequently in the deciduous and the permanent dentition, but there is a lower rate of incidence in children under three years of age.[73] Apparently, it is closely associated with pulpal inflammatory change and can precede either pulpal repair or pulpal abscess.[70] Complete necrosis develops as normal pulpal elements disintegrate, leaving the pulp canal predominantly filled with dead leukocytes. Frequently, the radiographic evidence is insignificant and the electric pulp tester is the only helpful diagnostic tool available.

Other sequelae of pulpitis due to trauma are chronic and acute *abscesses*, both periapical and gingival, occasionally with extraoral fistula. These abscesses are named in accordance with their location. An apical abscess is a localized infection arising at or near the apex of the root.[24] Histopathologic demonstration and radiographic interpretation of this are practically impossible and therefore unavailable.

Clinically, a cutaneous abscess appears as a hard localized swelling that is red and tender. Microscopically, a large number of neutrophils are found infiltrating the chronic inflammatory tissue; also present is an abundance of pus cells and other necrotic matter.

Cellulitis is another condition that may develop from trauma to hard tissues. The term refers to purulent inflammation of the loose subcutaneous tissue.[24]

Clinically, the cheek tissue is light red, semifluctuant, and sensitive to touch.

The pathogenesis of this entity is in the abundance of periapical inflammation that is characterized by a large amount of serous exudation into the loose tissues.[53] This edema may resolve or become suppurative; the latter is indicative of a true cellulitis.

Actinomycosis is a chronic infectious disease of cattle that is sometimes transmitted to man and is characterized by the formation of granulomatous lesions that break down and form abscesses, discharging a pus that contains yellow sulfur granules through numerous sinuses.[24] Other than being a sequela of tooth injury, this disease has been associated with tooth extractions.[27]

Microscopic examination reveals granulation tissue with fibrosis; the central portion is necrotic, and there is focal abscess formation. Examination of the pus reveals irregular lobulated actinomyces colonies in which the accumulation of the organisms appears granular in texture. (This disease is also discussed under Iatrogenic Factors in Oral Trauma.)

Osteomyelitis is also a sequela of oral trauma. (The influence of this disease on oral structures was discussed previously.)

Crown Fractures. There is a wide disparity in the reports concerning the incidence of crown fractures occurring in dental trauma. The range is from 26 to 76 per cent in the permanent dentition and from 4 to 38 per cent in deciduous teeth.[11, 14] It is believed that the most common causes of crown fractures are falls, bicycle and automobile accidents, and foreign bodies.[11]

Crazed lines are readily visible under indirect light and are manifested as cracks in the enamel that do not extend past the dentoenamel junction. These are frequently observed in cases in which there has been direct forceful contact with the labial surface of the tooth. This finding is suggestive of luxation trauma.

In the permanent dentition, there is a greater incidence of crown fractures extending through the *dentoenamel junction* than the more serious fractures with pulpal involvement.[54, 55] Crown fractures involving the dentoenamel junction frequently occur in the maxillary central incisors, since they are positioned most anteriorly in the normal dentition, where they are more accessible to impact. Consequently, the mesioincisal angle is the surface of these teeth most frequently traumatized (Fig. 3–VI–33*A*).

Occasionally, the center part of the *labioincisal edge* is involved, depending primarily on the point of traumatic contact (Fig. 3–VI–33*B*). When this type of fracture occurs, it is frequently in conjunction with injury of the supporting periodontal tissues and is often due to high-velocity impact by a small mass. It has been noted that the incidence of this type of fracture and of the more serious crown fractures is approximately the same in the deciduous dentition.[11]

When a fracture of this nature occurs, nu-

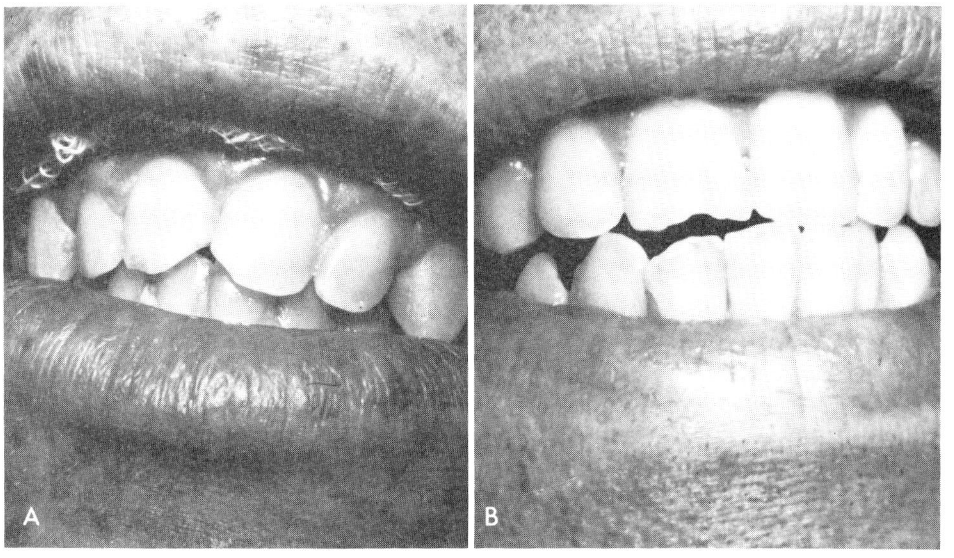

Figure 3–VI–33. Mesioincisal angle fractures. *B.* Labioincisal fracture.

merous dentinal tubules that lead toward the pulp are exposed. This renders the pulp most accessible to external stimuli such as thermal changes, toxic bacteria, and caustic chemical agents. Therefore, this condition often predisposes to pulpal inflammation.

Crown and Root Fractures. Comparatively speaking, *fractures involving enamel, dentin,* and *cementum* in permanent teeth occur infrequently (Fig. 3–VI–34*A*). These are commonly referred to as crown root fractures, and when they do occur there is usually pulpal exposure, and retention of the tooth presents a serious problem.

It has been observed that fractures of this nature are usually due to direct impact from a small object moving at relatively high velocity and making contact from a lateral direction. These teeth are usually very sensitive to acids, thermal changes, and pressure. If they are untreated, pulpal proliferation followed by degenerative changes (as previously described) will occur.

Root Fractures. Fracture of the root is a relatively infrequent finding in both the adult (1 to 7 per cent of injuries) and primary dentitions (2 to 4 per cent of injuries).[11, 14, 54, 55, 57] These fractures involving the dentin and cementum and pulp frequently occur in the middle third of the root[58] and may appear in any angle (Fig. 3–VI–34*B*). Many fractures of this nature are the result of fights.

Frequently these fractures heal without therapy. When this occurs, Kornfield explains, the void between the two fractured parts is filled with blood, fibroblasts, and tissue fluids.[29] Then

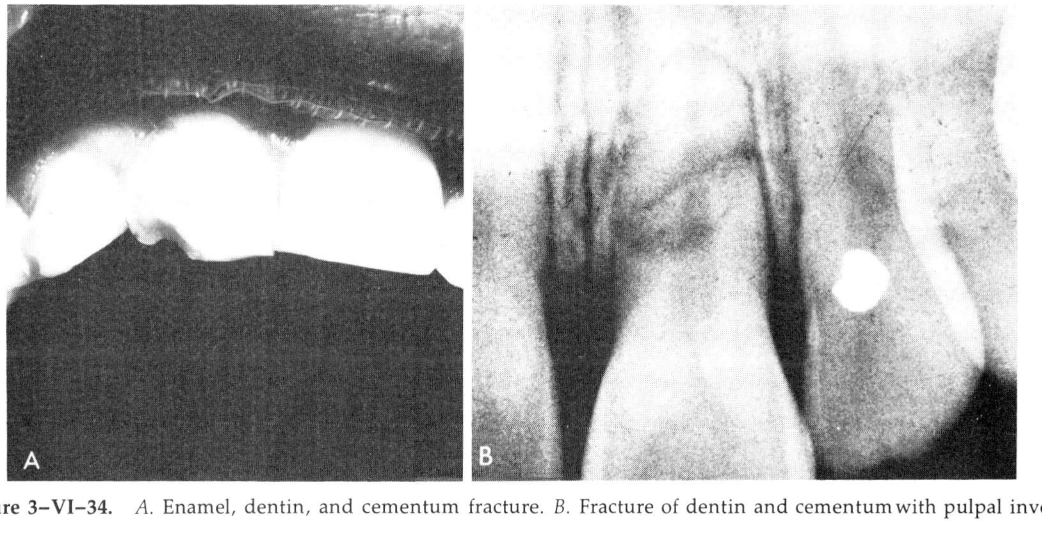

Figure 3–VI–34. *A.* Enamel, dentin, and cementum fracture. *B.* Fracture of dentin and cementum with pulpal involvement.

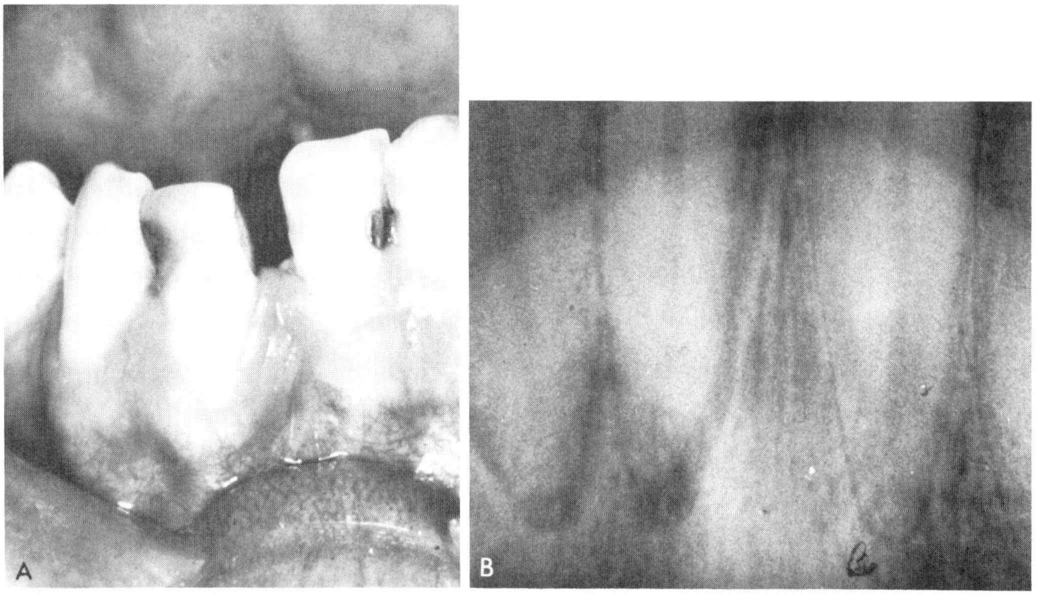

Figure 3–VI–35. Extrusive tooth luxation. *A*. Clinical appearance. *B*. Radiographic appearance.

there is a phase of dentin resorption due to an ingrowth of connective tissue. This is followed by cementum deposition and the development of collagen fibers, resulting in complete union in cases of small fractures. In other situations, the connective tissue remains, often with bone spicules interspersed.

Luxation. It has been reported that tooth luxations account for 62 per cent of oral injuries in deciduous teeth and 20 to 40 per cent affecting the permanent dentition (Fig. 3–VI–35*A*).[11] In this situation, the tooth is usually loose, malpositioned, and tender to touch. In permanent teeth the most common cause of this entity is fights. Falls are the most frequent etiologic agents in the deciduous dentition.[11] Also, it has been observed by the author that luxation by indirect impact occurs frequently. The maxillary central incisors are the most commonly involved teeth in both the deciduous and permanent dentitions.[60]

Radiographically, the picture varies with the type of luxation. In cases of extrusive luxation, there is a large, definite increase in width of the space in the apical area (Fig. 3–VI–35*B*). On the other hand, intrusive luxation reveals no

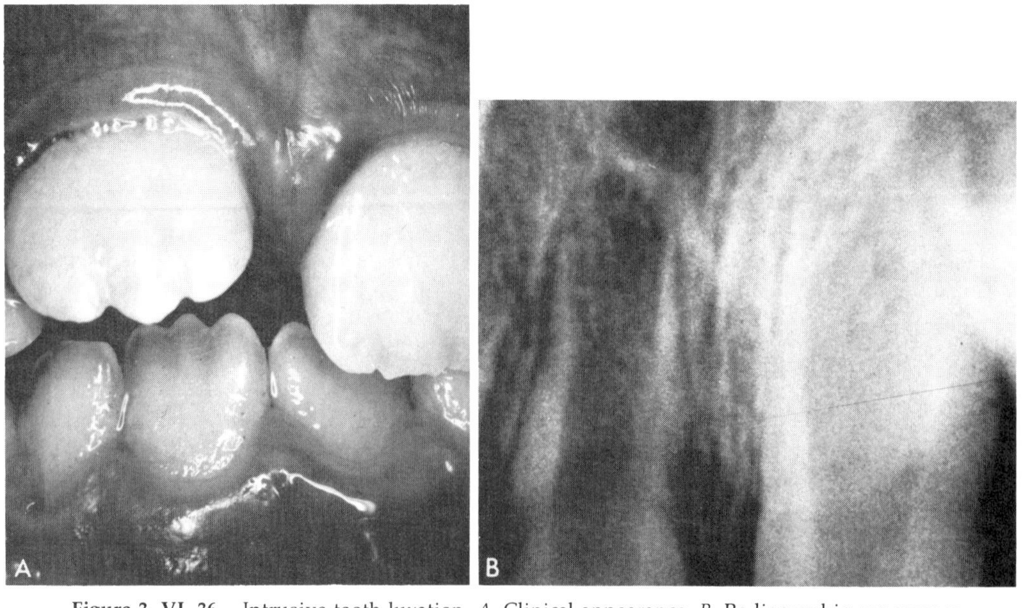

Figure 3–VI–36. Intrusive tooth luxation. *A*. Clinical appearance. *B*. Radiographic appearance.

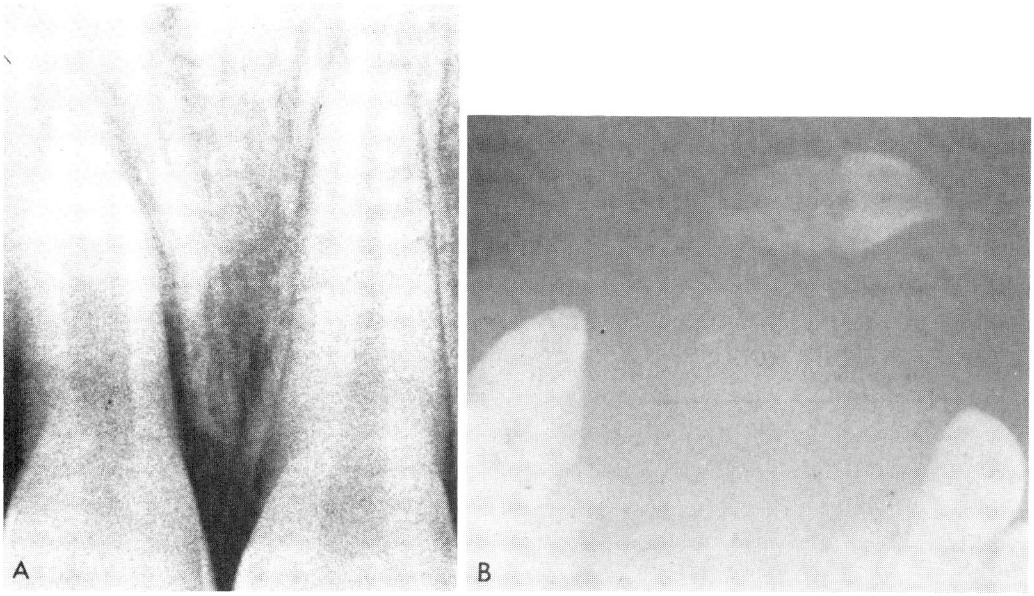

Figure 3–VI–37. *A*. Radiographic appearance of lateral luxation. *B*. Radiographic appearance of a tooth embedded in the tongue.

periodontal space around the displaced tooth (Fig. 3-3-VI-36*A* and *B*).

In lateral luxation there is a marked widening of the periodontal space apically on either side of the tooth depending upon the direction of impact (Fig. 3-VI-37*A*).

Microscopically, edema of the pulp occurs shortly after the trauma, and it has also been suggested that perivascular hemorrhage may be seen in the apical area.[23]

Avulsion. Complete avulsions in which the tooth is forced out of the socket are similar to luxations, from a statistical point of view, in that the etiologic factors and the oral area most often affected are the same.[11, 61, 62] According to the literature, the incidence varies from 7 to 13 per cent of injuries in the deciduous dentition and from 1 to 16 per cent in the permanent dentition.[11, 54, 57, 63, 64] It has also been noted that this type of injury occurs more frequently in the age group of 7 to 10 years.[62]

Fractures of the alveolus are not an uncommon finding in these cases, and diagnostic radiographs are of extreme importance. Extraoral films may be necessary to locate the tooth, since frequently it may be embedded in surrounding oral structures (Fig. 3-VI-37*B*). When these teeth are endodontically treated and replanted, frequently the radiographic picture appears to be one of healing, with the cementum of the root being surrounded by normal periodontium.

Clinically, the teeth have a normal sound to percussion, and it is not uncommon for them to be slightly discolored. Shortly after reimplantation of a permanent tooth, there is a resorptive process on the surface of the cementum that is occasionally demonstrated radiographically. This may be followed by ankylosis, but quite often there is pulpal degeneration, and resorption becomes more active, which results in disintegration of the root.

A favorable prognosis is given if the tooth is in the developing stage. The outlook is less favorable, however, for one that has completely developed, and pulpal necrosis is a common result.

It has been observed, clinically, that all pulps do not react to the same stimuli in the same manner. The injury to one tooth may set up a reparative and protective tissue reaction. On the other hand, the same injury to the adjacent tooth may initiate degenerative changes and pulpal necrosis. Occasionally, the one tooth will remain in status quo while the other will radiographically demonstrate repair (Fig. 3-VI-38*A*).

Ankylosis. Ankylosis is a union of the cementum of the tooth to bone, and is an occasional occurrence following oral trauma. It is commonly found in cases of tooth reimplantation. Apparently, this procedure causes extensive root resorption; the alveolar bone grows into these resorbed areas and is very likely to become united with the cementum.[65]

Radiographically, the root and bone appear to be one, and the periodontal space is absent (Fig. 3-VI-38*B*). There is a normal clinical ap-

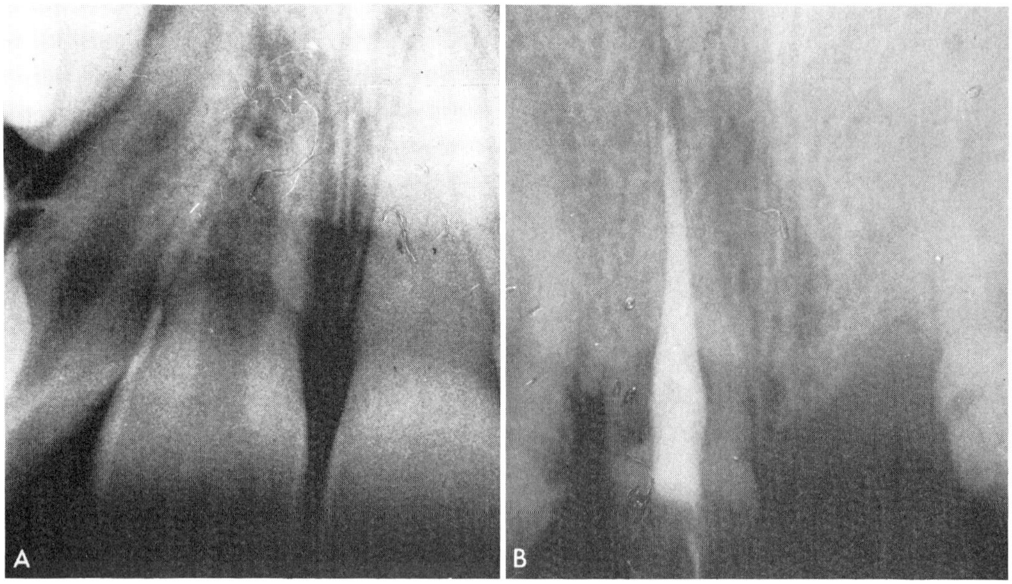

Figure 3–VI–38. *A*. Radiographic appearance of replanted central incisors (two and a half years postoperatively). *B*. Ankylosis.

pearance, so therefore radiographs are imperative since this entity becomes quite significant in cases of extraction.

Root Resorption. Root resorption, external and internal, may occur subsequent to oral trauma in both the deciduous and the permanent dentition. This condition is most frequently noted after intrusive luxations. Contrarily, this entity has the lowest rate of occurrence from subluxations.[66]

It has been suggested that the probable cause of *external resorption* is chronic inflammatory tissue that is developed in periodontal pockets (See Fig. 3–VI–3*A*).[66] Apparently this inflamed tissue comes in contact with the cementum, which then undergoes calcific degeneration. If allowed to continue, the resorption of dentin reaches the pulp and, if not treated, usually results in pathologic fracture or periapical pathosis or both.

Internal resorption has been reported in only approximately 2 per cent of reexamined teeth having a history of luxation (see Fig. 3–VI–3*B*).[60] Other writers have noticed this same trend toward infrequency.[68, 69]

The condition is apparently associated with trauma either from an impact or from cavity preparation in dental treatment. When this occurs, localized hemorrhage possibly leads to the pulpal metaplasia.[70] The destruction of dentin usually continues until there is communication with the oral fluids, which allows the invasion of the pulp by microorganisms and the resulting pulpal infection or pathologic fracture.

Discoloration. Tooth discoloration is a frequent consequence of oral trauma and is due to hemorrhage into the pulp chamber. There is hemolysis of red blood cells whose breakdown products penetrate the dentinal tubules and cause this discoloration.[70]

Bone Injuries

Trauma without Fracture. *Traumatic cysts* (or hemorrhagic extravasation) may be a result of injury to the jaws. They cause resorption of bone, swelling, and temporary pain. It has been demonstrated that intermedullary hemorrhage resulting from various types of trauma was the cause of bone resorption and cyst formation in six cases.[76] Although the etiology is unknown, a theory concerning the pathogenesis is that trauma that is of sufficient magnitude to cause intermedullary hemorrhage of arteries of the jaw results in the formation of an intraosseous hematoma. There is resorption of bone owing to the irritating influence of the decomposing fibrin, leaving a large cavity. There is a fibrous lining at the cystic wall that is formed from adjacent marrow spaces.[76]

Radiographically, the cyst appears as a well-defined irregular radiolucency (Fig. 3–VI–39).

Microscopically, there is an appearance of cellular, edematous granulation tissue. No epithelial lining is present.

Trauma with Fracture. Alveolar fractures may be classified as either associated with mandibular and maxillary fractures or associated with partial or complete avulsion of teeth with the alveolus attached.[74] It is reported that in a series of cases, there were 16 per cent with

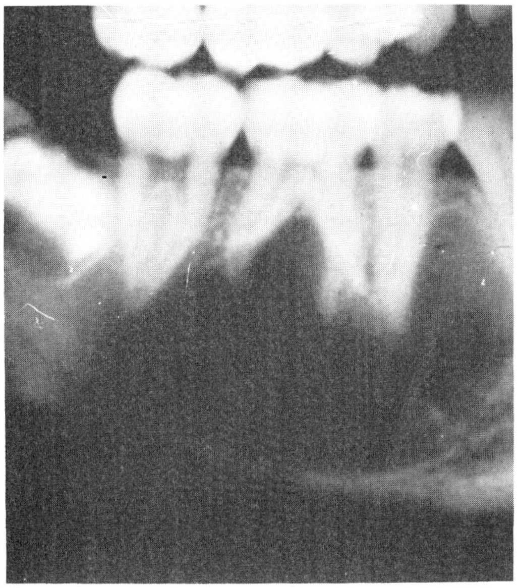

Figure 3–VI–39. Radiographic appearance of a traumatic bone cyst.

fractures affecting the alveolar bone in the permanent dentition and 7 per cent with such fractures in the deciduous dentition.[11] Fights and automobile accidents are the most frequent etiologic factors in these cases.[11, 75]

Clinically, they frequently appear as a displacement of several adjacent teeth; they can usually be diagnosed by palpation. It is also common for the bone fragment to be mobile. Radiographically, these fractures may appear at any level from the crest of the alveolar ridge to the area of the tooth's apex.

Jaw Fractures

Fractures of the maxilla and mandible are usually associated with either disease or trauma. Comparatively speaking, bone fractures associated with oral trauma are infrequent. When these are sustained, however, the incidence of fractures of the mandible is much greater (approximately 8 to 1) than that of fractures of the maxilla, probably because the mandible is more exposed.[78]

The pathologic aspect of fractures has been previously discussed (under predisposing factors). The external traumatic forces may be from gunshot wounds, fights, athletics, falls, occupational or automotive or aircraft accidents, or of iatrogenic nature. Of all these factors, the writer has observed that fist fights are the predominant cause of jaw fractures.

Oral trauma associated with truck tires is not an infrequent finding. This is usually due either to air blowing the rim off or to an actual "blowout" in which the air is released under pressure.

Of these two situations, the former appears to be more serious. These rims have been known to strike the jaws with sufficient impact to inflict fractures (Fig. 3–VI–40*A* and *B*).

In cases in which there is an actual "blowout," usually the trauma is external and superficial, and therefore healing is usually uneventful.

The type of injury produced is influenced by the velocity and direction of the force and also by the area upon which the force is exerted.

Incidence of Maxillary Fractures. According

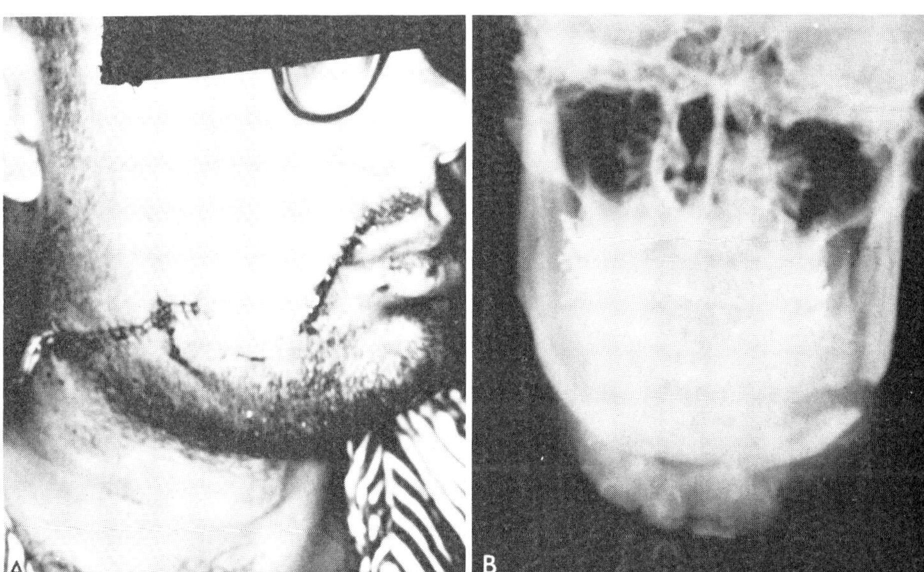

Figure 3–VI–40. *A*. Clinical appearance of injury from tire rim. *B*. Radiographic appearance of mandible fractured by a tire rim.

to Archer, maxillary fractures occur in the following order of frequency:

1. Segmental fracture of the alveolar process in the tuberosity region.
2. Segmental fracture of the anterior maxilla containing teeth.
3. Transverse fractures through the maxillary sinuses and nasal cavity.
4. Compound comminuted fractures.[81]

Incidence of Mandibular Fractures. Mandibular fractures are listed according to the frequency of occurrence at the following areas:

1. The area of the angle, where there is an unerupted or impacted third molar.
2. The mental foramen area.
3. The area of the symphysis.
4. The horizontal ramus (body).
5. The area between the angle and the cuspid.
6. Through the ramus.
7. Between the angle and the sigmoid notch.
8. The area of the coronoid process.
9. The anterior segment of the alveolar process without involvement of the horizontal ramus (body).[81]

Dingman and Natvig have noted that 36 per cent of all mandibular fractures occur in the weakest portion of the condylar process; 21 per cent occur in the region of the angle of the body, and 14 per cent occur in the symphysis area.[77]

It is further suggested that the direction of force is a very significant factor in determining the location of fracture. For instance, one might suspect bilateral fractures of the condylar neck when a severe force is applied to the symphysis and a subcondylar fracture on the side opposite to the impact when the trauma is to the side of the mandible.

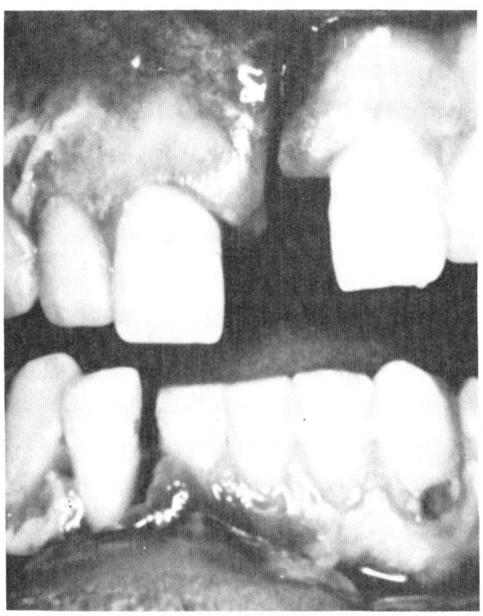

Figure 3–VI–41. Clinical appearance of a fractured mandible and maxilla.

The clinical impression of fractures is one of malocclusion, pain, swelling of soft tissues, ecchymosis, movement of fractured parts, grating noise during mandibular movements, and facial distortion, depending on the area affected (Fig. 3–VI–41).

Radiographic examination is imperative to determine the exact location, the extent of the fracture, and the condition of the teeth in the suspected area. The angulation of the x-ray depends upon the area under suspicion (Fig. 3–VI–42*A* and *B*).

Classification of Maxillary Fractures. At this time the Le Fort classification of maxillary fractures is widely accepted. The nomenclature was derived from results of experiments that were reported by Le Fort in 1900 and 1901.[79, 80]

A *Le Fort I* fracture is a transverse fracture through the maxilla that involves the alveolar process, the palate, parts of the maxillary sinus wall, and lower portions of the pterygoid processes. This type of fracture is the result of trauma to the lower region of the maxilla.

The *Le Fort II* fracture is caused by trauma to the upper maxillary area and is generally pyramidal in shape. The force is of such nature as to cause fractures of the nasal bones and frontal processes of the maxilla. The fractured areas may include the lacrimal bones, the inferior rim of the orbit, the zygomaticomaxillary suture, and the pterygoid plates.

Le Fort III fractures result from trauma that is sufficient to cause the entire maxilla and at least one of the facial bones to be separated from the craniofacial skeleton. Areas that are commonly affected are the maxillofrontal, zygomaticofrontal and nasofrontal sutures; the floors of the orbits; and the areas of the ethmoid and sphenoid attachments. These injuries are frequently accompanied by multiple fractures of the facial bones.

Classification of Mandibular Fractures. The classification of Dingman and Natvig is a practical system, since it is based on location and correlates anatomical and clinical nomenclature.[77] This method is as follows:

1. *Symphysis area:* the region that is bounded by vertical lines and is just distal to the lower cuspid teeth.
2. *Body area:* the area from the cuspid line to a line coinciding with the anterior border of the masseter muscle.
3. *Angle area:* a triangular region that is bounded by the anterior border of the masseter muscle and an oblique line that

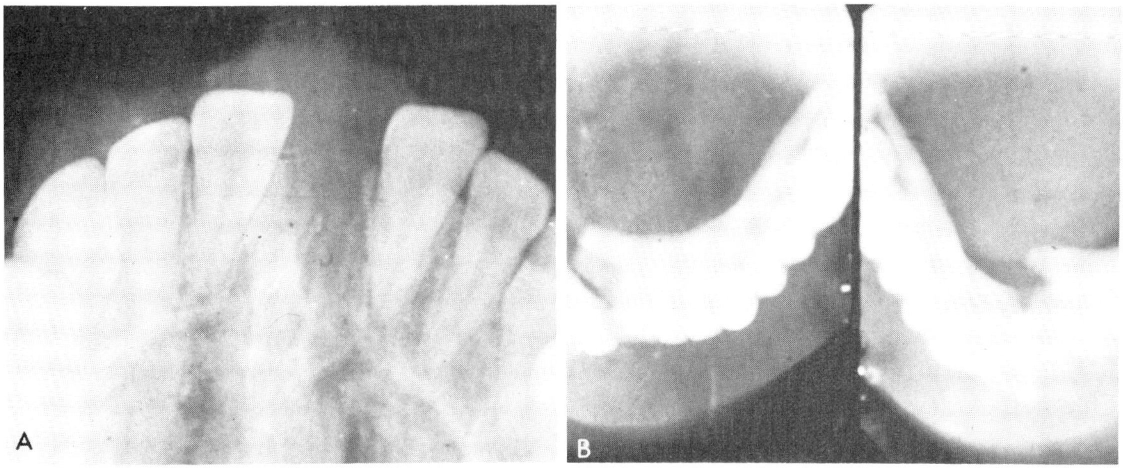

Figure 3–VI–42. *A.* Radiographic appearance of the fractured maxilla. *B.* Radiographic appearance of the fractured mandible.

extends from the third molar area to the posterior superior attachment of the masseter muscle.

4. *Ramus area:* bounded inferiorly by the angle region and superiorly by two equal lines that form a 90-degree angle at the midpoint of the sigmoid notch.
5. *Condylar process area:* located above the ramus region and including the neck and the condyle.
6. *Coronoid process area:* comprises the coronoid process above the ramus region.
7. *Alveolar process area:* may occur in the symphysis area or the body area, or may include fractures in both areas but limited to the alveolar bone.

Complications associated with fractures may be classified by their time of occurrence.

Early complications include hemorrhage, numbness, airway obstruction, and infection such as osteomyelitis and cellulitis.

Late complications include malunion, nonunion, malocclusion, chronic sinusitis, and anesthesia.

Pathosis of Untreated Fractures. Cases in which the fractures are not treated, for various reasons, frequently result in disfigurement and malfunction of the regions involved. Quite often these conditions lead to psychologic and functional disturbances.

Psychologically, the individual may undergo an alteration of his personality that results in lack of social acceptance, which frequently leads to financial problems.

Functional disturbances may alter one's respiration, vision, and speech. Mastication and swallowing are frequently affected, which influences one's ability to digest foods properly.

According to the author's observations, open bite deformities and various forms of malocclusion are the most frequent results of untreated jaw fractures (Fig. 3–VI–43).

Temporomandibular Joint Trauma. Extrinsic trauma is a very important factor in the etiology of *traumatic temporomandibular joint arthritis* (or arthrosis, according to most European nomenclature). It has been reported that approximately 20 per cent of patients with such disturbances present with a history of extrinsic trauma.[83] Such trauma is of further importance in this entity when one considers the results of a healed fracture that is in poor alignment and the possibility of permanent damage to the meniscus.[84]

It has been further observed that 1 of every 20 patients who have received a neck injury in

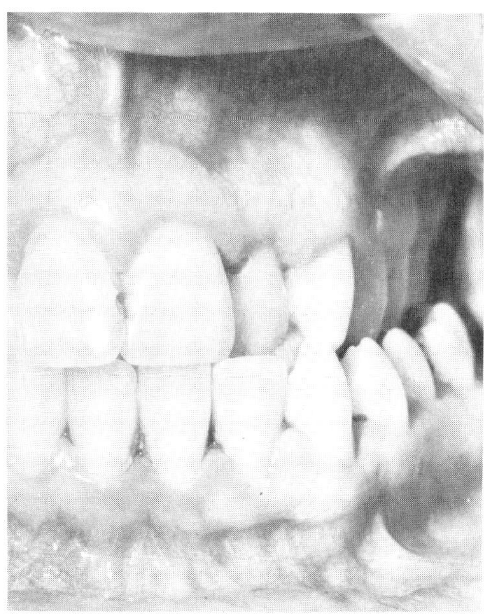

Figure 3–VI–43. Clinical appearance of malocclusion resulting from an untreated mandibular fracture.

a rear-end auto collision will develop *temporomandibular joint symptoms*.[85] Such manifestations are crepitation (a clicking noise), deviation of the mandible, pain during mastication, tenderness in the area upon palpation, restriction of mandibular movements, and pain upon yawning.

The explanation for this entity lies in the forward acceleration of the motorist's body while his head is snapped backward. Frequently, the jaw's inertia causes the mouth to open suddenly; then the stretch reflex of the masseters, which are the main muscles of mastication, causes the jaw to snap shut. This action, the force and speed of opening and closing, may be of sufficient intensity to stretch, strain, or even tear the ligament fibers. After an auto accident of this nature, the patient may complain of neck pain, restriction of head movement, dizziness, headache, and difficulty in swallowing.

The pathogenesis of traumatic temporomandibular joint disturbances is in controversy, but a popular explanation is the theory of "distal displacement" in which the mandible is thrust backward, encroaching on the auditory apparatus and producing pressure on nerve endings.[86, 87]

Another concept is that of the "temporomandibular joint pain dysfunction syndrome" in which, it is believed, muscle dysfunction and fatigue are the source of this entity.[88-90]

A third concept of the pathogenesis of traumatic temporomandibular joint arthritis is that it is a form of other types of arthritis of unknown etiology.[91]

Chronic Mechanical Trauma to Dental Hard Tissues

Frequently, this is a type of occupational trauma and the dental manifestations appear after a long period of time. Some of the more common conditions noted are small notches due to the constant biting of thread or holding of pins and needles between the teeth, and half-moon shaped abrasions from the playing of a musical instrument. Similar findings frequently appear in the glass blower's dentition. Notching of incisors from holding nails is a frequent finding in carpenters (Fig. 3–VI–44*A*).

Uncommon *dental abrasions* not directly associated with occupations are from the injudicious use of dental floss with toothpaste, shown in Figure 3–VI–44*B*, and from a pipestem being held between the teeth.

Pathologic findings include enamel loss and sclerosis of the adjacent dentin. Frequently, there is a build-up of irritation dentin in the area of the pulpal wall, but for all practical purposes the pulpal tissue appears normal.

Acute Mechanical Trauma to Soft Tissues

Types of Wounds

An *incision* is the simplest wound in which there is a clean cut by a sharp object with no tissue loss.

Laceration refers to a condition in which the

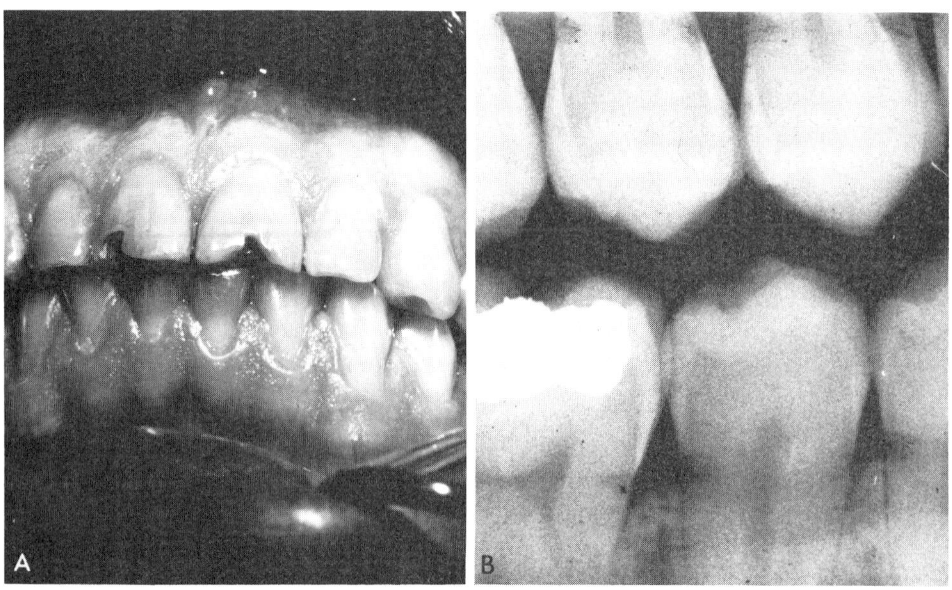

Figure 3–VI–44. *A*. Notching of enamel due to holding nails between teeth. *B*. Radiographic appearance of abrasion of bicuspids.

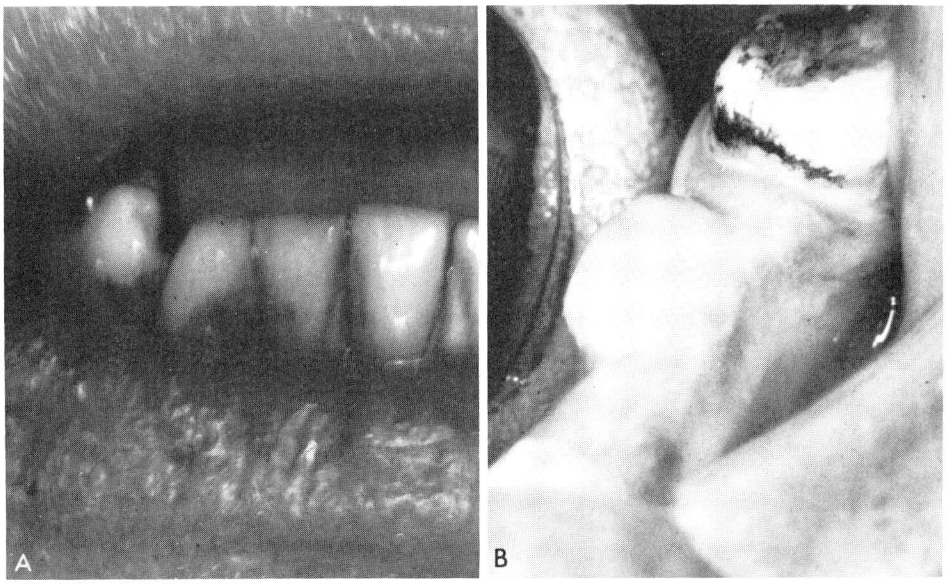

Figure 3–VI–45. *A.* Clinical appearance of a traumatic granuloma of the lip. *B.* Clinical appearance of a traumatic neuroma.

tissues are torn apart leaving irregular margins. This injury is also frequently caused by a sharp object, and infection is a frequent occurrence in this entity.

Abrasion is characterized by a raw, slowly bleeding surface that is denuded of skin. This is frequently caused by an object with a rough surface, and infection is common.

Contusion refers to a bruise resulting from crushed tissue and is frequently caused by a blunt object.

Pathosis of Soft Tissue Trauma

Tooth Brush Trauma. A not infrequent occurrence when a hard brush is used vigorously, tooth brush trauma affects the gingivae by causing puncture wounds. Clinically, this often appears as a small area that is red in appearance when not covered by a grayish yellow membrane. The pathologic picture of injury is one in which the epithelium is destroyed and the remaining area is invaded by numerous leukocytes.

Tongue Bites. Frequently associated with falls, these are characterized by an ulceration with a necrotic center and an erythematous border. They usually heal rapidly with good oral hygiene.

Granuloma and Neuroma. *Traumatic granuloma of the lip* clinically appears as a firm swelling of the lower lip (Fig. 3–VI–45*A*). The patient in the case illustrated had had multiple posterior extractions10 days prior to onset.

Histologically, the striated muscle appears infiltrated with lymphocytes, histiocytes, and a few polymorphonuclear leukocytes.

Traumatic neuroma occurs when nerve regeneration is unsuccessfully attempted after severence, and proliferation continues. Clinically, it appears as a firm, movable, nodular swelling that is light pink in color (Fig. 3–VI–45*B*). Microscopically, there is an intermingling of nerve elements and a varying amount of scar tissue.

Traumatic granuloma of the tongue may occur when the patient sustains injury to the area during a fist fight. In the case illustrated, there was localized ulceration and swelling of the tongue of approximately one week's duration (Fig. 3–VI–46*A*). Microscopically, this appears as an ulceration covered by neutrophils, eosinophils, and fibrin.

Pyogenic granuloma occurs as an individual response to minor trauma. Clinically it appears as an elevated reddish purple mass located in the approximate area of injury (Fig. 3–VI–46*B*). Ulceration is frequently associated with this entity. Microscopically, there is the appearance of inflammatory cells, proliferating capillaries, and granulation tissue with fibroblasts. The area gives the impression of marked vascularity.

Cat Scratch Disease. This regional lymphadenopathy is characterized clinically by a pustule arising at the site of contact approximately 10 days after the minor trauma (Fig. 3–VI–47*A*). There is pain in the parotid area. Microscopically, there is a build-up of histiocytes in the lymphoid tissue, and areas of necrosis are also present (Fig. 3–VI–47*B*).

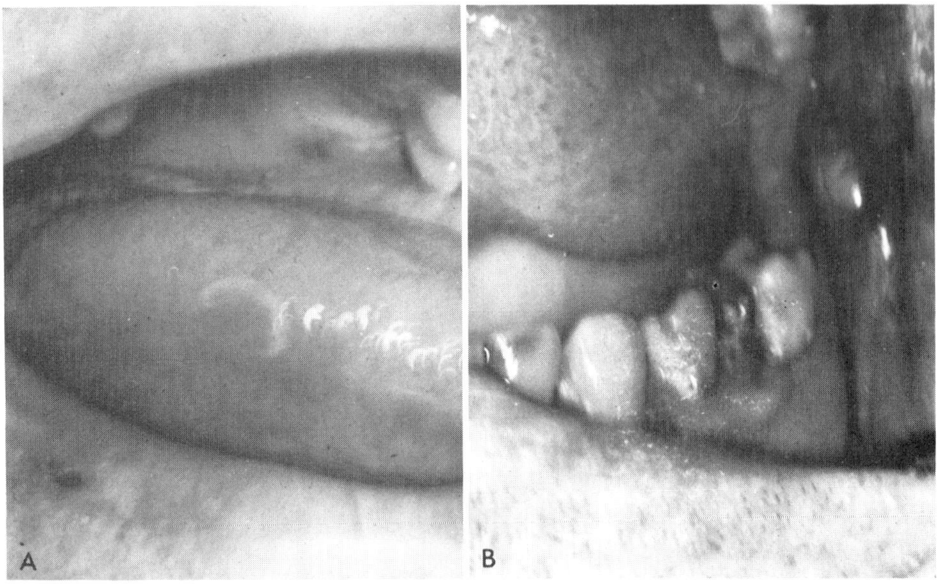

Figure 3–VI–46. *A.* Clinical appearance of a traumatic granuloma of the tongue. *B.* Clinical appearance of a pyogenic granuloma.

Nerve Injury. *Facial numbness* and *paralysis* are not infrequent findings that are associated with trauma to the seventh cranial nerve.

Frequently this injury is manifested clinically by unilateral paralysis of facial muscles. It has been observed that this entity occurs more frequently in middle-aged women than any other segment of our population. The duration of the numbness or paralysis depends upon the extent and location of the injury.

It has been noted that the inferior alveolar nerve regenerates in a relatively short time following surgery of the mandible or severance from a displaced fracture if the severed ends are in proximity to each other.[81] Regeneration of a severed mental nerve at the mental foramen area, however, is rare. This is believed to be because lip and cheek movement makes the approximation of the severed ends difficult.

Gunshot Wounds. Gunshot wounds of the mouth are infrequently seen. When they do occur, however, they are usually due to hunting accidents or are self-inflicted through accidental discharge. They are usually associated with low-velocity firearms.

Some of these shots remain dormant in the oral soft tissue for years. Others, however, instigate the typical inflammatory reaction to a foreign body.

The main problem arises in the actual loca-

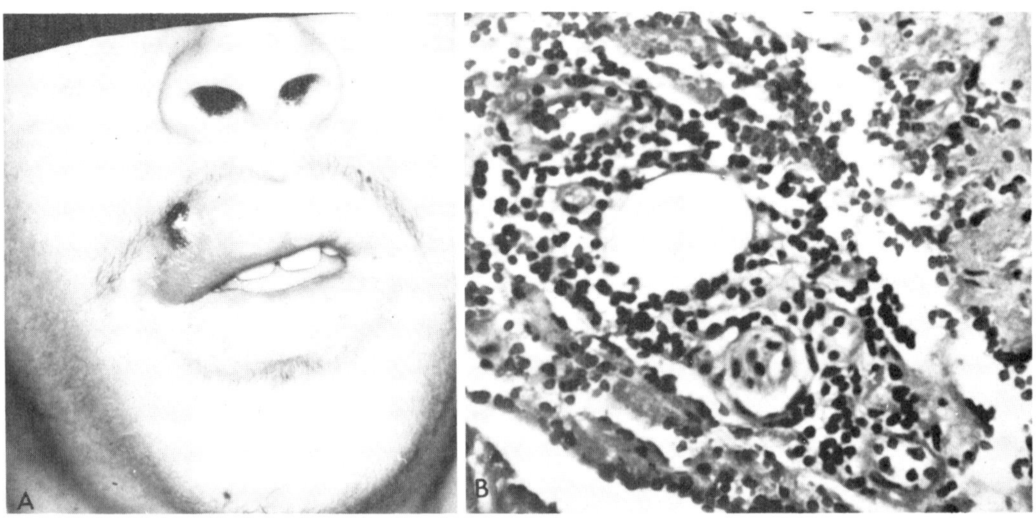

Figure 3–VI–47. Cat scratch disease. *A.* Clinical appearance. *B.* Microscopic appearance.

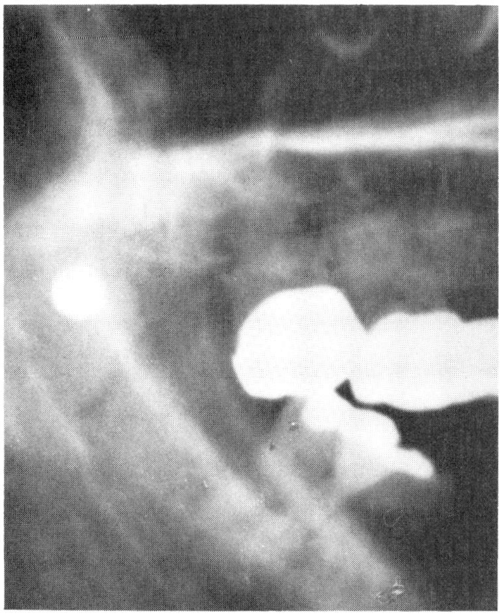

Figure 3–VI–48. Radiographic appearance of a BB shot in the cheek.

tion of these foreign bodies (Fig. 3–VI–48). Their removal is usually uneventful.

Chronic Mechanical Trauma to Dental Soft Tissues

Frequently, the extrinsic factors associated with this entity are oral hygiene devices. The sequelae of their misuse are briefly mentioned since they could possibly be mistaken for pathosis of a more serious nature.

Gingival Recession. Gingival recession due to tooth brushing is frequently associated with faulty use of a new or hard toothbrush over a relatively long period of time.

Clinically, the gingiva has moved away from the necks of the teeth, and the cementum of the root is exposed. Gingival clefts are also a frequent finding in this condition. There is atrophy and sloughing of the epithelium along the cementum owing to the trauma, and cleft formation occurs when this pattern becomes uneven.

Cleft Formation. Clefts caused by the overzealous use of dental floss are more frequently found at present because of current emphasis on preventive dentistry.

Clinically, this entity appears as a groove between the teeth that is caused by the trauma due to the faulty use of the floss (Fig. 3–VI–49). Pathologically, there is gingival inflammation, and the papillary projections have grown down into the subepithelium and anastomosed, thereby causing isolated sloughing of the tissue.

Gingivitis. Gingivitis caused by a broken toothpick appears clinically as localized redness and swelling between two teeth. This is the result of exudation and congestion from the area's reaction to the foreign body.

Microscopically, there are inflammatory cells that are predominantly lymphocytes and plasma cells.

INTRINSIC FACTORS IN ORAL TRAUMA

Acute Mechanical Trauma to Dental Hard Tissues

Most of the entities discussed in this section possibly have only minor forensic implications. They are important, however, because one could be misled in the interpretation of these findings.

Root fracture may be predisposed by *external* or *internal resorption*, as previously mentioned.[23, 29, 53, 93-95]

Chronic Mechanical Trauma to Dental Hard Tissues

Periodontal disturbances, hypersensitivity, tooth fracture, or all three may be associated with traumatic occlusion.[29, 53, 70, 93-95]

Other factors in this category would be *bruxism* and *tongue thrusting*.

Acute Mechanical Trauma to Dental Soft Tissues

It is observed that trauma from "foodstuffs" during the process of mastication is predomi-

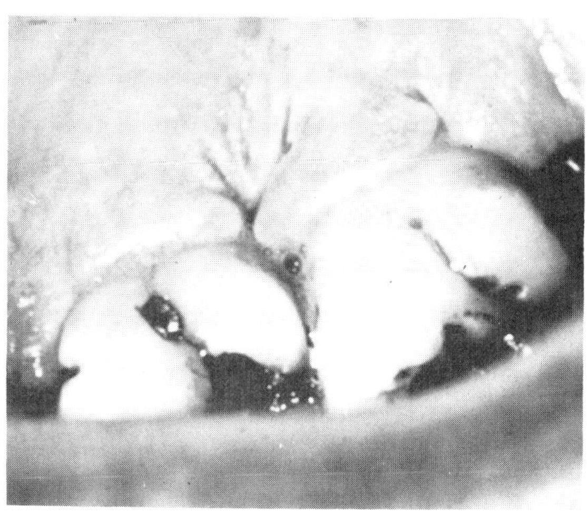

Figure 3–VI–49. Clinical appearance of cleft formation. (Courtesy of J. R. O'Neil, D.D.S., U. S. Public Health Service.)

nant in this category. Frequent food culprits are fish bones, shellfish, popcorn, nuts, and hard bakery products.

Accidents are another cause of this entity, e.g., tongue biting is frequently associated with falls.

Chronic Mechanical Trauma to Dental Soft Tissues

The most common finding in this category is tissue injury through *calculus build-up.*

Cheek biting due to malpositioned teeth or bad habits or iatrogenic in nature is not an infrequent finding.

Pericoronitis is found frequently during tooth eruption and is most especially noted in the third-molar areas.[29, 81, 94]

Chronic trauma to the tongue often occurs in cases in which there is a crown or restoration fracture or a rough prosthetic appliance.

Mucocele. A mucocele is a freely movable cyst that is filled with fluid and occurs in areas where salivary glands are present. Mucoceles constitute 2.8 per cent of oral biopsies.[28]

The lesion appears clinically as a bluish colored ovoid enlargement (Fig. 3–VI–50*A*). This entity is related to an injury that results in the rupture of the salivary duct, causing an accumulation of saliva in the area.

Microscopically, it appears as a cyst lined with thin epithelium and filled with mucus and fibrin.

Papilloma. A papilloma is a benign epithelial lesion that appears clinically as a soft, white cauliflower-like growth above the surface epithelium (Fig. 3–VI–50*B*). These neoplasms account for approximately 2 per cent of oral biopsies.[28]

Microscopically, sections demonstrate a plantlike appearance, with a narrow stalk and projections that are covered by stratified squamous epithelium.

Irritation Fibroma. A localized elevation where hypertrophy and hyperplasia of fibrous connective tissue proliferate in response to continuous mild trauma. Clinically, it appears normal in color, and it may occur anywhere in the oral cavity (Fig. 3–VI–51*A*). This entity constitutes approximately 7.5 per cent of all oral biopsies.[28] Microscopically, there is the appearance of generalized fibrous hyperplasia, and frequently there is some evidence of calcification.

Pregnancy Tumors. These are benign gingival enlargements that are localized between teeth and are a response to mild trauma and poor oral hygiene.[95] They are believed to occur in approximately 25 per cent of pregnancies. Clinically, they often appear as large red proliferations that are soft and bleed on slightest stimulation (Fig. 3–VI–51*B*).

Microscopically, there is an appearance similar to that of a pyogenic granuloma with the outgrowth of granulation tissue characterized by a large amount of endothelial proliferation. There is young connective tissue and many vascular spaces near the surface.

Hyperkeratosis. In this condition the horny cells of the stratum corneum either fail to be desquamated or are so rapidly produced

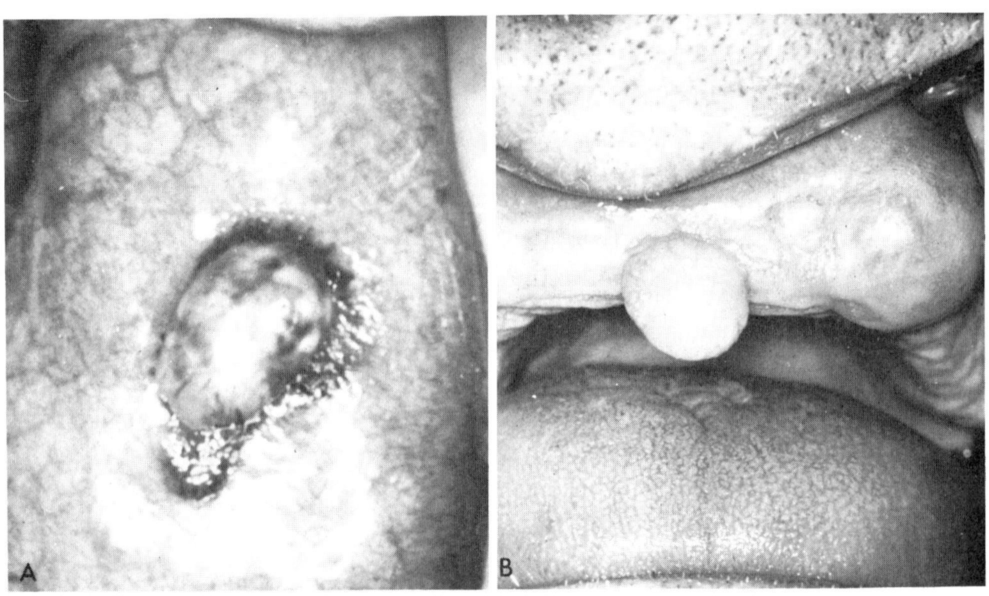

Figure 3–VI–50. *A*. Clinical appearance of a mucocele. *B*. Papilloma and cyst of the maxilla.

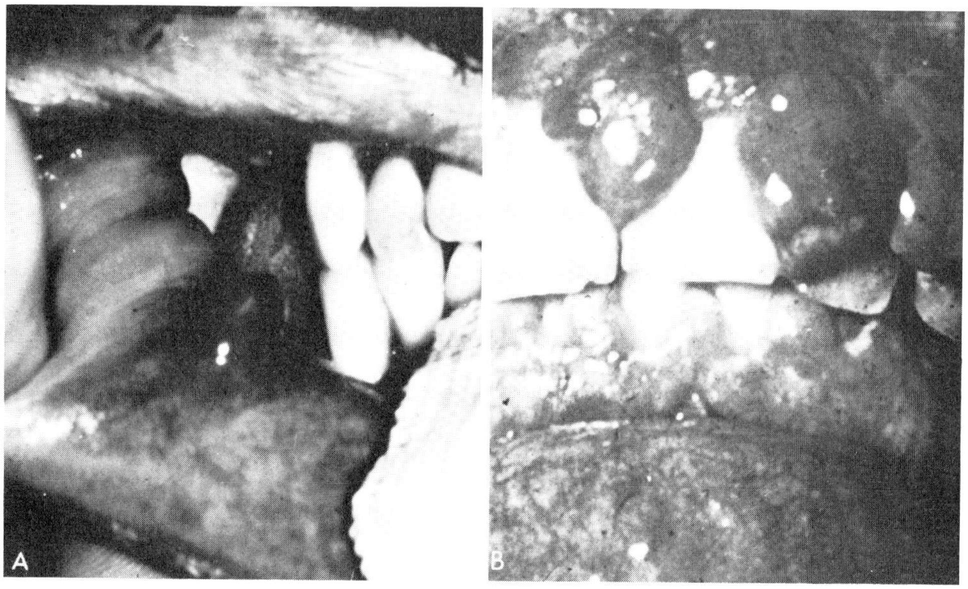

Figure 3–VI–51. *A*. Clinical appearance of an irritation fibroma. *B*. Clinical appearance of a pregnancy tumor.

that the cornified layer is thickened. This benign entity constitutes approximately 71 per cent of all white oral lesions and about 7.5 per cent of all lesions examined by biopsy.[28] Clinically, this lesion appears white and irregular (Fig. 3–VI–52*A*). It may be either flat or elevated, rough or smooth, depending on the amount of thickening of keratin.

Microscopically, there is a thickening of the keratin layer from cells that are devoid of nuclear detail. The underlying epithelium appears normal.

Leukoplakia. Leukoplakia is a precancerous condition in which there are hyperkeratotic changes in the oral epithelium, frequently as a response to chronic irritation. This entity makes up approximately 13 per cent of all white oral lesions and about 1 per cent of all dental lesions for which biopsy is performed.[28]

It has been noted that rough teeth with jagged edges are frequently the etiologic agent in this entity.[98, 99]

Clinically, the lesion appears as a white patch similar to hyperkeratosis (Fig. 3–VI–52*B*).

Microscopically, there is also a similar appearance except that in leukoplakia there is

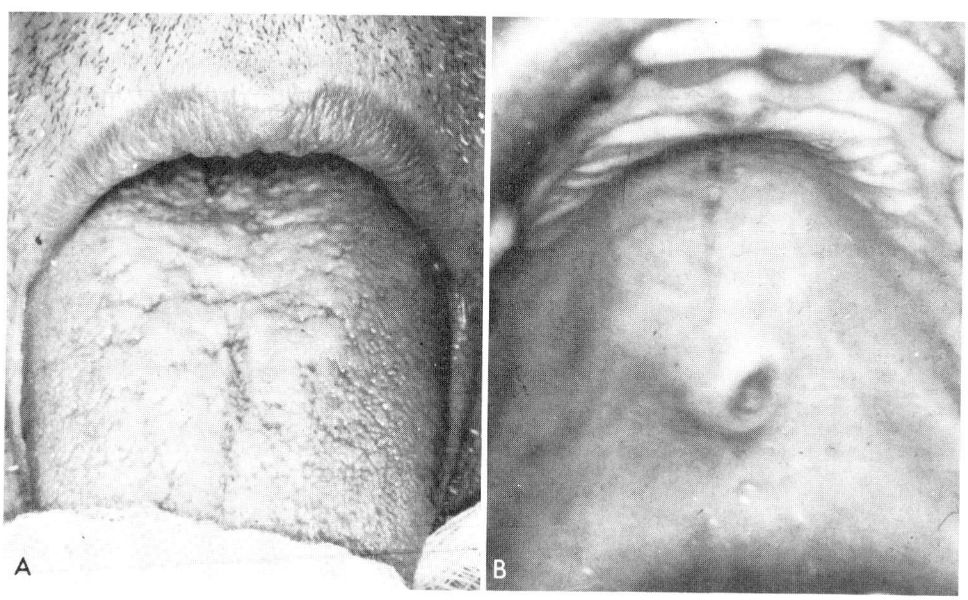

Figure 3–VI–52. *A*. Clinical appearance of hyperkeratosis of the tongue. *B*. Clinical appearance of leukoplakia of the palate.

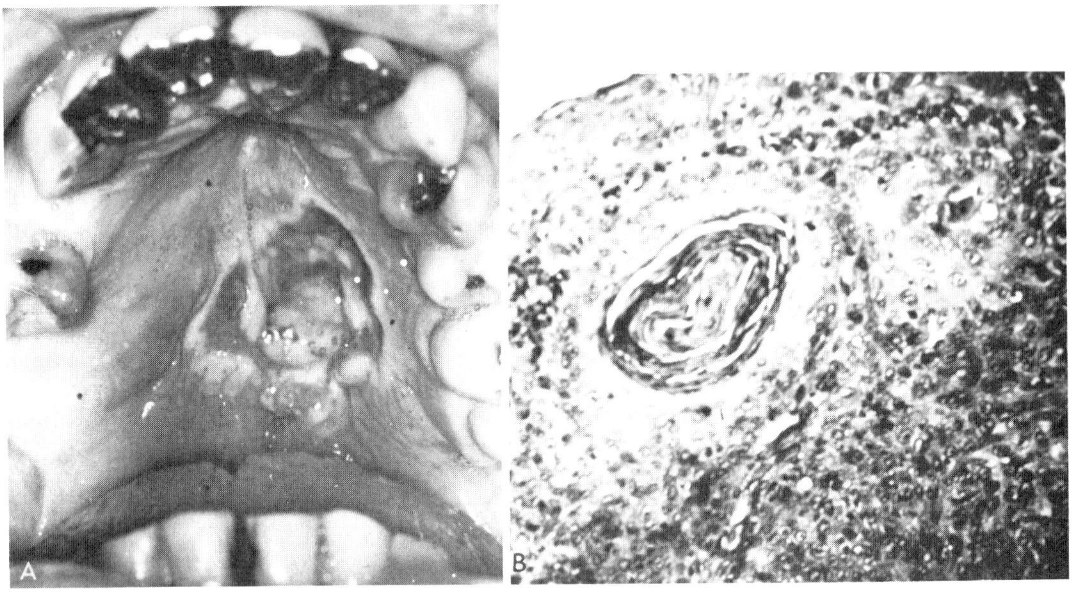

Figure 3–VI–53. *A*. Clinical appearance of epidermoid carcinoma of palate. *B*. Microscopic appearance of epidermoid carcinoma.

dyskeratosis (the presence of abnormal keratinocytes) demonstrated in the cells of the epithelium.

Epidermoid Carcinoma. This entity comprises basal cell, squamous cell, and transitional cell carcinomas and the like.[95] Of these, squamous cell carcinoma represents approximately 90 per cent of all oral malignant tumors and frequently shows evidence of ulceration located in traumatized areas.[95] Clinically, the diseased area appears white with a raised border around a depressed center with marked induration of the surrounding tissue (Fig. 3–VI–53*A*).

Microscopically, there are large, disorganized cancerous cells that vary greatly in appearance from their original form and structure (Fig. 3–VI–53*B*).

IATROGENIC FACTORS IN ORAL TRAUMA

Mechanical Trauma to Dental Hard Tissues

Iatrogenic dental injury is a disturbance of oral structure or function or both that is a result of the action, nonaction, or statements of a dentist. Some of the more common causes are faulty technique, misinterpretation leading to misdiagnosis, unnecessary therapy, failure to "follow up" treatment, and the adverse effect of drugs.

The most frequent finding in an iatrogenic dental condition is the *faulty restoration*, whether it has an opened contact, an overhanging margin, poor contour, malocclusion, or the like. Clinically, many of these defects are recognized because of food impactions. Radiographically, the results of opened contact and overhang demonstrate bone loss and proximal tooth decay due to the trauma of continuous food impaction (Fig. 3–VI–54*A*).

Trauma from Preparation

It is believed that the greatest single cause of pulpal damage is the *heat generated* by grinding procedures in tooth preparation. This damage is manifested by inflammation that is followed by reversible or irreparable changes.[100–102]

It has been noted that the use of air-water coolant is more important when high-speed instruments are used, and that the human pulp is traumatized less at speeds of 50,000 rpm and above with such coolant, than when 6,000 and 20,000 rpm were utilized with an inadequate coolant.[103]

Trauma from Insertion

Malleting Trauma. Pulpal irritation due to malleting trauma is not an infrequent finding during gold foil insertion. This, as well as crown fracture due to the placement or removal of a gold inlay, has also been observed. It has been noted that the pulp is much more irritated from foil insertion than from the placement of other dental filling materials.[104]

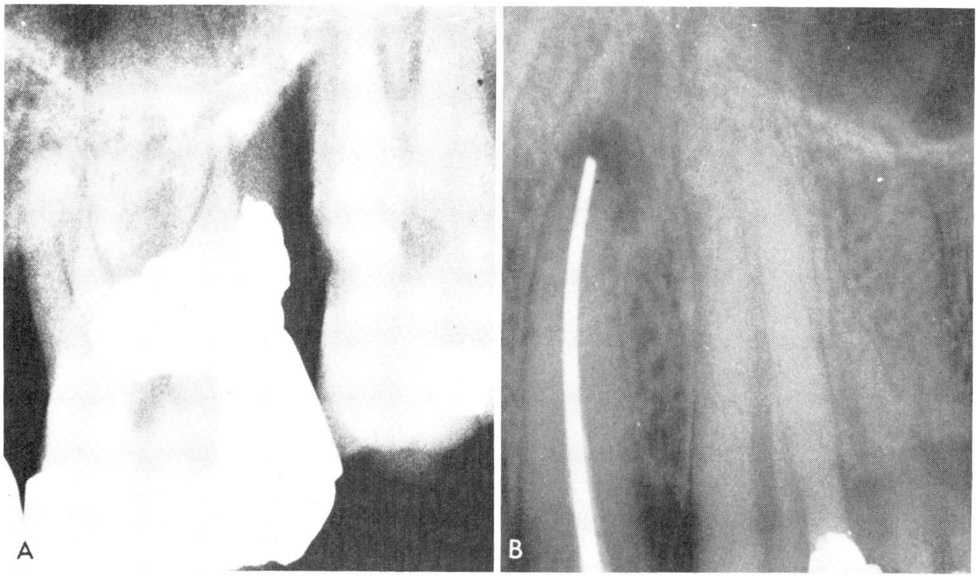

Figure 3–VI–54. *A.* Radiographic appearance of bone loss and tooth decay associated with a faulty restoration. *B.* Radiographic appearance of an overfilled root canal.

Root Canal Filling. Inflammation of the alveolar bone and, in many instances, resorption are found in cases in which there is trauma from a grossly overfilled root canal (Fig. 3–VI–54*B*). The author has noted that the association of intraoral implants with pathosis is not infrequent. This is an example of the human body's rejection of foreign material (Fig. 3–VI–55*A* and *B*).

Prostheses. A frequent finding is root resorption and pathosis from the insertion of an ill-designed prosthetic appliance. In cases of this nature, the supporting roots and alveolar bone are inadequate to withstand the traumatic forces of mastication (Fig. 3–VI–56*A* and *B*).

Orthodontic Appliances. *Root resorption* associated with *tooth movement* from the insertion of orthodontic appliances is not infrequent (Fig. 3–VI–57*A*).[53, 65, 82, 93, 94, 107] A review of the literature concerning the large amount of research on tooth movement reveals considerable controversy about root resorption. Certain writers have described varying degrees of root resorption regardless of the type of appliance, length of treatment, and force intensity utilized.[108-110] It has been reported that root resorption

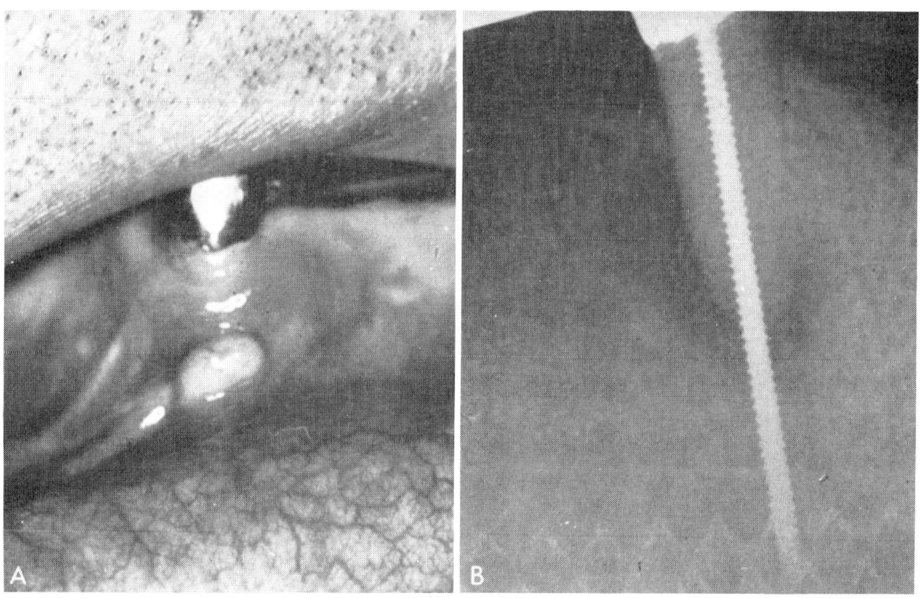

Figure 3–VI–55. *A.* Clinical appearance of the reaction to a foreign body in an endosseous implant. *B.* Radiographic appearance of the reaction to the endosseous implant.

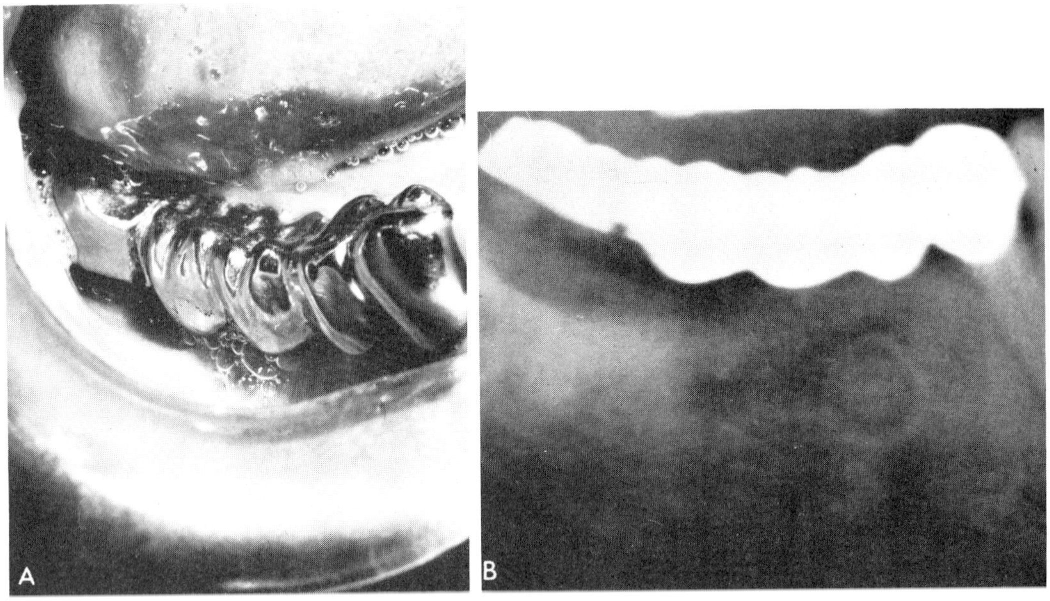

Figure 3–VI–56. *A.* Clinical appearance of an ill-designed bridge. *B.* Radiographic appearance of root resorption and bone loss in the third-molar area. Note the residual cyst in the bicuspid area.

occurs in at least 12 per cent of all patients undergoing treatment by competent orthodontists.[106] Clinically, these teeth appear normal except for the mobility that is often observed.

The pathosis of this entity is described as compression of the soft tissue of the periodontal membrane, resulting in a reduction of its blood supply.[65] This causes vascular thrombosis and asphyxia in the tissues that leads to necrosis. The necrotic areas between the cementum and bone are obvious.

Enamel decalcification due to orthodontic therapy is not infrequently observed. It may be due to poor construction of the appliance, poor oral hygiene, large carbohydrate intake, loose bands that have become uncemented, and failure of the dentist to make periodic examinations every four to six months.

These situations are likely to initiate the condition, which appears clinically as white lines located in the banded area (Fig. 3–VI–57*B*). These white areas are permanent and are as-

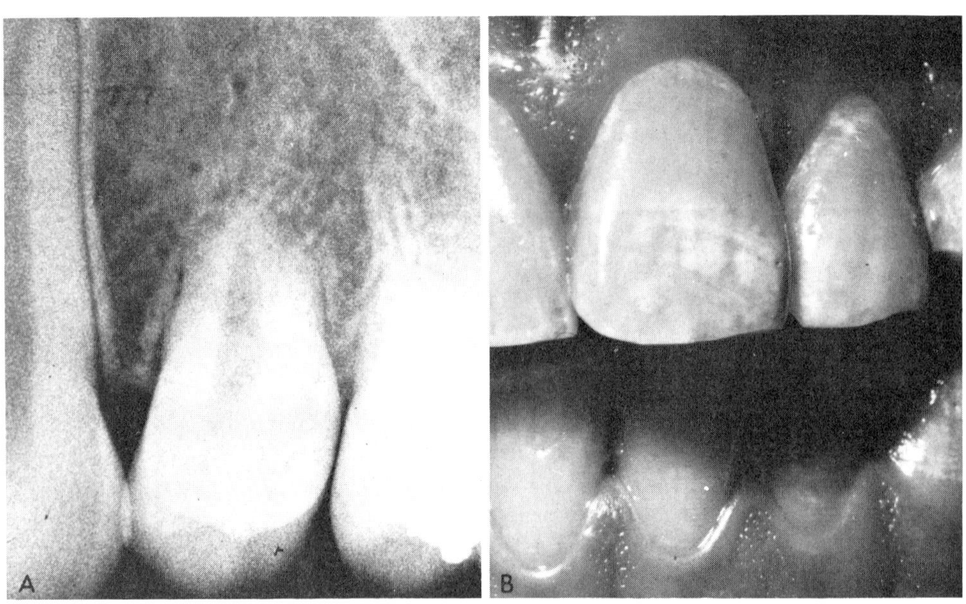

Figure 3–VI–57. *A.* Radiographic appearance of root resorption. *B.* Clinical appearance of enamel decalcification.

sociated with the findings of the early stages of dental caries, which will develop in cases in which there is no interception.

Trauma from Instrumentation

Broken Dental Instruments. These accidents are usually the result of misuse of the instrument or faulty technique of the dentist. Endodontic instruments are probably the ones most frequently broken (Fig. 3–VI–58*A*). Quite often, these cannot be retrieved, and surgical procedures must then be implemented. Oral surgical instruments break less frequently, but when they do, the injury can be quite severe.

Root Fracture. Fracture due to overinstrumentation of a root canal may occur when oversized endodontic instruments are used. This condition also may necessitate oral surgical procedures.

Some of the more common accidents to teeth during dental procedures are fracture of the crown or restoration of the adjacent tooth, bone loss due to overuse of electrosurgery, tooth loss due to the extensive loss of supporting bone from a previous extraction as shown in Figure 3–VI–58*B*, and the extraction of the wrong tooth.[81] This last procedure leads to more lawsuits than any other dental mishap.

Accidental perforation of the maxillary sinus and forcing of the extracted tooth into it is a possibility during the extraction of maxillary teeth (Fig. 3–VI–59*A*). This is basically due to the anatomical features of the area and the close proximity of the sinus to the surgical site. When it occurs, further oral surgical procedures such as the Caldwell-Luc operation must be performed. If not, an antrooral fistula is a likely sequela (Fig. 3–VI–59*B*).

Inexperience. Sometimes trauma to dental hard tissues results from inexperience. This is demonstrated in a case in which a mandibular fracture in a three-and-a-half-year-old boy who fell was treated with K pins by a plastic surgeon. This "treatment" violated the tooth buds and subsequently distorted the occlusion (Fig. 3–VI–60). An extraalveolar reduction of the fracture was indicated.

Unnecessary Procedures. Another cause of iatrogenic dental disease is found in cases in which a thorough treatment plan has not been considered. This situation is demonstrated in the case of the avulsion of a deciduous tooth in a girl of three and a half who fell. The treatment was the placement of *gutta-percha* in the root canal; the tooth was then replanted. Clinical oral manifestations were the results of tissue rejection of this replantation; perhaps a foreign body reaction (Fig. 3–VI–61). The procedure of replanting deciduous teeth is unsound, since failure could involve the permanent tooth bud. Furthermore, a resorbable material should always be used when filling a primary tooth that has a successor.

Mechanical Trauma to Dental Soft Tissues

A *traumatic vesicle* due to a cotton roll is caused by irritation when the dentist inserts

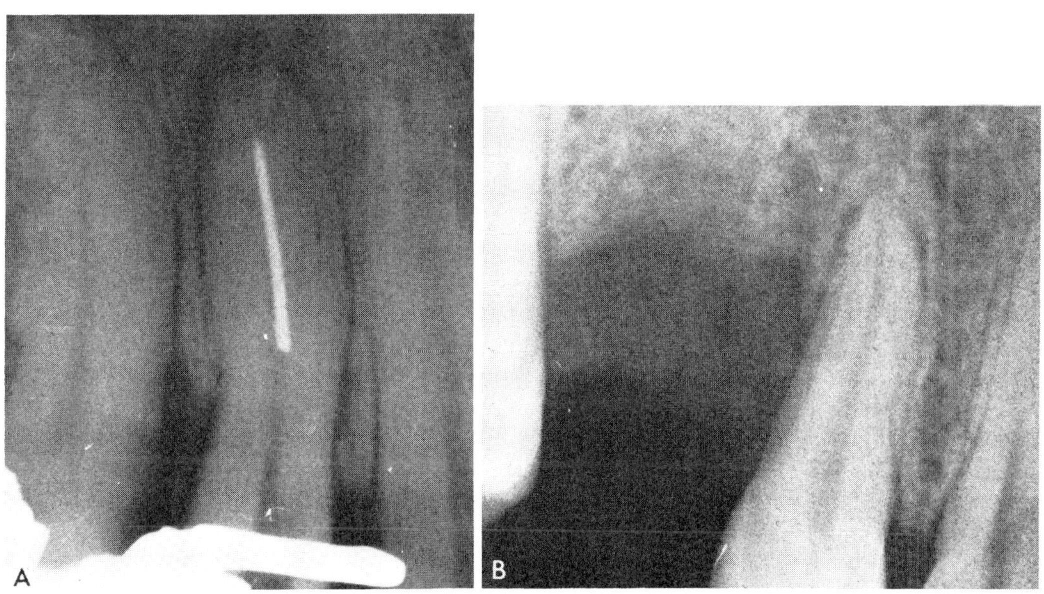

Figure 3–VI–58. *A.* Radiographic appearance of a broken endodontic instrument. *B.* Radiographic appearance in extensive bone loss after prior indicated tooth extraction.

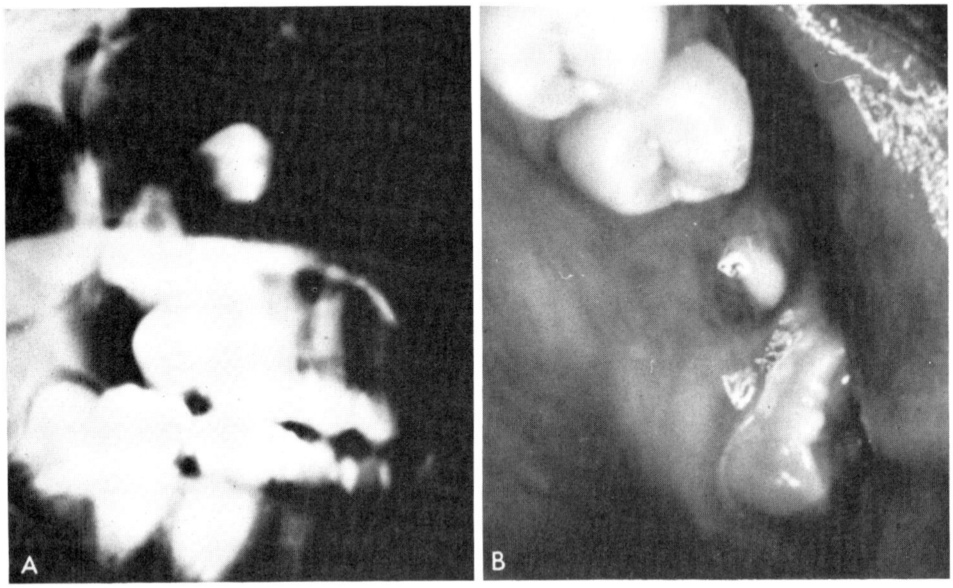

Figure 3–VI–59. *A.* Radiographic appearance of a tooth in the maxillary sinus. *B.* Antrooral fistula.

this material in the mouth in an attempt to create and maintain a dry operative field. Frequently, cotton rolls adhere to the oral mucosa, and the tissue is traumatized when they are changed, causing sloughing and ulceration that may be quite painful. Clinically, areas of white ulceration are surrounded by redness that is indicative of the inflammatory reaction. The healing of these areas is usually uneventful, but secondary infection is of primary concern.

Denture Sores. Acute denture sores are usually due to overextended denture borders. These may vary in size, usually depending upon the amount of overextension. This occurs most frequently after the insertion of new dentures and appears clinically as a white ulcer surrounded by red, inflamed tissue. Microscopically, there is a breakdown of the epithelial layer, exposing inflamed connective tissue.

Primary Herpetic Gingivostomatitis. This is an acute inflammatory condition characterized by small oval vesicles that are elevated and may appear anywhere in the oral cavity. These vesicles are yellowish gray in color, surrounded by red edematous tissue (Fig. 3–VI–62*A*). Clini-

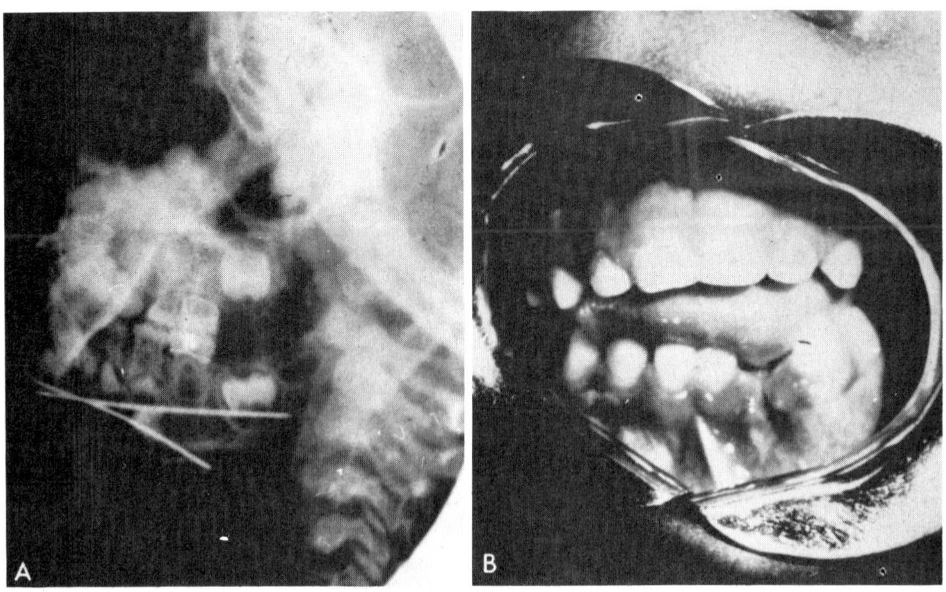

Figure 3–VI–60. *A.* Radiographic appearance of K pins used to treat a mandibular fracture. *B.* The resulting malocclusion. (Courtesy of Richard Resnick, D.M.D.)

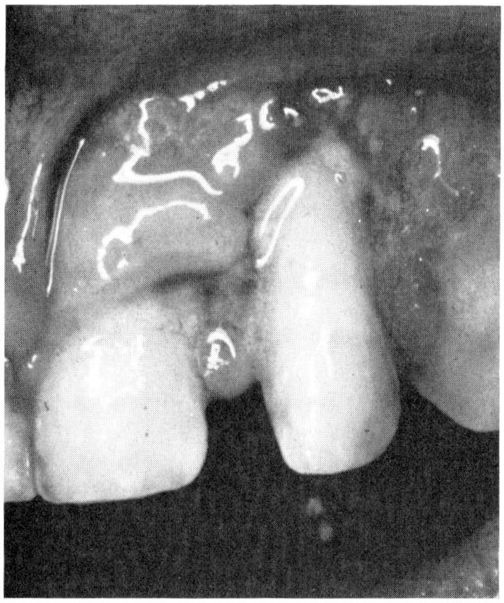

Figure 3–VI–61. Clinical appearance of an unsuccessful replantation. (Courtesy of Melvin N. Oppenheim, D.M.D.)

cally, it is believed to be present in 40 per cent of the population.[28]

The etiology may involve a condition in which an asymptomatic person is infected by herpes simplex virus. The trigger for the onset is, frequently, local injury during dental treatment, which lowers the resistance of the tissues that are then attacked by the preexisting virus.

Microscopically, there is a breakdown of the epithelial cells from the fluid accumulations in the epithelial covering. The subepithelial tissue is edematous and hyperemic.

Ulcerations. Ulcerations may be due to the insertion of new dental appliances. They appear round and superficial and affect the mucous membrane anywhere inside the oral cavity (Fig. 3–VI–62*B*). These ulcerations are caused by the trauma inflicted as the patient constantly rubs this foreign object with the tongue and cheeks. They start as small erythematous areas that are followed by necrosis. Secondary infection is of primary concern in this entity.

Exogenous Deposition of Dental Materials. This occurs frequently and may be misleading to the nondentist. This deposition is usually due to amalgam being incorporated into the tissue when a tooth is fragmented during an extraction. Clinically there appears to be a bluish discoloration on the gingiva and radiographically there are small radiopaque areas (Fig. 3–VI–63*A*).

Microscopically, these metallic particles are scattered in the collagenous fiber tissue, with no apparent inflammatory reaction. The overlying epithelium appears normal.

Occasionally, one will find dental cement deposited in the gingivae (Fig. 3–VI–63*B*). This is the result of faulty technique in cementing crowns. Both these foreign bodies are considered harmless, since the body tolerates amalgam and the dental cement is usually dissolved. When there is an adverse reaction to these foreign bodies, however, it is frequently the condition of epulis granulomatosa.[81]

Emphysema. Emphysema is an infrequent finding during dental treatment; its recognition, however, is important. In this condition

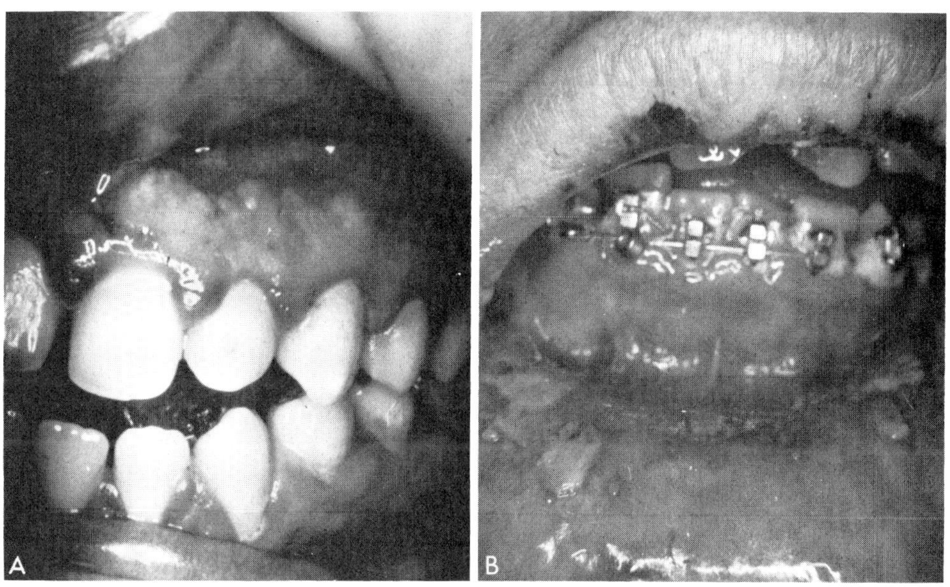

Figure 3–VI–62. *A*. Clinical appearance of primary herpetic gingivostomatitis. *B*. Ulcerations associated with orthodontic appliances. (Courtesy of Neal R. Riesner, D.D.S.)

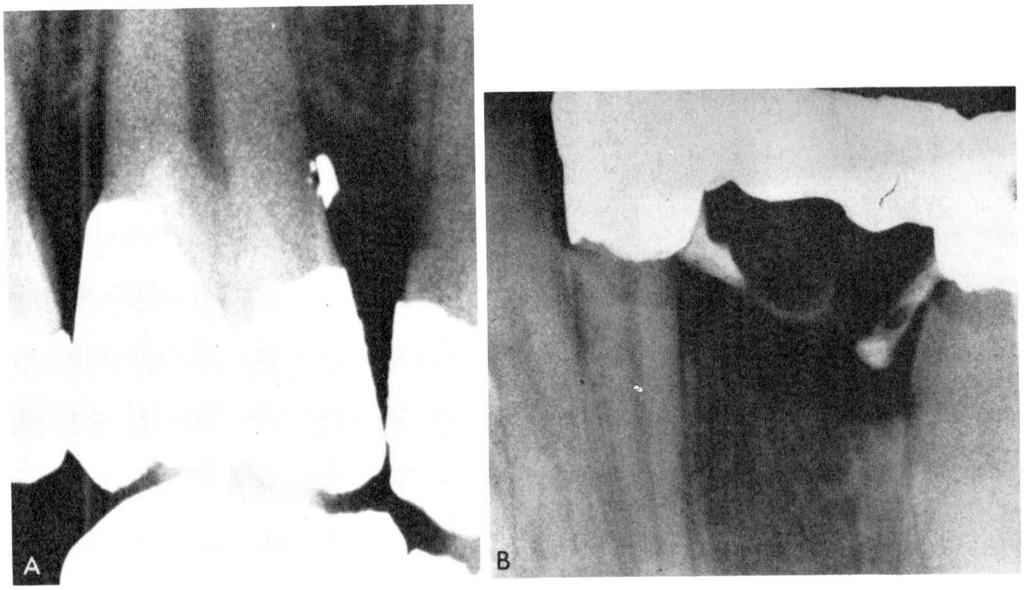

Figure 3–VI–63. *A.* Radiographic appearance of exogenous deposition of amalgam with bone loss in bicuspid area. *B.* Radiographic appearance of exogenous deposition of dental cement.

swelling results from the presence of air in the interstices of the connective tissue. There is crepitation upon palpation of the area.

My own experience with this condition occurred during the removal of a maxillary first molar. There was apparently an opening through the antral mucosa, and air was blown into the sinus through the extraction site and was forced into the facial tissue. Fortunately, this air was reabsorbed in several days with no significant consequences.

Injuries Related to Anesthesia. *Lip and tongue bites* resulting from local anesthesia during dental treatment occur most frequently in the younger age group. Quite often the patient does not understand the numbness and constantly bites the affected area. This condition appears clinically, as a large ulcerated area; when it is superficial, rapid healing is noted (Fig. 3–VI–64*A*). Occasionally, however, the teeth penetrate deeper into the tissue, causing vascular damage followed by thrombosis. Necrosis and secondary infection cause these more extensive bite areas to heal very slowly.

Needle infections are the most common oral manifestation of bacterial sensitization, and it

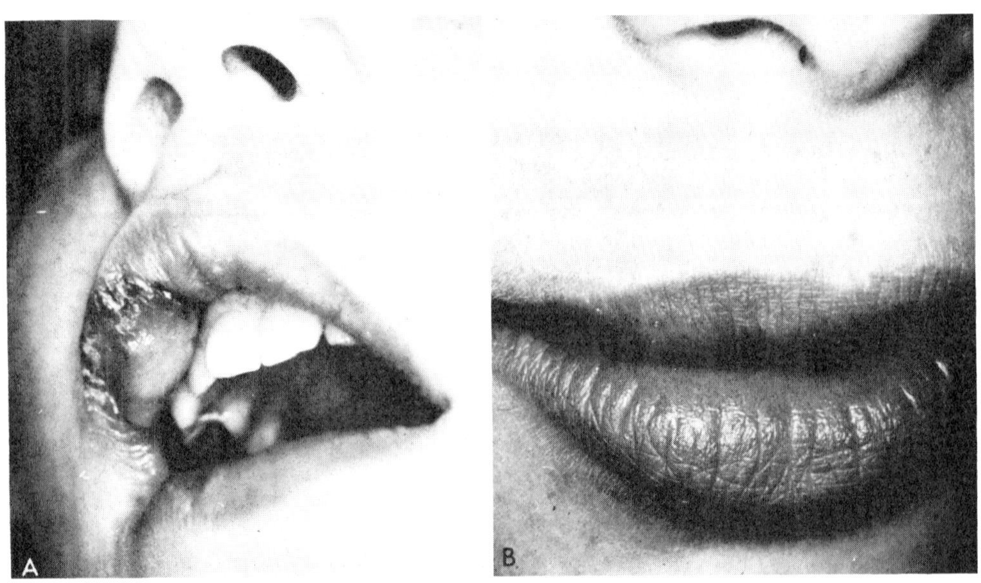

Figure 3–VI–64. *A.* Clinical appearance of a lip bite during local anesthesia (one day after dental treatment). *B.* Clinical appearance of angioneurotic edema.

has been suggested that these might be due to the increased intensity of traumatic inflammation.[95] Clinically, the lesion appears as a light yellow ulceration with regular margins that vary in size. This is surrounded by erythematous tissue that is suggestive of inflammation in the area. The microscopic appearance is one of breakdown of the epithelium with ulceration. There are also numerous inflammatory cells present in the underlying connective tissue.

Injury due to *overinjection* of local anesthetic is not infrequent. Clinically, shallow, irregular ulcers occur at the site of injection after several days. They are caused by the local anesthetic with a vasoconstrictor being forced into the dense connective tissue, which leads to pressure necrosis and ulceration.

Allergies to local anesthetics are also not infrequent. The reaction may appear on first contact with the drug or several days later, or the patient may become sensitized so that future contact may produce a reaction that varies from mild inflammation to necrosis of the area. Clinically, this begins as redness and swelling with vesicle formation that may appear in the oral cavity or on other parts of the body. Microscopically, the inflamed areas appear edematous and hemorrhagic and show eosinophil infiltration.

Angioneurotic Edema. This is a condition characterized by painless swelling that is localized frequently in the area of the upper lip (Fig. 3–VI–64*B*). It may be either familial or nonfamilial. In familial cases there is a recurring edema in the tissues that is frequently triggered by trauma, which instigates the release of histamine causing vasodilation and passage of fluid into the surrounding area.[111] Fatalities have been reported after tooth extractions in persons with this condition.[112]

Broken Instruments. *Broken injection needles* occurred more frequently before the advent of stainless steel. When this takes place, they usually break between the shaft and hub during the manidibular block procedure, usually because of faulty injection technique (Fig. 3–VI–65*A*). Broken needles that are not removed will usually instigate an inflammatory reaction to the foreign body. Deaths due to migration of needles have been reported; therefore their removal is imperative.

Fortunately, oral surgical instruments break less frequently than other more fragile dental tools. When they do break, however, the consequences can be more serious. Figure 3–VI–65*B*) demonstrates the tip of a *broken elevator* left in the socket of the third molar area for nine months. Note the radiolucency, suggestive of pathosis, in the reaction to this foreign body.

Faulty Instrumentation. Trauma resulting from pinching the lip between the handles of forceps and the teeth is occasionally seen and is an example of faulty instrumentation. Most of these conditions are manifested by a *bruised lip* that subsides in several days. In other instances, in response to this type of minor trauma, there may be an overgrowth of granulation tissue, frequently a *pyogenic granuloma*. This accounts for approximately 1.8 per cent of all oral biopsies.[28] (This has been discussed previously as a sequela of soft tissue trauma.)

Unsupervised Orthodontia. Lack of supervi-

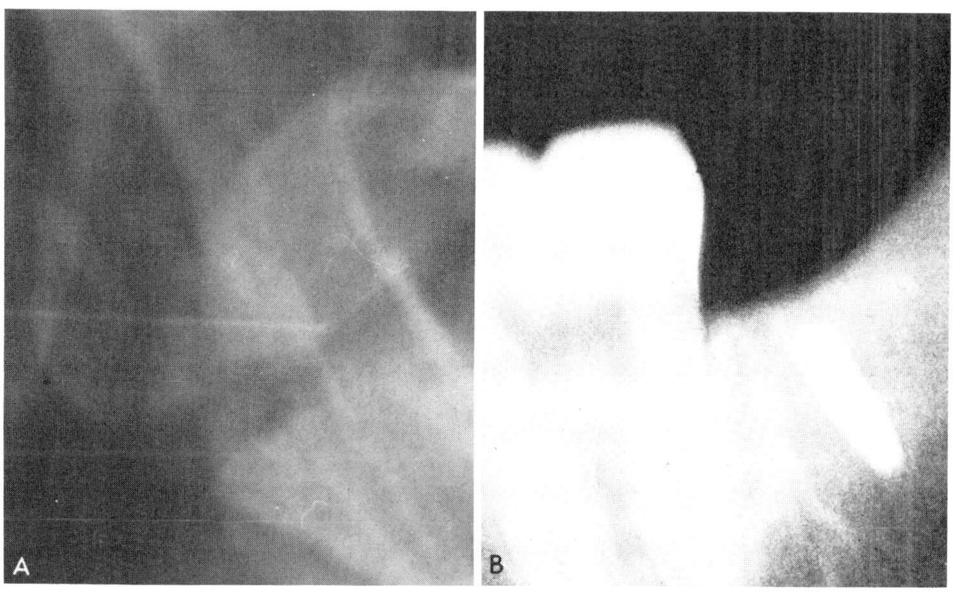

Figure 3–VI–65. *A*. Radiographic appearance of a broken injection needle. *B*. Radiographic appearance of a broken elevator.

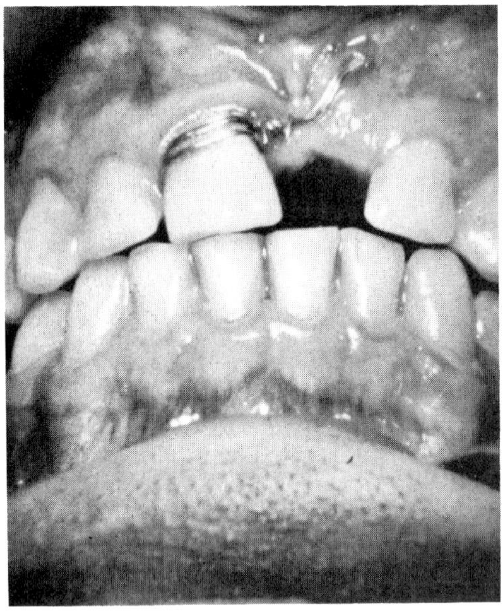

Figure 3–VI–66. Clinical appearance in a case of unsupervised orthodontic treatment.

sion can present serious problems. An example of this is seen in the case of a 19-year-old man who had a wire placed on his maxillary right central incisor and looped up around the left central incisor so that the eruption of the right incisor would pull the left down with it (Fig. 3–VI–66). This wire was placed when the patient was nine years old and had not been seen by a dentist for 10 years. Note the wire around the right incisor and the other end going up into the gingiva. A small fistula with a minute amount of drainage is noted in the entrance area. Figure 3–VI–67*A* shows the right central incisor with wire loop attached; Figure 3–VI–67*B* shows the left central incisor, with the other end of the wire around it, still unerupted.

Because of this lack of supervision the space allowed for the eruption of the left central incisor had closed, making the case a very difficult one to restore satisfactorily.

Sialography. The injection of radiopaque medium in sialography may have serious adverse effects.

Figure 3–VI–68 demonstrates widely diffuse radiopacities in the left parotid salivary gland area. Clinically, there was swelling in the area that was hard, immobile, and warm. The patient had a 102° temperature. He stated that one week previously he had swelling at which time the injection was made and x-rays were taken. The record indicated he had swelling, fever, and slight bleeding of unknown origin in the oral cavity. It further indicated that an iodized oil (Lipiodol) was injected, which apparently was not reabsorbed. Its injection is contraindicated in inflamed areas where bleeding has occurred. Deaths due to cerebral oil embolism, in similar cases, have been reported.[113]

Infection and Inflammation. *Actinomycosis* is a deep fungus infection that is characterized by granulomatous lesions that ultimately become suppurative. Cervicofacial actinomycosis, the most common form (approximately 50 per cent of all cases), involves the jaw and upper neck and is supposedly due to local trauma such as tooth extraction or jaw fracture.[28] Clinically, nodules form, slowly enlarge, break down, and drain a yellowish pus.

Microscopically, there is granulation tissue and focal abscess formation that is surrounded by numerous polymorphonuclear leukocytes.

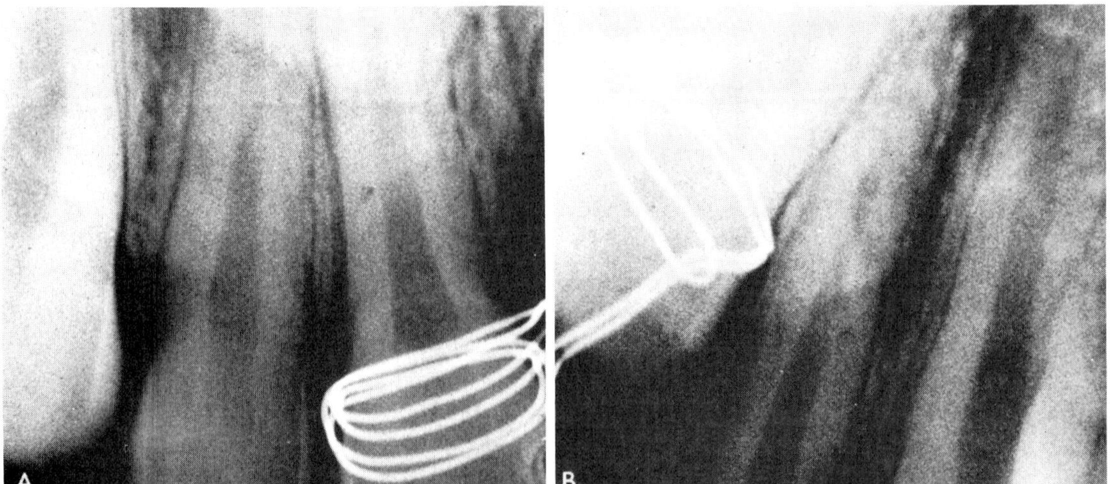

Figure 3–VI–67. Radiographic appearance in a case of unsupervised orthodontic treatment. *A*. Right central incisor. *B*. Left central incisor. (Courtesy of G. P. Barnes, D.D.S., U. S. Army Institute of Dental Research.)

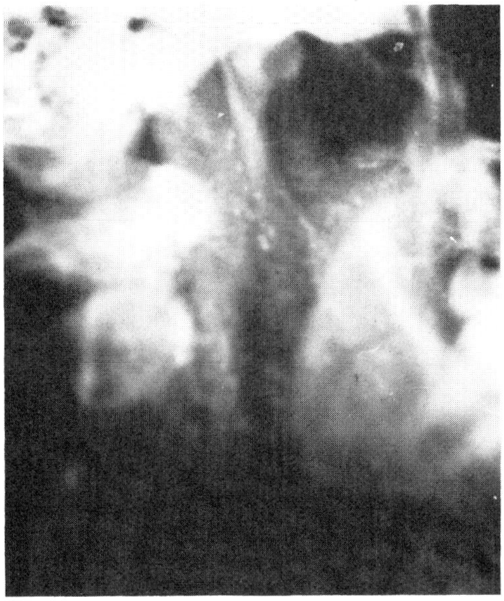

Figure 3–VI–68. Radiographic appearance one week after injection of radiopaque medium in sialography.

These polymorphs plus fungus granules help to make the suppurative exudate.

Chronic inflammatory papillary hyperplasia is a condition in which hyperplastic tissue is produced in response to chronic irritation. This condition constitutes approximately 1.5 per cent of all oral lesions.[28] The polyplike tissues appear red and soft and are freely movable (Fig. 3–VI–69*A*). The most frequent cause of this condition is the prolonged wearing of an ill-fitting denture. Microscopically, the section appears hyperplastic and very vascular with numerous inflammatory cells infiltrating. Numerous lymphocytes and plasma cells are present in the subepithelial connective tissues.

Epulis fissuratum is a tumorlike enlargement of soft, flabby, movable tissue that bleeds easily and is frequently associated with wearing ill-fitting dentures. Approximately 2.8 per cent of all oral biopsies are performed because of this condition.[28] Clinically, this entity is most frequently seen in the anterior maxillary region and most especially in patients with natural lower teeth (Fig. 3–VI–69*B*). It appears microscopically as a deep ulcerated crevice with heavy inflammatory cell infiltration in the fibrous connective tissue.

A form of *Ludwig's angina* has been noted in trauma due to ill-fitting lower dentures. Clinically, one patient had a temperature of 101°F and swelling below the mandible that increased to the extent that it made swallowing difficult. Drainage of yellowish-red, thick fluid with an unpleasant odor accompanied this swelling. This condition would have been fatal, owing to airway obstruction, had it not been for proper therapy.

Faulty Construction of Temporary Replacement. Another frequently seen example of iatrogenic dental injury is probably due to the dentist's belief that a replacement will be used for only a short period of time, so no adverse effects should arise. Most of the time, this thinking is correct; however, in our mobile society, it is not always true. This is demonstrated by the placement of a temporary bridge in which the embrasure space, which is imperative for proper oral health, was faulty. The temporary bridge obliterated the embrasure space

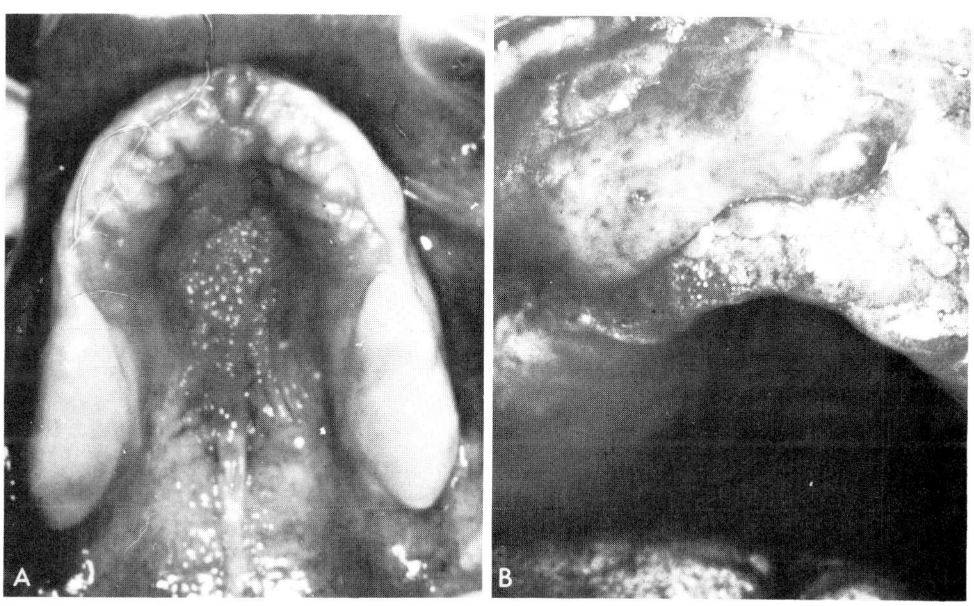

Figure 3–VI–69. *A*. Clinical appearance of chronic inflammatory papillary hyperplasia. *B*. Clinical appearance of epulis fissuratum.

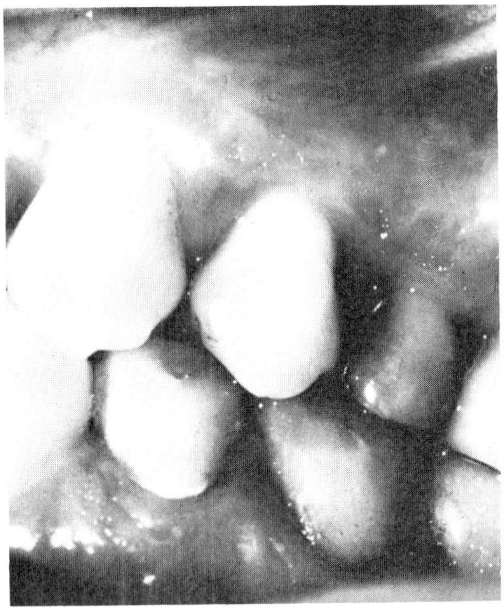

Figure 3–VI–70. Clinical appearance of the results of faulty construction of a temporary bridge. (Courtesy of J. R. O'Neil, D.D.S., U. S. Public Health Service.)

and displaced the papilla laterally in the bicuspid area and compressed the papilla in the first molar area, making it impossible for the patient to cleanse the teeth (Fig. 3–VI–70). This condition could progress to hypertrophy.

Injury was manifested in this case by gingivitis, papillary inflammation, and hemorrhage in proximal gingival areas.[114]

Other conditions that are occasionally associated with iatrogenic dental injury are *epidermoid carcinoma, traumatic neuroma,* and *facial numbness* and *paralysis,* all of which have been discussed previously. *Chemical* and *thermal burns* that could be due to iatrogenic cause are discussed later.

TRAUMA RELATED TO ABNORMAL HABITS

This subject has little forensic significance and is briefly mentioned to introduce the reader to sequelae of trauma that might resemble other entities. Therefore, only the more common conditions and pertinent references are listed. Outstanding discussions of habits are given by Goldman and by Graber.[82, 94] Additional references are:

Nail biting: Colby,[53] Ramfjord[93]
Bruxism: Ingle,[70] Hill,[115] Ramfjord,[93] Colby[53]
Tongue thrusting: Kelsten[116]
Bobby pin biting: Colby,[53] Ramfjord[93]
Eye glass biting: Sorrin[117]
Thumb sucking and biting: Kelsten[116]
Pencil biting: Ramfjord[93]
Chronic lip and cheek biting: Orban,[27] Colby,[53] Ramfjord[93]

MISCELLANEOUS FACTORS CAUSING INJURY OF A MECHANICAL NATURE

Chemical Injury

Soft Tissue Injury

Chemicals, whether ingested for pleasure, in the form of drugs for therapeutic use, or in conjunction with occupations, are associated with oral findings that vary from a minor burn to carcinoma. They are such a part of today's life that a thorough discussion of their possible hazards is appropriate.

Antibiotics. *Black hairy tongue* is an infectious, inflammatory condition that is characterized by an elongation of the filiform papillae that gives them the appearance of hair. This entity is frequently associated with the use of chemotherapeutic agents, usually antibiotics, or overuse of mouthwash.

Its pathogenesis may be that the papillae are invaded by fungi or bacteria or both. These, sustained by various foodstuffs, instigate continued enlargement and create an ideal environment for multiplication of microorganisms.

Moniliasis (thrush) is an infectious, inflammatory condition that is characterized by white patches that resemble curdled cream and may be found anywhere in the oral cavity (Fig. 3–VI–71*A*). It is believed that prolonged use of antibiotics is a predisposing factor. Microscopically, there appears to be abscess formation and necrosis of the epithelium. Fungus growth is noted in the epithelium, which is also infiltrated by leukocytes.

Allergies. *Toothpaste allergies* are infrequent, but when they do appear, it seems that the antigen is often related to oil of anise. Clinical features are redness of the tongue, a burning and stinging sensation, and vesicular lesion formation. The histopathologic aspects have been discussed previously.

Contact allergy is a type of reaction in which a lesion of the skin or mucous membrane occurs at a localized site after repeated contact with the causative agent.[118] In the case illustrated, a routine examination revealed a gingival color ranging from white to a pale pink (Fig. 3–VI–71*B*).[119, 120] The patient was asymptomatic. The cause of this condition was the overuse of mouthwash (used four times a day, held in the mouth for 15 minutes each time). When the cause was removed (the patient discontinued

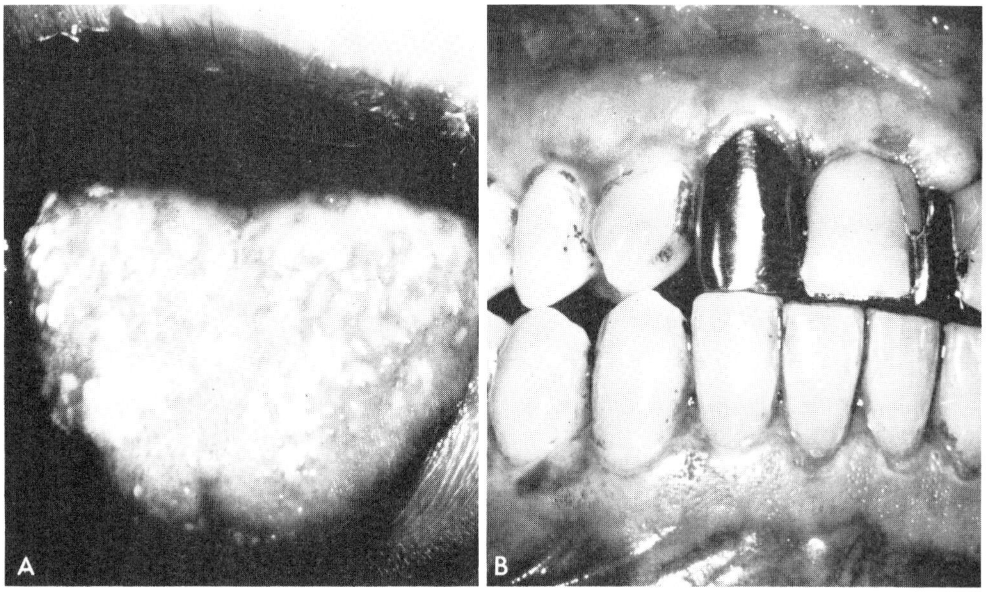

Figure 3–VI–71. *A.* Clinical appearance of moniliasis. *B.* Clinical appearance of contact dermatitis. (Courtesy of J. R. O'Neil, D.D.S., U. S. Public Health Service.)

the mouthwash), the gingival color appeared normal in one week.

Dilantin Hyperplasia. Dilantin gingival hyperplasia is an idiopathic condition in which there is gross enlargement of the gingiva associated with continuous intake of Dilantin Sodium for the control of epilepsy. It is observed in 10 to 30 per cent of epileptic patients who receive Dilantin.[28]

Clinically, the highly stippled gingivae have a granular appearance and firm consistency, and slowly begin to cover the teeth (Fig. 3–VI–72*A*). This condition is usually generalized. Microscopically, there are proliferation, increased keratinization, and fibrous hyperplasia of the connective tissue (Fig. 3–VI–72*B*).

Caustic Substances. *Aspirin burn* through self-medication or misunderstanding of professional advice is one of the most common chemical burns observed in the oral cavity. Clinically, this appears as an irregular white patch that is usually superficial (Fig. 3–VI–73*A*). It occurs most frequently in the mucobuccal fold where the patient holds it in the area while attempting to obtain relief from a toothache. Microscopically, there is a peeling off of the surface

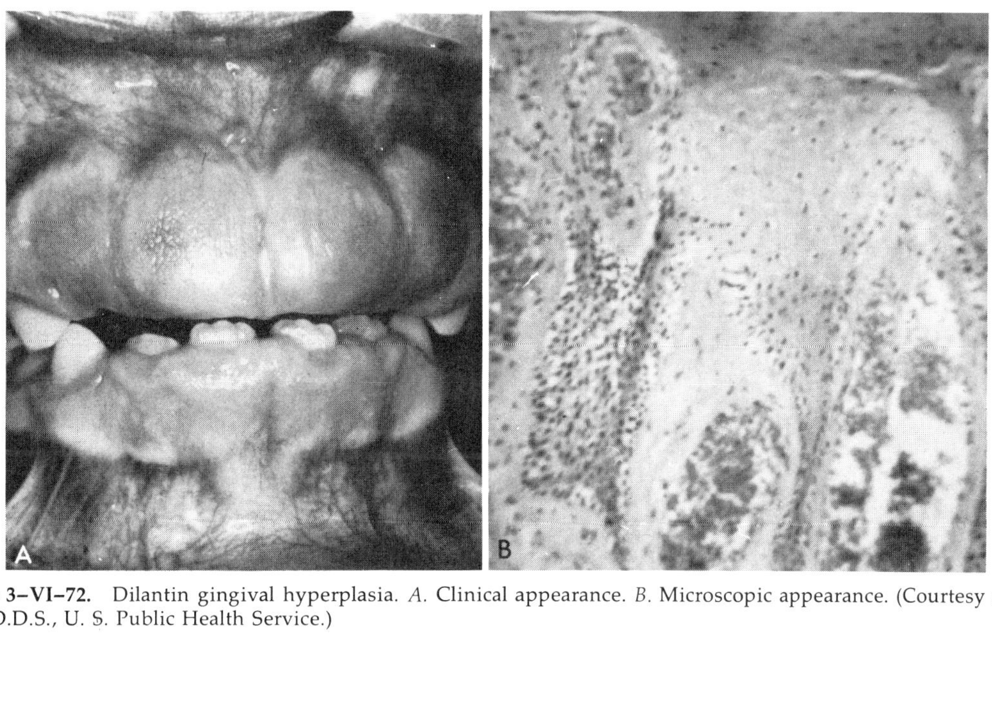

Figure 3–VI–72. Dilantin gingival hyperplasia. *A.* Clinical appearance. *B.* Microscopic appearance. (Courtesy of W. O. Engler, D.D.S., U. S. Public Health Service.)

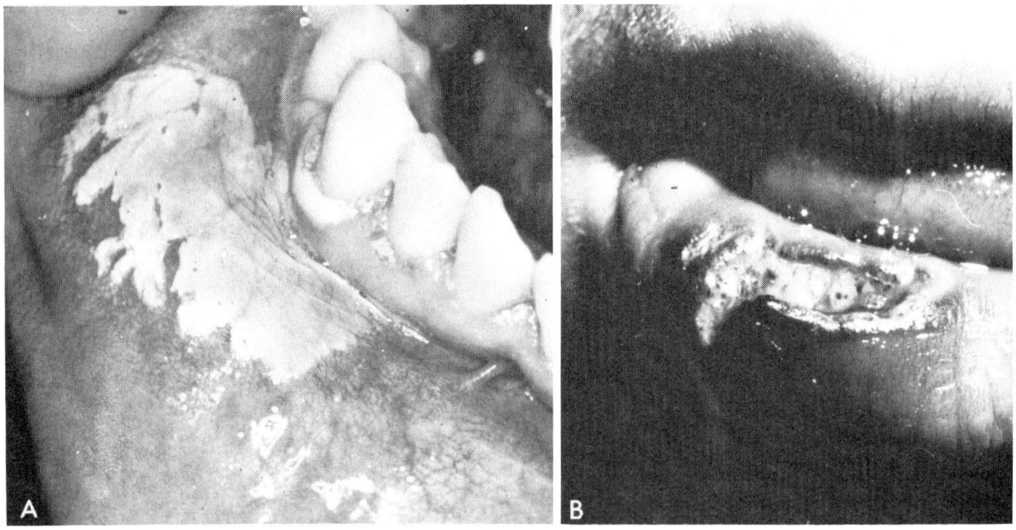

Figure 3–VI–73. *A.* Clinical appearance of an aspirin burn. *B.* Clinical appearance of a lip laceration to which silver nitrate had been applied.

layer owing to epithelial destruction, an infiltration of numerous leukocytes in the affected area, and areas of necrosis.

Silver nitrate is a very caustic chemical preparation and is capable of producing deep severe burns in certain conditions. Figure 3–VI–73*B* shows laceration of the lower lip in a three-year-old who was injured in a fall. Several applications of silver nitrate were made by the father, a paramedic, in order to stop the bleeding. There was deep ulceration with extensive sloughing in the area. Clinically, the healing process took 23 days and resulted in scarring.

Phenol is another caustic preparation that is used in dental treatment, and burns due to its accidental application are not an infrequent observation. Occasionally, a cotton pellet saturated with phenol is accidentally dropped to the floor of the mouth, causing a superficial, irregular whitish area at the place of contact (Fig. 3–VI–74). An inflammatory reaction with edema and hyperemia is the body's usual response to this caustic agent. The histopathologic characteristics are similar to those of aspirin burns.

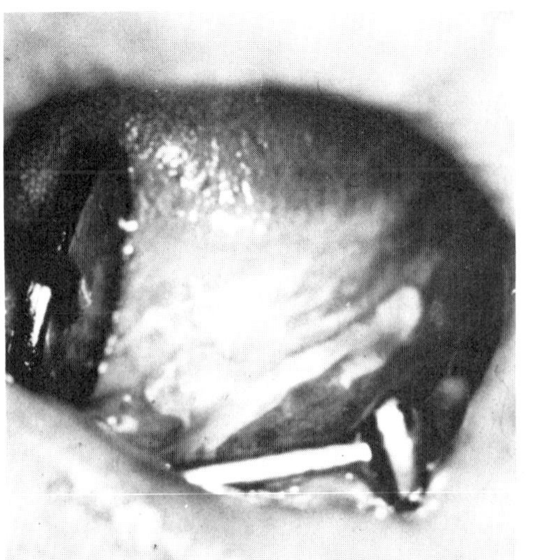

Figure 3–VI–74. Clinical appearance of a phenol burn.

Other widely used chemical preparations that have been noted to cause oral burns are Pyrozone, sodium perborate, zinc chloride, commercial toothache drops, and Superoxol.[53, 70] Both the clinical and histopathologic features are similar for all these caustic agents.

Chemicals used in numerous occupations create environmental hazards and are noteworthy. The possible oral manifestations range from a "dry mouth" to osteomyelitis and necrosis.[29] Some of the more common oral findings are gingivitis and the metallic line observed at the edge of the gums.

Chronic mercury poisoning has been observed in photographic workers and in persons working around mercury products. This entity is caused by the inhalation of mercury vapor or through skin absorption. The oral manifestations are increased salivation and usually a painless red gingivitis (Fig. 3–VI–75*A*). Cases of glossitis in this condition have also been reported in the literature.[28, 29, 95] This entity will develop into Vincent's infection, in which the gingiva is painful, if the condition is allowed to continue.

Histopathologic findings are frequently those of chronic inflammation in the corium. Deposition of the compound is noted around the walls of the distended blood vessels.

It is also interesting to note that in the litera-

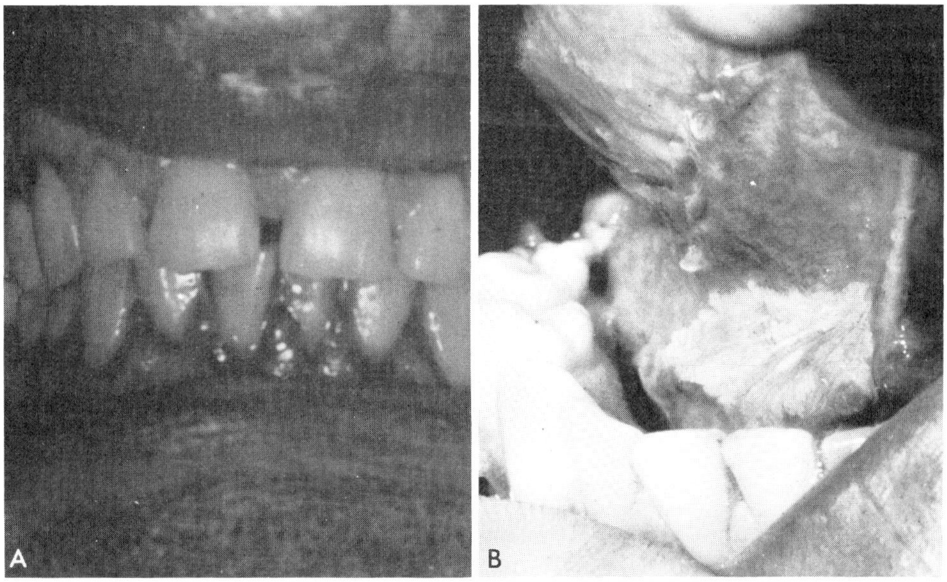

Figure 3–VI–75. *A.* Clinical appearance of gingivitis associated with chronic mercury poisoning. *B.* Clinical appearance of a titanium tetrachloride burn.

ture there are numerous reports of mercury sensitivity when dental amalgam is used as a filling material.[121-124] The clinical and pathologic reactions in this condition are similar to those of an allergy, as previously described.

Certain chemicals used in occupations cause burns by direct contact when introduced into the oral cavity. An example of this is titanium tetrachloride, which is a colorless liquid with a sharp odor that liberates heat and hydrochloric acid upon contact with moisture.

Clinically, the lesion usually appears as a large, irregular light gray area; frequently it is superficial (Fig. 3–VI–75*B*). The severity and appearances, however, depend upon the amount of the chemical and the length of time that the tissues are exposed to it. Therefore, these burns range from a superficial burn of the mucosa to a third-degree burn affecting deep connective tissue. Microscopically, its appearance is similar to the previously described aspirin burn, depending on the severity.

Bismuth Stomatitis. Bismuth stomatitis is characterized by the deposition and accumulation of bismuth sulfides along the marginal gingiva. Clinically, this is manifested by black areas in the gingiva around the necks of the teeth. It is caused by the use of bismuth preparations in the treatment of syphilis or open wounds. Microscopically, there are fine black deposits in the area of the free gingivae. Inflammatory cells are evident in the deeper connective tissue.

Alcohol. Frequently used in an undiluted state, alcohol has been considered by many writers to be one of the etiologic factors in leukoplakia.[29, 95, 115] It is, apparently, a significant factor in oral carcinoma.[125] Another study has shown that persons who consume more than 6 ounces of alcohol per day are 10 times more susceptible to oral cancer than moderate drinkers.[126] Clinically, chronic alcoholism is manifest in the oral cavity as a generalized redness of the soft tissues. Frequently, there are small white ulcerations present, probably owing to the person's low resistance to infection.

Nicotine. Excessive use of nicotine is associated with pathologic changes in dental soft tissues. The most common entities reported are nicotine stomatitis, hyperkeratosis, leukoplakia, and epidermoid carcinoma.

Nicotine stomatitis is a condition in which the orifices of the salivary ducts are inflamed and are very apparent because of the paleness of the surrounding mucosa that accompanies this entity. It constitutes approximately 3.5 per cent of all white lesions of the oral mucous membrane.[28] This condition may be manifested elsewhere in the oral cavity, but the most frequent site by far is the palate. Clinically, the appearance depends upon the stage of the condition. At early onset, the mucosa is covered with numerous small red dots. These later enlarge and become very pale and elevated (Fig. 3–VI–76).

Hyperkeratosis and leukoplakia have been previously discussed, but the writer would like to give a classic example of clinical leukoplakia

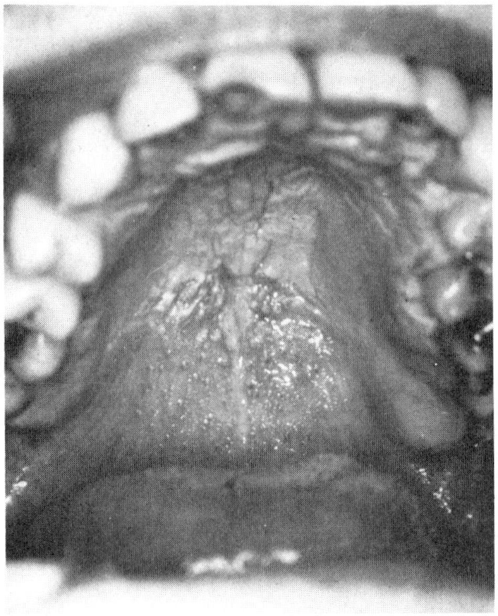

Figure 3–VI–76. Clinical appearance of late nicotine stomatitis of soft palate and clinical leukoplakia on hard palate.

associated with continued use of snuff. The lesion was white and elevated, with irregular borders, was slightly fissured, and was located in the mucobuccal fold in the lower anterior area (Fig. 3–VI–77*A*). The history of this 72-year-old man revealed that this was the area where the snuff had been placed over approximately 20 years after he had been told to stop smoking. A biopsy was performed and leukoplakia was diagnosed.

Numerous writers have noted the association between oral carcinoma and excessive use of nicotine.[28, 53, 81, 127, 128] An excellent example of this relationship is shown in the lesion on the buccal mucosa in the area of the commissure of the lips illustrated in Figure 3–VI–77*B*. Clinically, it appeared grayish white, irregular, rough, and slightly raised; there was a small amount of ulceration. The history revealed that this 48-year-old man had been a heavy smoker for approximately 30 years. He also had the habit of holding cigarettes and pipe in the same area as the lesion. The microscopic appearance was as has already been described under Chronic Mechanical Trauma to Dental Soft Tissues—Epidermoid Carcinoma. Squamous cell carcinoma was diagnosed.

Hard Tissue Injury

Fluorosis. *Mottled enamel* (endemic dental fluorosis) refers to a developmental abnormality that results from the ingestion of toxic amounts of fluoride during the time of tooth calcification. Clinically, the tooth enamel is marked with brown, yellow, and white areas (Fig. 3–VI–78*A*). This entity is geographic in nature and the etiologic factor is practically always excess fluoride in drinking water.

It has been noted that when the fluoride content of drinking water is 6 to 8 parts per million, nearly 100 per cent of the population reflects this condition.[115] The areas where it is most commonly found are Colorado and Northwest Texas, Arkansas, Arizona, California, Idaho, Illinois, Minnesota, New Mexico, North Dakota, South Dakota, Iowa, Virginia, Kansas, Nevada, North Carolina, Oregon, Washington, Bahama Islands, Barbados, Island of Brava,

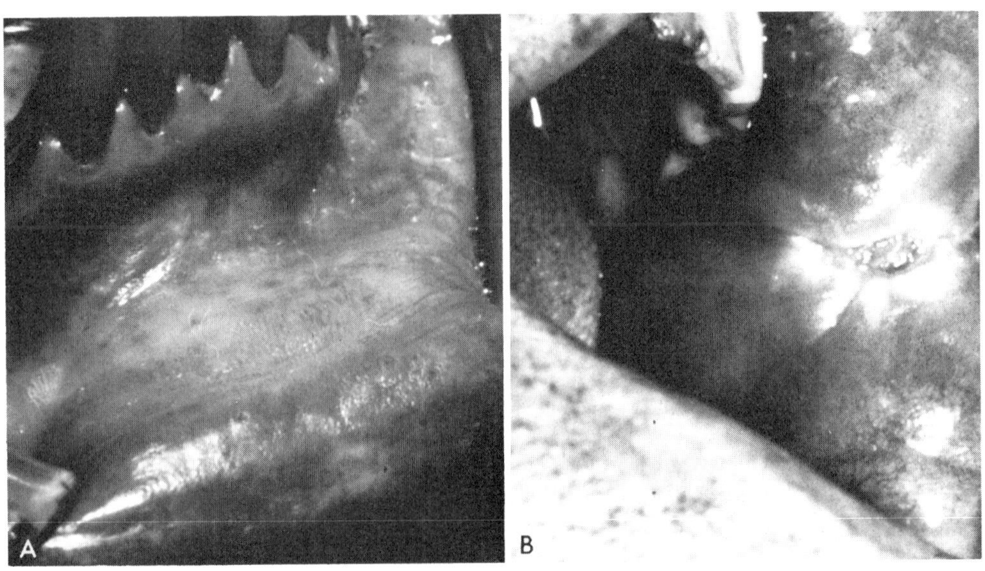

Figure 3–VI–77. *A*. Clinical appearance of the effects of long-term use of snuff. *B*. Clinical appearance of squamous cell carcinoma.

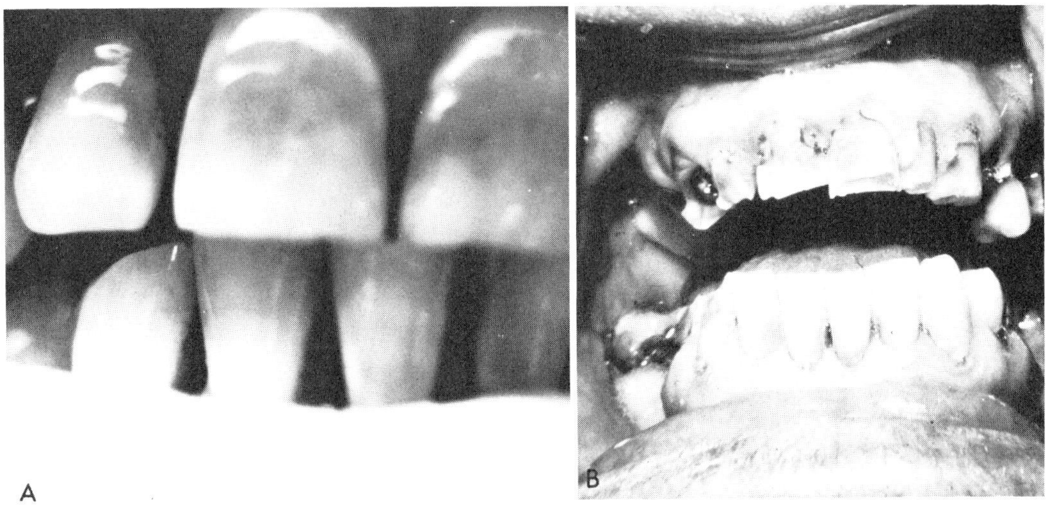
A B

Figure 3–VI–78. *A.* Clinical appearance of mottled enamel. *B.* Decalcification from excessive use of acid.

China, The Netherlands, Italy, Mexico, Spain, England, Africa and South America.[29]

Microscopic investigation has shown that the fluoride affects the interprismatic cementing substance, which is absent in the affected area, and causes the imperfect and atypical arrangement of enamel rods.[29] The affected area is quite porous and stains easily.

Acid. Excessive use of acid frequently causes decalcification of enamel in the areas that it first touches (Fig. 3–VI–78*B*). It has been noted that people who habitually use lemons may exhibit acid erosion, usually on the labial surface of the anterior teeth if they suck the lemon, and on the lingual surface if they chew it.

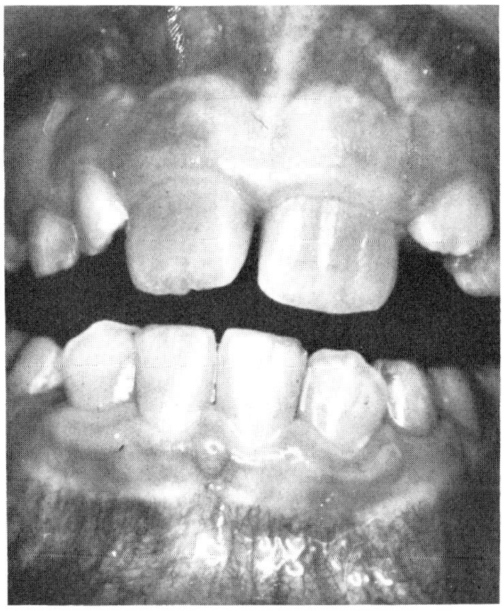

Figure 3–VI–79. Clinical appearance of tetracycline stain.

Tetracycline Stain. This has become more prevalent in the past decade. Clinically, this is manifested in children as a generalized grayish brown pigmentation of the teeth (Fig. 3–VI–79). This is a permanent condition and is due to the administration of tetracyclines during the developmental stage of crown formation. No treatment is required, except for esthetic reasons.

Thermal Injury

Extensive thermal burns in the oral cavity are very rare because it is relatively inaccessible and is surrounded by thick soft tissues, which act as an insulator.

The most common cause of minor burns in the oral cavity is hot food or liquid. Recently, pizza has been a popular culprit. This happens with such frequency that this entity is termed the "pizza palate." In the case illustrated, this is demonstrated by a generalized white area on the hard palate, with a definite border that appears to be normal mucous membrane (Fig. 3–VI–80*A*). This normal area was protected from the burn by an upper partial denture (Fig. 3–VI–80*B*). The pathosis of this injury may include infection if precautions are not taken. Histopathologic findings in thermal burns are similar to those in the previously discussed chemical burns. Other causes of thermal burns may be iatrogenic in nature, occurring during tooth bleaching, taking an impression, the use of electric cautery, or from the dropping of hot wax or dental instruments in the oral cavity.[53, 70]

Electrical Burns. Electrical burns of the oral

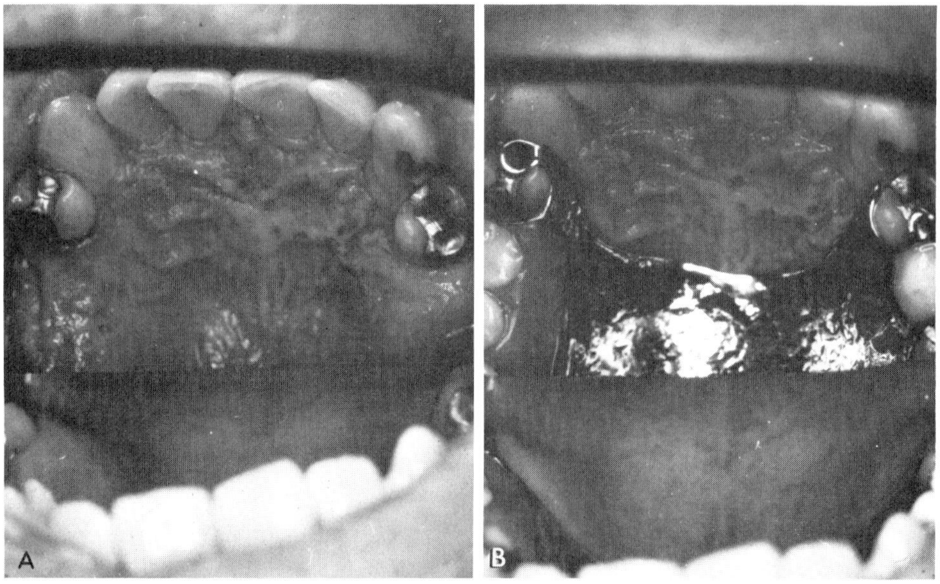

Figure 3–VI–80. *A*. Pizza palate. *B*. Pizza palate with partial denture.

cavity are infrequent and could easily be mistaken for other conditions. They occur predominantly in the infant or very young child. In most cases the child was left unattended and bit into an electrical cord. Clinically, the tissue appears erythematous with vesicles that later break down into a grayish sloughing area. The effects depend upon the area of contact and the severity of the burn. Figure 3–VI–81*A* demonstrates healing with deforming scar tissue limited only to the lip. The injury in this case was inflicted at the age of 10 months when the victim had no teeth. Figure 3–VI–81*B* shows scarring contractions that extend to the gingiva, indicating that the victim actually bit into the cord. The history reveals this child to have been 18 months old, with teeth present, at the time of the injury.

Radiation Injury

Solar Cheilosis. Certain persons, especially those with fair complexions, experience degenerative changes in the vermilion area of the lips from prolonged or intensified exposure to

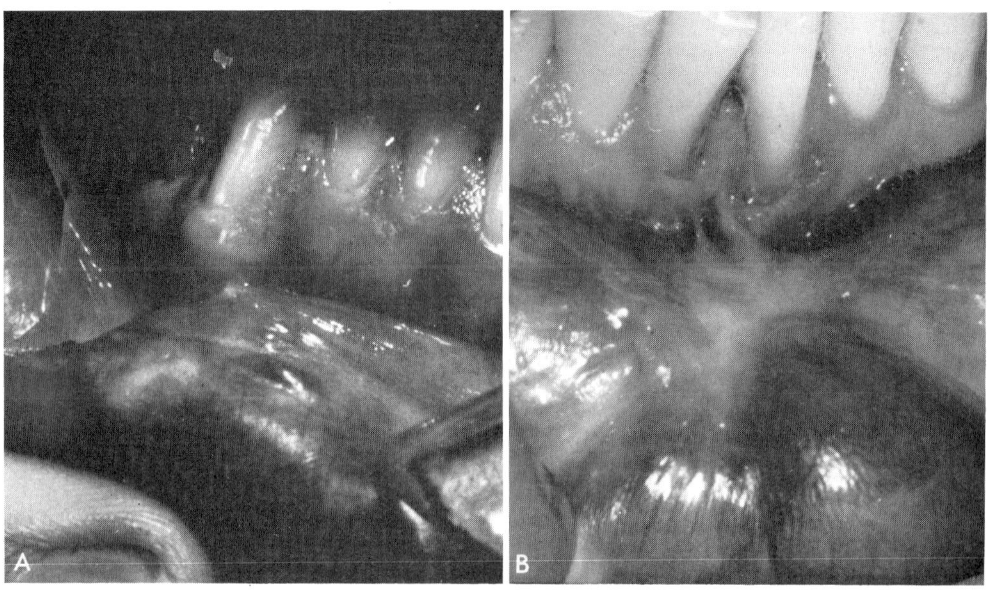

Figure 3–VI–81. Clinical appearance of an electrical burn. *A*. Injury occurred before the victim (aged 10 months) had teeth, and scar is limited to the lip. *B*. Scarring extends into the gingiva indicating that the victim (aged 18 months) actually bit into the cord.

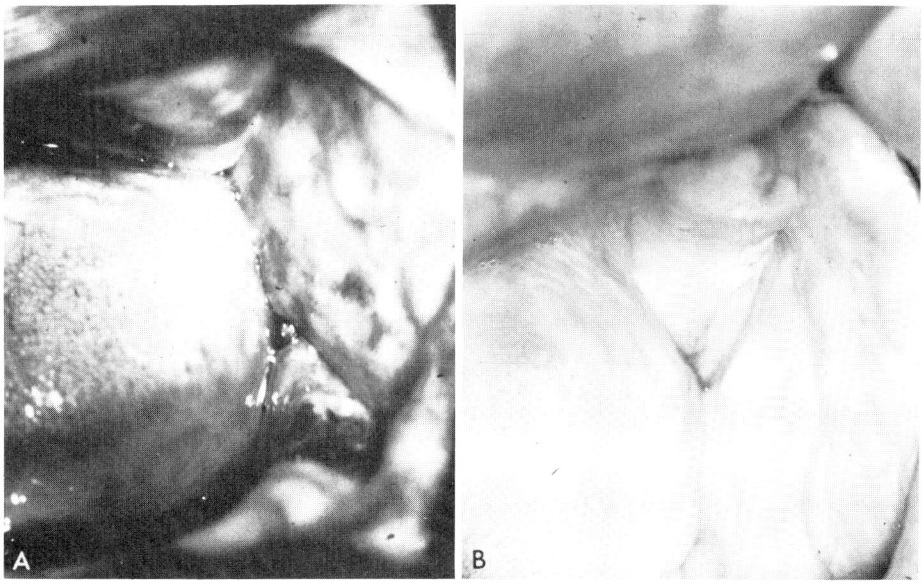

Figure 3–VI–82. *A*. Clinical appearance of erythema due to radiation. *B*. Postradiation clinical appearance of the denuded mucosa.

the sun's rays. Clinically, the lips appear very pale, with small red dots present. Advanced cases of this entity are considered to be precancerous.

Microscopically, there is a definite proliferation of the epithelium into the corium layer. Beneath this there are large areas of degenerating connective tissue.

Radionecrosis. Radiation utilized in the treatment of neoplasms usually causes injury to the adjacent normal tissue. The extent of such injury depends upon the susceptibility of the patient, the amount of shielding, the type and amount of radiation, and the division of the dosage.

There is usually no indication of any alteration to the soft tissues immediately following radiation, except occasionally there is a slight redness in color (Fig. 3–VI–82*A*). This disappears, but usually the erythema reappears within 30 days. More extensive radiation may result in denudation of the skin (Fig. 3–VI–82*B*). Xerostomia (dry mouth) is another frequently observed side-effect when salivary glands are irradiated.

Radiation alters the blood supply to the oral

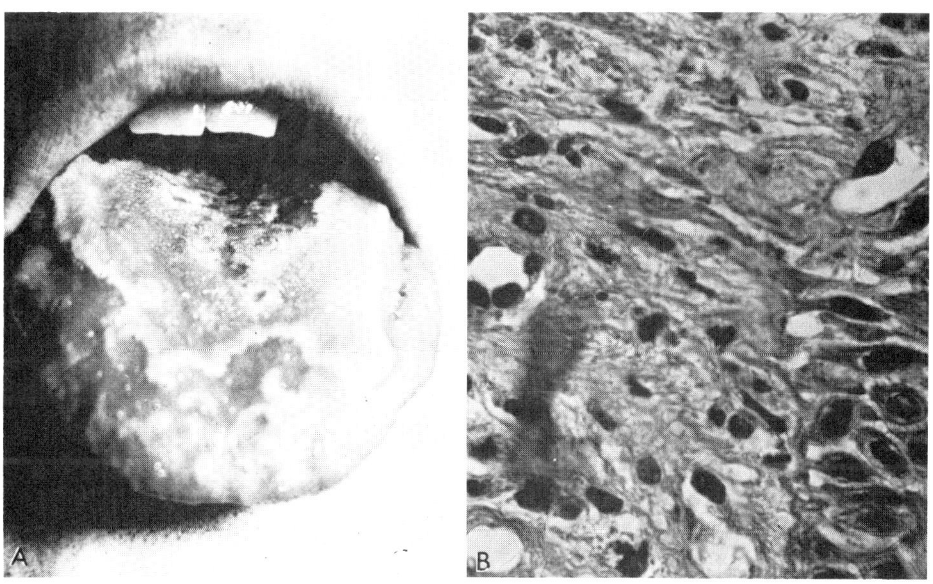

Figure 3–VI–83. *A*. Clinical appearance of slough and necrosis of the tongue. *B*. Microscopic appearance of the effects of radiation on the oral soft tissue.

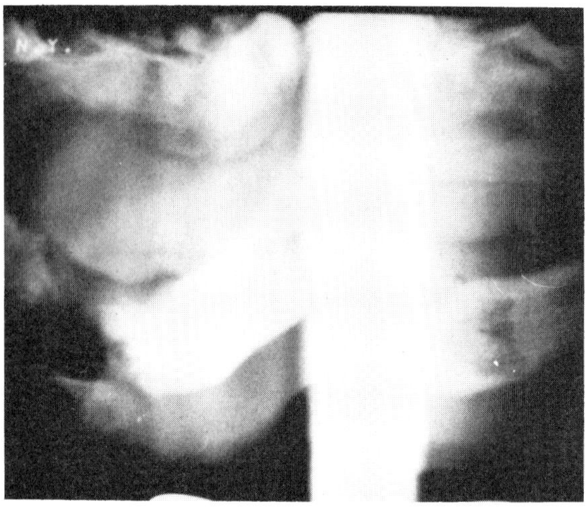

Figure 3–VI–84. Radiographic appearance of osteoradionecrosis with a pathologic fracture.

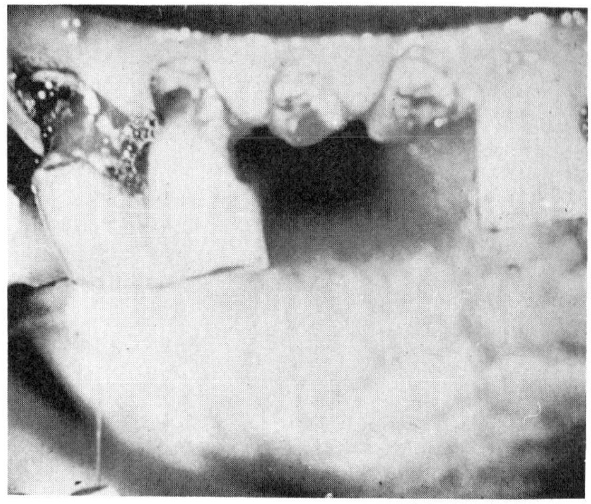

Figure 3–VI–86. Clinical appearance of radiation caries.

epithelium. This tissue frequently becomes atrophic, and sloughing and necrosis may result (Fig. 3–VI–83*A*). Microscopically, there appears to be numerous spaces formed in the epithelial cells, with nuclei smaller than normal (Fig. 3–VI–83*B*). This tends to give a bizarre shrinking appearance. The collagen content of the underlying connective tissue looks normal.

Osteoradionecrosis is a chronic, painful condition in which irradiated bone undergoes necrosis along with fibrosis or abnormal proliferation into the marrow spaces. Its pathogenesis is in the damage that radiation does to veins and lymphatics, which results in a diminished blood supply (ischemia) to the area.

Necrosis develops with bacterial invasion, which leads to thrombosis of the major arteries that carry the necessary oxygen to the area. This produces more areas of necrosis, owing to the further diminished blood supply. The bones become very brittle, and pathologic fractures occur frequently (Fig. 3–VI–84). Oral surgical procedures on patients with this condition are dangerous for obvious reasons. Therefore, it is generally agreed, that these procedures (such as tooth extractions) should be performed prior to radiation therapy.[53, 81, 127]

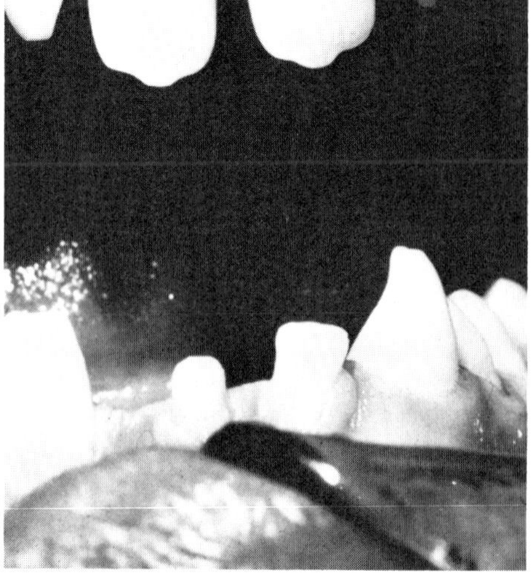

Figure 3–VI–85. Tooth malformation and ectopic eruption associated with radiation.

Radiation to areas where tooth development is taking place may result in the alteration of dentin formation, tooth form and structure, and tooth eruption (Fig. 3–VI–85).

Radiation caries is the demineralization of erupted teeth that have experienced irradiation (Fig. 3–VI–86). This is a common observation that is difficult to distinguish from dental caries, except the former tends to affect predominantly the tooth cervical area.

REFERENCES

1. Kessler, W.: *Kinder-Zahnheilkunde und Jugendzahnpflege.* 3rd Ed. Munchen, Carl Hanser Verlag, 1953, p. 144.
2. Akpata, E. S.: Traumatised anterior teeth in Lagos school children. J. Nigeria Med. Assoc., *6*:1, 1969.
3. Kessler, W.: Fratture dentarie Nell' infanzia. Riv. Ital. Stomatol., *14*:251, 1959.
4. Grundy, J. R.: The incidence of fractured incisors. Br. Dent. J., *106*:312, 1959.
5. Ellis, R. G.: *The Classification and Treatment of Injuries to the Teeth of Children.* 4th Ed. Chicago, Year Book Medical Publishers Inc., 1960.
6. Wallentin, I.: Zahnfrakturen bei Kindern und Jugendlichen. Zahnärztl. Mitt., *57*:875, 1967.
7. Buttner, M.: Die Häufigkeit von Zahnun fallen im Schulalter. Zahnärztl. Prax., *19*:286, 1968.
8. Beck, J. J.: Dental Health Status of the New Zealand

Population in late Adolescence and Young Adulthood. Department of Health Special Report Series 29. Wellington, N.Z., R. E. Owen, Government Printer, 1968, pp. 65–69.
9. Schutzmannsky, G.: Unfallverletzungen an jugendlichen Zahnen. Dtsch. Stomatol., *13*:919, 1963.
10. McEwen, J. D., McHugh, W. D., and Hitchin, A. D.: Fractured maxillary central incisors and incisal relationships, J. Dent. Res., *46*:1290, 1967.
11. Andreasen, J. O.: Etiology and pathogenesis of traumatic dental injuries. A clinical study of 1,298 cases. Scand. J. Dent. Res., *78*:329, 1970.
12. Woolridge, E. D.: Legal problems of the forensic odontologist. J. Forensic Sci., *18*:43, 1973.
13. Ravn, J. J., and Rossen, I.: Hyppighed og fordeling af Traumatiske beskadigelser af Taenderne hos kobenhavnske skoleborn 1967/68. Tandlaegebladet, *73*:1, 1969.
14. Magnusson, B., and Holm, A. K.: Traumatized Permanent Teeth in Children—A follow-up. I. Pulpal Complications and Root Resorption. Sven. Tandlak. Tidskr., *62*:61, 1969.
15. Kulowski, J.: Facial injuries: a common denominator of automobile casualties. J. Am. Dent. Assoc., *53*:32, 1956.
16. Woolridge, E. D.: Odontology in Identification. Inter. Micro J. of Legal Med. Vol. 9.
17. Picozzi, A., Dworkin, S. F., Leeds, J. G., and Nash, J.: Dental and Associated Attitudinal Aspects of Heroin Addiction: A Pilot Study. IADR Abst. No. 309. 1971, p. 130.
18. Wikstrom, L.: Narcotics and Teeth. Oral Res. Abst., *6*:460, 1971.
19. Thaller, J. L., Rosen, G., and Saltman, S.: Study of the relationship of frustration and anxiety to bruxism. J. Periodontol., *38*:193, 1967.
20. Vernalis, F. F.: Teeth-grinding: some relationships to anxiety, hostility, and hyperactivity. J. Clin. Psychol., *11*:389, 1955.
21. Lewis, T. E.: Incidence of fractured anterior teeth as related to protrusion. Angle Orthod., *29*:128, 1959.
22. Eichenbaum, I. W.: A correlation of traumatized anterior teeth to occlusion. J. Dent. Child., *30*:229, 1963.
23. Andreasen, J. O.: *Traumatic Injuries of the Teeth.* St. Louis, C. V. Mosby Co., 1972.
24. *Dorland's Illustrated Medical Dictionary:* 25th Ed., Philadelphia, W. B. Saunders Co., 1974.
25. Adkanazy, M.: Ueber Ostitis deformans ohne osteoides Gewebe. Arb. Geb. Pathol. Anat. Inst. Tubing, *4*:398, 1904.
26. Albright, F.: A page out of the history of hyperparathyroidism. J. Clin. Endocrinol., *8*:637, 1948.
27. Orban, B. J., and Wentz, F. M.: *Atlas of Clinical Pathology of the Oral Mucous Membrane.* St. Louis, C. V. Mosby Co., 1955.
28. Bhaskar, S. N.: *Synopsis of Oral Pathology.* 3rd Ed. St. Louis, C. V. Mosby Co., 1969.
29. Thoma, K. H.: *Oral Pathology.* 5th Ed. St. Louis, C. V. Mosby Co., 1969.
30. Brothwell, D. R. (Ed.): *Dental Anthropology.* Proceedings. Society for the Study of Human Biology. Elmsford, N. Y., Pergamon Press Inc., Vol. 5. 1963.
31. Oschinsky, L., and Smithurst, R.: On certain dental characteristics of the Eskimo of the eastern Canadian Arctic. Anthropologica N. S., *2*:105, 1960.
32. Hrdlicka, Al.: Shovel-shaped teeth. J. Phys. Anthropol., *3*:429, 1920.
33. Woolridge, E. D., and Ward, G. T.: The incidence of shovel-shaped incisors in the Mongoloid race. Presented at the meeting of the National Health Service Corp., Williamsburg, Virginia, June 1, 1973.
34. Ward, G. T., and Woolridge, E. D.: Some Clinical Applications of Adhesives in Restorative Dentistry. Paper presented at Dental Adhesive Materials Symposium, Nov. 8–9, 1973, New York City.
35. World Health Organization: *International Classification of Diseases—Application to Dentistry and Stomatology.* International Classification of Diseases—Dental Application. Copenhagen, 1969.
35. Woolridge, E. D., and Ward, G. T.: The incidence of shovel-shaped incisors in the Mongoloid race. Presented at the meeting of the National Health Service Corp, Williamsburg, Virginia June 1, 1973.
36. United States Department of Health, Education and Welfare, Public Health Service, National Health Center for Health Statistics: *Eighth Revision International Classification of Diseases, Adapted for Use in the United States.* Vol. 1, Tabular List. (Public Health Service Publication No. 1693.) Washington, D.C., U. S. Government Printing Office, 1967.
37. Federation Dentaire Internationale: *Dental Lexicon: A Lexicon of English Dental Terms with Their Equivalents in Espanol, Deutsch, Français, Italiano.* The Hague, Sijthoff, 1966.
38. Andreasen, J. O., and Ravn, J. J.: The effects of traumatic injuries to primary teeth on their permanent successors. II. A clinical and radiographic follow-up study of 213 injured teeth. Scand. J. Dent. Res., *79*:284, 1971.
39. Andreasen, J. O., Sundstrom, B., and Ravn, J. J.: The effect of traumatic injuries to primary teeth on their permanent successors. I. A clinical and histologic study of 117 injured permanent teeth. Scand. J. Dent. Res., *79*:219, 1971.
40. Via, W. F.: Enamel defects induced by trauma during tooth formation. Oral Surg., *25*:49, 1968.
41. Peckert: Ein Fall von Zahmissbildung durch Trauma. Korresp. Bl. Zahnärzte, *41*:58, 1912.
42. Gagliani, N.: Malposizioni e malformation dentarie consequenti a trauma in dentatura decidua. Dent. Cadmos, *35*:1393, 1967.
43. Hitchin, A. D.: Traumatic odontome. Br. Dent. J., *126*:260, 1969.
44. Rushton, M. A.: Partial duplication following injury to developing incisors. Br. Dent. J., *104*:9, 1958.
45. Arwill, T.: Histopathologic studies of traumatized teeth. Odontol. Tidskr., *70*:91, 1962.
46. Ball, J. S.: A sequel to trauma involving the deciduous incisors. Br. Dent. J., *118*:394, 1965.
47. Field, G. S.: Case of repair after injury to developing permanent incisors. N.Z. Dent. J., *24*:125, 1931.
48. Wallenius, B., and Granse, K. A.: Eruption disturbances: two cases with different etiology. Odontol. Revy, *5*:297, 1954.
49. Lenstrup, K.: On injury by fractures of the jaws to teeth in course of formation. Acta Odont. Scand., *13*:181, 1955.
50. Carmichael, A. F., and Nixon, G. S.: Two interesting cases of root resorption. Dent. Rec., *74*:258, 1954.
51. Beveridge, E. E., and Brown, A. C.: The measurement of human intrapulpal pressure and its response to clinical variables. Oral Surg., *19*:655, 1965.
52. Langeland, K.: Tissue Changes in the Dental Pulp. Norwegian Institute of Dental Research. Oslo, Oslo University Press, 1957, p. 134.
53. Colby, R. A., Kerr, D. A., and Robinson, H. B. G.: *Color Atlas of Oral Pathology.* 3rd Ed. Philadelphia, J. B. Lippincott Co., 1961.
54. Gelbier, S.: Injured anterior teeth in children. A preliminary discussion. Br. Dent. J., *123*:331, 1967.
55. Hardwick, J. L., and Newman, P. A.: Some observations on the incidence and emergency treatment of

fractured permanent anterior teeth of children. J. Dent. Res., *33*:730, 1954.
56. Ennis, L. M. et al.: *Dental Roentgenology*. 6th Ed. Philadelphia, Lea & Febiger, 1967.
57. Down, C. H.: The treatment of permanent incisor teeth of children following traumatic injury. Aust. Dent. J., *2*:9, 1957.
58. Andreasen, J. O., and Hjorting-Hansen, E.: Intraalveolar root fractures: radiographic and histologic study of 50 cases. J. Oral Surg., *25*:414, 1967.
59. Austin, L. T.: A review of forty cases of retained fractured roots of anterior teeth. J. Am. Dent. Assoc., *17*:1930, 1930.
60. Andreasen, J. O.: Luxation of permanent teeth due to trauma. A clinical and radiographic follow-up study of 189 injured teeth. Scand. J. Dent. Res., *78*:273, 1970.
61. Andreasen, J. O., and Hjorting-Hansen, E.: Replantation of teeth. I. Radiographic and clinical study of 110 human teeth replanted after accidental loss. Acta Odontol. Scand., *24*:263, 1966.
62. Lenstrup, K., and Skieller, V.: A follow-up study of teeth replanted after accidental loss. Acta Odontol. Scand., *17*:503, 1959.
63. Sundrall, H. I.: Olycksfallsskador pa tander och parodontium under barnaaren. Nord. Klin. Odontol., *3*:1, 1964.
64. Ravn, J. J., and Rossen, I.: Hyppighed og fordeling af traumatiske beskadigelser af taenderne hos kobenhavnske Skoleborn 1967/68. Tandlaegebladet, *73*:1, 1969.
65. Boyle, P. E.: *Kornfield's Histopathy of the Teeth and Their Surrounding Structures*. 4th Ed. Philadelphia, Lea & Febiger, 1955.
66. Skieller, V.: The prognosis for young teeth loosened after mechanical injuries. Acta Odontol. Scand., *18*:171, 1960.
67. Deeb, E.: Idiopathic resorption of permanent teeth. J. S. Calif. State Dent. Assoc., *28*:210, 1960.
68. Cohen, S.: Internal tooth resorption. J. Dent. Child., *32*:49, 1965.
69. Menyel, G.: Seltene Folgen eines Traumas an 2 Zahnen. Dtsch. Zahnärztl. Wochenschr., *45*:249, 1942.
70. Ingle, J. I.: *Endodontics*. Philadelphia, Lea & Febiger, 1965.
71. Anehill, S., Lindahl, B., and Wallin, H.: Prognosis of traumatised permanent incisors in children. A clinical-roentgenological after examination. Sven. Tandlak. Tidskr., *62*:367, 1969.
72. Weiskopf, J., Gehre, G., and Graichen, K.-H.; Ein Beitrag zur Behandlung von Luxationen und Wurzelfrakturen im Frontzahngebiet. Stoma (Heidelb.), *14*:100, 1961.
73. Dobrzanska, A., and Szpringer, M.: Obserwacje Zebow Mlecznyck, dotknietych urazem Mechanicznym. Czas. Stomatol., *19*:167, 1966.
74. Kingsbury, B. C.: Alveolar fractures. J. Oral Surg., *27*:530, 1969.
75. Huelke, D. F., and Harger, J. H.: Maxillofacial injuries: their nature and mechanisms of production. J. Oral. Surg., *27*:451, 1969.
76. Pommer, G., and Hampton, H. O.: Zur Kenntnis der Progressiven Hamatomund Phlegmasieveranderungen der Rohrenknochen. Arch. Orthop., *17*:17, 1919.
77. Dingman, R. O., and Natvig, P.: *Surgery of Facial Fractures*. Philadelphia, W. B. Saunders Co., 1964.
78. Clark, H. B.: *Practical Oral Surgery*. Philadelphia, Lea & Febiger, 1955.
79. Le Fort, R.: Fractures de la machoire supérieure. Cong. Internat. Med. C. R., Paris, 1900, Sect. de chir. gen., pp. 275–278.
80. Le Fort, R.: Etude experimentale sur les fractures de la machiore supérieure. Rev. Chir., Paris, *23*:208, 360, 479, 1901.
81. Archer, W. H.: *Oral and Maxillofacial Surgery*. 5th Ed. Philadelphia, W. B. Saunders Co., 1975.
82. Graber, T. M.: *Orthodontics: Principle and Practice*. 3rd Ed. Philadelphia, W. B. Saunders Co., 1972.
83. Hankey, G. T.: Temporomandibular arthrosis. An analysis of 150 cases. Br. Dent. J., *97*:249, 1954.
84. Gerry, R. G.: Effects of trauma and hypermotility on the temporomandibular joint. Oral Surg., 7:876, 1954.
85. Frankel, V. H.: Temporomandibular joint problems due to auto accidents. Ohio Dent. J., *44*:120, 1970.
86. Monson, G.: Occlusion supplied to crown and bridgework. Nat. Dent. A. J., 7:399, 1920.
87. Monson, G.: Impaired function as a result of closed bite. Nat. Dent. A. J., *8*:833, 1921.
88. Freese, A. S.: The myofascial trigger mechanism in temporomandibular joint and allied disturbances. Oral. Surg., *14*:933, 1961.
89. Schwartz, L.: Temporomandibular joint syndromes. J. Prosthet. Dent., 7:489, 1957.
90. Schwartz, L.: Conclusions of the Temporomandibular Joint Clinic at Columbia. J. Periodontol., *29*:210, 1958.
91. Boman, K. A.: Temporomandibular joint arthrosis and its treatment by extirpation of the disc, a clinical study. Acta Chir. Scand., Suppl. 118, 1947.
92. Trotter, M., et al.: Dentistry of select bones in human skeleton. Am. J. Phys. Anthropol. (New Series), *16*:197, 1958.
93. Ramfjord, S., and Ash, M. M.: *Occlusion*. 2nd Ed. Philadelphia, W. B. Saunders Co., 1971.
94. Goldman, H. M., and Cohen, D. W. (Eds.): *Periodontal Therapy*. 5th Ed. St. Louis, C. V. Mosby Co., 1973.
95. Bernier, J. L.: *The Management of Oral Disease*. 2nd Ed. St. Louis, C. V. Mosby Co., 1959.
96. Hopkin, E.: Deficiency of maxillary development with absence of anterior nasal spine, presumably from early accident. Br. J. Plast. Surg., *19*:73, 1958.
97. Thoma, K., and Goldman, H.: *Oral Pathology*. 5th Ed. St. Louis, C. V. Mosby Co., 1960.
98. Hazen, H. H., and Eichenlaub, F. J.: Leukoplakia buccalis. J.A.M.A., *79*:1487, 1922.
99. Bloodgood, J. C.: The facts in regard to cancer of the tongue. J.A.M.A., *85*:537, 1925.
100. Lefkowitz, W., Robinson, H., and Postle, H.: Interpretation of histologic sections of pulp. Ohio Dent. J., *31*:24, 1957.
101. Stanley, H. R., and Swerdlow, H.: Reaction of the human pulp to cavity preparation: results produced by eight different operative grinding technics. J. Am. Dent. Assoc., *58*:49, May, 1959.
102. Langland, K.: Histological Evaluation of Pulp Reactions to Operative Procedures. Oral. Surg., *12*:1235, 1959.
103. Stanley, H. R., and Swerdlow, H.: Reaction of the human pulp to cavity preparation: results produced by eight different operative grinding technics. J. Am. Dent. Assoc., *58*:49, 1959.
104. James, V. E., and Schour, I.: Early dentinal and pulpal changes following cavity preparations and filling materials in dogs. Oral. Surg., *18*:243, 1964.
105. Ritchey, B., Mendenhall, R., and Orban, B.: Pulpitis resulting from incomplete tooth fracture. Oral. Surg., *10*:665, 1957.
106. Rudolph, C. E.: An evaluation of root resorption occurring during orthodontic treatment. J. Dent. Res., *19*:367, 1940.

107. Ketcham, A. H.: A progress report of apical root resorption of vital permanent teeth. Int. Jour. Orthol., *15*:310, 1929.
108. Herzberg, B. L.: Bone Changes Incident to Orthodontic.
109. Stuteville, O. H.: Injuries caused by orthodontic forces and the ultimate results of these injuries. Int. J. Orthod., *24*:103, 1938.
110. Oppenheim, A.: Human tissue response to orthodontic intervention of short and long duration. Am. J. Orthod., *28*:263, 1942.
111. Irby, W. B., and Baldwin, K. H.: *Emergencies and Urgent Complications in Dentistry*. St. Louis, C. V. Mosby Co., 1965.
112. Richards, R., and Crombie, H. M.: Familial angioneurotic edema: two fatal cases after dental extractions. Br. Med. J., *5215*:1787, 1960.
113. *American Medical Association Drug Evaluations*. 2:757, 1973.
114. Amsterdam, M., et al.: Provisional splinting principles and techniques. Dent. Clin. North. Am., Mar. 1959, p. 75.
115. Hill, T. J.: *A Textbook of Oral Pathology*. 4th Ed. Philadelphia, Lea & Febiger, 1949.
116. Kelsten, L. B.: *Pedodontics for the General Practitioner*. Brooklyn, N.Y., Dental Items of Interest Publishing Co., Inc., 1956.
117. Sorrin, S.: Habit, an etiologic factor of periodontal disease. Dent. Dig., *41*:290, 1935.
118. Shafer, W. G., Hine, M. K., and Levy, B. M.: 3rd Ed. Philadelphia, W. B. Saunders Co., 1974.
119. Goldman, H., et al.: *Periodontal Therapy*. St. Louis, C. V. Mosby Co., 1973.
120. Grant, D., Stern, I., and Everett, F.: Orban's Periodontics. 4th Ed. St. Louis, C. V. Mosby Co., 1972.
121. Fernstrom, A. I. B., et al.: Mercury allergy with eczematous dermatitis due to silver amalgam fillings. Br. Dent. J., *113*:204, 1962.
122. Lippman, D. S.: Ans Fehlern Lernen. Quintessenz, *12*:53, Oct. 1961.
123. Frykholm, K. O.: On mercury from dental amalgam. Its toxic and allergic effects and some comments on occupational hygiene. Acta Odont. Scand., *15*:7 (Suppl. 22), 1957.
124. Engleman, M. A.: Mercury allergy resulting from amalgam restorations. J. Am. Dent. Assoc., *66*:122, 1963.
125. Keller, A. Z.: Cirrhosis of the liver, alcoholism and heavy smoking associated with cancer of the mouth and pharynx. Cancer, *20*:1015, 1967.
126. Wynder, E. L., Bross, I. J., and Feldman, R. M.: A study of the etiological factors in cancer of the mouth. Cancer, *10*:1300, 1957.
127. Gardner, A. F.: *Pathology in Dentistry*. Springfield, Ill., Charles C Thomas, 1968.
128. Pindborg, J. J.: *Atlas of Diseases of the Oral Mucosa*. 2nd Ed. Philadelphia, W. B. Saunders Co., 1968.

VII. The Thorax

by Mark M. Sherman, John R. McCormick, and Robert L. Berger

Since the bony thoracic cage contains the vital centers of circulation and respiration, trauma to the chest challenges the integrity and even the viability of the entire organism. Unfortunately, thoracic trauma is a serious matter, not only in terms of the individual patient, but also in terms of the numbers affected, since injuries to the thorax are common occurrences. In war, between 20 and 40 per cent of wounds involve the chest, and rapid, accurate diagnosis by the surgeon is mandatory for effective treatment. At examination of patients who die, the alert and knowing forensic pathologist is in a strategic position to uncover mode of injury and mechanism of death. For example, if pneumothorax is suspected, a small area of the chest wall should be opened under water to demonstrate air bubbles. With deceleration accidents, transection of the aorta or avulsion of the arch branches should be sought. The pathway of all penetrating instruments or missiles in the heart must be thoroughly studied so that multiple wounds are not overlooked. Particularly with intracardiac wounds, valvular or septal penetrations as well as coronary artery injuries should be noted. In a death from thoracic injury, the exact mechanism can usually be determined by the forensic pathologist. Unexpected sudden death due to occult intrathoracic pathologic conditions does occur, but not from wounds.

Most traumatic tissue wounds are produced by sudden exposure of the body to a force it cannot dissipate or absorb. The severity of the injury is related to the magnitude of the kinetic energy delivered, which can be expressed by the formula $KE = 1/2\ MV^2$, where KE is kinetic energy, M is mass, and V is velocity. From this formula, it is apparent that the velocity of the wounding object is the most important factor in determining the extent of the tissue destruction produced. When velocity is doubled, kinetic energy or the destructive force is quadrupled. The kinetic energy may be exerted by a moving or accelerating object on a stationary victim, e.g., a missile finding its human target. Just as frequently, the injury is of the deceleration type in which a moving victim collides with another moving or stationary object, e.g., an automobile accident. In general, injuries of all types are produced either by penetration of the body or by collision with a blunt object.

Penetrating injuries are produced either by sharp instruments (stab wounds) or missiles (gunshot wounds). The tissue damage inflicted by a stab wound is largely determined by the size of the instrument and the pathway it travels. Penetration of a specific organ results in a characteristic physiologic disturbance determined by the structure and function of that organ. With gunshot wounds, the trajectory is only a partial determinant of the severity of tissue damage. Another important element is the velocity of the bullet, which influences the perpendicular dissipation of destructive energy, resulting in injury beyond the trajectory of the bullet. As a general rule, low-velocity bullets tend to confine their destructive effect to the trajectory, whereas high-velocity missiles produce far greater tissue injury.

With blunt trauma, the extent of tissue damage inflicted by collision injuries is a function of the velocity and the mass of the object producing the injury. In the chest, low-velocity blunt injuries, such as a blow with a club, cause soft-tissue contusion with or without rib fractures. Higher-velocity collisions (automobile and airplane) may produce a wide variety of deceleration injuries. The nature of the trauma in the chest may range from soft-tissue contusion, to rib fractures and flail chest, to transection of the aorta or rupture of the heart.

Other mechanisms of thoracic trauma involve crush, blast, thermal extremes, and chemical agents. They are discussed subsequently in this chapter.

INJURIES OF CHEST WALL, HEMOTHORAX, AND PNEUMOTHORAX

Superficial Soft-Tissue Injuries

Superficial injuries to the soft tissues of the chest wall include abrasions, contusions, lacerations, hematomas, and burns. In the absence of through-and-through penetration of the chest wall, these injuries do not interfere with circulatory and respiratory functions and require only local wound treatment.

Rib Cage Injuries

Traumatic fractures of the bony rib cage are usually produced by blunt trauma and occasionally by a missile. The severity of these injuries ranges from simple fracture of a rib to the involvement of several ribs at multiple points, producing the so-called flail chest with severe cardiopulmonary dysfunction.

Simple rib fractures are common and are caused mainly by blows or by collisions with moving or stationary objects. The most commonly fractured ribs are 2 through 10. The site of fracture is usually in the lateral portion of the rib.

Simple fracture of one or two ribs produces little physiologic disturbance. The fracture heals without specific therapy in four to eight weeks. Comminution, displacement, and angulation are unusual. Rib fractures are painful and require analgesics or intercostal nerve blocks. The need for adequate pain relief should not be underestimated, particularly in the geriatric patient in whom inadequately treated pain often leads to splinting of the involved hemithorax and consequent atelectasis and pneumonia.

Flail, or "crush," chest is the result of fracture of several ribs in more than one place or simultaneous fracture of the sternum and several ribs. A portion of the chest wall is thereby detached, loses connection with the rest of the rib cage, and moves independently and paradoxically from the intact portion. During inspiration, when the chest expands, the negative intrapleural pressure exerts a sucking influence on the detached portion of the rib cage ("paradoxical plate"), which then moves inward. During expiration the opposite sequence of events takes place. This paradoxical motion of a portion of the chest wall results in inefficient ventilation and collapse of the underlying lung, producing respiratory insufficiency. In addition, the to-and-fro motion of the chest wall with each respiratory cycle is accompanied by similar excursions of the mediastinum. This pendular swing of the heart and mediastinal great vessels reduces venous return to the right cardiac chambers and decreases the output from the left side of the heart. Thus a flail chest involving a large portion of the chest wall can be lethal because of the combined cardiac and pulmonary dysfunction.

The diagnosis of flail chest is based on an appropriate history and on simple inspection of the area of paradoxical chest wall movement. Respiratory distress is usually marked, and circulatory collapse may be present. A roentgenogram demonstrates the fractured ribs and may show an associated hemothorax or pneumothorax. Specific therapy of flail chest consists of endotracheal intubation or tracheostomy, and mechanical ventilation. This treatment deals effectively with both the respiratory and circulatory dysfunction by eliminating the paradoxical respiration and stabilizing the mediastinum. Over a 10- to 20-day period the rib cage stabilizes and heals sufficiently to allow discontinuation of mechanical ventilation.

Hemothorax

Hemothorax is a collection of blood in the pleural cavity and may be due to injuries of the chest wall, the lungs, the pulmonary vasculature, the heart, or the major vessels. Penetrating trauma from a stab wound or a missile is the usual cause of hemothorax, although on occasion, blunt trauma may produce it also. External bleeding is usually minimal. Chest wall bleeding sufficient to cause a clinically significant hemothorax usually arises from intercostal or internal mammary artery disruption caused by a penetrating wound or the sharp ends of fractured ribs or sternum. Hemothorax also results from laceration of the lung or major pulmonary vessels. Indeed, injury to the latter may cause exsanguinating hemorrhage and requires prompt thoracotomy for control. The same is even more true of wounds in the great arteries of the thorax. Penetration of the heart, in those surviving the immediate episode, more often presents as cardiac tamponade than as hemothorax. Blunt trauma produces hemothorax either through laceration of soft tissues by fractured ribs or through avulsion of a major intrathoracic blood vessel.

Physical examination and a chest roentgenogram should demonstrate the presence of a hemothorax of any significant volume (400 to 500 ml). Massive bleeding results in shock, and the associated large volume of blood in the pleural space compresses the lung and causes respiratory embarrassment.

The initial treatment of hemothorax is volume replacement and closed tube thoracotomy. The tube drains the intrapleural blood, allows the lung to expand, and permits monitoring of the rate of bleeding. In 80 to 90 per cent of cases of hemothorax, tube thoracotomy provides definitive therapy. In the remaining 10 to 20 per cent, rapid or persistent bleeding necessitates thoracotomy and control of the bleeding site. If blood is allowed to remain undrained within the pleural cavity it may resorb spontaneously; may become infected, causing an empyema; or may form a constrictive "peel" over the affected lung, leading to loss of pulmonary function.

Pneumothorax

Pneumothorax is an air collection in the pleural cavity. There are three different types—simple, open, and tension. Pneumothorax may be caused by penetrating or blunt trauma, or iatrogenically during procedures such as thoracentesis, subclavian vein catheterization, or percutaneous pleural or lung biopsy.

With simple or closed pneumothorax, a wound in the chest wall or in the lung allows air to escape and to collect in the pleural cavity. The air leak usually stops spontaneously as the wound becomes sealed. Simple pneumothorax greater than 25 per cent necessitates tube thoracotomy with water-seal drainage. Occasionally, a persistent air leak from the lung may require surgical closure.

Open pneumothorax is usually associated with a large defect in the chest wall that allows air to enter freely from the atmosphere into the pleural cavity. An open pneumothorax is often referred to as a "sucking chest wound" because of the audible sucking sound created by attempted breathing. The situation is far more urgent than that with closed pneumothorax. Cardiorespiratory function can be severely compromised because of the total collapse of the lung and the instability of the mediastinum. The free movement of air through the open chest into the pleural cavity during inspiration prevents expansion of the ipsilateral lung and shifts the mediastinum toward the contralateral hemithorax, which in turn interferes with expansion of that lung. The reverse sequence occurs during expiration, and thus pulmonary function is severely disturbed. In addition, the pendulumlike motion of the mediastinum curtails venous return to the heart and produces serious cardiopulmonary dysfunction. Open pneumothorax is a serious emergency that has to be treated promptly. Initial treatment consists of sealing the wound with an airtight dressing and water-seal drainage. Definitive therapy is surgical debridement of the wound and closure of the chest wall.

Tension pneumothorax exists when air is under extreme pressure within the pleural cavity. The air may enter the pleural cavity through the chest wall, from the lungs, or from the tracheobronchial tree. Whatever the site, the wound acts as a one-way valve allowing air to enter the pleural space without an avenue for escape. Thus, with each respiratory cycle, more air is introduced and trapped in the pleural space and gradually builds up ever-increasing intrapleural pressure. The clinical presentation is that of severe dyspnea and cyanosis, and the chest roentgenogram reveals the pneumothorax with mediastinal shift. Tension pneumothorax requires treatment without delay since it is associated with compression of both lungs and mediastinal shift, causing both ventilatory insufficiency and shock due to impaired venous return to the heart. Closed tube thoracotomy with water-seal drainage provides both immediate relief and definitive therapy. In an occasional instance repair of the site of the air leak may be necessary.

INJURIES OF THE LUNG AND TRACHEOBRONCHIAL TREE

Pulmonary Lacerations

Pulmonary lacerations are usually produced by penetrating chest injuries and rarely by blunt trauma. The disruption of the visceral pleura and the pulmonary parenchyma may lead to a pneumothorax, which may be small or large, either under tension or not. The treatment is closed tube thoracotomy, which allows the lung to expand. The pulmonary wound, unless it is quite large, usually seals itself spontaneously in from minutes to a few days and does not require operative repair. Occasionally a lung wound is associated with a persistent air leak requiring drainage for several days. If a laceration of the lung is encountered during thoracotomy for an associated injury, it should be repaired to expedite recovery. Lung laceration may also result in minimal to massive bleeding. When the peripheral portion of the lung is injured, the blood loss tends to be modest and usually stops spontaneously. Wounds of central pulmonary arteries and veins bleed profusely, and the bleeding is unlikely to stop without surgical intervention. Emergency thoracotomy and control of the bleeding site is lifesaving. The treatment of bleeding from lung laceration is discussed in the section on hemothorax.

Pulmonary Contusion

Pulmonary contusion is usually produced by severe blunt trauma and is encountered most frequently in association with rib fracture. Occasionally, however, the lung is contused by a contrecoup force in the absence of rib cage injury. Penetrating injuries from missiles can also produce contusions of the pulmonary parenchyma. Rupture of a contused lung results in pneumo-, hemo-, or hemopneumothorax. Hemoptysis is a common symptom and may be brisk initially, only to subside with passage of time. With large lung bruises, respiratory insufficiency may develop. The diagnosis may be made on the basis of an appropriate history of chest trauma and a characteristic radioopacity on chest x-ray. Pathologic changes consist of intraalveolar hemorrhage, micro- and macroatelectasis, edema of varying degree, and distortion of pulmonary architecture. The treatment is supportive and in the more severe cases includes mechanical ventilation. Pulmonary contusions usually resolve over a period of days to weeks. In some instances, they may lead to diffuse interstitial pulmonary edema and the so-called adult respiratory distress syndrome. Occasionally the contused lung may become infected and form a lung abscess. Suture repair of a tear in a contused lung is hazardous because of possible disruption of the suture line; with extensive lacerations in a heavily contused lung, resection of the involved lobe or the entire lung is indicated.

Blast and Inhalation Injuries of the Lung

Blast injuries of the lung are produced by the shock waves occurring in close proximity to an explosion. A similar injury is caused by an underwater detonation near an immersed person. The pulmonary lesion is usually bilateral and consists of diffuse petechial hemorrhages and disruption of the alveoli. The process tends to be progressive, the lung becomes edematous and stiff, and relentless respiratory insufficiency is the usual course. Supportive treatment with mechanical ventilation is employed, since no specific therapeutic agent is available at the present.

Inhalation injuries of the lungs are seen frequently in our increasingly urbanized, industrial society. Smoke inhalation has been, and continues to be, a leading cause of morbidity among fire victims. Smoke inhalation is often compounded by thermal injury of the airways producing varying degrees of tissue destruction and edema. Thermal injuries of the tracheobronchial tree are suspected when the history of exposure to fire is accompanied by evidence of burns in the visible portions of the upper respiratory and digestive tract on physical examination. The upper airway may be obstructed by laryngeal edema, necessitating emergency tracheostomy. The ventilatory embarrassment may be compounded by bronchospasm secondary to the pulmonary burn. In addition, inhaled smoke contains a variety of noxious agents that may be absorbed and produce metabolic acidosis. Furthermore, smoke is also rich in carbon monoxide, which may be inhaled and absorbed, and will block the transport of oxygen by hemoglobin. If at autopsy the blood carboxyhemoglobin level is greater than 8 to 10 per cent, one may deduce that the victim was alive for some time during the fire.

All but the most severe cases of smoke inhalation are managed successfully with supportive measures.

A large number of chemical agents are readily absorbed across the alveolar-capillary membrane, each of which may be injurious or even fatal through its own specific mechanism of action. Inhaled carbon monoxide blocks oxygen binding sites on hemoglobin, cyanide gas blocks cellular metabolic pathways, and inhalation anesthetic gases may depress the central nervous system. Other noxious chemical agents can be inhaled and produce physical injury to the lungs.

Tracheobronchial Injuries

Disruptions

Disruption of the tracheobronchial tree can be produced by several different mechanisms. Penetrating injuries may traverse any part of the airway and result in defects of varying sizes. Blunt trauma from steering-wheel or other deceleration injuries, and from sharp blows by heavy objects, wires, cables, and swings, may produce partial or circumferential lacerations and even avulsion of the trachea from the cricoid cartilage or larynx. A blow to the chest when the glottis is closed may generate sufficient pressure to result in tracheal disruption. Hyperextension of the neck and other movements that stretch the trachea may produce similar damage. Explosion of anesthetic gases may cause rupture anywhere in the tracheobronchial tree. Instrumental perforation of the tracheobronchial tree is encountered in rare instances, during attempts at endoscopic removal of foreign bodies.

The extent of tracheobronchial injuries varies from small tears in the membraneous portion to fractures of cartilage and circumferential separation of the trachea or bronchus. Because of their elasticity, the large vessels running along the bronchi are seldom involved in these airway injuries.

The patient with injury of the tracheobronchial tree usually presents with dyspnea, rapidly progressive subcutaneous emphysema, and hoarseness. Although associated unilateral or bilateral pneumothorax and rib fractures are commonly present, they can also be absent. The diagnosis is made on the basis of the history, physical signs, chest x-rays, and bronchoscopy. The latter is essential to confirm the diagnosis and identify the site of the injury. Treatment consists of water-seal pleural drainage for evacuation of the air, and operative repair of the injury.

Asphyxiation

Asphyxia refers to cessation of effective respiration. Strangulation is asphyxia produced by mechanical obstruction of the upper airway. The cervical trachea can be compressed by hands or by a ligaturelike object such as a piece of rope or a necktie. At autopsy, strangulation can usually be diagnosed by skin marks, abrasions, and lacerations in the neck as well as by hematoma and laryngeal or tracheal cartilaginous fractures. In ligature strangulation, the identifying mark of the ligature may be present on the skin, e.g., the braid burn of a rope.

A special form of strangulation is hanging, in which ligature strangulation is carried out with the weight of the victim's body supplying the force to tighten the ligature. Legal (judicial), homicidal, suicidal, ritual, and accidental hangings occur. In all but judicial hanging, the mechanism of death is acute asphyxia. If legal hanging is properly performed, high cervical spine fracture with spinal cord transection caused by the snap of the laterally placed noose is the mechanism of death. Failing this, the victim is asphyxiated by ligature strangulation.

Another mechanism of asphyxia is simple obstruction of the upper airway from within the lumen by a foreign body.

Traumatic asphyxia, a misnomer, results from sudden compression of the chest or upper abdomen by a heavy object. This compression is not always lethal. Death, when it occurs, is most likely due to cerebral edema and not to asphyxia. The victim may have been run over by an automobile, trampled in a human or animal stampede, or crushed in the collapse of a building. Physical findings include cyanosis of the head, neck, upper part of the chest, and upper extremities associated with petechial hemorrhages in the eyelids, conjunctivae, and skin of the neck and chest.

Drowning is also a form of asphyxia. Acute respiratory insufficiency ensues when the tracheobronchial tree fills with fluid. While the medium is usually water, people occasionally drown in beer, dye, or other chemical solutions. A significant difference exists between drowning in fresh and salt water. It has been suggested that the mechanism of death from drowning in water may be sudden large shifts of fluids and electrolytes rather than acute asphyxia. Fresh water has a low salt concentration, and large volumes of water move into the vascular space, causing massive hemodilution, hemolysis, circulatory overload, hyperkalemia, and hyponatremia. In salt-water drowning, there is massive withdrawal of water from the circulating blood into the alveoli, causing pulmonary edema, hemoconcentration, increase in blood viscosity, hypernatremia, and myocardial anoxia. These factors all lead to heart failure and death. At autopsy, drowning as a cause of death is suggested by several findings. Water-dwelling microorganisms, such as diatoms, may be present in the tracheobronchial tree or in the blood. The cooling of the body occurs twice as fast in water as in air, or about 5°F per hour. Foam at the mouth or nostrils is from acute pulmonary edema. In drowning deaths, this foam presents as a white or pink balloon or mushroomlike mass, the "champignon de mousse."

The lungs of a drowned person are bulky or ballooned, have a doughy feel, pit on pressure, and are heavy. The picture has been described as "emphysema aquosum" or "emphysème hydroaérique" and is presumptive evidence of death by drowning. Emphysema aquosum is produced by aspiration of water, which stimulates the production of mucus by the respiratory epithelium. The ventilatory motion of the air in the bronchi and bronchioles churns up the mucus into a foam that ultimately acts as a check valve. Inspiratory motions bring air in, but expiratory efforts cannot expel the air, mucus, water, and foam.

INJURIES OF THE HEART

Penetrating Wounds of the Heart

Penetrating wounds of the heart are inflicted either by sharp instruments or by missiles. The majority of penetrating cardiac wounds result in serious hemorrhage, but an occasional laceration may be either too superficial or too small to produce significant bleeding. Approximately 60 per cent of the victims of penetrating cardiac injuries die from exsanguination into one of the pleural cavities. In the remaining 40 per cent, massive bleeding is prevented because the pericardial wound is sealed by clotted blood. If bleeding into the pericardium continues, intrapericardial pressure rises, compressing both ventricles during diastole. Ventricular filling is thus impaired, and stroke volume, or the blood ejected from both sides of the heart, is proportionately reduced. The hemodynamic result is referred to as cardiac tamponade and is manifested by low cardiac output, arterial hypotension (shock), and venous hypertension.

In penetrating cardiac wounds in which the pericardium does not become sealed, exsanguination usually occurs in a matter of minutes, and the victims do not reach a medical facility alive. In instances in which the pericardial wound seals itself, the patient usually presents in shock from cardiac tamponade. The triad for making this diagnosis is: (1) a penetrating wound anywhere in the chest or upper part of the abdomen, (2) arterial hypotension, and (3) venous hypertension in the absence of preexisting heart disease. Other signs of acute cardiac compression such as pulsus paradoxus, enlarged cardiac silhouette on x-ray, and low voltage on the electrocardiogram are helpful but not essential for establishing the diagnosis. A positive pericardial tap confirms the diagnosis.

The treatment of acute cardiac tamponade from penetrating injury is emergency thoracotomy, decompression of the pericardium, and suture repair of the myocardial wound. In a few institutions, penetrating heart wounds are treated by pericardiocentesis alone. The salvage rate with operative approach is in the vicinity of 70 per cent.

The right ventricle is the most commonly injured chamber; the left ventricle and the right and left atria follow in that order. In addition, the coronary arteries, the atrial or ventricular septae, the conduction system, and any one of the four heart valves can be involved.

Blunt Injury to the Heart

Blunt trauma to the heart is relatively infrequent. It is encountered mostly following steering-wheel injury in which the heart is compressed between the chest wall anteriorly and the rigid spine posteriorly. A blow on the chest with a heavy object can also damage the heart. Sudden compression or crushing trauma to the abdomen during cave-in accidents or falls from great heights also predispose to cardiac injury. At times the heart may be punctured by fractured ends of the ribs or sternum. Large explosions produce blast injuries of the heart.

The myocardial damage from blunt trauma ranges from superficial contusion to full-thickness rupture. In addition to the free wall of the ventricles or atria, the ventricular septum, the papillary muscles, the chordae tendineae, and the valve leaflets may be involved.

The most usual cardiac lesion caused by blunt trauma is myocardial contusion, and the damage ranges from the small and inconsequential to the massive and fatal. The diagnosis is suspected because of a history of trauma, electrocardiographic changes consistent with myocardial injury, and elevation of appropriate serum enzyme levels. The treatment and clinical course are similar to those after myocardial infarction from coronary artery disease. If the contusion is extensive, rupture, fibrosis, and aneurysm formation may follow.

Instantaneous rupture of the heart is rare, but nevertheless it is the most common form of lethal cardiac injury from blunt trauma. The right ventricle is the most common site of rupture. After that, the other cardiac chambers are involved with equal frequency. Cardiac rupture is usually discovered at autopsy, but an occasional patient, especially one with an atrial tear, may survive and reach a medical facility. These patients present with cardiac tamponade; early surgery could conceivably be lifesaving.

Rupture of the ventricular septum results in a left-to-right shunt. If there are no associated lethal lesions, the victim may survive. The mode of presentation depends on the size of the shunt; small ventricular septal defects, may be associated with impressive murmurs but are of little hemodynamic or clinical consequence, while large ventricular septal defects usually result in congestive cardiac failure.

Rarely, a papillary muscle, the chordae tendinae, or a valve leaflet may be injured during blunt trauma. More often than not, these lesions are associated with other lethal injuries and are discovered at autopsy as incidental findings. All these injuries lead to varying degrees of valvular insufficiency. The severity of the congestive heart failure is determined by the degree of valvular insufficiency. On rare occasions the pericardium ruptures from blunt trauma. If the defect is large enough, the heart may herniate and strangulate.

Electrocution

A form of violent death in which the heart is implicated is electrocution. In electrical shock or lightning, the danger is directly related to amperage, voltage, duration of contact, and the resistance of the skin. The mortality rate from electrical shock is reported at 5 to 50 per cent. It naturally varies with the type of shock. There is disagreement whether ventricular fibrillation or respiratory failure causes death, but the former mechanism is accepted by most. Salvage after hours of resuscitative effort has been reported. A physical sign of electrocution is the electric mark, joule burn, or endogenous thermal burn. Delayed effects of electrical injury include hemorrhage, gangrene, neurologic changes, and eye injuries.

GREAT VESSEL INJURIES

Blunt injuries of the intrathoracic great vessels are probably more common than penetrating ones.

Blunt Trauma

The intrathoracic great vessels are most commonly injured because of sudden deceleration in an automobile collision, a fall from a height, or an airplane crash. The injury results from the disparate speeds of a fixed and a mobile portion of the involved vessel. The fixed portion comes to an abrupt halt while the mobile segment continues on its course. A shearing force develops and disrupts the vessel. The thoracic aorta is involved with overwhelming frequency in this type of injury, while the arch vessels may also be affected, but less commonly.

Traumatic disruption of the thoracic aorta occurs most often at the aortic isthmus just distal to the origin of the left subclavian artery, where the aorta is fixed by the ligamentum arteriosum. Rarely, the disruption is at the aortic root or at the diaphragmatic aortic hiatus. Usually the vessel wall is circumferentially transected and the two ends retract and the victim dies from exsanguination. In a small percentage of cases, continuity of the vessel may be maintained by the adventitia, a mediastinal hematoma, and the mediastinal pleura. The lumen remains patent and blood flow to the organs distal to the transection site continues. If the traumatic aneurysm ruptures, immediate exsanguination follows.

The diagnosis of traumatic aortic disruption should be suspected in all cases of severe deceleration-type injury when the chest x-ray shows a widened mediastinum. A thoracic aortogram should be obtained immediately. This study either confirms or rules out the diagnosis with an almost absolute certainty. If traumatic transection of the aorta is present, immediate operation is indicated. The repair of a traumatic transection of the aorta usually consists of thoracotomy, proximal and distal control of the aorta, and interposition of a synthetic graft between the two retracted ends of the transected vessel.

Eighty-five per cent of patients sustaining traumatic aortic transections die within minutes of the injury from exsanguination. An additional 5 to 8 per cent succumb during transport and preparation for surgery. For the fortunate few who survive long enough to have an operation, the mortality rate is 5 to 20 per cent. Finally, in 2 to 3 per cent, the diagnosis is overlooked and the mediastinal hematoma organizes. Years later a calcified pseudoaneurysm may be discovered, to everybody's surprise, on a routine chest x-ray.

Avulsions or transections of the arch vessels due to deceleration injuries are rare. In general, the nature and mechanism of the lesion are similar to those described for aortic disruptions. A high index of suspicion should attend the absence or diminution of peripheral pulses coupled with a widened mediastinum seen on the chest x-ray and should lead to an arteriogram that confirms or denies the diagnosis. These lesions require prompt surgical repair.

Penetrating Trauma

Penetrating great vessel injuries may result from either missile or stab wounds. They may lead to massive hemorrhage. In a rare instance, however, a clot may temporarily seal the defect and stop the bleeding. The wound itself may vary from a clean, near-surgical type of stab wound to a jagged, large defect with loss of tissue substance. If the intrathoracic portion of the vessel is involved, the clinical presentation is massive hemothorax. Extrathoracic subclavian injuries usually present with a supraclavicular subcutaneous hematoma, distal pulses that may be normal or diminished or absent, and a to-and-fro bruit from an arteriovenous fistula. Injuries to the intrathoracic great vessels should be suspected whenever a penetrating chest wound presents with gross hemothorax and unrelenting bright red blood drainage from the chest tube. Although routine arteriography is advocated by some, frequently there is not enough time for such a diagnostic study and emergency thoracotomy is necessary to control the hemorrhage. With extrathoracic subclavian injuries the surrounding soft tissues may temporarily contain the bleeding, and contrast studies can be performed. Some traumatologists, however, recommend routine exploration of all suspected subclavian injuries without resorting to arteriography.

INJURIES OF THE ESOPHAGUS

Penetrating injuries of the thoracic esophagus are rare because of the small size of the organ and its protected position in the posterior paravertebral area. The cervical esophagus is in a more exposed location and therefore slightly more prone to be involved with penetrating injuries. Perforation of the esophagus during endoscopy occurs in less than 1 per cent of the examinations. Crushing injuries of the chest and abdomen are occasionally associated with esophageal perforation due to a sudden increase in intraluminal pressure. This type of injury may go unrecognized for days and be discovered only at autopsy. Foreign bodies frequently lodge in the esophagus, especially in children, elderly people, and psychotic patients. Blunt objects such as a poorly chewed meat bolus or a coin usually obstruct the lumen, whereas sharp or pointed items such as a fishbone or open safety pin may burrow through the wall and perforate it. Diagnosis is made from the history of ingestion of the object and symptoms of dysphagia or pain. Plain chest x-rays readily demonstrate radiopaque objects in the esophagus, whereas contrast swallow studies distinguish between obstruction and perforation. Certainly the patient with a perforated esophagus is much sicker and his condition more toxic than one with only an obstruction. The treatment is endoscopic removal if the foreign body is nonperforating. If the esophagus is perforated, operative intervention for retrieval of the foreign body, suture of the lacerated esophagus, and drainage of the mediastinum are necessary.

Caustic chemicals are ingested accidentally by children or during suicide attempts by adults and are responsible for varying degrees of burns and even perforation of the esophagus. The diagnosis is suspected from the history and the presence of burns in the mouth. Esophagoscopy to the area of the burn but not beyond is indicated to confirm the diagnosis. The pathologic changes consist of edema and inflammation of the tissues and thrombosis of the vessels. The mucosa may slough, and varying degrees of necrosis of the wall, up to full thickness, may take place. Healing is by cicatrization and reepithelization, and the final result may be a stricture. These burns are classified from first to fourth degree, corresponding to from minimal erythema to full-thickness destruction of the esophageal wall. Unfortunately it is not clearly established what constitutes the most effective treatment. Steroid therapy in combination with antibiotics or serial bougienage are employed most commonly. In a significant number of cases of corrosive esophagitis, strictures ultimately form, requiring dilatations or surgical reconstruction. The surgical procedures involved may be extensive, including esophagotomy, jejunal interposition, or colon by-pass. Many patients may require regular dilatations for years.

INJURIES OF THE DIAPHRAGM

Rupture of the diaphragm from blunt trauma is most commonly caused by deceleration-type injuries. In addition, a blow to the abdomen or chest, a crushing injury, or jackknifing of the body may cause a sudden increase in intraabdominal pressure and produce disruption of the diaphragm. The most common site of the tear is in the central portion of the left side of the diaphragm. Rupture may be followed by herniation of intraabdominal viscera through the defect into the thorax. The stomach, spleen, splenic flexure of the colon, and the left lobe of the liver are most frequently involved. If the diaphragmatic rupture is not repaired at the time of injury, a chronic hernia results with progressive ventilatory difficulty and intermittent bowel obstruction or strangulation. Occasionally, however, a traumatic diaphragmatic hernia may remain asymptomatic for years.

Diaphragmatic injuries are also sustained from penetrating trauma. Both leaves of the diaphragm are involved with approximately equal frequency, but herniation of abdominal viscera is more frequent with injuries of the left leaf. The possibility of diaphragmatic injury should be considered in all penetrating wounds of the lower thorax and upper abdomen, since there is usually no way to predict the exact pathway of any penetrating object.

Diaphragmatic injury should be suspected whenever a small irregularity in the contour of the diaphragm is seen on chest x-ray. With larger ruptures in the diaphragm, herniation of the abdominal viscera is commonplace; consequently the roentgenogram may show gas-filled stomach or intestine in the chest, decreased lung volume, obliteration or distortion of the diaphragmatic contour, or an actual air-fluid level in the chest consistent with a simple left hydropneumothorax. Insertion of a nasogastric tube makes it possible to outline the herniated viscera on the roentgenogram and verify the presence of a traumatic rupture of the diaphragm with gastric herniation. Furthermore, aspiration of the tube may change the gas pattern seen on chest x-ray. The treatment consists of operative exploration of the chest, reduction of the herniated viscera, and suture repair of the defect in the diaphragm. Although a transthoracic approach is usually preferable, occasionally the presence of associated injuries necessitates an abdominal or thoracoabdominal incision.

A chronic posttraumatic diaphragmatic hernia may first become evident weeks to years after the original injury. The patient develops either progressive respiratory insufficiency or intermittent or progressive gastrointestinal tract obstruction, most often involving the stomach or splenic flexure of the colon. The diagnosis is usually made from the history and appropriate plain and contrast radiologic study of the chest and gastrointestinal tract. Repair of a chronic posttraumatic diaphragmatic hernia is done by the same technique as that of the acute variety.

FOREIGN BODIES

Foreign bodies may lodge anywhere in the thorax. They can be ingested or aspirated, or can enter as missiles. Retained objects that enter the chest by penetration of the thoracic cage are usually bullets or missile fragments. If a thoracotomy is performed for treatment of the damage produced by a bullet wound, the foreign body is removed if it is readily accessible. The presence of a foreign body within the thorax, of itself, does not usually constitute an indication for thoracotomy for its removal. With time, the foreign body becomes encysted and fixed by fibrous tissue, precluding its migration. Thoracotomy is indicated, however, if a foreign body is in the vicinity of a major blood vessel, or if secondary symptoms or signs may be attributed to it, e.g., recurrent pneumonitis, abscess, hemoptysis, or atelectasis.

Aspiration of foreign bodies into the tracheobronchial tree occurs mainly in children, especially those aged one to three years. Peanuts, marbles, and pins are among the frequently aspirated items. Occasionally, an adult, debilitated or intoxicated, may aspirate a solid object into the tracheobronchial tree. Occlusive foreign bodies in the trachea are likely to cause death by asphyxiation. In the bronchi, total obstruction is followed by collapse and, frequently, by secondary pneumonia of the involved segment, lobe, or even lung. If the offending object is not removed, the affected pulmonary parenchyma may be completely destroyed through abscess formation and fibrosis. Partially occlusive foreign bodies in the airway may behave as one-way valves, allowing air to enter, but impeding exhalation. This type of air trapping causes hyperinflation of the lung. Organic foreign objects in the tracheobronchial tree absorb water, swell progressively, and once they attain a certain size become impacted in one location. Nonorganic materials, on the other hand, do not change size and, unless they are wedged, tend to move freely and cause paroxysms of coughing. The diagnosis is suspected from physical signs and radiologic evidence of collapse or hyperinflation in the involved lung. Confirmation of the diagnosis and treatment of foreign bodies in the tracheobronchial tree are carried out by bronchoscopy. Occasionally, transbronchoscopic removal may not be feasible; then thoracotomy and extraction by incision of the involved bronchus are required.

Foreign bodies within the cardiovascular system are usually bullets or missile fragments lodged in an artery, vein, or the heart. They may remain fixed at the site of penetration or embolize. Missiles entering veins embolize centrally through the right side of the heart and lodge in a pulmonary artery. At this site, they can remain innocuous or can cause a pulmonary infarct or abscess. Foreign bodies in the right ventricle can cause life-threatening arrhythmias and therefore should be removed. The indications for removal of objects from other sites in the lesser circulation, however, are not clearly defined. The procedure for extraction of foreign bodies may involve an operative approach. Alternatively, a variety of grasping instruments introduced through a peripheral vein and advanced into the great veins, the right side of the heart, or the proximal pulmonary arteries may be used to extract the foreign body. A significant degree of success has been obtained with these instruments, and the need for thoracotomy to remove foreign bodies from the right side of the circulation has been lessened.

Foreign bodies occasionally lodge within the heart itself. Fluoroscopy or even contrast dye study may be necessary to demonstrate the exact site of lodgment and the presence of any associated intracardiac pathologic changes. Recommendation for operation must be individualized. Possible sequelae of intracardiac foreign bodies are endocarditis and embolization.

If a missile embolizes to the arterial side of the circulation, it usually lodges at a point of bifurcation. In a gunshot injury, if no exit wound is found, the location of the bullet must be demonstrated by x-ray. Identification of the bullet at a site far removed from the entry wound may indicate distal embolization. A foreign body lying within an artery is clearly hazardous. The dangers include ischemia of the affected part, local infection, and delayed hemorrhage. Accordingly, these foreign bodies require surgical removal.

Air embolism to the right side of the heart and pulmonary arteries may occur after laceration of a large vein draining into the superior vena cava system. An increase in negative intrathoracic pressure sucks air through the opening; the air then migrates to the right side of the heart, where it causes mechanical obstruction of the right ventricular outflow tract and acute, severe, right ventricular distention, frequently with fatal consequences. Treatment of air embolization to the right side of the heart involves positioning the patient in a right lateral decubitus and head-down position. This maneuver displaces the air bolus from the outflow tract to the body of the right ventricle and thereby relieves the obstruction and restores pulmonary blood flow. Air may then be aspirated from the right side of the heart.

IATROGENIC THORACIC INJURIES

Modern medicine has become increasingly complex and aggressive. Invasive diagnostic and therapeutic procedures are employed with great frequency, and in this atmosphere, inconsequential as well as serious iatrogenic complications are encountered.

The incidence of catheter embolization has increased with the widespread use of plastic tubings for fluid infusion and venous pressure measurement. A host of different types of catheters available commercially have different degrees of propensity for breaking off inside the venous system. Once a portion of the catheter breaks from its extracorporeal connection it usually migrates centrally to lodge along its route in the great veins, the right side of the heart, or the pulmonary artery. More rarely, however, it may remain in a peripheral vein where it is accessible through a simple "cut down." Most of these catheters are radiopaque and can readily be located by roentgenograms. For centrally situated catheters, retrieval with specially designed grasping instruments through a transvenous nonoperative approach is clearly justified in all cases. If this method is without success, the indications for removal through thoracotomy are not clearly defined. It is generally agreed that catheters lodged in the right ventricle should be removed, since they can cause serious and lethal arrhythmias. Thoracotomy for removal of catheters lying in the distal pulmonary arteries is probably not justified, since they are unlikely to produce the serious problems of sizeable pulmonary infarction and local or systemic infections.

Perforation of any of the cardiac chambers may occur during cardiac catheterization. Implantation of a transvenous cardiac pacemaker may be associated with perforation of the right ventricle. Laceration of both ventricles and of the coronary arteries is encountered occasionally during pericardiocentesis, or from intracardiac injections of drugs during attempts at cardiopulmonary resuscitation. All these complications require close observation of the patient. In the rare instance when cardiac tamponade develops, it is usually managed successfully by pericardiocentesis alone. Occasionally operative decompression of the pericardium and suture repair of the cardiac wound is necessary.

Thoracentesis and percutaneous pleural or lung biopsy is occasionally complicated by hemo- or pneumothorax. Physical examination and a roentgenogram of the chest should be routine after any of these procedures. If a greater than 25 per cent pneumothorax or significant hemothorax is present, tube thoracotomy is indicated.

Rarely, insertion of a chest tube may, itself, be the cause of hemothorax, from laceration of an intercostal artery or other major vessels. With even lesser frequency, the trochar introducer may traverse the diaphragm and penetrate the liver, spleen, stomach, or colon. Awareness of the possibility of these mishaps should reduce their incidence to a minimum, and early recognition followed by appropriate therapy obviously decreases the seriousness of the complications. Intercostal artery aneurysms or intercostal arteriovenous fistulae have been reported to occur years after the occurrence of the injury.

A special note is in order about the complications of percutaneous subclavian vein catheterization, a procedure that is being practiced with steadily increasing frequency. It is fair to say that in experienced hands mishaps are minimal, but when the procedure is performed by the uninitiated, a host of complications are encountered. They include hemothorax, simple or tension pneumothorax, laceration of the subclavian artery, infusion of fluid or blood into the pleural space or mediastinum, pseudoaneurysm at the site of the puncture, and the like. Some of these complications are readily treatable, while others are more serious and potentially lethal. Percutaneous access to the subclavian vein is an important part of our therapeutic armamentarium, but the procedure should be performed with appropriate precautions and only by people who are proficient in the technique.

Perforation of the esophagus occurs in 1 per cent of esophagoscopies with the rigid esophagoscope and in 0.25 per cent of the procedures performed with the flexible fiberoptic scope. The most common sites of perforation are at the cricopharyngeus, at the diaphragmatic esophageal hiatus, and at the site of an obstructive lesion. The esophagus can also be perforated during bougienage and pneumatic dilatations. Involvement of the thoracic esophagus is far more serious than that of the cervical portion. Treatment consists of general supportive measures, antibiotics, drainage, and surgical closure, especially with perforations of the thoracic esophagus. Diversional or even resectional operations may be required when significant esophageal disease, such as neoplasm, achalasia, or stricture is present.

SELECTED READINGS

Adelson, L.: A microscopic study of dermal gunshot wounds. Am. J. Clin. Pathol., *35*:393, 1961.

Alfano, G. S., and Hale, H. W., Jr.: Pulmonary contusion. J. Trauma, *5*:647, 1965.

Battersby, J. S., and Kilman, J. W.: Traumatic injuries of the tracheobronchial tree. Arch. Surg., *88*:644, 1964.

Beall, A. C., Jr., Patrick, T. A., Okier, J. E., Bricker, D. L., and DeBakey, M. E.: Penetrating wounds of the heart: changing patterns of surgical management. J. Trauma, *12*:468, 1972.

Blades, B.: Ruptured diaphragm. Am. J. Surg., *105*:501, 1963.

Blair, E., Topuzlu, C., and Deane, R. S.: Major blunt chest trauma. Curr. Probl. Surg., May, 1969.

Bland, E. F., and Beebe, G. W.: Missiles in the heart. N. Engl. J. Med., *274*:1039, 1966.

Bloomfield, D. A.: Technique of nonsurgical retrieval of iatrogenic foreign bodies from the heart. Am. J. Cardiol., *27*:538, 1971.

Bogedain, W., Carpathios, J., Van Suu, D., and Moots, M. F.: Traumatic rupture of myocardium. J.A.M.A., *197*:1102, 1966.

Cohen, H., and Biskind, G. R.: Pathologic aspects of atmospheric blast injuries in man. Arch. Pathol., *42*:12, 1946.

Cordice, J. W. V., Jr., and Cabezon, J.: Chest trauma with pneumothorax and hemothorax. J. Thorac. Cardiovasc. Surg., *50*:316, 1965.

DeCandole, C. A.: Blast injury. Can. Med. Assoc. J., *96*:207, 1967.

DeMuth, W. E., Jr., Baue, A. E., and Odom, J. A., Jr.: Contusions of the heart. J. Trauma, 7:443, 1967.

Huller, T., and Bazini, Y.: Blast injuries of the chest and abdomen. Arch. Surg., *100*:24, 1970.

Inkley, S. R., and Barry, F. M.: Traumatic rupture of interventricular septum proved by cardiac catheterization. Circulation, *18*:916, 1958.

Jones, F. L., Jr.: Transmural myocardial necrosis after non-

penetrating cardiac trauma. Am. J. Cardiol., *26*:419, 1970.
Levine, R. J., Roberts, W. C., and Morrow, A. G.: Traumatic aortic regurgitation. Am. J. Cardiol., *10*:752, 1962.
Meyer, J. A., and Millar, K.: Perforation of the right ventricle by electrode catheters. Ann. Surg., *168*:1048, 1968.
Randolph, H., Melick, D. W., and Grant, A. R.: Perforation of the esophagus from external trauma or blast injuries. Dis. Chest, *51*:121, 1967.
Reul, G. J., Jr., Mattox, K. L., Beall, A. C., Jr., and Jordan, G. L., Jr.: Recent advances in the operative management of massive chest trauma. Ann. Thorac. Surg., *16*:52, 1973.
Spencer, F. C., Guerin, P. F., Blake, H. A., and Bahnson, H. T.: A report of fifteen patients with traumatic rupture of the thoracic aorta. J. Thorac. Cardiovasc. Surg., *41*:1, 1961.
Sugg, W. L., Rea, W. J., Ecker, R. R., Webb, W. R., Rose, E. F., and Shaw, R. R.: Penetrating wounds of the heart. J. Thorac. Cardiovasc. Surg., *56*:531, 1968.

VIII. The Liver, Pancreas, Spleen and Gallbladder

by Frederick W. Ackroyd

Since the origins of recorded history, abdominal trauma has had dire implications for survival. Like the Greek warrior at the walls of Troy, the American Marine in Vietnam wore body armor to minimize the effects of this dreaded event. Today seat belts are to auto collisions what athletic equipment is to sporting events. Whatever the cause of the trauma, the results are the same: grievously injured victims require prompt enlightened care to avoid catastrophic end results. Deaths are occurring every day, in many different settings, from injuries to the upper abdomen and lower rib cage that produce damage to the liver, spleen, and pancreas. Which organ or combination of organs is affected is determined by the location and severity of the blow and the position of the victim when injured. These are life-threatening injuries. The stakes are high for the patient, and the demands on the surgical team are great. It is axiomatic that the early recognition and effective management of these injuries are essential for survival and the prevention of far-reaching complications.

The history of the management of abdominal trauma from Greek and Roman times until the development of anesthesia in the nineteenth century was characterized by a conservative, nonoperative approach. Baudens, in 1836, was the first to report the survival of a patient with gunshot wound of the upper abdomen who was treated by a "Bold Operation."[1] The debate concerning nonoperative management versus more aggressive surgical exploration turned on the fact that in the latter part of the nineteenth century, the mortality rate from exploration of the abdomen alone was about 75 per cent to 80 per cent, yet only about 50 per cent of the penetrating wounds were associated with visceral organ injuries that would benefit from exploration, and so the risks of exploration were greater than those of the trauma itself.[2]

In 1899, during the Boer War, the British Medical Service abandoned an earlier policy of operating on casualties with penetrating abdominal injuries because those who were operated on had a higher mortality rate than those who were not. It was not until the early phases of World War I, with improvements in surgical anesthesia and antiseptics, that the bulk of opinion favored operative intervention. It was also at this time that larger-caliber and higher-velocity missiles were introduced to trench warfare, and these were associated with a staggeringly high mortality rate. Surgical intervention in the latter phases of World War I reduced the death rate for abdominal wounds from 85 to 56 per cent. The military casualty statistics of ensuing conflicts reflect the improvements in management of these penetrating abdominal injuries with aggressive techniques.[3] The death rate from penetrating abdominal wounds in World War I was 56 per cent; in World War II, 25 per cent; in the Korean War, 12 per cent; and in the Vietnam Conflict, 10 per cent.[4]

GENERAL CONSIDERATIONS

The goals of exploration are (1) control of hemorrhage, (2) repair or removal of damaged organs, (3) evacuation and drainage of hematomas, and (4) cleansing of the contaminated peritoneal cavity of chemical and bacterial soiling to avoid subsequent severe sepsis and abscess formation. Surgery should be carried out as soon as it is obvious or suspected that there has been injury to one of the intraabdominal viscera and the patient is deteriorating. A blow severe enough to tear the spleen may also have fractured the pancreas or torn the fourth portion of the duodenum; therefore a thorough abdominal exploration is essential to rule out other injuries. Beware of the patient with lower rib fractures on either side. A compression injury severe enough to fracture ribs exerts tremendous force on the underlying organs and can produce tears of the splenic capsule on the left side or of the liver parenchyma on the right side, or fracture of the body of the pancreas and tear of the duodenal wall in the midabdomen. Replacement of third-space sequestration losses must be aggressively attended to both before and after surgery. They are sure to occur because of the chemical and enzymatic irritation caused by the extravasation of digestive juices into the surrounding tissues after injury to the organs where they are produced. A study of abdominal trauma in 301 severely injured patients from the Detroit General Hospital revealed the presence of splenic injury in 30 per cent, hepatic injury in 19 per cent, and pancreatic injury in 9 per cent.[5] Protocols for dealing with injuries to individual organs and regions of the abdomen that have evolved from the experience in the military combat zones and civilian trauma centers deserve individual attention so that the most favorable outcome will be achieved.

MULTIPLE SYSTEM INJURIES

The full extent of injuries must be accurately appraised early in the management of a casualty. Associated injuries of the thorax, diaphragm, lungs, heart, and great vessels must be identified and, therefore, must be thought of and looked for. The trajectory of a penetrating missile or the location and direction of blunt trauma as surmised from bruises, fractured ribs or vertebrae or pelvic bones, and wounds of exit and entry are important clues in the search for the extent of injury. Often the site of bleeding or the location of pain as perceived by the patient will distract the attention of medical personnel away from other more devastating unsuspected injuries. Thoracic through-and-through missile wounds can crease the domes of the diaphragm, lacerating either the liver or spleen or stomach, particularly if the victim was in a crouched position when hit. Sometimes, unless the injury is suspected initially, no clues are available to suggest this diagnosis until bile is observed coming out of the patient's chest tube, or peritoneal irritation develops and he bleeds into shock with the passage of time.

In those patients with head, thoracic, abdominal, or extremity wounds, a system of priorities must be established. Two or three teams of specialists may be involved, working simultaneously to increase the diagnostic efficiency and shorten the duration of anesthesia. A multidisciplinary approach is to be preferred, with the most life-threatening injuries taking precedence over others.

Injury to both liver and spleen in the same patient is rather unusual because these organs are located on opposite sides of the abdomen, but it does occur, particularly in through-and-through missile wounds, and requires urgent intervention because both are vascular organs and exsanguinating hemorrhage will occur unless control by splenectomy and surgical suture or lobectomy of the liver is carried out. The spleen and the body and tail of the pancreas may be injured together; injury to one requires inspection of the other lest an associated injury be overlooked.

Patients with splenic rupture bleed to death. Patients with severe liver rupture involving major vessels in the liver may bleed to death, but they also run the risk of severe protracted sepsis and subphrenic abscesses from collections of bile and infected hematomas under the diaphragm. Pancreatic injuries produce delayed septic and hemorrhagic problems, sometimes a number of days after the injury. Pancreatic pseudocyst, lesser sac abscess with pancreatic necrosis and peritonitis, and finally massive bleeding from hemorrhagic pancreatitis may sometimes occur despite the best of care and often occur without it.

INJURY TO SPECIFIC ORGANS

Spleen

In those patients with blunt trauma of the upper abdomen and fractured ribs on the left, beware of a ruptured spleen. It is the intraabdominal organ most frequently injured in blunt trauma. In those patients in whom only the spleen is involved, the mortality rate is around 2 per cent, but with other organs involved, the mortality rate can rise to around 10 per cent. The injury can result from athletic contests, fights, or falls from horses or bicycles. Delayed rupture of the spleen can occur up to about two weeks after the injury; it has, however, been reported as late as six months after the trauma.[6]

The diagnosis is made from the signs and symptoms of blood loss as well as peritoneal irritation from the presence of blood in the abdomen. Pain due to associated rib fractures and pain radiating to the top of the left shoulder occur in about 20 per cent of the patients. Abdominal pain, nausea and vomiting, and hypotension constitute the most frequent combination of symptoms seen. Laboratory studies may reveal a high white cell count, but the hematocrit and hemoglobin values may not accurately reflect the intraperitoneal hemorrhage for a matter of hours, and frequently do not accurately reflect the degree of hypovolemia (blood loss) caused by the rapid bleeding associated with splenic rupture.

X-ray studies may reveal fractures of the lower left ribs and scalloping of the gastric shadow along the greater curve where the hemorrhage has extravasated along the short gastric arteries, causing an extraluminal hematoma on the gastric wall. When there is a question of delayed rupture or a slow leak from the capsule, angiography can often be helpful by revealing subcapsular hematomas or extravasation of dye. Isotope scintiscanning may reveal an abnormal splenic contour due to subcapsular hematoma; this technique is not as invasive as angiography but sometimes not as accurate. Whenever splenic injury is strongly suspected, exploratory laparotomy is indicated, and the spleen should be removed if damaged. A most important principle in the management of suspected splenic injury is careful observation over a period of time with serial hematocrit determinations and vital sign and vital function measurements so that the signs of hemorrhage and hypovolemia can be picked up early and exploration undertaken promptly before irreversible hemorrhagic shock occurs. The combination of left upper quadrant tenderness, peritoneal irritation, and left shoulder pain and a bloody tap obtained by abdominal paracentesis in two locations are the hallmarks of a ruptured spleen and mandatory indications for abdominal exploration.

The spleen is occasionally injured during needle aspiration of fluid from the left chest cavity for diagnostic purposes in cases of pleural effusion of unknown etiology or for therapeutic reasons in congestive heart failure patients who are having severe difficulty breathing. Usually there is an elevated diaphragm and the tap is carried through the diaphragm and into the spleen in search of fluid. With respiratory movements and a needle fixed at the intercostal space, tears occur across the splenic capsule and parenchyma, producing severe bleeding. Aspiration of ascites in the left subcostal and left lateral abdominal region of the peritoneal cavity for diagnostic purposes, when malignancy is suspected, may sometimes penetrate an enlarged spleen, tear the capsule, and produce hemorrhage.

The injection of radiopaque dye into the splenic pulp, a splenoportogram, is occasionally carried out as a mean of studying the portal venous system in preparation for surgically constructing a portosystemic shunt to relieve portal hypertension. Not all splenic punctures continue to bleed, but all must be followed carefully, and splenectomy is indicated whenever evidence of continued bleeding occurs.

Following splenectomy there is often a rebound rise in the platelet counts from normal levels of about 200,000 to levels of 750,000 or more. If the platelet count rises over one million, it is thought that anticoagulation with heparin, or salicylate therapy, or both may be indicated to prevent thrombotic complications. The level of platelets eventually drifts down to normal levels over weeks or months and the anticoagulation therapy can be discontinued.

Liver

Patients with blunt abdominal trauma and fractured lower ribs on the right or penetrating injury in the right upper quadrant have a high probability of liver injury. Because of its large size, extending as it does from the fourth interspace on the right, sometimes down into the iliac crest, the liver is a very commonly injured intraperitoneal organ. At the Detroit General Hospital between 1961 and 1971, mortality rates for patients with liver injuries were: stab wounds, 2.4 per cent; gunshot wounds, 16.7 per cent, and blunt trauma, 29.7 per cent. Simple lacerations from knife wounds not involving major vessels rarely require much surgical intervention. Wounds from small-caliber missiles of low kinetic energy involving peripheral liver tissues also require little surgical intervention. Stab wounds involving major vessels in the hilum or the major hepatic veins near the diaphragm, however, or high kinetic energy missile wounds producing an implosion effect with destruction of large areas of liver architecture, require exploration of the liver injury and control of the major vessel disruption. The cause of death in such cases is exsanguinating hemorrhage, and local suture or ligation of major vessels may be instrumental in controlling this hemorrhage. In the event that a large-scale disruption of a lobe has occurred, lobectomy may be the only means of controlling major vessel injury deep in the hepatic parenchyma, particularly in the region of the liver hilum or the hepatic veins under the diaphragm.

The patient who presents with right lower rib fractures, hypotension, tenderness in the right upper quadrant, and evidence of peritoneal irritation (blood in peritoneal lavage or abdominal paracentesis) requires mandatory exploration. Like those with a ruptured spleen, these patients die from exsanguinating hemorrhage, and the overriding concern is to stop the massive bleeding that this very vascular organ can produce. The postoperative convalescence of patients with liver injury is characterized by sepsis that is usually due to infection of devitalized liver tissue or infection of intrahepatic or subdiaphragmatic hematomas. Subsequent drainage of septic collections is frequently necessary, but these patients usually survive the septic complications of liver injury.

Injury to the diaphragm is common among patients with liver injury as well as among those with splenic injury, and a careful inspection of the diaphragm must be included in the abdominal exploration for injury of these two organs. A careful documentation of the wound of entry and the wound of exit for penetrating wounds and an identification of the location and direction of the blunt trauma is extremely helpful in determining the presence or absence of liver and spleen injury. Selective hepatic angiography, like selective splenic artery angiography, is frequently helpful in identifying the injury and its extent. If there is reasonable suspicion of hepatic injury, exploration should be carried out to rule out gallbladder rupture, bile duct disruption, or major vessel bleeding (which frequently goes on to exsanguination). If a patient with hepatic injury and upper abdominal penetrating wounds is to undergo exploration, care must be taken to rule out pneumothorax or pulmonary parenchymal injury on the same side lest a tension pneumothorax occur during endotracheal anesthesia for the abdominal exploration and produce cardiovascular collapse. In severe, unremitting bleeding, ligation of the hepatic artery should be considered, and packing of the hepatic injury may be necessary to control it if it is persistent. If a major vessel is injured, this vessel will have to be controlled. Formal hepatic lobectomy, except in experienced hands, carries a high risk because it produces further hemorrhage in an already hypovolemic patient. In order to get the damaged and bleeding liver segment or lobe out, however, it may, in desperate situations, be the only effective means of controlling major vessel injury deep in the right or left lobe of the liver.

Percutaneous needle biopsy of the liver is a well-established means of diagnosing various types of liver disease as well as the nature of metastatic liver nodules. Post needle biopsy hemorrhage occurs but usually will stop if the clotting factors are within normal limits. Patients with thrombocytopenia associated with hypersplenism of portal cirrhosis and portal hypertension are a greater risk, as are patients with hepatitis or cirrhotic patients with deranged clotting factors. In these cases attention to restoring the diminished clotting mechanism will prevent bleeding problems. Open liver biopsy by means of mini-laparotomy in the right upper quadrant over the liver, utilizing direct vision and suturing of the biopsy site, is thought to be safer than closed percutaneous needle biopsy in these high-risk cases.

Gallbladder

Gallbladder injuries are best treated with cholecystectomy or, if the anatomy is disrupted and there are widespread hematomas, cholecystostomy. Common duct disruptions should be carefully closed with interrupted synthetic suture material over a T-tube that is then left in place for at least six weeks. Portal vein injuries must be repaired, and hepatic artery injuries should be reanastomosed wherever feasible, but if this is not possible, ligation seems to be well tolerated.

Pancreas

Pancreatic injury is rarely an isolated phenomenon and is usually associated with injuries to adjacent organs such as the duodenum. The pancreas as a rule tolerates injury poorly. Local injuries such as a biopsy site or small penetrating knife wound may evolve into a large pseudocyst or pancreatic abscess, and larger, more profound injuries such as fractures or large-scale disruptions may evolve into massive hemorrhagic pancreatitis and death from exsanguination. The unforgiving nature of pancreatic injuries is related to the powerful digestive enzymes, which digest the pancreatic lobules with devastating consequences. The objectives of management are early diagnosis and surgical treatment designed to control the flow of these enzymes and remove severely contused and devitalized tissues. Because the pancreas lies across the vertebral column, it is fixed in position and thus trapped by compressing abdominal trauma. Fractures frequently occur across the midportion of the body of the gland at the junction of the head and tail. The duct system is disrupted, and extravasated enzymes produce an extensive retroperitoneal phlegmon with fat necrosis and abscess formation, and digest surrounding tissues. Implosive missile injuries that destroy pancreatic parenchyma have devastating consequences and, unless resected early, almost invariably evolve into hemorrhagic pancreatitis and exsanguination. Pancreatic injuries are associated with a large-scale fluid sequestration and third-space loss. Vasoactive substances that are metabolic by-products of the enzymatic breakdown of the substrate of pancreatic tissues may result in far-reaching hemodynamic changes, characterized by severe vasodilation, hypotension, and reduced perfusion of vital organs. The main causes of death in these patients are exsanguinating hemorrhage and sepsis. The pancreatic pseudocyst can be later drained, and pancreatic fistulae can be controlled. Sepsis can be drained in stages, but hemorrhage seems to be the final common pathway in the severely injured patients who develop hemorrhagic pancreatitis and die.

The most helpful diagnostic clue to pancreatic injury is an elevation of the serum amylase level. When pancreatic injury is suspected and exploration carried out, a thorough inspection of the lesser sac is absolutely essential and requires dividing the greater omentum near the greater curve of the stomach as well as a wide Kocher maneuver of the duodenum to inspect the head and uncinate process of the pancreas. These procedures also permit a careful inspection of the vena cava, aorta, both renal fossae, and the superior mesenteric vessels to rule out injury to them.

Surgical management again should be individualized and depend on the extent of the injury. When there has been minor injury to the pancreas, widespread drainage and resection of a contused tail is indicated; when there is widespread disruption of the architecture of the gland, a wide resection of destroyed tissues may be necessary.

Biliary tract decompression with some type of intubation such as a small T-tube in the common bile duct is thought to be helpful because the secretory pressure in the biliary tree is higher than in the pancreatic duct system and, with edema of the ampulla of Vater, bile may be forced into the injured pancreatic duct system, further aggravating the autodigestion of the pancreas.

Internal drainage of a fractured segment of proximal pancreas after the distal fragment has been resected can be accomplished with a Roux-en-Y technique. When the head of the pancreas has been shattered with concomitant duodenal injury, a pancreaticoduodenectomy is indicated. Pancreatic fistulae can be temporarily controlled with drainage, and should they fail to close, a Roux-en-Y patch technique can be used to drain them internally. All variations of surgical treatment are possible, depending upon the degree of injury of the pancreas, but when widespread injury to the pancreas has occurred, aggressive resection probably offers the best chance for survival of the patient.[8]

Pancreatic insufficiency resulting from resection of a portion of the gland is rare, and oral supplements are available in the event that it occurs. Insulin deficiency is also rare and, if necessary, can be replaced with exogenous insulin. The major complications of pancreatic injury are fistulae, pseudocysts, abscesses, and hemorrhage. Of these, hemorrhage seems to be the most lethal, with the other complications responding well to staged surgical intervention.

SUMMARY

Trauma to the upper abdomen in which the liver, spleen, pancreas, or adjacent viscera are damaged is a dangerous and grievous injury requiring prompt, highly individualized surgical treatment. Metabolic antibiotic support and staged surgical intervention are essential for survival of these patients. Approximately half the patients with duodenal injury, for example, have associated pancreatic injury, and association of pancreatic injury with duodenal injury raises the mortality rate from 5 per cent to 40 per cent.

It is sometimes extremely difficult to make the diagnosis of injury to these organs immediately after the trauma, but delays in diagnosis result in a tremendous increase in the mortality and morbidity rates associated with them. Duodenal injuries operated upon within the first 24 hours after admission had a 5 per cent mortality rate in one series. In those cases in which a 24-hour or greater delay occurred, in another series, a 65 per cent mortality rate was reported. When catastrophic injuries are involved, timely and aggressive remedies are required or the patient is lost.

REFERENCES

1. Loria, F. L.: Collective review—historical aspects of penetrating wounds of the abdomen. Internatl. Abst. Surg., *87*:521, 1948.
2. Loria, F. L.: *Historical Aspects of Abdominal Injuries.* Springfield, Ill., Charles C Thomas, 1968, pp. 134–138.
3. Anderson, C. B., and Ballinger, W. B.: Abdominal injuries. In *The Management of Trauma.* Edited by W. B. Ballinger, R. B. Rutherford, and G. D. Zuidema. Philadelphia, W. B. Saunders Co., 1973, pp. 396–397.
4. Pridgen, J. E., Herff, A. F., Jr., Watkins, H. O., Halbert, D. S., D'Avila, R., Crouch, D. M., and Prud'Homme, J. L.: Penetrating wounds of the abdomen: analysis of 776 operative cases. Ann. Surg., *165*:901, 1967.
5. Walt, A. J., and Grifka, T.: Blunt abdominal trauma: a review of 301 cases. In: *Impact Injury and Crash Protection.* Edited by E. S. Gurdjian, W. A. Lange, W. M. Patrick, and L. M. Thomas. Springfield, Ill., Charles C Thomas, 1970.
6. Shirkey, A. L., Wukasch, D. C., Beall, A. C., Jr., Gordon, W. B., and DeBakey, M. E.: Surgical management of splenic injuries. Am. J. Surg., *108*:630, 1964.
7. Ackroyd, F. W., Pollard, J., and McDermott, W. V., Jr.: Massive hepatic resection in the treatment of severe liver trauma. Presented, New England Surgical Society, September, 1968. Am. J. Surg., *117*:442, 1969.
8. Northrup, W. R., III, and Simmons, R. L.: Pancreatic trauma: a review. Surgery, *71*:27, 1972.

IX. Gastrointestinal Tract

by Herbert B. Hechtman

The progress of civilization has been an important factor in determining the prevalence of agents most likely to induce injuries to the gastrointestinal tract. During periods of peace, crush wounds, blunt trauma, and automotive deceleration injuries assume prominence in suburban surroundings. In large cities automotive speed limits reduce the incidence of blunt injury, while the availability of knives and hand guns makes penetrating injuries of the abdomen commonplace.

The gunshot wounds of civilian life are caused by medium- to low-velocity projectiles, in distinction to the destructive wounds from the high velocity missiles of modern warfare. An example of the latter is seen in the case of a 19-year-old infantryman who suffered a gunshot wound of the left side of the chest. The 1.5-cm wound at the point of entry was high in the left portion of the epigastrium, and there was a 15-cm exit wound in the posterior axillary line at the level of the left sixth rib. Radiologic examination showed fractures of the fifth to seventh ribs and hemopneumothorax on the left. The abdomen was silent and rigid. After insertion of a thoracostomy tube, exploratory laporatomy revealed approximately 1 liter of intraperitoneal blood, a ruptured spleen, and four small holes in the splenic flexure of the colon. The diaphragm was intact. Injury to the abdominal organs was related to the concussive force of the bullet and the perpendicular dissipation of energy far beyond the trajectory of the bullet. Civilian low-velocity bullet wounds produce destruction in a region much more confined to the trajectory of the bullet.*

DIAGNOSIS OF GASTROINTESTINAL INJURY

The diagnosis of injury to the gastrointestinal tract may at times be extremely difficult. Most surgeons routinely explore a gunshot wound of the abdomen. It is anticipated that in 15 to 20 per cent of these explorations the findings will be negative and in fewer than 1 per cent will be falsely negative.[1] Intestinal perforations when they are missed usually result in a fatality. The overall mortality rate of civilian gunshot wounds is 13 per cent. If the injury is restricted to the stomach and small intestine the mortality rate is less than 3 per cent.[1]

Other forms of injuries, stab wounds and blunt trauma, offer more of a diagnostic challenge. The diagnosis of bowel injury is based on the usual findings associated with damage to abdominal viscera. These include abdominal pain, signs of peritoneal irritation, absence of bowel sounds, a positive abdominal tap, and abdominal x-rays showing ileus. Occasionally the x-rays show free air in the peritoneal cavity. The absence of these findings, however, does not exclude bowel injury.

*The amount of kinetic energy or work that a bullet will dissipate in coming to rest is $\frac{1}{2}\ mv^2$, where m is mass and v is velocity. Thus, if one doubles velocity, kinetic energy is quadrupled.

Several additional diagnostic techniques may be employed. In stab wounds, proof that the instrument has entered the peritoneal cavity may be obtained by an x-ray study of the wound, a sinogram, using contrast material. Positive results usually lead to operative exploration; negative results require continued close patient observation to guard against an error in diagnosis.

A second diagnostic technique that has been popularized in the past few years is peritoneal lavage. Blunt abdominal trauma is often complicated by the presence of associated multiple system injury. Head trauma in particular limits the value of the history and physical examination. Diagnostic needle paracentesis is the first procedure advocated for routine use in blunt abdominal trauma. A negative result, that is, an absence of bloody return, calls for peritoneal lavage. In one large series, lavage yielded 3.5 per cent false positive results and 3.1 per cent false negative results.[2] The complication rate was 4.5 per cent. Another series showed 1 per cent false positive results, 2 per cent false negative results, and a complication rate of 1 per cent.[3]

A somewhat more aggressive approach is advocated in cases of blunt abdominal trauma in children.[4] Regardless of test results, surgical exploration is advocated if any suspicion of intraperitoneal injury exists or if the patient is difficult to evaluate. A negative result rate of 10 per cent for exploration is considered reasonable.[5] Injuries to children have increased by 250 per cent in the most recent decade, with 68 per cent being in the five- to nine-year-old group. Bicycle handlebar injuries have become extremely common.

A large review of patients suffering blunt abdominal trauma has shown that the overall mortality rate is 9 per cent.[6] Thirteen per cent of these fatalities are related to the gastrointestinal tract.

SEAT BELT SYNDROME

Seat belts save lives but may themselves be responsible for a characteristic pattern of injury.[7, 8] With abrupt deceleration, the seat belt compresses the contents of the abdominal cavity. There follows an explosive action within this cavity that causes rupture of musculature and often of the left hemidiaphragm. In addition, shear forces lead to bowel injury. Applied against adjacent structures, such forces cause bowel transection, particularly near points of fixation, such as the ileocecal valve and the ligament of Treitz. One author has reported four patients with colonic injuries secondary to shearing of the intestine between the vertebral bodies and the anterior abdominal wall.[9] This injury is more apt to occur if the patient is sitting on a soft seat or if the belt is applied loosely. In addition to abdominal wall contusions and intraabdominal visceral injuries, the seat belt may cause a fracture of the lumbar spine.[10] The presence of any of these injuries recommends a search for the others.

INJURIES OF THE STOMACH AND DUODENUM

High-speed motor vehicle accidents account for the increasing incidence of blunt abdominal trauma to the upper gastrointestinal tract. It is now well documented that impact against the steering wheel is the main cause of hollow viscus injury proximal to the ligament of Treitz. The protection afforded the stomach by the rib cage and the mobility of the stomach itself make injuries of that organ exceedingly rare. Up until 1936 only 68 cases of gastric rupture had been reported in the world's literature.[11]

The trauma necessary to rupture the stomach may be severe or trivial. One case occurred in a 25-year-old woman who simply had done 10 push-ups.[12] Two types of gastric injury are of clinical importance. The first is laceration of the mucosa, which causes hematemesis and may occur following closed chest cardiac massage.[13] The second is transmural perforation whose clinical presentation is similar to that of a perforated peptic ulcer. Combined injuries, particularly severe central nervous system injury, may mask all abdominal signs and symptoms. It is under these circumstances that routine peritoneal tap and lavage are of benefit. Other diagnostic tests include nasogastic aspiration, Gastrografin x-ray studies of the stomach, and gastroscopy.

Duodenal injuries from blunt trauma may be divided into two categories: intramural hematoma and rupture. The fixed position of the duodenum against the lumbar spine makes it susceptible to a crushing force directed anteroposteriorly, or to a shearing force applied tangentially.[12] In addition, a blowout may occur if the pylorus is closed and the duodenojejunal angle acutely flexed.[14] The majority of injuries are caused by the steering wheel or by a blow or kick to the upper abdomen.

The onset of signs and symptoms may be delayed for hours or days. An intramural duodenal hematoma is often an isolated lesion. It may manifest itself as pain and tenderness in the right upper quadrant. Occasionally a mass is palpable, and if the ampulla of Vater is obstructed there is jaundice. As 90 per cent of duodenal perforations are retroperitoneal, most patients complain not only of abdominal but also of back and flank pain. Plain x-rays show retroperitoneal air (Fig. 3–IX–1). Gastrografin studies are helpful in localization of the injury (Fig. 3–IX–2). Once the diagnosis of duodenal injury is made, an operative exploration is usually required. The rare exception in which conservative management may be considered is an intramural hematoma. Many authors, however, argue for surgical evacuation of this blood.[12]

INJURIES OF THE SMALL BOWEL

The vast majority of intestinal injuries result from automobile accidents and impact against the steering wheel. Approximately 5 to 10 per cent of patients with blunt abdominal trauma suffer injuries of the small bowel, and the portion most often injured is that which occupies a midline position at the moment of impact.[15] One mechanism of injury involves crushing of the bowel, usually against the lumbosacral spine.[16] A second mechanism of injury involves shearing of the bowel and its mesentery at points of fixation. The most common sites are the first portion of the jejunum and the terminal portion of the ileum. Pathologic fixation of the bowel by adhesions from previous surgery or fixation within a hernial sac have also led to perforations.[17] Bursting of a distended or

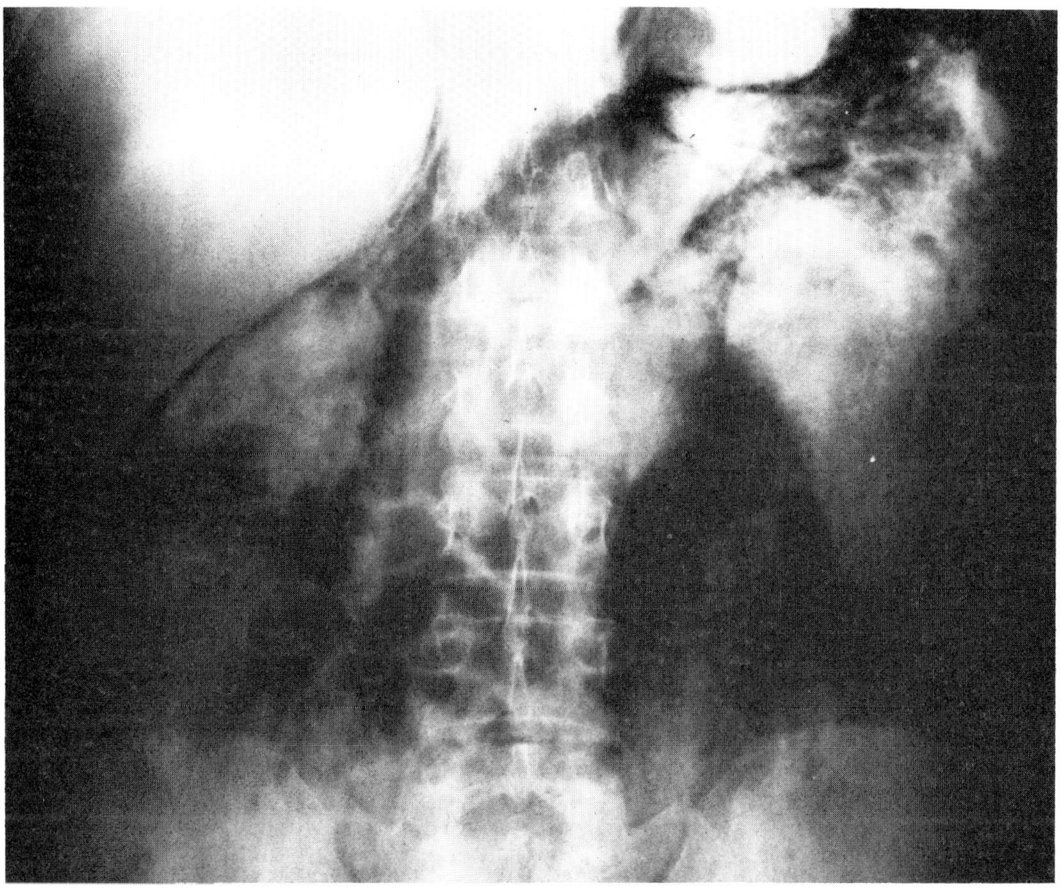

Figure 3–IX–1. Plain film of the abdomen demonstrates retroperitoneal air whose source was the retroperitoneal colon. Duodenal injuries may demonstrate a similar appearance. The air dissects around and outlines the kidneys and pancreas. (From M. Burrell, R. Toffler, and R. Lowman: Blunt trauma to the abdomen and gastrointestinal tract. Radiol. Clin. North Am., *11*:561, 1973. Reprinted by permission.)

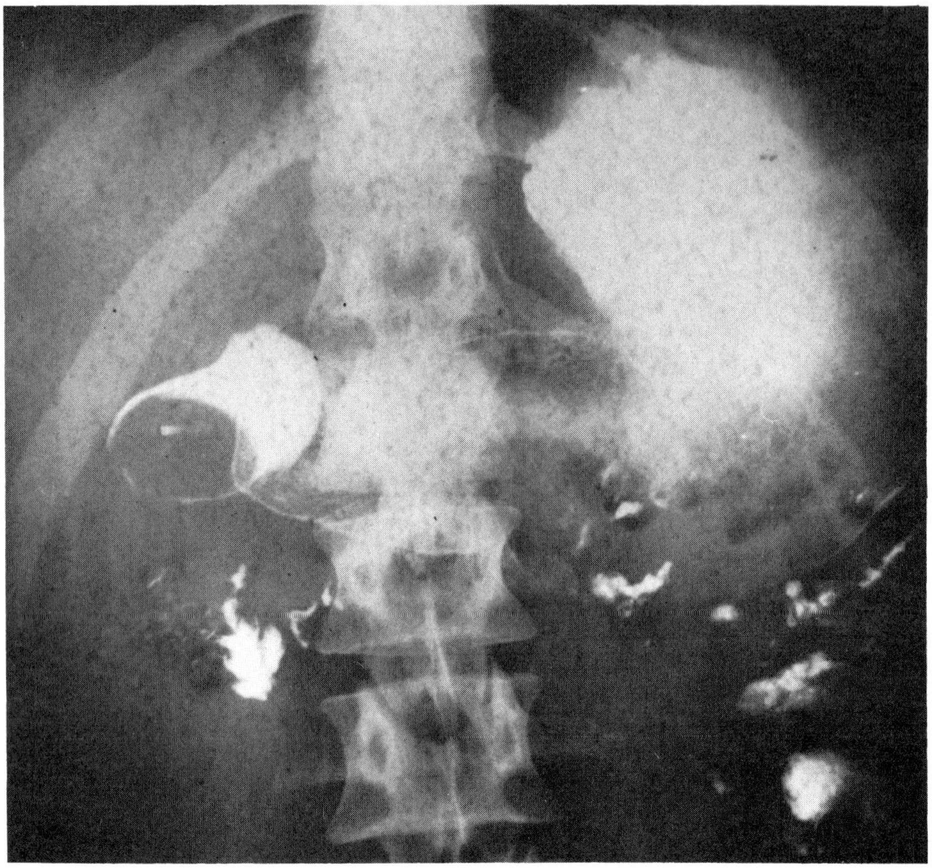

Figure 3–IX–2. This upper gastrointestinal contrast study demonstrates a large filling defect in the duodenum—a typical duodenal hematoma.

kinked loop of intestine is a rare mode of jejunal or ileal injury.

Blunt wounds of the intestine range from perforations and avulsions to intramural hematomas and serosal tears. Diagnostic techniques are standard and have been discussed. Again, negative findings, particularly during the first 24 hours after trauma, do not exclude bowel injury.[18]

The treatment of these injuries is surgical, but again there is some controversy regarding intramural hematomas. Most authors argue that large hematomas should be resected, since delayed perforation of such lesions has been reported.[19] It is essential that the condition of the mesenteric vessels be ascertained during operation. Rarely, laceration or avulsion of the major vessels occurs; direct repair of these injuries and successful revascularization are possible.[20]

In the absence of associated injuries of other organs or systems, blunt wounds of the small intestine have a mortality rate of less than 5 per cent.[15] The death rate increases strikingly with each additional organ involved in the trauma.

RETROPERITONEAL HEMATOMA

Retroperitoneal hematoma is a common complication of pelvic and spine fractures, and of injuries to the pancreas, duodenum, and urinary tract. As an isolated phenomenon, retroperitoneal hematoma occurs in only 1 to 2 per cent of nonpenetrating abdominal injuries.[15] About half of all patients with retroperitoneal hematomas have associated intraperitoneal injuries (Fig. 3–IX–3).

Blood loss into the retroperitoneal space may be massive. Experimentally, it has been shown that this space can accommodate up to 4 liters of blood injected under arterial pressure.

Most surgeons agree that nonexpanding retroperitoneal hematomas should not be explored, except for those that form adjacent to the duodenum and pancreas and those that en-

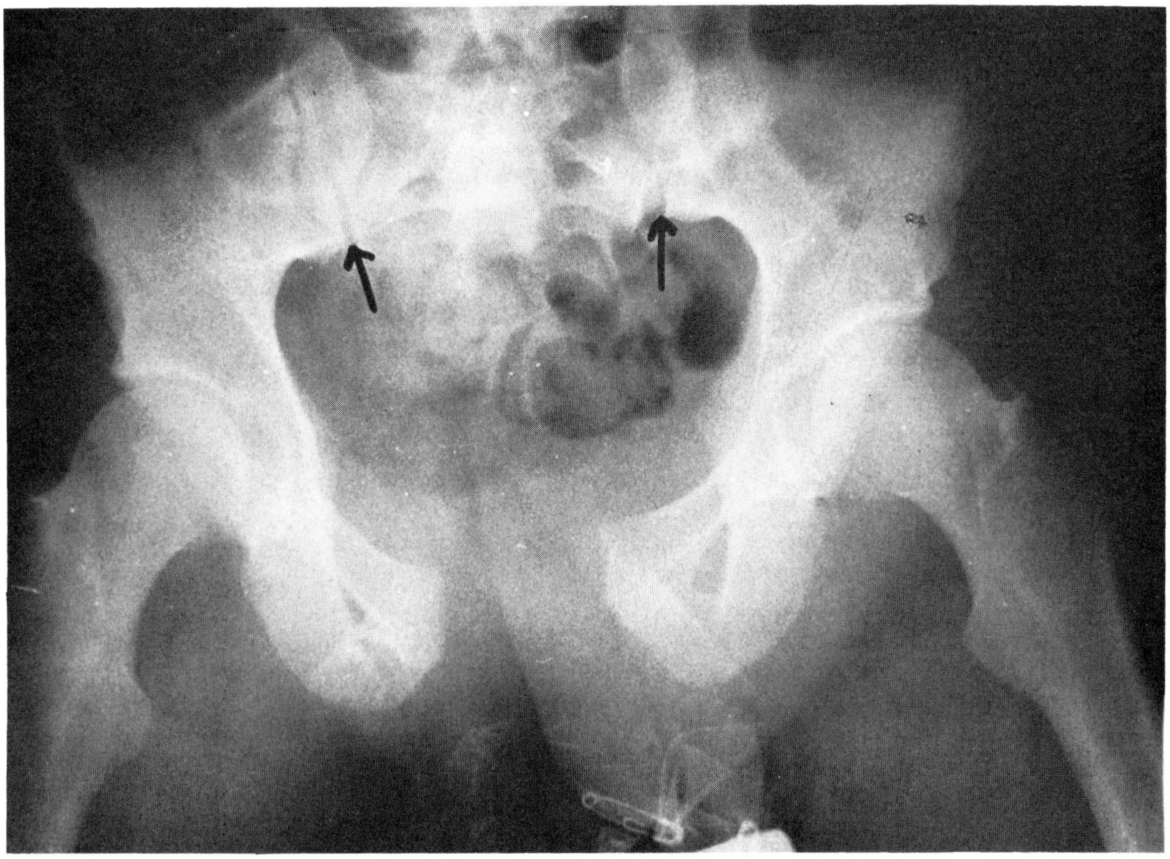

Figure 3–IX–3. This young man was struck by a car while riding a motorcycle, was thrown 30 feet, and struck his perineum against a guard post. The x-ray illustrates fracture dislocations of both sacroiliac joints (arrows) and a very wide disruption of the pubic symphysis. Three liters of blood were required to replace the blood lost into the retroperitoneal space.

velop the retroperitoneal surfaces of the colon. In these circumstances exploration is required to rule out injury to adjacent viscera.

The overall mortality rate associated with retroperitoneal hematomas has ranged between 19 and 38 per cent.[15] Most of the deaths have been due to accompanying visceral injuries both inside and outside the abdomen.

INJURIES OF COLON AND RECTUM

Perforating Injuries

In the past decade a dramatic increase has been noted in the number of patients with perforating wounds of the colon. These wounds are usually the result of crimes of violence among young men. In one large series, there were gunshot wounds in 84 patients, stab wounds in 43, and shotgun wounds in 10. The anatomical distribution of these injuries was fairly uniform with 31 per cent involving the right colon, 28 per cent the transverse colon, 33 per cent the left colon, and 8 per cent the extraperitoneal rectum and anus. The overall mortality rate was 15 per cent; half the patients died of hemorrhage.

In intraperitoneal injury of the colon, prognosis related to age of the patient, type of wounding agent, presence of hematomas adjacent to the perforations, and undue delay between the time of injury and that of operation.[21-23] The prognosis of anorectal injuries, however, is dependent on local pelvic conditions, rather than on the factors just listed. The morbidity of these wounds is extraordinary. More than half the patients with anorectal wounds spend over 50 days in the hospital.[24]

The treatment for colon injuries is operative. Primary suture is recommended for small perforations in the right or transverse colon in good-risk patients, and primary anastomosis is indicated after right colectomy in favorable instances.[23] Primary suture or anastomosis should be avoided in patients manifesting unfavorable prognostic signs or in patients with injuries of the left colon.

Nonperforating Injuries

Blunt trauma to the colon and rectum is usually the result of a motor vehicle accident and constitutes only 3 to 5 per cent of all blunt abdominal injury.[25-27] The force required to damage the large bowel is considerable, and it follows that the incidence rate of associated injuries is very high.

A variety of mechanisms is considered responsible for injuries of the intraperitoneal large bowel.[28] The bowel may be compressed against the vertebral column or burst by a sudden blow against a distended loop. Sudden deceleration may cause a tear of the bowel or disruption of its mesentery. Injury of the extraperitoneal rectum is usually incidental to fractures of the pelvis. This portion of the rectum is more or less fixed to the pelvis and thus may sustain severe injury simultaneously with pelvic fractures. Extensive comminution of the sacrum should suggest the possibility of rectal injury.[29]

A wide range of damage to the intraperitoneal large bowel may result from blunt trauma. The site of injury is usually near the junction of mobile and fixed portions of the bowel, such as the junction of the sigmoid and descending colon, or at the junction of the cecum with the ascending colon. The injury may be to the bowel itself or to the mesentery. Damage to the mesentery may result in hemorrhage, or may in addition affect the circulation of the bowel, with resultant infarction. Most of these injuries are recognized clinically and dealt with as acute problems. In a few cases, the acute injury may be unrecognized, and the patient may present later with such difficulties as colocutaneous fistula or posttraumatic stenosis.[30, 31] The former problem is a rarity, and the incidence of the latter is unknown. It may occur weeks or years after colonic injury and usually affects the left colon. Two mechanisms for formation of the stenosis are suggested. The first relates to an initial subserosal hematoma leading then to scar formation. The second postulated mechanism is that of local ischemia due to mesenteric injury with subsequent fibrosis.[32] Histopathologic study has revealed an infiltrative fibrosis with relatively normal appearing mucosa.

Injuries of the extraperitoneal rectum are relatively difficult to diagnose and more difficult to treat than injuries of the intraperitoneal colon.[33] The high degree of morbidity of these injuries relates to the associated fractures, crush, devitalization of tissue, massive hematoma formation, and presence of fecal material. Careful examination of the anorectum is vital in making a diagnosis, particularly in the presence of a sacral fracture. If blood is found in the rectum, proctoscopic examination should be added. Gross injuries are obvious, but small lacerations may be missed, with disastrous consequences.

Treatment of blunt colonic trauma follows many of the principles established for penetrating injuries of the colon. Particular care must be exercised in managing injuries of the extraperitoneal large bowel.[34, 35] Avulsion of the anorectum is a particularly difficult problem. Reconstruction of the rectal support and the sphincter mechanism should be attempted if conditions are favorable. Drainage must be liberal. When avulsion is complete, little can be done except to establish a permanent colostomy, debride, and drain.

REFERENCES

1. Taylor, F. W.: Gunshot wounds of the abdomen. Ann. Surg., *177*:174, 1973.
2. Thal, E. R., and Shires, G. T.: Peritoneal lavage in blunt abdominal trauma. Am. J. Surg., *125*:64, 1973.
3. Jahadi, M. R.: Diagnostic peritoneal lavage. J. Trauma, *12*:936, 1972.
4. Richardson, J. D., Belin, R. P., and Griffen, W. O.: Blunt abdominal trauma in children. Ann. Surg., *176*:213, 1972.
5. Schuster, S. R., Eraklis, A. J., and Trump, D. S.: Urgent surgical problems in childhood. Surg. Clin. North Am., *46*:747, 1966.
6. Aho, A. J., and Rastima, R. O.: Closed abdominal injury; Observations of changes in material and activation of treatment. Acta Chir. Scand., *137*:429, 1971.
7. Doersch, K. B., and Dosjev, W. E.: The seat belt syndrome. The seat belt sign, intestinal and mesenteric injuries. Am. J. Surg., *116*:831, 1968.
8. Traylor, F. A., Morges, W. W., Lucero, J. I., and Owen, J. C.: Abdominal trauma from seat belts. Am. Surg., *35*:313, 1969.
9. Towne, J. B., and Coe, J. D.: Seat belt trauma of the colon. Am. J. Surg., *122*:683, 1971.
10. Ritchie, W. P., Ersek, R. A., and Bunch, W.: Combined visceral and vertebral injuries from lap type seat belts. Surg. Gynecol. Obstet., *131*:431, 1970.
11. Wolf, N. J.: Subcutaneous rupture of the stomach. Review of the literature and report of a case. N. Y. State J. Med., *36*:1539, 1936.
12. Harrison, R. C., and Debas, H. T.: Injuries of the stomach and duodenum. Surg. Clin. North Am., *52*:635, 1972.
13. Lundberg, G. D., Davis, C. J., and Nelson, D. E.: Hemorrhage from gastroesophageal lacerations, following closed chest cardiac massage. J.A.M.A., *202*:123, 1967.

14. Coche, W. M., and Meyer, K. K.: Retroperitoneal duodenal rupture. Proposed mechanism, review of literature and report of a case. Am. J. Surg., *108*:834, 1964.
15. Orloff, M. J., and Charters, A. C.: Injuries of the small bowel and mesentery and retroperitoneal hematoma. Surg. Clin. North Am., *52*:729, 1972.
16. Williams, R. D., and Yurko, A. A.: Controversial aspects of diagnosis and management of blunt abdominal trauma. Am. J. Surg., *111*:477, 1966.
17. Weiss, M., and Dreiling, D. A.: Small bowel perforation in blunt trauma. Its relationship to previous laporatomy. Am. J. Gastroenterol., *50*:279, 1968.
18. Evans, J. P.: Traumatic rupture of the ileum. Br. J. Surg., *60*:119, 1973.
19. Hicken, W. F., and Carlquist, J. H.: Traumatic rupture of the gastrointestinal tract by non-penetrating forces. Am. J. Surg., *64*:209, 1944.
20. Killen, J. A.: Injury of the superior mesenteric vessels secondary to nonpenetrating abdominal trauma. Am. Surg., *30*:306, 1964.
21. Beall, A. C., Jr., Bricker, D. L., Alessi, F. J., Whisennand, H. H., and DeBakey, M. E.: Surgical considerations in the management of civilian colon injuries. Ann. Surg., *173*:971, 1971.
22. Chilimindres, C., Boyd, D. R., Carlson, L. E., Folk, F. A., Baker, R. J., and Freeark, R. J.: A critical review of management of right colon injuries. J. Trauma, *11*:651, 1971.
23. Christensen, N., Ignatrus, J., and Mathewson, C., Jr.: Treatment of injuries of the large bowel in civilian practice. Am. J. Surg., *89*:753, 1955.
24. Schrock, T. R., and Christensen, N.: Management of perforating injuries of the colon. Surg. Gynecol. Obstet., *135*:65, 1972.
25. Morton, J. H., Hinshaw, J. R., and Morton, J. J.: Blunt trauma to the abdomen. Ann. Surg., *145*:699, 1957.
26. Nance, F. C., and Crowder, V. H.: Intramural hematoma of the colon following blunt trauma to the abdomen. Am. Surg., *34*:85, 1968.
27. Welch, C. E., and Giddings, W. P.: Abdominal trauma: clinical study of 200 consecutive cases from Massachusetts General Hospital. Am. J. Surg., *79*:252, 1950.
28. McKenzie, A. D., and Bell, G. A.: Nonpenetrating injuries of the colon and rectum. Surg. Clin. North Am., *52*:735, 1972.
29. Morgan, C. N.: Wounds of the rectum. Surg. Gynecol. Obstet., *81*:56, 1945.
30. Wightman, J. A. K.: Delayed traumatic rupture of the colon with colocutaneous fistula. Br. Med. J., *2*:93, 1967.
31. Mays, E. T., and Noer, R. J.: Colonic stenosis after trauma. J. Trauma, *6*:316, 1966.
32. Altner, P. C.: Constrictive lesions of the colon due to blunt trauma to the abdomen. Surg. Gynecol. Obstet., *118*:1257, 1964.
33. Wanebo, H. J., Hunt, T. K., and Mathewson, C.: Rectal injuries. J. Trauma, *9*:712, 1969.
34. Lovenson, G. S., and Cohen, A.: Management of rectal injuries. Am. J. Surg., *122*:226, 1971.
35. Armstrong, R. G., Schmitt, H. J., Jr., and Patterson, L. T.: Combat wounds of the extraperitoneal rectum. Surgery, *74*:570, 1973.

X. Vascular System

by Robert C. Davis

Trauma to a major blood vessel is a disaster that may immediately imperil the life of the patient or the viability of the limb. Arterial injury is infrequently seen, even in a practice that deals with trauma, and because of its infrequency, in civilian practice the experience of the individual surgeon tends to be limited. The event is usually unexpected and often ends in crippling disability, amputation, or a fatal sequence of complications. Satisfactory results can be obtained in most cases by early diagnosis and expeditious management. The earlier effective treatment is instituted, the greater the probability of good results. Disappointing results are usually attributable to delays in diagnosis and sometimes to inadequate treatment.

HISTORICAL NOTE

Throughout the recorded history of man, the wounds of war have provided ample opportunity for physicians to apply themselves to salvage of life and limb by the treatment of blood vessel injuries. Ambrose Paré in the sixteenth century introduced the ligature for the life-saving control of arterial hemorrhage. Wounds were still submitted to astringents, boiling pitch, compression dressings, or heated cautery in the eighteenth century. Ligation was not fully accepted, probably because of late bleeding as a result of almost universal wound infection. The advent of the period of antisepsis brought a decline in incidence of secondary hemorrhage and gangrene of the extremity, and established ligation as the treatment of choice.[1] In the early years of the twentieth century Guthrie and Carrel achieved consistently good results with experimental vascular repairs and grafts in animals.[2] Matas described the technique for direct repair of aneurysms by endoaneurysmorrhaphy in clinical cases.[3] These direct repair techniques were employed, during World War I, in sporadic attempts to repair acutely injured arteries. German surgeons preferred reconstruction to ligation on theoretical grounds, but their experience was limited. Allied surgeons preferred ligation. Large numbers of false aneurysms and arteriovenous fistulae were successfully repaired.

During World War II, ligation for acute arterial lacerations remained as the standard therapy for acute arterial injury even though a high amputation rate resulted.[4] Around the end of World War II, great strides were made in vascular surgery in association with developments in blood banking, anesthesia, and antibiotics—leading to successful repairs of arterial wounds during the Korean War. The policy during the Vietnam War was to perform arterial repair whenever possible. This and helicopter transportion direct from the battlefield to fully equipped hospitals reduced amputation rates to less than 10 per cent, which compares favorably with the reported amputation rates in large series of civilian injuries.[5]

ACUTE VASCULAR INJURY

Penetrating Wounds

Acute injuries are lesions that are evaluated within a few hours of the time of injury. They can be caused by direct or indirect trauma to the artery. In most cases, pulsatile external bleeding does not occur. Instead, a periarterial hematoma develops. The primary consideration in diagnosing an arterial injury is to determine whether the traumatic agent and the location of the wounds suggest an arterial injury. A large hematoma, continued bleeding from the wound edges and distal ischemia would confirm the existence of an arterial wound. Ischemic signs can, infrequently, result from arterial spasm; in cases of distal ischemia that might have resulted from traumatic spasm, however, further evaluation by arteriography or surgical exploration of the artery should be undertaken. The absence of a peripheral pulse may not necessarily indicate an arterial injury since the peripheral pulses can be diminished in association with hypotension and may be absent in patients with preexisting chronic vascular occlusion. In addition, neither the absence of ischemia nor the presence of distal pulses excludes a major arterial injury, since a lateral wound of a peripheral vessel may not occlude the vessel and closed transection of a large vessel does not necessarily obliterate peripheral pulses.[7, 8]

A completely transected artery may stop bleeding spontaneously, particularly in avulsion wounds, crushing injuries, and wounds due to high-velocity missiles. Transected vessels retract and develop vascular spasm. This associated with intimal injuries and perivascular blood clotting leads to occlusion of the vessel lumen by thrombosis. A laterally lacerated vessel often bleeds more extensively than a transected one, since retraction of the edges leads to enlargement of the opening in the vessel wall.

In arterial wounds from high-velocity missiles, a grossly intact vessel can conceal an underlying thrombosis resulting from injury to the arterial intima. These injuries are caused by the pressure forces generated by high-velocity missiles. The thrombosis rate following primary repair declined significantly during the Korean War, in part because of recognition of the intimal injury in vessels surrounding high-velocity missile wounds and the resultant practice of excising 1 cm of normal vessel at each end of these arterial wounds.

Several factors are important in evaluating the prognosis of a patient with an arterial wound. The elapsed time between injury and treatment directly affects the results. In the Korean War, no amputations resulted from major arterial wounds repaired within nine hours, while in those repaired after nine hours the amputation rate was 25 per cent. Repairs made as late as 18 to 48 hours after injury, however, sometimes succeed. Undoubtedly collateral circulation plays a role in maintaining viability of these limbs. Extensive soft tissue wounds cause greater destruction of collateral circulation, leading to extensive distal small-vessel thrombosis, which can result in an irreparable injury.

The location of an arterial wound contributes significantly to the outcome. Arterial injuries of the lower extremity have a higher amputation rate than injuries of the upper extremity. Failure to repair a damaged popliteal artery usually results in loss of the extremity.[9, 10]

The upper extremity is particularly amenable to salvage by arterial repair and grafting techniques. Rich and co-workers report amputation rates between 5 and 6 per cent for injuries of axillary and brachial arteries.[5, 11] Injuries to both radial and ulnar arteries, which usually do not endanger the viability of the upper extremity, often cause symptomatic ischemia that should be corrected. Injury of either artery at the wrist can result in ischemia of the hand if the vascular arches are incomplete.[12] Vessels less than 1 mm in diameter can now be repaired. Amputated fingers have been salvaged in some cases.[13] Blood supply to a devascularized finger can be reestablished by island pedicle transfer techniques. In addition, digital artery transfer can correct chronic ischemia of a digit.[14]

Hypovolemia further reduces perfusion in a wounded extremity with a major arterial wound. In shock, thrombosis and tissue ischemia that can lead to the requirement for amputation of the limb occur earlier. There is a better possibility that tissue perfusion can be maintained in a limb distal to an arterial injury if blood volume and cardiac output are maintained.

Associated injuries can affect the results of an arterial injury. In patients with multiple injuries there is a greater shock and more opportunity for delay in operative treatment of a vascular wound because of the necessity for resuscitation or for treatment of other wounds and because of a greater chance of missing the diagnosis of arterial injury. The extent of arterial injury will affect the prognosis; arterial lacerations without complete transection when properly treated have excellent results, but if lateral repair is attempted following a high-velocity missile injury or injury associated with extensive periarterial injury, early necrosis of the arterial wall employed in the repair can be anticipated and will contribute to the thrombosis of the vessel and a poor result.

Soft tissue coverage is mandatory after a successful arterial repair. The failure to surround the entire artery with subcutaneous tissue or muscle is likely to lead to exposure and erosion of the exposed artery and the suture line. In severely contaminated wounds, primary closure of the skin may not be appropriate under these circumstances. Repaired blood vessels should be covered with viable muscle or subcutaneous tissue. An alternative is a bypass graft, which circumvents the wounded area, and proximal and distal ligation of the injured vessel.

Development of an infection following vascular repair is usually catastrophic. Sepsis of an arterial suture line invariably leads to its disruption, initiating a series of hypotensive and septic complications with fatal consequences. Aggressive debridement, flap transposition, local application of antibiotics, massive administration of systemic antibiotics, and circumventing bypass grafts have been successful.[15] Prevention of infection by adequate debridement, delayed primary wound closure when indicated, and antibiotic therapy is ideal.

The severity of the ischemic response following arterial injury varies with the tolerance of the different tissues to anoxia. In the extremity, peripheral nerves are most sensitive to anoxia; hence, paralysis and anesthesia quickly develop when arterial blood flow is seriously decreased. Striated muscle is almost equally sensitive to anoxia and usually becomes necrotic if arterial blood flow is decreased to such a degree that anesthesia and paralysis are present. Skin, tendon, and bone all have a great tolerance to anoxia and may survive ischemic injury that has produced extensive irreversible muscle necrosis. This is seen in the extremity in which an arterial repair is performed several hours after injury. The skin may appear viable but the extremity is anesthetic and paralyzed. After a period of time it will be found to have widespread necrosis of the muscle.

Nonpenetrating Wounds

In almost any fracture or dislocation, a major artery may be injured. Contusion and intimal injuries with thrombosis occur more frequently than laceration or transection.[16, 17] Soft tissue damage may be extensive, and collateral vessels may also be injured. A frequent error is to conclude that arterial spasm is the cause of a cold pulseless extremity and, therefore, to long delay arterial exploration. If limb perfusion does not return following reduction of the bone or joint deformity and reestablishment of blood volume and cardiac output in severely injured patients, arterial exploration should not be delayed.

Dislocation of the knee is frequently associated with popliteal artery injuries. In one series of 22 dislocated knees, 13 had associated popliteal injuries.[18] This is an important injury, since the amputation rate is high if repair of the popliteal artery is not performed early. Posterior dislocation of the elbow frequently causes brachial or radial ulnar artery injuries.[19] In a series of 24 cases, four amputations and one Volkmann's contracture resulted.[20] Anterior dislocation of the shoulder may produce axillary artery injury.[21] This can be serious, since important collateral vessels are injured. Dislocation or subluxation at the radioulnar joint may, in rare instances, cause transection of the radial artery in addition to medial nerve injury. Fractures of the clavicle may injure the subclavian artery, subclavian vein, and brachial plexus. Fracture of the neck of the humerus may lacerate the axillary or brachial artery. Fracture of the femur at the midshaft or lower third has produced laceration of the superficial femoral artery. Fracture of the tibia and fibula from the midshaft down to the malleoli has resulted in injury to the posterior tibial and anterior tibial arteries. The iliac arteries have been injured by pelvic fractures. Intravertebral disk surgery has resulted in aortic, vena cava, and common iliac artery and vein injuries.[22]

Repairs should be performed in all these cases regardless of the time since injury despite reports of the 50 per cent amputation rate with more than a 12-hour delay when the limb is ischemic. A seven-year-old boy whose femoral artery was injured at the time of a femoral fracture had vascular reconstruction 25 hours after injury. At that time, the toes were black, and bullae had developed over the foot and pretibial region. Four centimeters of the contused artery was resected and replaced by a vein bypass graft. This was successful, and only toe amputations were required. Failure to explore and repair fracture- or dislocation-related arterial injuries of the lower extremity with ischemia frequently results in amputation.[23, 24]

Occasionally an artery may be injured by direct blunt force.[25, 26] These injuries produce contusions, spasms, or intimal lacerations. Intimal laceration is associated with distal intimal dissection and prolapse of the intima with resultant occlusion and thrombosis of the vessel.[27, 28]

COMPLICATIONS OF DIAGNOSTIC PROCEDURES

Medical progress has resulted in precise methods of arteriographic localization of peripheral arterial lesions and complete anatomical diagnosis of cardiac and great vessel anomalies. In addition, arteriography aids in the diagnosis and localization of neoplasms and other space-occupying masses and is extensively used in neurosurgery for this purpose. The local complications of arteriographic studies include: hematoma formation, false aneurysm formation, hemorrhage, guide wire or catheter perforation of the artery remote from the puncture site, guide wire or catheter breakage with retention, intimal dissection and thrombosis and embolism.

Local pressure over the puncture site following removal of a needle or catheter usually suffices to prevent bleeding. The presence of an extensive hematoma overlying a peripheral artery following one of these diagnostic procedures should alert one to the possibility of persistence of the arterial puncture defect and false aneurysm formation.

Arterial perforation by guide wire catheter remote from the site of introduction into the arterial system rarely results in difficulty if recognized immediately. Usually the operator is immediately aware of the problem because there is sudden pain at the site of perforation. Guide wire breakage and catheter retention can result from defective equipment and can be prevented by careful testing of equipment. These foreign bodies can either be removed by open exploration or retrieved by a wire loop passed through a sheath under fluoroscopic control.

Small intramural injections are usually not accompanied by any difficulty. Extensive intimal dissection, however, can result in immediate occlusion of the arterial lumen and subsequent thrombosis. Subintimal injections or subintimal placement of guide wires or catheters can be avoided by tests made under fluoroscopic control. Vessel thrombosis can occur from trauma associated with needle or catheter insertion at the puncture site. Vessel size plays an important part in the incidence of thrombosis. The brachial artery is particularly prone to thrombosis following retrograde catheterization. The collateral circulation in the arm usually assures viability, but disabling forearm arterial insufficiency often persists. There are probably many more cases of forearm arterial insufficiency due to brachial artery thrombosis than are recognized. When forearm and hand ischemia follow brachial artery puncture, if any doubt exists, surgical repair or angiography should not be delayed. If treated early, the patency can be restored by thrombectomy with lateral suture repair or vein patch angioplasty. Delayed repair may require bypass reconstruction. Owing to the difficulty experienced with use of the brachial artery for retrograde catheterization studies, the femoral artery or the axillary artery approach may be preferred because of the larger diameter of these vessels.[29]

CHRONIC VASCULAR INJURIES

Repetitive Injury

Axillary and brachial artery lesions can be induced by prolonged use of axillary crutches. Fourteen such cases have been described in which the crutches were employed for many years.[26, 30] Lesions consist of complete thrombosis, mural embolism with distal embolism, and aneurysm formation with distal embolism.

A clinical syndrome occurring in air hammer and other laboratory tool operations has been described.[31, 32] Symptoms are usually those of distal ischemia. The most likely cause is thrombosis of the digital artery rather than a problem of the sympathetic nervous system. Thrombosis of the digital artery also occurs in baseball players and handball players. For baseball players, this usually occurs in the index finger of the catching hand, where the major force of the baseball is received. The fingers are cold and sensitive, and there are atrophy of the pulp, slow-healing ulcers, and trophic changes. Frequently cold sensitivity is exhibited with sensory impairment and cyanotic mottling. The usual cause is chronic repetitive trauma, but occasionally it may be acute injury from a direct blow to the bare hand. Handball players who develop symptoms as a result of repetitive trauma to the palm usually have ischemia to the index and middle fingers. Arteriograms reveal short blocks to the digital arteries of the index and middle finger.[33]

Axillary artery thrombosis in baseball pitchers has recently been reported. Year after year the throwing arm has moved with great force from a position of exaggerated hyperadduction down an arc to which various inward and outward twisting motions are added. Complete thrombosis of the axillary artery with distal filling through collateral vessels develops. This is the result of either an intimal tear due to repetitive stretching and twisting or to compression by a well-developed pectoralis minor tendon and development of the hyperadduction syndrome.[33]

False Aneurysms

In 1888 Rudolph Matas described his operation of endoaneurysmorrhaphy in which proximal and distal arterial control was established, the aneurysm widely opened, and communications into the artery sutured. This became the standard treatment for aneurysms for half a century. It was still in use for traumatic aneurysms following World War II. As techniques of vascular reconstruction developed, reconstruction of arterial continuity became the preferred form of treatment.

A traumatic aneurysm usually results from tangential laceration of the wall of an artery. Continuity of the blood flow through the lacerated artery is usually maintained. Following laceration, blood extravasates into the soft tissue surrounding the artery, forming a hematoma that compresses and seals the point of injury. The hematoma may be small enough to escape initial detection. After several days or weeks, the hematoma can liquefy, becoming a pulsating hematoma as a result of the communication with the blood vessel lumen. Usually, a traumatic aneurysm progressively enlarges, compressing adjacent nerves to produce pain and paralysis or eroding through to the skin or a body cavity with hemorrhage unless treated appropriately.

As the hematoma begins to enlarge, the tissues become tense, tender, and warm, leading to the not uncommon incorrect diagnosis of abscess. This erroneous diagnosis can lead to incision in order to drain the abscess, with resultant violent hemorrhage. In addition, a small traumatic aneurysm can become stable for many years and mimic a neoplasm, since these aneurysms are usually partially filled with thrombus and closely resemble a solid tumor. Attempted biopsy of such a lesion can also lead to massive hemorrhage.

Usually there is no disability from a traumatic aneurysm except for the local symptoms caused by the enlarging mass. The peripheral circulation is usually normal. An exception to this is peripheral embolization of thrombi from an aneurysm, which occurs infrequently. Intermittent compression of a subclavian aneurysm by motion of the shoulder may dislodge emboli; these patients can present with ischemia of the arm, and a subclavian artery traumatic aneurysm is found by angiography.

Treatment of traumatic aneurysms by resection and vascular reconstruction has had uniformly good late results.[15, 34] In the past, false aneurysms occurred frequently at the point of anastomosis of plastic prosthetic grafts when sutures of insufficient long-term tensile strength were employed. Modern suture material has greatly reduced this problem. Currently, false aneurysms of prosthetic grafts usually result from sepsis.

Traumatic Arteriovenous Fistulae

Hunter, in 1757, apparently first recognized an arteriovenous fistula to be a direct communication between the artery and vein and described the marked dilatation and tortuosity of the arteries and veins associated with the fistula. Later it was recognized that the pulse rate slowed upon temporary closure of a fistula; this has since become the classic test for evaluating the effect of an arteriovenous fistula on cardiac output. Proximal ligation of the artery invariably led to gangrene as a result of diversion of collateral blood supply from the distal artery. Modern treatment consists of excision of the fistula and arterial reconstruction when indicated.

A traumatic arteriovenous fistula is produced by a penetrating wound that lacerates the artery and adjacent vein, but it can also follow closed trauma. Communication develops either directly between the openings in these vessels or by way of a false aneurysm sac.

The immediate effects of an arteriovenous fistula are a decrease in blood flow to the tissue distal to the lesion and an increase in the venous pressure. Peripheral vascular resistance is lowered as a result of the fistula. This causes an increase in systolic and diastolic blood pressure and in cardiac output. Gradually the blood volume increases. Systolic blood pressure increases, causing an increase in pulse pressure. The pulse rate gradually decreases. Locally there is progressive development of extensive collateral circulation. The decreased peripheral resistance is a potent stimulus for the development of collateral circulation, and blood flow to the distal extremity may approach normal. The heart, the arteries leading to the fistula, the fistula, and the venous channels leading from the fistula gradually enlarge. After months or years, the arteries distal to the fistula may also enlarge and involved veins become markedly enlarged and tortuous. In the lower extremity, chronic venous congestion may lead to skin ulceration and other signs of venous stasis. In growing children, there may be hypertrophy of the involved limb with increased growth of bone and soft tissue. Progressive heart failure can develop from large fistulae. Usually the volume of blood in an arteriovenous fistula of an extremity is insufficient to produce heart failure. When major vessels are involved, however, cardiac failure can occur in a matter of days as a result of increased cardiac output due to flow that may develop through these fistulae.

Arteriovenous fistulae have resulted from operative procedures such an intravertebral disk removal, nephrectomy, and splenectomy. Arteriovenous fistulae have followed needle biopsy of the kidney, and intervertebral artery fistulae have followed arteriography of the vertebral artery. When major vessels are involved, the artery should always be repaired and the vein repaired when possible.

INADVERTENT INTRAARTERIAL INJECTIONS

Many medications routinely employed intravenously produce catastrophic results when injected intraarterially. These accidents are not only iatrogenic but also caused by intraarterial injection of drugs by addicts. Amphetamine is probably the drug most frequently causing serious loss of tissue, but meperidine, promazine hydrochloride, sodium pentobarbital, thiopental sodium, sodium sulfobromophthalein, chlorpromazine, and tetracycline have been reported to cause serious injuries.[35] The usual site of injection is the brachial artery in the antecubital fossa. There develops severe burning pain in the hand with blanching, paralysis, and sensory loss, but with pulses at the wrist remaining present. Later edema develops and is followed by gangrene.

These agents probably cause chemical injury to the intima of small blood vessels, resulting in microthrombus formation, ischemia, and gangrene of the vessel. Attempts to treat the injury have not been particularly successful.

REFERENCES

1. Halsted, W. S.: The effect of ligation of the common iliac artery on the circulation and function of the lower extremity. Report of a cure of iliofemoral aneurism by the application of an aluminum band to that vessel. Bull. Johns Hopkins Hosp., *23*:191, 1912.
2. Guthrie, C. C.: *Blood Vessel Surgery and Its Applications.* Pittsburgh, University of Pittsburgh Press, 1959.
3. Matas, R.: Operation for the radical cure of aneurysm based upon arteriorrhaphy. Ann. Surg., *37*:161, 1903.
4. DeBakey, M. E., and Simeone, F. A.: Battle injuries of the arteries in World War II. Ann. Surg., *123*:534, 1946.
5. Rich, N. M., and Hughes, C. W.: Vietnam Vascular Registry: a preliminary report. Surgery, *65*:218, 1969.
6. Morris, G. C., Beall, A. C., Roof, W. R., and DeBakey, M. E.: Surgical experience with 220 acute arterial injuries in civilian practice. Am. J. Surg., *99*:775, 1960.
7. Perry, M. O., Thal, E. R., and Shires, G. T.: Management of arterial injuries. Ann. Surg., *173*:403, 1971.
8. Drapanas, T., Hewitt, R. L., Weichert, III, R. F., and Smith, A. D.: Civilian vascular injuries: a critical appraisal of three decades of management. Ann. Surg., *172*:351, 1970.
9. Sullivan, W. G., Thornton, F. H., Baker, L. H., LaPlante, E. S., and Cohen, A.: Early influence of popliteal vein repair in the treatment of popliteal vessel injuries. Am. J. Surg., *122*:528, 1971.
10. Rich, N. M., Baugh, J. H., and Hughes, C. W.: Popliteal artery injuries in Vietnam. Am. J. Surg., *118*:531, 1969.
11. Rich, N. M.: Vascular trauma in Vietnam. J. Cardiovasc. Surg., *11*:368, 1970.
12. Ortner, A. B., Berg, H. F., and Lebendiger, A.: Limb salvage through small-vessel surgery. Arch. Surg., *83*:414, 1961.
13. Horn, J. S.: The reattachment of severed extremities. In *Recent Advances In Orthopaedics.* Edited by A. G. Apley. Baltimore, Williams & Wilkins Co., 1969.
14. Meagher, S. W.: Correction of digital ischemia by arterial transfer: a new indication for the neurovascular island transfer. Arch. Surg., *93*:139, 1965.
15. Crawford, E. S., DeBakey, M. E., and Cooley, D. A.: Surgical considerations of peripheral arterial aneurysms: analysis of 107 cases. Arch. Surg., *78*:226, 1959.

16. Collins, H. A., and Jacobs, J. K.: Acute arterial injuries due to blunt trauma. J. Bone Joint Surg., *43-A*:193, 1961.
17. Makin, G. S., Howard, J. M., and Green, R. L.: Arterial injuries complicating fractures or dislocations: the necessity for a more aggressive approach. Surgery, *59*:203, 1966.
18. Kennedy, J. C.: Complete dislocations of the knee joint. J. Bone Joint Surg., *41-B*:878, 1959.
19. Kilburn, P., Sweeney, J. G., and Silk, F. F.: Three cases of compound posterior dislocation of the elbow with rupture of the brachial artery. J. Bone Joint Surg., *44-B*:119, 1962.
20. Eliason, E. L., and Brown, R. B.: Posterior dislocation at the elbow with rupture of the radial and ulnar arteries. Ann. Surg., *106*:1111, 1937.
21. McKenzie, A. D., and Sinclair, A. M.: Axillary artery occlusion complicating shoulder dislocation. Report of two cases. Ann. Surg., *148*:139, 1958.
22. DeSaussure, R. L.: Vascular injury coincident to disc surgery. J. Neurosurg., *16*:222, 1959.
23. Gardner, C.: Traumatic vasospasm and its complications. Am. J. Surg., *83*:468, 1952.
24. Miller, D. S.: Gangrene from arterial injuries associated with fractures and dislocations of the leg in the young and in adults with normal circulation. Am. J. Surg., *93*:367, 1957.
25. Gibson, J. M. C.: Rupture of the axillary artery. J. Bone Joint Surg., *44-B*:114, 1962.
26. Rob, C. G., and Standeven, A.: Closed traumatic lesions of the axillary and brachial arteries. Lancet, *270*:597, 1956.
27. Morris, G. C., Jr., Creech, O., Jr., and DeBakey, M. E.: Acute arterial injuries in civilian practice. Am. J. Surg., *93*:565, 1957.
28. Pick, T. P.: On partial rupture of arteries from external violence. St. George's Hospital Reports, *6*:161, 1873.
29. Newton, T. H.: The axillary artery approach to arteriography of the aorta and its branches. Am. J. Roentgenol., *89*:275, 1963.
30. Stammers, F. A. R.: Peripheral arterial disease: some points of common interest to general and orthopedic surgery. J. Bone Joint Surg., *36-B*:209, 1954.
31. Barker, N. W., and Hines, E. A., Jr.: Arterial occlusion in the hands and fingers associated with repeated occupational trauma. Proc. Staff Meet. Mayo Clin., *19*:345, 1955.
32. de Takats, G.: *Vascular Surgery.* Philadelphia, W. B. Saunders Co., 1959.
33. Cooley, D. A.: Personal communication.
34. Hughes, C. W., and Jahnke, E. J., Jr.: The surgery of traumatic arteriovenous fistulas and aneurysms: A five year followup study of lesions. Ann. Surg., *148*:790, 1958.
35. Engler, H. S., Purvis, J. G., Kanavage, C. B., et al.: Gangrenous extremities resulting from intra-arterial injections. Arch. Surg., *94*:644, 1967.

XI. Genitourinary Tract

by Carl A. Olsson and Robert J. Krane

Several basic facts pertaining to genitourinary tract trauma should be mentioned first. On a large trauma service, injuries to the genitourinary tract account for only 2 to 3 per cent of admissions.[1] These injuries can be separated into two main groups: internal and external. Internal injuries involve the kidney (and its pedicle), the ureter, the bladder, and the urethra. A large percentage of them are associated with intraabdominal, intrathoracic, or pelvic trauma, which may initially mask the damage that has been sustained by the urinary tract. External injuries involve the external genitalia, primarily in men. These injuries affect the penis and the scrotum and its contents. In this section, the types of genitourinary injuries are reviewed, special attention is paid to mechanisms responsible for them, and the clinical manifestations of and general principles regarding trauma to particular genitourinary tract organs and their ultimate effects are discussed.

MANIFESTATIONS OF GENITOURINARY TRACT TRAUMA

Hematuria is almost always seen with injury to the genitourinary tract. This may be apparent on gross inspection of the urine or may only be discovered by microscopic examination. It should be stressed, however, that the absence of hematuria does not rule out trauma to the urinary tract (for example, in certain major injuries of the kidney or its pedicle as well as in avulsion injuries of the ureter, no urine is delivered to the bladder from the injured side, and therefore hematuria is absent). Although the degree of hematuria has traditionally been described as correlating with the severity of damage to urinary tract organs, this notion should be dispelled.

A deficiency in urinary output may be a manifestation of genitourinary tract trauma. There are, however, many explanations for such a deficiency in the injured patient, and its presence or absence is not helpful in establishing a clinical diagnosis. A decreased urinary output (oliguria) may occur if there has been interruption of urethral continuity, rupture of the urinary bladder, or trauma to both ureters or to a ureter draining a solitary kidney. Low urinary output may also indicate damage of both kidneys or even minor damage of a solitary kidney. Finally, deficient urine production may result from acute tubular necrosis of the kidneys (with no direct renal trauma) related to the clinical state of shock seen with severe trauma in general.

One should suspect genitourinary tract trauma when there are injuries to other structures known to be associated with injuries to genitourinary organs. It should be obvious that flank injuries are frequently associated with renal or ureteral damage. Penetrating abdominal injuries involve the kidney in about 8 per cent of cases.[2] Various bony fractures are associated with injuries to the urinary tract. Patients with pelvic fracture also have bladder or urethral injuries in approximately 15 per cent of cases.[3, 4] Fractures of the lower ribs or lumbar transverse processes are not uncommonly associated with damage to the kidney or ureter. Fractures of the os calcis or lumbar vertebrae (with the implied deceleration forces) may be associated with injuries to the renal pedicle (due to shearing effect). Finally, injuries of the rectum should lead one to suspect damage to the bladder or urethra, particularly in the male. Vaginal injuries in the female are not uncommonly associated with bladder or urethral injuries.

Diagnostic Procedures

The various diagnostic procedures employed in documenting urinary tract injuries should be defined for better understanding of the subject. The plain film of the abdomen (KUB; kidney, ureter, and bladder) allows examination of the bony structures just noted. In addition, one should inspect orientation of the lumbar spine. Scoliosis with concavity directed toward the side of injury is not uncommon after renal or ureteral trauma. The renal outline and psoas shadows should be inspected; these frequently are altered in renal or retroperitoneal trauma. A soft tissue flank mass, as well as dilatation (ileus) or displacement of bowel loops, is not infrequently seen with retroperitoneal injuries.

Intravenous pyelography (IVP) consists of the intravenous injection of radiopaque material that is concentrated and excreted by the kidneys, providing visualization of the renal parenchyma, renal collecting system, ureters, and bladder. High dosages of contrast medium or so-called infusion pyelography increases the yield of positive findings when one is dealing with injuries of the kidney or ureter. The use of nephrotomography along with intravenous pyelography enhances detection of renal parenchymal injuries.[5, 6] It should be noted that, since these studies are dependent upon circulatory integrity to deliver contrast medium to the kidneys, they may not yield renal visualization when clinical shock is present. When inspecting the intravenous pyelogram, one should be certain to document the presence and condition of the kidney on the side contralateral to the injury. Renal or ureteral injuries may be present with perfectly normal pyelographic studies. Usually, however, there is some delay in excretion of the contrast material on the injured side. Blood clots, represented by collecting system filling defects, may also be found. More severe trauma presents as extravasation of contrast material (clearly demonstrating a parenchymal or collecting system laceration). A reduction in the renal outline size is suggestive of major vascular injuries sustained by the kidney; nonvisualization of the kidney is complete in this instance as well as in severe parenchymal damage.

Retrograde urethrography (RUG) is performed by injecting contrast material in a retrograde fashion through the urethral meatus to outline the integrity of the urethra from this point to the bladder neck. Lacerations or interruptions of continuity of the urinary tract in this area can be easily demonstrated by contrast medium obstruction or extravasation or both.

Cystography involves the injection of contrast material through a urethral catheter into the bladder. Bladder shape may be altered by the presence of a pelvic hematoma. Extravasation of contrast material may be seen into either intraperitoneal or extraperitoneal structures when bladder lacerations are present.

Retrograde pyelography involves injection of contrast material through catheters placed directly into the ureteral orifices at cystoscopy. This study is of little value in outlining a renal injury, but is of great value in documenting the integrity of the ureter, the renal pelvis, and the collecting system of the kidney.

Arteriography is a study that involves the passage of an arterial cannula via femoral arterial puncture into the abdominal aorta. Subsequent injections of contrast material may be made within the aorta or selectively delivered to a variety of main arterial branches, including the renal artery (selective renal angiography). This study is valuable in documenting the presence of extrarenal hematoma (by capsular vessel displacement), traumatic arteriovenous fistula, thrombosis of arterial branches, discontinuity of major vessels, and discontinuity of renal parenchyma (as in major renal lacerations).[7, 8]

Renal scanning techniques involve the intravenous injection of radioactive material that is delivered to and excreted by the kidneys. By placing a scintillation counter over the renal fossa, assessment of renal vascular integrity and renal function, as well as an anatomical demonstration of renal parenchymal outline, may be obtained in a noninvasive manner. Technetium-99 pertechnetate is usually employed to demonstrate vascular supply to the kidney; radioactive iodinated Hippuran may be used to demonstrate functional integrity.[9]

RENAL PEDICLE INJURY

Injuries to the renal pedicle are seen in four circumstances, the most common being a penetrating abdominal or back wound traversing the anatomical site of the renal artery and vein. Because of the greater length of the left renal vein and the fact that this structure crosses the midline, this vessel is the one most commonly injured in such penetrating wounds.[10] Blunt trauma accounts for approximately 20 per cent of all pedicle injuries, the mechanism of injury usually being one of acceleration-deceleration, leading to shearing of the renal vessels with resultant intimal damage, dissection, and thrombosis.[11] Rapid deceleration may be implicated in fractures of the os calcis and lumbar vertebral bodies, as outlined earlier, accounting for the association of these injuries with renal pedicle injuries. During rapid deceleration, the kidney continues to move in a downward direction, limited only by its vascular attachments. A spectrum of vascular pathologic changes may be seen with such deceleration injuries. Total vascular avulsion may occur; an intimal tear of an artery may result in vascular thrombosis; finally, stretching of the artery may produce reflex vasospasm.[11] The third clinical circumstance in which renal pedicle injuries are encountered is electrical trauma, wherein it is not unusual for high-voltage electricity to be transmitted along the abdominal aorta, resulting in renal arterial thrombosis. Lastly, iatrogenic damage to the renal pedicle is encountered during closed renal biopsy (by needle technique) or in conjunction with surgery performed in the region of the major abdominal vessels (abdominal aneurysm resection, retroperitoneal lymphadenectomy, and the like).

Patients with renal pedicle injuries usually present in clinical shock secondary to blood loss. Flank pain and an expanding flank mass may be additional features. Hematuria, when present, is usually microscopic. It should be emphasized that hematuria may be absent in patients with the most severe avulsion injuries, as urine is not produced at all by the severed kidney.

With such a clinical presentation, preliminary radiologic studies often cannot be obtained and immediate operation is usually the treatment of choice if loss of life or kidney is to be avoided. If the clinical situation permits (shock is easily reversed by intravenous blood and fluid replacement), a variety of diagnostic measures can be undertaken. If the systolic blood pressure is in excess of 90 mm of mercury, infusion intravenous pyelography may be performed. This will demonstrate, by means of only a few abdominal films, the following findings: scoliosis of the lumbar spine away from the involved side, obliteration of the psoas shadow due to blood accumulation in the retroperitoneum, nonfunction of the kidney and decreased renal size on the involved side, and displacement of bowel gas by an expanding retroperitoneal mass.

Other studies may also be employed to document the lack of vascular integrity of the kidney involved by pedicle injury. Renal scanning employing technetium-99 pertechnetate will demonstrate that there is an absence of blood flow to the involved kidney.[9] Arteriography will demonstrate extravasation of contrast material from the involved vessels; if the vessel involved is an artery, there will be interruption of flow to the renal parenchyma. In penetrating injuries, arteriography may be of special use in documenting other intraabdominal lesions that may be associated with renal pedicle trauma, such as splenic or hepatic lacerations.

As already noted, the left renal vein is the most frequently injured component of the renal pedicle. Following this, the right renal vein is the next most frequently injured; finally the renal arteries are equally injured to an extent somewhat less than either vein. About 65 per cent of patients suffering from renal pedicle injuries have damage to more than one renal vessel; the remaining 35 per cent sustain damage to a single vessel.[10] Frequently there is associated damage to one or both of the major abdominal vessels (aorta and vena cava). Visceral injuries of the liver, stomach, pancreas, colon, spleen, and small bowel frequently accompany renal pedicle injuries and contribute to the prominent mortality rate seen with these injuries.[10]

The death rate and the rate of incidence of nephrectomy are much higher with vein injuries than with arterial injuries, a fact that is indicative of either the greater hemorrhage or the higher percentage of concurrent major vessel injuries associated with venous trauma. Overall, the mortality rate for renal pedicle injuries is approximately 30 per cent. This figure varies from 17 per cent in patients with injury of one vessel up to 100 per cent if all four vessels are traumatized.[10]

RENAL INJURY

The kidney, although a relatively fragile organ, is well protected by surrounding bony and soft tissue structures. Therefore, renal trauma in severe accidents is relatively infrequent. Anatomically, the kidneys are partially situated within the confines of the thoracic cage and are protected from injury by the lower ribs, lumbar vertebrae, strong paraspinal musculature, and enveloping Gerota's fascia.

Causes and Incidence of Renal Injury

Young men are most susceptible to renal injuries, indicative of their greater involvement in sports and vehicular accidents. Approximately 80 per cent of renal injuries occur in males, and the overall age median is 30 years.[12] Both kidneys are equally affected by trauma. Children under 15 years of age are particularly susceptible to renal trauma, owing to the larger size of the kidneys (relative to body size), underdevelopment of perirenal fat and Gerota's fascia (formed after 10 years of age), and lack of total ossification of the lower ribs (not complete until age 25).[13,14] An additional factor leading to an increased susceptibility to renal trauma in children is the ease with which abnormal kidneys can be injured. About 25 per cent of children with renal injuries are found to have preexisting renal disease.[15] Congenital hydronephrosis, renal ectopia, Wilms' tumor, megaureter, and other childhood kidney diseases predispose to renal trauma.[15,16]

Injuries to the kidney may be categorized as open (due to penetrating trauma) or closed (due to nonpentrating or blunt trauma). The latter category accounts for approximately 90 per cent of renal trauma seen in most series.[17] When consideration is limited to wartime renal trauma, however, there is a much greater incidence of penetrating wounds (caused by either high- or low-velocity missiles). Also, in center-city hospitals servicing communities where there is a high rate of criminal activity, penetrating injuries due to gunshot wounds or stabbing may account for up to 30 per cent of all renal trauma.[17,18] Approximately 7 per cent of all penetrating abdominal wounds demonstrate some involvement of the kidneys.[19] Conversely, 80 per cent of all penetrating renal injuries have associated intraabdominal injuries (the majority of these involving the liver, colon, spleen, and stomach).[19,20]

Blunt or closed renal trauma largely results from vehicular accidents (55 per cent). Eighteen per cent of blunt renal injuries result from falls. Sports injuries and direct blows to the flank region sustained during altercations account for approximately 6 to 7 per cent of renal trauma.[21] Eighty per cent of patients with blunt renal trauma have associated injuries to other organs or the skeletal system. About 61 per cent of patients have skeletal damage; about 20 to 25 per cent sustain injuries to intraabdominal or intrathoracic organs.[17]

In children, falls account for the largest proportion of closed renal injuries (20 per cent); other causes are traffic accidents (22 percent), direct blows (17 per cent), sports injuries (9 per cent), and sled accidents (6 per cent).[13] Open or penetrating injuries are rare in children. It should always be remembered that approximately 20 per cent of childhood renal trauma is associated with a preexisting renal anomaly that in itself predisposes to injury.[13,14] Bearing this in mind, along with the lack of protection afforded to the kidney in the child, one can easily see how childhood renal injury may be suffered after relatively mild trauma. Thus it should be emphasized that investigation is imperative in all children with even minimal signs or symptoms of kidney trauma.

The majority of blunt injuries to the kidneys result from direct blows to the renal area. When a patient is hit from behind, his kidney may strike against the liver. Direct blows anteriorly may cause laceration and contusion of the kidney against the lower ribs, which act as a central fulcrum in absorbing the energy of the blow. Another mechanism by which injury to the kidney is sustained is seen in association with osseous fractures; a fractured lumbar transverse process or lower rib may lacerate the kidney as easily as a bullet or knife blade.

Iatrogenic renal injury should be mentioned. These are injuries resulting from either ureteral catheterization (during retrograde pyelography) or biopsy of the kidney by needle technique. Fortunately, such trauma secondary to ureteral catheterization or percutaneous renal biopsy is usually minimal and handled easily by conservative means without the need for operative intervention.

Manifestations of Renal Injury

Trauma to the region of the kidney presents a spectrum of findings from minimal perirenal hemorrhage to total fragmentation or avulsion. For purposes of classifying renal trauma, the kidney can be divided into four distinct components: the renal pedicle (which injuries have already been discussed), the collecting system (the renal pelvis and calyces), the renal parenchyma, and the renal capsule and pericapsular tissues. Trauma to the pericapsular tissues is usually manifested by the development of a perirenal hematoma. The fatty and areolar tissues surrounding the renal capsule (and confined with Gerota's fascia) are traumatized, leading to hemorrhage and hematoma within Gerota's fascia. There may be no actual damage of the kidney in this injury. Renal contusions are mild injuries of the renal parenchyma with lacerations of either the renal capsule or collecting system, but not of both structures. This is the most common injury sustained by the kidney, accounting for close to 75 per cent of all renal trauma.[17, 18] Renal lacerations are linear injuries traversing the collecting system, parenchyma, and renal capsule together. Renal rupture or fragmentation is indicative of parenchymal laceration in which the portions of kidney are separated from each other. It should be emphasized that the foregoing classification is, in large part, an artificial one. Most frequently, patients with renal injuries do not undergo surgical exploration, nor do they often die, allowing postmortem examination. Thus, the classification is based primarily upon clinical and radiologic features, and is devoid of pathologic confirmation. The more severe renal injuries, such as laceration or rupture, more frequently require surgical intervention, and therefore, anatomical confirmation of the injury may be obtained in these instances.

The immediate effects of renal trauma are due to hemorrhage from the kidney combined with the effects of associated organ injuries. Patients may present in clinical shock, requiring rapid replacement of blood and intravenous fluids. Flank or loin pain may be present; these symptoms, however, are often masked by the presence of injuries to other structures. A flank mass may be palpable if the degree of retroperitoneal hemorrhage is severe. Abdominal pain and tenderness are usually present overlying the injured kidney. Rebound tenderness, indicative of peritoneal irritation, may be present, even in the absence of intraabdominal injuries. Pain may be referred to the chest, reflecting rib injury. Care should be taken to detect the occasional patient who has associated intrathoracic trauma (pneumothorax), which may require immediate therapy.

Hematuria is present in almost all cases of renal trauma. The degree of hematuria, however, need not be related to the degree of injury. In cases of relatively minimal trauma, gross hematuria may not be detected immediately following injury, owing to lack of urine output by the traumatized kidney. In such cases, hematuria may be seen some 24 to 48 hours later. An additional point to bear in mind is that bleeding from a damaged kidney may initially cease and then recur as delayed hemorrhage some two to three weeks later. The blood thrombus formed in the kidney during initial healing may become dislodged at this time.

Diagnostic Evaluation of Renal Injury

A flat plate of the abdomen will show scoliosis of the spine away from the side of the injury along with obliteration of the psoas margin when hemorrhage is severe. Fractures of the lower ribs or lumbar transverse processes may be noted. Reflex ileus is nearly always present. An expanding flank mass may cause displacement of bowel structures.

Further diagnostic evaluation may be performed to ascertain the degree of trauma sustained by the kidney. Intravenous pyelography should be performed, but the results of this study may be misleading. For example, even relatively mild renal contusions may cause delay in function of the involved kidney suggestive of more severe trauma. It should be emphasized again that in patients with clinical shock perfusion of the kidneys is not adequate to allow visualization of even normal kidneys by this technique. Enlargement of the size of the renal outline may indicate perinephric hematoma. It should be realized, however, that perinephric hematoma may also be an attendant finding with renal rupture, and therefore, visualization of the kidney should be strived for in all instances. Definition of renal outline should be obtained, in all cases of renal trauma, to document the presence or absence of parenchymal tears. Extravasation of contrast material is indicative of renal laceration or damage to the calyceal system alone. Renal contusions present in a variety of fashions radiographically. There may be delayed or decreased concentration of contrast material owing to reflex vasospasm, incomplete filling of a renal calyx in the region of the trauma, filling defects within the collecting system (indicative of blood clot), and changes in the renal contour secondary to subcapsular or intrarenal collections of blood. These findings may be present either alone or in combination in patients with simple renal contusion. On the other hand, these findings do not rule out more extensive renal damage.

Other diagnostic studies may provide more information about the status of the traumatized kidney. Renal scanning with radio isotope–tagged materials will give rapid and accurate information about the vascular supply to the kidney. In addition, parenchymal separations are easily detectable.[22, 23] Also, some assessment of renal function may be obtained by using radioactive iodine–labeled Hippuran scanning. An additional advantage of renal scanning techniques is that they may be employed even when the patient is in a state of marginal tissue perfusion. Finally, arteriography will yield very accurate anatomical evaluation of both vascular and parenchymal integrity.[8, 24–26] Arteriography is indicated in patients in whom it has been impossible to visualize the kidney by intravenous pyelographic studies.[1] Opinion on this matter is divided.[27, 28] Some authors feel that immediate angiography is appropriate to define the exact pathologic condition, while others feel that the renal salvage rate in these patients is too poor to warrant the potential risks of arteriography.[12] Arteriography should be recommended when there is an expanding flank mass (if time permits) or when the intravenous pyelogram shows extravasation of contrast material. It is interesting to note that, when renal scan studies are negative, arteriography rarely reveals any additional significant pathologic change.[9] It should be repeatedly emphasized that, during all these studies, the most important information to obtain is confirmation of the presence and function of the contralateral kidney.

A few additional notes should be made of the associated injuries experienced by patients with renal trauma. It should be stressed that approximately 25 to 35 per cent of patients with renal trauma also have injuries to intraabdominal or intrathoracic viscera.[17, 29] Death from renal trauma is often related to the extensiveness and location of these additional injuries. This is particularly true when the associated structures damaged are in the region of the hepatoduodenal ligament (liver, gallbladder, common bile duct, duodenum).[19]

Sequelae of Renal Injury

There are various delayed effects of renal trauma. These have often been reported in case reports and there are no firm incidence figures for delayed complications. There are many reasons for this failure in reporting. The patient who sustains renal trauma is often treated at an institution where he does not receive his usual medical care (often in a completely different geographic locality). Additionally, patients who sustain injuries in the course of criminal activities often do not return for follow-up studies. Therefore accurate statistics for delayed complications are not available in most trauma series.

Perhaps the most common situation in which delayed complications occur is that of the patient who has extensive urinary extravasation that is not surgically drained. In such cases, periureteral fibrosis may develop with associated hydronephrosis, pyonephrosis, and renal calculus. Another sequel of failure to drain urinary extravasation (especially when the urine is infected) is development of perinephric abscess. At times a perinephric hematoma will be reabsorbed, leaving a posttraumatic pararenal pseudocyst. This cystic structure may impinge upon the ureter, impeding drainage and causing hydronephrosis with its attendant complications. Secondary hemorrhage has been discussed previously. Renal arterial injuries in which the arterial wall remains intact are prone to delayed occlusion because of intimal damage and dissection of blood beneath the severed intima. In such cases renal atrophy may result. If the occlusion is within a segmental vessel, hypertension may develop because of hypoperfusion of a portion of kidney. Arteriovenous fistulae may result after healing of parenchymal tears. These, along with segmental vessel occlusions (described earlier) and compression of renal parenchyma by fibrous capsular thickening (after resolution of a perinephric hematoma), may all be responsible for the occasional development of hypertension.[30]

URETERAL INJURY

Ureteral trauma is most commonly due to injuries sustained during the course of a variety of operative procedures. For example, fewer than 100 reported ureteral injuries were found in the entire experience of World War I, World War II, and the Koream conflict.[31, 32] Nonoperative ureteral injuries are primarily caused by penetrating wounds of the flank or abdomen (gunshot or stabbing). Fewer than 10 per cent are due to blunt trauma.[33] In the child, however, because of deficient musculature attaching the ureter to the renal pelvis and the renal pelvis to the renal parenchyma, avulsion of the ureter or renal pelvis is not infrequently seen as a result of blunt injury.[34] Ureteral injuries sustained nonoperatively are usually unilateral, with right and left sides being equally affected. When ureteral injuries occur in the adult secondary to blunt trauma, frequently a fracture fragment is found as the cause of the ureteral damage (fracture of lumbar transverse processes). In the child, avulsion injuries, as already described, occur fairly specifically during vehicular accidents.[34]

Ureteral injury is often masked by the associated trauma that these patients sustain. Because of the anatomical protection afforded to the ureter, it is rarely injured alone; frequently trauma to the skeletal system or abdominal viscera accompanies ureteral damage.[35] Therefore, ureteral injury is immediately recognized in approximately one third of cases only.[32] This factor is of great significance in the ultimate outcome for the patient, since, when recognition is delayed, ultimate treatment by nephrectomy is required three times as frequently as when ureteral damage is recognized immediately.[32] The usual presentation of ureteral injury is in this delayed fashion. In the postoperative period, after treatment of associated injuries, the patient presents with flank pain, fever, or urinary fistula. At times there is palpable expanding flank mass, or urinary ascites. Perinephric abscess may herald the presentation as well. The best means for detecting the presence of ureteral injuries are intravenous and retrograde pyelography. The latter examination, while not terribly useful in the documentation of renal trauma, is of inestimable value in the definition and location of ureteral injuries.

Intraoperative Trauma to the Ureter

The majority of ureteral injuries are incurred during the course of various operative procedures.[36] The incidence of operative ureteral injuries is highly variable in different series. One of the primary reasons for this difference is that preoperative intravenous pyelograms have not been compared with postoperative pyelograms in all series, making the recognition of otherwise "silent" ureteral injuries impossible in some reports. The incidence figures are, of course, higher in those series in which these studies have been performed. The overall incidence of operative ureteral injuries in gynecologic procedures is 3 per cent.[37] In surgery performed for benign disease, the figure varies from 0.8 to 2.5 per cent.[38–40] On the other hand, after radical operations, such as the Wertheim procedure, the incidence rate varies from 9 to 14.6 per cent, depending upon the series reviewed.[41, 43] Ulfelder stated that it was impossible to reduce the incidence of ureterovaginal fistula formation below the 5 to 8 per cent level if surgery was adequately performed for removal of carcinoma of the cervix.[44]

In general surgical procedures the incidence rate is much lower.[45, 46] Some workers have stated that the right ureter is perhaps more often injured than the left because the surgeon's attention is directed more assiduously toward the preservation of the left ureter.[46] This statement has not proved true in a review of the surgical literature, however. Unilateral injuries are six times as common as bilateral ones, the left ureter being injured nearly twice as often as the right.[47]

Since gynecologic procedures are most commonly associated with operative injuries to the ureter, the female-to-male ratio of these injuries is 4 to 1. The average age incidence in the female correlates with the age incidence for a number of gynecologic operations (39 years).[47]

Few operations performed in the lower abdomen or back are exempt from the possibility of inadvertent ureteral injury. Abdominal gynecologic procedures are associated with ureteral injuries six times as frequently as are vaginal procedures, for the obvious reason that a longer portion of ureter is at risk during an abdominal approach. This is true even when the same operation is performed via the two routes (abdominal hysterectomy versus vaginal hysterectomy).[47] By far the most common of all surgical procedures in which the ureter is injured is abdominal hysterectomy.[38, 48] The second most common is abdominal salpingo-oophorectomy.[47] Ovarian cyst removal, myomectomy, anterior repairs of the urethra, and surgery for vesicovaginal fistula are less frequently associated with ureteral injury. Laparoscopy with tubal ligation should be mentioned as a recently developed operative procedure in which ureteral damage has already been reported.

Obstetrical procedures are much less implicated in ureteral injuries now than in the days when high forceps deliveries were common practice. The distortion of pelvic structures and ureteral course, however, along with the increase in size of the ureters during pregnancy (hydronephrosis of pregnancy), still makes the problem not totally uncommon. The obstetrical procedures associated with ureteral injury are high forceps delivery, cesarean section, vaginal hysterotomy, and episiotomy.[47]

The urologist might be looked upon as the surgeon least likely to damage the ureter inadvertently, since he is most intimately familiar with its anatomical variation. Such is not the case, however. Ureteral damage caused by urologists is understandable in those procedures that directly involve the ureter, such as ureteral catheterization, ureterolithotomy, basket extraction of ureteral calculi, or ureteropelvic repair. Inadvertent injuries may also be caused by the urologist during procedures in which the ureters are not clearly involved in the operative field (bladder diverticulectomy, radical prostatectomy, pyelolithotomy, and colovesical fistula repair).

The ureter is also at risk in the hands of the neurosurgeon or orthopedist. Although a rare complication, ureteral injuries have been reported during surgery for a ruptured intravertebral disk.[49, 50] The ureter is dangerously close to the L4–L5 interspace in many individuals and can be damaged during laminectomy carried out at this level.[51]

General surgical procedures implicated in operative injuries to the ureter are usually, but not confined to, operations for colorectal disease.[36] Sigmoid resection, anterior-posterior resection, and total colectomy are the procedures most frequently associated with ureteral damage. A retrocecal appendix may be quite close to the ureter (which may be mistaken for the former structure), and the ureter may be damaged by this error in identification during appendectomy.[47] The ureter may also prolapse into a hernia defect, at times sustaining inadvertent injury during herniorrhaphy.

Ureteral injuries are also sustained in the course of vascular procedures. Abdominal aneurysm resection, placement of bifurcated bypass grafts, caval plication, and sympathectomy are the operations most commonly associated with ureteral damage.[49, 52, 53] For example, the distal limbs of a Y-graft should be placed behind the ureters to avoid ureteral obstruction. Ureters have been mistaken for sympathetic chains or otherwise damaged during lumbar sympathectomy.[53]

The concluding point here is that the ureter can be injured during the course of diverse procedures. Surgeons should be totally familiar with various "danger points" in the course of these procedures in order to avoid ureteral trauma. The proximity of the ureter to the uterine artery and infundibulopelvic ligament should be borne in mind when doing either abdominal or vaginal gynecologic procedures. During abdominal gynecologic procedures, special attention should be paid to the relation between the ureter and uterosacral ligament. When there are abdominal masses, it should be recalled that the course of the ureter may be distorted by the mass. During vaginal gynecologic procedures, the ureter's course will become altered by traction on the cervix, and this should be borne in mind. During colorectal procedures, the relationships between the ureter and the inferior mesenteric artery should be recalled. The proximity of the ureter to the rectovesical pouch and lateral ligaments of the rectum should also make the surgeon wary. Most of these danger points are well known and diligently respected by well-trained surgeons. It should be noted, however, that it is during the simple task of reperitonealization that operative ureteral trauma frequently occurs. At the end of a difficult operative procedure, when performing this seemingly easy job, the surgeon's guard is somewhat relaxed and the ureter is damaged. The ureter, indeed, demands full respect until the dressing is on the wound.

A final point to be remembered is that the blood supply to the ureter, although extensively anastomotic and from multiple sources, is fragile. The supply arises from six different sources (renal artery, gonadal vessels, aorta, hypogastric vessels, vesical arteries, and uterine vessels), but because of its fragility, one should take care during surgery not to mobilize more than the length of ureter necessary for identification. Further, one should take care not to strip the ureter of its adventitia, as is often done during the course of lymphadenectomy. In the female, a large proportion of the pelvic blood supply to the ureter comes from the uterine artery in this area. Therefore the uterine artery should be ligated medial to the ureter in order to preserve ureteral branches.

Prevention of Operative Ureteral Injuries

A number of preventive measures can be used by the surgeon to avoid ureteral injury.

First, preoperative renal function studies and intravenous pyelography will give valuable information as to the number of kidneys present, their functional ability, and their position. Infusion pyelography will give a clearer definition of the course of the ureters than will routine studies. It should be recalled that branching or bifidity of ureters occurs in 1 of 150 patients and renal ectopia in 1 of 1,000 patients.[54, 55] Both these anomalies are crucial to recognize in order to avoid ureteral injuries. Preoperative intravenous pyelography is becoming a legal necessity because it has become a community practice standard in many regions of the country and because it is useful to have for comparison should the need for postoperative pyelography arise.

Ureteral catheters placed before surgery are useful for identification of but not for protection of the ureters. Many ureters have been cut even with ureteral catheters in place.[56] When catheters are used, it should be routine practice for the surgeon (not the scrub nurse or nursing aide) to remove them following surgery. If resistance is met to catheter removal, one must assume the possibility of inadvertent ligation of the ureter, and the catheter should be left in place until radiographic studies confirm or disprove this. If a very short ureteral catheter segment is retrieved, the cause is obvious. A recent modification of the ureteral catheter used in preventing operative ureteral trauma is the fiberoptic ureteral transilluminator, which causes the ureter to "glow" with light transmitted along the length of a fiberoptic catheter.

Operative ureteral injuries can be classified according to three factors: type of injury, location of injury, and time of recognition. The types of injury that might be sustained by the ureter include ligation, crushing, angulation, devascularization, incision, division, excision, and avulsion. To categorize them by position, ureteral injuries are usually described as upper third, middle third, or lower third. The classification according to time of recognition divides them into those injuries immediately recognized and those recognized after a delay.

Repair of Ureteral Injuries

A few factors in ureteral regeneration are of importance to a discussion of operative ureteral injuries. A longitudinal incision in a normal ureter will heal without scar or stricture formation, often without the need for suturing at all. A longitudinal defect will also heal by good mucosal regeneration (which is complete by seven days) and somewhat poorer smooth muscle regeneration (which is complete by four to six weeks). Regeneration of smooth muscle usually does not occur over a transverse defect. Such defects heal with fine linear scars. Peristalsis will still be synchronous across the scar, however, especially with a spatulated or otherwise beveled anastomosis.

Important to any ureteral repair is adequate drainage of urine. Ureteral anastomoses almost always leak after repair. In order to avoid the consequences of this leakage (which include periureteral fibrosis, sepsis, and heterotopic bone formation), proximal urinary diversion and the liberal use of drains to the anastomotic area are valuable adjuncts to the repair of a ureter. A final technical stratagem to be considered in the repair of ureteral injury is an attempt to surround the ureteral anastomosis with fatty tissue. This will prevent fixation of the ureter to the muscle of the retroperitoneum. (Such fixation will impair peristalsis of the ureter.) If free fat is not available in the retroperitoneum, omentopexy may be carried out, surrounding the ureter with a pedicle of fatty omentum.

By far, the most important single factor in the repair of ureteral injuries is the time the injury is recognized.[33, 36] The time of recognition to a great extent determines not only the treatment that will be required but also the ultimate outcome of the injury. The problems caused by delayed recognition of the injury are all those of septic versus clean wounds, well-oriented operative fields versus reoperative surgery with fibrosis and edema, and the like. Less ureteral length will be lost in an immediately discovered ureteral transection than in a delayed recognition situation in which "freshening" of ureteral ends may be required.

Higgins has often stated that the venial sin is to damage a ureter but that the mortal sin is the failure to recognize it.[57] That this recognition is not a simple task is proved by the fact only 30 per cent of operative ureteral injuries are recognized immediately. Even urologists are not much better in this regard, since only 50 per cent of ureteral injuries caused during urologic procedures are immediately diagnosed.[47]

An important factor in the immediate detection of ureteral injuries intraoperatively is the surgeon's willingness to admit that such injuries can occur in his hands. Intravenous dyes (e.g., indigo carmine) can be administered, and the fact that urinary extravasation has occurred can be ascertained by the staining of a sponge placed in the wound. The site of injury can sometimes be better localized (if suspected) with intravenous administration of diuretic agents to cause a sustained diuresis. With injuries that cause ureteral obstruction, e.g., from ligatures, ureteral dilatation may be accentuated, allowing identification of the point of obstruction. On the other hand, if the ureter has been incised or otherwise lacerated, the increased urine flow will make detection of the point of leakage easier. In some cases, the site of an obstructing ureteral injury can be found by catheterizing the ureter (from below by opening the bladder; from above by opening the renal pelvis). A final method of detecting ureteral injuries intraoperatively is the use of operative pyelography. This can be performed by the intravenous route (using a high dosage of contrast material and a single film taken at the 10- to 20-minute time interval) or by directly injecting 5 to 8 ml of contrast material into the ureteral lumen via needle or cannula. Both obstruction and extravasation can be detected in this manner.

Delayed Recognition of Ureteral Injuries

A special problem is posed by the diagnosis of ureteral injuries that are not recognized during surgery. Such delayed recognition of ureteral trauma is heralded by symptoms of urinary obstruction, urinary extravasation, or sepsis. Symptoms of obstruction include decreased urinary output, flank pain, and azotemia. Anuria may occur if both ureters are obstructed or if the ureter draining a solitary kidney is damaged. It should be emphasized that unilateral ureteral obstruction does not always announce itself by flank pain. Indeed, such lesions (so-called "silent" operative ureteral injuries) are often not discovered until years after the offending surgical procedure.[58] Extravasation is usually manifested as fistula. At times a cystic flank mass develops without actual fistula formation. Prolonged ileus is a common manifestation of such extravasation of urine in the retroperitoneum. Ureterovaginal fistulae are the kind most commonly encountered following gynecologic procedures. In general surgical procedures ureterocutaneous (through the operative incision) and ureteroperitoneal fistulae are the most common. If a fistula develops within the first two days after surgery one can assume that the ureteral injury was of the lacerating variety; if it appears a week to 10 days following surgery, that usually indicates that the injury was of a crushing or devascularizing nature, and that resultant necrosis, having led to ureteral sloughing, is the source of the fistula. Finally, postoperative fever of unknown origin should always prompt investigation for unrecognized ureteral injuries, especially following pelvic surgery. Such septic presentations are often due to gram-negative organisms, and therefore, attendant shock is not uncommon.

The overall incidence of "silent" ureteral injuries is approximately 25 per cent of large series.[40] An additional diagnostic maneuver that may be of value in detecting ureteral damage with extravasation following surgery is to measure the ammonia level in free peritoneal fluid. If this level is more than 3 μg per 100 ml, it usually indicates urinary ascites.[59] The overall incidence of delayed presentations of operative ureteral trauma is as follows: ureterovaginal fistula, 50 per cent; hydronephrosis, 30 per cent; ureterocutaneous fistula, 12 per cent; and anuria, 8 per cent.[36]

BLADDER INJURY

Although the bladder, a pelvic viscus, is protected anteriorly and laterally by the pubic arch, it is not uncommonly injured by penetrating and blunt trauma delivered to the lower abdomen and pelvis; occasionally operative trauma is the mechanism of injury.[3, 4] Bladder trauma, for the most part, is caused by blunt injury to the aforementioned regions in automobile accidents. Nearly 70 per cent of these injuries are associated with pelvic fractures.[31] The diagnosis and management of vesical trauma is usually straightforward, but unrecognized bladder rupture can occur in comatose patients and result in fatality.

Certain classic symptoms such as hematuria, low abdominal pain, urinary urgency, and inability to void should alert one to the possibility of bladder injury. In many patients, however, the symptoms of associated intraabdominal and pelvic trauma mask the symptoms of bladder injury.

The diagnosis of vesical rupture or perforation is made by visualizing extravasated contrast medium cystographically. It is important to remember that only a high-dosage cystogram (250 to 350 ml of dye) will detect smaller bladder perforations. The cystogram is performed by infusing contrast medium into the bladder through a urethral catheter. Films are taken and the bladder is then drained and a postdrainage x-ray is obtained. Occasionally smaller extravasations are not seen when the bladder is filled with contrast medium; hence the need for postdrainage x-ray. Cystoscopy has little value in the diagnosis of vesical injury and may even be hazardous if large amounts of irrigation solution escape extravesically.

Bladder Contusions

Bladder injuries are classified as contusions or ruptures. A bladder contusion is a minimal injury and implies some degree of hemorrhage from the bladder wall. The wall itself is intact, preventing urinary extravasation. It is essentially a diagnosis of exclusion; hematuria is present in the patient with lower abdominal or pelvic trauma, but the cystogram shows no evidence of extravasation. This type of injury is seen with blunt trauma to the lower part of the abdomen, pelvic fractures, obstetrical trauma, and some endoscopic procedures. Treatment is simple urethral catheter drainage to allow healing of the bladder wall until bleeding stops.

Bladder Rupture

A more seriously traumatized bladder may rupture either intraperitoneally or extraperitoneally, the latter being more common (75 per cent).[60] The distended bladder is decidedly more susceptible to injury. When the bladder enlarges, its walls become thinner and less able to withstand injury. A full bladder may rupture without pelvic fracture and usually ruptures intraperitoneally through the weakened dome. The empty bladder still enjoys the relative protection afforded to it by the pubic arch and is usually perforated extraperitoneally in association with pelvic fracture. Only 18 to 20 per cent of vesical ruptures associated with pelvic fracture are intraperitoneal.[60] In these cases it is likely that the same trauma causes two independent effects: a crushing force to the bony pelvis and a bursting force to the bladder.

A few points should be made regarding intraperitoneal bladder ruptures. A continuous flow of urine into the peritoneal cavity irritates the peritoneum and causes generalized peritonitis within 24 to 48 hours. Therefore, early appreciation of this injury is absolutely necessary. Cystography shows extravasated contrast medium outlining the bowel wall or lying in the dependent paracolic recesses. If the patient is turned during the examination the contrast medium will shift also. When intraperitoneal vesical rupture has occurred prompt operative intervention is required.

Conversely, vesical rupture is extraperitoneal in more than 80 per cent of those cases associated with pelvic fracture.[61] The fractures associated with bladder injury most commonly involve the pubic rami and symphysis pubis.[62] Almost all these perforations occur on the anterior surface of the bladder and are caused either by stresses placed on the lateral ligaments anchoring the bladder base or by direct perforation by bony spicules. The urine, in this type of injury, enters the space of Retzius (prevesical space) and from there may dissect along the abdominal wall into the inguinal canal and scrotum, through the obturator foramen into the thigh, or through the sciatic notch into the buttock region.[63] With cystography, contrast medium extravasated into perivesical tissues may be seen involving any of the areas just named. Because of the many potential routes for urinary extravasation and resultant secondary tissue necrosis, this injury must also be diagnosed and treated with dispatch. In certain cases in which slight extraperitoneal extravasation occurs, especially when the urine is known to be sterile, it may be acceptable to treat solely with urethral catheter drainage. This type of treatment can also be employed in cases of bladder perforation caused during transurethral resections when the perforation is immediately recognized and, again, the urine is sterile. When one chooses not to explore such an injury, the patient must be carefully watched and treated with antibiotics and catheter drainage; if signs or symptoms of pelvic inflammation or infection occur, operative intervention is mandatory. In some cases of penetrating trauma to the bladder rupture may be both intra- and extraperitoneal. This is usually seen with bullet or grenade wounds of the lower abdomen, buttocks, or perineum. The diagnosis of this combined injury is similar to that outlined for other forms of bladder rupture.

A word should be said concerning iatrogenic bladder trauma. Obviously this usually occurs in procedures involving the pelvic organs, such as obstetrical and gynecologic procedures, colorectal surgery, and transurethral resections of the bladder or prostate. Occasionally, a bladder contusion or perforation may occur during operative fixation of a fractured hip and aortofemoral bypass graft procedures. Vacuum curettage (abortion) may cause bladder perforation, as the organ may be exposed to extremely high negative pressures during this procedure. The diagnosis of bladder injury may be delayed because the sudden outpouring of urine is easily mistaken for amniotic fluid.

A particularly distressing complication of gynecologic surgery with inadvertent bladder injury is vesicovaginal fistula. This usually occurs in transabdominal hysterectomies, although it is also seen with other gynecologic and obstetrical procedures (especially with pelvic dystocia).[64] This fistula should be initially treated with urethral catheter drainage for up to six months.

The prognosis for patients with traumatic bladder rupture is largely dependent on prompt recognition and treatment. The mortality rate for untreated vesical rupture approaches 100 per cent, as evidenced by the 87 per cent mortality rate cited in older literature, before surgical management was common.[65] At present, the rate is approximately 20 per cent.[1] These cases represent either death due to delay in recognition and therapy or death from associated pelvic or intraabdominal trauma. One group of patients (those with bladder perforations and no history of antecedent trauma, so-called "spontaneous bladder rupture") still experiences a 50 per cent mortality rate, largely because of delay in therapy.[66] These patients usually have intrinsic bladder disease (neurogenic bladder dysfunction, tuberculosis, bladder tumor, outlet obstruction, or diverticula) that probably increases the susceptibility of the bladder to rupture with lesser degrees of trauma.[66]

URETHRAL INJURY

The major portion of this section deals with the male urethra, for by virtue of its greater length and anatomical position it is more susceptible to trauma than the female urethra. The female urethra is rarely injured except during birth trauma or gynecologic surgery.

The urethra is anchored at its membranous portion to the urogenital diaphragm. Injuries to the urethra are classified as posterior when they are at the level of the urogenital diaphragm or above, and anterior when distal to this point. Urethral injury ranges from contusion (without urinary extravasation) to partial and complete tears.

The diagnosis of urethral trauma should be entertained in any patient with pelvic fracture or straddle injury who has blood visible at the urethral meatus, hematuria, or inability to void. The diagnosis is confirmed by retrograde urethrography (although the distinction between complete and partial tears is usually impossible to make). Some authors prefer to attempt urethral catheterization first and, if this fails, resort to urethrography.[31] Others, however, stress the need for initial retrograde urethrography to avoid further damage to the urethra by catheterization.[60, 67]

Posterior Urethral Injury

Injury to the posterior urethra almost always occurs in the region of the membranous portion; rarely, in children, the posterior urethra may rupture in the region of the bladder.[67] These injuries are nearly always seen with pelvic fractures, especially those involving the pubis. This type of fracture forces the prostate posteriorly, causing the urethra to rupture from its prostatic attachments at the urogenital diaphragm. Rectal examination commonly reveals a displaced prostate (superior and freely mobile). When urinary extravasation occurs with this injury it follows the same route seen with extraperitoneal bladder perforations.

The sequelae of posterior urethral injuries depend, to some extent, on the primary treatment used. With attempts at primary surgical repair, there has been a large percentage of complicating urethral strictures (50 to 100 per cent), as well as a modest number of patients who became incontinent (50 per cent) or impotent or both (50 per cent).[68, 69]

More recently workers in this field have recommended that the initial treatment of posterior urethral trauma whatever the extent should be simple suprapubic cystostomy for six to eight weeks, with repairs, when necessary, delayed for six to twelve weeks.[68, 70, 71] Early reports on this type of treatment have been encouraging in that the sequelae of strictures, impotence, and incontinence have been greatly reduced.[68]

Anterior Urethral Injury

The anterior urethra may be traumatized iatrogenically or by straddle injury.[72] The mechanism for the latter injury is trauma to the perineum incurred during falls on railings, fences, or bicycle saddles, causing the bulbous urethra to be crushed between the object and the pubic arch.[73] Like other urethral injuries, the urethral tear may be partial or complete. Clues to this type of injury, on physical examination, are the presence of perineal hematoma or evidence of urinary extravasation into the perineum, scrotum, or penis. Diagnosis is confirmed by retrograde urethrography. It must be remembered that urine extravasating from this type of bulbous urethral injury may dissect not only into the penis and scrotum but also into the abdominal wall and even as high as the upper part of the chest. This dissection occurs below Scarpa's fascia and is only stopped in the region of the coracoclavicular fascia superiorly and the fascia lata inferiorly. If there is any suspicion of this type of urinary dissection, ample drainage of all areas involved should be provided.[31] If there is any evidence of extravasation into the perineum, this region is explored and liberally drained. Without such drainage, sequelae of subcutaneous and cutaneous necrosis and gangrene are common.

Iatrogenic trauma to the urethra remains the most common cause of anterior urethral injury and usually occurs during urologic manipulations. An indwelling urethral catheter may cause trauma to the urethra with delayed inflammatory stricture. The region most involved is the penoscrotal portion of the pendulous urethra, although such inflammatory response may occur over the entire length of the urethra (a similar penoscrotal urethral injury may also be seen following routine transurethral surgery, due to traction on the urethra by the resectoscope against the resistance of the suspensory ligaments of the penis).

Trauma resulting from urethral dilatation with sounds, passage of urethral catheters using a stylet, or passage of endoscopic instruments usually occurs in the region of the bulbous urethra and ranges from mild contusion to perforation. In most cases there is no permanent damage of the urethra resulting from these injuries. At times, permanent false passages or urethral strictures result.

As stated earlier, the female urethra is relatively immune to trauma. Although several cases of urethral rupture secondary to pelvic fractures have been reported in the female it remains a rare clinical occurrence.[74] Trauma to the female urethra almost exclusively occurs secondary to obstetric and vaginal procedures.[75] Birth trauma, especially in cases of pelvic dystocia with resultant prolonged labor, may in fact cause urethral necrosis due to pressure of the unborn child's head against the pubis. These injuries are seen most frequently in countries where obstetrical attendance is unavailable. Procedures such as anterior colporrhaphy or urethral diverticulectomy in the female may result in urethral trauma. Secondary urethrovaginal fistulae are the common sequelae of urethral injuries in the female. Patients whose fistulae arise from the upper urethra proximal to the continence preserving mechanisms present with continual urinary leakage; conversely, those with distal fistulae remain continent.

EXTERNAL GENITAL INJURY

Trauma to the external genitalia is not unusual.[1] In wartime injuries, for example, 30 to 50 per cent of all genitourinary injuries involve the external genitalia.[76, 77] This figure rose remarkably during the Vietnam Conflict, owing to the prevalence of "booby-trap" land mine devices employed in that war.[78] In other wartime series, the common mechanisms by which the genitalia were injured were gunshot (68 per cent), mine injuries (16 per cent), and mortar or grenade injuries (8 per cent). Fifty per cent or more of genital injuries involve the penis.[78]

Penile Injuries

Penile injuries may be classified as follows: strangulation, cutaneous injuries, circumcision injuries, penile skin avulsion, penile fracture, and penile amputation.

Strangulation

Penile strangulation is due to voluntary or involuntary placement of a constricting apparatus around the penis. Various constrictions have been reported. In the infant, it is not unusual for a piece of string or hair to be placed on the penis to prevent wetting. Additionally, when the infant's mother has long hair, a hair falling into the diaper area may be wound around the penis by the child's own manipulations.[79] Adolescents and young adult males employ a number of devices for masturbatory activities. Rings, other metal bands, or bottles have been found incarcerating the penis.[80] The more elderly male may employ such constricting devices to increase potency. Once the penis is incarcerated, subsequent edema of the distal portion may develop, preventing removal of the constricting device. If the incarceration is left untreated, violaceous changes in the skin will develop, and cutaneous gangrene is not unusual. Infarction usually involves the superficial tissues only. The corpus spongiosum and its contained urethra may also become necrotic, however, and a urethral fistula may result. The corpora cavernosa usually maintain their blood supply despite incarceration. The therapy of penile strangulation consists of removal of the constricting agent. In the case of nonmetallic objects, this problem is easily solved. With metallic rings or bands the string technique designed for removal of an incarcerated ring from the edematous finger may be used after draining the distal tissues by needles placed into the corpora and subcutaneous tissues.[81] Various saws and grinding devices have been used, as well, to remove such metal constricting bands.

Cutaneous Injuries

Penile skin injuries include simple lacerations, zipper injuries, circumcision injuries, and vacuum cleaner trauma. Simple lacerations of the penis may occur during the course of civil altercations, the most common weapon employed being the knife. Simple superficial lacerations are managed as any other cutaneous laceration. If the injury to the penis involves the corpora cavernosa, closure of the tunica albuginea is necessary prior to skin closure. If the urethra has also been transected, reanastomosis of the severed ends should be carried out and either urethral or suprapubic catheter drainage instituted. The zipper represents a frequent source of cutaneous injuries. The trouser zipper often entraps penile skin (usually in the region of the foreskin).

Vacuum cleaner injuries are experienced by young adult males during masturbatory activity. If the penis has been placed in the vacuum cleaner hose alone, simple incarceration may be the only damage. In order to increase the amount of suction, however, some men insert the penis into the vacuum cleaner suction aperture directly. Depending upon the brand of vacuum cleaner employed, the fan blades creating the suction may be fairly close to this aperture so that, when erection is complete, the blade will engage the glans penis or the skin of the penis and cause a variety of injuries including skin avulsion, glans laceration, and partial amputation.

Circumcision Injuries

Circumcision injuries are not infrequently seen. Hemorrhage following circumcision occurs in approximately 10 per cent or more of cases.[81] It has been estimated that, in 4 per cent of all circumcisions, reoperation may be required to control hemorrhage. In the infant, meatal ulcers may occur in as many as 31 per cent of children and meatal stenosis in 8 per cent, owing to the exposure of the fragile skin of the glans to a constantly wet and urea-soaked diaper.[81] Loss of penile skin may occur in either the child or the adult because of overzealous traction on the prepuce prior to excision of the foreskin. Glans amputation has been seen when circumcision has been performed after only simple external palpation of the position of the glans. When any form of surgical instrument is used, including the various clamp devices employed for circumcision, it should always be ascertained that the glans penis is not caught within the clamp prior to excision of the foreskin. Complete penile amputation has been reported in circumcision in the infant.[81] This is the most extensive injury that occurs with circumcision. It has been suggested that, if the amputated penis cannot be sutured into place, the child should be reared as a female, after further transsexual surgery.

Skin Avulsion

Penile skin avulsion is a common feature of power take-off injuries. Usually a trouser leg is caught in the power take-off of an industrial or farm machine (46 per cent of these occur on the farm).[82] After trouser engagement in the power take-off, scrotal and penile skin may become engaged with the trousers with resultant avulsion from the penis, scrotum, or both structures along the dartos and Colle's fasciae. The presence of the cremasteric reflex almost always preserves the testes. The skin of the glans is tightly adherent to its subcutaneous structures and, therefore, the glans remains covered with skin in power take-off injuries.

Fractures and Amputations

Penile fractures are infrequently seen. They always are caused by blunt trauma to the erect penis. Approximately one third of these injuries occur during coitus; two thirds are noncoital.[83] There is a sudden cracking sound that is easily heard, followed by immediate pain, detumescence of the penis, distortion and angulation of the penis to the side opposite the injury, and extravasation of blood into the subcutaneous tissue of the penis, perineum, and thigh. Shock may result if a large amount of blood is lost. The mechanism of injury is a rupture of the tunica albuginea. The urethra may be involved in the fracture in about 20 per cent of cases. Management of penile fractures is divided between conservative and surgical means. Surgical therapy usually results in a shortened hospital stay and fewer subsequent problems with potency.[1]

Penile amputation occurs with vacuum cleaner injuries (usually partial), or after self-inflicted trauma. These patients often have a history of psychosis and extreme guilt or a history of erotic sexual practices in which the amputation has occurred. The therapy for amputation is to attempt to reanastomose the amputated penis whenever possible.[84] It should be strongly stressed that psychiatric consultation is required in all patients who suffer penile amputation. This is true for two reasons: many of the patients suffering penile amputation are psychiatrically abnormal to begin with, and even if they were perfectly normal psychiatrically prior to their penile injuries, a failure of anatomical restoration will undoubtedly result in subsequent psychic trauma to the patient.

Testicular and Scrotal Injuries

Testicular and scrotal injuries usually occur in the young adult. Scrotal lacerations may result from gunshot or knife wounds. They are managed easily in the same way as lacerations elsewhere. Care should be taken to insure that scrotal contents have not been damaged by such penetrating wounds. Trauma to the scrotal contents includes traumatic hydrocele, hematocele, testis fracture, testis laceration, and testicular dislocation. It should be stressed that patients with testicular neoplasms frequently recall incidents of scrotal trauma. Whether the patient's attention has been drawn to the scrotum after trauma and the testicular mass is palpated on self-examination, or whether the testis in which a neoplasm already exists is more prone to injury is uncertain. Blunt trauma resulting in testicular contusion, fracture, or dislocation commonly occurs during sports activities, falls, or saddle injury (e.g., from bicycles or motorcycles). When the testis has been fractured, the damaged tunica albuginea should be closed after debridement of any protruding testicular tissue to avoid the possibility that the patient develop autoantibodies to his own sperm. Testicular dislocation results from blunt, squeezing injury to the region of the scrotum. The testis is pushed from the scrotum in one of two directions: it may follow the course of the spermatic cord and be found along the inguinal canal or actually in the retroperitoneum, or it may be forced along fascial planes to various subcutaneous locations along the lower abdominal wall and penis. Because great pressures are required to produce this injury, pelvic bony injuries such as fractures of the pelvis or dislocations of the hip are not uncommonly associated with dislocated testes. The testis usually remains intact although some degree of disjunction with its epidydimal attachments may occur.

REFERENCES

1. Waterhouse, K., and Gross, M.: Trauma to the genitourinary tract: A five-year experience with 251 cases. J. Urol., *101*:241, 1969. [Chap. 2.]
2. Scott, R, Jr., Carlton, C. E., Jr., and Goldman, M.: Penetrating injuries of the kidney. J. Urol., *101*:247, 1969.
3. Peltier, L. F.: Complications associated with fracture of the pelvis. J. Bone Joint Surg., *47-A*:1060, 1965.
4. Wiggishoff, C. C., and Kiefer, J. H.: Pull-through reconstruction of the posterior urethra. J. Urol., *93*:233, 1965.
5. Kazmin, M. H., Brosman, S. A., and Cockett, A. T. K.: Diagnosis and early management of renal trauma: a study of 120 patients. J. Urol., *101*:883, 1969.
6. Mahoney, S. A., and Persky, L.: Intravenous drip nephrotomography as an adjunct in the evaluation of renal injury. J. Urol., *99*:513, 1968.
7. Elkin, M., Meng, C. H., and de Paredes, R. G.: Correlation of intravenous urography and renal angiography in kidney injury. Radiology, *86*:496, 1966.
8. Halpern, M.: Angiography in renal trauma. Surg. Clin. North Am., *48*:1221, 1968.
9. Freeman, L. M., Kay, D. J., and Meng, C. H.: The contribution of renal scanning in the evaluation of renal trauma. Radiology, *86*:102, 1966.
10. Guerrier, W. G., Carlton, C. E., Jr., Scott, R., Jr., and Beall, A. C., Jr.: Renal pedicle injuries. J. Trauma, *11*:53, 1971.
11. Evans, A., and Moggs, R. A.: Renal artery thrombosis due to closed trauma. J. Urol., *105*:330, 1971.
12. Persky, L., and Hoch, W.: Genitourinary tract trauma. Curr. Probl. Surg., 1–64, 1972.
13. Smith, M. J. V., Seidel, R. F., and Bonacarti, A. F.: Accident trauma to the kidneys in children. J. Urol., *96*:845, 1966.
14. Morse, T. S., Smith, J. P., Howard, W. H. R., and Rowe, M. I.: Kidney injuries in children. J. Urol., *98*:539, 1967.
15. Persky, L., and Forsythe, W. E.: Renal trauma in childhood. J.A.M.A., *182*:709, 1962.
16. deBear, L., and Heise, V. E. : Hydronephrosis and renal trauma. Br. J. Surg., *53*:532, 1966.
17. Nation, E. F., and Massey, B. D.: Renal trauma: experience with 258 cases. J. Urol., *89*:775, 1963.
18. Gleen, J. F., and Harvard, B. M.: The injured kidney. J.A.M.A., *173*:1189, 1960.
19. Scott, R., Jr., Carlton, C. W., Jr., and Goldman, M.: Penetrating injuries of the kidney: an analysis of 181 patients. J. Urol., *101*:247, 1969.
20. Carlton, C. E., Jr., and Scott, R., Jr.: Penetrating renal injuries: an analysis of 100 cases. J. Urol., *84*:599, 1960.
21. Scholl, A. J., and Nation, E. F.: Injuries of the kidney. In *Urology*. Edited by M. F. Campbell and J. H. Harrison. Philadelphia, W. B. Saunders Co., 1970, p. 785.
22. Woodruff, J. H., Jr., Cockett, A. T. K., Cannon, R., and Swanson, L. E.: Radiologic aspects of renal trauma with the emphasis on arteriography and renal isotope scanning. J. Urol., *97*:184, 1967.
23. Smith, M. J. V., Seidel, R. F., and Bonacarti, A. F.: Ac-

cident trauma to the kidney in children. J. Urol., *96*:845, 1966.
24. Rous, S. N.: The value of serial selective renal angiography in the delayed management of renal trauma. J. Urol., *107*:345, 1972.
25. Flaster, S. L., and Bush, I. M.: The use of intraoperative renal arteriography in evaluating renal injuries. J. Urol., *109*:763, 1973.
26. Lang, E. K.,Trichel, B. E., Turner, R. W., Fontenot, R. A., Johnson, B., and St. Martin, E. C.: Arteriographic assessment of injury resulting from renal trauma: an analysis of 74 patients. J. Urol., *106*:1, 1971.
27. Chovnick, S. D., and Newman, H. R.: Management of renal injuries. J. Urol., *83*:330, 1960.
28. Holland, M. T., Hurwitz, L. M., and Nice, C. M., Jr.: Traumatic lesion of the urinary tract. Radiol. Clin. North Am., *4*:433, 1966.
29. Peterson, N. E., and Norton, L. W.: Injuries associated with renal trauma. J. Urol., *109*:766, 1973.
30. Girl, J., and Tyky, J.: Development of hypertension after rupture of a kidney. Circulation, *32*:992, 1965.
31. Peters, P. C.: Trauma to the genitourinary system. In Shires, G. T.: *Care of the Trauma Patient.* New York, McGraw-Hill Book Co., 1966.
32. Grant, R. P., Jr., Gifford, R. W., Jr., Pudvan, W. R., Meaney, T. F., Straffon, R. A., and McCormack, L. J.: Renal trauma and hypertension. Am. J. Cardiol., *27*:173, 1971.
33. Walker, J. A.: Injuries to the ureter due to external violence. J. Urol., *102*:410, 1969.
34. Halverstadt, D. B., and Fraley, E. E.: Avulsion of the ureter secondary to blunt trauma. Br. J. Urol., *39*:588, 1967.
35. Choithani, C. H., Evans, G. H., and Scardino, P. L.: Nosocomial ureteral injuries. South. Med. J., *60*:1180, 1968.
36. Higgins, C. G.: Ureteral injuries during surgery: a review of 87 cases. J.A.M.A., *199*:118, 1967.
37. Solomons, E., Levin, E. J., Bauman, J., and Baron, J.: A pyelographic study of ureteric injuries sustained during hysterectomy for benign conditions. Surg. Gynecol. Obstet., *111*:41, 1960.
38. Rusche, C. F., and Bacon, S. K.: Injury of ureter due to surgery, intra-ureteral instrumentation, external violence and foreign bodies. J.A.M.A., *114*:201, 1940.
39. Herman, L., Greene, L. B., and Hayllar, B. L.: Ureteral injuries. J. Urol., *56*:688, 1946.
40. St. Martin, E. C., Trichel, B. E., Campbell, J. H., and Locke, C. M.: Ureteral injury in gynecologic surgery. J. Urol., *70*:51, 1953.
41. Liu, W., and Meigs, J. V.: Radical hysterectomy and pelvic lymphadenectomy. Am. J. Obstet. Gynecol., *69*:1, 1955.
42. Calame, R. J., and Nelson, J. H.: Uretero-vaginal fistula as a complication of radical pelvic surgery. Arch. Surg., *94*:876, 1967.
43. Wertheim, E.: Ein neuer Beitrag zur Frage der Radikaloperation Beim Uteruskrebs. Arch. Gynaekol., *65*:1, 1901.
44. Kickham, C. F. E.: Urologic problems in carcinoma of the cervix. Surg. Gynecol. Obstet., *112*:27, 1961.
45. Feiner, D.: Operative injuries of ureter. Surg. Gynecol. Obstet., *66*:790, 1938.
46. Bandler, C. G., and Roen, P. R.: Urologic complications of left colon surgery. Ann. Surg., *128*:80, 1948.
47. Rusche, C., and Morrow, J. W.: Injury to the ureter. In *Urology.* Edited by M. F. Campbell and J. H. Harrison. Philadelphia, W. B. Saunders Co., 1970.
48. Newell, Q. U.: Injuries to ureters during pelvic operations. Ann. Surg., *109*:981, 1939.
49. Baird, H. H., and Justis, H. R.: Surgical injuries of the ureter and bladder. J.A.M.A., *162*:1357, 1956.
50. Borski, A., and Smith, R. A.: Ureteral injury in lumbar disc operation. J. Neurosurg., *17*:925, 1960.
51. Kern, H. B., Barnes, W., and Malament, M.: Lumbar laminectomy and associated ureteral injury. J. Urol., *102*:675, 1969.
52. Badenoch, A. W.: Injuries of the ureter. Proc. R. Soc. Med., *52*:101, 1959.
53. Culp, O. S., and Bernatz, P. E.: Urologic aspects of lesions in abdominal aorta. J. Urol., *86*:189, 1961.
54. Campbell, M.: Anomalies of kidney. In *Urology.* Edited by M. F. Campbell and J. H. Harrison. Philadelphia, W. B. Saunders Co., 1970, p. 1456.
55. Campbell, M.: Anomalies of ureter. In *Urology.* Edited by M. F. Campbell and J. H. Harrison. Philadelphia, W. B. Saunders Co., 1970, p. 1488.
56. Beare, J. B., Wittenberg, C. A., and Parsons, R. P.: Ureteral injury. J. Urol., *96*:885, 1966.
57. Higgins, C. C.: Ureteral injuries. J.A.M.A., *182*:225, 1962.
58. Spring, W. B.: Management of injuries to lower ureter. Can. Med. Assoc. J., *75*:806, 1956.
59. Mansberger, A. R., Jr., and Young, J. D., Jr.: The value of ammonia levels as an aid in the diagnosis of urinary extravasation. J. Urol., *94*:125, 1965.
60. Morehouse, D. D., and MacKinnon, K. J.: Urological injuries associated with pelvic fractures. J. Trauma, *9*:479, 1969.
61. Prather, G. C., and Kaiser, T. F.: The bladder in fracture of the bony pelvis. The significance of "teardrop bladder" as shown by cystogram. J. Urol., *63*:1019, 1950.
62. Flaherty, J. J., Kelley, R., Burnett, B., Bucy, J., Surian, M., Schildkraut, D., and Clarke, B. G.: Relationship of pelvic bone fracture patterns to injuries of urethra and bladder. J. Urol., *99*:297, 1968.
63. Prather, G. C.: Injuries of the bladder. In *Urology.* Edited by M. F. Campbell and J. H. Harrison. Philadelphia, W. B. Saunders Co., 1970.
64. Everett, H. S., and Mattingly, R. F.: Urinary tract injuries resulting from pelvic surgery. Am. J. Obstet. Gynecol., *71*:502, 1956.
65. Quain, E. P.: Rupture of the bladder associated with fracture of pelvis. Surg. Gynecol. Obstet., *23*:55, 1916.
66. Thompson, I. M., Johnson, E. L., and Ross, G.: The acute abdomen of unrecognized bladder rupture. Arch. Surg., *90*:371, 1965.
67. Mitchell, J. P.: Injuries to the urethra. Br. J. Urol., *40*:649, 1968.
68. Morehouse, D. D., Belitsky, P., and Mackinnon, K.: Rupture of the posterior urethra. J. Urol., *107*:255, 1972.
69. Gibson, G. R.: Impotence following fractured pelvis and ruptured urethra. Br. J. Urol., *42*:86, 1970.
70. Turner-Warwick, R.: The repair of urethral strictures in the region of the membranous urethra. J. Urol., *100*:303, 1968.
71. Waterhouse, K., Abrahams, J. I., Gruber, H., et al.: The transpubic approach to the lower urinary tract. J. Urol., *109*:486, 1973.
72. Blumberg, N.: Anterior urethral injuries. J. Urol., *102*:210, 1969.
73. Sterioff, S., Jr., Izant, R. J., Jr., and Persky, L.: Perineal injuries in children. J. Trauma, *9*:56, 1969.
74. Jameson, R. M.: Foreign bodies and damage to the female urethra and bladder. Br. J. Urol., *39*:506, 1967.
75. Turner-Warwick, R.: Observations on the treatment of traumatic urethral injuries and the value of the

fenestrated urethral catheter. Br. J. Surg., *60*:775, 1973.
76. Kimbrough, J. C.: War wounds of the urogenital tract. J. Urol., *55*:179, 1946.
77. Young, H. H.: Wounds of the urogenital tract in modern warfare. J. Urol., *47*:59, 1942.
78. Busch, F. M., Chenault, W., Jr., Zinner, N. R., and Clarke, B. G.: Urological aspects of Vietnam war injuries. J. Urol., *97*:763, 1967.
79. Beck, A. R., and Wesser, D. R.: Constrictive digital injuries in infants, caused by human hair. Plast. Reconstr. Surg., *49*:420, 1972.
80. Hoffman, H. A., and Colby, F. H.: Incarceration of the penis. J. Urol., *54*:391, 1945.
81. Preston, E. N.: Whither the foreskin? J.A.M.A., *213*:1853, 1970.
82. Kendall, A. R., and Darafin, L.: Repair of the denuded penis. J. Urol., *98*:484, 1967.
83. DeWeerd, J. H.: Management of injuries to the bladder, urethra and genitalia. Surg. Clin. North Am., *39*:973, 1959.
84. McRoberts, J. W., Chapman, W. H., and Ansell, J. S.: Primary anastomosis of the traumatically amputated penis. J. Urol., *100*:751, 1968.

XII. The Female Genital Tract

by David Charles and Joel Rankin

The phrase "injuries of the female genital tract" immediately focuses the attention of the physician on the topic of rape. It is, however, erroneous to consider these as synonymous; trauma to the female genital tract has a much wider scope. Lacerations of the vulva and perineum are sometimes the result of falls astride a bar or the edge of a bathtub, or not so infrequently, are secondary to motorcycle accidents. A hematoma of the vulva may result from a blow even when there is no laceration, or may be due to rupture of a varicose vein caused by violent exertion. The fact that exertion alone, without direct trauma, can lead to rupture of a vulvar varix must be remembered and appreciated by physicians and attorneys alike, especially when evaluating the individual who has allegedly been raped. Despite these possibilities, one cannot deny that in the majority of patients brought to a doctor's office or the emergency room of a hospital, genital tract injuries are related to sex and sexual matters.

The medical and legal implications of rape are fully discussed in Chapter 37; in this section, the authors describe in a more general and comprehensive manner those injuries of the female genital tract that occur primarily in the nonpregnant state, both those related to the individual's sexual being and those that have no relationship to sexuality. At the same time, one must remember that obstetric injuries constitute by far the greatest number of insults in this region of the body, and it is worth pointing out that evidence for this type of trauma may be important in determining whether a woman has concealed a pregnancy, especially if she has been accused of infanticide.

In every land and in every generation, human sexuality has been and still is regarded as one of the outstanding problems of the day. With the passage of time it has become no longer accepted that human sexuality defies understanding, and the recognition that its mechanisms are complicated merely stimulates inquiry into a matter that is to be examined and explained.

The percentage of injuries attributable to rape must be on the increase, since it is known that sexual offenses against females have increased enormously during the past decade.[1] Unfortunately they still involve a great deal of the time of medical and legal authorities. One would have imagined that with the increase in sexual freedom and the sexual mores of the present era, there would have been a decrease in rape and sexual assault. Haymann and Lanza feel that the current trend is a symptom and expression of an aggressive and violent society rather than an augmented sexual drive of individuals.[2] This type of violence can be considered as allied to and accompanied by the rampant, compulsive behavior and social unrest of the present era.

FUNCTIONAL ANATOMY AND PHYSIOLOGY

In the evaluation of the extent of any injury, an appreciation of the anatomical and physiologic factors is extremely important. In addition, when considering reproductive system trauma, one must be cognizant of the effects of age, prior sexual activity, marital status, and parity on the female genital tract. Incomplete from the point of view of the anatomist and the physiologist, the following descriptions comprise the rudiments that are pertinent in eliciting the effects of traumatic insults to the various segments of the genital tract.

External Genitalia

The term "vulva" is synonymous with the external genitalia, and includes the mons veneris, the labia majora and minora, the vaginal orifice, the hymen, the clitoris, and the vestibule (Fig. 3–XII–1). The perineum is the descriptive term for that part of the body between the vaginal orifice and the anal canal. A further anatomical relationship to be considered is the close proximity of the urethral orifice to the vagina, which means that trauma directed at the vaginal orifice may involve the urinary tract.

This area of the female anatomy has an extensive vascular supply derived predominantly from the internal pudendal artery (Fig. 3–XII–2). The venous drainage is via the internal pudendal veins, but veins from the clitoris also drain into the vesical and vaginal plexuses. The anastomotic nature of the vascular channels in this region readily explains why injury can result in hematoma formation that can diffuse over the anterior abdominal wall or inferiorly to the medial aspect of the thigh. The extravasation of blood following trauma to the perineum can readily be explained by the fact that the superficial perineal fascia is continuous with Scarpa's fascia of the abdominal wall.

Surrounding the vaginal orifice is the sphincter vaginae muscle, and deep to it on either side are the bulbs of the vestibule, which consist of loosely encapsulated erectile tissue and which converge anteriorly to form the glans clitoridis. At the posterior end of each vestibular bulb is Bartholin's gland, a compound racemous structure enclosed in a fibrous capsule, which under normal conditions cannot be palpated but which can be involved in hematoma formation after perineal injury.

The labia majora are not well formed until puberty, at the time when pubic hair appears. The labia enlarge during adolescence and meet in the midline, overlapping the intervening

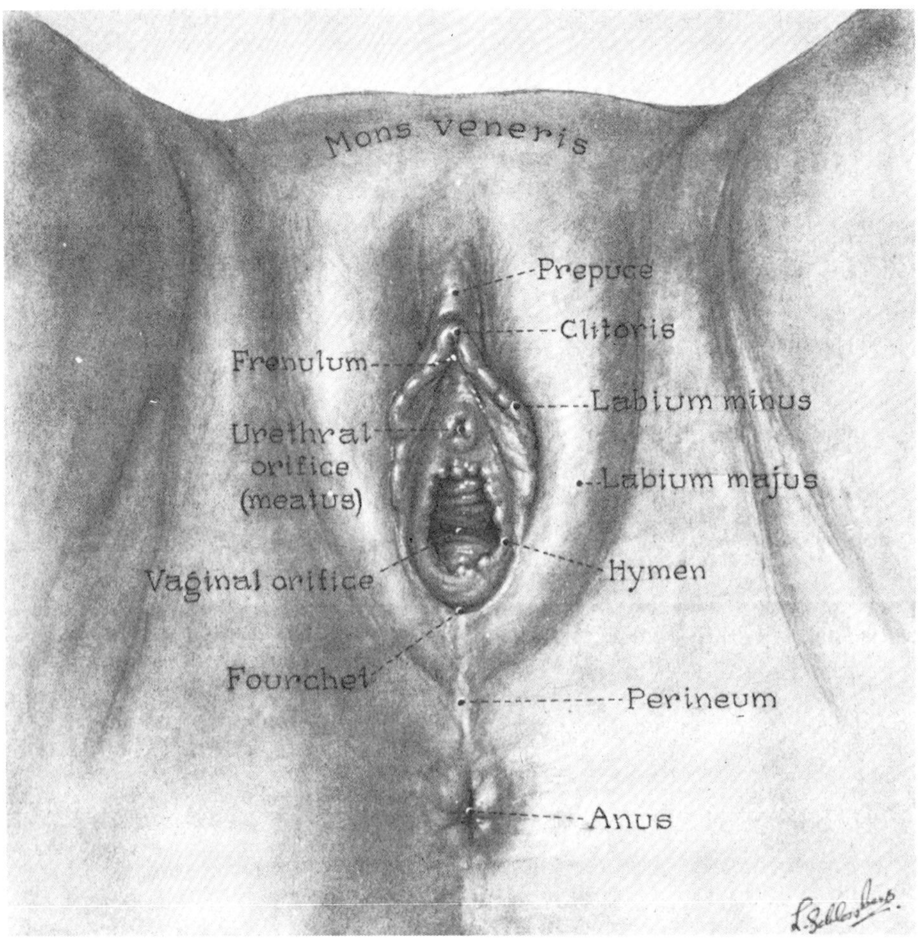

Figure 3–XII–1. The female external genitalia. (From L. M. Hellman, and J. A. Pritchard (Eds.): *Williams Obstetrics.* 14th Edition. Englewood Cliffs, N. J., Appleton-Century-Crofts, Publishing Division of Prentice-Hall Inc., 1971. Reprinted by permission.)

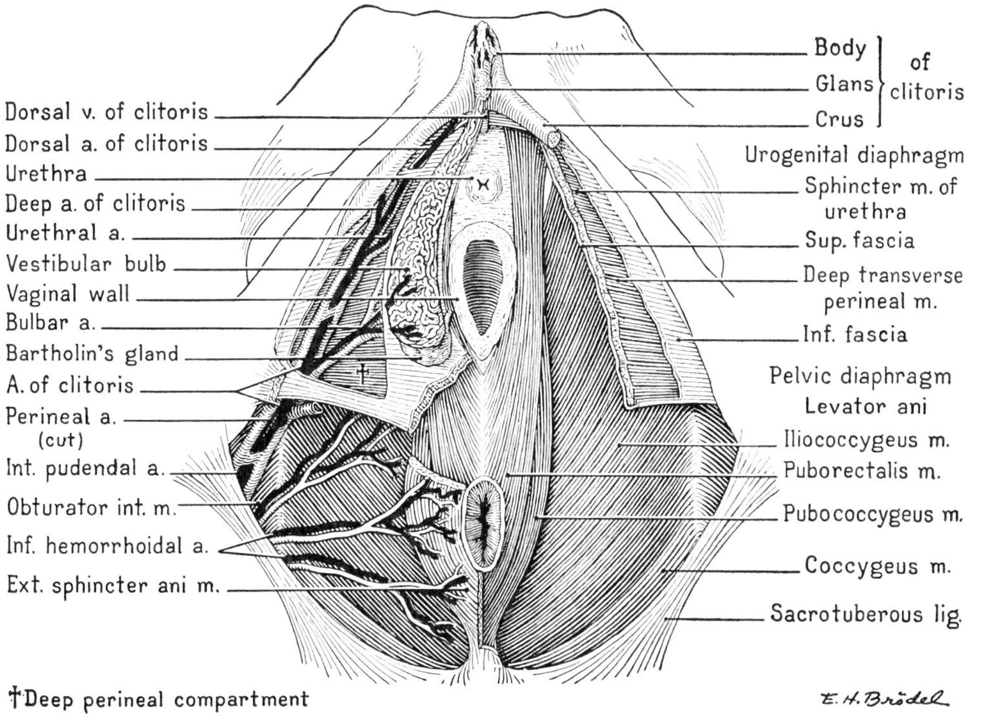

Figure 3–XII–2. The muscles and blood supply of the perineum. (From L. M. Hellman, and J. A. Pritchard (Eds.): *Williams Obstetrics.* 14th Edition. Englewood Cliffs, N.J., Appleton-Century-Crofts, Publishing Division of Prentice-Hall, Inc., 1971. Reprinted by permission.)

structures. After childbirth the labia majora tend to remain somewhat apart, and after the menopause they have minimal amounts of subcutaneous fat and hair.

The labia minora or nymphae are a pair of thin cutaneous folds of soft tissue that lie within the greater labia and form the lateral boundaries of the vestibule.

The vaginal orifice is the entrance to the vaginal canal and is partially covered by the hymen. The latter is composed of connective tissue covered on both the vaginal and vulval surfaces by stratified squamous epithelium. In the virgin, the hymen is little more than half a centimeter in thickness and attached to the posterior half or two thirds of the vaginal orifice. The membrane may, however, sometimes be attached to all margins of the vaginal orifice or may have either a central aperture or two lateral apertures separated by an anteroposterior bridge. At times, it takes the form of a cribriform plate, and in other instances is entirely closed, the so-called imperforate hymen. The strength and dilatability of the hymen are variable; it may be so elastic as to stretch without laceration during intercourse, or on the other hand, may be so resistant that its surgical removal is necessary before intercourse can ensue. Conception does not always imply penetration of the hymen, since pregnancies have been reported in women in whom the hymen was intact or had merely a pinpoint aperture in the membrane. Normally, after intercourse, the hymen is found stretched or lacerated, and subsequent to this, access to the vagina is simplified. During the first coitus, tearing occurs at several points, usually in the posterior portion. The edges soon heal, and the hymen then becomes permanently divided into two or three portions separated by narrow slits extending down to the base. Although the vasculature at the base of the hymen is rather extensive, the hymen itself is a relatively avascular structure. Thus in rupture during first coitus, a few drops of blood may exude but heavy bleeding is rare.

The function of the external genitalia is less important than their anatomy in delineating the effects of trauma. On the other hand, Masters and Johnson have described the marked vascular engorgement that occurs in the labia majora and to a lesser extent in the labia minora during the plateau phase of the human sexual response.[3] This attests to their extensive vasculature. Similarly, the clitoris undergoes vasocongestive increase in diameter during the excitement phase.

The Vagina

Several considerations are of paramount importance in the effects of trauma to the vagina. One must pay particular heed to the introitus, the vasculature, the relationship of the vagina to other structures, and the physiologic response of the vagina to sexual excitement.

The vagina is a fibromuscular canal that passes upward and backward from the introitus at an angle of approximately 45 degrees. It is lined by stratified squamous epithelium, which rests on connective tissue surrounded by involuntary muscle and a fascial sheath.

Anterior to the vagina lie the urethra, bladder, and uterovesical pouch. Lateral to this canal are the levatores ani muscles, the endopelvic fascia, and the base of the broad ligaments. The posterior relationships are with the perineal body, the rectum, and superiorly, the pouch of Douglas (Fig. 3–XII–3). The extensive vascularity of the vagina can be appreciated from Figure 3–XII–4.

The arterial supply comes from the hypogastric arteries via the vaginal, uterine, internal pudendal, and middle hemorrhoidal branches. It has a vast anastomotic plexus of veins, which connect with the vesical and rectal veins to drain into the internal iliac veins.

It is well to bear in mind that the principal muscles that impede entrance to the vagina are the levatores ani. This fact is best appreciated when one considers the syndrome of vaginismus, in which there is involuntary spasm of these muscle groups. Vaginismus is the most common and most important cause of dyspareunia and is a protective mechanism. In its severe form, it is occasionally accompanied by spasm of the abductor muscles of the thigh so that the vulva is inaccessible. Indeed, although the syndrome is usually psychogenic in origin, many women have been injudiciously subjected to surgery because the clinical picture has not been properly evaluated. It does occur, however, whenever there is marked tenderness associated with an organic lesion in the perineum or pelvis, and in such instances surgical treatment can be curative. Other factors must always be considered in the evaluation of vaginismus, specifically ignorance, lack of sex education, initial painful attempts at coitus, assault, or in some cases, a history of the administration of an enema in childhood. In the latter context proctalgia fugax may occur; similarly, a degree of rectal spasm and pain may ensue following trauma to the levator muscle, especially in the presence of contusion of the paravaginal tissues.

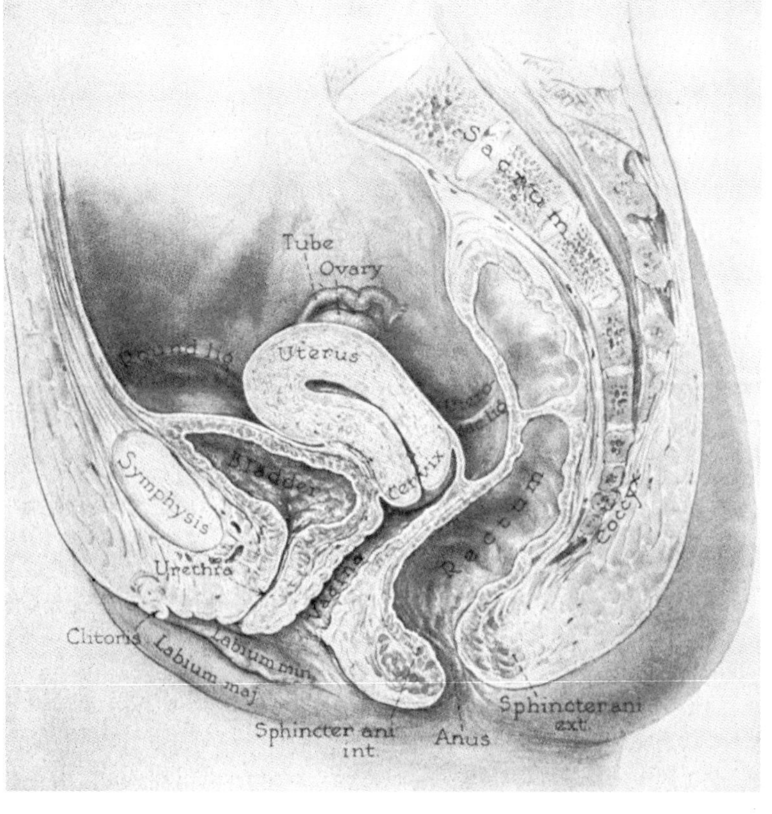

Figure 3–XII–3. Sagittal view of the female pelvis. (From A. H. Curtis and J. W. Huffman: *A Textbook of Gynecology.* 6th Edition. Philadelphia, W. B. Saunders Co., 1950. Reprinted by permission.)

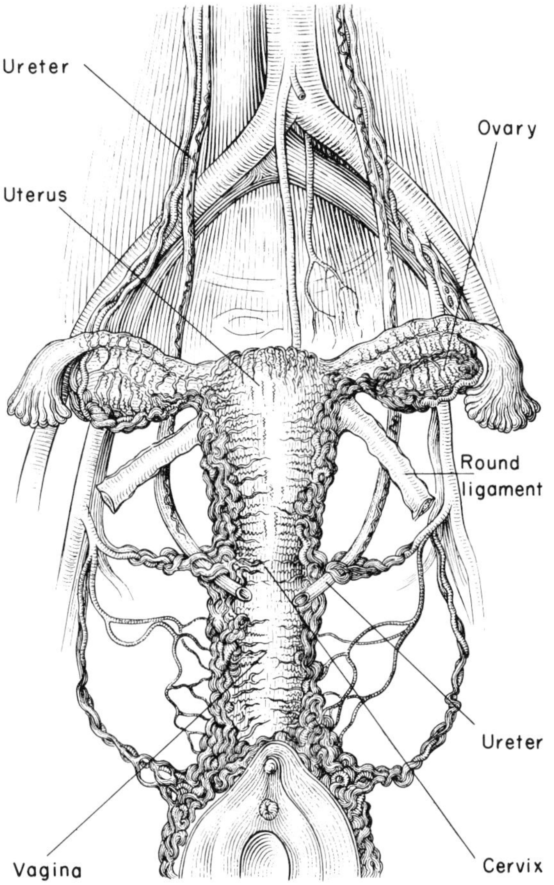

Figure 3–XII–4. The major vascular supply to the lower genital tract.

The work of Masters and Johnson has been of inestimable value, from both the theoretical and practical points of view, in elucidating the participation of the vagina in the human sexual response and at the same time explaining why coital injuries may result during both voluntary and forced coitus.[3] These authors have demonstrated that the physiologic responses to sexual excitement in females conform to a pattern. Successful sexual stimulation elicits an identical response no matter what the source or location of stimulation, but any psychologic intrusion rapidly reduces the level of excitation. The extensive vascularity of the vagina is well illustrated by the vasocongestive response that occurs during the excitement as well as the plateau phases.

More impressive still, physiologically, is the response of the vaginal barrel to sexual stimulation (Fig. 3–XII–5). The length of the unstimulated nulliparous vagina is from 7 to 8 cm, but during the excitement phase vaginal length increases to 9.5 to 10.5 cm. There appears to be unlimited distensibility, so that the more the vagina dilates, the more dilatation becomes possible; with excitement, vaginal length extensions to 11 to 12 cm have been observed. At the level of the cervix, there is also transverse expansion of the vaginal barrel. In the unstimulated state, the width averages 2 cm, but with excitement it expands to transverse measurements of 6.75 to 7.25 cm.

The implications of the investigations are striking: the vagina is capable of enlargement during sexual excitment to accommodate the male organ regardless of size. These studies also demonstrated that the artificial vagina, whether fashioned surgically or by mechanical means, undergoes the same response to sexual stimulation as the normal vagina, although to a lesser degree. Thus, lengthening and transverse enlargement of the vaginal barrel is a

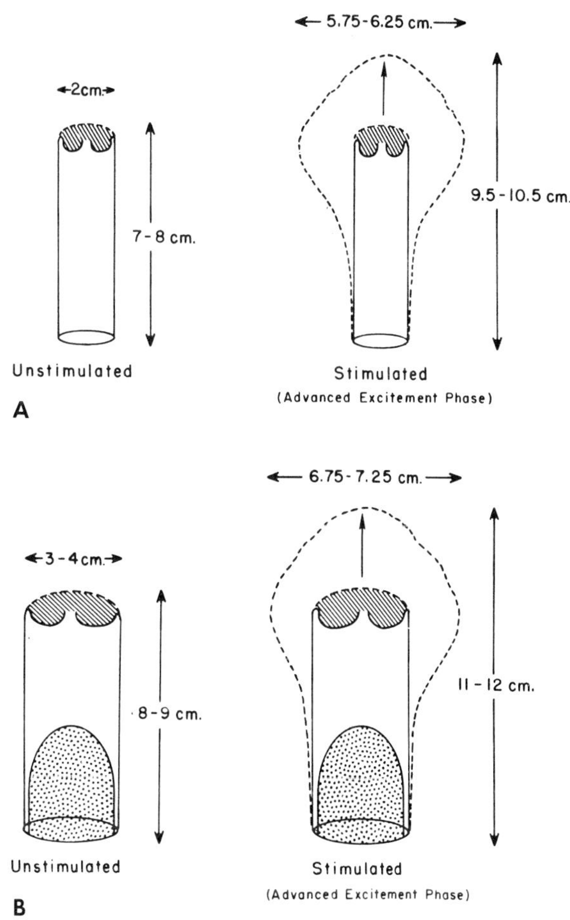

Figure 3–XII–5. The response of the human vagina to sexual excitement. *A.* Baseline measurements. *B.* Measurements after prior speculum dilatation. (From W. H. Masters and V. E. Johnson: *Human Sexual Response.* Boston, Little, Brown and Co., 1966. Reprinted by permission.)

normal expected concomitant of sexual excitement and the human sexual response. It is also worthy of note that enlargement of the barrel is further enhanced by uterine elevation, which occurs during the excitement and plateau phases, producing a tenting effect in the mid-vaginal plane.

On the other hand, the distensibility is not evoked in the absence of sexual excitement. Difficulties in coitus may occur if mounting takes place early in the excitement phase before expansion in length and transcervical diameter have developed. Under these circumstances, a woman may experience some difficulty in accommodating an erect penis, particularly a large organ. Women who have not been sexually active, especially those who are postmenopausal, experience some shrinkage of the vaginal barrel. Their vaginal response to sexual stimulation is slow, and thus distention of the vaginal barrel to an adequate degree may not occur until the advanced stages of female sexual tension.

The Cervix and Uterus

The uterus in the nonpregnant patient is relatively well protected from potential trauma because it is located within the confines of the bony pelvis. When the uterus rises out of the pelvis, as it does in the gravid state, it is more vulnerable to injury. Nevertheless, when considering injuries to the pelvic organs, it is well to bear in mind the vasculature and the relationships of the uterus to other structures.

The uterine blood supply is derived from the uterine arteries, which arise from the anterior division of the hypogastric arteries. In its course, the uterine artery crosses above the ureter approximately 1 cm lateral to the cervix and then divides into an ascending and a descending branch. The ascending division anastomoses with the tubal branch of the ovarian artery as well as its counterpart from the opposite side. The descending branch is the cervical artery, which in turn anastomoses with the vaginal arteries. As is well known, there is far less tendency to extensive hemorrhage in cervical injuries. It should, however, be borne in mind that the cervicovaginal tributaries of the uterine artery descend on the lateral aspects of the cervix; suitably placed sutures here will obviate bleeding when extensive operative procedures are performed on the cervix.

The uterus is relatively mobile, and its supravaginal cervical portion is the most fixed part, owing to the endopelvic fascial attachments. Anterior to the upper part of the uterus is the uterovesical pouch of peritoneum; the lower part is in close proximity to the bladder. The pouch of Douglas is posterior to the uterine body, and the posterior fornix lies behind the cervix. On each side of the uterus is the broad ligament, which contains the uterine vessels.

TRAUMATIC LESIONS OF THE VULVA AND VAGINA

Vulval and vaginal injuries do not account for many hospital admissions to a gynecologic service and, in fact, in comparison to other entities encountered in clinical practice, occupy a very small percentage of the time of the physician. In the report of Metsälä and Nieminen, only 0.02 per cent of more than 300,000 patients seen for obstetrical or gynecologic consultation required hospital admission for traumatic lesions of the vagina.[4] Similar figures have been recorded by Hakanson and also by Rush and Milton.[5,6] One cannot, however, negate the importance of such injuries as far as the physical and emotional well-being of the afflicted patient are concerned. Similarly, the fact should not be minimized that these lesions may be associated with massive hemorrhage, necessitating blood transfusion.[4,7,8] Infection and death from exsanguination and overwhelming sepsis have been recorded.[9,10] Recognition of traumatic lesions is of prime importance, not only to the patient for her own peace of mind but also to the physician and the legal authorities in order to establish or refute allegations of rape. But perhaps the major reason for discussing this topic, as far as the physician is concerned, is that these lesions are all too frequently omitted from consideration in the differential diagnosis of bleeding and pain, and as a result, appropriate therapy is delayed. Furthermore, in this context the clinician must appreciate the fact that vulvovaginal trauma may relate to sexuality, but also may in many instances bear no relationship to the individual as a sexual being.

Injuries Related to Sexuality

Coital Trauma

There is no doubt that the vast majority of traumatic lesions of the vulva and vagina are sexually related, although not always the result of coitus. Metsälä and Nieminen evaluated 76 patients who were admitted to the hospital with vaginal lacerations, and discovered that 88 per cent of the injuries resulted from coitus.[4] Sixty-nine per cent of the 36 cases summarized by Rush and Milton had a similar causation.[6]

It may come as a surprise to the casual observer that a substantial number of coitally acquired injuries result from intercourse with consenting partners. When one attempts to ascertain the percentage of these injuries resulting from rape compared to those unrelated to sexual assault, it is immediately apparent that the statistics vary so much that any conclusion is meaningless. Of the 37 patients studied by Wilson and Swartz, 7 had vaginal injuries as a result of rape.[8] This report encompassed all such injuries admitted to Harlem Hospital in eight and one quarter years. Chandra and Rathee noted that only 1 of 10 coital injuries could be ascribed to rape, while Diddle found that sexual assault was the precipitating factor in only 2 of his 133 cases (1.5 per cent).[10, 11] On the other hand, at District of Columbia General Hospital in Washington, admissions for vulvovaginal injuries as a result of rape probably constitute a much larger percentage, and this undoubtedly also holds true for the Philadelphia General Hospital, as both institutions provide emergency facilities for victims of alleged sexual assault.[2, 12] Nevertheless, regardless of the statistics, it is important to recognize that coital injuries of the vagina are not solely due to rape. Similarly, these injuries are not restricted to the prepubertal, virginal, or postmenopausal female. In fact, Wilson and Swartz, in summarizing their 37 cases, found that 24 of the individuals were in the reproductive age group and sexually active, and 6 were virgins.[8] Seventy per cent of the 76 patients reported by Metsälä and Nieminen ranged in age from 18 to 40 years, and the majority were sexually active.[4]

A great many factors have been claimed as predisposing or contributory causes of vulvovaginal injury as a result of coitus. (Table 3–XII–1).[4, 5, 7-11, 13-15] In light of the data accumulated by Masters and Johnson, one must seriously question any direct relationship of many of the so-called etiologic factors to the injury. Indeed, their description of the vaginal ballooning that accompanies sexual excitement in the female would almost negate the significance of genital disproportion. Furthermore, the concept of vaginal enlargement applies both to the normal female and to the individual with an artificial vagina. The latter statement implies that the patient with pathologic changes of the vagina would not be expected to suffer undue trauma if properly and adequately

TABLE 3–XII–1. PREDISPOSING AND CONTRIBUTING CAUSES OF VULVOVAGINAL COITAL INJURIES

Rape
Prepuberty
Virginity
Postmenopause
Pregnancy
Recent vaginal surgery
Multiple consorts
Alcoholic intoxication
Heroin addiction
Genital disproportion
Clumsiness
Male brutality during coitus
Violent male passion during coitus
Excessive active involvement of the female
Pathologic changes of vulva and vagina
Vaginal attenuation
Post–potassium permanganate scarring
Congenital anomalies
Postradiation atrophy
Renewed sexual activity after prolonged abstinence
Vaginismus
Exceptional coital positions
Uterine retroversion
Paravaginal inflammation

aroused. The dorsal decubitus position with the thighs hyperflexed predisposes to deep penetration by the male, a fact that has frequently been recorded as a contributory factor in vaginal vault laceration, but again, such a posture should be of minimal import in the sexually aroused female.

Probably very few of the factors enumerated in Table 3–XII–1 operate in isolation in promoting or producing traumatic lesions of the female genital tract. In the unprepared and unaroused tense individual, damage is much more likely to occur than in the one who has at least reached the excitement phase of the human sexual response. It is well to consider most of the items listed as predisposing or contributory rather than absolute etiologic antecedents.

In the virgin experiencing her initial coitus, hymenal lacerations are not infrequent because the hymen presents an anatomical barrier to penetration. Some virgins, however, experience vaginal lacerations instead of or in addition to hymenal tears. One therefore wonders whether such vaginal insults are related solely to the state of preparedness. The concept of vaginal vault muscle spasm with a concomitant reduction in vaginal volume resulting from intense sexual feeling on the part of the woman should also be considered sub judice in light of the work of Masters and Johnson.[3] Be that as it may, there is little doubt that the virgin is prone to lacerations, but there is no unanimity in the literature as to the true incidence of trauma accountable to virginity per se.

On the other hand, there does appear to be a significant relationship between the postparturient state and vaginal injury. The latter is well illustrated by the report of Wilson and Swartz in which they noted four puerperal women among their 37 patients with vulvovaginal lacerations.[8] In addition, in the series reported by Fish, 4 of the 14 individuals sustained vaginal injuries within several weeks of parturition.[7] Similarly, Diddle noted that 13 of his series of 133 patients developed vulvovaginal lacerations and contusion at the time of their first sexual contact after childbirth.

The postmenopausal woman also appears to be prone to this type of injury. Six of the thirty-seven patients in the series of Wilson and Swartz had completed the climacteric, as had 8 of the 133 individuals reported by Diddle.[8, 10] In fact, Speert claims that coital trauma must be considered in the differential diagnosis of postmenopausal bleeding in elderly women who resume sexual activity after prolonged abstinence.[15]

The extent and location of coital injuries vary, as exemplified by the fact that a minimal hymenal laceration may result in only minimal blood loss in one virgin, whereas another might, at defloration, experience an extensive tear accompanied by profuse hemorrhage and even a state of shock. Similarly, vault injuries vary from minimal mucosal trauma to extensive lacerations that can result in death from sepsis or hemorrhage.[4, 10] In the majority of instances, vault injuries present as mucosal lesions approximately 3 cm in length.

In general, injuries to the vulva are most often encountered in young women at the time of initial intercourse or in rape. Vaginal vault lacerations are usually found in women who have had previous coital experience but who have had only a few well-spaced pregnancies.[6, 7, 8] Of the 57 coital injuries reported by Metsälä and Nieminen, 14 per cent involved the introitus, 21 per cent the lateral vaginal wall, and 65 per cent the vault of the vagina.[4] It should also be brought to the attention of the clinician that in 18 of the 37 patients reported by Wilson and Swartz, multiple injuries were observed in the lower genital tract.[8] This fact further emphasizes the necessity for careful clinical evaluation in order to appreciate the full extent of the trauma.

As already stated, minor injuries to the hymen are almost inevitable with defloration and are associated with minimal bleeding in most instances. On the other hand, occasionally a relatively large vessel is severed; if not properly dealt with, this can result in exsanguination.[16] Hymenal lacerations may be accompanied by lateral vaginal wall injuries, especially in the young child. Sulcus tears may be present in the absence of contusion or laceration of the vulva, and they require immediate investigation and treatment. Examination should be performed under general anesthesia in order to determine the extent of the trauma.

Nevertheless there is little doubt that the majority of vaginal coital lesions involve the fornices.[4, 6, 8] The preponderance of these lacerations are located in the posterior fornix, more specifically, on the right side of the vault. Less frequently the left fornix is involved, and from the literature it would appear that the anterior fornix is well nigh immune to this type of injury.[4, 6, 8] The fact that the right fornix is usually larger than that on the left side may explain the greater incidence of lacerations at this site.[4, 8]

In view of the close proximity of the vagina to the other pelvic viscera, bowel complications may follow any severe coital injury. Penetration of the cul-de-sac can result in peritonitis, intestinal prolapse, or even a rectovaginal fistula.[10, 11] Likewise, urethral or vesical complications have been reported.[5, 7] In such instances, cystoscopy is mandatory to determine the extent of the trauma. All these complications, although infrequent, are potentially lethal and require immediate investigation.

As is well known, vulvovaginal injury is a common concomitant of sexual assault. In 501 rape cases referred to Philadelphia General Hospital in 1968, demonstrable genital tract lacerations were noted in 5.2 per cent.[12] It is undoubtedly true that a great many of the assaults on women are related to sexuality, and consequently, in cases of rape, the obligations of the physician warrant some discussion.

The physician has innumerable responsibilities toward a patient and at no time will he find it more difficult to gain good rapport with an individual than when she has been raped. There are several ways a physician can evaluate the patient both from the general and local physical examination, but above all he must remember that all must be documented for members of the legal profession.

The date and time of the examination must be recorded, as the interval between the alleged incident and the appearance of the patient in his office or in the hospital is of supreme importance. An interval of undue length requires clarification and explanation, as after a few days, if injury has occurred, the reparative process will have obscured any evidence of rape. In fact, if a few days have elapsed, one should expect the findings at the time of examination of an adult female to be negative, especially if she is married or has an active sexual life. The physician should observe the gait of the victim as she enters the office, and her general demeanor. He should ascertain whether walking produces the type of pain likely to result from trauma to the genital tract, and note whether there is any evidence of mental disturbance due to drug abuse. Finally, the patient's physique will inform the doctor about her capacity to resist violent assault.

One must reiterate that if the patient is accompanied by parents or friends, the physician should document their opinions in the absence of the victim. Likewise, all details must be elicited from the victim and these should include her name, age, social and marital status, menstrual history, and whether she is taking an oral contraceptive or has an intrauterine device for the same purpose. The time, date, and place of the incident and the steps taken by the individual to resist the assailant are of major importance. Specifically, the woman must be asked if she had any loss of consciousness during or subsequent to the attack on her person. It must be emphasized that only after consent has been obtained can the victim be examined, and this consent must be obtained by the physician in the presence of a witness. In the case of a child, the consent of a parent or guardian should be obtained, and this individual should preferably be in attendance at the time of the examination. Again, one must emphasize that in all cases, historical documentation is essential, and any abnormalities that are subsequently found on examination must be correlated with the history.

Brutality

The genitalia of the female can also serve as the focal point for assault. In a given instance, it is probably difficult to ascertain whether the damage inflicted represents sheer sadism or sadism related to sexuality. In any event, the resulting damage can be severe. Metsälä and Nieminen described a vault laceration that resulted from the introduction of a man's fist into the vagina.[4] This produced a 10-cm longitudinal rupture in the left vaginal wall associated with numerous minor tears in the area of the vulva. Kiel recounts the gory death of a 25-year-old woman who was found completely nude in a field outside her home. Eventrated between her legs were her uterus and several loops of intestine that had been avulsed through the vagina.[17] On the other hand, it is perhaps surprising how often victims of rape or other sexual assaults manifest evidence of trauma to other parts of the body in the absence of demonstrable damage to the genital tract.[2]

Foreign Bodies

Whether foreign bodies in the vagina have a sexual connotation is open to question, and consequently to various interpretations. There is little doubt that in the adult female the insertion of various objects into the vagina is not always a chance happening, but bears some overt or subconscious relationship to the individual's sexual function. Nymphomania can become an obsession and can result in self-inflicted injury of the vagina by a foreign body. One of us has encountered such a patient who had an excessive sexual drive during the climacteric. She was admitted to the hospital with a sulcus laceration that extended up to the base of the broad ligament. She claimed the injury was the result of rape, but later, after evaluation of the damage under general anesthesia had revealed a fractured test tube in the posterior fornix, she stated that it was the orgasmal response to masturbation that was responsible for the injury. The traumatic role of foreign bodies inserted into the vagina was noted in 2 of the 37 cases of coital injury reported by Wilson and Swartz.[8] In cases of multiple lacerations, Hakanson considers that foreign bodies should always be suspected as the causal agent.[5]

Foreign bodies should always be searched for, and radiologic assistance is considered mandatory in order to delineate such items. All manner of objects have been removed from the vagina, and they all too frequently tax the imagination of the most avant-garde physician. Howkins and Bourne quote the famous case of Bland Sutton, which involved the removal of a small bust of Napoleon from the vagina, presumably introduced as a supreme act of hero worship.[16]

It would be erroneous to assume that all objects removed from the vagina are related to sexuality. In the past, severe vaginal lacerations occurred in the procurement of abortion by unskilled individuals who used a variety of household devices, which were frequently recovered from the vagina at the time of hospital admission. In the adolescent female, the presence of a persistent vaginal discharge should always alert the physician to the possibility that a foreign body might be the precipitating cause for this symptom. Out of mere curiosity, younger children not infrequently insert candy, toys, and pencils into the vagina. Likewise, during the last of the seven ages of woman, foreign bodies, including neglected pessaries, may be retrieved from the lower genital tract.

Genital Self-Mutilation

Self-mutilation is extremely rare in both the male and female, and to many physicians the term brings to mind an entity encountered only in the demented individual. Certainly in the past a great many women inadvertently injured themselves attempting to procure abortions. If, however, one restricts the term to situations in which the female injures her genitalia deliberately for conscious or subconscious gain, then indeed it is rarely seen in clinical practice. Reich and Wehr feel that these patients manifest a hostile-dependent relationship with others, including their physicians.[18] The symptoms so produced serve the purpose of attracting attention, and in addition, may express hostility directed at the physician for failure to relieve or cure her complaint. French and Nelson described a patient who presented with anorexia and bulimia, in whom self-injury occurred in the form of superficial lacerations of the lower genital tract.[19] The trauma was felt to indicate hostility toward her husband, whose interest in her was largely or wholly sexual to the exclusion of her other attributes. Goldfield and Glick described the case of a 19-year-old patient in which the diagnosis of self-mutilation was finally established by painting the vaginal wall with gentian violet at night.[20] The presence of the dye under the patient's fingernails the following morning established the cause of her "unexplained" vaginal bleeding. Reich and Wehr also described a patient who was pregnant and in whom vaginal bleeding was the result of intravaginal manipulation with a nail file. Although this woman had a distinct desire to rid herself of the pregnancy, self-mutilation also played a role in her psychologic reaction to the gestation.

The physician would do well to recognize the existence of this syndrome and to consider it in the differential diagnosis whenever a patient presents with unexplained vaginal bleeding. Undoubtedly, many more examples exist and have been overlooked. Although there is a potential danger to life, as self-mutilation can theoretically do extensive damage, perhaps the main reason for calling this entity to the attention of members of the medical profession is the realization that vast numbers of unnecessary surgical procedures are performed on such patients in search for the cause of the abnormal bleeding.

Vulvovaginal Injury Unrelated to Sexuality

Although the majority of traumatic lesions of the female genital tract that occur in the nonpregnant state are related to sexuality, and especially to coitus, many examples can be sited in which coitus and sexuality play no role. It is important that the gynecologist or practicing clinician appreciate the fact that trauma must be considered in the differential diagnosis of gynecologic disease, and also recognize that this trauma need bear no relationship to the individual as a sexual being.

Direct Trauma

Noncoital vulval injuries as the result of direct trauma are frequently seen. Children appear to be especially prone to such injuries, which generally originate from falling astride gates, chairs, bars, or sharp objects. In fact, in this age group, astride injuries make up the majority of cases.[21] The lesion may involve only the vulva or may extend into the vagina. Although the vascularity of the vulva and perineum is less in a child than in a postadolescent, extensive bleeding can occur, and on occasion blood transfusions are required. Since it is essential to ascertain the full extent of the damage, anesthesia is frequently necessary because during childhood the structures involved are small and complete cooperation is essential to obtain adequate exposure. In the experience of Ezell and associates, the most common agents responsible for such injuries are the open dresser drawer and the tricycle.[21]

Direct trauma to the vulva in the adult female is apt to be complicated by the development of a large hematoma because of the presence of the large venous plexuses and the loose areolar tissue. Injury with a sharp object may lead to extensive hemorrhage, especially if the laceration involves either the region of the clitoris or the erectile tissue around the vaginal orifice. Thus, a blow with a blunt instrument may produce extravasation of blood into the loose connective tissue, while injury with a sharp object is more apt to produce external bleeding. Direct trauma to the external genitalia may also take the form of gunshot or stab wounds. The absence of any external evidence of trauma, however, does not exclude injury to the pelvic viscera. Hakanson illustrates this point by describing a 5-year-old child who inadvertently sat down on a pointed phonograph spindle.[5] The child presented with hematuria, but with no evidence of external injury. During detailed examination under anesthesia it was discovered that the spindle had entered the anal canal, perforated the rectovaginal septum, and proceeded through the vagina to enter the bladder.

The foregoing discussion has centered on trauma directed at the vagina and perineum. The physician must also remember that vaginal injury may result from severe accidents in the absence of direct trauma to the vulva or vagina. Automobile accidents may lead to fractures of the pelvis, and vaginal avulsion has been reported as a complication of such an injury.[22] Abdominal trauma associated with a sudden increase in intraabdominal pressure may also result in vaginal tears in the adolescent.

Spontaneous Rupture of the Vaginal Vault

Many reports in the literature have dealt with spontaneous rupture of the vagina in the absence of any direct injury to this portion of the female genital tract.[4, 6, 23-29] The vaginal rupture is almost always located in the posterior fornix and confined to postmenopausal women.

The lesion varies from a simple vault laceration to total disruption of the cul-de-sac and evisceration. It is of interest to note that the majority of individuals so afflicted have undergone previous vaginal surgery.

In most instances the incident is preceded by some exertion that increases intraabdominal pressure, for example, lifting or coughing.[23, 24, 29] Purnell postulates that vaginal rigidity, which may result from previous vaginal operative procedures, does not allow for abrupt changes in intraabdominal pressure.[23] Undoubtedly, the loss of tissue elasticity that characterizes the postmenopausal state also predisposes to rupture of the vaginal vault in elderly women.

Hemorrhage is rarely profuse in these cases because of the atrophic state of the tissue, but the clinician should always consider the existence of such an entity in the differential diagnosis of postmenopausal bleeding.

Instrumentation

It is not within the scope of this chapter to discuss the damage that can accrue from the use or misuse, intentional or otherwise, of instruments in the course of legal or illegal gynecologic procedures. Certainly, this could serve as the basis of a chapter in itself. Nevertheless, it is somewhat frightening to note that four of the nine noncoital lesions summarized by Metsälä and Nieminen were produced by the simple introduction of the speculum into the vagina.[4] One would imagine that the postmenopausal subject is particularly prone to such damage, and indeed one of their patients was an 88-year-old widow in whom a vaginal speculum produced a 4-cm rupture of the vaginal vault.[4]

Gynecologic Complications of Water Skiing

Several reports have appeared in the literature describing the gynecologic hazards of water skiing.[30-33] Every sport has its risks, and in the woman engaged in athletic endeavors, the most common gynecologic lesion is undoubtedly the "astride" injury. Although gynecologic injuries encountered in water skiing are quite rare, the nature of these lesions is unique and warrants a limited discussion.

The element in water skiing responsible for gynecologic injury is the sudden markedly elevated hydrostatic pressure to which the vagina is exposed if the perineum strikes the water under inappropriate circumstances. The force created can result in laceration of the lateral wall of the vaginal vault and profuse hemorrhage. In addition to hemorrhage, this high-pressure "vaginal douche" can also give rise to pelvic inflammatory disease.[30, 32] Whether this implies forceful entry of water not only within the vagina but into the Fallopian tubes per se is unknown. The possibility that miscarriage can be caused by water skiing also has been recorded.

Most of the reports regarding the gynecologic hazards of water skiing emanate from Australia and warmer climes. It should also be mentioned that the majority of complications occur in women who use standard swimsuits. Water skiers in cooler climates are less susceptible to these complications because they are more likely to wear rubber wet suits, thereby obviating the possibility that water under high pressure can reach the perineal area and enter the vagina.

Chemical Trauma to the Female Genital Tract

There are undoubtedly countless chemical agents that have caused injury to the female genital tract in the nonpregnant patient. Various douche solutions can act as irritants, and in this era of feminine hygiene spray deodorants, we have seen many examples of erythema and irritation of the external genitalia secondary to the use of such preparations.

Perhaps the most notorious injurious chemical agent is potassium permanganate. The use of this substance as a mild solution for douching dates back to the turn of the century. If properly diluted, little danger (and perhaps less good) results from its use as a cleansing douche or as therapy for various forms of vaginitis and pelvic inflammatory disease.[34] In the late 1940s and in the 1950s, the medical literature was inundated with reports of injuries resulting from the use of potassium permanganate in the form of a solid tablet as an abortifacient.[34–41]

Potassium permanganate is generally sold in the form of 300-mg tablets and owes its antiseptic action to its power of oxidation. When this chemical is in contact with organic material, it is reduced to manganese dioxide with the liberation of nascent oxygen. A superficial brown staining of the tissue takes place and is almost pathognomonic of a potassium permanganate reaction. Extensive injury may take place, however, especially at sites where there are high concentrations of the agent, owing to the formation of the caustic potassium hydroxide, which penetrates into the deeper tissues, eroding blood vessels and thereby producing hemorrhage, which is in essence the major complication of the destructive process.

The use and abuse of potassium permanganate was reported in the French and Italian literature long before its corrosive properties were recognized in North America. In all probability, the first report in North America of complications due to this chemical emanated from the Boston City Hospital in 1941, when Shull described 17 cases treated in that insitution in the preceding five years.[42] By 1945, 65 cases had been seen at Boston City Hospital.[43] In 1954, Steward and Webster summarized the findings in 105 patients reported to that date, and up to 1966 there were 319 cases reported in the medical literature.[44]

Undoubtedly, an occasional individual has been the victim of incomplete dissolution of the permanganate tablet in a double solution, so that fragments emerged from the douche nozzle, with resulting injury to the vaginal mucosa. In most instances, however, the tablet has been inserted into the vagina with intent to procure abortion. Generally, vaginal bleeding ensues about 20 hours after insertion of one or more tablets.[38, 44] The patient is apt to interpret such bleeding as the successful initiation of abortion, and as such, or because of the severity of the bleeding, presents herself at the physician's office or the hospital.

The diagnosis should be suspected when the bleeding is profuse and painless and the blood is bright red and contains no tissue, especially in a woman during reproductive life with secondary amenorrhea suggestive of pregnancy.

The findings on physical examination are pathognomonic. Classically, punched-out craters in charred brown mucosa are seen in the vaginal fornices or on the cervix. The craters are generally from 2 to 7 cm in diameter, and the extent of bleeding bears no relationship to the size of the lesion. The ulcers are often of the "kissing" variety and may diffuse over the vaginal cervix and upper third of the vagina.

All too frequently, these patients are the unfortunate victims of misdiagnosis because the pelvic examination is too hastily performed or because the physician fails to entertain the possibility of potassium permanganate burns in his differential diagnosis.[35, 38, 44] It is important to remember that the open speculum can hide the crater, and pressure from the instrument may arrest bleeding from an eroded vessel. Steward and Webster point out that the tendency to assume that any vaginal bleeding in a pregnant patient is due to a threatened abortion has been responsible for the failure to recognize the existence of polyps, carcinoma, foreign bodies, and chemical burns.[35]

It should be reiterated that the vagina has an extensive blood supply, which is accentuated in pregnancy. Therefore it can readily be appreciated that any erosion produced by a caustic burn can eventuate in extensive damage and severe vaginal bleeding necessitating blood transfusion. Deaths have been reported as a result of hemorrhage and shock.[36]

Although hemorrhage and shock are the major sequelae of the injudicious use of potassium permanganate tablets, other complications have been reported. Owing to the caustic nature of the material and its tendency to necrose tissue, it is not surprising that fistula formation may occur. Erosion into the parametrial tissue may lead to secondary bacterial invasion and pelvic cellulitis, peritonitis, and the formation of tuboovarian abscesses. Jetter and Hunter reported hemorrhagic necrosis of the uterus, pigmented casts in the renal tubules, and alkaline methemoglobinemia subsequent to the use of concentrated potassium permanganate vaginal douches.[45]

On occasion, termination of the pregnancy does ensue. Nine of the one hundred and twenty-eight cases reviewed by Steward and

Webster aborted.[35] In two it was proved that the abortion was due to other factors, but the causes of the remaining seven could not be determined. Vandergriff and Diddle state that the incidence of abortion after potassium permanganate instillation is almost identical to that for spontaneous abortion.[44] It is even more discouraging to note that a great many of the victims had erroneously assumed they were pregnant when they resorted to the use of this chemical as an ecbolic agent only to discover later that their amenorrhea was due to other causes.

The injudicious and inappropriate use of potassium permanganate as an abortifacient was not infrequently seen at Boston City Hospital as late as the mid-1960s. Whether as a result of an increase in patient awareness, a better educated populace, or greater access to therapeutic and elective abortion, not a single case of vaginal burns from potassium permanganate has been seen at this institution in the past five years.

UTERINE INJURIES

So far in this chapter, the major emphasis has been on injuries of the lower genital tract, but trauma to the cervix and uterine corpus warrants some discussion. The majority of such lesions are the direct result of factors incidental to pregnancy, labor, or abortion and are fully considered in obstetrical textbooks.

Automobile Accidents

Automobile accidents may result in direct violence to the gravid uterus, especially in the last trimester when uterine rupture may occur. If the uterine rupture is complete, it is associated with all the symptoms and signs found in the presence of severe intraperitoneal hemorrhage. When the rupture is incomplete, a broad ligament hematoma freqently occurs, and in such instances, shock may not be evident for several hours.

Therapeutic Abortion

Perforation of the uterus is a well-recognized hazard of gynecologic procedures and may be produced by the uterine sound, the cervical dilator, or the curette. In former years, before the introduction of legislation designed to liberalize both the attitude to and the practice of pregnancy termination, uterine injuries due to a variety of instruments—knitting needles, hairpins, and so forth—used to procure illegal abortions were frequently encountered in departments of gynecology in general hospitals. Such injuries were always serious because of the grave risk of infection within the peritoneal cavity.

Abortion always indicates some type of failure. It is now widely accepted that there is an urgent need to control population expansion and improve the living standards for individual families and the communities in which they reside. There still remains a wide divergence of opinion concerning the role of liberal abortion in relation to the control of human reproduction. In medical education, greater emphasis should be placed on the issues of contraception and abortion in relation to the lives of the patients and the community.

The consequences of therapeutic abortion are often minimized, specifically when a community believes that induced abortion is both a minor and a safe surgical procedure. In 1932, Whitehouse wrote:

> The procuring of abortion is not always safe, even in experienced hands. With all the care possible, and with all the surgical precautions of hospital practice, I have lost a patient from sepsis, whose uterus I had evacuated of its contents for therapeutic reasons. On another occasion I had to perform an immediate hysterectomy on a patient whose uterus I perforated in spite of every care as I thought.[46]

Although we recognize that the preceding statement was made when very few gynecologists had had much experience with therapeutic abortion, the identical complications occur in this decade. Nathanson in a recent review of 30,000 therapeutic abortions, reported that the incidence of uterine perforation was 0.8 per 1,000 (24 cases). Ten of the patients with this complication were nulligravid. Furthermore, in 50 per cent of the cases, the perforation was located in the anterior wall of a retroposed uterus. In fact, uterine position and the inexperience of the physician were the most common etiologic factors.[47] Inept handling of the instruments should also be considered as a causative factor, especially as 10 of the perforations were due to the uterine sound and 5 due to the suction tip.

Trauma to the cervix is a well-recognized complication of therapeutic abortion. What is not widely appreciated is that such injuries or even suction curettage per se may result in subsequent reproductive failure because of either an incompetent cervix during the second trimester or premature rupture of the membranes and premature labor at or around 28 to 30 weeks in a planned gestation.

The gynecologist's primary interest is the health and well-being of his patient, and from this point of view much good has resulted to individual patients from the present liberal attitude to pregnancy termination. On the other hand, the demographer, who does not have to deal with the problems that may arise, all too often regards abortion as a major method of attaining population control. Surely he should institute a more widely accepted positive approach to contraception, including male and female sterilization.

Intrauterine Devices

The intrauterine device has had widespread acceptance as a method of contraception during the past 15 years. It also has inherent risks to the individual that are now becoming more widely recognized. The German gynecologist Gräfenberg popularized in 1929 a device that could be completely placed within the uterus for contraceptive purposes.[48] His original device was in the form of a ring made of silkworm gut. In due course he replaced the silkworm gut with coiled silver or gold. Initially, this intrauterine device never found general acceptance in clinical practice because it was associated with a relatively high rate of incidence of pelvic inflammatory distress. As recently as 1955, MacLeod and Read wrote,

> Many instances of salpingitis, peritonitis and intramural abscess formation have been traced to their use, and one of us has seen a Gräfenberg ring which had ulcerated through the uterine wall. The authors wholeheartedly condemn their use and would like to see their use prohibited by law.[49]

Their wish was not granted, but there was very little interest in this form of contraception until the appearance in 1959 of a paper by Oppenheimer.[50] He recorded that he had encountered no pelvic inflammatory disease in 329 women who had used the intrauterine device.

During the past 15 years there has been a marked revival in this form of contraception, and a variety of polyethylene and metal devices have been used. Some devices, such as the Birnberg bow, were soon discarded because of the relative frequency of uterine perforation and, in some instances, bowel obstruction. With respect to uterine perforation, there is no doubt that the complication occurs at the time of insertion when the device is pushed into or completely through the uterine wall. Complete perforation of the uterus results in the deposition of the device in the peritoneal cavity. On the other hand, impaction at the time of insertion also can result in extrusion of the device into the abdominal cavity as the result of uterine contractions. The majority of such perforations can be avoided if the physician gives due consideration to the position, mobility, and consistency of the uterus.

At the time the Gräfenberg device was introduced into clinical practice, physicians were still concerned with the morbidity and mortality rates associated with beta-hemolytic streptococcal infections. Today we are confronted by life-threatening infections caused by the obligatory anaerobe *Bacteroides fragilis*, and these are seen in patients with the intrauterine devices. The majority of the untoward effects of the device, reported both in the medical and lay press, have been bleeding, expulsion, pain, perforation, and pregnancy, but rarely has pelvic inflammation been mentioned. The presence of plasma cells in the endometrium and an increase in secretory immunoglobulins in uterine fluid (as recently reported by Chandra and associates), in women using an intrauterine device, indicate a relationship between this form of contraception and infection.[51] To be more specific in this regard, during the past few months one of us has encountered three patients with severe infection in association with intrauterine devices.

Case A

The patient was a 23-year-old nulligravid individual who had had a Dalkon shield inserted two years previously. Except for occasional intermenstrual bleeding during the first six months, she was well satisfied with the device. As she was desirous of a pregnancy she visited a physician's office to have the device removed. The attempt at removal was unsuccessful and profuse bleeding ensued. The patient was admitted to the hospital with a temperature of 102.4°F, chills, and moderate vaginal bleeding. Both aerobic and anaerobic bacteria were grown from cultures obtained from the endocervix and blood. While the culture specimens were being obtained, a laceration of the cervix extending into the broad ligament was observed, and the device was located at this site. Operative removal of the device and repair of the laceration was performed. The anerobic cultures of both cervical secretions and blood revealed the presence of *Bacteroides* infection, which responded to suitable antibiotic therapy.

Case B

This patient was 26 years of age and had had one child who was delivered by cesarean section because of cephalopelvic disproportion. Two months post partum a size C Lippes loop had been inserted without any difficulty. For the following 18 months she was symptom free. She presented at the emergency floor of the hospital with acute abdominal pain and a temperature of 103°F. The pulse rate was 120 beats per minute, and abdominal pain was maximal in the right lower quadrant. A diagnosis of "acute abdomen" possibly due to acute appendicitis was considered. The leucocyte count was 22,600 with 80 per cent polymorphonuclear cells; when the count was repeated in two hours, similar results were obtained. On pelvic examination a tender swelling could be felt to the right of the uterus. Cultures of blood and cervical secretions were obtained, and a diagnosis of an acute tuboovarian abscess was made. Gram-stained slides of material from the vagina and cervix did not reveal any evidence of intracellular gram-negative diplococci. Antibiotic therapy was commenced, but after 24 hours the clinical findings were compatible with diffuse peritonitis. At laparotomy, pelvic peritonitis and a tuboovarian abscess on the right side were discovered. The Lippes loop was partially extruded from the uterus and involved in the medial wall of the abscess. Further cultures were obtained, and a total hysterectomy and bilateral salpingo-oophorectomy were performed. All cultures were positive for *Bacteroides,* and clindamycin was substituted for the original antibiotic. Except for some cellulitis of the abdominal wound, the patient had an uneventful postoperative course.

Case C

This woman, aged 25 years, had had three full-term normal deliveries. After her last confinement, a Dalkon shield was inserted and she was symptom-free for 16 months, when she missed a period. In due course pregnancy was confirmed. At 12 weeks' gestation, she had a low grade fever and slight vaginal bleeding. The fever and the bleeding increased. Uterine colic and the passage of blood clots necessitated admission to the hospital. Blood and cervical secretion cultures were obtained, and the device was found to be in the cervical canal. Further culture specimens were obtained from the device, and all were positive for *Bacteroides.* A diagnosis of septic abortion was made, and ampicillin and clindamycin therapy was instituted. Coagulation studies revealed the presence of fibrin degradation products, but no full-blown disseminated intravascular coagulopathy accrued. After evacuation of the retained products of conception from the uterus, she made an uneventful recovery. Mention should be made that this patient had three sons and was desirous that the pregnancy should continue, in the hope that she might have a daughter.

These three cases illustrate the potentially lethal hazards of the intrauterine device encountered in private practice. Uterine trauma was present in two, but pregnancy was the complication that accounted for the systemic infection in the third patient. With regard to the latter statement, many physicians consider that removal of the device in early pregnancy will in itself initiate an abortion, but it is only too well known that such an assumption is incorrect. The inherent dangers of such action include septic abortion, septicemia, disseminated intravascular coagulopathy, and septic thrombophlebitis, as well as the pulmonary and renal complications of shock. One of the authors recently encountered such a sate of affairs when a patient who had had intermittent bleeding for 10 days after removal of the device was admitted to the hospital with acute pelvic inflammatory disease and peritonitis, which necessitated ablation of the uterus and adnexa. It behooves the physician who removes a device in early pregnancy to terminate the pregnancy, and in view of our experience in private practice, we consider that removal of the device and termination of the pregnancy are mandatory in all instances.

There is no doubt that the intrauterine device should and will play a role in family planning. Its effective acceptance, however, will only be achieved in conjunction with the prompt recognition and management of complications in order to circumvent some of the potentially serious problems that arise from uterine perforation and sepsis.

SUMMARY

Injuries to the genital tract in the nonpregnant female are infrequent. The majority of lesions are related in some way to sexuality and are usually sustained during voluntary or nonvoluntary coitus. On the other hand, it is well to bear in mind that not all genital tract injuries in the nonpregnant patient are the result of sexual intercourse.

Although trauma is a rare cause of vaginal bleeding and pain in gynecologic experience, nevertheless the gynecologist must constantly be aware of the fact that bleeding and pain may be traumatic in origin and trauma requires due consideration in the differential diagnosis. Indeed, as Speert pointed out, advanced age does not preclude sexuality, and trauma must be included in the differential diagnosis of postmenopausal bleeding.[15]

The attorney must be aware of the fact that traumatic lesions of the female genital tract are not limited to those resulting from rape and other sexual assaults. Bleeding as a result of coitus does not imply rape or sexual assault, since this can occur during coitus with consenting partners. In addition, vaginal lacerations with bleeding in the postmenopausal female cannot be equated with rape, sexual assault, or even sexual intercourse, since such bleeding can occur in the absence of direct trauma.

REFERENCES

1. Kelley, C. M.: Crime in the United States (Uniform Crime Reports). Washington, D.C., U. S. Government Printing Office, 1973.
2. Hayman, C. R., and Lanza, C.: Victimology of sexual assault. Medical Aspects of Human Sexuality, 5:152, 1971.
3. Masters, W. H., and Johnson, V. E.: *Human Sexual Response*. Boston, Little, Brown and Co., 1966.
4. Metsälä, P., and Nieminen, U.: Traumatic lesions of the vagina. Acta Obstet. Gynecol. Scand., *47*:482, 1968.
5. Hakanson, E. Y.: Trauma to the female genitalia. Lancet, *86*:287, 1966.
6. Rush, R., and Milton, P. J. D.: Injuries of the vagina. S. Afr. Med. J., *47*:1325, 1973.
7. Fish, S. A.: Vaginal injury due to coitus. Am. J. Obstet. Gynecol., *72*:544, 1956.
8. Wilson, F., and Swartz, D. P.: Coital injuries of the vagina. Obstet. Gynecol., *396*:182, 1972.
9. Blair, R.: A fatal injury of the vagina. Br. Med. J., *1*:828, 1925.
10. Diddle, A. W.: Rupture of the vaginal vault during coitus. West. J. Surg. Obstet. Gynecol., *56*:414, 1948.
11. Chandra, S. P., and Rathee, S. D.: Coital injuries. J. Obstet. Gynecol. India, *14*:930, 1964.
12. Massey, J. B., Garcia, C-R., and Emich, J. P.: Management of sexually assaulted females. Obstet. Gynecol., *38*:29, 1971.
13. Daw, E.: Coital vaginal vault laceration. Obstet. Gynecol., *40*:451, 1972.
14. Nicholls, R. B.: Rupture of the posterior vagina during normal coitus. Am. J. Obstet. Gynecol., *52*:500, 1946.
15. Speert, H.: Vaginal lacerations resulting from coitus. Am. J. Obstet. Gynecol., *53*:539, 1947.
16. Howkins, J., and Bourne, G. (eds.): *Shaw's Textbook of Gynecology*. 9th Ed. Edinburgh and London, Churchill Livingstone, 1971, pp. 270–271.
17. Kiel, F. W.: The psychiatric character of the assailant as determined by autopsy observations of the victim. J. Forensic Sci., *10*:263, 1965.
18. Reich, L. H., and Wehr, T.: Female genital self-mutilation. Obstet. Gynecol., *41*:239, 1973.
19. French, A. P., and Nelson, H. L.: Genital self-mutilation in women. Arch. Gen. Psychiatry, *27*:613, 1972.
20. Goldfield, M. D., and Glick, I. R.: Genital self-mutilation of the female genitalia: a case report. Dis. Nerv. Syst., *31*:843, 1970.
21. Ezell, W. W., Smith, E. I., McCarthy, R. P., Thompson, I. M., and Habib, H. N.: Mechanical traumatic injury to the genitalia in children. J. Urol., *102*:788, 1969.
22. Ikpeme, J. O., and Morison, C. R.: Vaginal avulsion complicating pelvic fracture. Br. J. Surg., 57:317, 1970.
23. Purnell, L. W.: Spontaneous rupture of the vaginal vault. J. Obstet. Gynaecol. Br. Commonw., *72*:799, 1965.
24. Rolf, B. B.: Vaginal evisceration. Am. J. Obstet. Gynecol., *107*:369, 1970.
25. Heys, R. F.: Ileal prolapse through ruptured vagina. Complication of Manchester operation. Br. Med. J., *2*:223, 1963.
26. Galloway, R. K., Edmond, P., and Hamilton, T.: Vault rupture with bowel prolapse after Manchester repair. J. Obstet. Gynaecol. Br. Commonw., *76*:1035, 1969.
27. Hunter, R. E., Jahadi, M. R., and Chandler, J. P.: Spontaneous rupture of enterocele. Obstet. Gynecol., *36*:835, 1970.
28. Beebe, R. A., and Edwards, E. A.: Lesions of the vaginal vault following complete hysterectomy. Am. J. Obstet. Gynecol., *62*:1034, 1951.
29. Morrison, J.: Vault lacerations due to sneezing. J. Obstet. Gynaecol. Br. Commonw., *74*:773, 1967.
30. Pfanner, D.: Salpingitis and water-skiing. Med. J. Aust., *1*:320, 1966.
31. McCarthy, G. F.: Hazards of water skiing. Med. J. Aust., *1*:481, 1969.
32. Morton, D. C.: Gynaecological complications of water-skiing. Med. J. Aust., *1*:1256, 1970.
33. Tweedale, P. G.: Gynaecological hazards of water-skiing. Can. Med. Assoc. J., *108*:20, 1973.
34. Lammert, A. C., and Scott, R. B.: Hazards in the intravaginal use of potassium permanganate. Am. J. Obstet. Gynecol., *68*:854, 1954.
35. Steward, M., and Webster, A.: Vaginal hemorrhage from potassium permanganate burns. Obstet. Gynecol., *3*:169, 1954.
36. Wanamaker, F. D.: The lay use of potassium permanganate as an abortifacient. Am. J. Obstet. Gynecol., *69*:259, 1955.
37. Kobak, A. J., and Wishnick, S.: Potassium permanganate burn of the vagina followed by bowel obstruction. Am. J. Obstet. Gynecol., *70*:409, 1955.
38. Carney, B. H.: Vaginal burns from potassium permanganate. Am. J. Obstet. Gynecol., *65*:127, 1953.
39. O'Donnell, R. P.: Vesicovaginal fistula produced by potassium permanganate. Obstet. Gynecol., *4*:122, 1954.
40. Miller, J. C.: Potassium permanganate as an abortifacient. Br. Med. J., *1*:526, 1951.
41. Bookrajian, E. N., and Wagner, V.: Chemical burns of the vagina with severe hemorrhage. Am. J. Obstet. Gynecol., *64*:681, 1952.
42. Shull, J. C.: Vaginal bleeding from potassium permanganate burns. Am. J. Obstet. Gynecol., *41*:161, 1941.
43. McDonough, J. F.: Vaginal bleeding from potassium permanganate as an abortifacient. N. Engl. J. Med., *232*:189, 1945.
44. Vandergriff, W., and Diddle, A. W.: Intravaginal use of potassium permanganate as an abortifacient. The error in diagnosis. Obstet. Gynecol, *28*:155, 1966.
45. Jetter, W. W., and Hunter, F. T.: Death from attempted abortion with potassium permanganate douche. N. Engl. J. Med., *240*:794, 1949.
46. Whitehouse, B.: A paper on the indications for the induction of abortion. Br. Med. J., *2*:337, 1932.
47. Nathanson, B. W.: Management of uterine perforations suffered at elective abortion. Am. J. Obstet. Gynecol., *114*:1054, 1972.
48. Gräfenberg, E.: *In Geburtenretelung: Vortrage und Verhandlungen des Arzterkursus.* Edited by K. Bendix. Berlin, Selbstverlag, 1929.
49. MacLeod, D. H., and Read, D. C.: *Gynaecology*, 5th Ed. London, J. and A. Churchill, 1955, p. 175.
50. Oppenheimer, W.: Prevention of pregnancy by the Graefenberg ring method. Am. J. Obstet. Gynecol., *78*:446, 1959.
51. Chandra, R. K., Malkani, P. D., and Bhasin, K.: Levels of immunoglobulins in the serum and uterine fluid of women using an intrauterine contraceptive device. J. Reprod. Fertil., *37*:1, 1974.

XIII. Musculoskeletal System

by Ronald F. Kaplan, Barry C. Dorn, J. Sudler Hood, and Peter D. McGann

GENERAL CONSIDERATIONS

Response to Trauma

Trauma to the skeletal system has local and systemic effects. The prognosis is influenced by the degree of injury to the skeletal system and by associated injury to other organ systems. Some of the potential systemic effects are shock, respiratory insufficiency, infection, and renal insufficiency, as well as psychologic difficulty. The patient's overall general medical condition is a prime consideration in treatment. Associated soft-tissue injury can include varying degrees of skin injury and loss, damage to nerve and vascular structures, muscle strains, and contusions. The local effects on the skeletal system include fractures, dislocations, subluxations, sprains, and internal derangements of joints. A *fracture* can be defined as a complete or incomplete break in the continuity of a bone. *Dislocation* is the complete and persistent displacement of the articular surface of one of the bones entering into the formation of a joint from that of its fellow. A *subluxation* is an incomplete dislocation. A *sprain* is a partial or complete disruption in the continuity of a ligament. A sprain is to be distinguished from a *strain*, which is the partial or complete disruption of muscle or fascia or both. Pain is a response to local injury, frequently immediate, oftentimes delayed. This is also true of spasm, although spasm is more often a delayed effect. Loss of function of the injured part, also, is often immediate but, depending upon the trauma, is frequently delayed. Tissue swelling is a delayed effect. Hematoma formation is swelling secondary to the disruption of blood vessels, and is more immediate.[1-6]

General Principles of Trauma Treatment

The primary goal of treatment is to return a patient to the best level of function possible for that particular patient after that particular injury. Goals of restoration depend on the demands of the patient's occupation and avocation; for example, the demands on a knee differ markedly for the professional athlete and for the sedentary worker. A careful clinical evaluation, often assisted by anesthesia, is essential. This should include not only attention to the local wound but also attention to effects produced in distal structures by the local insult. A complete history should be obtained, and it should include the mechanism of injury as well as the circumstances under which the injury occurred. A past history of the patient is important. A pertinent physical examination completes the clinical evaluation.

X-rays are of considerable value in determining the extent of bone injury. It is important to note that x-rays must be inclusive to evaluate the effect of injury fully. Specialized radiographic studies can be especially helpful to the surgeon in his appraisal of patients. Such studies include spot views, stress views, laminagrams, arthrograms, myelograms, and vascular studies.[7-10] Electromyographic studies may assist him to draw conclusions about a nerve lesion or muscle damage. They are also useful in following improvement progress, and offer reasonable evaluation of ultimate prognosis.[11,12] Arthroscopy, a percutaneous visualization of the joint interior, may also be helpful in ascertaining the extent of injury.[13-15]

In the initial handling of a fracture patient, one has to be careful not to convert a simple problem into a more serious one. Immobilization of the injured part by the simplest means at hand is essential. One should not convert a closed wound to an open one, allow a clean wound to become a dirty one, or allow a fracture to cause neurovascular damage. As with all major trauma, attention should be directed to the maintenance of adequate respiration and adequate perfusion of all vital organs. The maintenance of normal blood pressure by hemostasis is essential. Transportation need not be hurried, but should be relatively swift. Again, the injury should not be aggravated in the course of transportation from the scene of the accident to an appropriate medical facility.

There are few true orthopedic emergencies. These include vascular or neurologic embarrassment. Priority in treatment depends upon the severity of injury, and orthopedic treatment is often deferred until the patient's general condition is stabilized. The patient should be evaluated thoroughly, and treatment of underlying conditions should be instituted. One should take into account that a patient has been receiving steroids or anticoagulants, has a heart condition, is diabetic, or has other systemic difficulties. For example, if a patient is being treated with a corticosteroid drug, the clinician should allow for the increased need for corticosteroids by the body in time of stress, and should accordingly increase the patient's steroid dosage. One of the major pitfalls in the treatment of the critically injured patient is the failure to recognize a serious but occult injury while directing attention to a less serious but more obvious problem. Conversely, small injuries are often missed when the attention is focused upon a patient's primary injury. For example, a potentially dangerous injury to the spine without neurologic deficit may be overlooked while attention is directed to a comminuted compound fracture of a long bone that is quite obvious. Postoperative management in the hospital must continue for as long as the patient needs this intensive form of care. The stay must be long enough to insure that the patient can care for himself or be cared for at home or in an extended-care facility. After discharge from the hospital, follow-up continues until the condition has been resolved or until clinical judgment indicates that no further treatment is required. In some cases a patient must be followed for much of his life. It may be necessary to ask for consultations from other disciplines for further treatment of his condition. Overall treatment of a patient depends upon his injuries, the patient himself and his socioeconomic situation, and the patient's physician's assessment of the situation. The direction of the rehabilitation efforts is determined by the doctor. He alone has the scope of knowledge to decide what the needs of the individual patient are and which ancillary services will best aid this patient in his recovery.

Principles of Treatment of Musculoskeletal Injury

In the initial treatment of musculoskeletal injury, one has to be careful not to increase the degree of injury; the age-old principle, "splint them where they lie," is valid. Splint the fracture before moving the patient. Whenever possible, splinting should include some degree of traction—not only to immobilize the injured part but to prevent excessive pain, damage to neighboring soft tissue, hemorrhage, and shock. If there is a skin opening at the site of the deformity, one should realize that the deformity may be due to an open fracture. Care should be taken not to cause further contamination. In most situations an attempt at closed reduction is appropriate. When closed reduction fails, open reduction is usually indicated. An exception to this is a severely comminuted fracture that can neither be anatomically reduced closed nor satisfactorily fixed by open methods. The best result obtained by closed methods may have to be accepted. When the decision has been made to open a fracture or dislocation and a surgical incision has been made, every possible means should be used to obtain the best possible reduction in that particular situation. For example, after open reduction of a long bone, one should use internal fixation when applicable rather than merely opening the site, reducing the fracture, closing the wound, and hoping that plaster immobilization alone will be sufficient. There are exceptions to this such as dislocations in which it is unnecessary to fix the affected joint internally.

Generally, anatomical reduction is the goal of treatment; there are, however, many situations in which anatomical reduction is either impossible or not actually desirable. A case in point is a markedly unstable intertrochanteric fracture of the hip in which one would perform a medial displacement osteotomy in order to insure healing rather than attempt a strict anatomical reduction to achieve this purpose. There are several situations in which an anatomical reduction may be deleterious and a functional reduction is better. For example, a Colles' fracture in an elderly person is best treated to obtain a useful wrist rather than merely a cosmetically pleasing one. In this situation it is better for a patient to be able to use her hand and wrist well and to have some deformity rather than a purely cosmetic but stiff result. In elderly patients fracture treatment is sometimes different because of the ease with which older patients develop joint adhesions and stiffness.[16–18]

There are a number of mitigating circumstances that have a bearing on appropriate treatment. Delayed treatment is often mandatory because of skin lesions, such as blebs and excoriations. One often has to reduce swelling by elevation of the part before definitive treatment can be carried out. Some research has shown that delaying surgery on a fracture by one to two weeks in certain instances even promotes union.[19, 20] Closure would also be delayed in a grossly contaminated fracture; this is first thoroughly debrided and then left open to heal by itself, or later closed secondarily.

It is to the patient's best interest to have open

wounds attended to as swiftly as possible, within six hours after injury, the legendary "golden period."[2] This golden period can, however, be extended by the administration of antibiotics. Open fractures that come to treatment after the six-hour period are best treated open, under an antibiotic cover. It is best not to insert an internal fixation device in a long-standing open fracture. Recent work from the Vietnamese War experience indicates that internal fixation devices can be used in open wounds if adequate debridement has been accomplished.[21] There are other factors besides time that dictate the type of primary care given to a particular wound. For example, grossly contaminated wounds, particularly wounds caused by human or animal bites or those contaminated by human or animal excrement, should never be closed primarily. In general, the amount of foreign material and the degree of contamination dictate whether the wound can be closed primarily.[22]

THE UPPER EXTREMITY

The Shoulder Girdle and Upper Arm

Brachial Plexus Injury

Open injury to the brachial plexus may occur in penetrating wounds of the neck, shoulder, and chest. Closed injury, usually a traction injury, may result from a fall from a moving vehicle, a fall while walking, or an air or automobile crash. The plexus may also be injured in other ways, such as by a direct blow on the shoulder or hyperabduction of the arm.[23, 24]

Injuries to the brachial plexus may also be associated with skeletal injuries. In closed injury to the brachial plexus, pathologic elongation of the nerves results from traction on them (Fig. 3–XIII–1). These injuries are much more difficult to treat than open ones because an open laceration of a nerve can be repaired with some expectation of improvement. Depending on the nature of the injury, the prognosis for traction injuries of the brachial plexus is considered to be poor despite surgical attempts at repair. Although anatomical continuity may remain, most efforts at surgical correction tend to result in the return of only the sensory component of the nerve.[25–27] Complete recovery is sometimes found when the injury to the brachial plexus is minor. In general, the more severe the injury, the greater the resultant deficit. A minor injury to the brachial plexus, for instance, to the axillary nerve, can resolve well to complete recovery. Severe traction injury to the entire brachial plexus has a grave prognosis, however, and may result in a completely flail upper extremity.

Musculotendinous Injuries of the Shoulder

The shoulder is a very mobile joint with a loose articulation. For stability, it depends upon its supporting muscles, tendons, and ligaments; therefore injury to these structures can result in significant disability to overall shoulder function.[28–30]

Pectoralis Major Muscle Rupture. Rupture of the pectoralis major muscle is an uncommon injury.[31, 32] It follows extreme muscle tension, direct trauma, or a combination of both. Fifty-

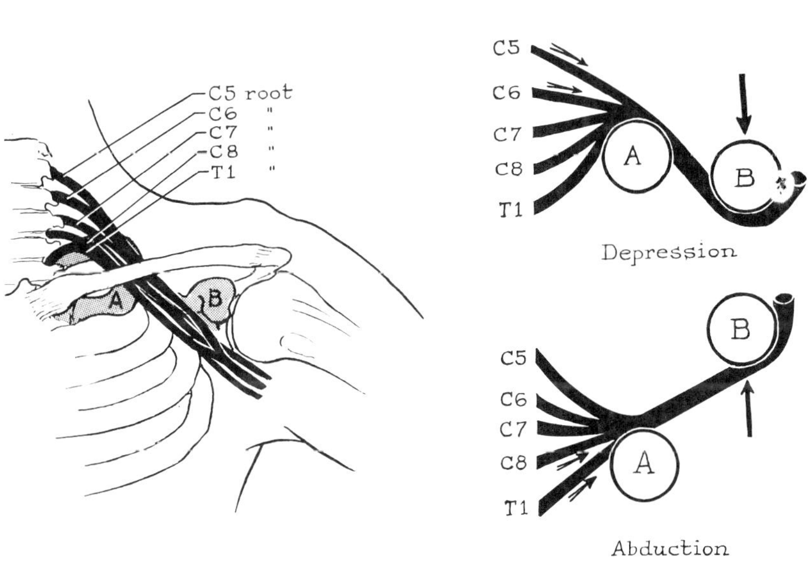

Figure 3–XIII–1. Stretch injury of the brachial plexus. The nerve roots, C5 to T1, of the brachial plexus are snubbed to the transverse processes of the respective vertebrae and are fixed by the clavipectoral fascia between the clavicle and first rib. The first rib (A) and the coracoid process (B) act as pulleys over which traction injuries to the nerve are produced. When the shoulder is depressed violently, the upper elements of the brachial plexus receive the brunt of the stretching impact; conversely, when the arm is forcibly hyperabducted, the nerves are pulled taut under the pulley of the coracoid process and the lower elements are likely to be injured. Most traction injuries produce a mixed type of upper and lower brachial plexus lesion. (From H. L. McLaughlin: *Trauma.* Philadelphia, W. B. Saunders Co., 1959. Reprinted by permission.)

six cases were reviewed by McEntire, in July 1972, and in 33 of the 56, he questioned the diagnosis because only 22 injuries were confirmed at surgery and one other at autopsy. Some cases may have been congenital absence of the pectoralis major erroneously labeled. Surgical correction is important to restore function and appearance, but some cases respond to conservative treatment with only minor loss of strength. The pectoralis muscles rupture at specific locations in particular injuries. Wrestlers seem to rupture only the upper sternoclavicular portion, while persons preventing a fall from a height disrupt the humeral insertion or avulse the musculotendinous junction. Tearing of the fibers of the muscle belly is due to direct trauma. There has been evidence that portions of the deltoid muscle can be ruptured with the pectoralis major, as well as the pectoralis minor and the rotator cuff.

Biceps Tendon Injury. Trauma about the shoulder can result in *bicipital tendinitis* and *tenosynovitis, dislocation of the biceps tendon* out of the intertubercular groove, and *rupture of the tendon* itself. A study of 92 shoulders with bicipital tenosynovitis revealed that 31 per cent had a history of unusual physical activity, direct trauma to the shoulder, a fall on the extended arm, lifting or pulling, or other traumatic incidents. In 40 per cent of the shoulders, the tenosynovitis was found in conjunction with some other lesion and may or may not have been caused by this lesion. In 43 per cent of the shoulders no specific cause for the affection could be found.

Attritional processes that occur with aging may well weaken the biceps tendon and predispose it to rupture from relatively minor trauma. Biciptal tenosynovitis can be a complication of *calcareous tendinitis* when a calcium deposit is close to the bicipital groove (Fig. 3–XIII–2). The biceps tendon and its sheath may be secondarily involved in the inflammatory reaction surrounding the deposit. An indirect force, such as forceful contraction of the biceps, causes most of the ruptures of the biceps tendon. Such an injury occurs following moderately severe trauma in younger people, but in those in the older age group minor trauma can be the cause. This injury is seen especially in workmen. The typical patient is a middle-aged workman who lifts a heavy load in front of him. The extent of disability resulting from this injury is related both to the severity of the injury and to the occupation of the injured. With regard to dislocation of the biceps, following the initial dislocation, recurrences occur relatively frequently. Repeated dislocations produce bicipital tenosynovitis.

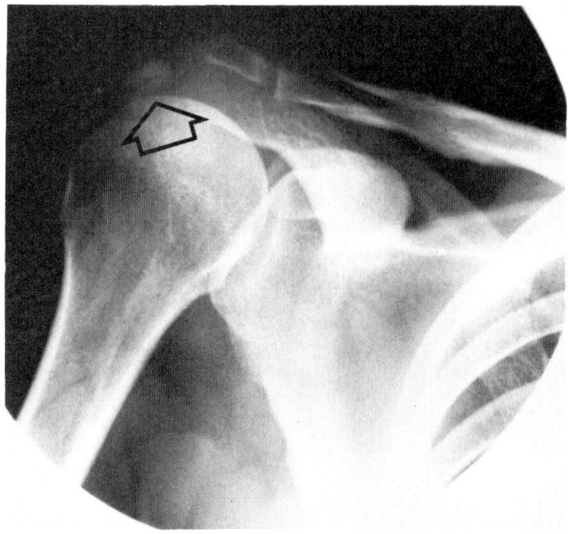

Figure 3–XIII–2. Calcareous (calcific) tendinitis of the shoulder.

The natural history of degenerative arthritis of the shoulder can be applied to many types of injuries that are a result of wear and tear in the shoulder region. For example, workers who are required by their occupation to spend much of their time working above their heads, such as painters or file clerks, are predisposed to successive microinsults to the tendinous, bony, and capsular regions of the shoulder. As degenerative alterations progress, calcifications may develop in the biceps tendon as well as in the other tendons constituting the shoulder joint capsule. This could lead secondarily to bursitis or tendinitis. As a consequence, these changes may predispose to further rupture of the shoulder capsule or rupture of the biceps tendon itself.

Injury to the Rotator Cuff. Calcific deposits in the tendons of the rotator cuff are frequently the cause of painful and stiff shoulders and a predisposing factor in rupture of the rotator cuff. Disruption of the rotator cuff, the major dynamic stabilizing force of the glenohumeral joint, occurs at any age, but especially in middle-aged workmen such as carpenters, painters, paper hangers, and plasterers. The trauma can be direct, indirect, acute, or chronic (Fig. 3–XIII–3). Incomplete or minor tears can progress without further trauma because of the divergent pull of the muscular components of the cuff. Any cuff tear can subject the biceps tendon to the aforementioned conditions. Diagnosis is often difficult, but is aided by arthrography, as demonstrated by Kernwein,

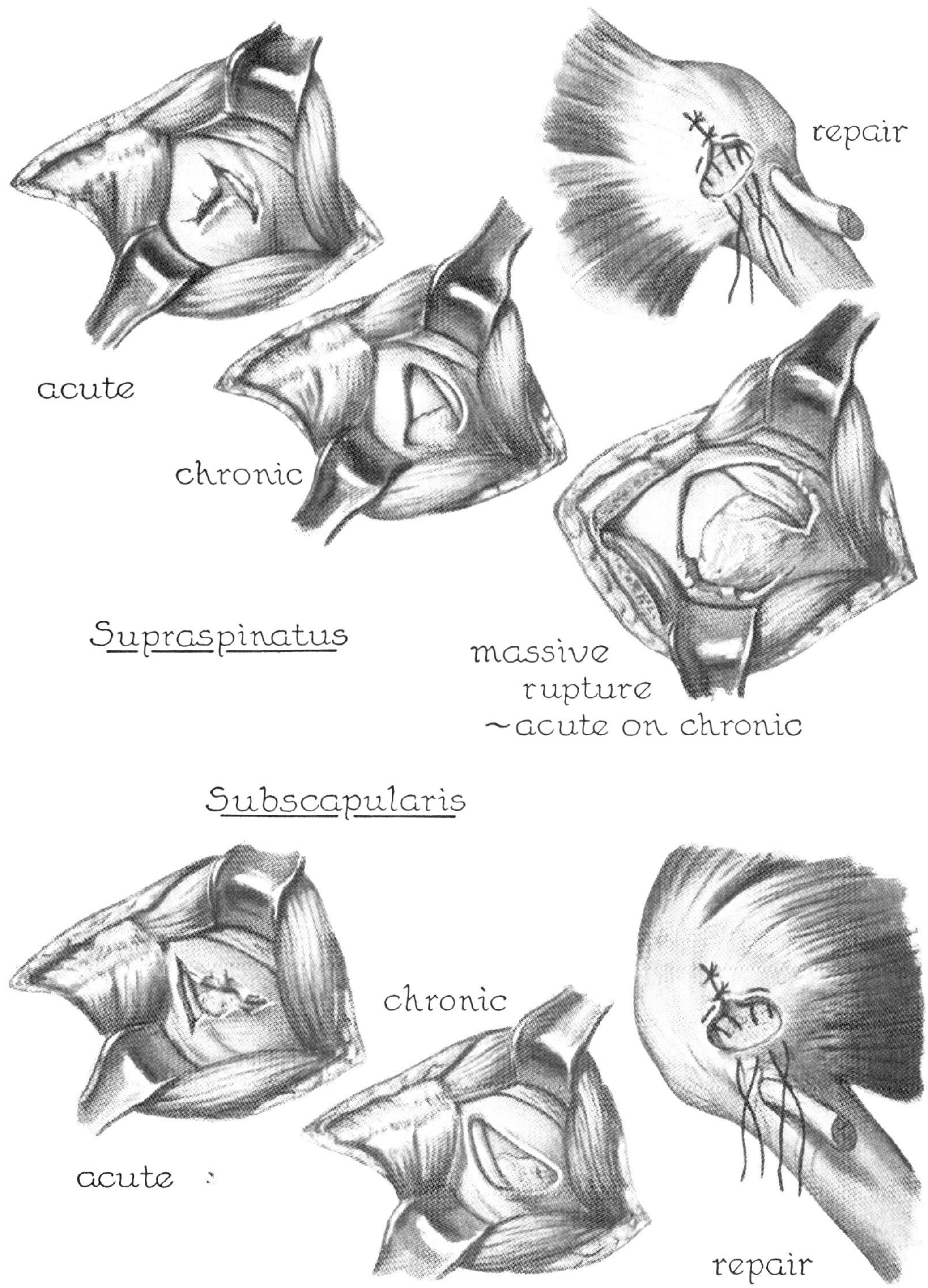

Figure 3–XIII–3. Acute and chronic rupture of the rotator (musculotendinous) cuff of the shoulder. The humerus is rotated laterally to expose the subscapularis tendon rupture medial to the biceps tendon. (From F. F. Moseley: *Ruptures of the Rotator Cuff.* 1952. Courtesy of Charles C Thomas, Publisher, Springfield, Ill.)

Samilson, Neviaser, and Debeyre and their associates (Figs. 3–XIII–4 to 3–XIII–6). Initial treatment is usually conservative, but operative treatment is advised for massive tears. Tears are not always symptomatic, however; in an autopsy study there was a 20 to 30 per cent incidence of asymptomatic tears.[34-37] The prognosis for incomplete ruptures of the musculotendinous cuff is good, as opposed to that for complete ruptures of the cuff. There may be limitation of initiation of abduction, limitation of elevation, or weakness of elevation against resistance.

Scapulocostal Syndrome. One often encounters pain in the shoulder at the medial inferior border of the scapula. Digital pressure upon this "trigger zone" reproduces pain radiating into the shoulder musculature, particularly the trapezius. The syndrome is usually caused either by a traction injury of the upper arm or by direct trauma to the area, but can also be caused by local environmental changes such as cold drafts.[38] Cervical discogenic disease may refer pain to this area, as well as to the shoulder, but in the absence of specific neurologic deficit in the upper extremity, the pain can be unrelated to the cervical spine. It is frequently relieved by antiinflammatory medication or local infiltration of anesthetic, and possibly by the instillation of steroids. This scapulocostal syndrome can also be caused by inflamed, distended bursae in the scapulothoracic interval.[39]

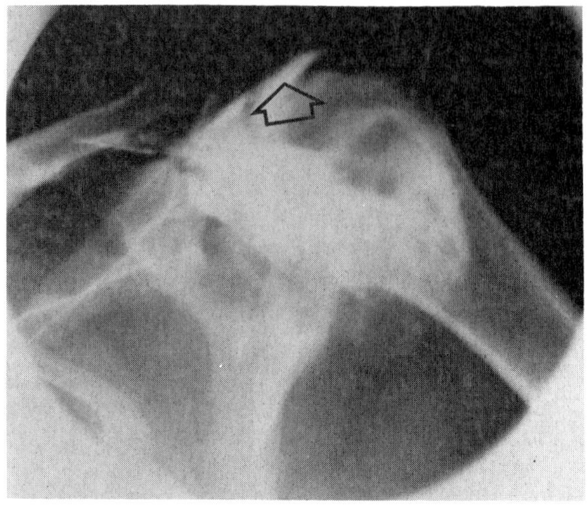

Figure 3–XIII–5. Small rotator cuff tear. The point of leakage of the dye is evident. There is some haphazard extension of the dye throughout the joint inferiorly.

Shoulder-Hand Syndrome. The shoulder-hand syndrome usually develops after trauma to the upper extremity, but in some cases there may have been no trauma. It is also called reflex dystrophy or causalgia and is characterized by a painful shoulder with limited movement and swelling, pain, stiffness, sweating, and color changes in the hand. The local pain is "burning," and the vasomotor changes of coldness and perspiration may often develop into coldness and stiffness in which the skin appears white, puffy, and thickened. Muscle atro-

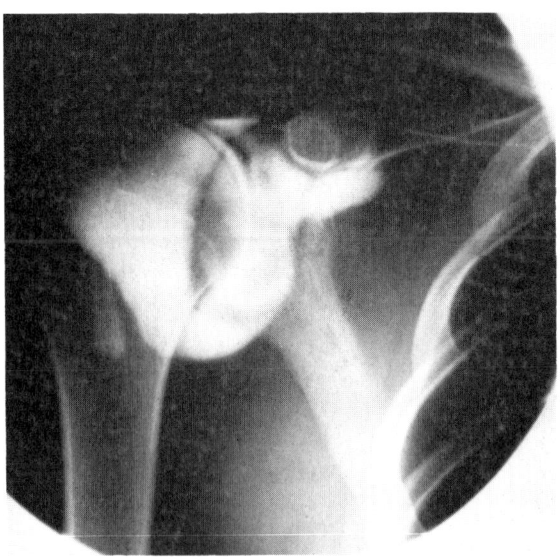

Figure 3–XIII–4. Normal shoulder arthrogram. The central area of the joint is outlined, and there is an extension of the dye into the subscapular recess.

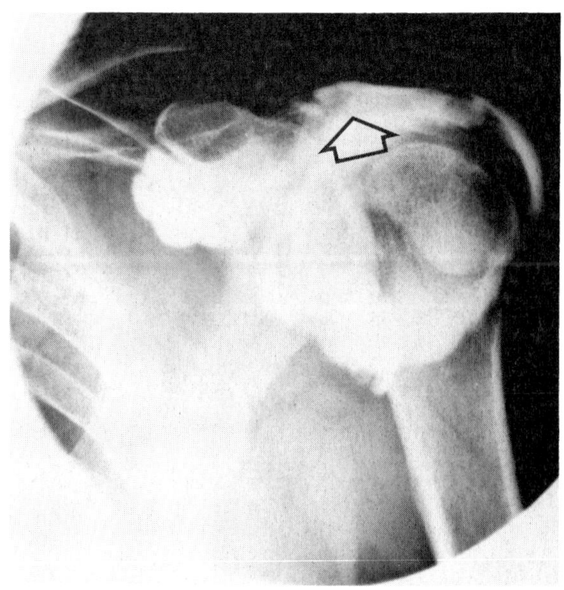

Figure 3–XIII–6. Large rotator cuff tear. The dye escapes through the defect in the capsule and lies under the acromion.

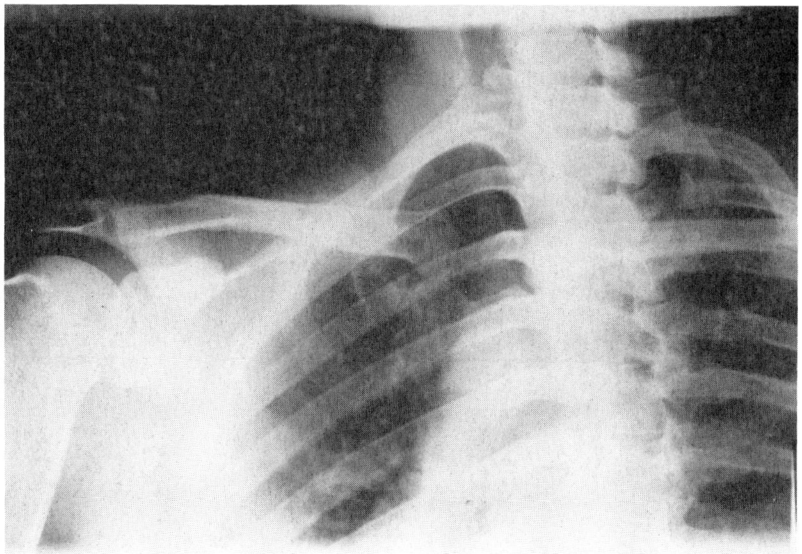

Figure 3–XIII–7. Sternoclavicular separation. (Courtesy of Dr. Robert E. Leach.)

phy appears, and joints lose range of motion. In later stages, osteoporosis is seen on x-rays. This is called Sudeck's atrophy. The prognosis depends in large part on the motivation of the patient. This syndrome often leads to a frozen shoulder.[40]

Dislocations of the Shoulder Joint

Sternoclavicular Joint Lesions. Lesions of the sternoclavicular joint, shown in Figure 3–XIII–7, occur infrequently. Most injuries are the result of an indirect mechanism, and a great deal of force is necessary to produce the injury. The force is applied to the lateral aspect of the shoulder or along the abducted arm. Retrosternoclavicular dislocations, however, are generally caused by a severe direct blow to the area and occur frequently in athletes such as wrestlers and football players.[41, 42] Retrosternoclavicular dislocations deserve special consideration because of the serious complications that may accompany them. Although difficult, manipulative reduction should be attempted in all fresh lesions (under 48 hours).[28]

Open reduction and internal fixation are indicated if closed reduction cannot be achieved or cannot be maintained (Fig. 3–XIII–8). Some of the anatomical structures located in the vicinity of the sternoclavicular joint are the

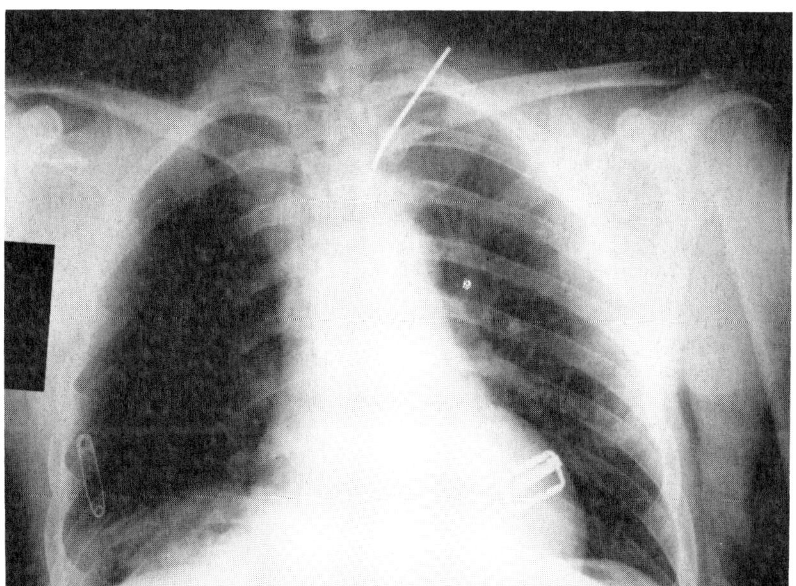

Figure 3–XIII–8. Postoperative radiograph following open reduction and internal fixation of sternoclavicular separation. (Courtesy of Dr. Robert E. Leach.)

dome of the pleura, the trachea, and the esophagus as well as the great vessels in the neck. Any one of these may be injured in sternoclavicular dislocations of the retrosternal type.

In a series of cases reported by Salvatore, there were a number of complications of a serious nature in those cases in which surgical repair was carried out. These complications included infection, tracheal compression, and migration of the wire (one death resulted from migration of the wire into the heart).[43]

Anterior sternoclavicular dislocations do not have the same life-threatening potential as do posterior (retro) dislocations.[44] The disability from this kind of dislocation is primarily pain or cosmetic deformity. Neglected or recurrent sternoclavicular dislocations may not cause any disability other than an altered appearance. A tear of the sternoclavicular meniscus can be produced by the same mechanism of injury that causes dislocation when the force is less severe. This type of injury can cause chronic pain and posttraumatic arthritis of the sternoclavicular joint. Surgery may be indicated.

Acromioclavicular Joint Lesions. Injuries to the acromioclavicular joint are usually the result of direct trauma, particularly in athletes (Figs. 3–XIII–9, 3–XIII–10, and 3–XIII–11). Differentiation between complete and incomplete disruption is important. This is often difficult and can best be done with an anteroposterior x-ray view of both joints with the patient holding weights in his hands. The type of treatment in acromioclavicular injuries depends upon the severity of the injury and the needs of the patient.[45] A patient's occupation is indeed a determining factor in treatment. A follow-up of 116 cases of acromioclavicular joint injuries for as long as 35 years showed that 51 per cent of the patients treated nonoperatively or not treated had symptoms; 54 per cent of the surgically treated patients also had symptoms.[46] Therefore, in deciding which method of treatment is most applicable, one should consider carefully all the possible complications, the most frequent of which is residual subluxation. As Allman notes, it should be remembered that a patient with a poor result anatomically may be asymptomatic, whereas perfect anatomical restoration of the joint does not always relieve the symptoms.[44]

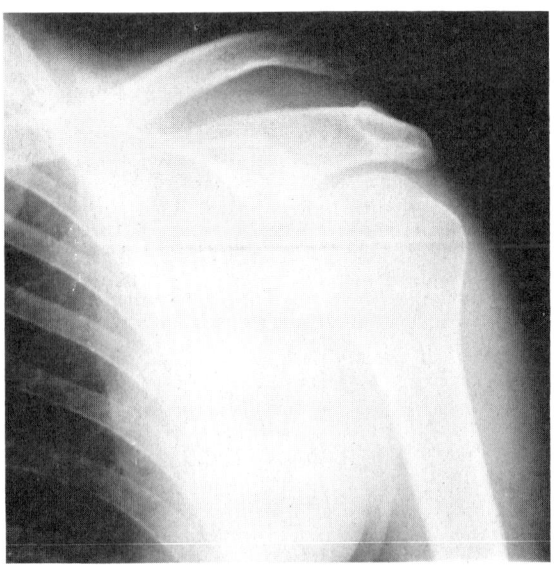

Figure 3–XIII–9. Acromioclavicular separation. Patient is holding weights in both hands. Separation is evident in this, the affected shoulder.

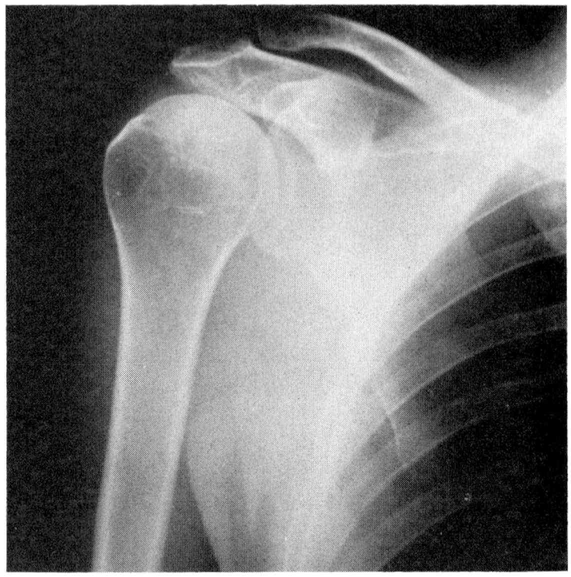

Figure 3–XIII–10. The opposite normal shoulder while the patient was holding weights.

Glenohumeral Dislocations. Subluxation of the shoulder can occur after there is tearing of the capsule and ligaments or tearing of either the capsule or the ligaments alone. This tearing is incomplete and may actually be minimal. Subluxation can also occur after traction or pulsion injuries in which there is a loss of normal muscle tone. It is this normal muscle tone that provides the stability of the shoulder joint. With rest, subluxations usually resolve in a short time.

Anterior Dislocations. Although a small number of acute dislocations of the shoulder (6 per cent) are atraumatic, the vast majority (94 per cent) are due to significant trauma.[30] The following classification describes the relation-

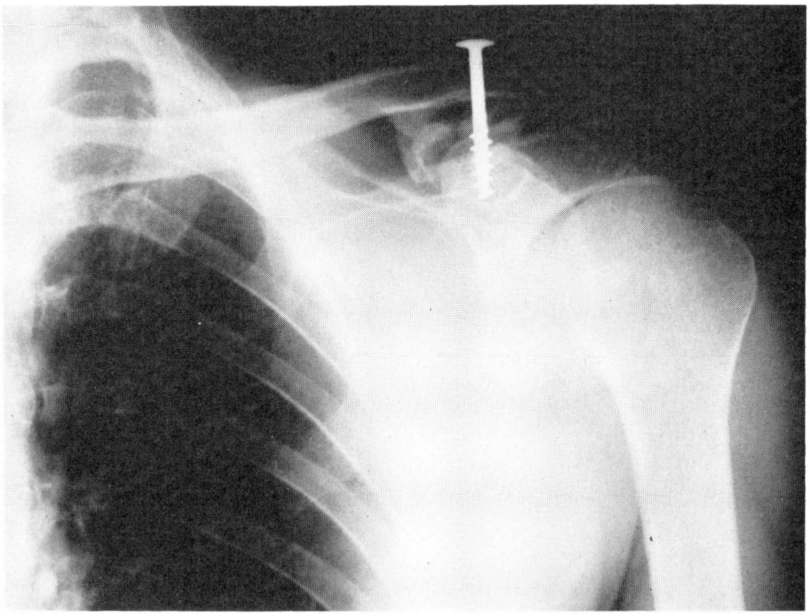

Figure 3–XIII–11. Acromioclavicular separation after operative reduction.

ship of the dislocated humeral head to the glenoid fossa: (1) *anterior or subcoracoid*, (2) *inferior or subglenoid*, (3) *posterior or subspinous*.[47] By far the greatest number of shoulder dislocations are anterior (Fig. 3–XIII–12). Most acute anterior shoulder dislocations do well. There are, however, a number of significant complications that can alter the prognosis of this injury. The most common encountered by the orthopedic surgeon, but not necessarily the most disabling, is recurrence of the dislocation. The factors affecting the recurrence rate are age, amount of trauma, and duration of initial immobilization following the injury. In a series reported by McLaughlin and Cavallaro, 90 per cent of the patients under the age of 20, 60 per cent of the patients between 20 and 40 years of age, and only 10 per cent of the patients over the age of 40 years developed recurrent dislocations.[48] In the experience of Rowe, the less trauma causing the initial dislocation, the greater the incidence of recurrence. The explanation offered for this apparent contradiction is that only mild to moderate force is required to dislocate joints in patients who have preexisting laxity of those joints, whereas people with joints of normal stability require greater force for dislocation. The latter heal with more scarring, which may limit their motion somewhat but does confer some protection from recurrent dislocation.[49] Rowe has also shown that the shoulder should be immobilized for three weeks. In older people, however, it is often better to immobilize a freshly dislocated shoulder for less time to avoid a frozen shoulder. Rupture of the rotator cuff is an uncommon complication of a fresh shoulder dislocation. It does occur frequently after middle life and in the elderly. Fractures of the bony elements of the glenohumeral joint occur in approximately 25 per cent of all dislocations.[28] Recurrence of dislocation does not occur frequently in patients with fractures. The exception to this is fracture of the anterior and inferior glenoid rim.[50] Rupture of the axillary artery is considered to be an uncommon complication of anterior dislocation of the shoulder. Of interest is

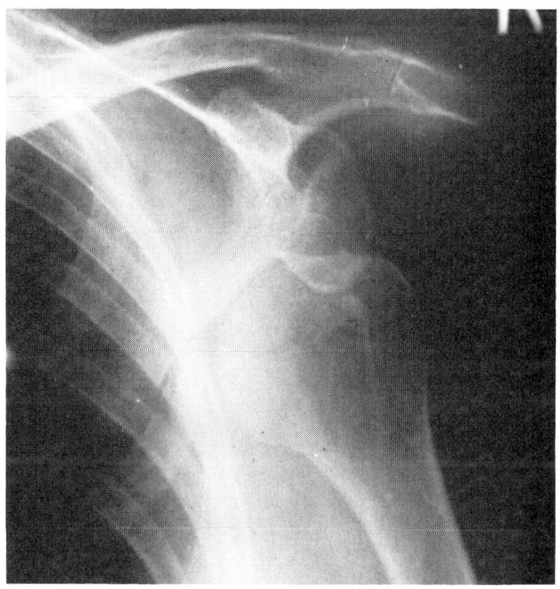

Figure 3–XIII–12. Anterior subglenoid dislocation of the shoulder.

the fact that, since 1825, fewer than 100 cases have been reported in the literature. In a large series studied by Calvé and associates, 90 cases were described, most of which occurred during the nineteenth century and were complications of the reduction procedure itself. Modern reduction techniques with the use of anesthesia require considerably less force than was formerly employed. Consequently the incidence of this complication has been reduced. Fewer than 1 case in 10 has been ascribed to the dislocation itself with absolute certainty.[26, 51-53]

Inferior dislocations of the shoulder were described by Bankart in 1938. In this dislocation the head of the humerus is forced out of the joint capsule at its weakest point between the subscapularis and triceps muscles. This lesion, it is said, always heals and therefore inferior dislocations are not complicated by recurrence.[54] *Superior dislocation*, a very rare form of dislocation of the shoulder, can only be seen with a coincident fracture of the acromion. Often when this fracture is seen on x-ray the shoulder appears to be relocated owing to the effects of gravity. A special form of this dislocation is luxatio erecta; in this the arm is forcibly abducted and the head of the humerus is thus inferior to its normal articulation. Also, the humeral head is found outside the capsule in this form of dislocation.

Posterior Dislocations. Posterior dislocations of the shoulder constitute about 3 per cent of all shoulder dislocations (Figs. 3–XIII–13 and 3–XIII–14). They are frequently found in patients who have a violent seizure disorder and in those patients who have sustained severe electrical shock.[55–57] Surgical intervention is necessary for the correction of recurrent posterior subluxations and old unreduced posterior dislocations.

Shoulder Fractures

Fractures of the Clavicle. The late complications of fractures of the clavicle are uncommon and restricted almost entirely to adults. Malunion and exuberant callus can lead to compression of the adjacent neurovascular structures. Nonunion of the clavicle occurs infrequently. Less than 2 per cent of clavicle fractures treated by closed reduction go on to nonunion; about 3 per cent of those treated by open reduction go on to nonunion. Nonunion of the clavicle must be distinguished from congenital pseudarthrosis of the clavicle. Of interest is a man with congenital pseudarthrosis of the clavicle who fraudulently claimed to have nonunion of a clavicle fracture after having been struck by a car. In fact, this medicolegal opportunist successfully sued three different motorists before he was exposed. Of historical note is a case reported by Watson-Jones regarding Sir Robert Peel, who is famous for creating the police force of Great Britain in the first half of the nineteenth century (so that we still refer to English policemen as Bobbies or Peelers). He died of a fractured clavicle. The pathology report indicated that his death was caused by laceration of the subclavian vein by splinters of the fractured bone.[53]

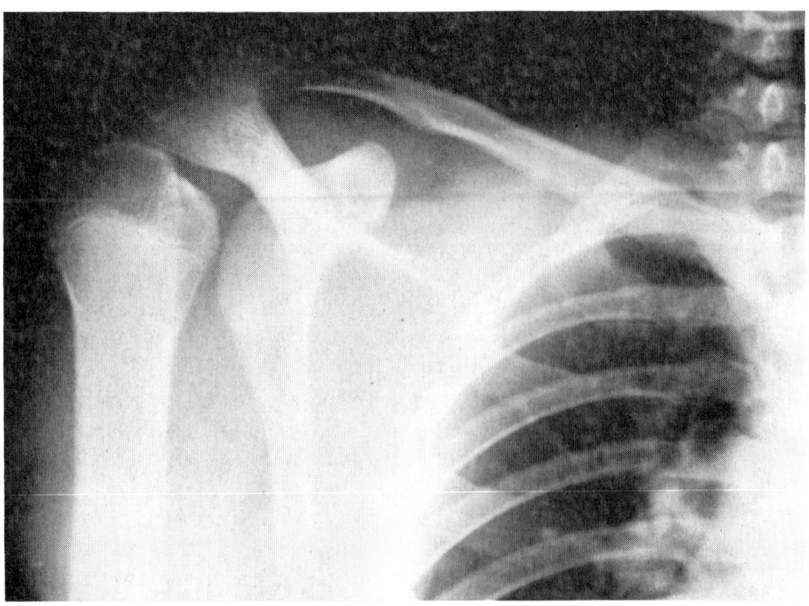

Figure 3–XIII–13. Posterior dislocation of the shoulder, anterior view.

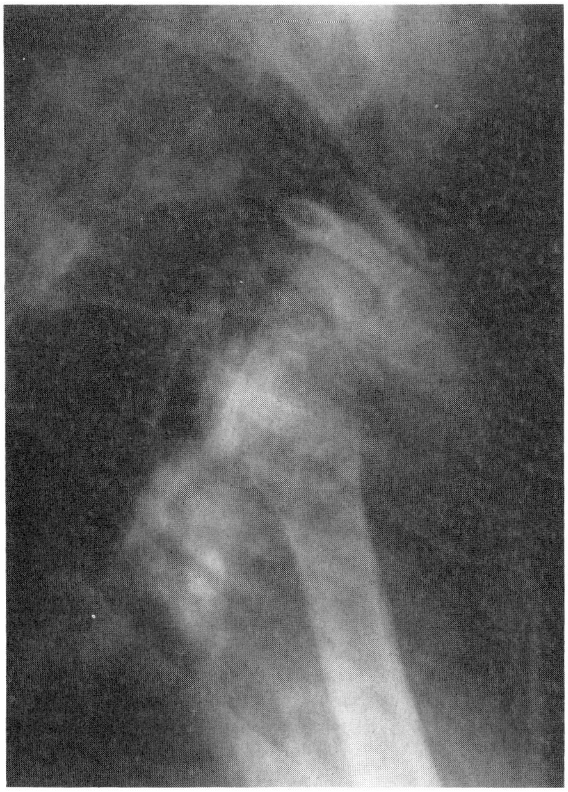

Figure 3–XIII–14. Posterior dislocation of the shoulder, lateral view.

Fractures of the Scapula. Fractures of the body of the scapula are usually caused by direct crushing injury and are sometimes associated with rib fractures. Usually the only treatment indicated is strapping. The discomfort is relieved, and in most cases healing is uneventful. If, however, the fracture should go on to nonunion, then the consequences are significant because of the location of the scapula and the lack of interference with normal function. It should be noted that forces causing such fractures are great, and one should always look for additional injuries to the nearby spine and thoracic cage. Fractures of the neck of the scapula occur, usually, as the result of direct impact on the anterior or posterior region of the shoulder. The articular surface of the glenoid fossa remains intact, and the capsule and ligaments are not involved.[28] Fracture of the glenoid fossa results from direct injury to the side of the shoulder. It may range in severity from a simple undisplaced linear fracture running through the glenoid fossa to one of a most severe type, with explosion-like effect on the glenoid. It may be severely impacted.[58] Two cases of chronic shoulder dislocations reported by Kummel involved fractures of the rim of the glenoid not appreciated at the time of the injury. When the humeral head became redislocated, and axillary lateral roentgenograms revealed the traumatic lesion, internal fixation was necessary to stabilize the shoulder joint.[59] Chip fractures of the glenoid rim commonly accompany anterior dislocation of the shoulder caused by abduction and external rotation of the arm. Rather large fractures of the anterior glenoid result, however, when a dislocation occurs with the arm adducted.[60] In general, depending upon the degree of severity of the fracture, complete anatomical restoration in the severe type is impossible by any means of treatment and is not actually necessary for the restoration of adequate function. Attempts should probably not be made to restore anatomical alignment, especially in the elderly. Brief immobilization followed by active exercises is necessary to insure maximum functional recovery. In some cases, however, posttraumatic arthritis will ensue.

Avulsion of the inferior rim of the glenoid by powerful contraction of the long head of the triceps is seen in athletes, particularly baseball pitchers and tennis players. DePalma feels that progress in the rehabilitation period should be deliberately slow because one hard wrench can undo the entire healing process. Usually, healing by fibrous union occurs between the glenoid and the avulsed bony fragment, which is usually sufficient to meet the demands of normal activity. In an athlete, however, this injury can limit the player's performance.

Fracture of the coracoid process constitutes a rather rare type of fracture usually caused by indirect violence such as that produced by muscle pull with the arm in abduction. This condition may also be found with multiple fractures about the shoulder region. McLaughlin feels that fibrous union of this fracture is common, and no treatment other than that for dislocation is needed.[2] No residual defect follows the fibrous union. Bateman states, however, that considerable disability may result from disruption of suspensory ligaments of the shoulder girdle.[29] *Fractures of the acromion* usually result from direct trauma to the tip of the shoulder. These fractures rarely require manipulation and usually heal following six weeks of immobilization. Occasionally, however, the acromion may be sufficiently depressed so that it impinges on the greater tuberosity of the humerus in the abducted position; in this case further measures are necessary. It should be noted that fractures of the coracoid process or the acromion may occur with dislocations.

These are rare lesions. The usual practice is to disregard the fracture and treat the patient as one would for an uncomplicated dislocation.

Fractures of the Proximal Humerus. One form of fracture of the proximal humerus is the fracture associated with dislocation of the shoulder. McLaughlin, in a study of over 1,700 cases of shoulder injury, states that only 1.1 per cent of these injuries resulted in a fracture-dislocation. Because the concept of what constitutes a fracture-dislocation is unclear, the literature is replete with many methods of treatment, and the results are indeed confusing. McLaughlin claims that in his experience, in a fracture-dislocation, the proximal humerus is divided into four major fragments: the humeral head, the shaft, and the greater and lesser tuberosities.[2] It is important to note that in the treatment of this fracture both open and closed methods are often unsuccessful. Avascular necrosis of the head of the humerus often results, leading to degenerative arthritis of the joint or severe stiffness and limitation of motion at the joint. In shoulder dislocations there are often fractures of the greater tuberosity. When the tuberosity is displaced 1 cm or more, it is indicative of severe soft-tissue disruption, particularly a tear of the rotator cuff. The fracture often involves the bicipital groove. Bicipital tenosynovitis and frozen shoulder are frequent complications.

Fractures through the anatomical neck of the humerus without impaction and with minimal displacement require no reduction or internal fixation. This is also true of valgus fractures through the surgical neck, provided that the head-neck angle does not exceed 160 degrees.[28] Surgical neck fractures of the humerus that are comminuted with moderate deformity are acceptable without reduction, as long as the fragments are in contact. Early mobilization is essential, particularly in elderly people, to avoid a frozen shoulder. The primary goal is mobility, and often one encounters a shoulder that is well healed but irreversibly stiff.

In the severely comminuted fracture of the proximal humerus, if one feels that mobility of the shoulder will be greatly limited, the decision for surgical intervention must be considered. Two options are available. One is the reconstitution of the fragments of the normal humeral head, and the other is the replacement of the fragments with a prosthesis (Fig. 3–XIII–15). Skeletal traction is sometimes necessary to reduce unstable fractures of the neck of the humerus.[61]

Frozen Shoulder

Turek describes the frozen shoulder as

> . . . a condition of unknown etiology characterized by gradually progressive painful restric-

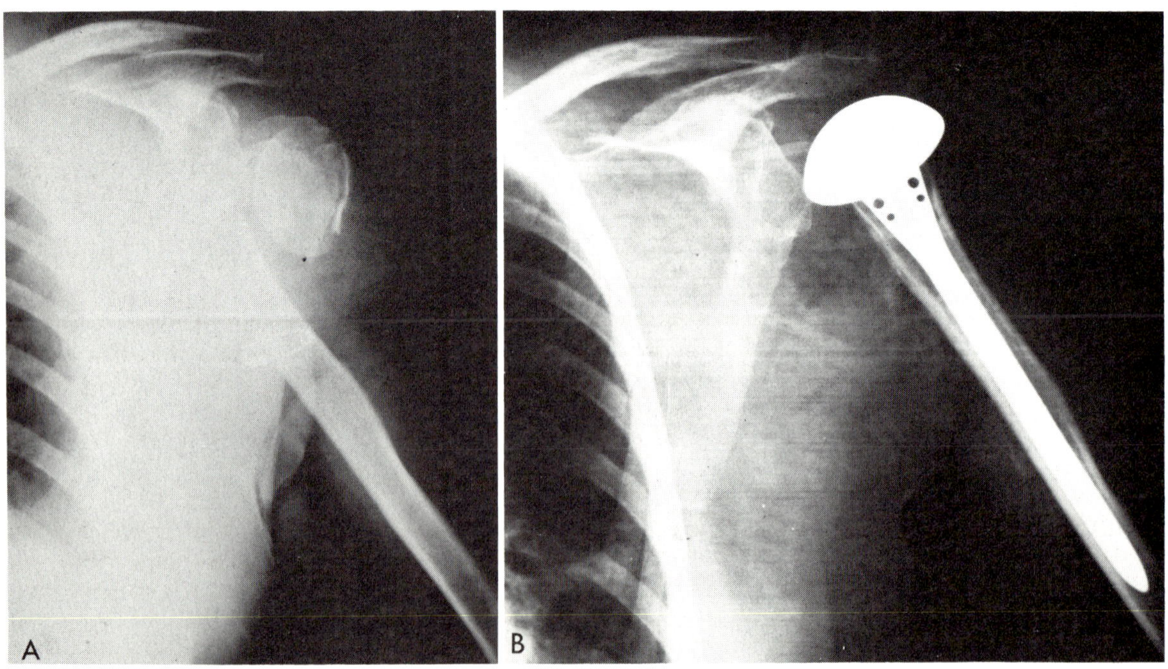

Figure 3–XIII–15. *A.* Severe fracture of the head of the humerus with marked displacement. *B.* Postoperative x-ray after excision of humeral head, and insertion of Neer humeral head prosthesis.

tion of all joint motion, chronicity and slow spontaneous restoration of partial or complete motion over months to years.[38]

"Frozen shoulder" is also known as adhesive capsulitis.

Limitation of motion of the shoulder joint secondary to any of the conditions already discussed may lead to stiffness. This must be differentiated from the classic "frozen shoulder," which, as has been stated, is a self-limiting and correctable process. Usually the limitation of motion secondary to trauma is irreversible. Also, the classic "frozen shoulder" may be the result of disease elsewhere in the body, examples of which are cervical arthritis and disk lesions, apical lung tumors, pulmonary tuberculosis, chronic epilepsy, cardiac disease, and even some inflammatory diseases in the abdomen.

Fractures of the Humeral Shaft

Humeral shaft fractures are generally treated in a closed manner, with good results and good return of function. Injury to the radial nerve can occur in these fractures, particularly in spiral fractures in the mid to distal third of the humeral shaft. The management of this problem is subject to some controversy in the literature. Ralston mentions that the nerve is usually contused as opposed to being completely divided. Therefore, the paralysis that is observed in this injury will usually clear within three months. Thus routine exploration of the nerve is not indicated.[58] According to Holstein and Lewis, there is a specific syndrome in which the nerve becomes entrapped in the fragments of a spiral fracture of the distal third of the humerus. In this particular syndrome the patient presents with a humeral fracture and normal nerve function. On reduction of the fracture, however, there is a loss of function of the radial nerve. This is an indication for exploration of the nerve.[62] Shaw and Sakellarides noted the clinical indications for nerve exploration. When paralysis occurs at the time of the accident and is associated with a closed fracture, exploration of the nerve is indicated when no recovery is noted within seven to eight weeks. If the paralysis occurs with an open fracture or a closed fracture requiring open reduction, or if the paralysis is progressive, immediate exploration is indicated. If paralysis occurs following manipulation of a fracture in the lower third of the humerus, with angulation and displacement of the fragments, this also requires early exploration.[63] In an article by Klenerman, reporting from London, England, a series of 98 fractures of the humerus was described in which there were found to be 10 radial nerve palsies. Seven recovered spontaneously and two were later explored. In one case the nerve was found to be lacerated, and in a second case the nerve was found entrapped within callus. The third person was lost to follow-up.[64] According to Sim, Kelly, and Henderson, correlation of the type of treatment with the time of onset and degree of palsy indicated that ultimately restoration of nerve function was better in the group with radial palsy who underwent early operation. Remediable lesions were encountered too frequently to ignore early nerve exploration.[65] It appears that the best course is to explore the radial nerve and extricate it from the fracture site or repair it if necessary. At the same time, the fracture can be stabilized by compression plating. Besides the radial nerve, median and ulnar nerves can be involved in rare instances. Distraction of bone ends during treatment predisposes to delayed union or nonunion, and for this reason DePalma discourages the use of a hanging cast.[4] Disability of humeral shaft fractures is due to delayed union, nonunion, and radial nerve palsy. Malunion is a rare sequela.

The Elbow

Medial and lateral views of the structure of the elbow are shown in Figure 3–XIII–16.

Conditions About the Elbow

Tennis Elbow. Lateral epicondylitis (tennis elbow) is a syndrome characterized by pain over the lateral aspect of the elbow that is aggravated by active extension of the wrist. This condition may be due to one or more causes, including radiohumeral synovitis, radiohumeral bursitis, and tendinitis of the conjoint extensor origin. In the latter, there is usually attritional degeneration in the conjoint extensor fibers secondary to repeated bouts of minor trauma. The literature on this subject contains a plethora of methods of treatment. It should, however, be noted that the majority of cases of tennis elbow will do well with conservative management. In studies from North Carolina and Tennessee evaluating over 1,000 cases of tennis elbow, it was found that the vast majority did well with conservative treatment.[66, 67] Patients resistant to conservative therapy may, however, require one or another operative procedure. Bosworth, who has had considerable experience treating tennis elbow, has inves-

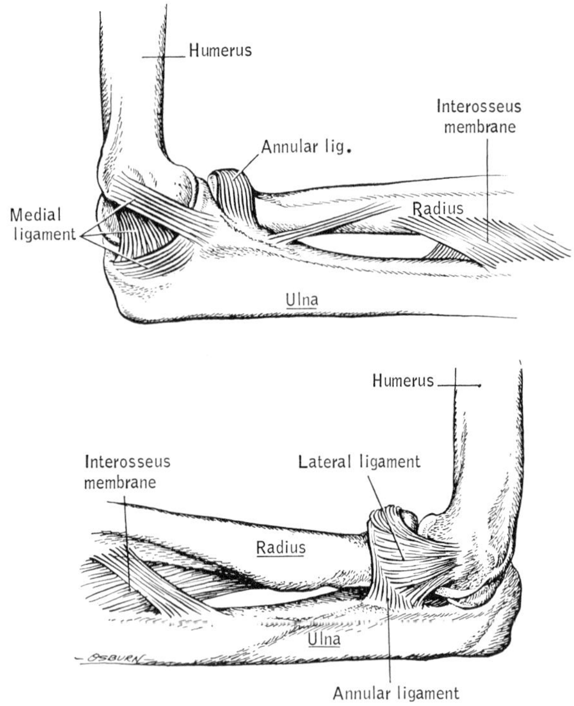

Figure 3–XIII–16. Medial and lateral views of the elbow showing bony and ligamentous structures. (From D. H. O'Donoghue: *Treatment of Injuries to Athletes.* 3rd Edition. Philadelphia, W. B. Saunders Co., 1976. Reprinted by permission.)

tigated a variety of surgical procedures used in its treatment. He now feels that removal of the orbicular ligament provides better results than division of the common extensor origin, either alone, or with removal of the synovial fringe. His results have provided a stable painless elbow without evidence of recurrence of symptoms.[68, 69] Roles and Maudsley from England reported in 1972 on 38 cases in which they felt that the cause of pain was entrapment of the radial nerve and its branches about the elbow. With selective release of this nerve and its branches they were able to show excellent results in 18 cases, good results in 17 cases, fair results in 2 cases, and poor results in 1 case.[70]

Medial Epicondylitis. Another process almost identical in pathologic characteristics to lateral epicondylitis, or tennis elbow, is medial epicondylitis. This process, classically described in the baseball pitcher who snaps his wrist in flexion and supination in the act of throwing a curve ball, causes a similar pain along the medial epicondyle of the elbow. There is obviously no single solution to the problem of epicondylitis. The decision as to which surgical procedure may be necessary is obviously dependent upon the individual physician's assessment of the individual case.

Olecranon Bursitis. This is usually caused by either an episode of acute mechanical trauma or chronic repeated mechanical irritations. Actual bacterial sepsis may or may not influence the picture. Those cases secondary to acute trauma often subside spontaneously with conservative therapy. Those cases complicated by sepsis, or those secondary to repeated mechanical irritation that are refractory to treatment, may require surgical excision of the olecranon bursa.

Elbow Strain. Another condition seen infrequently about the elbow is elbow strain. This syndrome consists of either a sprain of the radial collateral ligament or the ulnar collateral ligament, or attenuation of the entire capsule. The majority of these injuries give minimal temporary disability and usually respond well to immobilization in flexion for a short period of time. This allows fibrous healing of the sprained ligament or stretched capsule, and usually no permanent disability ensues.

Biceps Tendon Rupture. Ruptures of the distal insertion of the biceps tendon are noted either in older patients with attritional changes of this tendon secondary to minor trauma, or in younger patients who are subject to more severe mechanical trauma. Conservative therapy without surgical intervention usually results in an arm that is functional for the activities of daily living, but more supination strength may be obtained by surgical intervention if necessary.

Dislocation of the Elbow. The dislocation may take place in any direction, with the forearm being driven posteriorly, anteriorly, laterally, or medially in relation to the articular surface of the humerus (Fig. 3–XIII–17). By far the most common displacement of the elbow is posteriorly. Some element of lateral or medial displacement of the proximal forearm bones may often accompany the posterior type of dislocation. Pure forms of the other types are rare. Most frequently this injury results from a fall on the hand with the elbow in extension. As a general rule severe concomitant soft-tissue injury occurs. One must consider the possibility of associated fractures. Because of the possibility of severe complications as a result of this injury, prompt reduction is necessary. If there are associated fractures they should be treated as they would have been treated had they occurred without the dislocation. Reduction of the fracture-dislocation should be done immediately.

Recurrent dislocations of the elbow are relatively uncommon. A variety of soft-tissue and osseous

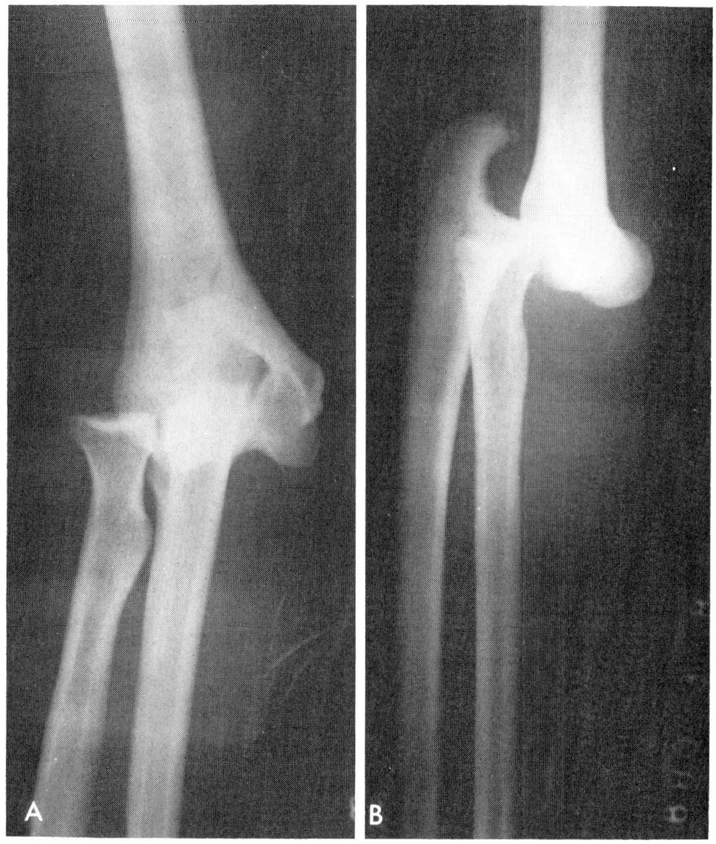

Figure 3–XIII–17. Elbow dislocation. *A.* Anterior view. *B.* Lateral view. An avulsion chip fracture from the olecranon is evident.

abnormalities may be found. Treatment is individualized, depending upon the exact nature of the pathologic changes. *Isolated traumatic dislocation of the radial head* at the elbow joint is a very rare lesion. It is usually associated with fractures of the upper portion of the shaft of the ulna. It behooves the examiner to check for evidence of a radial nerve deficit in these lesions. The radial nerve or its posterior interosseous branch may be injured. Failure to achieve reduction by manipulative maneuvers requires surgical exploration with repair or reconstruction of the orbicular ligament.[4]

Fractures of the Lower End of the Humerus

Fractures in this region may be due to hyperextension or hyperflexion. Lateral or medial displacement often occurs along with backward or forward displacement of the distal fragment (Fig. 3-XIII-18). These fractures exhibit varying degrees of outward or inward angulation of the lower fragment and the forearm (cubitus valgus, cubitus varus). Fractures in this area produce much hemorrhage, and one must be aware of compromise of forearm venous circulation. Indeed, the arterial blood supply may also be embarrassed. The median and ulnar nerves are rarely traumatized at the outset, but the ulnar nerve may be secondarily involved, particularly if there is healing malalignment. Occasionally, laceration or contusion of the brachial artery occurs at the time of injury or during manipulation. DePalma feels that these fractures should be reduced immediately, regardless of the amount of swelling, because the very nature of the displacement of the fragments may be a factor in causing vascular embarrassment and swelling.[4]

Distal humeral fractures usually result from direct trauma over the olecranon or posterior aspect of the elbow, and the force can be transmitted to the long axis of the forearm. Fractures may also occur from traction forces transmitted through the forearm muscles to the elbow. Approximately 95 per cent of fractures in adults involve the articular surface of the humerus. Such fractures may be unicondylar or bicondylar. The remaining 5 per cent are extraarticular fractures, either epicondylar or supracondylar. It should be noted that half the distal humeral fractures are bicondylar T or Y fractures, and less than one third are severely

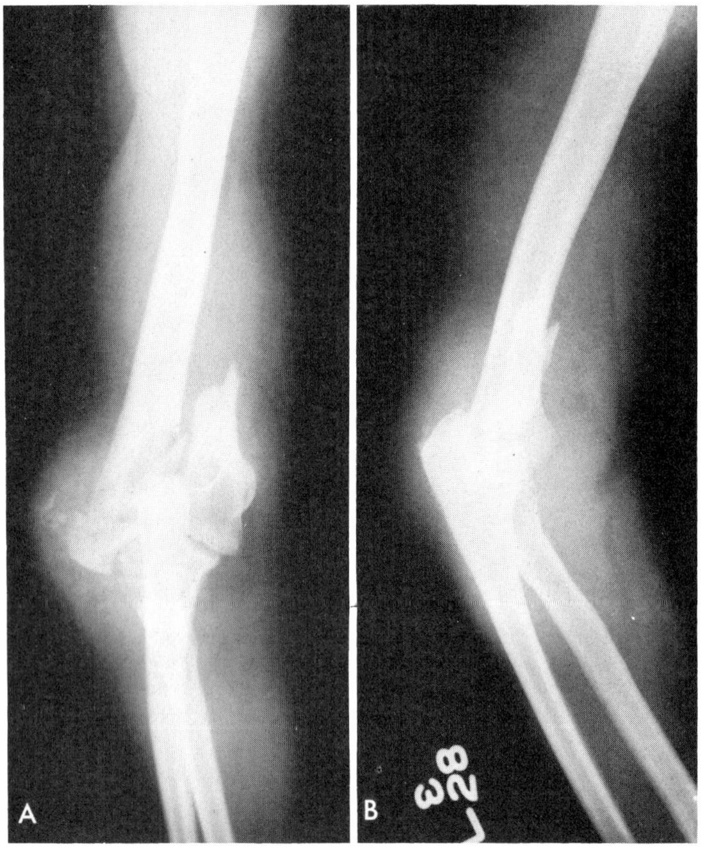

Figure 3–XIII–18. Markedly comminuted fracture of the elbow. *A.* Anterior view. *B.* Lateral view.

comminuted. These two types of fractures present difficult problems for the orthopedic surgeon.

Distal humeral fractures, in particular those with significant displacement, most often need open reduction and internal fixation.[73] Open reduction of such bicondylar fractures is directed toward the restoration of anatomical position. In cases of severe comminution this restoration is sometimes unachievable. If it is necessary to excise a fragment from a comminuted fracture, some lateral instability of the elbow joint may occasionally result, which may be quite disabling to a patient whose occupation requires elevation of his arms above the level of the shoulder. There is a dilemma peculiar to the supracondylar fracture of the elbow: when the elbow is placed in flexion to reduce the fragments, one notes that the radial pulse disappears; extension of the elbow results in return of the radial pulse, but there is subsequent loss of fragment position. This then necessitates either treatment with skeletal traction or open reduction and internal fixation of the fragments. One of the crippling residua of supracondylar fractures of the humerus may be Volkmann's ischemic contracture of the forearm.

Fractures of the Elbow Joint

A general premise by McLaughlin concerning severe fractures about the elbow is that prolonged immobilization of the elbow may lead to a fibrous ankylosis.[2] Therefore, early mobilization of the elbow is essential even if one has to except malunion with gross bony deformity. Here again is another dilemma: too active mobilization of an injured elbow may add to the predisposition toward myositis ossificans. With regard to intercondylar fractures, DePalma recommends that surgical intervention be avoided except in exceedingly rare instances.[4] Watson-Jones concurs with him on this.[53] Miller recommends open reduction and internal fixation as the treatment of choice, however, and he "has no regrets."[73] Ralston agrees that open reduction may be indicated in some instances, especially in those cases in which there is a wide separation of fragments but minimal comminution. He cautions that even when reduction of the fragments with internal fixation is quite adequate, the final range of motion may be disappointing.[58]

Humeral Condylar Fractures. Fracture of the *medial* (internal) *epicondyle* of the humerus alone is so rare as to be "almost a curiosity" in adults, according to Smith, who reported that in a series of 143 consecutive fractures of this epicondyle treated at the Presbyterian Hospital, New York City, only two cases unassociated with other fractures or dislocations were found occurring in adults.[74] DePalma feels that before the age of 18, avulsion of the medial condyle following abduction strain of the elbow is relatively common.[4] The intensity of the abduction force determines the varying positions assumed by the avulsed fragment pulled off by the common flexor muscles. The ulnar nerve may be involved in lesions of this sort with subluxation and dislocations of the elbow joint. When the fragment is displaced into the elbow joint, manipulative measures rarely achieve adequate reduction. The treatment of choice is operative repositioning of the avulsed fragment. It is also beneficial to transpose the ulnar nerve anteriorly to preclude ulnar neuritis, according to DePalma.

Lateral condyle fracture with lateral displacement and rotation over the fragment is relatively common in children, but rare in adults. Manipulative reduction is difficult, and because of marked rotation of the fragment, operative intervention is usually necessary to achieve adequate reduction. *Lateral epicondylar fracture* is also seen in youngsters, but rarely in adults. Fracture of the capitellum is another childhood fracture rarely seen in adulthood. These lesions may be complicated by a fracture of the head of the radius. Intraarticular small fragments are best removed surgically. Large fragments should be preserved and anatomically reduced with internal fixation. Small intraarticular fractures of the capitellum may undergo avascular necrosis and cause posttraumatic arthritis within the elbow joint if not removed.[74] When intraarticular fragments in the elbow are removed shortly after injury, the elbow can be mobilized earlier and one can expect to recover a maximum range of motion.

Trochlear Fracture. A fracture involving only the trochlear process of the humerus is very uncommon. It is usually sustained in a fall on the olecranon, which wedges and splits the trochlear process from the medial condyle. These fractures are usually undisplaced, but a fragment of the trochlear process may become loose within the joint. Thorough removal of the intraarticular fragment and early mobilization, as in other intraarticular fractures, are recommended. The ulnar nerve is sometimes damaged along with this injury as in fracture of the medial condyle. In all elbow intraarticular fractures, the primary complication is limitation of joint motion due to irregularity within the joint or possibly to avascular necrosis following poor healing or even nonunion.

Fractures of the Olecranon. Fractures of the olecranon occur more frequently in adults than in children. They usually result from a fall on the forearm with the elbow in moderate flexion. Occasionally the fracture may occur as a result of a fall directly on the olecranon itself.[58]

The fractures are usually somewhat comminuted, but may show little displacement of fragments. The triceps attachment usually remains undisturbed. Considerable comminution may exist with no separation of the fragments because of the toughness of the fibrous covering of the olecranon process itself. Comminuted fractures of the olecranon in older patients are often best treated by excision of the olecranon. This is also true of high fractures in which only a small fragment is separated and displaced upward. This lesion is comparable to rupture of the triceps tendon.[4] It is worthy of note that a true anterior dislocation of the elbow is virtually impossible without fracture of either the olecranon or the lower humerus. Anterior fracture-dislocation is a very serious injury usually resulting from force applied directly to the posterior part of the flexed elbow. According to O'Donoghue, the olecranon breaks, the triceps attachment holds the proximal fragment posteriorly, the lateral ligament gives way, and the humerus moves backward and downward into the fracture line. The olecranon may act as a wedge and cause a condylar or T fracture when it is driven into the distal end of the humerus. In treatment of a fractured olecranon, a surprising amount of the olecranon process may be removed; the elbow will still function well if the triceps is repaired carefully. The triceps sling should give sufficient stability.[75] According to Watson-Jones, the essential feature of surgical repair of the olecranon is not the repair of the olecranon itself, but the repair of the triceps.[53] Early mobilization after treatment of a fractured olecranon is essential, as prolonged lack of motion may lead to unnecessary elbow stiffness.

Fractures of the Head and Neck of the Radius

Fractures of the radial head and neck are associated with strains of the medial collateral ligament and injury to the articular surface of the capitellum. Segments of the articular surface of the capitellum may be detached; fragments are then free bodies in the joints. Occasionally avulsion of the internal epicondyle is a concomitant lesion. DePalma states that all comminuted fractures and marginal fractures with any amount of displacement should be treated by total excision of the radial head. The functional results are far better with removal of the entire radial head than with removal of only the displaced fragment, a practice that should be discouraged.[4] Radin and Riseborough state that although inferior radioulnar subluxation does occur following excision of the radial head, it is of so little significance that it may be ignored when excision of the radial head is indicated.[76] Undisplaced radial head fractures are best treated with early motion after minimal immobilization. It is often advantageous to aspirate the elbow joint when this type of fracture is first seen, as the joint is a small one and a small amount of entrapment fluid prohibits flexion and, incidentally, is very painful. Again, mobilization of an elbow should be active, not passive, up to but not beyond the point of pain.

There are two points of view regarding operative intervention in radial head fractures. Watson-Jones states that the ideal time for a surgical procedure is within a few days or weeks of injury. He asserts that there is no liberty to adopt conservative treatment for several months in the belief that late excision will still be successful. Some improvement may be gained by late excision, but usually the joint will not regain normal function unless the operation is performed early.[53] On the other hand, McLaughlin believes that surgery should be performed either within 24 hours of the injury or after a lapse of several months but not during the intervening period. He favors an anterior approach, as he believes this less frequently results in secondary myositis ossificans.[2] Other eminent surgeons, however, favor a more posterolateral approach. In fractures of the radial head and neck, maximum restoration of function is attained only after many months. Progress is usually very slow.

Fractures of the Proximal Ulna

Coronoid Process Fractures. Isolated fractures of the coronoid process are very rare lesions. They are usually associated with posterior dislocation of the elbow. When fragments are displaced into the joint cavity, causing blocking of the joint, excision of the fragments is recommended.

Monteggia Fracture-Dislocation. The Monteggia lesion is a typical example of a double bone injury (Fig. 3–XIII–19). It has come to be defined as a radial dislocation combined with a fracture of the ulna. The most frequent site of fracture is at the junction of the proximal and the middle thirds of the ulna. This occurs in approximately 60 to 70 per cent of cases. Since the dislocation of the radial head can be anterior, lateral, or posterior, any dislocation found with an ulnar fracture constitutes the anatomical clinical picture of the lesion discussed by Monteggia. There are numerous possible combinations of injury that fall under the classification of the Monteggia lesion. These have been divided into four classes.[76, 77] Smith has provided a separate classification of these injuries.[74] Monteggia lesions are classified according to the pathologic anatomy of the fracture, which is determined by the mechanism of injury. For example, 60 per cent are type I lesions, which comprise those anterior dislocations of the radial head in union with fracture of the ulnar diaphysis at any level with anterior angulation. The mechanism of injury of a type I lesion is a fall on the hand with the forearm in pronation with a superimposed external rotation force applied. This exaggerates an already full pronation. The treatment of these lesions is determined by the mechanism of injury and the anatomy of the fracture that results from it.

Campbell's Operative Orthopedics states that in acute lesions in which the radial head can be reduced by closed methods, the ulna should be immobilized with a compression plate or fixed with intramedullary devices. If soft-tissue intraposition precludes replacement of the radial head, open reduction of the radial head is indicated along with secure internal fixation of the ulna. In an injury six weeks old or older the ulna should be securely fixed internally and the radial head should be excised.[1]

Chronic subluxation of the radial head occurs occasionally, possibly as the result of a lack of adequate correction of ulnar angulation at the time of operation or inadequate internal fixation. Sometimes the ulna fails to unite and requires subsequent bone grafting. Radial nerve paralysis has been noted, usually preoperatively. Four of five cases reported by Boyd and Boals recovered spontaneously. The other did not improve. The patient who did not improve had multiple injuries that had precluded open reduction of the Monteggia lesion.[78] Since the radial nerve usually recovers spontaneously, surgical exploration of the nerve is not indicated. Seven cases of posterior interosseous nerve palsy, three of which were

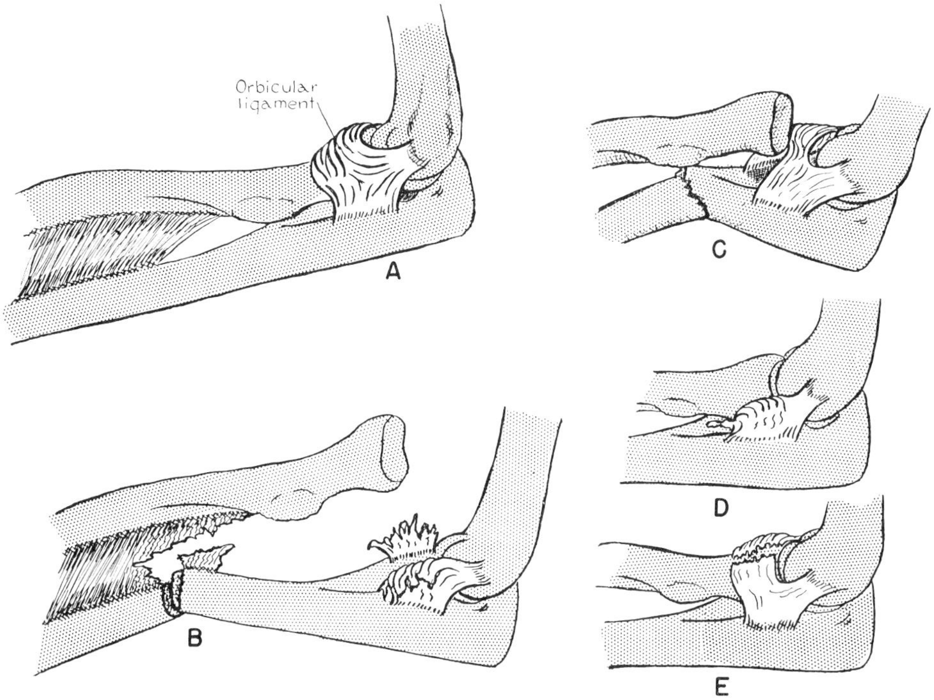

Figure 3–XIII–19. Variations in orbicular (annular) ligament injury in Monteggia fracture. *A.* Normal appearance. *B.* The radial head may disrupt the ligament. *C.* It may pull out from under the orbicular ligament. *D.* The radial head may return to position on top of the ligament. *E.* It may be replaced within the orbicular ligament. (From H. L. McLaughlin: *Trauma.* Philadelphia, W. B. Saunders Co., 1959. Reprinted by permission.)

associated with ulnar nerve palsy, as a complication of Monteggia lesions, were reported in an article by Stein and co-workers.[79] The posterior interosseous nerve may be stretched by the dislocated radial head or compressed against the aperture in the interosseous membrane. Ulnar nerve injuries are secondary to compression within the cubital tunnel. Surgical decompression of the nerves is recommended. In anterior Monteggia fracture, closed treatment may fail because interposed soft tissues prevent reduction of the radial head, and also because the surgeon fails to consider the appropriate pronation-supination position of immobilization. It is recommended that the arm be immobilized in a cast in 100 to 110 degrees of elbow flexion, with the cast molded over the lateral side of the ulna to prevent radialward bowing of the ulnar fracture.

The Monteggia lesion is very difficult to treat. DePalma lists complications as follows: malunion, delayed union, nonunion, angulation of the ulna toward the radius, dislocation of the radial head, synostosis between the ulna and the radius, and subluxation or dislocation of the distal end of the ulna. He states that in most instances the orbicular ligament is torn or disrupted completely, permitting anterior dislocation of the radial head.[4]

The elbow is a compact joint with precision-fit articulations. It takes little injury to this sophisticated mechanism to produce permanent derangement. It is a rare situation indeed in which an elbow is injured, particularly intraarticularly, and rehabilitation restores the joint to its preinjury condition. According to McBride, normal motion of the elbow is through an arc of 45 degrees from 180 degrees, or full extension, to an angle of 35 degrees, or full flexion.[81] This range of motion is rarely achieved after elbow injury.

The Forearm

Wringer Injuries. These injuries occur primarily in children, 50 per cent of them in children under the age of five years.[1] Similar injuries can be sustained in industry. According to Tachdjian, the maximum damage to the soft tissues is sustained in the antecubital fossa if the elbow is flexed as the forearm is drawn into the roller. If the elbow is extended, however, the maximum trauma is to the axilla.[82] A second crushing increases the extent of the injury when countertraction is applied or when the direction of the rollers is reversed. The crushing injury is primarily to the soft tissues. Bones are rarely fractured. There may be no break in the skin, but the patient may still have severe disruption of nerves or tearing of tendons. Vascular damage is also common. Prognosis is guarded, particularly early after the injury. Sloughing of the regional skin and devitalization of muscles can occur within one or two days after the initial injury.

Hospitalization is essential for the management of this potentially serious problem, which is best handled by thorough cleansing of the possibly abraded skin and soft tissues, splinting in the position of function, and careful observation to head off other possible complications such as Volkmann's contracture.[83] Edema often develops within 24 hours after the initial injury, and excessive swelling of the skin and soft tissues may require an extensive incision in the axis of the limb to relieve tension and to prevent death of skin and muscle.[84] Additional complications and sequelae of this injury include: skin destruction of varying degree, which may or may not require grafting; hematomas that may cause pressure on the structures; and impaired circulation to a digit of the hand. Volkmann's contracture is seen in rare instances. This complication has been managed successfully by the use of occlusive compression dressings. Depending upon the degree of injury, fibrosis of muscles with partial dysfunction of the hand may occur. In older patients, especially those over 50, partial or complete ankylosis of joints may be seen. Posttraumatic osteoporosis may also result. This syndrome has been cited as one of the major causes for prolonged loss of function and severe aching pain in or about the wrist joint.[85] Although true wringer injuries are seldom seen in the present-day practice of medicine, modern industrial equipment may produce similar injuries and even injuries that are more severe.

Forearm Fractures. The results of treatment of forearm fractures are difficult to evaluate and compare. Because of the complex structure of the forearm, the muscles of which may pull the bony fragments in many directions, normal length and rotational alignment must be reestablished. Owing to the action of the pronator teres, the pronator quadratus, the supinator, and the biceps musculature, fractures of the radius and the lower portion of the ulna should be immobilized in certain positions. In general, the more proximal the fracture, the more the arm should be placed in supination. The more distal the fracture, the more the forearm should be pronated. This classic positioning, although more difficult to determine for fractures in the middle third of the forearm, is important because the major disability of these fractures is lack of proper pronation and supination of the forearm. They may also lead to a rather marked cosmetic deformity. Many eminent sources in the field of orthopedics feel that most fractures of the diaphyseal portions of the bones of the forearm should be treated by open reduction and rigid internal fixation. *Campbell's Operative Orthopaedics* states that almost every diaphyseal fracture of the radius or ulna, or both, in adults should be treated by open reduction and rigid internal fixation.[1] Charnley, in his book entitled *The Closed Treatment of Common Fractures*, goes so far as to make the statement:

> There are many difficulties in treating the radius and ulna by closed manipulation; closed methods can give excellent results, but the element of luck is rather prominent, and for this reason I am in favor of operative treatment.[5]

In forearm fractures soft-tissue injury is always an accompaniment. There may be tearing of muscles, nerve injuries with subsequent derangement of muscle function, and vascular injuries. Volkmann's ischemic contracture may follow forearm fractures; this type of injury is the second most common cause of Volkmann's contracture.[58] Many methods of internal fixation have been employed. Excellent results have been obtained from intramedullary fixation, as well as from plating with bone grafting and from compression plating.[86-89] In cases in which shaft fractures of the radius and ulna fail to unite after bone graft procedures, prolonged fixation and impaction by external pins can be considered.[90]

The Wrist

Soft-Tissue Injuries

Sprains. A sprain, being a ligamentous injury, is relatively uncommon in the wrist. According to O'Donoghue, most of the so-called "sprains" are not sprains at all, but are strains of the tendon attachments or injuries to the bone.[75] In the very common dorsiflexion injury of the wrist, the damage is usually on the dorsal aspect. If there is tenderness over the carpus, careful x-ray study should be made, as there may be injury to the carpal bones, particularly the navicular. Injury to a carpal bone may not be demonstrable immediately after injury, but may become demonstrable on x-ray a week or 10 days thereafter. It is often good practice to re-x-ray a "sprained wrist" at that time to ascertain whether there is any fracture or dislocation of a carpal bone, in particular, of the navicular.

If a patient has tenderness and pain in the sulcus between the ulna and the carpus, but not on the ulnar styloid process, one must think of possible injury to the triangular cartilage that is the fibrocartilaginous extension of the radiocarpal joint lying between the ulna and the carpus. This is often injured in sprains of the wrist, and in fractures as well. Rupture of the fibers of this ligamentous and cartilaginous structure may result in hemorrhage and degeneration. Calcification is a late manifestation of this same condition. If conservative measures are not sufficient, excision of the triangular cartilage may be necessary.

Ganglion. A ganglion, which is actually a synovial hernia, has a predilection for the dorsum of the wrist, but it is often seen on the volar aspect as well. As a rule, a ganglion results from a defect in the fibrous sheath of the joint or tendon that permits a segment of underlying synovium to herniate through it. Direct trauma is often the cause. Even with careful surgical excision, the recurrence rate is 20 per cent.

Tenosynovitis. Overusage and chronic attrition can cause inflammation of tendon sheaths. Tenosynovitis is common in stitchers and in those in similar occupations in which there is constant repetitive use of tendons, particularly in peculiar positions, of the hand and wrist. Stenosing (constrictive) tenosynovitis of the first dorsal extensor compartment tendons, deQuervain's disease, is one of the most common of these entities. It is seen 8 to 10 times as frequently in women as in men.[85] Stenosing tenosynovitis is also seen in the wrist extensors. Steroid infiltration into the tendon sheath has been recommended and is often sufficient for short-term improvement. It often provides a definitive cure if the patient is seen early. Operative lysis of the tendon sheath usually results in complete relief of the symptoms.

Calcium Deposition. Calcium may be deposited in the tendons at the level of the wrist, resulting in a chronic tendinitis. The cause of calcium deposition may be related to minor trauma that produces a zone of poor blood supply into which the calcium salts are precipitated. The presence of calcium in tendons at wrist level is usually accompanied by a great deal of pain. This syndrome can mimic acute infectious processes at that level. Radiologic examination aids in confirming the diagnosis. Most cases occur in women between the ages of 30 and 60 years. The pain may be extremely disabling. Splinting the wrist in neutral position along with injections of steroids or local anesthetic may relieve the symptoms. Aspiration of the calcified mass may be carried out with some degree of success. This syndrome is analogous to the calcific tendinitis frequently seen in the shoulder. Occasionally surgical intervention is required for excision of the calcified mass, usually in cases of long duration.[91]

Pisiform-Triquetral Joint Sprain. Smith describes a sprain of the pisiform-triquetral joint as a specific entity. Trauma is either direct, as from a direct blow or fall against the bone, or indirect, as from excessive occupational use of the hand. Discomfort is localized at the insertion of the flexor carpi ulnaris. Treatment is conservative, although occasionally permanent relief may be obtained only by arthrodesis.[92] Removal of the pisiform for relief has also been described.

Carpal Tunnel Syndrome. This syndrome is common; in fact, it is the most common nerve entrapment syndrome.[93] Any condition that crowds or reduces the capacity of the carpal tunnel may initiate the symptoms. The median nerve is vulnerable to compression by the carpal tunnel or within the carpal tunnel. The syndrome may be initiated by direct trauma, such as a fall on the outstretched hand, or by tenosynovitis of the flexor tendons. It is seen also as a complication of Colles' fracture, or after lunate dislocation. The disability resulting from carpal tunnel syndrome is primarily the result of motor and sensory dysfunction of the branches of the median nerve. When dysfunction becomes significant, decompression is often indicated. Continued disability may result, however, even after surgical correction of the underlying problem. This is primarily for three reasons according to Langloh and Linscheid. These are incomplete sectioning of the compressive fibers of the carpal tunnel, tenosynovitis of the structures surrounding the median nerve, and fibrous proliferation within the sectioned carpal tunnel.[94] In Phalen's series, in which he treated 235 wrists surgically, 72 per cent regained normal function. Of those, however, 27 per cent, although improved, still had some impairment of nerve function.[93] This is important to note since this syndrome is often seen in workers in certain occupations such as stokers, blacksmiths, laundry women, and ironers. These patients need to retain full function in order to pursue their normal occupation.

Ulnar Nerve Entrapment. This is more often caused by chronic overuse of the wrist than by acute injury. *Campbell's Operative Orthopaedics* states, however, that usually a ganglion is the cause of compression.[1] Sometimes thrombosis of the ulnar artery or acute trauma such as fracture of the hamate with the accompanying hemorrhage can be the cause. This condition may produce atrophy of the intrinsic muscles of the hand, since the deep branch of the ulnar nerve supplies almost all these muscles. There may be no sensory involvement because the superficial branch of the ulnar nerve is relatively less vulnerable. Surgical release is usually sufficient for relief of symptoms. O'Donoghue recommends that the ulnar nerve or the overlying ligament not be injected with any local anesthetic, since this can only increase the pressure around the nerve.[75] Some authors, however, advocate injection if the symptoms have been mild and of short duration.[1]

Two iatrogenic conditions that may result from surgical incisions about the wrist are damage to the palmar cutaneous branch of the median nerve and damage to the recurrent motor branch of the median nerve. Damage to the motor nerve may result in motor dysfunction of the thenar muscles, and damage to the palmar cutaneous branch may result in continued pain in the area of distribution of the median nerve.[95]

Wrist Dislocations

Dislocation of the radiocarpal joint is extremely uncommon, although it has happened as a result of violent action. A complete carpal dislocation is also uncommon and is obviously a serious injury. It is recommended that careful x-ray study of the normal as well as the injured wrist in several positions be obtained in order to decrease the margin of error in diagnosis of this type of dislocation through the carpus. It is essential that these conditions be diagnosed early, as the longer the dislocation remains unreduced, the greater is the likelihood of recurrence and of permanent residual disability.[75]

There is an almost infinite variety of dislocations and fracture-dislocations of the carpus. Any carpal bone may be dislocated forward; or the rest of the carpus may be dislocated dorsally from one bone, which remains in its normal position.

Lunate Dislocation. One frequently occurring example of dislocation is that of the lunate (Fig. 3–XIII–20). This bone may be displaced by itself or it may remain in its normal position in relation to the radius while the rest of the wrist is dislocated from it. This is called perilunar dislocation of the carpus.[58] Failure to diagnose dislocation of the lunate is common and usually results from incomplete clinical examination and casual x-ray examination. It must be remembered that an extruded lunate compresses both the median nerve and the flexor tendons of the fingers within the volar carpal canal. As McLaughlin emphasizes, *a wrist sprain accompanied by numb fingers and a weak grasp must be considered a lunate dislocation until proved otherwise.* Early manipulative reduction is usually successful. When manipulative reduction fails, however, open reduction or excision of the lunate should be performed for relief of pressure in the carpal canal. Force applied to the hyperextended hand dislocates the other carpal bones on the lunate, whereas dislocation of the lunate results from a force applied to the palm of the moderately extended hand. McLaughlin stresses that classification of the many combinations of fractures and dislocations peculiar to the injured carpus is of "academic rather than therapeutic significance."[2] The capitate is the keystone of the carpal mechanism to which most of the carpals are firmly connected, directly or indirectly. All except the lunate tend to follow the capitate into a displaced position. In perilunate dislocations, reduction by manipulation is easier and more certain than in dislocations of the lunate, but the extensive ligamentous damage that facilitates reduction may also make maintenance of exact intercarpal relationships impossible. Small residual subluxations of one bone on another are common and are rarely controllable by external fixation. Long-term immobilization is often necessary. If there are continued instability of the subluxated elements and persistent severe pain and disability, excision of the offending carpals or wrist fusion may be necessary.[96–98]

Scaphoid Dislocation. Dislocation of the navicular (scaphoid) is rare as an isolated injury. It is frequently the residual of an incompletely reduced perilunar or intercarpal dislocation. Because of the complexity and number of small bones in a relatively small area of the carpus, there may be a multitude of different types of fractures or fracture-dislocations or both. Some of these may be transscaphoid-perilunate fracture-dislocations, periscapholunar dislocations, dislocations of the lunate and proximal half of the scaphoid, dislocation of the lunate and the scaphoid, backward and anterior dislocation of the metacarpal bones on the carpus, isolated dislocation of the greater multangular, and

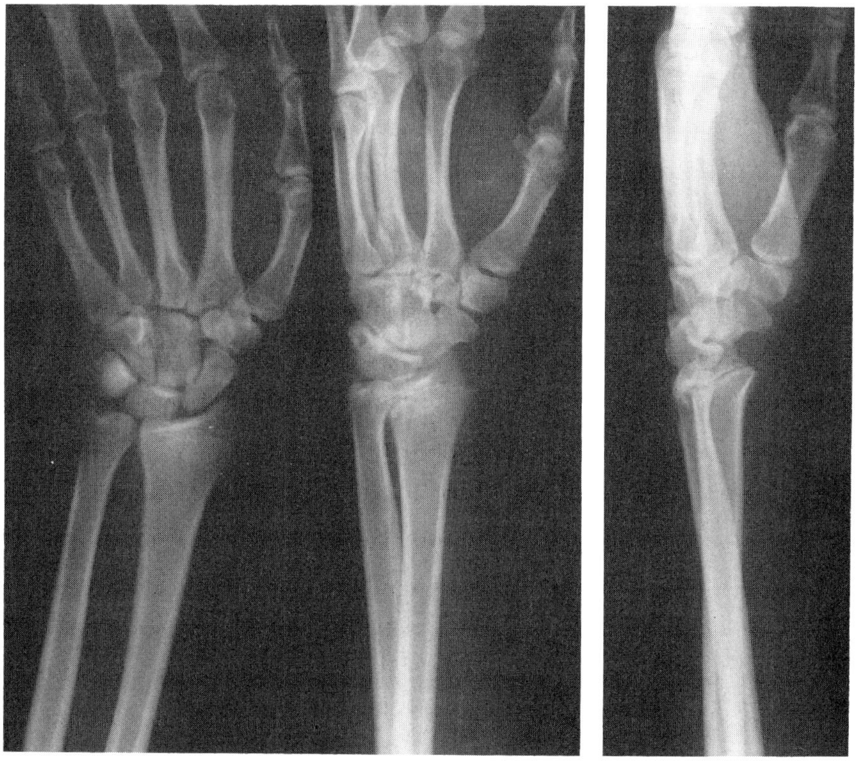

Figure 3–XIII–20. Dorsal dislocation of the navicular and lunate bones. There is also a transverse fracture through the most distal portion of the radius, the distal fragment being slightly posteriorly displaced.

carpal-metacarpal dislocation on the ulnar side of the hand.[4, 99-101] The disability following dislocations and fracture-dislocations in and about the carpus usually results from ligamentous injury leading either to stiffness and decreased range of motion of the wrist or to laxity and instability of the wrist. Disability may also be caused by avascular necrosis of one or more bones or parts of bones of the carpus. This results in eventual degenerative arthritis and disability secondary thereto. At the time of injury the eventual outcome is not predictable, although it may well be determined at the time of injury because of injury to the vascular supply of these bones.

Radioulnar Joint Dislocation. Dislocations of the distal radioulnar joint have not been frequently described in the literature. Up until 1972 there was no series larger than five patients. This may be a result of the difficulty of diagnosing these injuries. When diagnosed, this dislocation can usually easily be reduced by placing the arm in supination. The resultant disability is usually the result of an untreated dislocation of the radioulnar joint leading subsequently to difficulties in supination and pronation of the forearm at the radiocarpal joint.[102, 103]

Fractures of the Wrist

Colles' Fracture. Colles' fracture of the wrist is "a displaced fracture of the lower end of the radius within one and one half inches of the joint," according to Abraham Colles, 1814 (Fig. 3–XIII–21).[104] We usually include the fracture of the ulnar styloid process in our diagnosis of Colles' fracture today. Colles could not have known of this entity because he did not have the benefit of x-rays. There are various methods of treatment. The most recent article on this subject by Christopher Pool summarily states that all displaced Colles' fractures should be reduced. This was ascertained in a study of 239 Colles' fractures. He also recommends that a below-elbow plaster cast be used after reduction. It is his opinion that an above-elbow cast has no advantages and may have some disadvantages.[105] McLaughlin states that "there is no single or best method of reduction or fixation, nor is there any standard period of immobilization for a Colles' fracture."[2] Maintenance of reduction is difficult. Circular plaster dressings are a constant potential source of circulatory embarrassment, particularly in the first few days after application. "Sugar tong" splints have been recommended to obviate this prob-

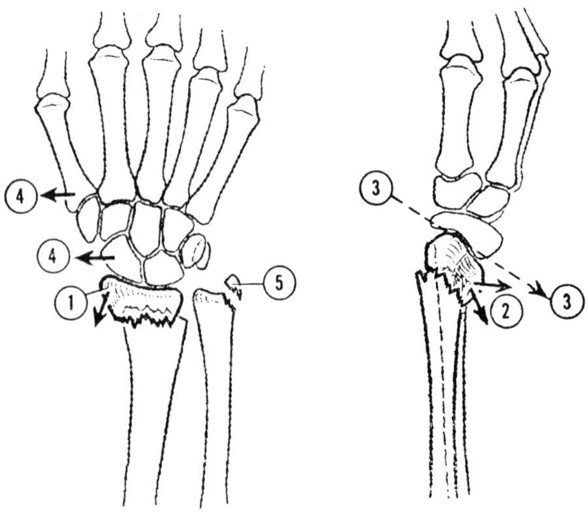

Figure 3–XIII–21. Colles' fracture of the wrist (extension fracture). 1. The distal radial fragment is displaced proximally (the radial styloid process may be on the same plane as the ulnar styloid process or proximal to it). 2. The distal radial fragment is displaced upward and backward. 3. The plane of the articular surface of the radial fragment projects backward (this angle varies greatly with each case). 4. The carpus and the hand deviate toward the radius. 5. The ulnar styloid process may or may not be fractured. (From A. S. DePalma: *The Management of Fractures and Dislocations—An Atlas.* 2nd Edition. Vol. 2. Philadelphia, W. B. Saunders Co., 1970. Reprinted by permission.)

lem with circularization. Many orthopedic surgeons prefer immediate application of a circular plaster cast, but it should be pointed out that this should be checked shortly afterward to detect vascular embarrassment. It is recommended that no matter what mode of immobilization is used, free interphalangeal and metacarpal-phalangeal joint motion should be allowed. It is recommended that the fingers, elbow, and shoulder be moved as much as possible after treatment, within the limits of the immobilization. This prevents stiffness, which is one of the long-term disabling effects of Colles' fractures.

The literature is replete with methods of treating Colles' fractures. In 1929, Böhler was the first to use skeletal traction to reduce the fracture and to use pins in plaster to hold the reduction. In 1949 Rush and Rush used intramedullary pins in the radius to hold the fracture. In 1952 DePalma treated 39 patients with skeletal traction and pinning of the distal radius and ulna. He was able to restore the normal articulation fairly well and hold the normal volar tilt of the radius, and showed 82 per cent satisfactory results in his patients.[108] Another method that is commonly used was described in 1966 by Cole and Obletz. They used proximal and distal pins, and were able to show 94 per cent satisfactory results in their cases.[109] In 1951 Gartland and Werley did a retrospective study of 60 cases treated only with dorsal and volar splints. They showed 84 per cent satisfactory results in simple Colles' fractures. With comminuted Colles' fractures involving the radial articulation with displacement, however, only 48 per cent of the results were satisfactory.[107] A more recent study in 1971 by Blichert-Toft and Jensen, who treated 92 patients with all types of Colles' fractures by placing the hand in ulnar deviation and severe pronation, showed that 30 per cent of the fractures became redisplaced.[109] Thus, it can be seen that this most common fracture has many variables. Because of this, the type of treatment used is dependent not only on the type of fracture but on the age of the patient in whom this fracture occurs and the occupation of the particular patient. For example, in the very elderly person, a considerable amount of displacement can be accepted for fear that longer immobilization would cause an undue amount of stiffness.

There are multiple complications of Colles' fractures. Avulsion of the ulnar styloid process occasionally can cause pain after the fractured radius has healed. There can be derangement of the triangular fibrocartilage. This manifests itself as pain in the inferior radioulnar joint. Excision of the ulnar head is the recommended treatment. Subluxation of the ulnar head may require excision of the distal ulna. Rupture of the extensor pollicis longus tendon is a rare complication, and trigger finger (stenosing tenosynovitis) is also seen. This latter complication appears more frequently in women than in men. Occasionally one sees subluxation of the extensor carpi ulnaris tendon because the annular fibers binding this tendon into its groove on the dorsal surface of the ulnar head are stretched or torn when the hand is driven backward and toward the radial side when a Colles' fracture occurs. According to McLaughlin, operative stabilization can be done, but ulnar head excision provides the most rapid and certain relief of the symptoms.[2] An exceedingly rare complication is nonunion. In Colles' fractures, one should be aware of a possible fracture of the navicular, which is occasionally seen concomitantly.

As previously mentioned, the degree of disability is often difficult to determine. Bacorn and Kurtzke evaluated 2,000 Colles' fractures for the New York State Compensation Board, however, and showed that the disability was directly related to the amount of residual deformity, and that the average disability was 24 per cent. They also made note in their article that only 3 per cent of all cases evaluated had no disability whatsoever.[110] An opposing point was made in the literature by Smaill, from Wellington, New Zealand, who after following 41 patients with Colles' fractures for five years, stated that the objective results were not as satisfactory as the subjective, but overall there seemed to be no reason to depart from plaster management of these fractures. He felt that Abraham Colles' belief, that in time these patients would regain full function irrespective of how the fracture was treated, is true.[111]

Smith's Fracture. In a Colles' fracture, the mechanism of injury is usually a fall on the outstretched hand; it is a pronation-extension injury of the wrist. In a Smith's fracture, the mechanism of injury is the reverse, and a Smith's fracture is often called a reverse Colles' fracture (Fig. 3–XIII–22). The mechanism of injury is a fall on the supinated and flexed wrist. In a Colles' fracture, there is dorsal displacement of the distal fragment of the radius, and in a Smith's fracture, there is volar displacement of the distal fragment. Charnley recommends, and it has been generally accepted, that a Smith's fracture is best held in the reduced position by applying a plaster dressing with the wrist in full supination. A Colles' fracture is usually treated with the wrist in some flexion, pronation, and ulnar deviation. Charnley feels in a Smith's fracture it is necessary to incorporate the elbow in plaster in order to hold the fully supinated position.[5] Open reduction and internal fixation with a buttress plate has been recommended for Smith's and Barton's fractures by Ellis, from Southampton, England.[112] On the other hand, Woodyard, from Exeter, England, followed 44 cases of Smith's fractures and seemed to be quite satisfied with treatment in plaster.[113] As with the Colles' fracture, dislocation of the extensor pollicis longus tendon has also been reported in Smith's fracture.[114]

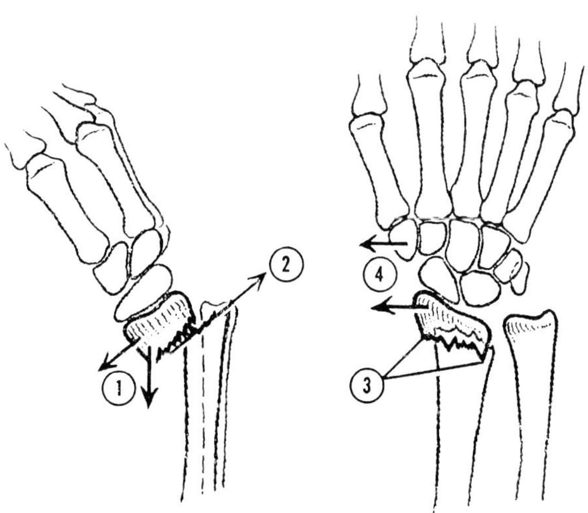

Figure 3–XIII–22. Smith's fracture (reversed Colles' fracture, flexion fracture). 1. The distal fragment is displaced forward and upward. 2. The fracture line runs obliquely from below upward and forward. 3. The distal fragment comprises the entire thickness of the shaft of the radius. 4. The distal fragment and the hand are deviated toward the radial side. (From A. S. DePalma: *The Management of Fractures and Dislocations—An Atlas.* 2nd Edition. Vol. 2. Philadelphia, W. B. Saunders Co., 1970. Reprinted by permission.)

Barton's Fracture. In 1838 Barton published his paper describing a fracture that now bears his name. The term "Barton's fracture" should be reserved for the anterior fracture-dislocation in which a wedge-shaped fragment of the radius of varying dimension is sheared off the anterior margin of the bone and displaced with the carpus forward and proximally.[115] It is De Oliveira's opinion that Barton's fracture-dislocation and Smith's fracture not only require distinctly different treatment but also have very different prognoses. Smith's fracture can be treated by manipulation and plaster immobilization, internal fixation being necessary in only a few patients. Good function can be expected once the reduction is achieved and maintained. Reduction of Barton's fracture-dislocation is very often impossible to achieve by manipulation, however, and open reduction is necessary to restore the correct alignment of the fragments. Even if manipulation is successful, redislocation occurs frequently no matter what kind of plaster cast is used. De Oliveira recommends the use of Ellis' buttress plate.

Malunion of fractures of the distal radius occurs. Osteotomy of the radius to restore cosmesis and function may be indicated. An essential preliminary is often excision of the subluxated lower end of the ulna, the Darrach procedure. Nonunion of fractures of the distal radius are exceedingly rare. This entity is usually due to an alteration in the process of bone repair because of concomitant factors such as infection.[53] Other exceedingly rare complications include ulnar nerve palsy as well as radial and median nerve dysfunction.[3, 116]

Styloid Process Fractures. *Fractures of the base of the radial styloid process* are often caused by falls on the outstretched hand; or as previously described by Watson-Jones, by early-in-the-century backfire injuries when the engine of a car was started with a hand crank.[53] This particular mode of injury is not seen today, but the process still occurs in industry. The carpus is driven backward and outward against the radius, but the impact is transmitted mainly by the scaphoid so that the fracture enters the wrist joint between the scaphoid and lunate bones.

Closed reduction is adequate. This fracture has been dubbed the "chauffeur's fracture." O'Donoghue recommends that, if the articular surface is deranged, the fracture must be perfectly reduced and firmly held until union is secure or the articular surface must be removed and the radiocarpal ligament sutured to the radius. Internal fixation is recommended.[75] In his discussion of this, O'Donoghue is referring to athletes, in whom maximum return of function is desired. *Avulsion of the ulnar styloid process* is also seen in athletes. The styloid process of the ulna may be pulled off by the ulnar collateral ligament. It usually heals by fibrous union without instability. If instability does occur, or if there is pain, excision of the ulnar styloid is recommended along with suturing of the ligament to the lower end of the ulna.

Fracture of the Navicular (Scaphoid). This fracture is often overlooked, either because x-rays are not taken or because the fracture is not seen on x-ray when the initial injury is presented (Fig. 3–XIII–23). McLaughlin feels that a *wrist sprain must be considered a fracture of the scaphoid until it is proved otherwise.*[2] Union can occur without treatment, but certainly better results are obtained with initial treatment by plaster immobilization. Failure to diagnose and treat an unstable scaphoid fracture will eventually result in painful arthritis of the radiocarpal joint. Immobilization of a wrist for two or three weeks is recommended after the diagnosis of "wrist sprain" when x-rays show no carpal fracture but the patient has a painful wrist. When there is localized point tenderness over the snuffbox, fracture of the carpal navicular should be suspected, and treatment should be instituted accordingly. Re-x-ray of the wrist after 10 days or two weeks will probably reveal a fracture line of the navicular if one exists, even though the fracture line was not seen on the initial roentgenograms. It should be kept in mind, however, that occasionally the surgeon will encounter a bipartite scaphoid. This, according to Waugh and Sullivan, is quite rare, and when a line is seen through the midportion of the scaphoid, the surgeon is most likely dealing with a fracture. This should be treated as such until proved not to be.[117] Stewart, who has studied a great number of fractures of the carpal navicular, states that as many as 95 per cent of the acute fractures may well unite when treated conservatively. A study of 100 fractures, which had been present an average of 38 weeks before any treatment was initiated, showed that after 20 weeks 73 per cent were proceeding to union or were already united.[118, 119]

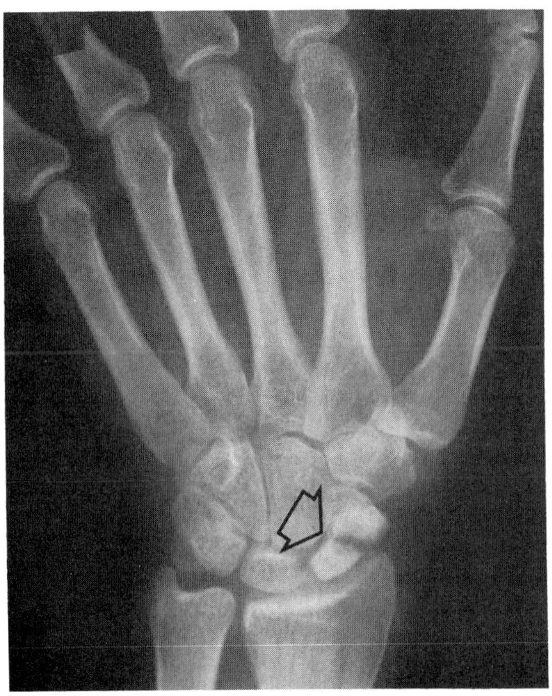

Figure 3–XIII–23. Nonunion of carpal navicular fracture.

As to length of time of immobilization, it is generally accepted that one immobilizes a fractured navicular until there is healing as ascertained clinically and by x-ray. Immobilization in plaster may be for as long as 18 months. O'Donoghue feels that there is little justification for continuing immobilization for many months if union does not appear to be progressing or if the fragment has become sclerotic or cystic. Prolonged immobilization has in some cases finally resulted in bony union, but in his experience and in the experience of many others, these are few and far between Surgical intervention is then recommended.[75] Bone grafting, internal fixation, excision of one or more fragments, and prosthetic replacement are all acceptable methods of treatment.[1, 2, 4, 119] Radial styloidectomy is indicated in localized radiocarpal arthritis. Excision of the proximal row of carpal bones also has been a treatment of choice for radiocarpal arthritis, as has wrist arthrodesis.

Compression Fractures of the Carpus. Many so-called sprains of the wrist that improve with time are compression fractures of one or more carpal bones. Diagnosis is virtually impossible by early x-ray, according to O'Donoghue.[75] Protection against motion that causes pain is recommended, either by a cock-up splint or a circular plaster dressing. Sometimes Ace bandage protection is sufficient. Avascular necrosis of a carpal bone can ensue as a late complication of compression fracture, particularly in the lunate. A fall on the heel of the hand may fracture the hook of the hamate bone. Fibrous union is likely. Persistent pain may require excision of the hook of the hamate. Delayed ulnar nerve palsy can occur.[121] Fracture of the pisiform can also cause ulnar nerve injury, particularly by compression. Pisiform fracture may be associated with fractures of the distal ulna or distal portion of the radius; or it may exist as an isolated fracture. In all fractures of carpal bones, posttraumatic arthritis can ensue, requiring either excision of fragments, excision of the injured carpal bone, arthrodesis, or prosthetic replacement.

THE LOWER EXTREMITY

The Hip

Soft-Tissue Injuries

Muscular strains in the vicinity of the groin are relatively frequent, the most frequent being that of the iliopsoas tendon.[75] It is caused by overactive contraction of the iliopsoas when the flexed thigh is forced into extension. It is recommended that careful x-ray study be made of the lesser trochanter to determine whether there has been avulsion of the bone. This is particularly true in the adolescent in whom the epiphysis of the lesser trochanter has not united with the shaft. Immobilization with the thigh flexed and externally rotated is sufficient to protect the limb. Susceptible to damage in this area is the abdominal muscle group that attaches along Poupart's ligament. Rest, heat, and protection are recommended.

Athletic injuries caused by direct trauma are often encountered in the area over the greater trochanter. Contusion may result in damage to the underlying musculature or to the bursa. Trochanteric bursitis may be caused by a direct blow. "Snapping hip" is due to chronic bursitis with thickening of the bursal walls; spasm of the tensor, as it slides back and forth over the trochanter on each step produces an audible and palpable snap. Turek states that the "snapping hip" syndrome is due to an overlying fascial band that snaps over the greater trochanter. This condition is usually pain-free but may become a source of annoyance when an underlying bursa is inflamed. Treatment of this condition can usually be successfully carried out by the injection of medication and, in resistant cases, by surgical intervention.[38] Strain of the muscles attached to the greater trochanter, particularly the gluteus medius, is often encountered. Conservative treatment is usually sufficient for resolution of this difficulty. Green reported a case of proximal avulsion of the iliacus with paralysis of the femoral nerve in a gymnast. Recovery occurred after decompression.[123] A few other cases have been presented.

Numerous bursae have been described about the hip. These bursae may become inflamed because of repeated chronic mechanical irritation. The three major ones that may be involved are the subgluteal bursa, the trochanteric bursa, and the ischiogluteal bursa. The iliopectineal bursa may also become involved. Inflammation of the ischiogluteal bursa is known as "weaver's bottom." Calcific deposits are quite frequently seen in bursitis of long duration. Indeed, as in the shoulder, calcium deposits may occur within the tendons about the hip. These may then in turn become irritating to the surrounding bursa, and produce secondary bursitis. Bursitis and calcific tendinitis about the hip usually respond better to conservative therapy than do similar conditions about the shoulder. Occasionally, surgical intervention may be required.

Hip Dislocations

Dislocations are seen almost exclusively in young adults or individuals in middle years of life. Trauma that produces dislocation in this age group would produce fractures of the hip in the very young and the elderly. McLaughlin lists three varieties of hip dislocation: posterior—the head of the femur rests behind the acetabulum; anterior—the head of the femur rests in front of the acetabulum; and central—the femoral head is forced through the floor of the acetabulum. These three types of dislocation are also known as sciatic dislocation, obturator dislocation, and intrapelvic dislocation.

Posterior Dislocations. These are more common than the others because the direction of injury is more often posterior, and because the posterior capsule is weaker than the anterior capsule. In fact, in Epstein's series of 559 dislocations of the hip, there was a 9 to 1 ratio.[123] All traumatic dislocations of the hip should be treated as emergencies. Severe complications of posterior hip dislocations are sciatic nerve damage and avascular necrosis of the femoral head (Fig. 3–XIII–24).[1, 2, 123] A long-term complication of this injury is myositis ossificans. Another complication, which is quickly apparent, is

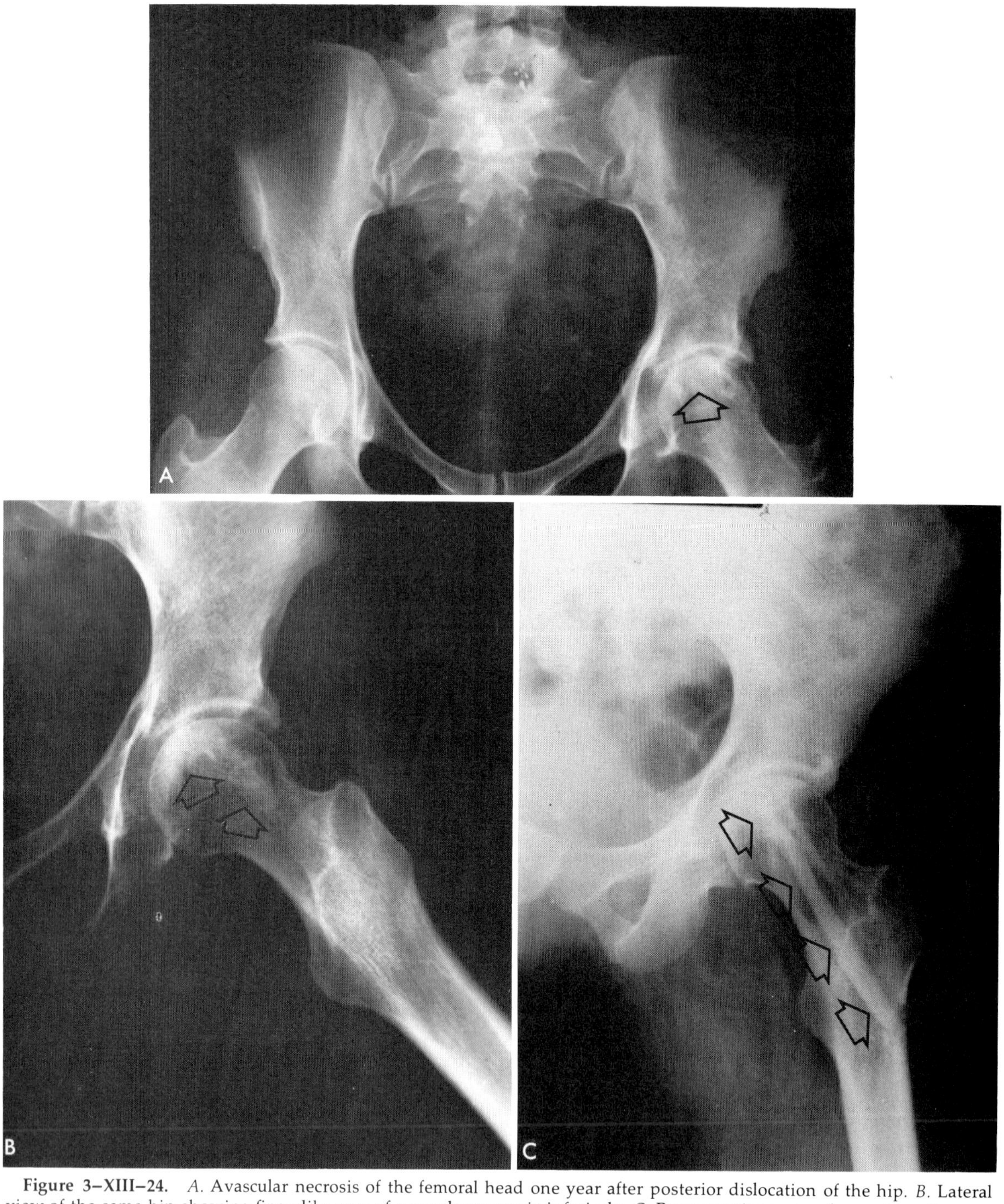

Figure 3–XIII–24. *A*. Avascular necrosis of the femoral head one year after posterior dislocation of the hip. *B*. Lateral view of the same hip showing fingerlike area of avascular necrosis inferiorly. *C*. Postoperative x-ray of same hip after cortical bone grafting with bone taken from the tibia.

damage to the peroneal nerve, probably due to injury to particular fibers of the peroneal nerve lying within the main body of the sciatic nerve. Eisenberg and associates reported a case of posterior dislocation of the hip producing lumbosacral nerve root avulsion. In this case the site of the neurologic lesion was ascertained by a careful neurologic examination with muscle testing and myelography.[124] Electromyography is another diagnostic tool useful two or three weeks after the injury. Discovery of lumbosacral nerve root avulsion means that an irreparable lesion exists; this is helpful prognostically, and it can also prevent unwarranted and futile exploration of the sciatic nerve.

When posterior dislocation of the hip is accompanied by fracture of the posterior rim of the acetabulum, it is necessary not only to reduce the displacement of the head, but also to replace the fragment of bone in its normal position if the fragment is of significant size (Fig. 3–XIII–25). Incomplete reduction of the joint or the fragment often is followed by rapid disintegration of the joint cartilage. It should be noted at this point that multiple attempts at closed reduction are contraindicated in both anterior and posterior types of dislocation. If the examiner cannot reduce the hip under adequate general anesthesia, open reduction is then indicated.[123] Watson-Jones advocates open reduction in cases of sciatic nerve palsy associated with fracture-dislocation of the hip in which manipulative reduction has been carried out with incomplete replacement of the acetabular fragment. He indicates that this acetabular fragment should then be replaced after it has been freed from the nerve.[53]

Occasionally posterior dislocation of the hip is accompanied by a fracture of the head of the femur. If the fragment is small and comes from the inferior quadrant of the head, it may be reduced satisfactorily by manipulation and may then unite in its proper position. If the fragment is a large one or comes from the weight-bearing portion of the head, it should be excised. If an attempt is made to replace it in its normal position, it will probably undergo avascular necrosis. Indeed, some authors advocate primary reconstruction of the hip such as cup arthroplasty or total hip arthroplasty for injuries of this type. Posterior dislocations of the hip associated with fractures of the femoral neck or of the femoral shaft fortunately are quite rare. When associated with fracture of the femoral neck, they should probably be treated by excision of the femoral head and a reconstructive operation on the hip. Those associated with femoral shaft fractures should do well. The dislocation should be reduced and the femoral shaft then treated as a separate entity.[126-128]

Recurrent posterior dislocations of the hip are quite rare although there are some case reports in the literature. At surgery in one case, a T-shaped rent in the posterior capsule was revealed along with separation of the labrum from the acetabulum. This pathologic change allowed a series of three recurrent posterior dislocations over a seven-year period.[129] In a case he described, Watson-Jones emphasized that the pathologic mechanism of the recurrent dislocation was a direct result of the failure to immobilize the patient for a length of time sufficient to insure healing about the joint. He

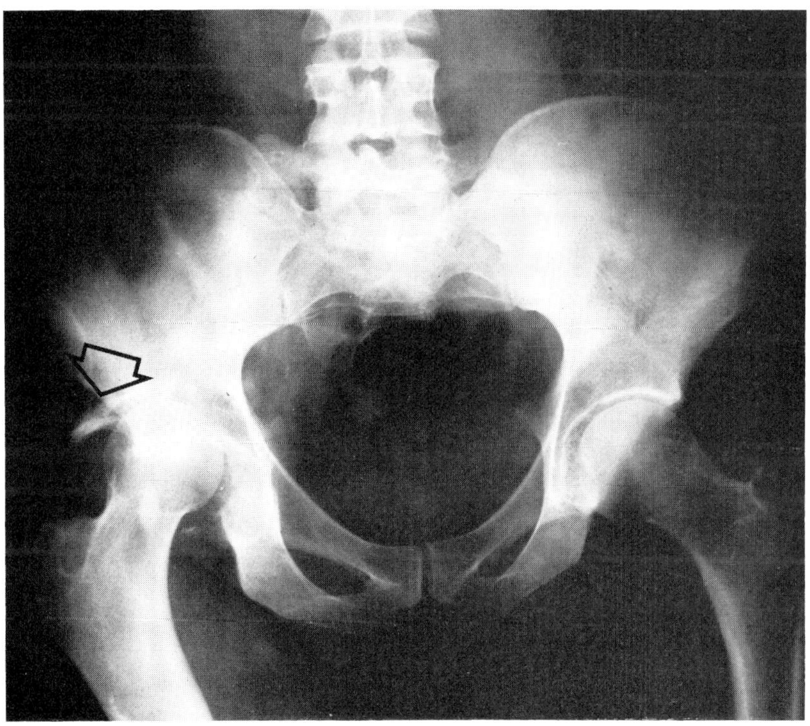

Figure 3–XIII–25. Hip dislocation with fracture of posterior acetabulum.

stressed that several weeks of immobilization with prolonged protected weight-bearing was essential to prevent recurrence of dislocation.[53]

Anterior Dislocations. Forced abduction is the mechanism of injury of anterior dislocation of the femoral head. McLaughlin cites the instance of a stevedore standing with one foot on the boat and the other on the dock as the boat moves away from shore, or a dancer doing the "splits," as situations that may cause this lesion.[2] The femoral head may produce pressure upon the femoral vessels. Anterior dislocations of the hip can further be subdivided according to the position of the femoral head, i.e., pubic, obturator, or perineal. In fact, there have been several case reports of perineal dislocations in which the femoral head presented in the scrotum.[130] Reduction can be accomplished by traction and internal rotation. Anterior dislocation may embarrass the femoral vein, and massive pulmonary infarction with sudden death following manipulation has been reported. McLaughlin suggests that, for this reason, vein ligation should precede reduction in neglected cases, particularly in those in which reduction was delayed more than 12 hours.[2] Epstein in his series of 55 cases of anterior dislocation of the hip found that only 70 per cent of the patients with anterior dislocations had excellent results. Eight dislocations were associated with compression fracture of the femoral head, two with acetabulum fractures. There was one patient with avascular necrosis and seven with traumatic arthritis.[131] Anterior dislocations may also damage the obturator nerve or the femoral nerve.[4]

Central Dislocations. This type of dislocation occurs when a blow upon the trochanter drives the femoral head medially against the floor of the acetabulum. The ischiopubic rami are rotated inward. There may be extensive comminution. It is recommended that when displacement is minimal, early motion be begun and increased within pain limits. Both McLaughlin and Watson-Jones agree on this.[2, 53] Weight-bearing is deferred from four to six months until a firm fibrocartilaginous repair has minimized discrepancies in the articular surface. Early motion is important to produce molding of the fragments. Skeletal traction is recommended for displaced lesions. Open reduction is indicated, especially in young people, when the head has become caught in the pelvis by fragments of the acetabulum, when closed reduction is impossible, or when the head or one or more large fragments of the dome of the acetabulum remain displaced or interposed despite the use of traction. In severe central fracture-dislocations of the hip the pelvic viscera may be severely damaged. One of the complications reported is protrusion of the small bowel through the central acetabular defect.[132, 133]

Otto pelvis (protrusio acetabuli, arthrokatadysis) is abnormal deepening of the acetabulum, and is usually caused by trauma (Fig. 3–XIII–26). Central dislocation of the hip is implicated.[134–136] In central acetabular protrusions, posttraumatic arthritis frequently develops in

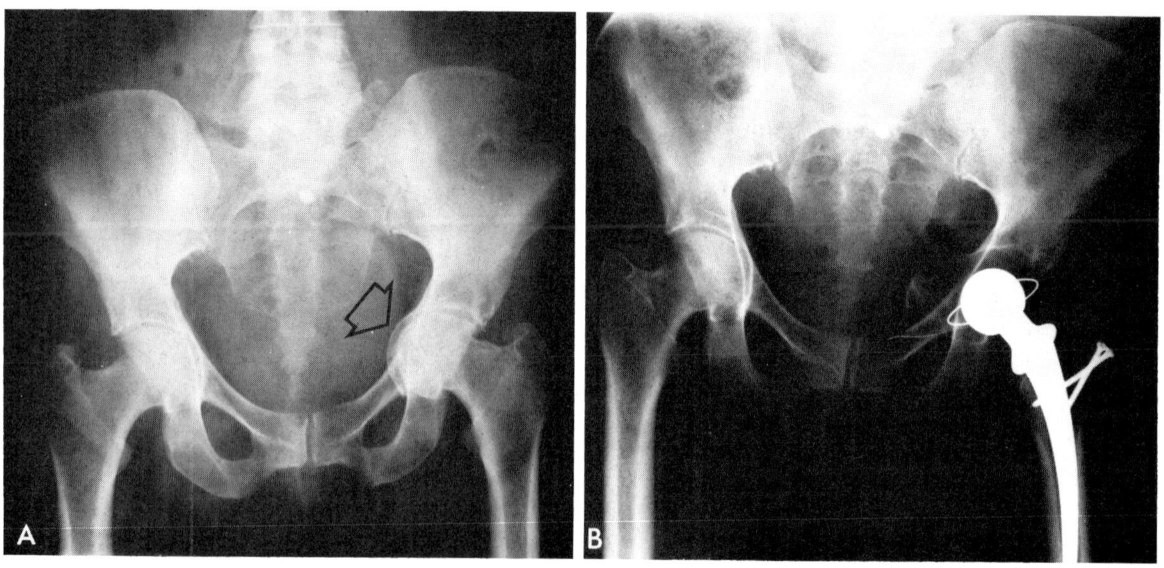

Figure 3–XIII–26. *A.* Otto pelvis (protrusio acetabuli, arthrokatadysis). *B.* After total hip replacement.

later months or years as a secondary consequence (Fig. 3–XIII–27). Surgical procedures may then be indicated such as arthrodesis or arthroplasty. Pickett states that

> . . . trauma sufficient to dislocate the hip may severely injure the articular cartilage, with the eventual occurrence of traumatic arthritis. These changes may be delayed for a number of years, and this presents a definite medical-legal complication, as a number of patients may develop severe disability sometime after the compensability of their injury has terminated.[125]

In almost 100 per cent of patients with central dislocations and fractures of the floor of the acetabulum, traumatic arthritis has developed.

Fractures of the Hip

Various classifications of hip fractures have been described by various authors. This has been done because treatment and prognosis depend upon how a hip is fractured. In general, intracapsular fractures produce less morbidity and fewer deaths than do extracapsular lesions, according to McLaughlin. He feels that the former lesions are splinted by the capsule. On the other hand, nonunion and avascular necrosis of the femoral head frequently complicate certain intracapsular frractures but are rarely seen in the extracapsular group. Extracapsular fractures include those involving the base of the femoral neck (within ligamentous attachments), as well as intertrochanteric and subtrochanteric lesions. These fractures cause little concern with regard to avascular necrosis and nonunion; however, the displaced fractures of this group produce severe systemic effects and a high mortality rate. In addition, McLaughlin notes, the unstable comminuted type often has a tendency toward varus rotation, resulting in significant shortening of the extremity. Displaced intertrochanteric fractures are serious injuries, unlike the simpler nondisplaced fractures. Soft-tissue trauma and bony comminution are the main reasons for this.[2] This is borne out by Boyd and Griffin's study of 300 trochanteric fractures. They found that the death rate the first three months after injury was 16.7 per cent, more than twice that for fractures of the femoral neck.[137]

Intracapsular Fractures. An early classification of intracapsular fractures was made by Pauwels.[138] He emphasized the importance of these categories insofar as the prognosis for union was concerned. Pauwel's type I was an impacted valgus fracture, his type II was a transcervical fracture, and type III he denoted as a vertical subcapital fracture (Fig. 3–XIII–28). Union decreases with the increase in the angle of incidence of the fracture line. An impacted valgus fracture heals much better than a type III vertical subcapital fracture.

Another classification for intracapsular frac-

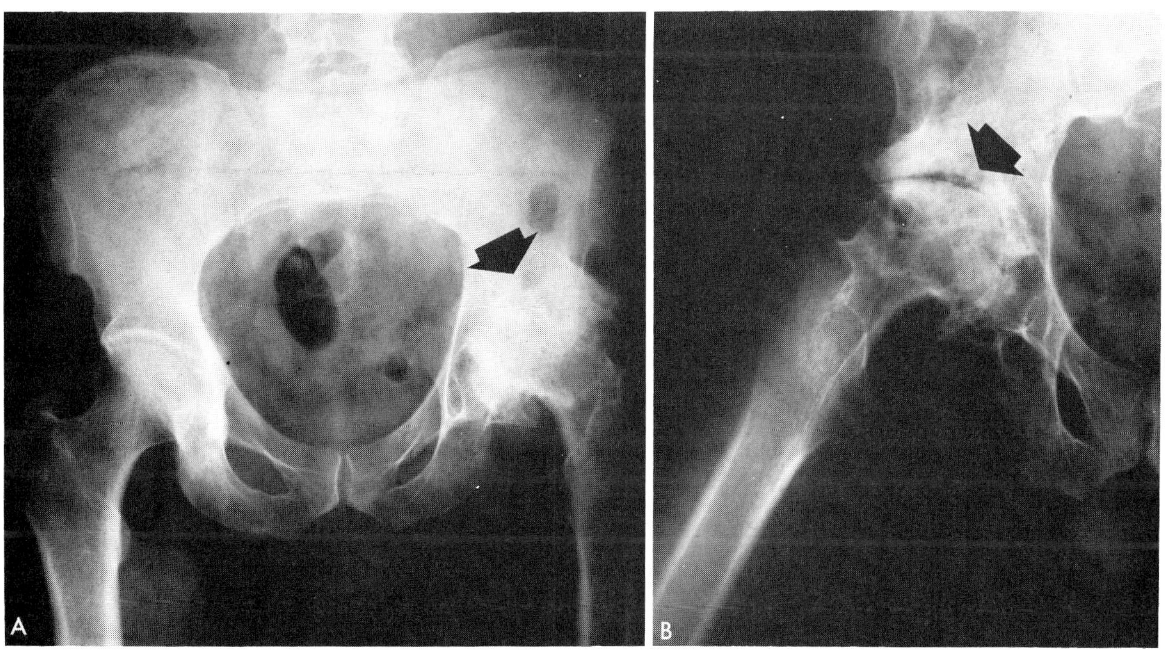

Figure 3–XIII–27. *A.* Severe posttraumatic arthritis of hip after dislocation, anterior view. *B.* Lateral view of same hip showing narrowed joint line.

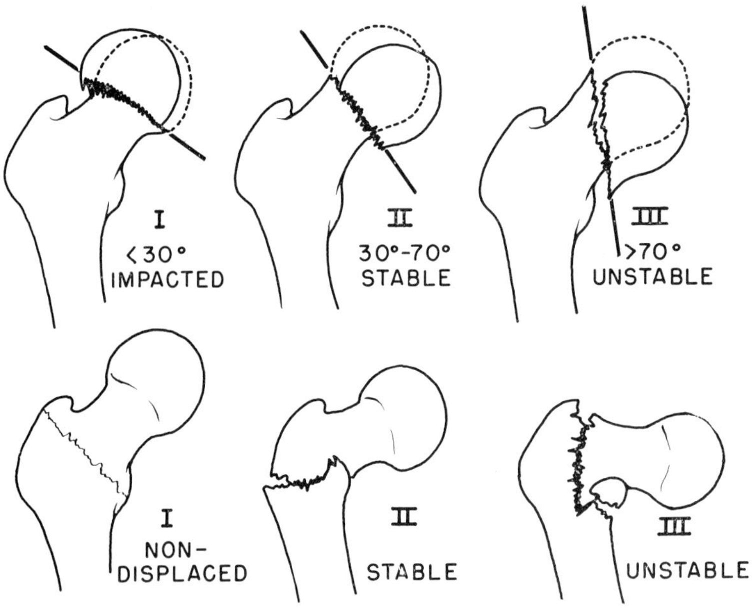

Figure 3–XIII–28. Classification of hip fracture. *Upper.* Intracapsular group (Pauwels' classification): type I, "impacted valgus" (10 per cent); type II, "transcervical" (25 per cent); type III, "vertical subcapital" (18 per cent). (Degrees indicate angle of incidence of fracture line.) *Lower.* Intertrochanteric group (McLaughlin classification): type I, "nondisplaced" (15 per cent); type II, "stable" (6 per cent); type III, "comminuted" (29 per cent). (From H. L. McLaughlin: *Trauma.* Philadelphia, W. B. Saunders Co., 1959. Reprinted by permission.)

tures, which the authors accept as a more realistic prognosticator of ultimate complications, is the classification described by Garden. In his system, Garden divides intracapsular fractures of the hip into four stages (Fig. 3–XIII–29). Stage 1 is an incomplete fracture. This basically is a greenstick fracture in a valgus position. Stage 2 is a complete fracture without displacement of the head from the neck. The line of the medial trabecular group is basically undisturbed. Stage 3 is complete fracture with partial displacement. The capital fragment is tilted into a varus position, and its medial trabeculae are out of line with their fellows in the pelvis. Stage 4 is a complete fracture with full displacement. The capital fragment has returned to its normal position in the acetabulum and its medial trabeculae are in line with the pelvic projections.[139] The reason the authors accept this as a better method of classification is that Garden takes into account not only the two-dimensional stresses exerted by weight-bearing on the head and neck, but also the rotatory and three-dimensional stresses that are exerted by external rotation of the distal fracture fragment. The important point in the differentiation between a stage 3 and a stage 4 fracture in the Garden classification is that in the stage 4 fracture the blood vessels contained in the ligament of Weitbrecht are disrupted. Thus, the blood supply to the femoral head is further compromised than it would be in stage 3. This may portend more serious late complications such as nonunion and avascular necrosis.

In young, vigorous adults an attempt should be made to restore normal anatomical relationships after a hip fracture. Multiple methods of internal fixation of intracapsular fractures exist. Prior to internal fixation, as nearly perfect an anatomical reduction as possible should be obtained. The blood supply to the femoral head is fragile, and less than anatomical reduction can result in nonunion and subsequent avascular necrosis of the femoral head. Resorption of the femoral neck can occur as well. On the other hand, in older persons one may want to reduce the hip into a slightly valgus position and impact it. Statistics have shown that the valgus-impacted fracture is less subject to avascular necrosis and is more stable to weight-bearing stresses. Too much valgus inclination, however, will compromise the blood supply to the femoral head and may result in avascular necrosis.[140]

Many types of apparatus have been designed for internal fixation of intracapsular fractures (Fig. 3–XIII–30). These include the Smith-Petersen nail, the Austin-Moore pin, the Knowles pin, the Hagie pin, the Henry screw, the Henderson lag screw, the Pugh sliding nail, the Massie sliding nail, the McLaughlin sliding nail, and the Deyerle pin apparatus as well as many others. The primary problems in intracapsular fractures are avascular necrosis of the femoral head and resorption of the femoral neck. Sir Astley Cooper in 1822 called the intracapsular fracture of the femur the "unsolved fracture," and it has been so denoted by many authors since. It remains thus. Many aspects of the "unsolved fracture" can, however, be solved by ac-

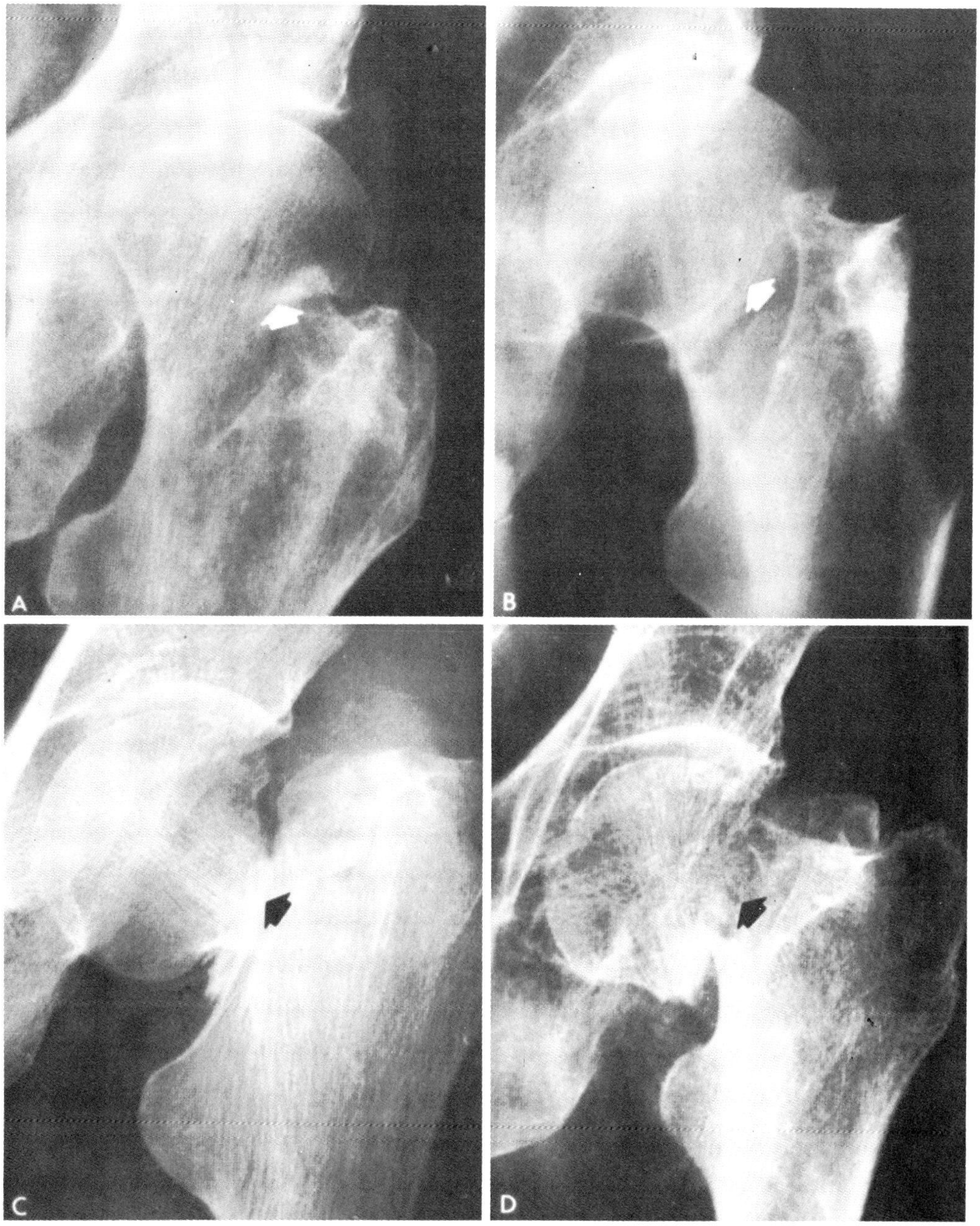

Figure 3–XIII–29. Garden classification of intracapsular fractures of the hip. *A.* Stage I: incomplete subcapital fracture. The "abducted" or "impacted" injury in which the fracture of the inferior cortical buttress is greenstick in nature, and a minimal degree of lateral rotation of the distal upon the proximal fragment creates the radiologic illusion of impaction. The medial lamellae of the internal weight-bearing system in the distal fragment lie in abduction as compared with those in the capital fragment, which is itself adducted. If unprotected, this fracture may at any time become complete. *B.* Stage II: complete subcapital fracture without displacement. The inferior cortical buttress has been broken, but no tilting of the capital fragment has taken place. As in the stage I fracture, the closely opposed fragments in this complete fracture may succumb to lateral rotation forces and show the classic displacement of "subcapital separation." *C.* Stage III: complete subcapital fracture with partial displacement. The two fragments retain their posterior retinacular attachment, and crushing of the posterior cervical cortex has not yet taken place. Lateral rotation of the distal fragment therefore tilts the capital fragment into abduction and medial rotation is shown radiologically by the direction of the medial weight-bearing lamellae in the femoral head. If the tendency for the limb to rotate laterally is not resisted by external or internal fixation, stripping of the retinacular attachment and crushing of the thin posterior cervical cortex will allow the full displacement of stage IV to occur. *D.* Stage IV: complete subcapital fracture with full displacement. This stage is reached when the retinacular hinge is detached from the posterior surface of the neck and collapse of the posterior cortical shell has taken place. The fragments are then divorced from each other, and the capital fragment at once returns to a more normal position in the acetabulum. Its medial weight-bearing lamellae are then seen radiologically to lie in alignment with their fellows in the pelvis. (From R. S. Garden: Low-angle fixation in fracture of the femoral neck. J. Bone Joint Surg., *43-B*:647, 1961. Reprinted by permission.)

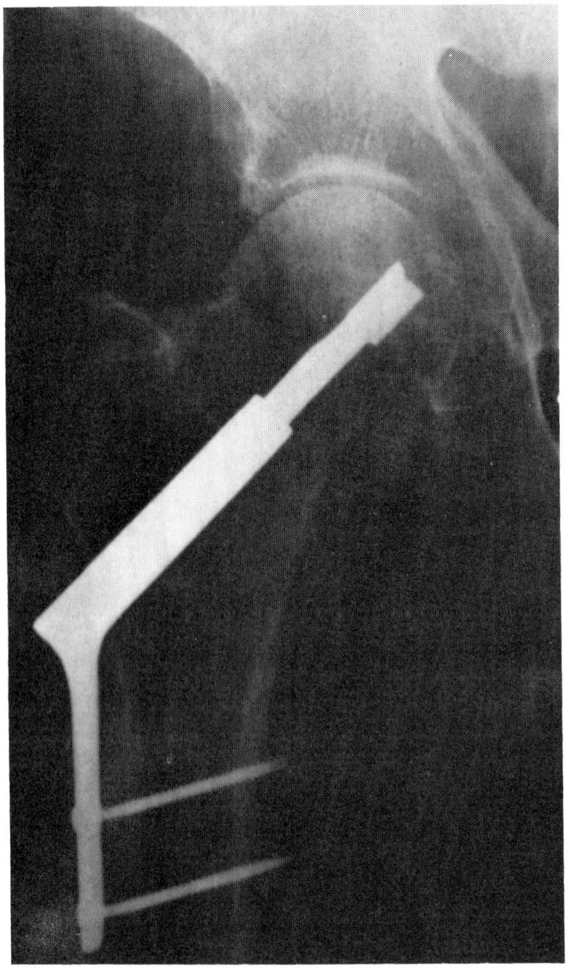

Figure 3–XIII–30. Internal fixation of intracapsular fracture of the hip with a sliding nail.

curate reduction, careful internal fixation, and closely supervised postoperative care.[141]

On the basis of concepts established by Judet and Garden, Meyers and associates have designed a new procedure to promote union in fractures of this type.[142,143] On the premise that a posterior wedge has been removed from the femoral neck, in this procedure an attempt is made to move a bone graft still attached to a muscle pedicle and place it in the posterior aspect of the femoral neck. The fracture is maintained in anatomical position by Hagie pins. The bone graft increases the incidence of union between the fracture fragments. In Meyers's hands this technique has met with approximately 89 per cent success in patients followed six months or more.

The use of a prosthesis, such as an Austin-Moore or a Thompson prosthesis, may be the procedure of choice when a fracture is more than one week old, is pathologic, or is so comminuted that adequate reduction and fixation is improbable.[144] Old age in itself is not an indication for its use. Hinchey and Day have reported satisfactory results in 84 per cent of their patients. Their indications were poor general health that contraindicated a second operation, Parkinson's disease, spastic hemiplegia, severe arthritis of the fractured hip, pathologic fractures, and the need to become ambulatory as soon as possible for reasons such as blindness and age over 70.[145] Another method of treatment that should be considered in the intracapsular fracture with concomitant serious degenerative joint disease is primary total hip replacement arthroplasty.[146] In the less common impacted valgus type of fracture, nonoperative management with frequent observation and radiologic examination is possible. Frequently, in well-chosen cases, nonoperative management of this fracture results in satisfactory union of the fragments.[147] Even in the best of hands, internally fixed intracapsular fractures that have been well reduced may fail to unite, or complications may develop. A salvage procedure such as prosthetic replacement is then indicated.

Extracapsular Fractures of the Hip. Basal fractures of the neck of the femur, intertrochanteric fractures, and subtrochanteric fractures occur through or outside the ligamentous attachments of the hip joint, and therefore the blood supply is good. Union can be expected provided the fracture is immobilized. Prior to the era of internal fixation, plaster immobilization and "well leg" traction were the methods used, and the results were good. Even now, there are situations in which conservative treatment is recommended, without the use of internal fixation. This would be when a fracture is minimally displaced or when a patient is too poor a risk for general anesthesia.

INTERTROCHANTERIC FRACTURES. Avascular necrosis and nonunion are of little concern in intertrochanteric fractures; however, displaced fractures of this group produce severe systemic effects and a high mortality rate. There is an overwhelming tendency toward varus rotation in the unstable comminuted type, resulting in significant shortening of the extremity. McLaughlin classifies intertrochanteric fractures as type I, nondisplaced; type II, stable; and type III, comminuted and unstable.[2] Massie uses the same classification for intertrochanteric fractures.[148] Boyd and Griffin in 1949 proposed another method of classification in which intertrochanteric fractures and subtrochanteric fractures are included (Fig. 3–XIII–31).[49] Evans in his classification of intertrochan-

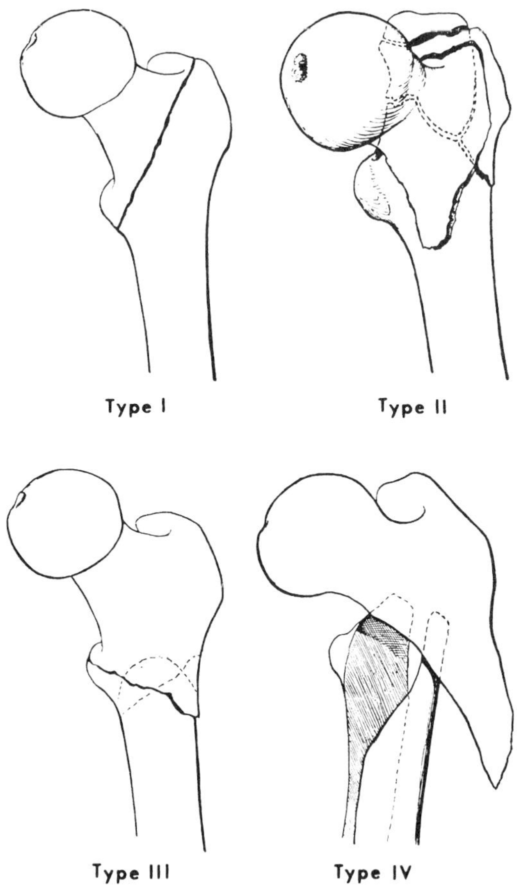

Figure 3–XIII–31. Boyd and Griffin's classification of intertrochanteric fractures of the hip. Type I designates fractures showing a more or less linear break extending along the general direction of the intertrochanteric line from greater to lesser trochanter. In this group reduction is usually simple and maintained with the least difficulty. Type II designates fractures that are comminuted, with the main line of fracture being along the intertrochanteric line but with multiple breaks occurring in the cortex. Reduction here is more difficult. Type III designates fractures that are essentially subtrochanteric, with at least one fracture line passing across the upper end of the shaft just below or in the region of the lesser trochanter. Various degrees of comminution may be associated with this type. The features seen in either type I or type II may be present in addition to the subtrochanteric fracture. Type III fractures are generally much more difficult to reduce and to maintain in reduction than either of the first two types. Type IV designates comminuted fractures that extend through the trochanteric region and usually on into the shaft, with fracture lines in at least two planes. In the event that open reduction and internal fixation are employed, these fractures require two-plane fixation. (From H. B. Boyd and L. L. Griffin: Classification and treatment of trochanteric fracture. Arch. Surg., *58*:853–866, June 1949. Copyright 1949, American Medical Association. Reprinted by permission.)

teric fractures found that 72 per cent were stable and 28 per cent were unstable (Fig. 3–XIII–32). His definition states that if the medial cortical buttress is intact, undisplaced, or restored by reduction the fracture is stable and the result inevitably good. The fracture is considered to be unstable when there is cortical overlap that is not corrected or destruction that cannot be restored.[150] Banks has pointed out additional factors of instability such as posterior comminution, iatrogenic fractures, metallic failure, and the possibility of telescoping of the proximal into the distal fragment.[151] There have been many internal fixation devices used for treatment of intertrochanteric fractures. These include the hardware recommended by Smith-Petersen, McLaughlin, Jewett, Massie, Holt, Sarmiento, and others (Fig. 3–XIII–33).[152-154] Dimon and Hughston have popularized the displacement osteotomy in unstable intertrochanteric fractures and report far more satisfactory results than with other types of treatment (Fig. 3–XIII–34).[155, 156] Harrington has used a sliding compression screw fixation device for unstable intertrochanteric fractures with good results.[157] He and his co-author, Johnston, agree with Dimon and Hughston that the stability at the fracture site should be gained by inserting the cortical spike of the proximal fragment within the medullary canal of the distal fragment. They also believe that the Harrington-Johnston device extends this principle logically by fixing the displaced fracture fragments with a device that maintains their alignment, yet encourages their physiologic impaction. Various authors have differing opinions as to when weight-bearing should occur. Holt recommends early weight-bearing in noncomminuted intertrochanteric fractures when his device is used.[153] Sarmiento allows for early weight-bearing when the fracture has been anatomically reduced, especially in the medial cortical buttress area.[154] There is, however, a limit to the usefulness of these ingenious devices. They do not replace bone, but only support it. Delayed weight-bearing is advisable when there is doubt as to the stability of fractures fixed internally. It is often better to be cautious and wait until there is clinical and radiologic evidence of healing before weight-bearing is attempted. Again, as stated previously, a decision such as this is the surgeon's, as he is most familiar with the individual patient and with the individual patient's fracture.

In intertrochanteric fractures, shortening may be one of the permanent residual effects. This occurs more often in severely comminuted unstable fractures, in osteoporotic older individuals, and when medial displacement osteotomies have been performed to restore stability.

SUBTROCHANTERIC FRACTURES. According to McLaughlin approximately 10 per cent trochanteric lesions are subtrochanteric fractures,

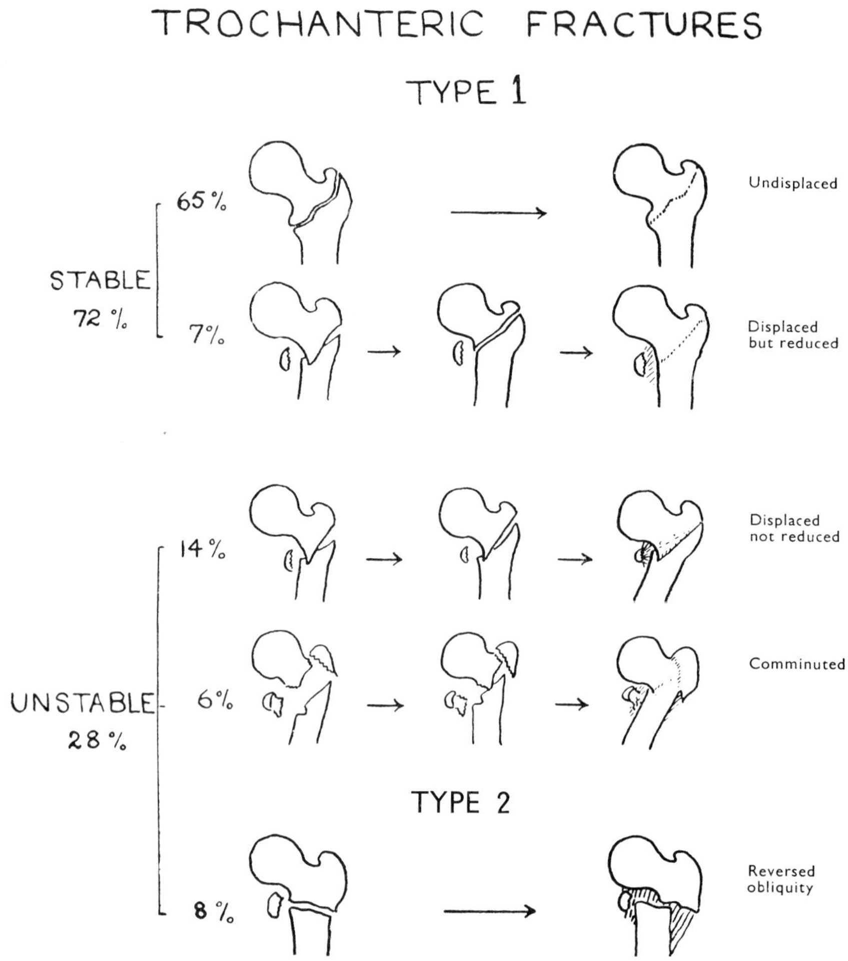

Figure 3–XIII–32. Evans classification of intertrochanteric fracture. (From E. M. Evans: Treatment of trochanteric fractures of femur. J. Bone Joint Surg., *31-B*:190, 1949. Reprinted by permission.)

and these result from severe trauma.[2] The patients are often active individuals from a younger age group, and the fracture is usually comminuted. The abductors, flexors, and external rotators of the hip act upon the proximal fragment, while the shaft is displaced upward and inward by the adductors. Interposition of soft parts occurs frequently, warranting open reduction. Poor immobilization or improper alignment of the fragments will lead to nonunion. Internal fixation is the favored method of treatment in adults. Secure internal fixation is often impossible to obtain because of comminution, however, and skeletal traction is often the treatment of choice in severely comminuted subtrochanteric fractures. A plaster hip spica cast has been used as treatment, but this of course has the disadvantage of keeping the patient immobilized. This leads to disuse atrophy of the muscles and disuse osteoporosis.

High subtrochanteric fractures are frequently fixed with a nail and long side plate, or with a blade-plate fixation device, as described by DePalma.[4] Intramedullary rod fixation has been recommended for subtrochanteric fractures that are more distal. Because standard nail-plate devices have not always been successful in the treatment of fractures of the proximal third of the shaft of the femur, Zickel has devised a new method (Fig. 3–XIII–35). Nail-plate combinations have often been inadequate for treatment of subtrochanteric fractures because of bending and breaking of plates or nails, loosening of screws, and medial migration of the femoral shaft. Postoperative traction was often necessary until the fracture healed. Although intramedullary rods are successful in low transverse fractures, they permit varus angulation in the higher subtrochanteric fractures because of inadequate fixation of the proximal fragment. Zickel's new device obtains an adequate anchor in both the proximal and

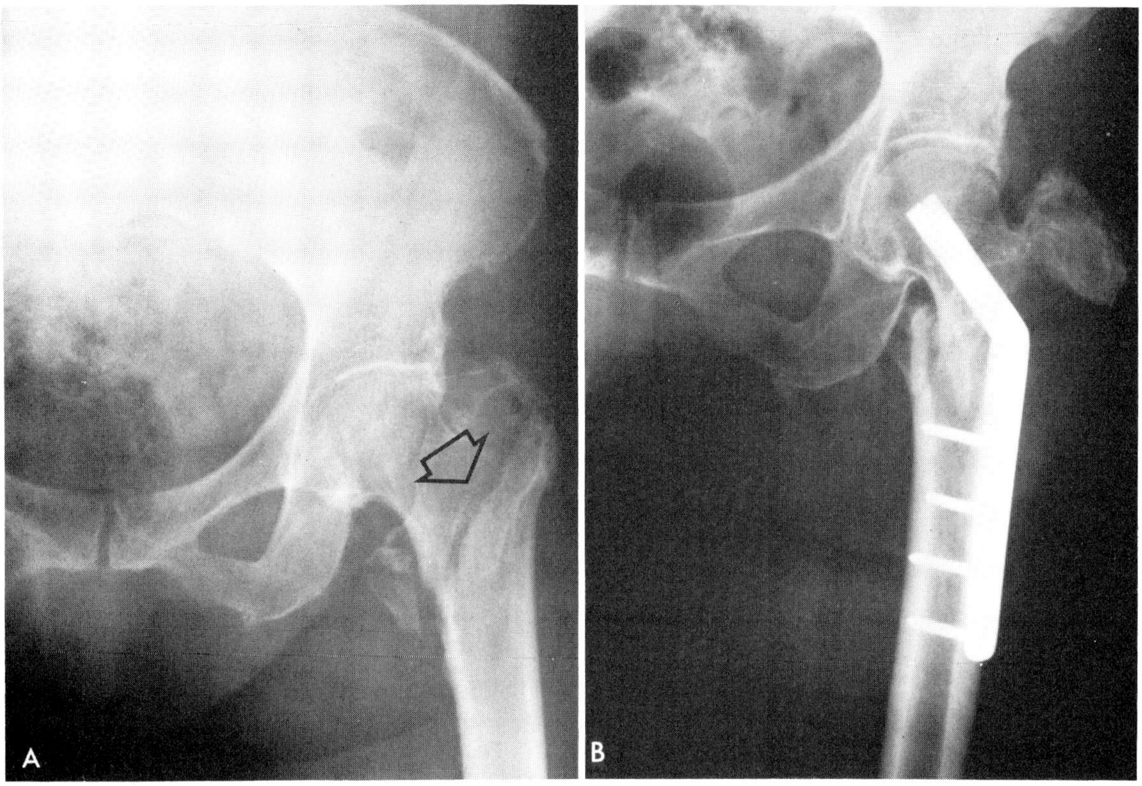

Figure 3–XIII–33. *A.* Comminuted intertrochanteric fracture of the hip. *B.* After medial displacement osteotomy with Jewett nail-plate fixation.

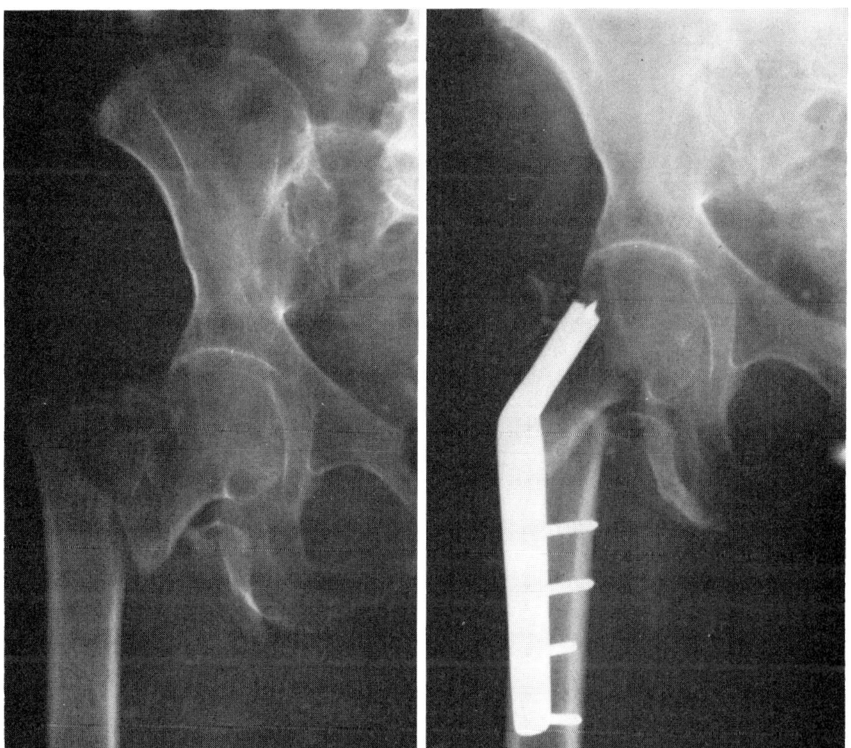

Figure 3–XIII–34. *A.* Markedly comminuted and displaced intertrochanteric fracture of hip. *B.* After medial displacement osteotomy with Jewett nail-plate fixation, with "cutting out" of nail from femoral head and neck superiorly.

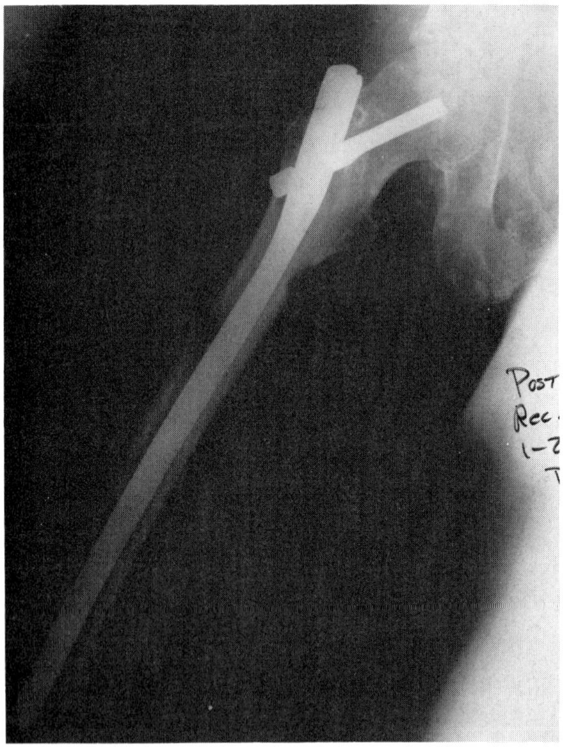

Figure 3–XIII–35. Zickel nail fixation in patient with subtrochanteric lytic areas from breast carcinoma metastases. (Courtesy of Dr. Malcolm Meyn, New England Medical Center.)

distal fragments of the femur. Immobilization is stronger than with conventional appliances. Patients with comminuted fractures are frequently permitted early ambulation because angulation and rotation of the fragments are controlled by the device.[158]

Uncomplicated subtrochanteric fractures generally heal well with little resultant disability.[3]

FRACTURES OF THE GREATER TROCHANTER. Generally fractures of the greater trochanter occur as a result of a direct blow on the subcutaneous bony prominence. Occasionally, however, the trochanter may be avulsed by the strong action of the hip abductor musculature. In children the separation will then occur through the epiphyseal line. Those fractures with minimal displacement can usually be treated nonoperatively with excellent return of function. If the fragment is severely displaced, operative intervention may be indicated.[4] Disability, if any, from this type of injury is minimal.

FRACTURES OF THE LESSER TROCHANTER. Avulsion of the lesser trochanter is seen in the adolescent athlete in whom the epiphysis of the lesser trochanter has not yet united with the shaft. Even if the avulsion is complete, surgical repair is rarely indicated. The trochanter reattaches by fibrous union and usually is not painful. If a painful union does occur, the attachment may be transferred to the anterior femur. Duration of protective treatment depends upon the symptoms. A patient's athletic activity should be terminated for several weeks until he is symptom-free. Otherwise, any effort to run or jump can cause excessive strain on the iliopsoas tendon, with resultant pain.[75] Dimon suggests that normal activities be resumed within 12 weeks after an isolated fracture of the lesser trochanter.[159]

Disability following severe injuries about the hip are manifest chiefly by pain, stiffness, and limp, which may be due to a variety of problems such as shortening of the extremity or muscle weakness. Because the hip is a major weight-bearing joint, derangements and disability about the hip may lead to subsequent problems in other weight-bearing joints owing to the mechanics of the gait. These may include difficulties with the lumbosacral spine, the knee, or the foot-ankle mechanism. Pain may be due to degenerative arthritis or to the subsequent formation and inflammation of bursae over bony prominences or prominent hardware. Localized pain about the hip may require treatment by secondary reconstructive measures. In deformity and disability of long duration that has subsequently influenced other weight-bearing joints, the disability may be severe indeed, and major surgery with significant morbidity and mortality rates may be necessary to alleviate the patient's pain and suffering.

The Thigh

Soft-Tissue Injuries

Thigh contusions occur frequently in contact sports such as football. Some degree of hematoma is probably present in any contusion of muscle, although the bleeding may be more in the nature of infiltration in the muscle than of pooled blood.[75] Zadek reports a case of an ossifying hematoma in the thigh. The terms "ossifying fibroma" and "myositis ossificans" have been used interchangeably in the literature, causing considerable confusion. Zadek feels that "ossifying hematoma" is appropriate only for oval masses of bone not attached to the skeleton developing in a previously traumatized area, as in the case he reported.[160] In myositis ossificans, the aberrant bone is usually adjacent to or actually attached to a nearby bone. It is usual practice to excise an area of myositis ossificans or ossifying hematoma only after the lesion has matured. The lesion may resolve spontaneously.[161]

A heavy blow to the front of the thigh while the quadriceps is tense often produces rupture of many muscle fibers over a poorly circumscribed area. Large, well-localized hematomas should be aspirated if seen within 36 hours after the injury, according to McLaughlin.[2] Rest and a compression dressing are recommended as well as relative immobilization. Frequently the hematoma organizes and is replaced by scar. Often it liquefies and remains entrapped within fascial planes, requiring subsequent aspirations. This is often inadequate, however, as a new seroma may replace the old one in the compressed space. A gross injury of this type may produce a massive muscle belly rupture. Operative repair is unwarranted except when the disruption has occurred at the musculotendinous junction of the quadriceps mechanism. It is usually impossible to suture muscle to muscle adequately – like suturing the torn ends of a paint brush. After thigh muscle rupture, there is occasionally persistent pain that remains. O'Donoghue cites a case in which careful surgical removal of the detached portion of the muscle relieved the pain caused by entrapment of a neurovascular bundle. The patient's symptoms were caused by traction on the nerve in the neurovascular bundle as the semitendinosus muscle contracted. O'Donoghue also cites a similar occurrence involving the adductor longus.[75]

Fascial hernia in the thigh is uncommon. It usually occurs along the anterolateral aspect of the thigh where the fascia becomes thinner anterior to the iliotibial band. Treatment is seldom necessary because pain is minimal. In severe cases, repair of the rent is recommended if the edges are well defined and reparable. If repair of the defect is impossible, O'Donoghue recommends enlarging the slit to a length of 3 or 4 inches.[75] This condition is ordinarily not disabling, and treatment can usually be postponed until a convenient time.

The lateral femoral cutaneous nerve of the thigh on occasion becomes entrapped where it emerges from under the lateral aspect of the inguinal ligament. This entrapment neuropathy may be initiated by direct trauma to the region or fracture of the anterior portion of the ilium. The symptoms are those of burning pain and paresthesia over the lateral aspect of the thigh. The diagnosis may be confirmed by infiltration of the nerve at its emergence from under the inguinal ligament with subsequent relief of symptoms. If conservative treatment does not relieve the symptoms, operative intervention may be necessary. There are two operative procedures for treatment of this condition. The first is neurolysis and the second is resection of the nerve. Following resection of the nerve there is mild disability from numbness over the anterolateral aspect of the thigh.

Fractures of the Femoral Shaft

According to McLaughlin, "the inevitable penalty of a fractured adult femur is stiffness of the knee."[2] This is because of the fibrous adhesions that form an inelastic checkrein between the femur and the patella. One can, however, sustain a fracture of the femur and have excellent healing without subsequent disability of the knee. Nevertheless, treatment of fractures of the adult femur should be planned to preserve as much knee joint mobility as possible. The more distal the fracture, the more likely is the patient to have knee stiffness. Union almost always occurs, if the fracture is adequately treated, unless the process of repair is overwhelmed by tissue destruction, infection, or distraction of the bone fragments. It is essential to neutralize the strong muscle forces influencing the fracture in order to obtain complete union.

Some of the earlier methods for treatment of femoral shaft fractures included the application of a plaster spica cast for undisplaced fractures; reduction by several different methods of traction for comminuted, multiple, moderately displaced, and certain oblique fractures; skeletal traction; and the use of the Hoke traction apparatus. These methods are nonsurgical choices for the treatment of fractures of the femur in those cases that can effectively be treated in such fashion. Other types of displaced, open or unstable spiral and oblique fractures may require open reduction and internal fixation. There are several methods used for internal fixation of bone fragments. These include metal screws, Roger Anderson pins, plates and screws, intramedullary rods, and other mechanical methods for obtaining stabilization.[16]

Holm and Embick treated and studied 110 cases, concluding that traction-suspension is indispensable in the overall management of fractures of the femur, and yet it is the most neglected and poorly understood treatment modality.[162] The usefulness of Russell traction in the treatment of comminuted and spiral fractures of the femur was reemphasized by

Anderson. He studied 39 fractures in children and 59 in adults, all treated without surgery and, for the most part, by Russell traction. The disadvantages inherent in the method were longer hospitalization, slow ambulation, and sometimes inadequate reduction. There were, however, no infections, negligible mortality rates, and infrequent delayed union.[163] Another form of nonoperative treatment was postulated by Kaufer in 1972. He used a walking hip spica cast in treatment of 60 patients who had fractures of the shaft of the femur. The infection rate was only 3.3 per cent, and the rate of other significant complications did not rise above 5 per cent. He postulated that this method allowed the patient to have a shorter hospitalization, while yielding results comparable to others published in reports of nonoperative as well as operative treatment.[164] Traction is well tolerated in the younger patients according to Martyn and McGoey. Unable to find any significant difference in the end-results obtained from traction or operative treatment, except for the longer hospital stay when traction was used, they suggested that the intramedullary fixation method may not stand critical scrutiny in peacetime civilian practice.[164] It must be noted, however, that Küntscher never advocated opening of the fracture site.[166] This is common practice with many surgeons in the United States today and may account for the higher rate of infection they encounter. In Küntscher's hands, blind nailing with x-ray control produced an infection rate significantly less than that found in the United States today. Many British parachutists who sustained fractures of the femur in World War II were treated by the Küntscher rod. They awakened from anesthesia and were surprised at being able to walk the following day. Schneider and other authors feel that closed intramedullary nailing is the method of choice when internal fixation is indicated in selected fractures of the shaft of long bones, particularly midshaft femoral fractures.[167]

Dencker compared results of various methods of treatment in 1,003 cases comprising fractures treated by medullary nailing, traction, encircling wire, and plate fixation. Of seven who died, four patients had been treated with medullary nailing, two with medullary pins, and one with a plate. Nonunion was more common following encircling wire fixation (8 per cent). Dencker expressed the view that skeletal traction should be the standard method of treatment for both closed and open fractures of the femoral shaft, no matter what the patient's age, the type of fracture, or the level of fracture, unless special circumstances call for the use of another method.[168] According to Smith, the optimal time for definitive operation, from many points of view, is between the tenth and fourteenth day following injury. This is because blood loss from a femoral shaft fracture is often severe, and delayed operation gives time for the vascular system to stabilize. Also, patients with femoral shaft fractures often have other severe injuries that require attention first. In situations in which the femoral shaft fracture is the only injury, definitive operation on the day of injury is suggested.[169]

Compression plating has been recommended by the Swiss. Experience with 14 closed fractures treated with the compression plate of the Association for the Study of Problems of Internal Fixation is reported by Gant, Shaftan, and Herbsman. Three instances of double plate breakage and one of plate disruption, screw breakage, and fracture angulation occurred. The authors recommended that the method be reserved for cooperative patients whose fractures cannot otherwise be treated.[170]

Nichols studied 181 patients who had been treated by various methods. He determined the duration of disability in each of these patients and showed that with early medullary nailing the average duration of disability was 26 weeks; with skeletal traction, 38 weeks; with closed reduction with plaster fixation, 40 weeks; with skin traction, 42 weeks; and after compression plating, 42 weeks. He also determined the percentage of knees regaining range of motion of 90 degrees or more and showed that with skin traction, 41 per cent regained this range of motion; while with skeletal traction, 51 per cent gained it; with plating, 53 per cent gained it; and with early medullary nailing, 78 per cent gained it. When he evaluated the percentage of these patients with shortening, he showed that with early medullary nailing, 20 per cent showed shortening, whereas only 17 per cent showed it with the delayed intramedullary nailing. With skin traction, 55 per cent showed shortening, and with skeletal traction, 53 per cent showed shortening. The incidence of adherence of the quadriceps was greatest in open reduction and plating with 27 per cent; while with intramedullary nailing it was 7 per cent; with skin traction, 5 per cent; and with skeletal traction, 3 per cent.[171]

Various articles have been written on vascular complications of femoral shaft fractures treated in an open manner.[172-174] Stabilization of the fracture is an absolute prerequisite to repair of arterial injury occurring with these fractures.

Functional cast-bracing as described by Mooney and associates, by Sarmiento, and by

Mital has evolved as a popular treatment of femoral shaft fractures (Fig. 3–XIII–36). In general, the incidence of complications and the length of disability are less if this method is used. Mital, who has treated femoral fractures from the level of the lesser trochanter to the level of the knee, shows an average healing time of approximately 10 weeks. He also has found that when patients come out of a cast-brace, they have 80 to 90 degrees of knee flexion. This is very significant because, as stated frequently in the literature, one of the greatest complications of a femoral shaft fracture is stiffness of the knee.[175–179]

Supracondylar Fractures of the Femur

A purely supracondylar fracture of the adult femur is uncommon, for the force required to break the massive lower end of this bone is so great that the condyles also are apt to be shattered or split apart. There is massive soft-tissue damage frequently accompanied by hemarthrosis. Posteriorly displaced fragments may damage the neurovascular structures in the popliteal space. Closed methods of treatment are preferred to open methods except when closed methods fail. Closed methods include skeletal traction with or without subsequent cast-bracing. There have been multiple methods of open reduction described, and a plethora of hardware exists for this (Fig. 3–XIII–37).[4]

In an important study of supracondylar fractures of the adult femur, Neer and associates selected 110 fractures for analysis. In treatment of these fractures a variety of techniques were used. They included blade-plate fixation, Rush

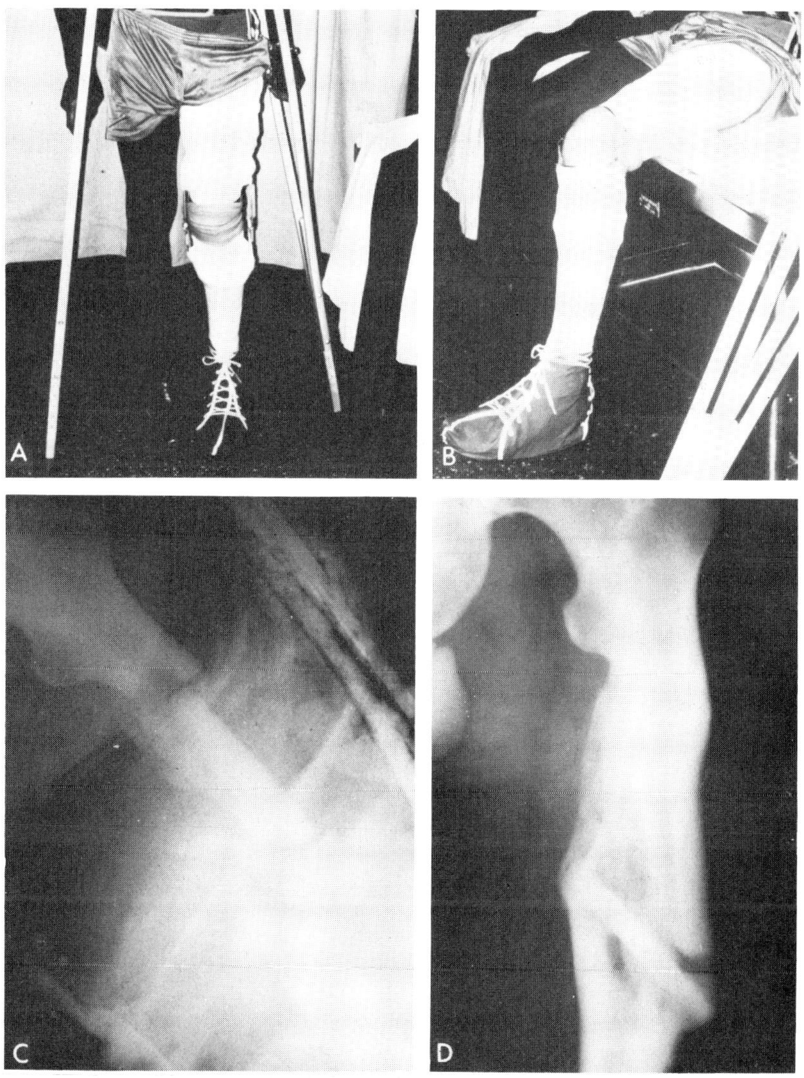

Figure 3–XIII–36. Cast-bracing for markedly comminuted and displaced subtrochanteric and mid-shaft fractures of the femur. *A*. The involved leg in extension. *B*. The leg in flexion at the knee and hip. *C*. The fracture immediately after application of the cast-brace. *D*. After the cast-brace has been removed and healing has occurred. (Courtesy of Dr. Mohinder Mital.)

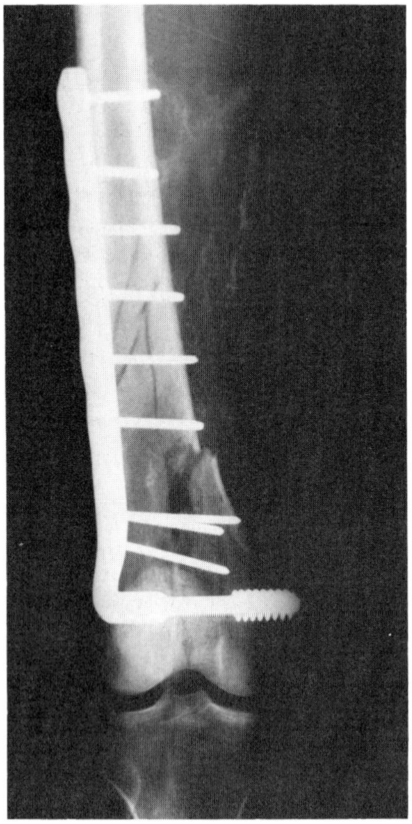

Figure 3–XIII–37. Comminuted fracture of distal femur with Richards supracondylar fixation apparatus.

nails, plates and bolts, and various combinations of bolts and screws. Many patients were also treated with traction and a plaster cast. Because of the variety of fractures, an artificial classification was drawn up to subdivide the types of fractures found in this series. The subdivisions were: fractures with minimal displacement, fractures with medial displacement of the condyle, fractures with lateral displacement of the condyles, and conjoint supracondylar and shaft fractures. The classification usually indicated the degree of trauma causing the fracture that the patient had sustained. This indirectly affected treatment and duration of hospitalization. The most common complications of treatment were varus deformity and internal rotation deformity. It should be noted that there were some instances in which vascular injuries sustained at the time of fracture necessitated amputation of the extremity distal to the fracture. The long-term results in patients treated by internal fixation were compared with those in patients treated by closed methods. Neer stated that no category of fractures appeared particularly well suited for internal fixation, and the fixation that was obtained rarely accomplished the goal of eliminating the need for external support or shortening convalescence. Most serious local complications occurred after open fixation. Of 29 patients so treated and evaluated, only 52 per cent had results that were rated satisfactory. Satisfactory results were obtained in 90 per cent of the 48 patients treated by closed methods, and in 84 per cent of those with supracondylar fractures that were displaced. It was Neer's thinking that replacement of irreducible segments of closed fractures could better be performed in traction after the initial reaction to injury had subsided. Perfect anatomical apposition of the fragments was rarely obtained and was not necessary for satisfactory results as long as articular congruity was present and rotation and angulation had been corrected within 5 degrees of normal.[180]

It is interesting to note that in a survey article by Riggins and co-workers in which 702 board-certified orthopedic surgeons selected at random answered a mail questionnaire concerning their preference of treatment for a specific closed supracondylar fracture of the femur, he showed that skeletal traction using a tibial pin for 8 weeks with weight-bearing beginning at 13 weeks was the preferred method of treatment.[181]

Disabilities following supracondylar fractures of the femur are joint stiffness and malunion, which impose abnormal stresses on the knee and lead to subsequent deterioration of that joint.

The Knee

Injuries of the Extensor Apparatus

The quadriceps extensor mechanism is the heart of good knee joint function. Knee joint stability depends upon it. Each of the four muscles that compose the quadriceps mechanism has an individual function. Together, they act as a synchronized unit to produce extension and stability of the knee. The quadriceps extensor mechanism can be injured by: (1) avulsion of the rectus femoris from or with the anteroinferior spine of the ilium, (2) rupture (usually incomplete) through the quadriceps muscle belly, (3) rupture through or avulsion of the quadriceps tendon from the upper pole of the patella, (4) rupture through or avulsion of the patellar tendon from the lower pole of the patella, (5) rupture through the patella, or (6) avulsion of the tibial tubercle.[2]

A common occurrence in athletes is rupture of a few fibers of the quadriceps, usually of the rectus femoris. Smillie feels that so-called "pulled muscles" are really nothing more than small intramuscular hemorrhages from ruptured veins, particularly when the injury is direct.[182] The physical disability is insignificant in ruptures of the rectus femoris. Operation is recommended only on cosmetic grounds. Repair of the rupture is technically difficult and likely to prove unsatisfactory, for it does not improve function. Injuries to the *vastus medialis*, when small, produce no ill effects whatsoever. These injuries are often not diagnosed. Injury to the muscle alone usually requires no treatment. When there is dysfunction of the vastus medialis, however, it is usually the result of a gross injury such as acute traumatic dislocation of the patella and usually requires operative intervention. *Vastus intermedius* injury also is usually sustained from a direct blow. It is this particular component of the quadriceps in which myositis ossificans may occur. The *vastus lateralis* is seldom subject to injury, as it is protected by the powerful iliotibial band. An iatrogenic difficulty that can occur is herniation through the vastus lateralis of the underlying musculature after a strip of fascia lata has been used for reconstructive procedures.

Avulsion of the Quadriceps from the Patella. Avulsion of the quadriceps muscles from the patella is an injury that occurs in patients past middle age or patients who are overweight; in younger age groups, injury in this area is usually a transverse fracture of the patella or avulsion of the patellar ligament. This fact is borne out by Ramsey and Muller in their evaluation of 17 patients with quadriceps tendon rupture in which they showed that 6 of the 17 patients were in the seventh decade of life. Quadriceps avulsion from the patella is sustained when the whole body weight is transmitted through the flexing knee, and the patient, in attempting to avoid a fall, contracts the quadriceps violently and tears the muscle from its attachment to the superior pole. This has been classified as a diagnostic trap by Ramsey and Muller, who noted that although the quadriceps may be ruptured, if examination is not done carefully, the knee may appear normal. For example, a quadriceps rupture may occur without knee swelling and with full ligament stability. Therefore unless the knee is tested for its active ability to extend, this injury may be misdiagnosed as a sprain.[183] Underlying diseases such as myxedema, rheumatoid arthritis, and gout can predispose to rupture of the quadriceps tendon. Bilateral spontaneous and simultaneous rupture of the quadriceps tendons have been reported.[184]

DePalma advocates immediate operative repair in all instances of avulsion of the quadriceps tendon from the patella. Turek, Campbell, and most other authors agree. L. D. Anderson in *Campbell's Operative Orthopaedics* notes that although stability is improved and a practical range of knee motion is regained when late ruptures are repaired, a full forceful extension is rarely restored. Old neglected cases exhibit a typical deformity of the knee joint in which the retracted distal end of the quadriceps muscle is prominent and a sulcus exists between the end of the quadriceps and the upper margin of the patella. The sulcus becomes more pronounced with contraction of the quadriceps.[1]

Avulsion of Patellar Tendon. Avulsion of the patellar tendon from the patella generally occurs in young patients participating in athletics. Frequently, when the tendon is torn from the lower pole of the patella, a small segment of bone is avulsed. Occasionally old cases are encountered in which there is marked shortening of the quadriceps muscle and formation of heterotopic bone in the interval between the patella and the tibial tubercle. Avulsion of the patellar tendon from the patella is caused by the same mechanism that injures any of the components of the extensor apparatus. The injury occurs at any point in the apparatus where it is weakest or the stress is greatest. "The weakest link of this chain may be at any point along this complicated mechanism at any given moment."[75] Nonoperative repair or delayed repair of this tendon meets with the same diminution of function as does the delayed treatment of an old rupture of the quadriceps tendon. For this reason and for best results, surgical intervention is recommended.

Fractures of the Patella. A transverse or avulsion fracture of the patella is a rupture of the quadriceps extensor mechanism. The bone fractures because it is weaker than the quadriceps and patellar tendon. The vastus tendons may escape injury, or may be ruptured by horizontal extensions of the patellar tear.

The patella should not be indiscriminately removed, as it plays an important role in the mechanical function of the knee joint. Previously it was erroneously suggested that the patella was inherited phylogenetically and was not a truly functional organ.[185] The patella protects the anterior aspect of the knee joint by increasing the strength of the quadriceps muscle. Permanent deformity of the joint occurs when it is lost. Fractures of the patella resulting from direct violence usually exhibit only minimal displacement of fragments, and the patellar retinaculum remains intact. Fractures resulting from indirect force are usually associated with rupture of the medial and lateral retinacula and separation of the fragments (Fig. 3–XIII–38).[4] Treatment of the fractured patella should provide relief from pain and protection against reinjury. Maintenance of function is also necessary. It is often sufficient to use a cylindrical plaster cast alone, but open reduction is often necessary when the fracture is transverse. Open reduction is indicated when there is obvious marked disruption of the patellar expansion.

McMaster disagrees with a number of writers who state that in falls on the knee the force is not taken on the patella but rather on the tibial tubercle. He examined a number of people, both children and adults, and found that almost invariably in the falling-kneeling position, the patella, not the tibial tubercle, was in direct contact with the ground. He reasoned that the toes and the forefoot on the ground cause the knee to be flexed at more than a right angle, thus placing the patella in the most vulnerable position. The tibial tubercle would strike the ground first and take the blow if the foot hung over a ledge in the fall, in which position the knee would be in essentially a right-angle position with the leg parallel with the ground.[186] Falls on the knee are a definite cause of fracture of the patella by direct force. Fractures produced by indirect force are usually transverse and may be somewhat comminuted. These may be centrally located, but are more often near the lower pole and occasionally near the upper pole. Quadriceps muscle pull causes separation of the fragments.

Smillie contends that treatment of a fractured patella should be early, especially if an operation is selected. The earlier the open procedure is performed, the more rapid the recovery and the better the end-result in terms of return of flexion.[182] When reconstitution of patellar fragments is the treatment of choice, care should be taken to get anatomical reduction, as steppage in the articular surface of the patella predisposes to patellofemoral arthritis. This will eventually lead to varying degrees of knee dysfunction. Quite frequently partial excision of the patella may be indicated in fractures involving the upper or the lower poles of the patella, but total excision should be re-

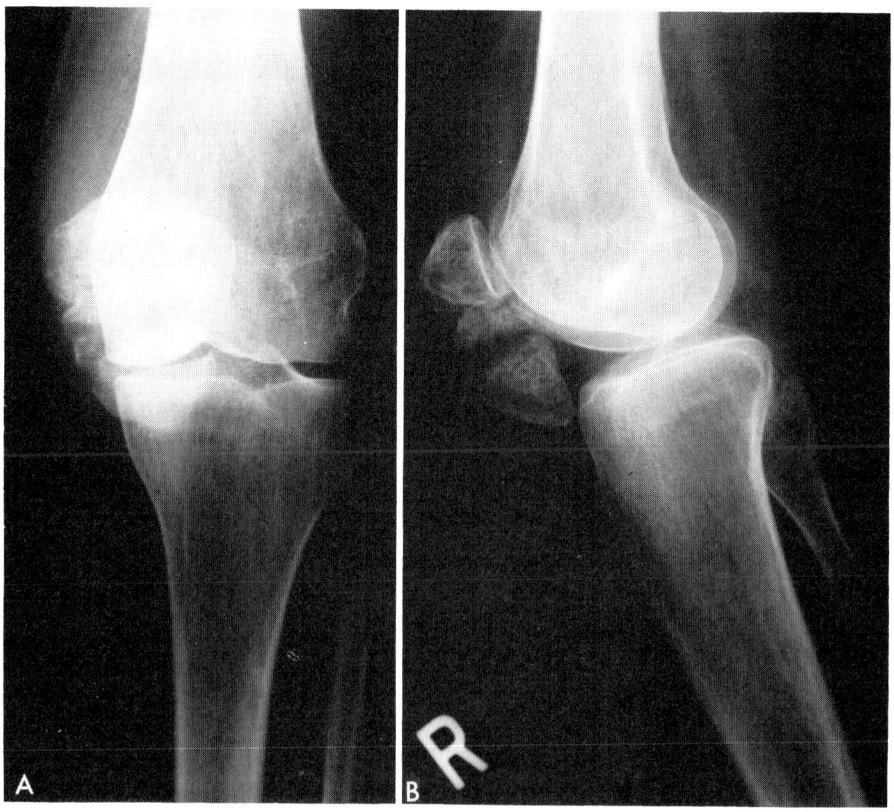

Figure 3–XIII–38. Comminuted fracture of the patella. *A.* Anterior view. *B.* Lateral view.

served for those cases in which comminution is excessive, in which compounding is severe, or in which infection of the bone is imminent or already present.[187] Quadriceps exercises started soon after surgery will help maintain muscle tone and prevent adhesions and stiffness. Some residual limitation in flexion is more apt to result than limitation of complete extension. O'Donoghue and associates, in a study of 34 patellectomies, confirmed the impression of another author that the strength of extension of the knee rarely approaches normal after patellectomy. The patients in his series had an average of 71 per cent of normal extensor strength.[188] West reviewed 83 patellectomies in 74 patients a considerable time after surgery and showed the result to be good or excellent in 82 per cent of the patients despite some quadriceps atrophy.[189] They both noted that poor results were most frequent when an adequate program of rehabilitation could not be carried out because of factors such as mental retardation, associated fractures, or lack of physical therapy. West pointed out there was no increase in arthritic changes of the femoral condyles after patellectomy.

Osteochondral fracture of the patella may be one source of *loose bodies* in the knee joint. According to DePalma, it results from forceful contraction of the quadriceps following subluxation or dislocation of the patella with engagement of the medial border of the patella under the edge of the lateral femoral condyle; the trapped portion of the articular surface is sheared off the main body of the patella. Excision of the loose body is recommended. Marginal fractures of the patella result from direct violence to the margin of the patella, which shears away a fragment of its periphery. Displacement is minimal. The retinacula of the quadriceps are intact. An osteochondral fracture should be distinguished from congenital bipartite patella. DePalma is of the opinion that excision of the fragment is essential because, if it is not excised, late degenerative changes occur in the patellofemoral joint.[4]

Chondromalacia of the Patella. This degeneration of the articular cartilage of the patella is frequent and is a precursor to degenerative arthritis of the knee. In fact, as noted in *Campbell's Operative Orthopaedics*, the patellofemoral joint is usually the first joint in the body to show degenerative changes and these may begin as early as the second decade.[1] Particular occupations, such as ballet dancing, predispose to this difficulty. Haliburton and Sullivan, in a review of 154 patellectomies for chondromalacia or degenerative arthritis, found a predisposing cause for this entity in 89 knees. These causes included recurrent subluxation or dislocation of the patella, fracture of the patella, a forceful blow on the anterior aspect of the knee, and torn meniscus.[190] O'Donoghue feels that any condition that disturbs the normal rhythm of the quadriceps mechanism, such as locking of the knee, may be a major cause of chondromalacia.[188] Chondromalacia of the patella, when caused by a particular lesion such as recurrent dislocation of the patella, can be cured by treating the cause of the chondromalacia. Small localized areas of chondromalacia can be treated by local débridement, but they should not be extensive. Small craters fill with fibrocartilage and cause little disability later. Patients who obtain a good result after débridement do so within a few months after surgery; those who do not, show no improvement later, according to the study by Wiles, Andrews, and Bremner. These authors conclude that if a good result is not achieved after a few months, patellectomy is indicated.[191] Patelloplasty has also been recommended by Cave and Rowe.[192] Convalescence is usually prolonged after patelloplasty, and improvement continues for at least a year under a supervised program of rehabilitation. Hypertrophic degenerative changes in the patella usually follow chondromalacia, particularly after trauma, with or without fracture, or they occur as part of the gradual aging process plus wear and tear.

Dislocation of the Patella. Traumatic dislocation of the patella in an adult is almost always accompanied by a significant rupture of the vastus medialis tendon at the medial joint capsule, and usually is complicated by an injury to the articular cartilage of the patella, the lateral femoral condyle, or both.[2] The edge of the lateral femoral condyle can be fractured by the displaced patella. Recurrent dislocation of the patella is most frequently seen in those patients who have a small, laterally placed patella with laxity of the medial part of the joint capsule and contracture of the lateral part of the joint capsule. Although trauma may cause resultant disability in these people, it was noted by MacNab that in recurrent dislocations of the patella the articular surfaces degenerate, not so much because the patella is often dislocated, but because its excursions are abnormal during any motion of the knee.[193] When dislocation does occur, there are usually underlying factors responsible. These include preexisting abnormalities of the articulating surfaces, which permit lateral displacement. The precipitating trauma is usually an outward thrust of the leg while the knee is fully extended. This carries the patellar tendon laterally with the dislocating patella. A typical first dislocation occurs in a young person. Pathologic changes follow, as outlined by MacNab, and the patella is increasingly susceptible to dislocation following the same type of precipitating trauma. With an increasing number of dislocations, the opposing aspects of the patella and the lateral femoral condyle become eroded and thin, and the structures around the patella are greatly stretched. Redislocations then occur with greater ease with less pain and effusion. For patients with these chronic recurrent dislocations, surgical correction is usually necessary to prevent recurrence and to eliminate disability.

Avulsion of the Tibial Tubercle. This rarely occurs as an isolated lesion in an adult, but is seen with a comminuted fracture of the upper tibia. Avulsion of the apophysis of the tibial tubercle may, however, occur as an isolated injury. Immobilization of the limb in extension is usually adequate treatment, but occasionally the loose fragment must be secured in position by some form of internal fixation. The resultant disability from this injury is similar to that from rupture of the patellar tendon. It should, however, be noted that since the healing here is bone to bone, as opposed to tendon to tendon, functional results should be somewhat better.

Bursal and Fascial Affections of the Knee

O'Donoghue, discussing the development of calcification about the knee following chronic strain with repetitive injury, states that it is most common at the attachment of the patellar tendon to the tubercle of the tibia. Conservative treatment is recommended, including splint immobilization or a walking cast. Steroid infiltration is sometimes necessary along with physical therapy. Occasionally surgical excision is required. Athletes often encounter this difficulty repeatedly and, because of chronic disability, have to stop playing ball professionally.[75]

Gliding synovial structures at each friction point in the knee permit friction-free motion betweeen contiguous moving parts (Fig. 3–XIII–39). These bursae are a potential source of pain and disability when they become inflamed. Bursitis occurs in response to direct trauma or repetitive occupational trauma. Any of the multiple bursae of the knee can be affected. The most constant and most important of them are: (1) prepatellar bursa, which lies between the skin and the patella; (2) the superficial infrapatellar bursa, between the skin and the patellar tendon; (3) the deep infrapatellar bursa, lying deep to the tendon; (4) the lateral four bursae, one between the lateral head of the gastrocnemius and the capsule, another between the fibular collateral ligament and the biceps tendon, a third between the fibular collateral ligament and the popliteal tendon, and the fourth, usually a synovial extension from the joint lying between the popliteal tendon and the lateral femoral condyle; and (5) the medial bursae, often communicating with the joint, one lying between the medial head of the gastrocnemius and the tendon of the semimembranosus, another lying superficially between the tibial collateral ligament and the tendons of the sartorius and gracilis and semitendinosus, and the third, which meets the tendon of the semimembranosus, at its attachment to the head of the tibia. There are other bursae beneath the tibial collateral ligament related to the meniscus and the capsule.

The prepatellar bursa is particularly susceptible to direct trauma. Recurrent minor injuries produce "housemaid's knee." Conservative treatment such as compression or aspiration is usually adequate, but as in other bursae, infection may ensue. Chronic prepatellar bursitis is common in tile setters and carpet layers. Thickening of the bursal wall occurs. Surgical excision is often necessary in this situation, and there is usually no resultant disability except for a barely noticeable hairline transverse scar. If the patient intends to continue occupationally traumatizing his prepatellar area, a knee pad is recommended.

Traumatic prepatellar neuralgia has been described by Gordon in which pain like a persistent toothache or like an electric shock becomes a source of constant annoyance to the patient. It is caused by direct trauma to the front of the knee. Slight pressure, even the contact of clothing, increases the pain. This syndrome is due to contusion of the neurovascular bundle just under the skin where it enters the prepatellar bursa. Fibrosis of the nerve ensues with adherence to the surrounding structures. Local anesthetic infiltration, or if necessary, excision of the neurovascular bundle, produces complete relief without any disability.[194] Smason reported a case of a posttraumatic fistula connecting the prepatellar bursa with the knee joint. This rare entity probably began as a rent in the quadriceps muscle immediately proximal to the patella, forming a communication between the prepatellar bursa and the joint, which communication was maintained by the pumping action of the knee in the presence of an effusion.[196] This possibility should be considered in any case of recurrent

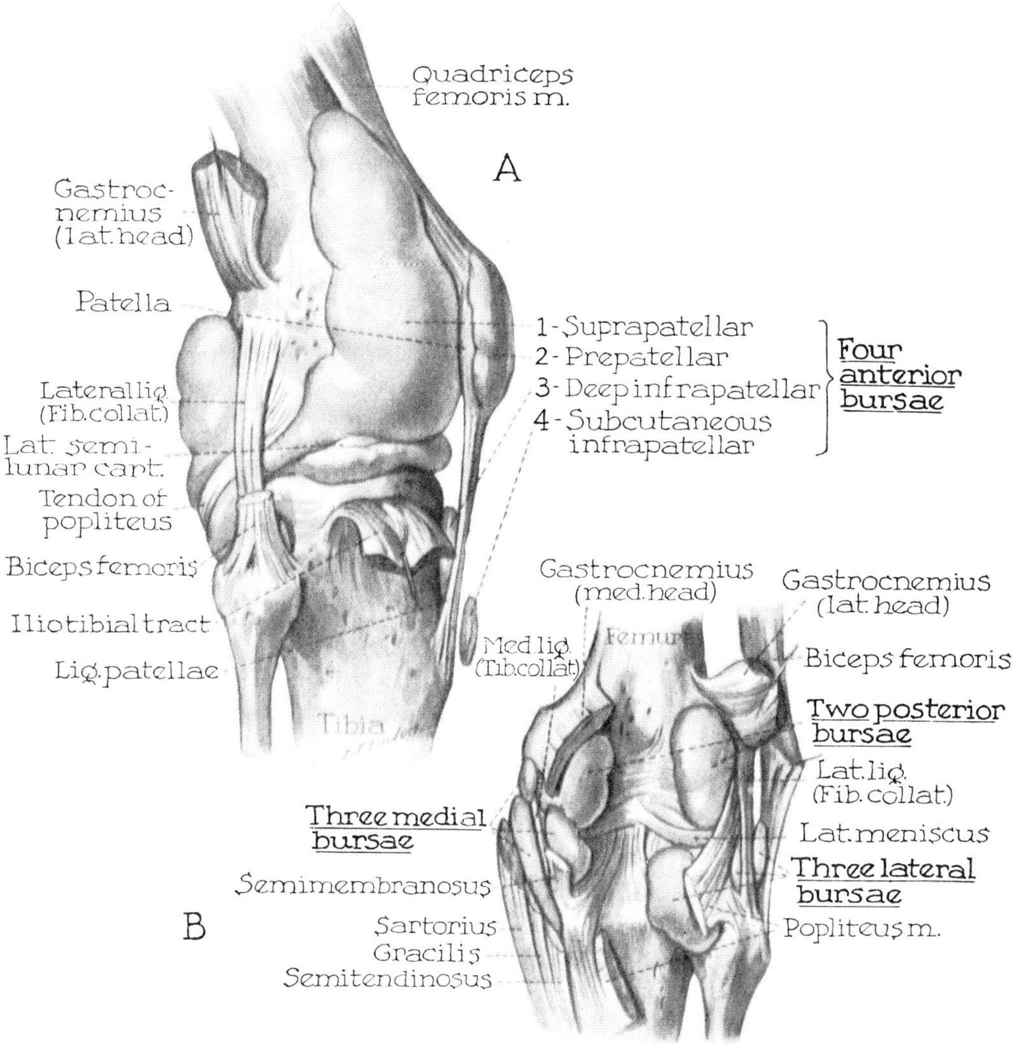

Figure 3–XIII–39. The 12 bursae around the knee joint. *A*. Lateral view of the right knee joint. *B*. Posterior view. (From P. Thorek: *Anatomy in Surgery*. 2nd Edition. Philadelphia, J. B. Lippincott Co., 1962. Reprinted by permission.)

noninfectious effusions following trauma involving the prepatellar bursa, particularly when there is no history of repeated direct trauma to the prepatellar area. In Smason's case, surgical excision of the bursa and capsular repair produced a cure, and there was no recurrence.

A direct blow over the patellar ligament causes bursitis of the deep infrapatellar space. Conservative treatment is usually sufficient, but if necessary, surgical excision is curative without producing any resultant disability. In the lateral or medial bursae, inflammation can result in deposition of amorphous calcific material similar to calcium deposits in the shoulder bursae or tendons. A classic area for this is the anserine bursa, which lies between the tendons of the sartorius, gracilis, and semitendinosus muscles. Adequate treatment generally leaves no residual disability.

A popliteal cyst, known also as a Baker's cyst, is due to effusion into the semimembranosus bursa. Turek feels that the very probable cause is the repeated trauma due to constant friction between adjacent muscles.[38] Another theory postulates a herniation of synovium through a defect in the posterior capsule. Occupational trauma can produce either of these causes. Excision of the distended bursa and closure of the communication with the knee joint cavity are recommended by McLaughlin to avoid recurrence.[2] Turek feels that it is unnecessary to close the opening in the capsule. Haggart recommends that in addition to completely excising the bursa, one should close its capsular orifice either by scarification of its edges and simple suture or, when this is impossible, by a graft from the tendinous part of the medial head of the gastrocnemius or from the semimembranosus tendon.[196] Burleson, Bickel, and Dahlin agree with Turek that it is not necessary to close any opening into the knee and that doing so does not decrease the incidence of recurrence.[197] The Campbell Clinic agrees.

Voshell and Brantigan observed bursae between the longitudinal part of the tibial collateral ligament and the capsule of the knee. They reported instances of calcification in one or more of these bursae and suggested that this might be identical with Pellegrini-Stieda disease. Proper treatment was curative.[198] An occult lesion of the lateral meniscus should be considered, however, when there are symptoms related to the tibial collateral ligament and these are not relieved by the usual conservative measures. Besides tibial collateral ligament fibrositis and bursitis, fibular collateral ligament bursitis is seen. Thickening of the bursal wall and effusion with local irritation may become severe enough to cause pressure on the peroneal nerve as it winds around the back of the fibular head. Peroneal palsy can develop. Subsequent to direct trauma, a cyst may develop within the sheath of the common peroneal nerve where it passes behind the head of the fibula; careful excision of this cyst, actually a ganglion, is no guarantee that it will not recur. Excision of the sac generally relieves the peroneal neuropathy, albeit sometimes only temporarily until the cyst recurs. Clark felt that the pedicle should be excised and the cyst decompressed by incisions, but that removal of the cyst was not necessary.[199] Attempts to dissect out the cyst from an extensively involved nerve or neurectomy are followed by poor results according to Parkes.[200] Acute avulsion of the fibular collateral ligament from the femur with a flake of bone has been described by O'Donoghue.[75] Surgical treatment is sometimes necessary if conservative measures fail.

Anserine bursitis is typically of the friction type, although it may be initiated by an external blow thrusting the bursa against the hard tibia beneath. Involvement in this area tends to be chronic, particularly if full activity is allowed too early. Athletes should not participate in their sport until motion of the knee joint has been eliminated for long enough to allow complete healing of the anserine inflammation. This is true of those engaged in other similarly demanding occupations such as ballet dancing.

Knee Ligament Injuries

Sprains. O'Donoghue defines a sprain of the knee as any injury to a ligament caused by abnormal motion (Fig. 3–XIII–40).[75] This in-

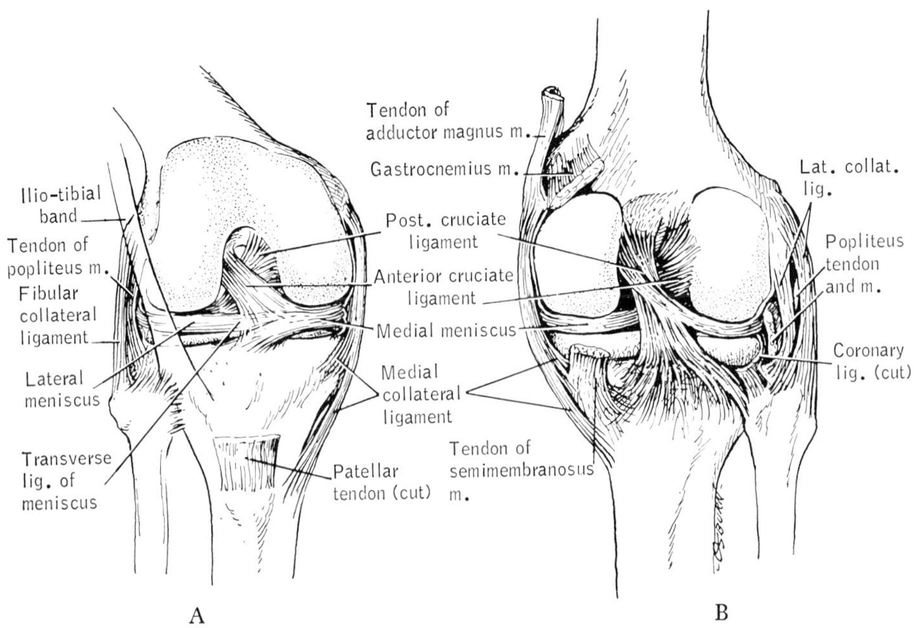

Figure 3–XIII–40. Ligaments of the knee. *A.* Anterior view. *B.* Posterior view, knee extended. (From D. H. O'Donoghue: *Treatment of Injuries to Athletes.* 3rd Edition. Philadelphia, W. B. Saunders Co., 1976. Reprinted by permission.)

jury can vary from a slight tearing of a few isolated fibers with no loss of function to a complete dislocation of the joint with total loss of integrity of the ligament. Abnormal motion of the knee producing ligamentous injury can be in any direction: adduction, abduction, hyperextension, excessive internal or external rotation, forward or backward displacement, or any combination of these. A violent abduction injury of the knee causes a disruption in the *medial collateral ligament.* The ligament may be avulsed from its attachment to the femur or from the tibia, or ruptured through the ligament itself at any point. McLaughlin feels that a concomitant rupture of the anterior cruciate ligament is the rule, and more often than not the medial meniscus is lacerated or pulled loose from its coronary ligament attachment. This is because the medial collateral ligament is attached to the medial meniscus.[2] When the ligament is avulsed from its bony attachment and carries a bony fragment with it, healing occurs with less disability than when the ligament itself is torn. When the medial collateral ligament is sprained, particularly if it is sprained repetitively, an ossification adjacent to the adductor tubercle within the ligament can develop. As previously mentioned, this is known as *Pellegrini-Stieda disease.* Particularly in an athlete, the medial collateral ligament can be weakened when an initial injury to the ligament has been underestimated and the knee inadequately protected against the strain of weight-bearing. This can also occur when there has been insufficient conditioning of the quadriceps after this injury. The ligament stretches and slightly elongates; this attenuation of the ligament is related to future disability. As characterized by Smillie, the resultant disability depends upon the ligamentous control surrounding the knee. He states that absolute perfection of ligamentous control is unobtainable following gross ligamentous lesions, and subsequent disability of the joint is determined by the capacity of the quadriceps to compensate for this disability.[182] Injury to the medial (tibial) collateral ligament is very common because trauma is more likely to occur from the lateral aspect of the limb, causing severe valgus distortion and subsequent medial ligament injury, than from the medial aspect, causing a varus injury to the knee and, with it, lateral collateral ligament injury. Rupture of the medial collateral ligament is caused by momentary subluxation of the knee joint when the injury occurs, the knee being flexed and the tibia fixed. The femur rotates internally.

Ruptures. Complete rupture of the *lateral (fibular) collateral ligament* is rare, not only because injury to the knee usually results from an external force, but also because the lateral collateral ligament does not have a rigid attachment to the lateral meniscus, as does the medial collateral ligament to the medial meniscus. A lesion commonly associated with complete rupture of the fibular collateral ligament is stretching or rupture of the common peroneal nerve, according to DePalma.[4] The prognosis is grave following injury to the common peroneal nerve, even when immediate surgical repair is achieved. This was borne out by Towne and associates in their article on the lateral compartment syndrome of the knee.[201] Because rupture of the lateral collateral ligament usually is caused by great violence, there is usually avulsion of a fragment of the fibular head by the ligament and the biceps tendon. The iliotibial band and the lateral knee joint capsule may also be torn. McLaughlin feels that neglected ruptures often do not incur a serious penalty in terms of knee joint instability or dysfunction.[2] As previously stated, the primary disability is due to the peroneal nerve injury.

Collins agrees with O'Donoghue that early surgical restoration (within the first 10 days after injury) offers the best chance of complete recovery.[202, 203] His studies have shown that even in the most severe injuries, early repair gives better results than late repair. Clayton and Weir have shown that surgical repair of the ligaments allows better healing.[204] This is borne out by the statement in *Campbell's Operative Orthopaedics* that all ligamentous injuries resulting in a varus-valgus opening of more than 10 degrees should be repaired immediately.[1] Stress films and arthrography are often helpful in confirming this diagnosis.

Injury to the medial collateral ligament, if severe enough, can be accompanied by a rupture of the *anterior cruciate ligament;* conversely, a *posterior cruciate injury* is associated with severe injury of the lateral collateral ligament. Isolated injury to either cruciate ligament can occur, however. Both cruciates can be torn if the injury, to either the medial side of the joint or the lateral aspect, is severe enough. Isolated lesions of the anterior cruciate ligament are rare, being caused by severe hyperextension of the knee or by a force driving the femur backward on the fixed tibia while the knee is flexed. The ligament may be avulsed either from the lateral femoral condyle or from the tibial spine. A portion of the tibial spine may be avulsed with the ligament attached. Authors generally agree that lesions of the anterior cruciate ligament are combined with lesions of the tibial collateral ligament and lesions of the medial meniscus as well, resulting from severe abduction or rotatory forces.

An isolated injury of the posterior cruciate ligament is rare, usually occurring when a direct force drives the tibia posteriorly while the foot and femur are fixed and the knee is flexed. Avulsion of the tibial attachment with a fragment of bone may be encountered, as may rupture of the femoral attachment of the ligament. DePalma feels that surgical repair is the treatment of choice. He feels this is true of the anterior cruciate ligament as well, but knee stability depends more on posterior cruciate ligament integrity.[4] Feagin and co-workers studied 64 cases of isolated tear of the anterior cruciate ligament and concluded that surgical repair can be effective in the large majority of cases. Repair was possible in 49 patients in his series. Reexploration as a result of subsequent trauma or internal derangement revealed that 8 of 16 repaired ligaments were intact and of good quality.[205] In comparison, Trickey evaluated conservative versus operative treatment of rupture of the posterior cruciate ligament of the knee. In 7 cases treated conservatively and 10 cases treated operatively, he noted that there was some posterior cruciate laxity in the more severe cases treated conservatively, but there was also laxity in those treated surgically. About an equal number of patients in each group had a loss of 10 degrees of knee flexion one year after injury. He also noted, in evaluation of late cases, that persistent posterior cruciate laxity can be as severe a disability as the rupture of the anterior cruciate ligament, and this laxity can be present whether or not there has been bone avulsion.[206]

When the severe disability caused by old rupture is considered, the importance of immediate repair of the damaged ligaments can easily be appreciated. With old ligamentous injury the knee becomes unstable, and therefore is injured repeatedly. With each successive injury there is greater instability of the knee and further atrophy of the thigh muscles. Thus a cycle is set up in which the thigh muscles, which are needed to protect the knee, become less and less effective in this protection. Also, the articular cartilages become involved in the degenerative process. This may lead to disabling degenerative arthritis of the knee, quite unrelated to the original ligamentous injury. Thus it becomes readily apparent why multiple operations have been described for late reconstruction of the torn ligaments of the knee. In deciding on repair of an old ligamentous injury, it is of utmost importance that not only the degree of disability, but the patient's occupation, be taken into consideration. For example, Nicholas has described what is known as the five-one reconstruction for anteromedial instability of the knee. Yet, in his article he makes the point that this operation is designed not for the patient with simple instability of the knee but rather for the individual who wishes to participate in competitive sports.[207] It is important to note that even when old ruptures are treated by reconstruction before the joint has been severely damaged, function of the knee will not be normal because the structure and function of the ligaments cannot be completely restored by such procedures.

Dislocation of the Knee

Complete dislocations of the knee are rare. They are often misdiagnosed because many of them are reduced at the scene of the accident, according to Kennedy. The most common type is anterior dislocation in which the tibia slips forward in relation to the femur. Kennedy reported involvement of the nerve or vessels in more than 50 per cent of cases. He recommends immediate treatment and closed reduction under spinal anesthesia, which has the added advantage of increasing the circulation to the leg. Circulation should be watched carefully after reduction. He advises against a circular cast. If the adequacy of circulation is in doubt, surgery is indicated.[208] Meyers and Harvey studied 18 traumatic dislocations of the knee and agreed that it is essential to perform immediate closed reduction with examination of the knee for stability under anesthesia. These authors recommend early operative repair of all torn ligaments, including the posterior cruciate ligament, and all capsular tears, especially of the posterior capsule. Arteriography is suggested if there is any doubt of the adequacy of the circulation.[209]

Meniscus Injuries

The most common serious injury to the knee is damage to the menisci. The medial meniscus is more frequently injured than the lateral, the ratio being 7 to 1. This is true for the same reason that the medial collateral ligament is more often injured than the lateral ligament: injury is more likely to occur from the lateral aspect of the knee, and the medial meniscus is attached to the unyielding medial collateral ligament, while the lateral meniscus is not attached to the lateral collateral ligament. A meniscus tear is usually not caused by a direct blow to the knee. Meniscal injury occurs if the patient twists the knee or falls as the result of a blow. When the femur is forcefully internally rotated while the knee is flexed and the tibia fixed, the menisci are swept into the interior of the joint. If the knee is extended, the menisci are crushed between the femoral condyles and the tibial plateaus. This mechanism of injury can also cause the menisci to be torn from their peripheral attachments. Meniscus tears can be extended by reinjury. Once a diagnosis of a tear is made, the meniscus should be removed. A torn meniscus disturbs the joint mechanics and can harm the articular cartilage and the chondral surface of the patella. It also causes stretching of the anterior cruciate ligament and subsequent laxity. After a meniscus has been excised, a new one may regenerate at the site of the old one. Microscopically, however, the new meniscus is fibrocartilage rather than hyaline cartilage. A new fibrocartilaginous meniscus can be torn by trauma in the same manner that a hyaline cartilaginous meniscus is torn. There has been much discussion of the temporary upset of joint mechanics following meniscectomy. This is related to the degree of alteration of the relationship of the opposing condyles and the rapidity of the change, i.e., the change will be far greater in the case of a thick, weight-bearing discoid meniscus than in that of a thin, degenerated meniscus that has undergone attrition over years of rubbing between the two condyles. In the latter form, no adjustment of mechanics is necessary following operation, for it has already taken place. Meniscectomy in a young patient is generally followed by no disability. One often encounters a postoperative numbness, however, either around the incision site or on the contralateral side, owing to injury to the infrapatellar nerve, the course of which generally is in line with the arthrotomy incision. The nerve often regenerates, but permanent localized numbness often occurs as well. This is usually not a disabling complication and goes relatively unnoticed by the patient. If, however, the diagnosis of neuroma of this nerve becomes established, the scar should be excised, the neuroma isolated, and the nerve traced in a more proximal direction and divided with a sharp scalpel. When both menisci are removed from a knee, disability, if any, is minimal in young patients, as when one meniscus is removed from a knee. In older patients, unilateral or bilateral meniscectomy of a knee may relieve most of the patient's symptoms, but the patient may continue to have pain and limitation of motion because of underlying degenerative arthritis. Postoperative quadriceps exercises are essential for complete rehabilitation of meniscectomy patients, and these exercises are usually performed well by the young. Older people often have difficulty complying with a vigorous postoperative exercise regimen, and this fact also contributes to greater disability in the older age group. According to *Campbell's Operative Orthopaedics*, the two most frequent complications that may occur immediately after meniscectomy and affect the final result are severe hemarthrosis and chronic synovitis.[1] Aspiration of the joint as necessary usually resolves the hemarthrosis, and vigorous rehabilitation of the muscles of the extremity improves the synovitis, particularly in the type of synovitis that does not respond favorably to rest.

Although a knee can function well without its menisci, late degenerative changes in the joint do occur after injury of a knee and meniscectomy.

Cysts of menisci can develop after injury, and are much more frequent in the lateral meniscus than in the medial cartilage. A large untreated cyst of the lateral meniscus may erode the tibial condyle inferior to the lateral margin of the articular cartilage. Excision of the meniscus and its cyst is recommended. "*Snapping knee*" is usually caused by a cyst of the lateral meniscus.[1] It may be caused by a *discoid meniscus*. A discoid meniscus is one that is discoid in configuration, rather than semilunar. It is more frequently seen laterally than medially. There have been no studies to date to indicate whether discoid menisci are more susceptible to injury than normal menisci. The results of excision of torn discoid menisci are comparable to those in which torn semilunar menisci are excised.

Acute Traumatic Synovitis and Traumatic Hemarthrosis

All types of knee injuries produce acute traumatic synovitis in which fluid accumulates slowly over 12 to 24 hours and the joint becomes tense. In traumatic hemarthrosis, the fluid accumulates swiftly. Intraarticular fractures produce traumatic hemarthrosis, which, according to DePalma, may also accompany maceration of the infrapatellar fat pad, rupture of one of the cruciate ligaments, tears of the synovium, or tears in the vascular peripheral attachment of the menisci. In both acute traumatic synovitis and traumatic hemarthrosis, one is obliged to ascertain and to correct the cause. In either of these entities, aspiration of the joint is recommended. Joint aspiration in the knee, as in joints elsewhere in the body, should be undertaken under the most aseptic conditions. Otherwise, infecting bacteria may be brought into the joint, causing sepsis, an unenviable iatrogenic situation.

Fractures of the Distal End of the Femur

Intercondylar Fractures. Massive hemarthrosis and severe soft-tissue damage accompany intercondylar fractures of the femur. It is often necessary to aspirate the knee joint before reduction and after reduction as necessary.[4] These lesions are usually treated with manipulation and skeletal traction. Open reduction and internal fixation with Rush rods or other devices has been done and is indicated if skeletal traction and manipulation are not adequate. According to McLaughlin, fractures of both condyles (T or Y fractures) are the most common fractures of the lower end of the adult femur. An associated wound is often present. The knee mechanism is grossly disorganized by the splitting of the femoral condyles by the shaft fragment. External immobilization is usually to no avail. Connolly and associates reported on 36 cases of femoral or tibial fracture. It was their opinion that fractures associated with arterial injury, such as those in the study, are best immobilized by 4.5 to 6.8 kg of skeletal traction.[210] The method of managing the fracture should not be allowed to take precedence over treatment of the related serious injury to the soft tissue. As in other similar fractures, traction immobilization should be continued for at least six weeks and probably for eight weeks to allow the fracture fragments to become "sticky."

Single Femoral Condyle Fractures. Fractures of a single condyle of the femur are usually the result of direct violence forcing the knee joint into varus or valgus position. The fracture line is usually in the sagittal plane and is vertical. The fractured condylar fragment is often undisplaced and is seldom displaced more than a small amount. Its soft-tissue attachments remain essentially intact, so that the broken fragment is usually quite stable. A fracture in the frontal plane rarely occurs. When it does, it is due to force applied with the knee moderately flexed. The collateral ligament on the affected side usually remains intact, while the contralateral collateral ligament is stretched or is partially or completely torn. In the rare fractures in the frontal plane, the "cracked-off" fragment may not be controlled by ligamentous attachments and may be a free body. Fractures of this type usually do well with a short period of immobilization after which progressive knee motion may be begun. Occasionally, internal fixation is necessary to prevent rotation of the displaced fragment or fragments. As in all injuries about the knee joint, quadriceps exercises are essential for restoration of the most nearly normal function of the knee possible. When reduction of single condylar fractures of the femur is accurate, a good range of motion of the knee is regained.

Chondral and Osteochondral Fractures of the Femoral Condyle. Chondral fractures are fractures involving the articular cartilage, and these are particularly prevalent in the knee because of the direct stresses and strains applied to the knee joint. A chondral fracture, according to O'Donoghue, may be extremely difficult to diagnose and may only be ascertained after arthrotomy of the knee.[75] Kennedy, Grainger, and McGraw pointed out in 1966 that osteochondral fractures of the femoral condyles should be operated upon. They felt that early surgery allowed a more correct diagnosis as well as the best chance for reconstruction of the fracture fragments. They did point out, however, that in a review of eight patients seen, on an average, for six years after removal of a large osteochondral fragment, although results were extremely satisfactory in seven patients, they felt that a 15-year follow-up would be more helpful in deciding whether or not to discard the fragment.[211] If an osteochondral fracture fragment or a piece of cartilage is loose in the knee, the patient will develop symptoms of a foreign body within the joint, requiring arthrotomy and removal of the foreign body. Chondral fractures that are completely unrecognized are usually those in which the fracture is incomplete and a fragment is not actually dislodged. O'Donoghue and others are quite sure that many cases of osteochondritis dissecans are in fact initiated by fractures of the cartilage.[75] Besides condylar damage, the patella is particularly vulnerable because it is common for an individual to fall upon the flexed knee. In a series of 15 cases of osteochondral fracture presented by Rosenberg, 13 patients had surgical treatment in which the fragment that was displaced was removed as soon as possible. All of those so treated had good results. In contrast, the two patients treated without operation continued to have recurrent episodes of pain, effusion, restriction of motion, or a tendency of the knee to give way. The follow-up on all these patients, at this time, is inadequate to allow assessment of possible future articular surface changes. The comment was made that it is unknown whether the fibrocartilage that fills the condylar defect will be sufficient to provide a lifetime of weight-bearing on the articular surface.[212] Whether this will result in the onset of degenerative arthritis in the knee joint remains to be seen. Proper treatment depends largely upon a proper diagnosis. If a subchondral fracture is present, protective immobilization will permit it to heal. If, however, the cartilage itself is fractured without subchondral bone, the healing potential is so poor that it probably will not heal in any event.[25] Arthroscopy and arthrography are often helpful in establishing the proper diagnosis.

Osteochondritis Dissecans of the Knee. Aichroth studied the relationship of osteochondral fractures to osteochondritis dissecans of the knee in 60 mature rabbits in which osteochondral fractures of various types were made in the medial femoral condyle. The fractures or fragments that remained stable united, but those in which movement occurred progressed to nonunion. An ununited osteochondral fragment resembled osteochondritis dissecans in the human both radiologically and histologically. Aichroth concluded that the fragment in osteochondritis dissecans follows an osteochondral fracture that remains ununited (Fig. 3–XIII–41). He also reviewed 100 patients with osteochondritis dissecans of the knee. The outstanding etiologic features were found to be direct injury to the joint surface (46 per cent), repeated injuries sustained in athletics, and mechanical abnormalities of the knee. Aichroth's management plan is to use conservative measures if symptoms are slight and the fragment remains in situ. Exploration of the knee is recommended if the symptoms are exacerbated and there is evidence of buckling or locking of the knee. Removal of the fragment is recommended if it is known to be loose initially, or is found so at arthrotomy. He suggests it is not enough simply to cut down on the loose body and extract it, because additional pieces may separate from the condylar defect.[213, 214] Smillie agrees.[182] The site from which the fragment comes must therefore be carefully inspected, and the crater cleared out. Drilling of the lesion is recommended if the cartilage appears intact, and also if there is incipient osteochondritis. Smillie has recommended internal fixation with his device, but internal fixation has the disadvantage that the pins may have to be removed and the fragment

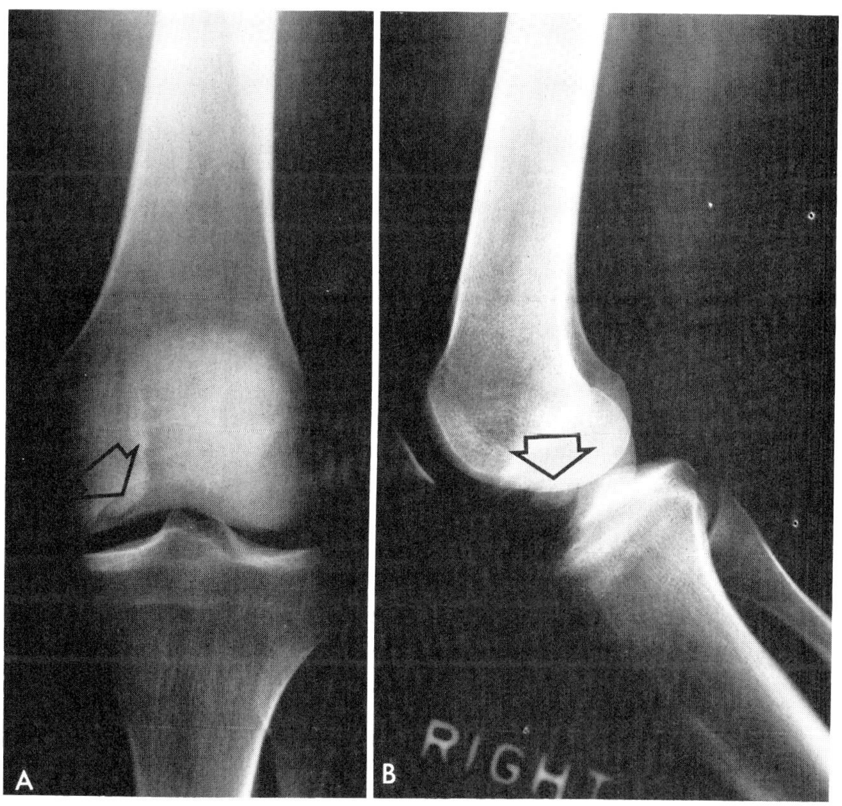

Figure 3–XIII–41. Osteochondritis dissecans of the knee, medial femoral condyle. *A.* Anterior view. *B.* Lateral view.

may remain ununited or may later again become loose.

Fractures of the Proximal End of the Tibia

Fractures of the Tibial Condyles. Avulsion fracture of the upper tibia is basically an avulsion of the anterior cruciate ligament and, according to O'Donoghue, should be treated as such, the main emphasis being placed on the restoration of the anterior cruciate ligament to its normal length and function.[75] Open repair is recommended. Normal function of the knee cannot be obtained when there is an unreduced displacement of the tibial spine on the superior surface of the tibia. Avulsion fracture of the upper tibia is produced by a severe shearing by the femur on the flexed knee.

Tibial condyle fractures are usually caused by severe abduction or adduction forces applied to the outer or inner aspect of the knee, particularly the former. These fractures can also be produced by forces acting in the vertical direction on the tibial plateau. These lesions are accompanied by damage to the ligamentous apparatus. Fracture is uncommon in young individuals, a rupture of the medial collateral ligament being the usual injury. In the middle-aged and older population, bones are more brittle, and femoral impact causes crushing of the tibial condyles. Lateral condylar injury is accompanied by damage not only to the medial collateral ligament but also to the anterior cruciate ligament and the lateral meniscus. Medial condylar fracture is associated with posterior cruciate injury as well as injury to the lateral collateral ligament and the medial meniscus. Lesions of the medial condyle are exceedingly rare. DePalma recommends that, in management of tibial condylar lesions, the anatomical alignment of the tibial plateaus should be restored to as nearly normal as possible. The limb should be immobilized long enough to allow adequate soft-tissue healing. As in all other injuries about the knee, quadriceps exercises should be continued throughout rehabilitation. Conservative management is recommended in tibial condyle fractures when there is no fragmentation or depression. The prognosis is excellent provided the postfracture care is adequate. In depressed fractures of the tibial condyle, however, open reduction is recommended, with elevation of the plateau and internal fixation if necessary. This was borne out by Meyers and McKeever in their article in 1970 on fracture of the inner condylar eminence of the tibia.[215] Frequency of deplorable end-results in fractures of the tibial plateau is due to failure to effect reduction, failure to furnish dependable immobilization, and failure to maintain maximum function. Anderson and Loughlen had good results with their assured fixation technique.[216] Another method of treatment, which has recently come into vogue as an effective means of resolving these difficult problems, is the cast-brace. This has also been effective in the treatment of distal femoral and intercondylar fractures of the femur. This method not only provides for fracture immobilization but also allows for motion at the knee, factors that have proved critical in rehabilitation of these patients.

Fracture of both tibial condyles is a relatively uncommon injury produced by femoral impact without valgus strain. The force of the femoral impact is distributed diffusely, and gross depression of the fracture fragments is uncommon. In the absence of comminution, the tibial condylar fragments tend to split apart; for this McLaughlin suggests the use of a transverse bolt.[2] When the upper tibia is comminuted, significant displacement is uncommon, and prolonged immobilization is the treatment of choice. Whenever there is prolonged immobilization, quadriceps exercises are essential, but even with assiduous exercising, knee stiffness to some degree is usually seen as a permanent disability. This was well demonstrated by Porter in his study of 137 patients who sustained 138 crush fractures of the lateral tibial table. He demonstrated that in those fractures that were depressed 10 mm or more, far better results were obtained with open reduction and realignment of the fracture fragments.[217] Roberts studied 100 cases of fracture of the condyles of the tibia. The study emphasized the vulnerability of the lateral tibial plateau to a valgus force on the extended knee. Roberts concluded that type I, nondisplaced, fractures can be successfully treated by an initial period of traction with early institution of active knee exercises and subsequent prolonged protection from weight-bearing. Type II, local compression, fractures of the lateral plateau are successfully managed by conservative methods recommended for type I fractures. Type III, displaced, fractures may require open reduction to restore joint stability. Postoperative care is based on principles followed in the treatment of type I and type II fractures. Early mobilization of the knee is the key to restoration of maximum joint function. The patients who had unacceptable results were those who had persistent pain in the knee, limited motion, and valgus deformity. One of the patients in the study had a poor result because of extensive calcification of the medial collateral ligament. Anteroposterior instability was found in 10 patients.[218] In fractures of the tibial condyles, there is every expectation that the cancellous bone, with its good circulation and osteogenic potential, will unite, but stability of the knee depends upon the amount of soft-tissue injury as well as on the amount of bone deformity.

T or Y Fractures of the Upper End of the Tibia. These fractures are usually due to a violent force acting downward on the tibia. Falling from a height and landing on the feet is a typical mechanism of injury. The tibial condyles are driven downward and the shaft is displaced upward. Mechanical traction is the method recommended for elevation of the condyles and restoration of tibial length. Operative intervention is indicated when closed methods fail. As in all other fractures about the knee, disability is less when the articular surface is not involved and is worse when the articular surface is involved.

Fractures of the Fabella

Fabella fractures are extremely uncommon. The fabella is a sesamoid bone frequently found in the tendon of the lateral head of the gastrocnemius muscle as it passes under the femoral condyle. O'Donoghue recommends excision of the fabella if it is fractured or if it is involved by osteochondritis or chondromalacia.[75] There should be no disability subsequently.

Weight-bearing and the accommodation that permits the folding action of the extremities in sitting, kneeling, and squatting are the chief functions of the knee. According to McBride, a stiffened but fully extended knee, or one that can be extended to within 15 degrees of full extension, will retain most of its capacity for strength, endurance, and security in weight-bearing.[81] The nearer the knee motion can approach full extension, the less the disability will be. The resultant disability after injuries of the knee depends upon intraarticular damage and alignment of the tibia with respect to the femur. Patellofemoral alignment is also important.

Fracture of the Head of the Fibula

The head of the fibula may be broken by a direct blow. However, any fracture below the head, actually involving the neck, should lead one to suspect ankle injury rather than primary injury of the knee. Fractures of the fibular head may involve the peroneal nerve, the biceps tendon, and the lateral collateral ligament. A simple fibular head fracture, without soft-tissue damage, produces minimal or no disability. Peroneal nerve damage can be permanent, however.

Dislocation of the Fibula from the Tibia

This rare injury is due to a twisting force, with resultant damage to the ankle joint.[75] Direct force against the fibular head can cause it, however, in localized trauma to the knee. Replacement should be accurate, and if there is instability of the fibula, internal fixation is recommended, the fixation device being removed as soon as ligament healing is complete (Fig. 3–XIII–42). Other authors have found that direct pressure over the fibular head with the knee flexed will reduce the joint in most cases.[219, 220] Crothers and Johnson have reported, however, that if the injury is more than two to three days old, reduction is often impossible and open stabilization is necessary.[221]

The peroneal nerve is extremely vulnerable to injury either posteriorly or laterally because it lies directly between the skin and bone. Contusion of the nerve is common without any attendant bony injury. A relatively minor blow may cause serious nerve injury.[75] Inversion of the foot with plantar flexion can pull the peroneal nerve taut against the fascial edge that delimits the opening in the origin of the peroneus longus muscle.[12] One or both branches of the peroneal nerve may be stretched by a varus strain of the knee and, secondarily to trauma, can be compressed by fibrous tissue or callus. According to McLaughlin, peroneal nerve palsy commencing immediately after injury usually recovers spontaneously except when it is due to stretch. It is recommended that the patient's foot be supported by a light spring brace; although spontaneous recovery is probable, it may not be complete for many months.[2] Bateman makes note of the fact that injury to the peroneal nerve causes significant disability of the lower limb. He also mentions that there is still a resultant disability even after successful reconstruction of the involved limb.[222]

The Lower Leg

Soft-Tissue Injuries

"Shin Splints." This is a term well known to athletes. The entity usually occurs early in an athlete's training period, after a layoff. It is frequently due to intensive athletic activity on

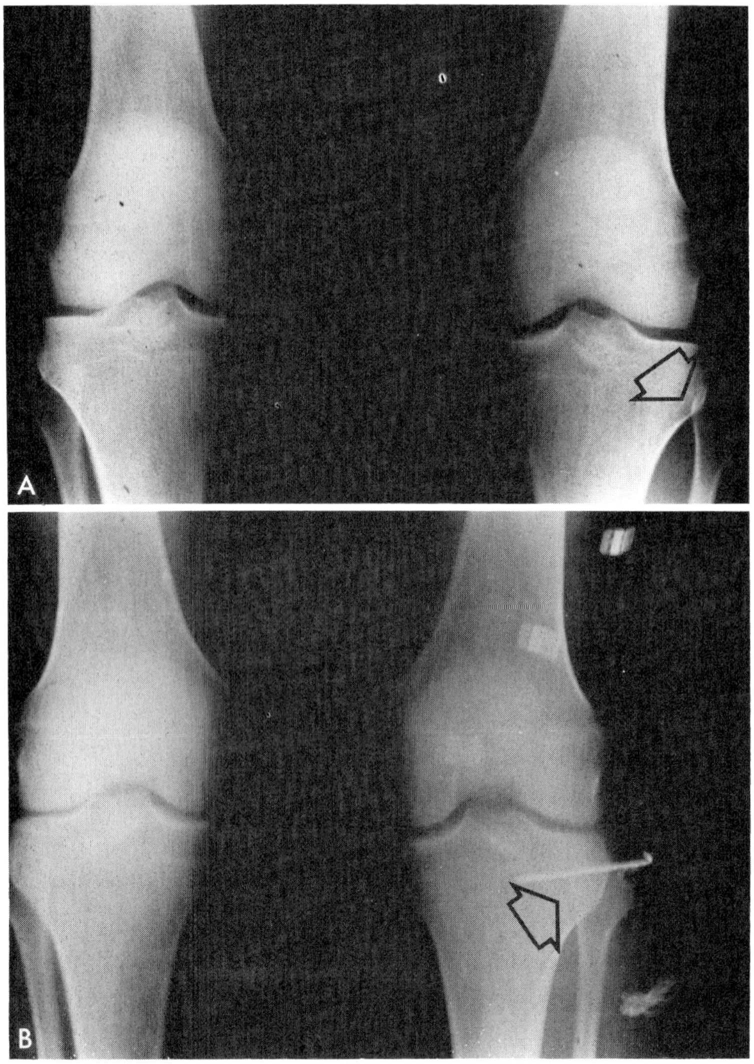

Figure 3–XIII–42. Dislocation of the fibula from the tibia. *A*. Preoperative x-ray. Note the diastasis in the involved side as compared to the normal fibula-tibia relationship in the uninvolved side. *B*. Postoperative x-ray after internal fixation. (Courtesy of Dr. C. Crothers, Maine Medical Center.)

hard ground in the early fall or the early spring. O'Donoghue mentions that this entity is a "waste basket including many different conditions." One of the conditions is irritation of the attachment of the posterior tibial muscle along the posterior face of the tibia with resulting periostitis. Another cause is the actual tearing of the attachment of the posterior tibial muscle along the tibia. The "shin splints" denotation is also used when there is irritation at the interosseous membrane in which the symptoms are somewhat more posterior and seem to be deeper in the muscles of the calf. Periostitis along the posteromedial angle of the tibia, as well as involvement of the anterior tibial muscle at the anterior border of the tibia and onto its anterolateral face, is also called "shin splints." This latter condition may progress to an anterior compartment syndrome.[75] Turek agrees with this contention.[38] Devas, however, believes that the condition is analogous to the "shin splints" in horses, which is actually a stress fracture through one tibial cortex. He maintains that radiographs can frequently show callus formation, the evidence of fracture.[223] The treatment for "shin splints" often involves the use of heat, particularly whirlpool therapy. O'Donoghue suggests that heat aggravates the tension within the anterior tibial compartment. Rest and strapping are preferred, and possibly the use of local heat. The condition has a great tendency to recur. A longer initial period of rest and protection will provide for a more complete recovery.

Anterior Tibial Compartment Syndrome. The anterior tibial compartment of the leg is tightly roofed by the anterior fascia of the leg (Fig. 3–XIII–43). In the anterior tibial syndrome there

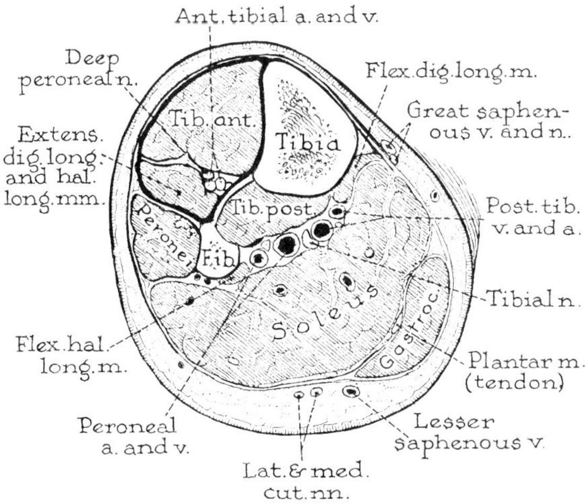

Figure 3–XIII–43. Cross section of leg showing its anterior compartment outlined by heavy line indicating muscles and vascular bundle within the compartment. (From D. H. O'Donoghue: *Treatment of Injuries to Athletes.* 3rd Edition. Philadelphia, W. B. Saunders Co., 1976. Reprinted by permission.)

is a rapid swelling of the muscle within this compartment. This syndrome may follow direct injury in which there is a great deal of swelling and hemorrhage into the anterior tibial space. It is important to note that the anterior tibial compartment syndrome differs from "shin splints" in that there is actual loss of muscle power in the former condition. This indicates damage to the muscle within the anterior tibial compartment and should alert the surgeon to institute prompt treatment. The differential diagnosis should include cellulitis, osteomyelitis, stress fracture, thrombophlebitis, intermittent claudication, and simple "shin splints." Although all the aforementioned conditions may be readily confused with the advanced stage of the anterior tibial syndrome, the critical finding in the acute syndrome is weakness or paralysis of the anterior compartment muscles. In none of the other conditions is this present.[224] Another variant of the anterior tibial compartment syndrome is the chronic form in which the patient complains of pain and disability after relatively minor exertion. This also must be differentiated from "shin splints," which usually occurs once in the active season of an athlete. The chronic syndrome is a repeated phenomenon that occurs with any slight exertion. This is important in those occupations in which ambulation is necessary. O'Donoghue mentions that occasionally the peroneal nerve may be involved in an anterior compartment syndrome with sensory loss, but the loss of muscle function is usually due not to nerve involvement but to pathologic change within the muscle itself. Ischemic necrosis of the muscles, often called Volkmann's ischemia of the leg, can ensue. Muscle tissue is replaced by fibrous scar, rendering the muscle group firm, inelastic, and noncontractile. In an ischemic situation, application of ice without pressure dressings is recommended. Anterior fasciectomy of the leg is recommended if the symptoms do not respond within a few hours. This situation is an extreme emergency when it occurs. O'Donoghue emphasizes that the danger lies in the similarity of the early symptoms of ischemia to "shin splints."[75] A late result of the anterior tibial syndrome is an intractable deformity of the foot due to pressure of the vessels in the anterior compartment of the leg.

Muscle Rupture. *Rupture of the plantaris muscle* is a frequent injury in tennis players and basketball players. When the muscle itself is completely ruptured, pain is deep in the calf and is quite disabling. The plantaris muscle is functionally insignificant, and repair is not recommended. After the inflammation subsides, there is usually no disability. Injury of the plantaris muscle or tendon is important in that it should be distinguished early from a possible injury to the gastrocnemius-soleus mechanism. The latter, when left untreated for a period of time, can cause permanent disability.

Rupture of the calf muscle may be partial or complete, anywhere from its origin to its attachment to the calcaneus. The tear is more frequently in the musculotendinous junction between the gastrocnemius and the conjoined tendon with the soleus. If it is seen early, repair is feasible, and most authors recommend surgical repair of the Achilles tendon after rupture, even if the case is seen late. Gillies and Chalmers, however, treated seven patients by immobilization with the foot in plantar flexion and six patients surgically with formal repair of the tendon. They demonstrated that there was no significant difference between the two groups in subjective symptoms, and that the differences in movement around the ankle and subtalar joints were minimal. They also demonstrated that gait was similar in both groups.[225]

Renne and Davis recently reported a case of bilateral detachment of gastrocnemius muscle bellies from the aponeuroses. A hospital maintenance man sustained this injury in his job, which required repetitive ascending and descending of stairs. No acute trauma could be ascertained in the history. Surgical repair produced excellent results.[226] Judet and associates reported a series of 12 patients with tears of the gastrocnemius. They emphasized the role of sudden trauma and hematoma formation, although one of their patients was said to have had spontaneous development of an "ascending calf." They recommended surgical repair and also reported excellent results.[227] In an unusual case report, Friedlander described a patient who, several years prior to seeing his physician, was injured in a basketball game and sustained a hematoma in the calf as a result of a muscle tear. The hematoma had become organized and encapsulated and, drawing fluid into it, became an expanding compressing mass in the calf. It was excised without residual deficit.[228]

Fascial Hernias. These may occur in various areas of the body, of which one of the most common is the anterior compartment of the leg. A small rent develops along the attachment of the anterior fascia to the tibia. Through this rent in the fascia, a small amount of muscle herniates, causing a significant amount of pain and discomfort. This most frequently happens in the anterior compartment but may happen in the calf muscle also. Usually symptomatic treatment is sufficient, but occasionally surgery is required. Surgical treatment usually involves either repairing the defect, which is accompanied by good results, or extending it further and allowing a larger area to bulge through, relieving the acute tension that causes the pain. Results are good with this method also.

Shaft Fractures of the Tibia and Fibula

Fractures of the shaft of the tibia and fibula are produced by either an angulatory force or a rotational force. Transverse or short oblique fractures of both bones at the same level are generally produced by angulatory forces. Rotational forces produce spiral fractures at different levels. The fibular fracture is usually at a higher level than the tibial fracture. Union is slow and nonunion is common. The fibular fracture is generally disregarded in treatment, and attention is directed to the tibial fracture. A recent review article by Quigley and coworkers drew important conclusions from the recent literature. Rotary stress at the fracture site, shortening, and moderate angulation do not seem to be as important as had been thought and appear to be outweighed by the considerable advantages of active ambulation and almost certain union. The concept that the intact or rapidly healing fibula holds the tibial fracture faces apart and contributes to delayed or nonunion is no longer tenable.[229] This has also been borne out in a large study of 705 cases by Nicoll in England.[230] All authorities agree, however, that there is no substitute for surgical decompression of increasing pressure in closed spaces, such as the anterior compartment of the lower leg, if viable functioning muscle is to be salvaged. Garrick and associates reported in October 1972 on 655 questionnaires returned by board-certified orthopedic surgeons on their hypothetical management of a specific closed fracture located in the midshaft of the tibia and fibula. Seventy-five per cent of the respondents indicated a preference for closed methods of treatment. The most popular closed method entailed manipulative reduction and the use of a long-leg cast. It was estimated that the patient so treated would be non–weight-bearing for an average of seven weeks, after which he would be allowed to ambulate in a long-leg cast. Surgeons who elected surgical stabilization of the fracture indicated that on the average they would not begin weight-bearing any sooner than those who preferred closed methods of treatment. Only 18 per cent of the orthopedists who indicated a preference for internal stabilization of the fracture would begin weight-bearing without supplemental external immobilization.[231] The realization that early ambulation and joint mobilization can be achieved by cast-bracing has made closed treatment methods more appealing than open methods.[230, 232, 233] Sarmiento, one of the foremost advocates of this technique, in a series of 100 consecutive cases of fresh tibial fractures, concluded that healing occurred more rapidly than would be expected with immobilization. He found that this method was successful, provided good alignment of the fragments, and resulted in minimal or no shortening of the extremity. He concluded that the treatment of tibial fractures by this method has the advantage of allowing extremity activity throughout the healing process. It eliminates the need for intensive rehabilitation of the knee and thigh muscles after healing has occurred, as is necessary when fractures are treated by immobilization.[232, 233]

Although the hazards and complications of open reduction have been well reported in the literature, Müller and his associates recommend open reduction and internal fixation with compression plates.[234] Many of the fractures they treat, however, result from ski injuries and are better suited for open reduction than those resulting from more severe trauma such as occur in road accidents. Nicoll feels that the important factors in prognosis are the amount of initial displacement, the degree of comminution, the presence or absence of infection, and the severity of the soft-tissue injury, excluding infection. He found that when these factors were considered, the age of the patient (except in children), whether the fibula was also fractured, and the level of the tibial fracture did not influence prognosis. He stated that in his patients, had open reduction been contemplated, this method would have been possible in only 280 of 674 fractures. He also compared the results of open reduction with closed methods and concluded that fractures most suitable for open reduction are the same ones in which prognosis would be best were they treated by closed methods, provided the four previously mentioned factors in prognosis were considered (Fig. 3–XIII–44).[230] Sakellarides and associates reviewed 100 cases of delayed union and nonunion of tibial shaft fractures and concluded that comminution impairs healing. In this series of fractures with delayed union and nonunion, 73 per cent were located in the distal third of the tibia compared with 53 per cent in this location in another series of unselected fractures studied at the same hospital.[235, 236] The authors concluded that an open

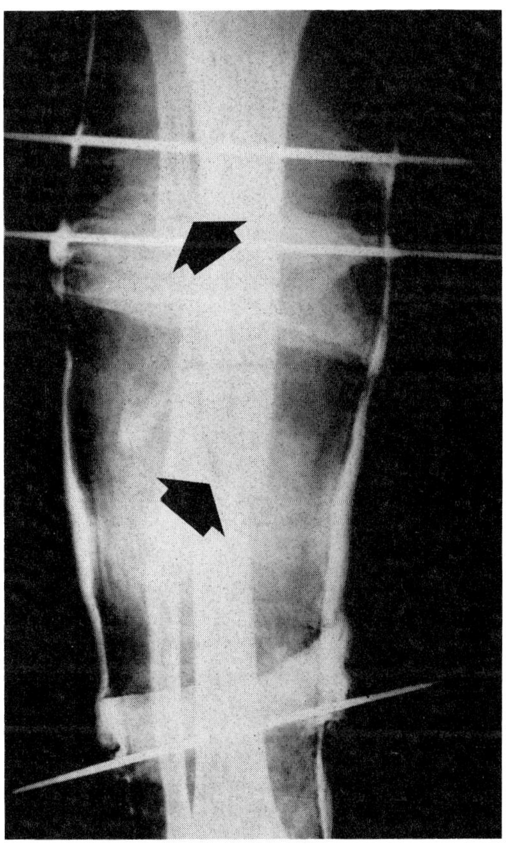

Figure 3–XIII–44. Pin in plaster immobilization of fracture of tibial shaft and proximal fibula.

fracture is a significant cause of delayed bone healing or of nonunion. Predisposing factors to nonunion in the primary management of the fracture include open reduction, infection, distraction of the fracture, and insufficient immobilization.

In a series of 60 patients with 63 open fractures of the tibial shaft treated at Fitzsimmons General Hospital, Brown and Urban concluded that early weight-bearing treatment of open fractures of the tibia produces good results. Concomitant wounds sustained at the time of fracture were allowed to heal under the cast after being dressed primarily. These authors considered wound closure less important than weight-bearing, and indicated that the final appearance of the wounds was superior or at least equal to that of wounds treated by skin grafting. Most patients achieved full weight-bearing within a few days of injury, but a few were forced to wait for as long as three weeks. The average number of cast changes required per patient was six. Brown and Urban felt that good control of correction of angulation as well as union was obtainable. All fractures united, and the shortening deformity was actually minimal compared with that associated with other forms of treatment, the average being 1 mm. In general, shortening of the fragments could not be attributed to weight-bearing. Persistent angulation or malrotation was somewhat more common, in that 44 of the 63 fractured tibiae had some residual angulation, but it was felt that with further experience with the technique, measurable angulation could be almost entirely eliminated. The average healing time was 19 weeks in this series, which compares favorably with other published series. After removal of the final cast, it was noted, significantly less time was required for rehabilitation, for building up muscle strength and tone, and for improving joint motion. The authors commented that this technique was used in a military population, but that it is certainly applicable to civilian fractures as well. The possibility of late degenerative changes of the knee or ankle, secondary to angulatory deformity of the healed fracture, must not be ignored. It will probably take many years for this to be evaluated thoroughly.

> The medical-legal aspects of shortening, angulation and rather bizarre roentgenograms are not to be discounted. It is important that the method be explained to the patient with an appraisal of possible complications in a comparison with those encountered with other methods.[237]

Patient acceptance of early weight-bearing has

been very gratifying, and, in this series, only seven patients have expressed any criticism of the end-result. This dissatisfaction was related to the cosmetic appearance of the scars.[237]

An alternative method of treatment that yields good results (other than plaster immobilization alone, cast-bracing, or internal fixation) is treatment of tibial fractures, particularly those with marked comminution, by skeletal traction in plaster. McLaughlin recommends this method even though various authors have felt that a delay in union of the fracture occurs because of distraction of the bone ends. He has felt that delayed union in tibial fractures treated by properly applied continuous traction is a

> . . . statistical figment which ignores the fundamental fact that fractures which are sufficiently shattered to require treatment by traction are likely to suffer from delayed union under any circumstances.[2]

Scudese and associates also believe in the treatment of tibial fractures by multiple pin fixation, but they advocate immediate weight-bearing and feel they obtain excellent results with this method. In their series they achieved 100 per cent healing, no shortening, and early functional recovery. There were only 3 of 75 patients who had some malrotation. The average healing time in this series was 18.5 weeks, and the authors comment that this technique is most applicable to those patients who are otherwise able to withstand the stresses of standing and weight-bearing for long periods of time each day.[238]

In fractures of the lower leg, neurovascular injuries can occur, and these should be taken into consideration in initial treatment. The method of managing the fracture should not be allowed to take precedence over treatment of neurovascular injury.[210] Ischemia in the calf gives rise to prolonged disability with joint stiffness and deformity.[239] Ellis analyzed disability after tibial shaft fractures and showed that 6 per cent of the patients had severe ankle and foot stiffness with deformity, mainly from ischemia.[240] Before arterial repair is undertaken, fractures should be fixed to facilitate immobilization and healing of the vascular repair.[241] This is true not only in the lower leg but anywhere there is peripheral vascular injury associated with fracture. Primary amputation is often the treatment of choice after severe injury to a limb, particularly the lower limb, if it appears that the patient, after a long time in the hospital and multiple reconstructive procedures, would be left with poor function or with impairment or even with absence of sensation.[242] A rare complication of closed fractures of the tibia and fibula is the formation of an arteriovenous fistula of the posterior tibial vessels.[244, 245]

After a fracture of the distal third of the tibia, a checkrein deformity of the great toe can develop. The flexor hallucis longus muscle adheres to callus at the fracture so that its tendon forms a bowstring between this point and the site of insertion of the tendon into the great toe. More common complications of fractures of the tibia and fibula not previously discussed are: traumatic arthritis of the knee, the ankle, and the tarsal bones; deformity causing painful arch strain or misalignment of weight-bearing; and ankylosis of the knee, ankle, or tarsal bones. Peroneal nerve paralysis is more apt to occur in proximal fractures or be caused by pressure of splints on the back of the head of the fibula. Weatherache at the fracture site is often a chronic recurring problem. Muscle wasting always occurs with disuse, but should cease, and strength should gradually return as function progresses. After a tibial shaft fracture has healed, if there is posterior bowing of the shaft, the tension of the calf muscles on the heel is decreased because the foot is plantar flexed. In anterior bowing, there is a bowstring effect on the heel cord, with a tendency to pull away from the lower fragment because the foot is dorsiflexed to bring it into the level of standing. McBride states that the lower the deformity of the tibial shaft, the less will be the deflection of the knee from the perpendicular weight-bearing line from the hip.[81] Deformity of the middle or the lower third of the shaft produces a misalignment that is more directly related to the ankle and the foot, but may also influence the knee or the hip.

Isolated fractures of the shaft of the fibula are rare, and displacement is seldom severe. The mechanism of injury is usually a direct blow against the outer side of the leg. If conservatively treated, these usually produce no disability. Oblique or spiral fractures are caused by some combination of leverage and rotation. These fractures, in the absence of a fracture of the tibial shaft, must be considered to be accompanied by disruption of the inferior tibiofibular syndesmosis until proved not to be, according to McLaughlin.[2] O'Donoghue feels that this is without doubt the most serious consideration in the fracture of the fibula. If a fibular fracture is accompanied by a tear of the tibiofibular ligament with resulting instability or separation of the ankle mortice, the outcome is a serious permanent disability. Stress fractures of the fibula are frequently seen, but stress fractures of the tibia are rare. Fibular stress fractures are seen in athletes early in their training period, and if found early, do well with immobilization. If the fracture is found after the time for immobilization has passed, careful muscular rehabilitation and other physical therapeutic measures should be carefully undertaken to avoid chronic muscular disability in the leg. Because the tibia is a weight-bearing bone, when a stress fracture is recognized in it, a protective cast worn until union has progressed to the point of good stability with no pain is recommended by O'Donoghue.[75]

O'Donoghue discusses *traumatic exostoses,* which frequently occur at the upper and lower ends of the tibia in athletes. He recommends a simple protective pad, and if this is not successful, surgical excision. There should be no resultant disability. If a small exostosis occurs at the upper end of the tibia directly under the pes anserinus, one of the tendons in this area may snap over the exostosis and may even catch on it. This entity should be recognized so that the condition not be misdiagnosed as a knee derangement.[75]

The Ankle

Soft-Tissue Injuries and Affections

Ankle injuries are due to the following mechanisms: abduction force, lateral rotational force, a combination of abduction and lateral rotation, adduction force, and vertical compression.[4] The last named may act singly or in combination with any of the foregoing mechanisms. The intensity of the acting forces of these mechanisms determines what injuries are produced. Moderate intensity of the acting force produces sprains in which the continuity of the ligament remains intact. Avulsion of a ligament with or without avulsion of a fragment of bone is produced by a greater intensity of the acting force. Dislocations and fracture-dislocations are produced by severe intensity of the acting force. All authors agree that the components of the ankle joint require restoration to their normal anatomical position after injury, as the ankle is a weight-bearing joint made up of many sophisticated interrelated bones and ligaments. Failure to obtain a normal anatomical position after injury results invariably in instability of the joint or posttraumatic arthritis. The arthritis is due to the incongruity of the articular surfaces. The majority of poor results follow ankle injuries because of failure to recognize and treat ligament injuries or failure to restore and maintain a normal relationship between the tibia and the talus.

Tenosynovitis. This is frequently seen about the ankle and frequently follows strain. It frequently affects the peroneal tendons and the anterior tibial tendon in ballet dancers. Irritation between the tendon and surrounding tissues causes loss of the smooth gliding pattern. Acute traumatic tenosynovitis results from acute stretching of a particular tendon. Applications of cold packs and rest of the part usually produce good results, but applications of heat and steroid infiltrations are often necessary. If the tenosynovitis becomes chronic and there is some thickening of the tendon sheath, causing stenosing tenosynovitis, the disability is more severe. Lysis of the tendon sheath may be necessary, particularly when there is constriction of the common peroneal tendons by adherence of the peroneal retinacular sheath. Release of the retinacular sheath produces relief of pain, but the peroneal tendons may be weak because they are looser than they were when the sheath was intact. This can be particularly disconcerting to dancers and athletes. After lysis of the retinacular sheath, with adequate rest, the peroneal tendons can function well. There have been many documented cases of recurrent tenosynovitis of the posterior tibial tendon. In a review of 21 cases treated at the Mayo Clinic, Ghormley and Spear found that 11 were the direct result of anomalies of the posterior tibial tendon. Accessory tendons were found that were implicated in the cause of this syndrome.[246] Tenosynovitis is seen in the sheath of the extensor digitorum longus beneath the inferior extensor retinaculum, but this tendon sheath is less frequently involved than the others previously mentioned. Repetitive occupational trauma may be so severe that acute traumatic synovitis will develop into stenosing tenosynovitis, which although relieved by conservative treatment or tendon sheath lysis, may prevent the patient from actively returning to an occupation such as professional dancing or athletics, which led to the condition.

Tendon Dislocations. *Dislocation or subluxation of the peroneal tendons* is produced by a severe blow behind the lateral malleolus while the peroneal tendons are taut in dorsiflexion and the foot is everted. One or both of the peroneal tendons pop out of the groove onto the lateral side of the malleolus when the peroneal retinaculum gives way. They usually return to place spontaneously. O'Donoghue recommends immediate surgical treatment if the diagnosis of an acute dislocation is made. He states that active athletics should not be permitted for eight weeks.[75] DuVries recommends plaster immobilization after an acute dislocation, and he feels that good results are obtained by this conservative method. Should recurrence ensue, however, he, like O'Donoghue, recommends surgical repair.[247] O'Donoghue and DuVries recommend surgical reconstruction of the groove and repair of the retinaculum when dislocation of the peroneal tendons is chronic, and they both feel that this is a very successful type of repair. Prompt relief can be expected, although six to eight weeks of immobilization is necessary for good stability.

Traumatic *dislocation of the posterior tibial tendon* at the ankle is an unusual lesion. This injury was sustained by a boy who was thrown from a motorcycle. The injury was thought to have been caused by forcible dorsiflexion of the ankle in slight inversion counteracted by a sudden pull of the tibialus posterior. No anatomical irregularities that would predispose to this injury were found at surgery. Surgical treatment involved replacing the tendon, repairing the torn retinaculum, and applying a plaster cast for 10 weeks. The final functional result was excellent.[248]

Rupture of Anterior Tibial Tendon. This rare tendon rupture usually results from a misstep that causes sudden forcible flexion or eversion of the foot. It almost always occurs at a weak point of degeneration in the tendon. McLaughlin recommends immediate operative repair. Failure to restore continuity and function of the anterior tibial tendon may produce a painful everted foot because there is no opposition to peroneal muscle action. McLaughlin states that a secure repair permits ambulation in a plaster boot during convalescence. Removal of the boot and progressive resumption of unsupported function may be allowed after two months.[2]

Calcium Deposits. Calcium deposition in tendons, particularly in the area of insertion of tendons, occurs in the ankle and foot as it does in the shoulder and arm. The most frequent location is in the peroneus longus tendon at its point of entrance into the groove on the plantar surface of the cuboid bone. Conservative treatment is usually adequate; rarely, surgical decompression is necessary.

Ganglion. A ganglion (synovial hernia) in the ankle is not particularly common, as it is in the foot or wrist. It usually occurs after direct trauma and can present itself within a week or after a long period of time—even six months after the trauma. An area of frequent ganglion formation is near the peroneal tendon distal to the lateral malleolus. Surgical excision should be complete and should include the base of the ganglion. Even with careful excision including the capsular origin, there may be recurrence.

Ligamentous Injuries of the Ankle Joint

Inversion Injuries. The ankle is functionally a hinge joint and normally permits only dorsal or plantar flexion (Fig. 3–XIII–45). Injuries to the ankle are primarily due to lateral or medial stresses that force it into positions of which it is not normally capable. Hyperflexion and hyperextension occasionally cause ankle injuries, but these are rare. O'Donoghue states that approximately 85 per cent of all injuries to the ankle are inversion injuries and are confined to ligament injury.[75] Sprains of the lateral ligaments are caused by inversion injury and are far more common than isolated sprains of the medial ligaments. Simple sprains of the lateral ligaments are relatively minor lesions, while avulsions of lateral or medial ligaments are serious lesions (Figs. 3–XIII–46 and 3–XIII–

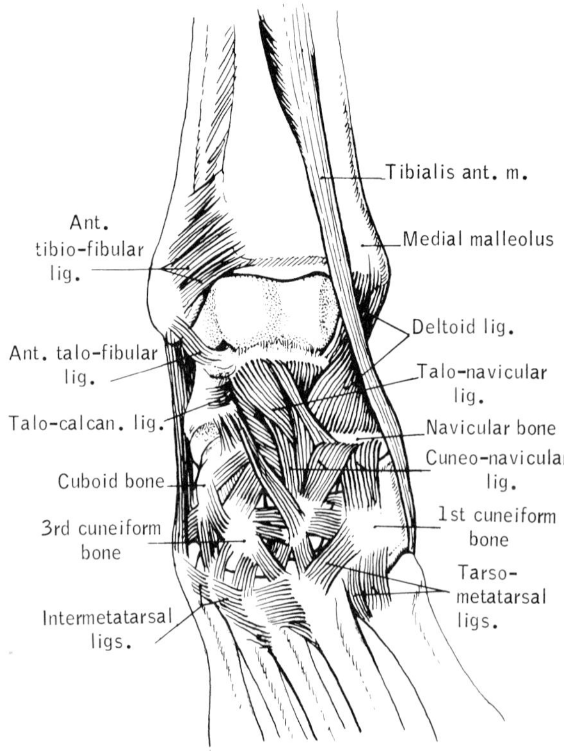

Figure 3–XIII–45. Ligaments of the ankle, anterior view. The joint capsule has been removed. (From D. H. O'Donoghue: *Treatment of Injuries to Athletes.* 3rd Edition. Philadelphia, W. B. Saunders Co., 1976. Reprinted by permission.)

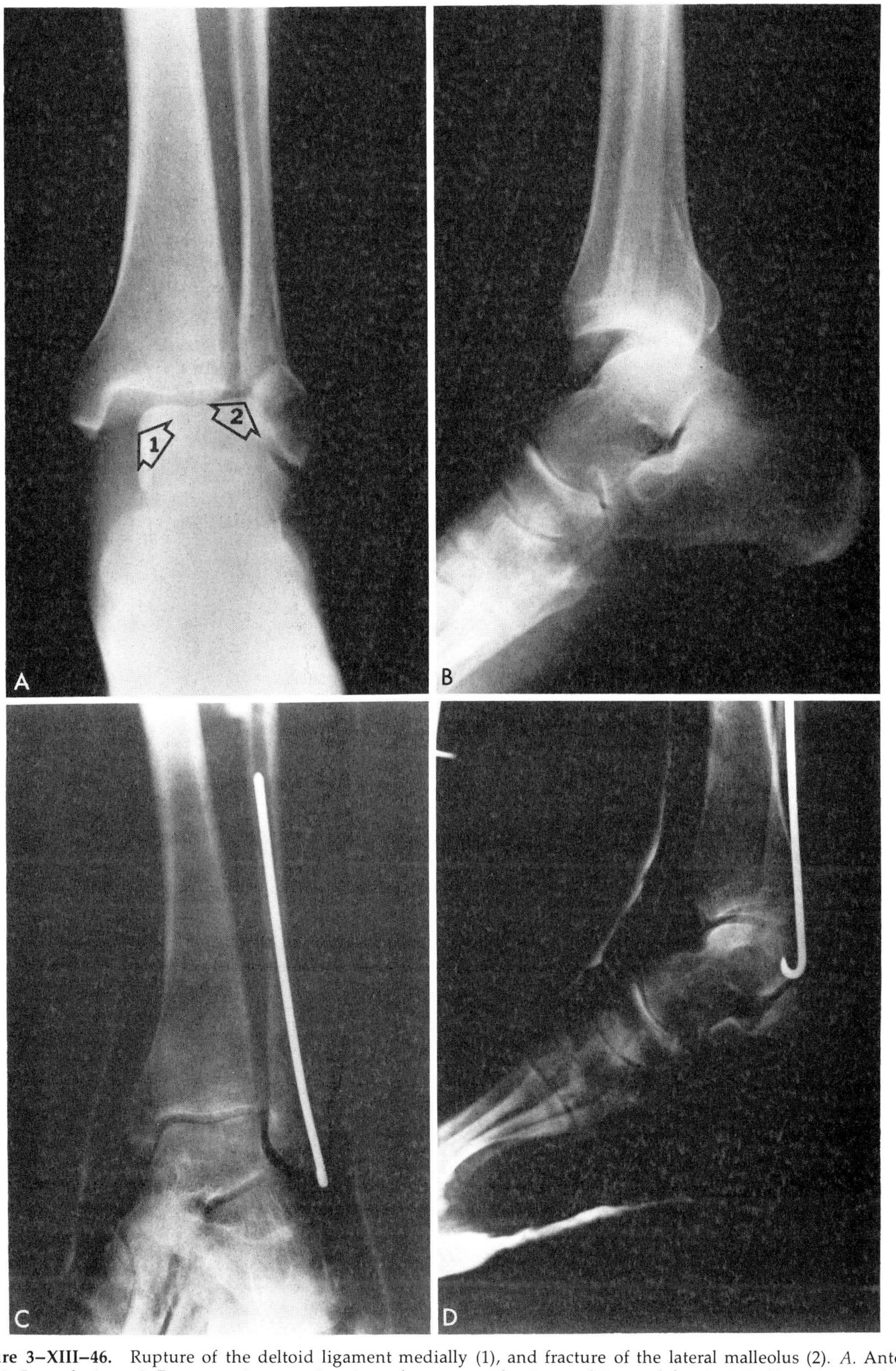

Figure 3–XIII–46. Rupture of the deltoid ligament medially (1), and fracture of the lateral malleolus (2). *A.* Anterior view. *B.* Lateral view. *C.* Postoperative anterior view after open reduction and internal fixation. *D.* Postoperative lateral view.

47). The range of ankle motion from the lateral to the medial side is greater than that from the medial to the lateral side; therefore lateral ligaments are more frequently implicated than medial ligaments. Also, as in the knee, injuries are more likely to occur from the outside, i.e., laterally, causing inversion, than from the inside, i.e., medially, causing eversion injury. Inversion injuries of the ankle, resulting in sprains of the lateral ligamentous complex, may vary from very mild to severe. The milder injuries may be treated with rest, elevation, ice packs, and ambulatory support with cane or crutches. More severe sprains may well necessitate a plaster cast for treatment. If the sprain is of the most severe type, with resulting instability of the ankle mortice and tilting of the talus evident in stress films, the ligament should probably be repaired surgically, especially in the younger patient.[1] Mild sprains, adequately

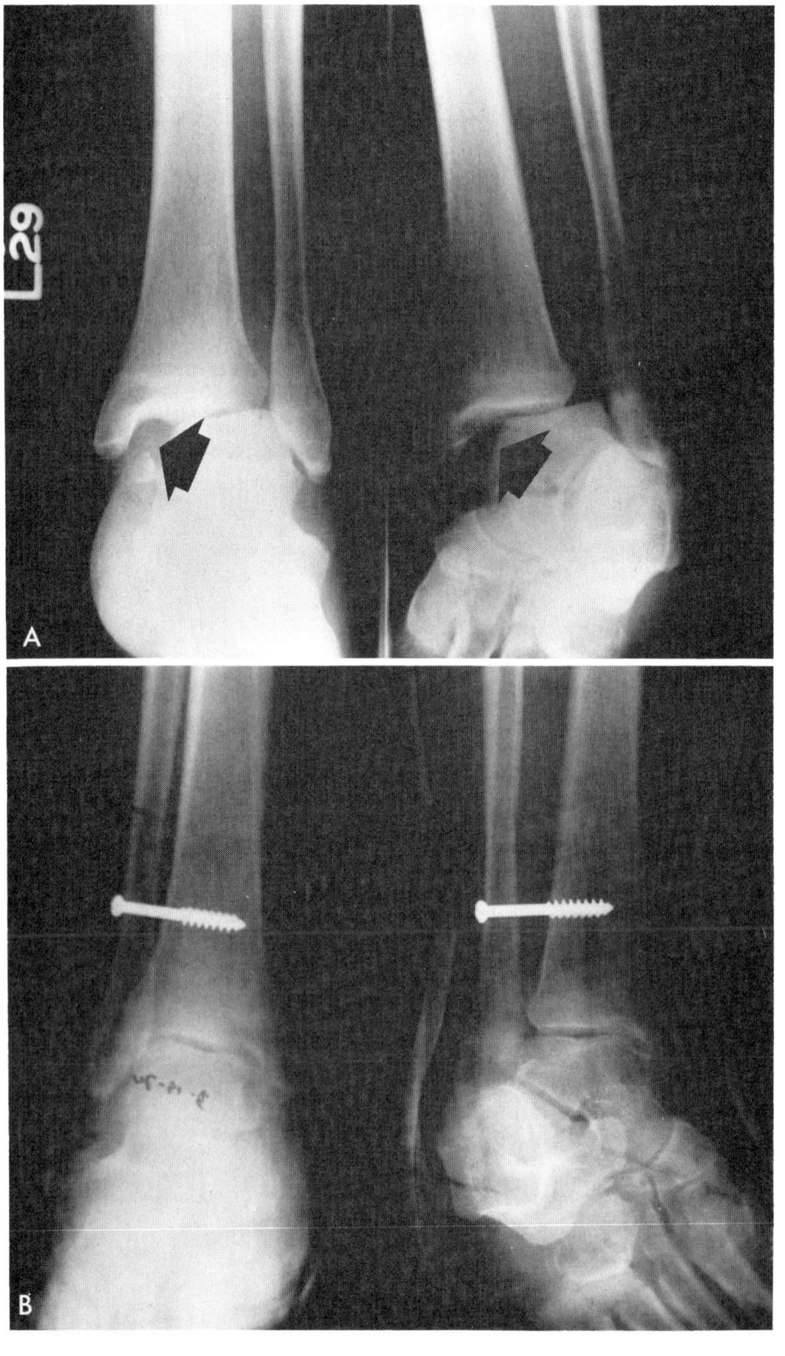

Figure 3–XIII–47. Avulsion fracture of medial malleolus with diastasis. *A.* Preoperative x-rays. *B.* Postoperative x-ray.

immobilized for sufficient time, heal without any disability. If the severity of a sprain is underestimated, however, and mobilization is too early or too active, chronic disability from weak ligaments can occur. Peroneal tenosynovitis can follow a sprain of the lateral collateral ligament. Recurrent episodes of sprain of ankle ligaments may leave these ligaments completely stretched or torn. Repetitive sprains of the ankle may result in an unstable joint. According to Bonnin, a sprained ankle can and often does lead to permanent disability.[249] Bosien and co-workers followed 133 cases of ankle sprains for over two years. Of their patients, 36 per cent had had previous injury to the same ankle, and one third of the total number of patients had continuous residual ankle symptoms.[250] The lateral ligament holds the talus against the lateral malleolus and prevents it from inverting within the mortice. When the continuity of the ligament is intact, as in a simple sprain, talar stability is not jeopardized. When the anterior band is ruptured, however, some excess mobility of the talus accompanies inversion of the foot, and slight subluxation of the talus on the tibia occurs. This is the cause of repeated sprains and patients' complaints that their ankles "turn" easily. When both the anterior and middle bands of the lateral ligaments are ruptured, the talus tends to tilt out of the malleolar mortice on inversion of the foot because the lateral stabilizers are not functioning. Failure to treat an acute *complete* rupture of the lateral ligament of the ankle correctly will result in chronic recurrent dislocations of the ankle joint. Operative reconstruction of the lateral ligament is necessary. McLaughlin states that maximal rehabilitation occurs within three or four months after this procedure, and the results are good if the operation is performed before arthritis has developed in the ankle. He states that reconstruction of the lateral ligament has consistently restored talar stability sufficient to allow a return to heavy labor. One of his patients resumed a career as a professional hockey player.[2]

Violent inversion combined with internal rotation and a forward thrust of the foot on the leg will wrench the talus from the mortice. Occasionally, this injury can cause extensive rupture of the anteroposterior and lateral ligaments and complete dislocation of the ankle without fracture. The circulation in the foot is acutely compromised, and immediate reduction is essential. Eight weeks of plaster immobilization is necessary, but there should be minimal or no disability if the injury is attended to early. If the dislocation is an open one, however, the disability can be very severe because of poor circulation, infection, or the need for skin grafting at a later date.

Eversion Injuries. Ligamentous injuries of the medial side of the ankle joint are not common. When they do occur, the injury is usually caused by sudden eversion of the foot, which subjects the deltoid ligament to a great deal of stress. If the deltoid ligament is torn, this tear is likely to be accompanied by a fracture of the tip of the medial malleolus. These injuries are most frequently accompanied by other ligamentous injuries, especially of the tibiofibular ligaments, or by fractures, usually involving the distal fibula. Accurate clinical and radiologic examinations, especially with stress x-rays, are essential to determine the nature of these injuries. With either severe inversion or eversion sprains of the ankle, the tibiofibular diastasis may be disrupted. This allows the fibula to spring away from the tibia and results in severe instability of the ankle mortice. One should be aware of possible herniation of the ankle capsule following a sprain of the anterior inferior tibiofibular ligament. This occurs particularly in severe skiing injuries. The injured anterior tibiofibular ligament may heal imperfectly, leaving a defect in the "arcuate veil" of ligaments supporting the anterior ankle joint capsule. The synovial membrane can herniate into the resulting hiatus to become pinched on dorsiflexion of the foot. Herniorrhaphy is the treatment of choice. Severe disruption of the tibiofibular syndesmosis resulting in instability of the ankle mortice should be treated by open reduction and internal fixation. McLaughlin states that early closed reduction and careful plaster immobilization produce excellent results; although the disability period is prolonged and full recovery seldom occurs within six months, he feels that closed reduction produces as good a final result as open reduction. He does state that open reduction and internal fixation of a recent diastasis reduces the period of disability.[2] The authors prefer open reduction and internal fixation for rupture of the interosseous ligaments. Colton emphasizes the need for anatomical reposition of the structures about the ankle. He notes that a displacement of the lower end of the fibula of the order of 2 to 3 mm in an anteroposterior or lateral direction can cause considerable alteration in the mechanics of the ankle joint and predispose to osteoarthritis. For this reason, he advocates open reduction and internal fixation for the best possible anatomical repositioning.[252]

O'Donoghue makes special mention of dorsiflexion injury of the ankle because it is an injury frequently seen in athletes. He states that it is a type of eversion injury and is significant because it accounts for a relative frequency with which calcification is noted between the tibia and fibula in x-rays of the ankle, because calcification is prone to occur where chronic irritation takes place. This chronic condition is discouraging because it carries permanent disability. O'Donoghue does not recommend excision of the calcification unless there is separation between the tibia and fibula, or intractable pain on ankle motion.[75]

Ankle Fractures

Isolated Fractures of the Medial Malleolus. Adduction stress will shear off the medial malleolus. Abduction stress will produce transverse fractures of the malleolus. DePalma and other authors mention that a periosteal flap often drops between the fractured surfaces, preventing reduction and bony union. Conservative methods are usually adequate, but operative intervention with internal fixation is recommended for displaced fractures or fractures of the medial malleolus at the level of the "shoulder" of the malleolus or above. After closed reduction of a simple medial malleolus fracture, fibrous union may occur, producing instability of the ankle medially. When this is symptomatic, operative intervention with internal fixation and excision of the fibrous tissue may be necessary. Bone grafting may be required. It should be noted that whenever there is an isolated malleolar fracture, one should look carefully for ligamentous injury on the other side of the ankle; such injury often accompanies a single malleolar fracture. When the medial malleolus is fractured, there is usually no injury to the deltoid ligament. One should suspect deltoid ligament injury when there is no medial malleolus fracture but there is an injury to the lateral side of the joint, particularly if the injury is a fracture of the distal fibula. If the tip of the malleolus is fractured, there is likely to be an attendant deltoid weakness because the deltoid ligament is attached to the fractured tip and loses its ability to maintain medial stability of the ankle. Nonunion of the avulsed tip with its attached intact deltoid ligament requires more plaster immobilization until healing occurs. If healing does not occur, surgical reconstruction may be necessary. Otherwise, there will be continuing medial instability of the ankle. Fibrous union of a malleolus allows for shifting of the talus: medially when there is fibrous union of the medial malleolus, and laterally when there is fibrous union of the lateral malleolus. Chronic pain ensues with eventual degenerative arthritis.

Isolated Fractures of the Lateral Malleolus. Fracture of the lateral malleolus alone is caused by an abduction force or more frequently by a lateral rotational force.[4] The lateral malleolus may often be avulsed by an adduction force. Abduction produces a spiral fracture at the level of the tibiofibular joint. The talus does not shift because the ligaments of the joint are intact. There is usually no displacement of the malleolar fragment. As in an isolated fracture of the medial malleolus, one should be aware of the possibility of rupture of contralateral ligaments, particularly when the fracture is unstable. McLaughlin states that the contralateral ligaments should be "considered ruptured until it is proved otherwise in every instance of an unstable fracture of one malleolus."[2] In a discussion of nonunion of malleolar fractures of the ankle, Mendelsohn reviewed much of the available literature on ankle fractures. In his studies he found that nonunion of the medial malleolus can be present in a stable painless ankle and that open surgery for such ununited fractures is rarely necessary. In his series of 253 ankle fractures, he found 10 nonunited fractures of the medial malleolus and two of the lateral malleolus. All were treated primarily by closed reduction and plaster immobilization. The two ununited fractures of the lateral malleolus were associated with severe pain and disability, requiring extensive reconstructive surgery. He concluded that failure of union of malleolar fractures can be related to loss of talotibial (foot-leg) alignment, early or late. This may be a source of persistent and profound disability.[253]

It is very common to have lateral displacement of the talus with a fracture of the lateral malleolus. The lateral malleolus sustains a spiral fracture at the level of the tibiofibular joint, and the medial ligament is ruptured. Mortice diastasis is evident on x-ray because there is a widening of more than 5 mm medially. In any ankle fracture it is imperative to ascertain the status of the mortice, as widening here is ample evidence of severe ankle injury and instability. Anatomical reduction is essential when there is widening of the mortice, and if closed reduction is not adequate, open reduction is recommended. If the widening is not recognized soon after injury and the fracture remains unreduced for some time, one cannot expect a satisfactory ankle, even after reconstructive procedures. Ligaments are torn or stretched, fibrous union occurs, and degenerative arthritis develops.

Bimalleolar Fractures of the Ankle. Bimalleolar, or Pott's, fractures of the ankle are unstable. Closed reduction may be sufficient for some of them; however, open reduction may well be necessary if closed reduction is unsuccessful because of either massive soft-tissue swelling or interposition of soft parts. A long-term follow-up of 55 patients with displaced bimalleolar fractures showed that the open and closed methods had the same incidence of degenerative joint disease.[154] The mechanism of injury of bimalleolar fractures may be either inversion or eversion; one of the malleoli is avulsed by traction on the ligaments, and the other one is fractured by direct pressure from the tilting talus. Closed reduction of bimalleolar fractures can be accomplished, but it is certainly much more difficult than closed reduction of unimalleolar fractures. If anatomical reduction is not accomplished, open reduction is necessary. The consequences of inadequate anatomical repositioning of the ankle bones are those mentioned previously: pain, instability, and degenerative arthritis.

When a patient sustains a fracture of the fibula above the level of the tibiofibular joint, and there is an associated medial malleolar fracture or deltoid tear, one should suspect diastasis of the tibiofibular joint. This lesion is the result of a severe abduction stress. The talus is displaced laterally. This fracture-dislocation is very unstable and is best treated by open reduction and internal fixation. In order to restore the proper dynamic stability of the ankle, the internal fixation device used for closure of the diastasis should be removed after the interosseus ligament has healed, usually after six weeks.

Colton studied 46 cases of closed Dupuytren fracture-dislocations of the ankle joint in adults. This injury is a disruption of the medial structures of the ankle (either a ruptured medial ligament or a traction fracture of the medial malleolus), together with total rupture of the inferior tibiofibular joint and an indirect fracture of the fibula above the syndesmosis (Fig. 3–XIII–48). Twenty of the cases were treated closed and 26 were treated by internal fixation. Colton's analysis revealed that the results of internal fixation were superior to those of closed treatment. As in other ankle fractures, production and maintenance of an anatomical reduction of the fracture fragments gave the best chance of achieving a good final result. Colton stated in his article that this series did not answer the question of whether it is harmful to insert a screw from the fibula into the tibia across the syndesmosis. Twenty-three patients underwent screw fixation, and all but one had the screw removed between 8 and 14 weeks after injury. One patient retained the screw in the fibula and tibia for three and a half years after injury and had no complaints whatsoever. None of the patients had synostosis of the inferior tibiofibular joint. X-rays showed evidence of loosening of the screw in the fibula. Colton quoted other authors who found little disability from leaving the screw, but it was his opinion that it is "probably prudent to remove the screw at a later date" after its insertion.[252] We agree.

Trimalleolar Fractures of the Ankle. Trimalleolar, or Cotton, fractures of the ankle are those in which both malleoli (medial and lateral) are fractured, as well as the posterior lip of the tibia (Fig. 3–XIII–49). Most of these fractures require open reduction and internal fixation. If the fractured posterior lip of the tibia constitutes less than 10 per cent of the articular surface, it may be left as is, and attention may be directed to repair of the medial-lateral instability of the ankle joint. If the posterior lip fracture involves 25 per cent or more of the articular surface, it must be anatomically reduced and internally fixed. If the portion of the articular surface involved lies between 10 and 25 per cent, accurate examination of the open ankle joint is necessary. If there is a tendency to subluxation of the talus in the mortice, repositioning of the posterior fragment and internal fixation are necessary. Occasionally the posterior tibial tendon may be found within the ankle joint. There is almost inevitably a subluxation of the talus within the mortice; and indeed, sometimes the talus may be completely dislocated. Because of the severe forces that produce this injury, as in bimalleolar fractures, multiple cartilaginous or osteocartilaginous chips are frequently avulsed from the dome of the talus. These may lead to subsequent degenerative arthritis of the ankle joint.

Compression Fractures of the Tibia. Vertical compression fractures of the distal end of the tibia are usually caused by a fall from a height. Hyper-plantar flexion or hyperdorsiflexion can also cause them—as seen in firemen who catch the heel on the rung of a ladder. Fractures of the calcaneus and the tibial spine are frequently concomitant injuries. In fractures of the anterior margin of the tibia with forward displacement of the foot, the prognosis is good with correct treatment. Severe comminution of the whole inferior articular surface of the tibia, however, has a poor prognosis, regardless of management. Fractures of the anterior surface of the tibia with forward displacement of the

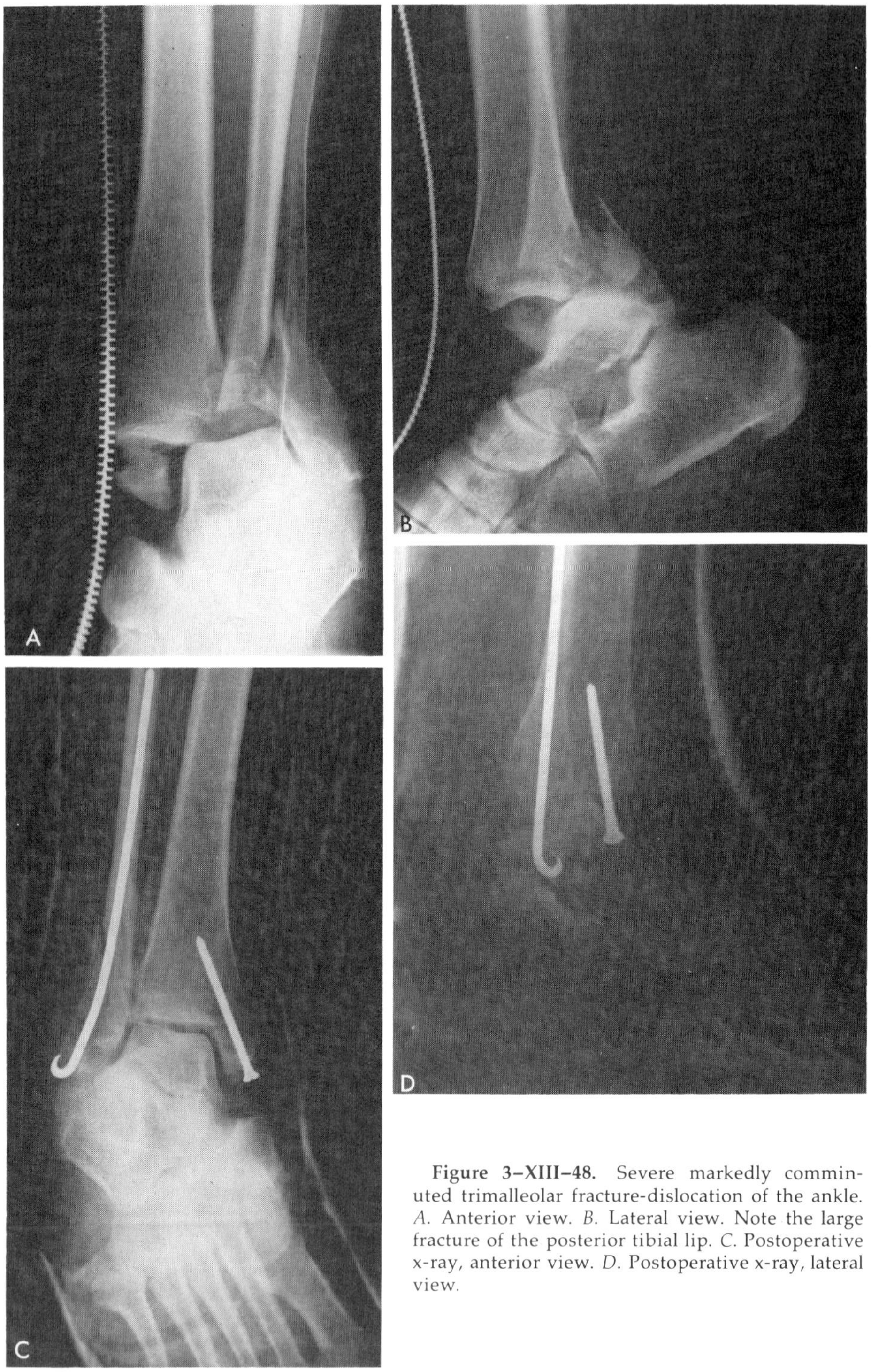

Figure 3–XIII–48. Severe markedly comminuted trimalleolar fracture-dislocation of the ankle. *A.* Anterior view. *B.* Lateral view. Note the large fracture of the posterior tibial lip. *C.* Postoperative x-ray, anterior view. *D.* Postoperative x-ray, lateral view.

talus are usually well treated by open reduction and internal fixation. Occasionally, manipulation alone produces a satisfactory result. It is imperative to replace the talus accurately in relation to the articular surface of the tibia. An "explosion fracture" of the distal tibia may include fracture of the lateral and medial malleoli. Severe comminution of the inferior articular surface of the tibia occurs, and restoration of a smooth articular surface is impossible by either closed or open methods. Fusion of the ankle joint is the procedure of choice.

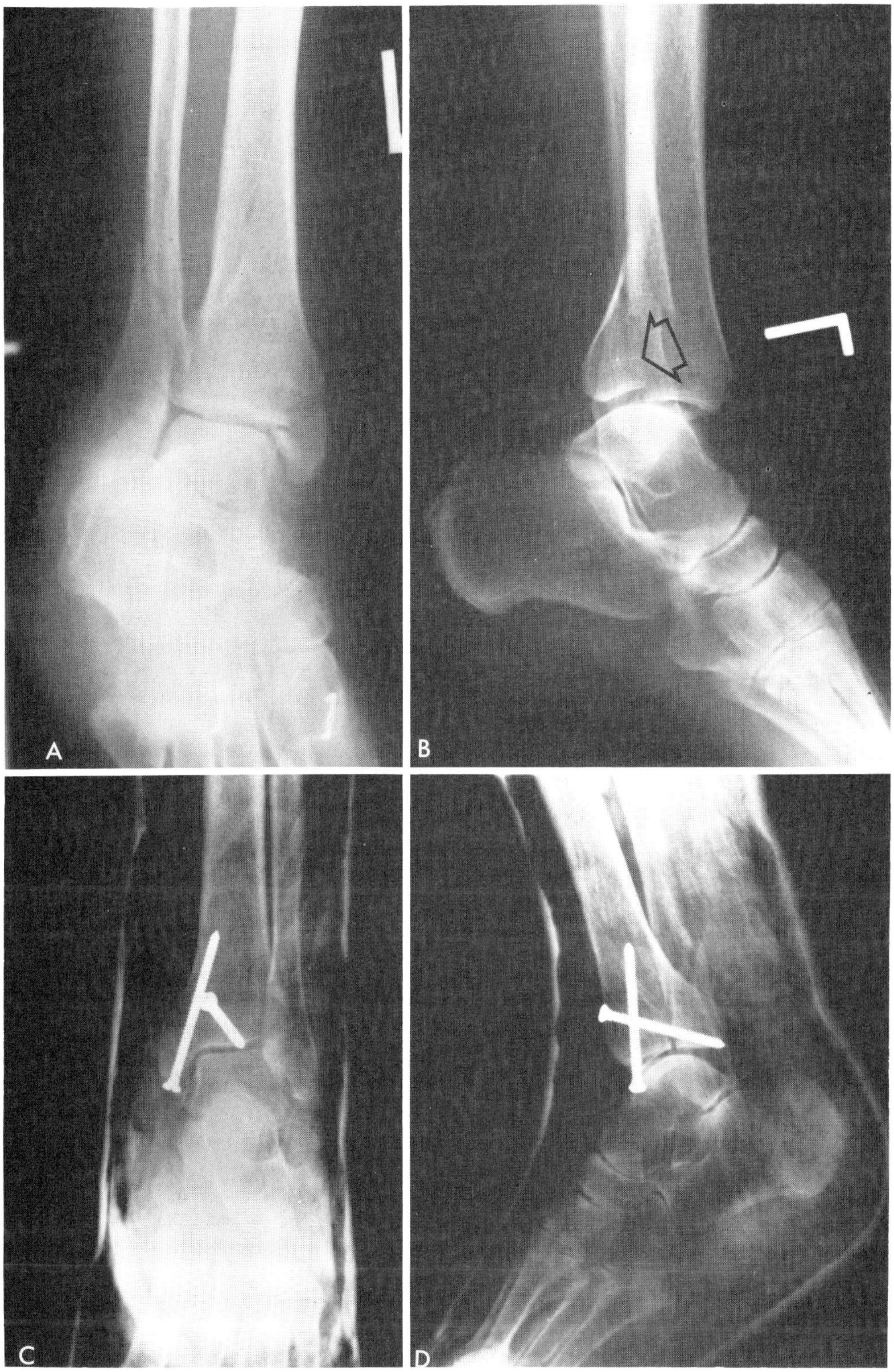

Figure 3–XIII–49. Trimalleolar fracture of the ankle. *A.* Anterior view. *B.* Lateral view. Note the large posterior lip fracture involving the articular surface (arrow). *C.* Postoperative anterior view. *D.* Postoperative lateral view. Although the reduction is good, the diastasis between the posterior lip fracture and the tibia predisposes to posttraumatic arthritis.

Compression fractures of the tibia are prone to ankle instability and degenerative arthritis.

Fracture of the Dome of the Talus. The dome of the talus is the part of the talus that articulates with the ankle mortice formed by the lower articular surfaces of the tibia and fibula. The injury usually results from an inversion injury of the ankle, and the possibility of its presence should be borne in mind whenever there is a strain of the lateral ligament of the ankle. A large dome fracture with displacement should be accurately reduced by open operation in order to preserve congruity of the joint surface.[255] Conservative treatment is sufficient for a small fracture with no displacement. A small fracture with marked displacement is best treated by early excision of the fragment to prevent further damage to the ankle joint. Chondral fractures of the talus are often unrecognized until osteochondritis dissecans ensues. Untreated, unrecognized chondral fracture can result in degenerative arthritis and severe disability, often requiring open intervention.

Complete Ankle Dislocation

Posterior dislocation of the ankle joint is a rare lesion but is the most common of all dislocations of the ankle joint. This lesion is the result of severe plantar flexion of the foot with a strong forward thrust of the leg. This dislocation is usually accompanied by a fracture of one or both malleoli or a posterior marginal fracture of the tibia. As in all dislocations of the ankle, vascular compromise is the major problem. Reduction should be performed as early as possible after the injury is sustained. Closed reduction is usually sufficient unless there are associated malleolar fractures that require open reduction. Anterior dislocation of the ankle joint is also rare, and is produced by forcible dorsiflexion of the foot or a fall on the heel with the foot in dorsiflexion. It is frequently accompanied by a fracture of the anterior margin of the tibia or of one or both malleoli. Lateral dislocation of the ankle joint is always associated with fractures of the malleoli and may be the result of adductive, rotational, or abductive stresses. Open reduction is usually necessary. Anatomical reduction is desired here as in other injuries of the ankle; otherwise, degenerative arthritis or instability may occur.

Exostoses of the Ankle Joint

An exostosis is an accumulation of bone at the site of an irritation and characteristically develops as a response to direct trauma. It is frequently seen at the top of the talus or in front of the tibia, and is described as a talotibial exostosis. It is less frequently seen anterior to the medial malleolus or the lateral malleolus, where it is due to impingement of the talus. Repeated hyperflexion, hyperextension, hyperinversion, or hypereversion of the ankle joint beyond the ordinary range produces posttraumatic exostoses. These can break off to become loose bodies superior to the talar neck or elsewhere. If exostoses are asymptomatic, nothing need be done. If they are disabling, however, excision is recommended. After removal, little or no disability should be expected. O'Donoghue distinguishes an exostosis from a marginal osteophyte. He states that a marginal osteophyte is an osteochondral ridge developing at the joint margin as a result of chronic synovitis or a chronic arthritic change. Débridement of marginal osteophytes has little effect on chronic arthritis that is present, and the results will prove disappointing.[75]

The Foot

Soft-Tissue Injuries

Strain of the foot is common, particularly in the Achilles tendon and the anterior tibial tendon. Less frequently there is strain of the peroneal tendons at their attachment, or of the posterior tibial and flexor tendons of the toes. Immobilization either by strapping or by plaster is necessary, and occasionally steroid infiltrations into a strained tendon may be expedient, particularly in an athlete or dancer who must continue his game or performance. Sufficient rest of the strained part is essential for complete recovery. Otherwise there will be continuous disability from the attenuated tendon. O'Donoghue distinguishes between static sprain and the acute traumatic sprain. He states that acute traumatic sprain is caused by violent overstretching of a ligament when the involved joint is forced through a wider range of motion than the ligaments will normally permit. Chronic traumatic sprain is caused by the same force being applied repeatedly. He defines static sprain as injury due to the constant stress of superimposed weight on the arch of the foot. This is most frequently manifested by pain along the plantar ligament from its attachment to the calcaneus to its attachment near the metatarsal heads. Static sprain is promptly relieved by elimination of weight-bearing. O'Donoghue recommends that traumatic sprain be treated as any other sprain, with compression, application of cold packs, and immobilization as necessary, followed by local heat application. Traumatic sprain usually takes longer to resolve than static sprain.[75]

Tenosynovitis and Bursitis. Tenosynovitis in the foot is common, and the cause is the same as in other locations—direct injury or chronic overuse. Treatment is as previously discussed, and once recovery is complete, strapping is important to prevent recurrence. If strapping is inadequate, a plaster cast may be necessary for complete immobilization to expedite recovery. Bursitis of the foot is infrequent. The only constant anatomical bursal sac in the foot is the retrocalcaneal bursa, which is situated between the posterosuperior surface of the calcaneus and the Achilles tendon. The etiology of this bursitis includes tension from a tight heel cord, friction, and pressure from the shoe counter, possibly followed by secondary infection. Conservative treatment is usually adequate, but if necessary, bursal excision is recommended. Results are excellent, but even after surgical excision, use of protective padding is recommended. Repetitive trauma can cause bursitis in other areas, such as above the tendo Achillis insertion or under the first metatarsal head. Again, whether treatment is conservative or surgical, adequate protection of the area after resolution of the bursitis has occurred is recommended. Otherwise, the patient will have continuing disability in the area and subsequent recurrence of his difficulty.

Fascial Hernia. DuVries discusses fascial hernia of the foot. When this occurs, there is a protrusion of the soft subfascial tissues. Fascial hernia may be asymptomatic, but if it is symptomatic, repair is recommended. The results are good. Fascial hernias have been found particularly on the dorsolateral aspect of the foot, especially over the tarsal bone, where the extensor brevis digitorum muscle may herniate. The herniation simulates a ganglion or lipoma. Ganglion of the foot is common because of the multiplicity of joints and tendons in the foot. Chronic sprain followed by weakness of the capsule and herniation of the synovium may occur. Foot ganglia are frequently seen near the peroneal tendon distal to the lateral malleolus and the dorsum of the foot in the long extensor tendons, where they may come off the tendon sheath or from the tarsal joints. The treatment and prognosis of ganglia are as previously discussed. Recurrence of ganglion formation in the foot is quite probable, because ganglia in this area are often multilocular and have ducts that lead to other sacs in the plantar fascial planes. This is particularly true of ganglia that occur in the metatarsal interspace.[247]

Neuralgia. *Plantar digital neuritis*, known also as Morton's toe, Morton's metatarsalgia, neurofibroma, and neurinoma, results from the development of a neuroma in a digital nerve just proximal to its point of bifurcation and is associated with severe neuralgic pain in the distal end of the sole and referred to the corresponding two toes. It can be caused by trauma, particularly repetitive trauma. Walking on hard floors or standing for long periods predisposes to this condition. Complete relief is obtained by excision of the entire involved nerve. *Causalgia* is a neuralgia characterized by constant intense local pain and burning, which may be accompanied by local skin changes such as redness and vesicle formation.[247] This syndrome is associated with lesions of the nerves that can result from accidental or surgical trauma to a peripheral nerve containing sensory fibers. Sudeck's atrophy, or severe osteoporosis, can be due to causalgia. A seemingly minor sprain of the foot or ankle can cause this entity. Sympathetic block is a valuable diagnostic and prognostic test as well as a therapeutic measure. Lumbar sympathectomy is often necessary for intractable causalgia. Sympathectomy performed at an early age produces good results, but the pain may still remain to some extent. Permanent trophic changes and deformity may develop if there is a delay in performing surgery, once the diagnosis of causalgia has been made.

Nerve Entrapment Syndromes

Entrapment of the *posterior tibial nerve* underneath the flexor retinaculum at the ankle has been called the tarsal tunnel syndrome.[255-262] Any surface trauma may trap the major cutaneous nerve trunks such as the posterior tibial nerve, or the entrapment may be secondary to any space-occupying lesion. It should be noted that space-occupying lesions may include scarring secondary to trauma. According to Kopell, the best-known example of involvement of the posterior tibial nerve occurs as a result of a regional "spacial alteration" caused by a fracture or a dislocation involving the malleoli, talus, or calcaneus.[12] Entrapment of this nerve causes burning pain involving the toes and sole of the foot. If the posterior tibial nerve is entrapped by scar tissue, and conservative treatment is not effective, surgical intervention may be indicated. The surgical intervention may give complete relief of symptoms, but the scar tissue may return and entrap the nerve again.

The *deep peroneal nerve* can be entrapped in its terminal portion on the dorsum of the foot.

This is a frequently unrecognized complication of a direct blow to the dorsum of the foot. The deep peroneal nerve lies on bone with very thin overlying tissue; therefore, direct trauma can easily injure it. Repetitive trauma from a poorly designed shoe or cast can cause entrapment. Pressure on the nerve can result from a ganglion arising from the tarsal bones. Rest and removal of external pressure are usually sufficient treatment. Otherwise, operative intervention is recommended.

Forced plantar flexion, or inversion twist of the ankle and foot, can cause entrapment of the *superficial peroneal nerve*. Conservative treatment is usually adequate, but as in other situations, surgery is sometimes necessary. A thorough local fascial release is usually recommended, but if this is inadequate, the involved portion of the nerve should be resected. An area of skin anesthesia results. Occasionally, branches of the sural or medial plantar nerves may be involved by subcutaneous scarring from direct trauma.

Metatarsalgia

Turek defines metatarsalgia as pain about the distal end of the foot at the metatarsophalangeal junctions.[38] This entity is caused by various factors. Trauma is certainly one of them. Prolonged walking can cause a sprain of the transverse metatarsal ligament; direct impact, as from a heavy object dropped on the foot or a fall from a height, can cause a contusion over the metatarsal heads dorsally or on the plantar aspect, depending upon where the impact occurs. Metatarsalgia can result from malunion of metatarsal fractures.

Plantar Fasciitis

Plantar fasciitis, also known as policeman's heel, deck feet, and other eponyms, is seen in people who spend a great deal of time on their feet. This disease is characterized by pain under the calcaneus at the origin of the plantar fascia. It is generally felt that it is due to microtears within the origin of the plantar fascia. The plantar fascia, in pulling away from its origin, may produce a traction spur that can be seen on roentgenograms. This entity frequently responds to conservative therapy. If the pain is unrelenting and conservative therapy is not effective, however, surgical intervention may be indicated. Results of treatment are usually satisfactory; however, repeated trauma may reactivate the condition. Fibromatosis of the plantar fascia *(Dupuytren's contracture)* is characterized by the invasion of fibromatosis in the plantar fascia. The cause is obscure. Skoog, in his 1948 review, listed multiple causes, one of which was trauma. Many others were suggested, however, and are probably more important in the etiology of Dupuytren's contracture than is trauma. These other causes include neuropathy, gout, rheumatism, endocrinopathy, local infection, and tuberculosis.[262]

Foot Sprain

Foot sprain usually consists of an injury to the ligaments supporting the intertarsal or tarsometatarsal joints. Overstretching of ligaments can cause avulsion of small bone chips; a wrenching or twisting injury causes sprain. Acute traumatic sprain of the foot is similar to sprain elsewhere and is usually caused by violent overstretching of ligaments. The involved joint is forced through a wider range of motion than the retaining ligaments will normally permit. O'Donoghue makes a distinction between chronic sprain of the foot and static sprain of the arch. He states that chronic sprain is due to frequent repeated episodes of overmotion, and static sprain is due to constant stress of superimposed weight on the arch of the foot.[75] Other authors refer to this syndrome as plantar fasciitis, as previously discussed. Another type of chronic sprain is produced by forces applied to the intermetatarsal ligaments by standing for a long time. Static stretching of the ligaments occurs between the metatarsal heads and results in a severe incapacitating type of pain.

Dislocations of the Foot

The Talus. *Total dislocation* of the talus is produced by forceful inversion-adduction and plantar flexion of the foot. According to DePalma, both the lateral ligaments of the ankle joint and the interosseous ligaments of the subtalar joint are ruptured.[4] In this rare injury, the circulation of the talus is markedly embarrassed, predisposing it to development of avascular necrosis. Closed or open dislocations must be reduced immediately to prevent further circulatory disturbance. *Anterior dislocation* of the talus occurs when the dorsiflexed foot is driven forward from the tibia. The talus, as it is displaced, usually fractures the anterior lip of the tibia. Avascular necrosis in this type of dislocation is an uncommon sequela. This is because the primary blood supply to the talus is subtalar and the subtalar joint is intact. *Lateral dislocation* of the talus is also uncommon; in this injury the medial collateral and the anterior and posterior capsular ligaments of the ankle are widely disrupted. The talus swings out of the malleolar mortice on the hinge of the intact lateral collateral ligaments. *Medial dislocation* is even more uncommon according to McLaughlin. In lateral or medial dislocations of the talus, all nutrient vessels to the talus except those entering the plantar surface, and possibly the intact dorsalis pedis branch, are completely disrupted. McLaughlin states that in a few cases that have been encountered in which reduction was immediately performed, avascular necrosis did not occur.[2] As previously stated, immediate reduction is essential, not only to preserve the talus but also to preserve the blood supply to the foot.

Subtalar dislocation is due to eversion, abduction, and forced plantar flexion of the foot, all acting simultaneously. The interosseous ligaments of the subtalar joint are ruptured and the foot is dislocated medially about the talus. The talus remains in the ankle mortice but is forced into equinus position. DePalma recommends checking for associated fractures of the head of the talus or of the navicular in subtalar dislocations.[4] The blood supply to the talus enters inferiorly through the subtalar ligaments; subtalar dislocations disrupt that blood supply, and there is a high rate of incidence of avascular necrosis of the talus following these injuries. If avascular necrosis of the talus does occur, surgery is probably indicated and may be either talectomy, bone grafting, or pantalar arthrodesis.[264]

Tarsal, Metatarsal, and Phalangeal Joints. The midtarsal joint is composed of the talonavicular and the calcaneocuboid joints. Partial or complete *dislocations of the midtarsal joint* occur after severe torsional stresses. Associated fractures of the tarsal bones are frequently seen, particularly of the navicular or cuboid bones. One should direct one's attention to reduction of the dislocation and pay little attention to the fracture in treatment. A primary surgical arthrodesis is occasionally necessary when there is severe disruption of the joints. As in previously mentioned dislocations, immediate reduction is recommended. Open reduction should be performed if manipulative reduction was not done immediately after the diagnosis was made and time has passed since the initial injury. Occasionally, open reduction may be indicated because the tendons to the foot become looped around the neck of the talus and the dislocation cannot be reduced in a closed fashion. Exceedingly rare injuries involving isolated dislocations of the navicular, cuneiforms, and cuboid are documented by individual case reports in the literature. These injuries must be individually assessed and treated.[265, 266]

Tarsometatarsal dislocation is usually the result of an indirect force that is exerted through the metatarsals with the foot in a plantar-flexed position. One or all of the metatarsal bones are then dislocated dorsally and subsequently displaced laterally or medially. This is potentially a particularly dangerous type of dislocation because of possible arterial spasm and thrombosis of the main plantar vessels. Frequently, good results can ensue from simple manipulative reduction, but if closed reduction fails, surgical reduction is indicated. Dislocations may occur also at any of the *metatarsophalangeal joints* or the *interphalangeal joints* of any of the toes. By far the most important joints are the metatarsophalangeal joint and the interphalangeal joint of the great toe. Most of the dislocations can be reduced in a closed fashion, but occasionally there is buttonholing of the capsule and open reduction may be necessary. Indeed, with complete dislocations of some of the minor interphalangeal joints, such as the distal joint of the fifth toe, there may be completely normal function of the foot with no disability.

Fractures of the Foot

The Talus. Fractures of the dome of the talus have been previously discussed. Fracture of the *posterior process* of the talus is usually the result of forceful plantar flexion of the foot. One has to be careful not to mistake the os trigonum, an anomalous bone, for a fracture of the posterior process. Closed reduction and plaster immobilization are usually satisfactory for treatment without subsequent disability.

Fracture of the *body of the talus* is rare and results from falling from a height. The talus is compressed between the tibia and the calcaneus. A vertical fracture is usually sustained, and occasionally the inferior or superior surfaces of the talus are disrupted. If there is no fracture into the joint, reduction and plaster immobilization are satisfactory. If there is fracture into the joint, however, as in any other fracture, posttraumatic arthritis may occur. The body of the talus may be fractured transversely as well as longitudinally. A tense hemarthrosis is usually present unless the joint capsule has been ruptured. Vascular embarrassment can occur and should be treated appropriately. Displaced fractures often require open reduction. Impacted fractures in reasonably good alignment should not be disimpacted, but should be immobilized in the position of impaction. McLaughlin states, however, that this impaction is an invitation to avascular necrosis of the posterior segment of the fracture.[2] The more posterior the fracture line, the greater is the danger of avascular necrosis of the posterior fragment. If this fragment is to survive, accurate reduction and secure fixation are necessary. Weight-bearing is best deferred until there is complete union. If there is evidence of progressing avascular necrosis, one should consider tibiotalar arthrodesis, because once avascular necrosis is established, it is probable that arthrodesis will be required at a later date. According to Parkes, the development of avascular necrosis is due to several factors. The blood supply to the body of the talus is derived primarily from the medial capsule of the ankle, where it attaches to the articular surface, as well as from the anterior capsule, where it attaches to the superior surface of the neck, and in the area of the sinus tarsi. If more than two thirds of the blood supply is interrupted, avascular necrosis is likely to occur.[267] If the fracture is associated with subtalar dislocation, more than 80 per cent of patients will develop avascular necrosis of the talus.[268] Mechanical incongruity of the ankle and the subtalar joint will occur if comminution or displacement is not accurately reduced. This will require pantalar arthrodesis. Even if there is anatomical alignment of the fragments, the prognosis is only fair.

Fractures of the talus at the neck constitute approximately 30 per cent of talus fractures (Fig. 3–XIII–50).[269] The basic cause is excessive extension. When the ankle joint reaches its maximum limit of extension, the talar neck is brought into contact with the anterior lip of the tibia. Further motion in this direction leads to fracture of the talar neck. The fracture will remain undisplaced if the force stops at this level. If the extension force continues, comminution of the fracture fragments ensues. A vertical fracture through the neck of the talus is produced by forcible dorsiflexion of the foot. This mechanism forces the neck of the talus against the anterior margin of the tibia. DePalma emphasizes that backward displacement of the body of the talus often occurs; in fact, "it is the rule rather than the exception."[4]

When there is no displacement of the fracture, plaster immobilization is adequate treat-

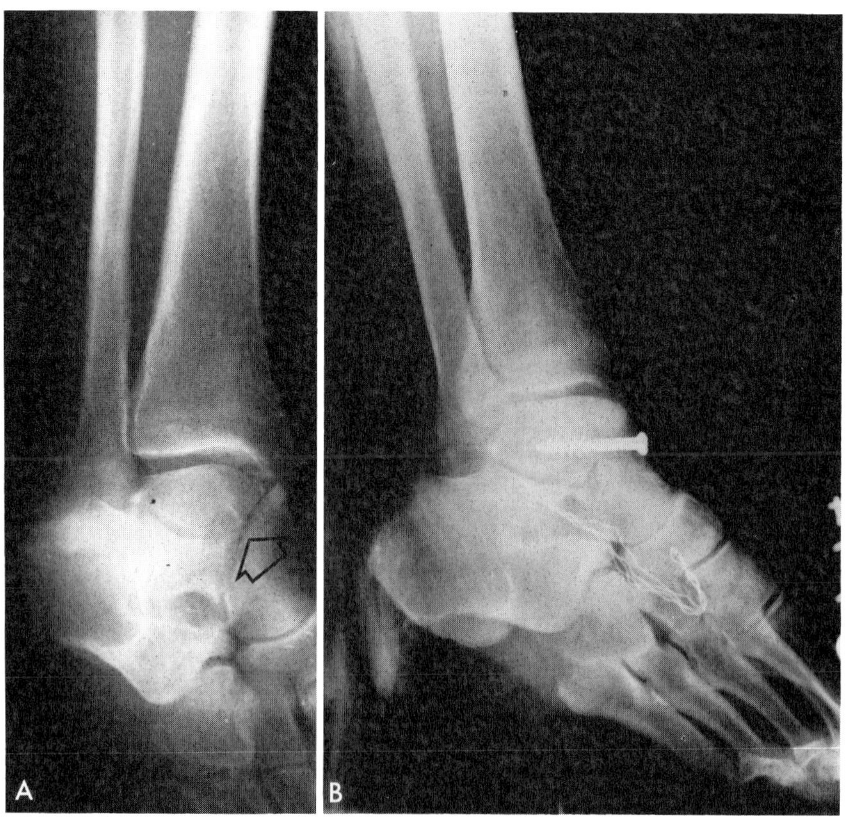

Figure 3–XIII–50. Fracture of the neck of the talus. *A.* Preoperative x-ray. *B.* Postoperative x-ray after internal fixation.

ment. Any radiographic evidence of avascular necrosis necessitates continuing non–weight-bearing and plaster immobilization. In automobile collisions, fracture of the neck of the talus is caused by the impact of a pedal against the plantar surface of the foot. If the impact is severe enough, displacement of the body of the talus occurs. This can be expected, since fracture of the neck of the talus results from a fall in which the patient lands on the dorsiflexed foot. Gross displacement causes ligamentous damage and subluxation of the calcaneocuboid joint. X-rays taken immediately after the injury may fail to disclose an undisplaced fracture in its early stages, as they do in fractures of the carpal navicular. If there is clinical evidence of talar fracture, the injury should be treated as a fracture until subsequent x-rays confirm absence of bone damage. Accurate reduction is essential in a displaced fracture. As previously stated, however, if there is severe comminution, and particularly if there is fracture into the joint, avascular necrosis or degenerative arthritis may occur. In fractures of the talar neck, there should be no delay; delay of three to five hours may make closed reduction impossible. Open reduction is indeed necessary when displacement and dislocation occur. Coltart recommends talectomy when there is talar contamination in an open fracture. Thirty per cent of his patients did well without a talus, and the remainder required a talocalcaneal fusion for relief of pain.[268] Garcia and Parkes prefer pantalar arthrodesis to astragalectomy, as it offers a better long-term functional result.[272] Dunn, Jacobs, and Campbell are optimistic about protection from weight-bearing by patellar tendon–bearing casts or braces for reconstitution of ischemic bone. They state that this may be necessary for two or three years.[270] McKeever, however, recommends primary early triple arthrodesis, feeling that it is too much to expect the articular cartilage of the ankle, subtalar, and talonavicular joints to undergo treatment by this lengthy method of bracing without developing severe degenerative arthritis.[271] Posterior tibial nerve involvement occurs in talar injury and can have serious consequences.[270] Clawtoe deformities from intrinsic muscle contracture and sensory defects in the sole of the foot have occurred.

Fracture of the neck of the talus with total posterior dislocation of the body occurs when extreme violence forces the foot into marked dorsiflexion. As the talar neck is fractured, the calcaneus is displaced and locked under the body of the talus. The body is ejected out of the tibiofibular mortice when the foot returns to plantar flexion. Avascular necrosis frequently follows this injury. Besides injury to the posterior tibial nerve, there may be injury to the posterior tibial artery from excessive pressure.

Hawkins, in 1965, studied 50 consecutive fractures of the talus and found that 13 of them were fractures of the lateral process. The mechanism of injury was usually that of dorsiflexion and inversion. The outcome in these cases was variable. Some of them went on to union with no problems, whereas others went on to nonunion and pain. There were also some cases of malunion with subsequent impingement and pain. Surgical intervention was usually of benefit to those patients with pain secondary to the aforementioned causes.[272]

Pennal states that fractures of the head of the talus constitute 10 per cent of the fractures and dislocations involving the talus. They are usually due to the impact of a fall on a completely dorsiflexed foot. The head of the talus is compressed by the force transmitted from the forefoot to the navicular. Prognosis is good in these fractures, but if there is severe comminution, there may be chronic pain because of either chondromalacia of the head of the talus or posttraumatic arthritis of the talonavicular joint. Triple arthrodesis may be necessary at a later date. In Pennal's series, 22 per cent of the injuries were fractures of the articular surface. Coltart stated that fractures of the articular surface were the most common fractures involving the talus. When it is violently compressed against the tibial plafond, the articular surface fractures. This is particularly true when the foot is inverted. Excision of loose fragments is recommended, with saucerization of the underlying bone. Mechanical incongruity of the joint will occur if there is an unremoved loose fragment, and degenerative arthritis and instability will follow. There is usually a good result after excision of loose fragments and saucerization, if they are done early.[268]

Larson, Sullivan, and Janes of the Mayo Clinic studied the incidence of avascular necrosis after fractures and dislocations of the talus. In their patients, they found the incidence of avascular necrosis in fractures of the talar neck to be only 57 per cent; in fractures of the body, only 83 per cent; in fractures of the head, 0 per cent; and in fractures of the neck and the body, 25 per cent.[274] Mindell and co-workers studied 40 patients and analyzed the disability and late results of severe injury to the talus. Patients with undisplaced fractures had 82 per cent satisfactory late results; those with dislocations, 73 per cent; and those with fracture-dislocations, 50 per cent. Only 65 per cent of the total series had satisfactory late results, and even the patients with the best results were rarely completely normal. Late operative procedures were necessary in a number of patients with unsatisfactory results. The authors felt that conservative treatment of patients with avascular necrosis seemed advisable. They advocated protection from weight-bearing until the necrotic bone had been sufficiently replaced with viable bone of adequate strength.[275]

The Os Calcis (Calcaneus). The os calcis is the largest bone of the foot, and its function is to transfer the body weight to the ground. It also is the site of attachment for the heavy calf muscles. Fractures most frequently occur from a crush injury secondary to a fall on the heel, and occasionally from an avulsion fracture of the tuberosity of the calcaneus by the Achilles tendon. There are many different fractures of the os calcis, and many attempts have been made to categorize them. There can be isolated fractures without joint injury; fractures with a slight amount of joint involvement; and severely comminuted fractures, with crushing of the articular surfaces and significant joint involvement. Isolated, undisplaced fractures of the calcaneus, if they do not penetrate into the joint, usually do well when treated conservatively. When there is displacement, it is recommended that the displaced fragments be restored to their anatomical position if possible. Extraarticular fractures are usually accompanied by little, if any, disability; but intraarticular fractures require a prolonged convalescence and, frequently, surgical intervention either at the time of the injury or at a later date (Fig. 3–XIII–51).

Fractures of the anterior process of the calcaneus are seen infrequently. Adduction and plantar flexion produce this injury and avulsion of the anterior process. Fractures of the *posterior process* of the tubercle are due to an avulsive force that occurs when the patient falls from a height with his knees and feet in extension. Instead of tendo Achillis avulsion, posterior process avulsion occurs. If the parts are displaced, open reduction is recommended with the foot placed in equinus position. The prognosis is generally excellent. Only 3 of 76 patients did poorly in a series of cases reported by Kleiger.[276] *Fractures of the medial and lateral processes* of the tuberosity are also uncommon injuries and are usually secondary to abductive or adductive force exerted when the patient's heel

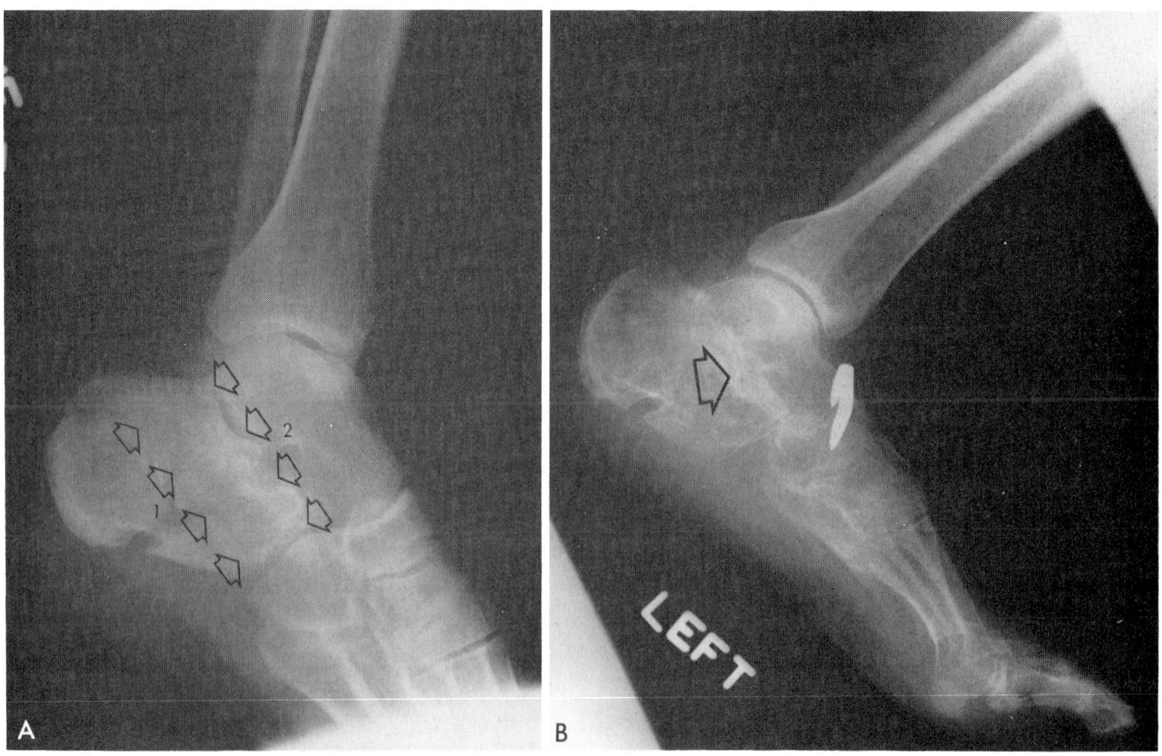

Figure 3–XIII–51. Os calcis fracture. *A.* (1) Fracture line; (2) subtalar joint. *B.* After healing of triple arthrodesis performed because of painful posttraumatic subtalar arthritis.

strikes the ground either in eversion or in inversion. The former produces fracture of the medial process, and the latter produces fracture of the lateral process. Nonunion in these fractures rarely occurs, and the prognosis is good. Occasionally the fracture fragment must be removed if there is nonunion. *Linear fractures of the body*, without involvement of the talocalcaneal or calcaneocuboid joints, should be treated by reduction of the fragments by whatever technique is most appropriate. Disability following these simple linear fractures is usually not serious. An extremely rare injury is fracture of the *sustentaculum tali*. It is usually caused by compression of the calcaneus by the talus with the foot in extreme inversion. The prognosis is good in these isolated fractures. In two papers, Carey, Lance, and Wade reported a series of 303 fractures of the os calcis of which extraarticular fractures constituted 25 per cent of the total. They generally did well as opposed to fractures involving the articular surface.[277, 278] Prolonged disability in these injuries is usually caused by inadequate diagnosis of avulsion fractures, particularly the anterior process fracture. This entity is often mistaken for a sprained ankle.

Intraarticular fractures of the os calcis constitute 75 per cent of the fractures of this bone.[279] Of these, simple linear fractures into the joint, without disruption of the normal anatomy, can usually be expected to do well. If there is minor displacement with resulting incongruity of the subtalar joint, the fragments can frequently be reduced by using either traction or open techniques. If the anatomical relationships are completely restored, these patients should have good results. Unfortunately, however, a large number of these fractures are severe crush injuries with multiple fragments and severe distortion of the anatomy. These fractures have been called "lover's heels." They are incurred by jumping from a height. Compression fractures of the lumbar vertebrae and associated rib fractures may be seen concomitantly. Anatomical reduction of these os calcis fractures is usually impossible, and severe disability may result. Secondary operative procedures such as subtalar joint fusion or triple arthrodesis are frequently necessary. Even after these secondary surgical procedures, a painful, stiff hindfoot may result. Late pain and disability after compression fractures of the calcaneus occur because of various factors. The tendo Achillis is lengthened because of malunion with upward displacement of the tuberosity. Therefore calf muscle power is reduced. The patient walks with a flatfooted gait and has eventual compensatory shortening of the calf muscles. Spastic flatfoot can occur from crowding of the peroneal mechanism under the lateral malleolus. The thickened calcaneus can impinge upon the lateral malleolus. Plantar fasciitis can occur from malunion, causing reversal of the plantar curve of the calcaneus. Derangement of the calcaneocuboid joint can be a significant source of pain as well. Because the supporting ligaments are involved in every compression fracture of the calcaneus, there is derangement of the subtalar joint. The joint itself is also deranged frequently. The potential of joint surface damage to produce pain is not directly proportional to the severity of the damage. On the contrary, the more damaged the joint, the more likely is the result to be a painless spontaneous fibrous ankylosis. Because this may not occur for a year or more, surgical arthrodesis may be recommended if the patient is having too much pain to bear.[280, 281]

Many long-term end-result studies of calcaneus fractures have appeared in the literature.[277, 282–287] Rowe and associates followed up 154 fractures for from 1 to 20 years. They reported that the overall treatment of 38 fractures extending into the subtalar joint failed completely in 27 per cent of the cases, and that closed treatment gave good or excellent results in 50 per cent. On the other hand, in 48 severely comminuted fractures with central depression, there were failures in only 15 per cent of the cases, with good or excellent result in 50 per cent. The authors recommended that the former type of fracture be reduced accurately and by open reduction if necessary. The latter type (central depression fracture with comminution) may best be treated by hand molding, supportive bandages, and early mobilization.[284] Brav followed 103 fractures for an average of 4.2 years and reported that, in general, the results with open reduction were only slightly better than those with no reduction but with early mobilization, except in severely comminuted fractures.[285] In a review of 50 cases of fractures of the os calcis sustained in industrial accidents, Deyerle evaluated them from 4 to 22 years following fracture. He found that, after the passage of 4 to 22 years, the two groups subjected to open reduction or triple arthrodesis had no better results in the final evaluation than the 10 patients who were treated conservatively. He stated that the numbers were small and probably not statistically significant, but the results were actually better in those treated conservatively. One amputation was necessary because of infection incurred during an operative procedure. The final average disability was 22 per cent loss of function of the foot in all his cases. The most frequent complaints in this series were those of patients who had residual stiffness of the foot and inability to control the foot and ankle. This led to an unstable gait on irregular surfaces. Most of the patients with comminuted fractures retained a permanent limp. Pain was infrequently mentioned as a sequel, but it was a secondary finding in a few cases. It was found that most of the patients who initially complained of pain experienced relief from it over the years. Among factors that the physician can control in treatment of these fractures are the degree of shortening of the os calcis and the degree of widening of the os calcis under the fibula. This spreading may tend to incarcerate or force the peroneal tendons out of their normal groove behind the fibula, resulting in peroneal dysfunction. The patients in whom this syndrome develops have an ankle instability and a lack of control to resist inversion. This problem can be corrected surgically, improving both inversion and eversion of the foot. One of Deyerle's conclusions in his series is that there is never a need for a triple arthrodesis, either primarily or secondarily, since the natural course of events in the severely displaced fracture produces the same amount of immobilization of the subtalar joint after the passage of several years. According to Deyerle, this makes surgical arthrodesis unnecessary.[288]

The Tarsal Navicular. Because the navicular is enveloped in strong ligaments, displacement of fragments of this bone is rarely more than minimal. Displacement occurs when fracture of the navicular is accompanied by talonavicular dislocation. Navicular fractures and fracture-dislocations are caused by forcible dorsiflexion of the foot. Fracture of the tuberosity of the scaphoid is an avulsion fracture produced by traction of the posterior tibial tendon. Avascular necrosis and posttraumatic arthritis are common sequelae to fractures or fracture-dislocations of the tarsal navicular, and may require arthrodesis of the dislocated joints. Tolerance of the talonavicular joint to posttraumatic arthritis without serious symptoms is great. Fracture of the body of the navicular is rare and is often due to direct trauma. Union of the body of the navicular usually occurs, but occasionally one encounters nonunion of the navicular tuberosity. Excision of the loose fragment can be performed, and it is advisable to resuture the posterior tibial tendon to the navicular for good results. In a review article, Eichenholtz and Levine reported that in those patients in whom the diagnosis was missed or the fracture was disregarded, symptoms persisted for prolonged periods, depending upon the degree of activity.[289]

The Cuboid and Cuneiform Bones. Fractures of the cuboid and cuneiform bones are associated generally with dislocation of the midtarsal or tarsometatarsal joint. Isolated injuries may occur as the result of direct violence. There is little or no displacement of the fragments in isolated fractures. Joint incongruity or late arthritis is rarely encountered because there is so little motion at these joints. Reduction is difficult and often impossible, except by open procedures when there is significant displacement. When cuboid and cuneiform injuries are caused by a direct blow from a heavy object falling on the foot, it is important to follow the patient because in some instances permanent soft-tissue damage will present itself in the form of necrosis of the skin and the underlying soft tissues 48 to 72 hours after the injury. A window cut in the dorsum of the cast after reduction permits inspection of the foot beneath it.

Metatarsal Fractures. These injuries are usually the result of direct violence. "March fractures," however, are caused by repeated stresses such as prolonged walking. There may be stress fractures in one or more metatarsal bones, usually the second or third. There is usually no displacement. To avoid serious disability of the foot, accurate reduction is recommended, particularly at the distal ends of the metatarsals. Manipulative reduction is usually adequate for treatment, but open reduction is justified if closed reduction fails. If metatarsal neck fractures are poorly reduced, the metatarsal heads are depressed toward the plantar surface of the foot. Malunion in this position creates an extremely painful area on the weight-bearing surface of the sole of the foot, often requiring excision of the metatarsal head. In "march fractures" (fatigue fractures), although the amount of callus formation may initially appear to be excessive, a considerable amount of callus is spontaneously absorbed as time passes, and there is no resulting disability. Rest of the foot, either by plaster immobilization or avoidance of weight-bearing, is good treatment. The most common of all metatarsal fractures is fracture of the base of the fifth metatarsal, usually caused by inversion stress leading to sudden increase in tension of the peroneus brevis tendon.[267] Avulsion of the styloid process of the fifth metatarsal occurs. A direct blow can cause this type of fracture. Immobilization produces a good functional recovery, but there are situations in which a patient will have pain for a year or more; this may or may not have any relationship to the degree of initial displacement.

The Phalanges of the Toes. The major concern in correcting fractures of the phalanges of the toes is angulation deformity. If this is not corrected, the toe continues to be clawed, and persistent pain and tenderness may result. If many toes are fractured, reduction should be carried out manually and the foot should be immobilized in a plaster cast. The most common mechanism of injury to the forefoot is the dropping of a heavy weight on the forefoot. This results in comminuted fractures of multiple phalanges. These can be dressed and treated in a firm soft boot, but occasionally casting is required. In extreme situations, arthrodesis of various joints may be indicated, and rarely, amputation of a phalanx may be necessary. Crushing injuries of the distal parts of the toes often produce nail problems. Part or all of a nail may require excision, and even though the nail bed is thoroughly curetted, subsequent growth of the nail may be irregular. This can be painful, although it is not necessarily so.

Sesamoid Bones of the Foot. Stress fractures of the sesamoids of the great toe occur (Fig. 3–XIII–52).[290] This is particularly true in modern ballet dancing in which performers are barefooted. Acute traumatic fracture of the sesamoids can also occur after a misjudgment in a terpsichorean leap. A fall can cause fracture of the sesamoids, as can the dropping of a heavy weight on the foot. Most commonly involved are the sesamoid bones under the first metatarsal head, and even more frequently, the medial sesamoid. Relief of pressure on the plantar aspect of the first metatarsal head by the application of a metatarsal pad in the shoe is good treatment, as is limitation of weight-bearing until the fracture heals. Symptoms may, however, persist because of nonunion or because of chondromalacia, which can develop on the articular surface of the sesamoid. Excision of the involved sesamoid is then necessary.

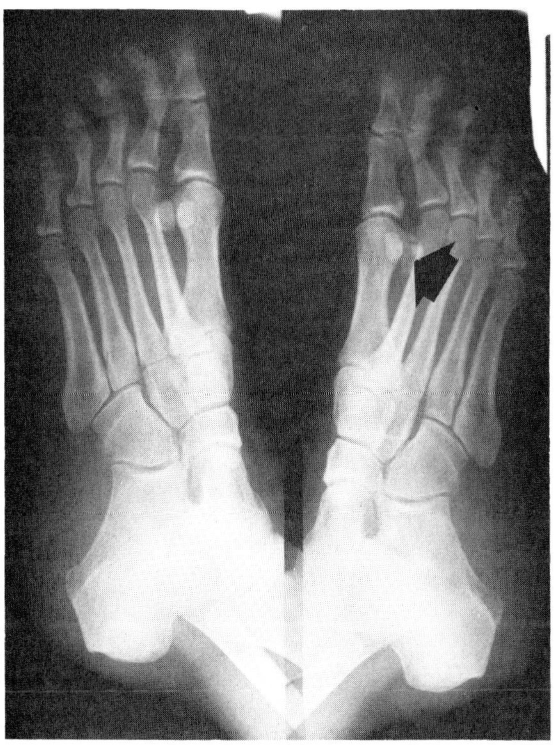

Figure 3–XIII–52. Fracture of a sesamoid bone of the foot.

Hallux rigidus is fixed ankylosis of the great toe at the metatarsophalangeal joint. This arises from a severe fracture extending into the joint or from repetitive trauma. It can also result from infection or from operations that involve the joint, or from degenerative arthritis or gout. Push-off is reduced, being accomplished by the outer four toes and the distal phalanx of the great toe, thereby protecting the first metatarsophalangeal joint from painful dorsiflexion. Painful calluses develop between the heads of the central three metatarsal heads and along the outer border of the heel. Keller arthroplasty, with or without the insertion of a Silastic prosthesis, and arthrodesis of the metatarsophalangeal joint are recommended surgical procedures.[291] Pain is relieved, but there is some permanent limitation of push-off ability.

THE PELVIS

Fractures of the pelvis can usually be treated successfully by closed methods except for fractures of the acetabulum associated with central dislocation of the hip. Disability is usually minimal even with rather gross displacement or with nonunion of one or more rami of the pubis and ischium. Extensive injuries such as separation of the symphysis pubis with fracture of the ilium or dislocation of the sacroiliac joint also usually go on to healing with little disability. When an injury is severe, however, open reduction may be necessary.[1] In all crushing injuries of the pelvis, intraabdominal and intrapelvic viscera may be injured. Minor pelvic fractures may be accompanied by serious visceral complications, and there may be severe fractures of the pelvis with minimal or no abdominal involvement. Injuries to the bladder and urethra are the most frequent complications in pelvic injuries. Urologic consultation and treatment should be prompt if there is any evidence of urinary tract injury. The pelvis is a virtually rigid structure, as the innominate bones and the sacrum form a circle of bone. Pelvic stability is assured, with no measurable motion at the symphysis pubis or sacroiliac joints, by the strength of the sacroiliac and interpubic ligaments. There is also good resilience to absorb some of the impact of direct or indirect trauma to the pelvis.

Injuries to the pelvis involving areas that bear no weight are rarely accompanied by vascular or urologic injury and need little treatment except rest until sitting and walking are comfortable. These include stable fractures of the ilium, undisplaced fractures of either pubic ramus, and occasional avulsion of the ischial tuberosity. Fractures involving major weight-bearing areas are unstable and are often accompanied by severe urologic injury and hemorrhage. These include complete diastasis of the pubic symphysis, disruption of the hemipelvis, and severe bilateral pubic rami fractures. Prolonged bed rest required in treatment of pelvic fractures, in company with pelvic congestion secondary to retroperitoneal hemorrhage, can produce deep vein thrombosis and pulmonary embolism.

Avulsion Fractures of the Pelvis

The pelvis is suspended between the trunk and locomotor muscles and serves as a fulcrum over which the upright position is maintained and the lower extremities are propelled.[2] Avulsion of the bony attachment of a muscle from the pelvis occasionally occurs after violent contraction against resistance, and occurs usually in youthful patients in athletics (Fig. 3–XIII–53). Because of strong fascial connections, gross displacement of the avulsed bone fragment does not occur and there is spontaneous sound healing. Exuberant callus about an avulsed ischial tuberosity may cause some inconvenience on sitting.

Avulsion of the Anterior Iliac Spines. Adolescents engaged in strenuous activity sustain this injury when powerful contracture of muscles avulses the anterior superior or anterior inferior iliac spine. Complete restoration of function with bony union can be expected, even though the fragments are not fully restored to their anatomical position. The avulsing muscles usually implicated are the sartorius and the rectus femoris. Bed rest with the hips and knees slightly flexed, followed by restricted activity and progressive ambulation, produces complete recovery.

Avulsion of the Tuberosity of the Ischium. Powerful contractions of the hamstring muscles produce this injury. If the fragments are widely separated, fibrous union may occur, but bony union is the rule. In most cases of fibrous union and in all cases of bony union, normal function can be expected. DePalma states that excision of the fragments is indicated ony in old cases of fibrous union with pain.[4] Bed rest is adequate treatment. Healing may produce a slightly oversized tuberosity. Schlonsky and Olix reported on two cases of avulsion fracture of the ischial epiphysis. The two patients were teen-age sprinters who sustained their injuries during track meets. The boys did well after conservative treatment and were able to go about their usual activities without difficulty. Their athletic ability declined, however. They objectively demonstrated decrease in hamstring strength, thigh girth, and athletic profi-

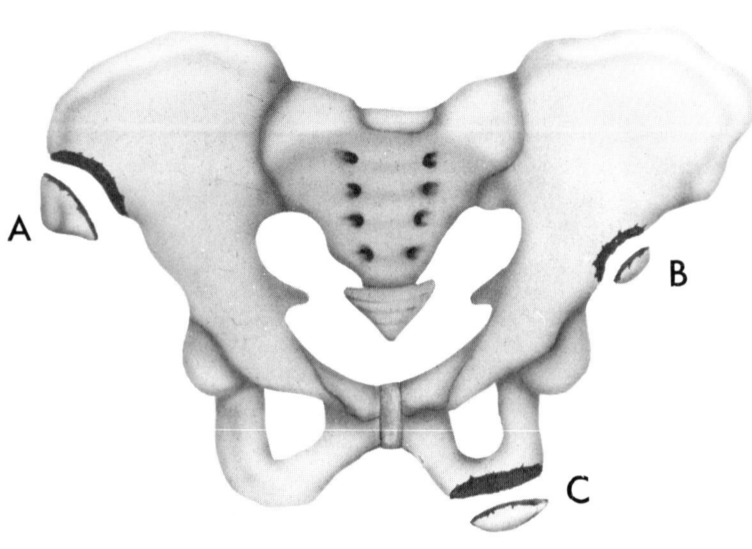

Figure 3–XIII–53. Avulsion fractures of the (A) anterior-superior iliac spine, (B) anterior-inferior iliac spine, and (C) ischial tuberosity. (From A. W. Dunn and H. D. Morris: Fractures and dislocations of the pelvis. J. Bone Joint Surg., *50-A*:1639, 1968. Reprinted by permission.)

ciency.[292] Schlonsky and Olix questioned the conclusion of Milch and DePalma that surgical reattachment is not recommended nor is repositioning of fragments necessary for a good result.[4, 293] Because of the functional disability in their two cases, the authors also questioned Sullivan's opinion that surgical intervention is not required even though x-rays reveal wide separation of the fragments.[294] In athletes, surgical repair may be indicated because of the enormous stresses placed on the pelvis by the locomotor musculature.

"Motorcycle Injury." Avulsion of the ilium by external violence occurs almost exclusively to motorcyclists, according to McLaughlin. The motorcyclist throws himself sideways from his seat at the moment of impact in a collision, and his forward momentum drives him against a steering handle, which hooks into the abdomen and against the abdominal surface of the iliac wing. Variable amounts of ilium are shattered and gouged toward the surface. The cecum or the descending colon may be damaged. Abdominal surgical repair may be necessary. The shattered fragments of ilium may be removed or left undisturbed according to the particular situation. An excellent result can be expected unless there is damage to the acetabulum, in which case reconstruction of the acetabulum is recommended.[2]

Stable Fractures of the Pelvis

There include fracture of a single pubic ramus, fracture of the wing of the ilium, fracture of the ischium, and fracture of the sacrum (Fig. 3–XIII–54). These fractures are either not displaced at all or are only minimally displaced. When there is displacement with an apparently isolated break in the continuity of the pelvic girdle, a second injury must be present, frequently a small disruption of one sacroiliac joint. This often cannot be ascertained by x-ray. Because the pubic ring is a rigid circle of bone, displacement cannot occur with fracture of a single pubic ramus. One can expect sound union and complete recovery. If the pelvic ring is broken in only a single plane, displacement cannot occur. This is true of unilateral fractures of both pubic rami. In this situation, weight-bearing strain is transmitted to the injured segment because of some relaxation of the sacroiliac ligaments. The bone fragments will not be displaced, but painful symptoms on weight-bearing may persist for four to eight weeks. It may be several months before there is complete recovery.

Subluxation of Sacroiliac Joints. Distortion of one sacroiliac joint often occurs when there are unilateral fractures of both pubic rami with a small amount of displacement. The ilium is displaced upward and backward in relation to the sacrum and is closer to the midline than the opposite ilium. This injury rarely produces early or late symptoms, even if there is gross disruption and prolonged sacroiliac instability. McLaughlin states that an isolated subluxation of a sacroiliac joint would probably be accompanied by a comparable small distortion of a relaxed symphysis pubis.[2]

Unstable Injuries of the Pelvis

Bilateral or Comminuted Fractures of the Pubis ("Straddle Injury"). These injuries do not affect the stability of the pelvic ring, but are considered unstable fractures because the bones themselves may be displaced upward by the abdominal muscles or into the thigh by the adductors (Figs. 3–XIII–55 and 3–XIII–56).

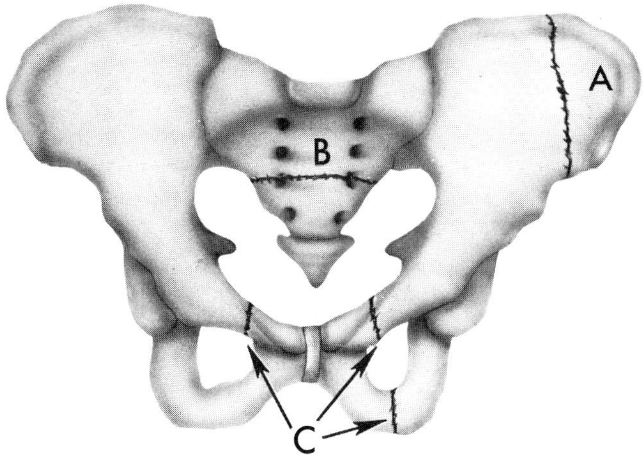

Figure 3–XIII–54. Stable fractures of the pelvic ring: (A) ala of ilium, (B) body of sacrum, and (C) one to three pubic rami. (From. A. W. Dunn and H. D. Morris: Fractures and dislocations of the pelvis. J. Bone Joint Surg., *50-A*:1639, 1968. Reprinted by permission.)

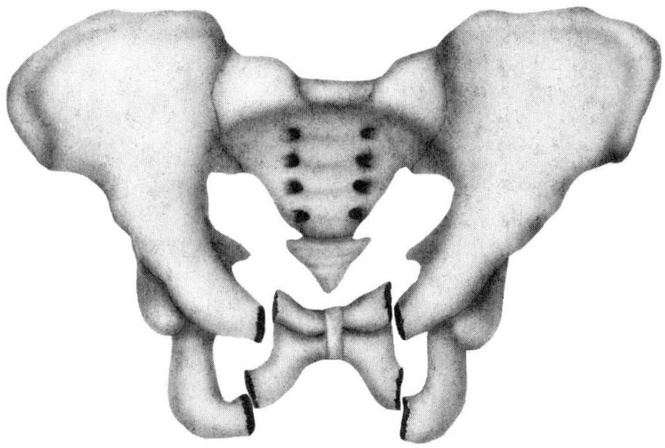

Figure 3–XIII–55. Straddle fracture. (From A. W. Dunn and H. D. Morris: Fractures and dislocations of the pelvis. J. Bone Joint Surg., *50-A*:1639, 1968. Reprinted by permission.)

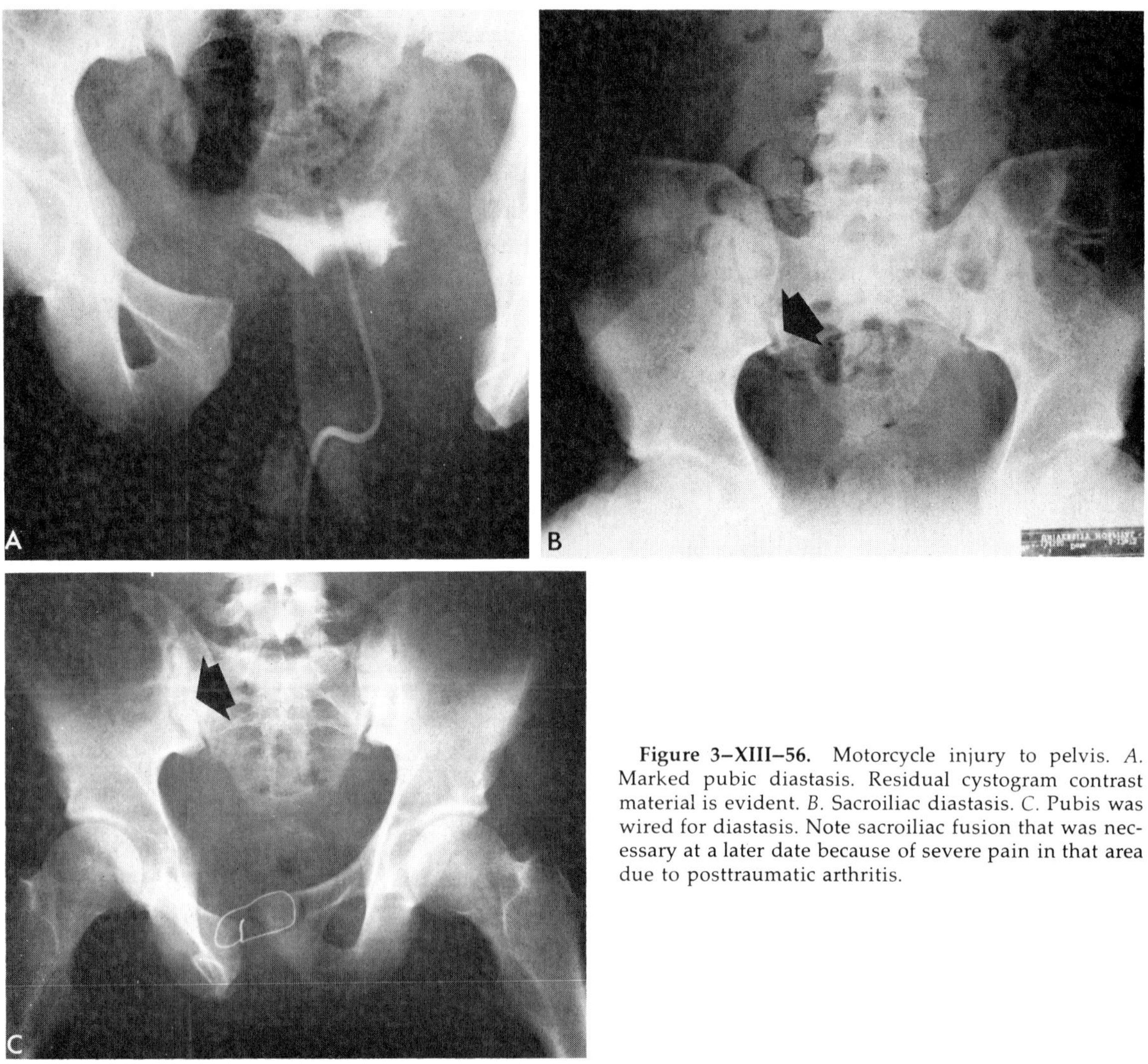

Figure 3–XIII–56. Motorcycle injury to pelvis. *A*. Marked pubic diastasis. Residual cystogram contrast material is evident. *B*. Sacroiliac diastasis. *C*. Pubis was wired for diastasis. Note sacroiliac fusion that was necessary at a later date because of severe pain in that area due to posttraumatic arthritis.

These fractures are nearly always associated with damage to the urinary tract. Recumbency is mandatory, but McLaughlin emphasizes a semisitting position because the supine position may cause silent displacement of the fracture fragments upward, as previously mentioned. Open reduction and internal fixation of the fracture or fractures may be necessary to improve urinary function. The anterior urethra is most commonly ruptured in a "straddle" injury, and the posterior urethra is usually lacerated by a displaced fragment of bone. *It should be noted here that injury to the genitourinary tract may be a complication of the simplest and most minor injury to the pelvis.* An empty bladder can be lacerated only by gross displacement of fracture fragments, but a full bladder may be ruptured easily by the impact to the pelvis of force that is insufficient to cause a fracture.[2] Hemorrhage from fractures of the pubis extravasates along the urogenital diaphragm to pool around the neck of the bladder. Sphincter spasm can occur. *The integrity of the urinary tract should be confirmed in every pelvic injury, no matter how minor it appears.*

Straddle fracture (comminuted fracture of the tie arch) was the most common type of unstable fracture in a series of 115 patients studied by Dunn and Morris and constituted almost 30 per cent of the group of unstable fractures. Rupture of the bladder was a complication in two patients. On the average, sufficient union had occurred to permit ambulation without redisplacement by seven weeks. None of these patients had permanent disability. In this same series, 77 patients had stable fractures of the pelvic ring; one of these had a urethral rupture. These so called "nonworrisome" injuries were accompanied by the following concomitant injuries: rupture of the bladder or spleen, renal contusion, rupture of the liver, perforation of the rectum, injury of the cauda equina, contusion of the bladder, hemothorax, thrombosis of the renal artery, and avulsion of the origin of the gluteus maximus.[295] These concomitant injuries emphasize how major stable pelvis fractures can be.

Vertical Shear Fractures of the Pelvis. The second most common unstable fracture or fracture-dislocation, according to Dunn and Morris, was the vertical shear fracture (Fig. 3–XIII–57). The fracture either occurred through the sacral or iliac alae or through the sacroiliac joint. Anteriorly, the superior and inferior ischiopubic rami fractured on the ipsilateral side, and one side of the pelvis was displaced either cephalad or posteriorly or both in combination. Skeletal traction was carried out for an average of six weeks, with gradual progression thereafter to crutch supported ambulation. None of these patients experienced redisplacement or residual disability.[295]

Dislocations of the Pelvis

Pelvic disruption by rupture of its great supporting ligaments results from rotation of one innominate bone in the sagittal plane while the remainder of the pelvic ring remains fixed. The primary force is leverage by the hyperextended femur. The pelvis splits apart at the symphysis when the femoral lever is also abducted. The two halves, released by disruption of the sacroiliac ligaments, swing open like an oyster shell on a posterior hinge. If the hyperextended femoral lever is adducted, the two pelvic segments telescope so that the pubic bones overlap (Figs. 3–XIII–58 to 3–XIII–61).

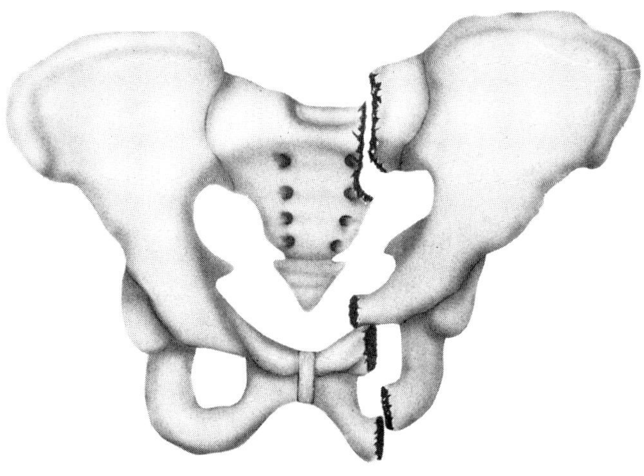

Figure 3–XIII–57. Vertical shear type of injury. (From A. W. Dunn and H. D. Morris: Fractures and dislocations of the pelvis. J. Bone Joint Surg., *59-A*:1639, 1968. Reprinted by permission.)

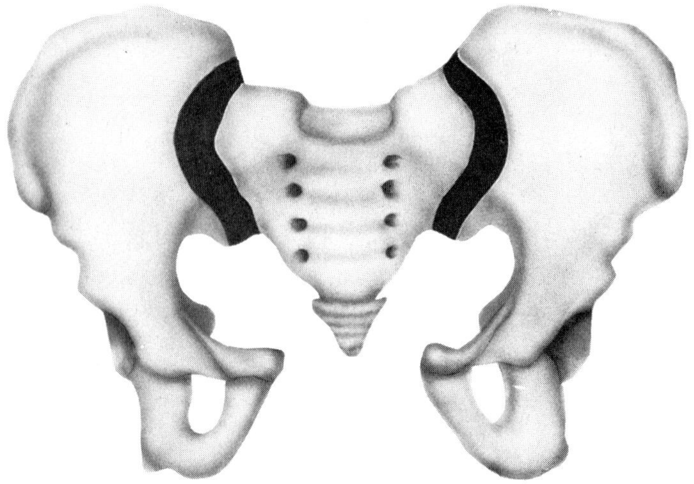

Figure 3–XIII–58. Dislocation of pelvis. (From A. W. Dunn and H. D. Morris: Fractures and dislocations of the pelvis. J. Bone Joint Surg., *50-A*:1639, 1968. Reprinted by permission.)

McLaughlin states that reduction of the displaced pelvic segment greatly facilitates repair of the associated visceral injuries.[2]

Total Dislocation of the Ilium. A case of total dislocation of the ilium after disruption through the triradiate cartilage in a girl of 13 years was described by MacKinnon and Lansdown. The injury was sustained when a heavy rock fell upon the patient. X-rays revealed fracture-dislocation of the left sacroiliac joint. The entire ilium was separated through the triradiate cartilage and rotated posteriorly and laterally. The sacral promontory was fractured as well. Open reduction and internal fixation were performed, and a short double plaster spica cast was applied. One year after injury the girl was free from disability. It was the conclusion of the authors that this injury could occur only in the immature skeleton before ossification of the triradiate cartilage. The force of the falling rock was applied to the anterior part of the ilium while the pelvis was in the supine position.[296]

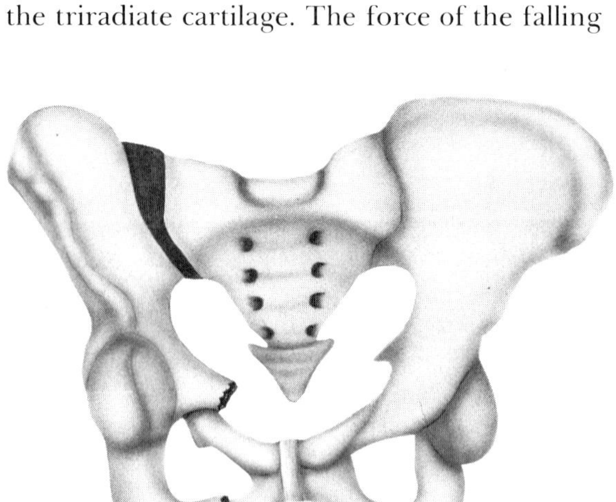

Figure 3–XIII–59. Lateral compression injury. (From A. W. Dunn and H. D. Morris: Fractures and dislocations of the pelvis. J. Bone Joint Surg., *50-A*:1639, 1968. Reprinted by permission.)

McLaughlin defines a "burst pelvis" as one in which there is separation of the symphysis pubis with opening of one or both sacroiliac joints. This is caused by violent hyperextension of the femoral lever with abduction. Rupture of the bladder or urethra, or avulsion of the urethra from the bladder, often occurs. Reduction should be performed as soon as possible, as little else can be accomplished until the bones are restored to as normal an anatomical position as possible. Plaster immobilization affords maintenance of reduction.[2] In Dunn and Morris's series, in two patients, ambulation was permitted at five and one half weeks and partial redisplacement resulted. Both had residual disability due to chronic sacroiliac pain, and one also had partial impotence from rupture of the membranous urethra.[295] Separations of the symphysis pubis were uncommon in Peltier's series of 186 cases; they accounted for 4 per cent of the cases. In two of the eight cases, the bladder was involved.[297] If closure of the symphysis pubis gap cannot be obtained or, if once obtained, cannot be maintained, internal fixation of the symphysis pubis may be necessary. Although the pubic symphysis is stable after internal fixation, there may be a cosmetic defect, a depression over one side of the pubic area, after healing has occurred. If there is diastasis of one or both sacroiliac joints along with pubic symphysis diastasis, and if one or both sacroiliac joints continue to be painful, sacroiliac fusion may be necessary. One can usually expect fibrous ankylosis of an injured sacroiliac joint or osseous fusion following injury, but the senior author has two cases in which sacroiliac fusion was necessary because of persistent pain

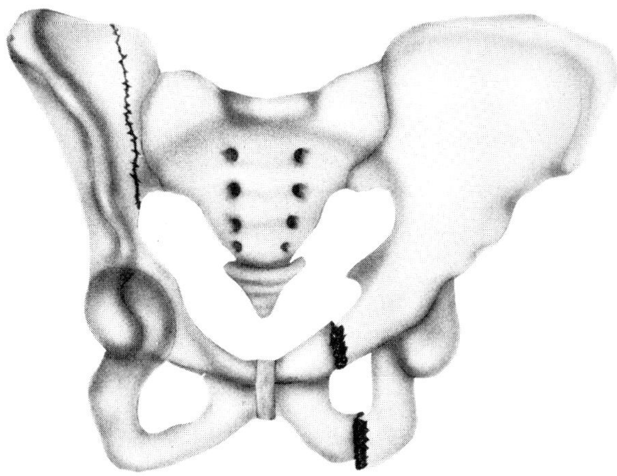

Figure 3–XIII–60. Bucket-handle injury. (From A. W. Dunn and H. D. Morris: Fractures and dislocations of the pelvis. J. Bone Joint Surg., *50-A*:1639, 1968. Reprinted by permission.)

due to sacroiliac diastasis. Shanmugasundaram reported a case of dislocation of the symphysis pubis with locking without injury to any other part of the pelvic ring. His patient did well after closed reduction and plaster immobilization. Urethral damage required reconstruction, and because of this the patient required considerable follow-up care. In this case there was roentgenographic evidence of osteitis pubis, but there were no clinical symptoms.[298] Chronic pubic pain can occur in this injury.

McLaughlin emphasizes the necessity for x-ray examination at least once a week for several weeks after reduction of a burst pelvis. Silent cephalad displacement of the unstable segment may occur. When this displacement remains unrecognized for even a short time, correction is made very difficult or impossible by repair of the soft tissues. If this displacement is observed, McLaughlin recommends continuous traction to the affected extremity.[2]

Fracture-Dislocations of the Pelvis

Multiple fractures throughout the pelvic ring with gross ligament disruption occur in massive crushing injuries. One can almost always expect visceral injury as well. There is usually disruption in both the anterior and posterior segments of the pelvic ring. Besides visceral damage, one can expect marked retroperitoneal hemorrhage and, possibly, profound shock. Various types of fracture-dislocations are encountered, such as lateral compression, in which both ischiopubic rami are fractured on the side of impact. Posteriorly there is disruption on the side of impact either through the sacral or iliac ala, or through the sacroiliac joint. "Bucket handle" injuries may occur in which both ischiopubic rami are fractured on the side opposite impact. Posteriorly, either the sacral or the iliac ala is fractured, or the sacroiliac joint is dislocated on the side of impact. The hemipelvis on the side of impact is displaced upward and inward, and is rotated. Urinary tract injury can be expected concomitantly.[295] Fractures involving major weight-bearing areas are unstable and are accompanied by hemorrhage and urologic injury.[297-303] Permanent sacroiliac instability or hypermobility is likely if the pubic symphysis remains separated. It does not usually cause significant pain, nor does it produce much difficulty in locomotion, except in the presence of cephalad hindquarter displacement. Chronic urinary difficulties are frequently seen after pubic symphysis disruption. McLaughlin mentions that the entire anterior wall of the pelvic girdle is functionally unimportant to locomotion, and, if

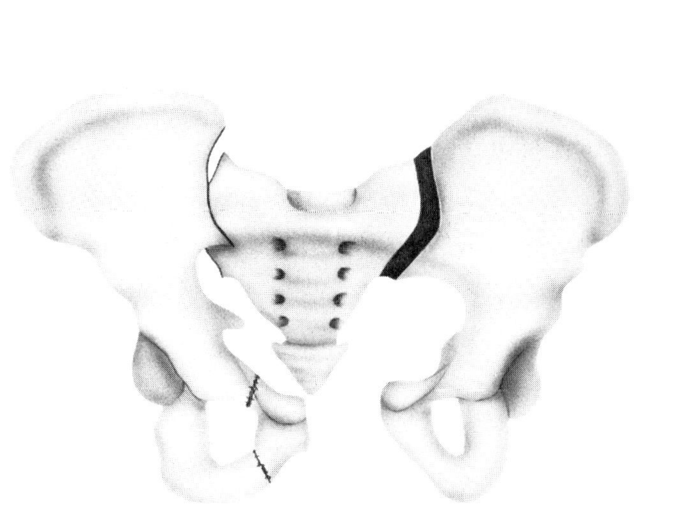

Figure 3–XIII–61. Total pelvic disruption. (From A. W. Dunn and H. D. Morris: Fractures and dislocations of the pelvis. J. Bone Joint Surg., *50-A*:1639, 1968. Reprinted by permission.)

necessary, late excision of a grossly displaced pubic segment can be performed.[2]

The visceral complications of pelvic fractures often assume more importance than the fractures themselves. Shock due to hemorrhage may require laparotomy and ligation of the hypogastric artery, but the results are discouraging.[304] Laceration or thrombosis of external iliac or femoral vessels with ischemia and gangrene of the lower extremities has occurred.[306, 307] Aneurysm of the superior gluteal artery in its course through the greater sciatic notch has been reported.[307] Besides paralytic ileus and acute gastric dilatation, injury to the intestinal tract, primarily lacerations of the rectum, occur all too frequently in pelvic injuries. Subsequent peritonitis, gas gangrene, or septicemia can ensue.[302] Genitourinary tract injury can cause chronic urethritis, cystitis, or epididymitis. Needless to say, obstetric and gynecologic injuries occur in patients with pelvic fractures, as does fetal death.[302] Avulsion of lumbar nerve roots in fractures of the pelvis was recently reported. Myelographic evidence of diverticula at the roots, dural scarring, or both were found. In each case, the pelvic injury included dislocation of or fracture adjacent to a sacroiliac joint. The presence of a diverticulum in a lumbar myelogram does not usually mean complete avulsion of the nerve root, however, and some recovery may be anticipated, according to the authors.[308] Other cases of avulsion of lumbar roots complicating fractures of the pelvis have appeared in the literature.[309–312] Injury to nerves, including complete or partial laceration of the sciatic nerve (most often the peroneal component), lateral femoral cutaneous nerve injury, injury to the superior gluteal nerve, and injury to the posterior branches of the sacral nerves, has been reported.[307] An isolated injury to the femoral nerve by proximal avulsion of the iliacus was reported by Green. A schoolgirl of 16 years sustained the injury in a gymnastic exercise that involved turning a somersault on a vaulting horse. Paralysis of the femoral nerve from pressure by the hematoma resolved after decompression.[122] Diaphragmatic rupture as an injury related to pelvic compressive forces has been reported, and the same explosive effect of abdominal compression can produce a rectal "blowout."[302]

Fracture of the Sacrum

Direct trauma, usually the result of a fall against a hard object, is the mechanism of injury in fracture of the sacrum. The fracture is usually transverse and can be displaced or undisplaced, depending upon the force of impact. Displaced fractures are uncommon; those that have been described are fractures in which the lower half is driven forward, sometimes with injury to the cauda equina, anesthesia of the perineum, and paralysis of the bladder. Purser has reported a fracture of the sacrum at the level of the first and second segments with forward displacement of the first segment. The line of cleavage was created by rupture of each fifth lumbar transverse process, with resulting avulsion by the iliolumbar ligaments. There was rupture of the upper part of each sacroiliac ligament, the fracture line across the ala of the sacrum entering the first sacral foraminae, then crossing the body of the sacrum at the level of the junction between the first and second segments. This injury occurred in a 19-year-old girl who was sitting with her legs at right angles to her trunk and her back against the side of the van in which she was traveling. The side of the van was struck by a bus. Purser surmised that sudden flexion possibly combined with an element of shear, as the trunk was driven forward on the pelvis, must have been responsible for the injury.[313] Traumatic spondylolisthesis, or forward slipping, at the lumbosacral junction of the sacrum is also a rare injury.[314] The mechanism of injury is similar to that in Purser's case. It occurs when there is a flexion injury when the knees are extended so as to fix the pelvis by tightness of the hamstrings, causing great stress to be exerted on the lumbosacral junction. The upper half of the sacrum is relatively protected by the posterior iliac spines and securely stabilized by the sacroiliac ligaments. Therefore, fractures that damage the second and third sacral nerves and create serious bladder and rectal complications are uncommon. Injury to the lower and relatively unprotected sacral segments is unlikely to be complicated by more than mild and transient neurologic complications. Transverse fracture of the sacrum, with displacement in the lower half of the sacrum above the sacrococcygeal junction, can be reduced by rectal manipulation. This fracture heals well if the area is protected from undue external pressure for four to six weeks. If early reduction is not performed, within two weeks fibrosis precludes manipulative replacement, and neurosurgical decompression of the cauda equina is necessary. McLaughlin states that in this situation, there is "rather forlorn hope for improvement."[2]

Injuries to the Coccyx

Coccyx injury occurs in direct trauma. Contusion of the coccyx without fracture can cause acute and chronic coccygeal pain, called coccygodynia. Conservative treatment includes protection from external pressure by correct sitting posture, sitting on a pillow or foam rubber doughnut, avoidance of constipation, sitz baths, and occasionally, anesthetic infiltration of the area. All too frequently these conservative measures fail, and coccygectomy is necessary. Even after rectal manipulation and reduction of an acutely fractured coccyx, with postreduction x-rays revealing anatomical position and alignment, coccygodynia may occur and require subsequent coccygectomy. The senior author has had excellent results with eight cases of long-term coccygodynia treated by coccygectomy. One patient treated by coccygectomy, however, continues to complain of chronic, intermittent pain, particularly in changeable weather, and still cannot sit in a hard chair.

COMPLICATIONS OF MUSCULOSKELETAL INJURY

Delayed Union

Delayed union may be defined as union of a fracture that takes longer than the expected time to heal. If a delayed union persists, it becomes a nonunion. Since different bones of the body heal at different rates, no specific time interval may be given. In general, delayed unions tend to have pain when the fracture site is manipulated, whereas established nonunions usually are painless. Some of the common sites of delayed union are: the clavicle, the humerus (especially the distal third), both bones of the forearm (the ulna more prevalently), and the cortical portion of the tibia.

The carpal navicular and the talus are also predisposed to delayed union because of their peculiar blood supply. The treatment for delayed union is continued immobilization until it has been decided that nonunion is present. Disability from delayed union is due to the prolonged immobilization necessary and the accompanying joint stiffness secondary to the prolonged immobilization. McBride states that one of the most frequent causes of delayed union is "continuous meddling."[81] Inadequate splinting, readjustment of the immobilization apparatus, frequent handling, and adjustment of the fragments tear down the continuity of the osteogenic process as fast as it can take place. Nevertheless, it is frequently necessary to readjust traction to avoid malunion, as in femoral fractures.

Malunion

A malunited fracture is one that has healed with the bones in abnormal position. There may be angular or rotatory deformity. It should be noted that malunion does not necessarily lead to functional impairment. Malunion may, however, block joint motion or cause disturbance of joint function, leading to secondary degenerative changes. There may also be some degree of cosmetic deformity. Malunion of interarticular fractures may lead to further degenerative changes, and almost always does so in the major weight-bearing joints. Malunion is less tolerable in the lower extremities than in the upper, because of the greater abnormal forces that are transmitted to weight-bearing joints. There is therefore greater predisposition to degeneration of the joints of the lower extremities. Surgery is not always indicated for malunion of a fracture, especially when the functional loss is slight. A certain degree of malunion of Colles' fractures in older patients is perfectly compatible with acceptable function. In the ankle, however, malunion produces severe difficulty, as the ankle is a precisely fitted joint and the malunion produces an incongruity of the articular surfaces. Therefore altered weight-bearing and posttraumatic arthritis always result. The degree of posttraumatic arthritis depends upon the severity of injury to the joint. The object of surgery for malunion is to restore function. It is rarely indicated for cosmetic purposes only. Surgery for malunion should be delayed until the area of injury has become biologically stabilized. Severe comminuted fractures of the subtalar joint may progress to spontaneous fusion and thus eliminate the need for surgery.

Malunion is usually due to inaccurate reduction or to ineffective immobilization during healing. Accurate reduction and adequate immobilization should obviate most malunions. Despite the most expert care, however, malunion may occur in certain instances. It is well known that fractures of different areas of a bone will angulate in different directions owing to the muscle pull involved on either side of the fracture site. This should be taken into account by the attending surgeon. In children, axial angulation of a fracture of a long bone can be accepted to a much greater degree than in an adult, because of the remodeling that occurs during growth. Rotational deformities, however, are not remodeled to such an extent and are less acceptable. Shearing injuries of the epiphyseal plate in children may undergo remodeling if the plate has not been functionally damaged. On occasion, surgical correction of a malunion may be necessary because of interference with the function of overlying muscles and tendons. This is seen in the Colles' fracture, which if left in an extremely malunited position may lead to degeneration and subsequent rupture of the extensor tendons. It is also seen in the femur, where malunion may interfere with quadriceps function. Malunion in severe valgus inclination at the elbow may produce traction on the ulnar nerve and subsequent tardy ulnar palsy.

Nonunion

The difference between delayed union and nonunion lies in the capacity of the bone fragments in the former condition to unite under adequate treatment, whereas in the latter condition, union is no longer possible. The distinctive features are readily seen in x-rays. They include marked sclerosis and rounding of the bone ends, closing of the medullary canal in each fragment, and a wide, well-defined gap between the fragments. Ray and associates, in 1964, evaluated 125 cases of delayed union and nonunion seen at the University of Illinois Research and Educational Hospital. They traced failure of union in these 125 fractures to one or more of the following factors: (1) inadequate initial reduction of the fracture, including interposition of soft tissues between the fracture fragments; (2) distraction of the fragments because of improperly applied traction or internal fixation devices; (3) loss of bone; (4) improper operative interference; (5) improper immobilization; (6) impairment of blood supply; (7) infection; (8) metabolic disturbances; and (9) local pathologic conditions.[315]

Once the diagnosis of nonunion is established, there are only two alternatives open to the patient and the surgeon. The first is acceptance of the nonunion; the second, surgical correction of same. Nonunion of the upper extremity may be accepted, especially in older patients who frequently are able to live with this condition. In bedridden patients, nonunion of fractures of the major bones of the lower extremities may be acceptable. Nonunion of a fracture of the distal third of the humerus may be compatible with the activities of daily living of an elderly, retired, inactive patient. Nonunion of the carpal navicular is sometimes discovered as an incidental finding on x-ray in patients who do heavy manual labor and who have no complaints referable to this nonunion. Surgical intervention for established nonunion, in general, consists of either open reduction and internal fixation, with or without bone graft, or prosthetic replacement. Even with surgical correction, however, the failure rate after the first procedure may approach 13.5 per cent, as reported by Boyd and associates.[316] These failed cases may require an additional surgical procedure to attempt to correct the nonunion. There are many bone grafting techniques and many methods of internal fixation. The choice of technique depends on the preference of the individual surgeon. The important factors in successful treatment of nonunion are firm fixation, apposition of the fragments, and the proper osteogenetic environment.

Nonunion is characterized by an abnormal flexibility without pain on movement or pressure according to McBride.[81] There is no tenderness or swelling about the region of the fracture. X-rays show clearly marked margins of the fragments, with tapering regular or irregular ends joined by fibrous union. The disability from nonunion is created by flexibility in a necessarily rigid lever. Pseudarthrosis can be present in an extremity, however, and that extremity can be used well. For example, a pseudarthrosis in the distal humerus of a patient with a markedly stiff elbow is often tolerated quite well; the patient learns to use the pseudarthrosis as his elbow joint. The muscles and fibrous tissue often approximate the bone ends in such a manner as to facilitate some function. One of the authors has two patients with pseudarthrosis of the distal third of the tibia. Both these pseudarthroses developed as a result of boot-top ski injuries. At present, both patients are functioning with relatively minimal disability in sedentary capacities.

Avascular Necrosis of Bone

Avascular necrosis of bone implies death of bone resulting from impairment or total loss of blood supply. Trauma is the most common cause. This complication frequently follows a fracture of a bone close to its articular end or a dislocation if the blood supply to the end of the bone is disrupted. Another reason for deprivation of blood supply may be infection. Avascular necrosis is a common cause of delayed union and nonunion. When necrosis involves the articular surface of a joint, osteoarthritis frequently is a sequela. Intracapsular fractures of the femoral head are often complicated by avascular necrosis. This is also true of segmental fractures of the tibia, fractures of the carpal navicular, and fractures of the talus. In the latter two bones, avascular necrosis frequently occurs because the blood supply to the navicular and talus enters these bones distally. Because pain is a clinical manifestation of avascular necrosis, surgical treatment for alleviation of this pain is indicated. Surgical treatment includes bone grafting, arthrodesis, or arthroplasty.

Osteochondritis Dissecans

Osteochondritis dissecans is a condition in which part of the articular surface of a joint separates, owing to a plane of cleavage through the subchondral bone (Fig. 3–XIII–62). This condition is found most frequently in the knee joint, although other areas can be affected, notably the elbow, ankle, and hip. The cause of the separation remains unknown. Theories that have been suggested fall into two groups; one supports the theory of ischemia, and the other advocates a traumatic etiology. Today, most authorities consider that trauma plays at least some part in the etiology, and there are those who believe that the two theories are not mutually exclusive. In 32 cases, Green found that more than 40 per cent of his patients had had an injury to the knee prior to the beginning of symptoms.[317] This tends to support the theory of trauma.

Adhesions and Joint Stiffness

Joint stiffness is a frequent complication of both fractures and the treatment of fractures. If a fracture is adjacent to the musculotendinous structures about a joint, such as the quadriceps mechanism of the knee, subsequent callus formation and healing of the fracture may involve the musculotendinous unit in adhesions and scar tissue. This leads to stiffness and limitation of motion of the joint. Plaster immobilization of a joint also inevitably leads to stiffness. The degree of stiffness is quite variable, and some must be accepted in order to get proper healing of the fracture. Fortunately, most of the joint stiffness secondary to immobilization can be resolved with post-immobilization physical therapy. Fractures into a joint and resulting hemarthrosis lead to adhesions within the joint itself. These are much more difficult to alleviate through physical therapy and may cause permanent loss of motion of the joint. It is important to note that the following factors may enhance the forma-

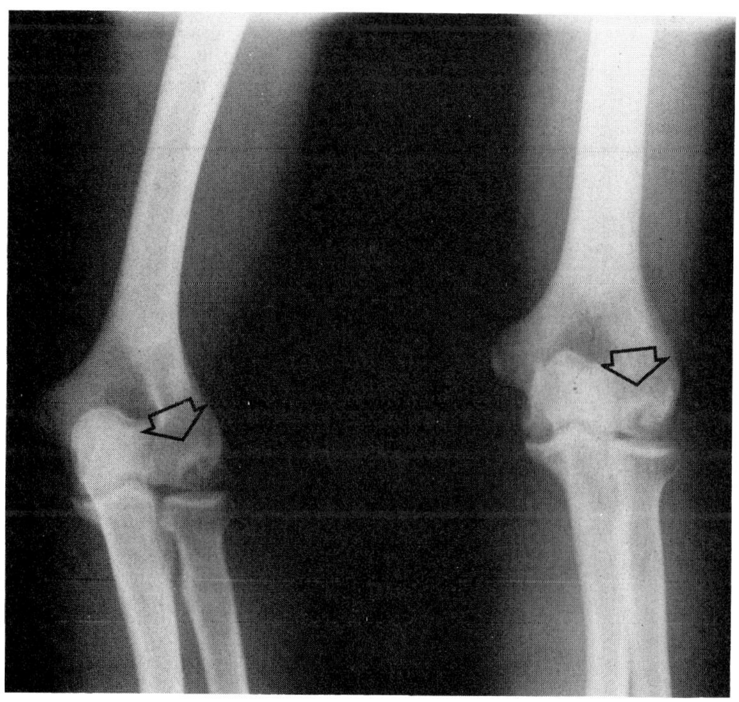

Figure 3–XIII–62. Osteochondritis dissecans of the elbow.

tion of periarticular adhesions: (1) inadequate immobilization of a fracture with persistent edema of the surrounding soft tissue, (2) failure to maintain maximal functional activity in the affected part as well as in the involved muscles and joints of the limb, (3) persistent and recurrent edema, (4) any form of passive manipulation of a stiff joint, (5) pin tract infection in the vicinity of a joint and, (6) infection adjacent to a joint.[4]

Myositis Ossificans (Posttraumatic Ossification)

This lesion is a relatively rare complication of injury, particularly fractures and fracture-dislocations in the vicinity of a joint. It consists of the formation of a mass of bone in soft tissue after trauma (Fig. 3–XIII–63). It is found more frequently in children and adolescents than in adults. According to Turek, the condition is alleged to be due to displacement of periosteum, which performs its bone-forming function in an abnormal location.[38] Hematoma formation seems to be a necessary prerequisite. McLaughlin states that "whether this is called ossifying hematoma or myositis ossificans is academic."[2] This condition is found in the brachialis muscle in the anterior aspect of the elbow, in the quadriceps mechanism just above the knee, in the deltoid muscle of the shoulder, and in the adductor musculature of the thigh. Myositis ossificans in the brachialis occurs after a markedly displaced fracture of the radial head or after a severe dislocation of the elbow. Quadriceps myositis ossificans is seen in linemen in football as a result of repetitive blocking. The deltoid ossification is seen in foot-soldiers who repeatedly carry rifles against their shoulders. Adductor ossification is seen in horseback riders and has been called "Prussian disease." It should be noted that the bony mass that forms is true trabeculated bone. One may also see small periarticular calcifications in the ligaments surrounding a joint following injury, but this should not be called myositis ossificans. Recently a case of triceps brachii ossification has been reported.[318] The reporter of this case used the term "fibrodysplasia ossificans" to denote the condition, as suggested by Searle.[319]

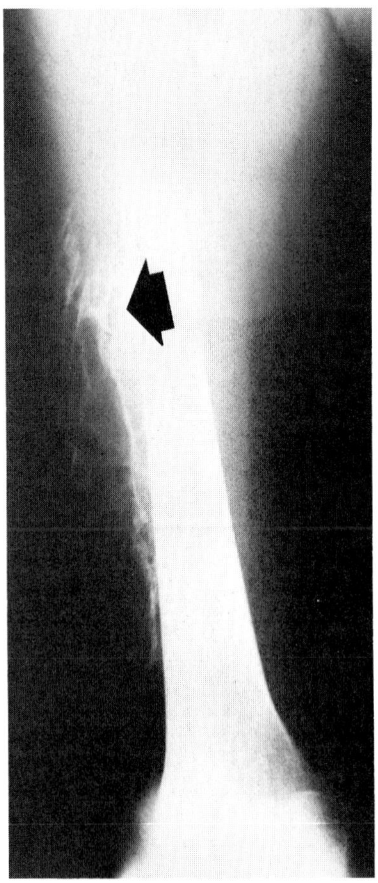

Figure 3–XIII–63. Myositis ossificans of the femur.

Treatment of this condition depends upon the symptoms present. Asymptomatic bony masses do not need to be excised. If the mass produces functional impairment, either of muscle or of joint, excision is probably indicated. One must be very cautious about the time chosen for excision, waiting until all evidence of ongoing ossification has ceased and radiographic studies show that the mass has become mature. If excision is performed before this time, there is a high rate of recurrence. The condition may even be aggravated. There is a dilemma in treatment. Absolute immobilization will probably minimize the amount of bone formed, but on the other hand, one does not want to develop a stiff joint because of prolonged immobilization. Therefore, a balance must be struck between mobilization and immobilization. One should never passively stretch a joint. Never perform active forceful exercises, and perform active assistive exercises only within the tolerance of pain.

Periarticular Calcifications

In contradistinction to myositis ossificans, one may see small periarticular calcifications following an injury. Radiographically, these calcifications do not have the structure of mature trabeculated bone as seen in myositis ossificans.

In contrast to myositis ossificans, which is seen within a muscle, periarticular calcifications are seen in the ligaments and other soft tissues surrounding a joint. One example of this is Pellegrini-Stieda disease, which is calcification in the medial collateral ligament of the knee. Other examples are calcifications within the rotator cuff; in the conoid and trapezoid ligaments; just proximal to the pisiform bone in the tendon of the flexor carpi ulnaris; and in tendon sheaths such as that of the first dorsal extensor compartment in the hand (DeQuervain's disease) and those of the peroneal, anterior tibial, and posterior tibial tendons in the foot. Treatment depends upon location and symptoms. Calcium deposits are often very painful and limit a patient's occupational activities. The size of the calcification is not always proportional to the amount of disability. Ectopic calcification can erode underlying soft tissues, for example, in the rotator (musculotendinous) cuff in the shoulder. Attrition ensues, and the cuff tears. Surgery may be necessary if conservative treatment fails. Particular occupations often produce particular calcium depositions; e.g., in "weaver's bottom" calcium is deposited adjacent to the ischial tuberosities.

Injuries to Overlying Soft Parts

There may be associated injury to overlying soft parts such as the skin, adjacent muscles and tendons, vascular structures, and nerves. The degree of injury to the structures is to a certain extent proportional to the amount of violence producing the injury. These complications of fractures must be individually assessed and dealt with in each patient. In some cases the injury to the overlying soft part is more significant than the actual fracture. Injury to overlying muscles may result in loss of function of a muscle or muscle group, and may require surgery such as tendon transfer or joint fusion. Injuries to overlying nerves may result in paralysis distal to the point of injury, and secondary surgical reconstructive procedures may be necessary.

Injury to overlying arteries may result in ischemia distal to the point of injury. The resulting ischemic fibrosis of the musculature is known as Volkmann's ischemic contracture. This may occur in either the upper or lower extremities. Surgical treatment of established Volkmann's ischemic contracture is extremely difficult and leads to only partial return of function. The disability associated with this condition is severe.

Sudeck's Atrophy and Causalgia

Sudeck's atrophy (acute traumatic bone atrophy, reflex sympathetic dystrophy) tends to occur when an extremity is immobilized. This is expected in all fractures requiring immobilization; however, when atrophy is severe and occurs swiftly, it may be acute traumatic bone atrophy (Fig. 3–XIII–64). Pain is out of proportion to that expected from the injury and persists after immobilization. There are swelling, dilatation of the superficial vessels, and purplish discoloration in a warm and moist extremity. Its exact etiology is unknown, but it appears to be a reflex sympathetic dystrophy.

Causalgia, as defined by Dorland, is a burning pain, often accompanied by trophic skin changes, due to a wound or other injury of a peripheral nerve.[320] This condition, particularly when it is associated with posttraumatic osteoporosis, may require surgical intervention. The pain can be severely disabling. Upper thoracic or lumbar sympathectomy may be necessary.[321] These procedures often produce a good deal of relief in some cases; the results may be disappointing in others.

Posttraumatic Arthritis

Degenerative arthritis almost always follows severe direct trauma to a joint. The greater the trauma, the worse the arthritis. One can expect degenerative changes whenever there are infractions of the articular surface of a joint. Avascular necrosis is another cause of posttraumatic arthritis. In the lower extremity malalignment of a long bone such as the tibia leads to abnormal stresses on major weight-bearing joints, particularly the knee, and may cause degenerative arthritis even though the knee itself was not injured at the time of the accident. The degree of tearing of soft-tissue structures about a joint determines the degree of secondary traumatic arthritis. The more instability in a joint, the greater the likelihood arthritis may occur. Preexisting degenerative arthritis may worsen after trauma with posttraumatic arthritis superimposed. Loose bodies (joint mice) can be caused by arthritis and can cause arthritis.

Infection

Infection, as a complication of a fracture, may be caused by bacteria introduced from without when the skin overlying the fracture

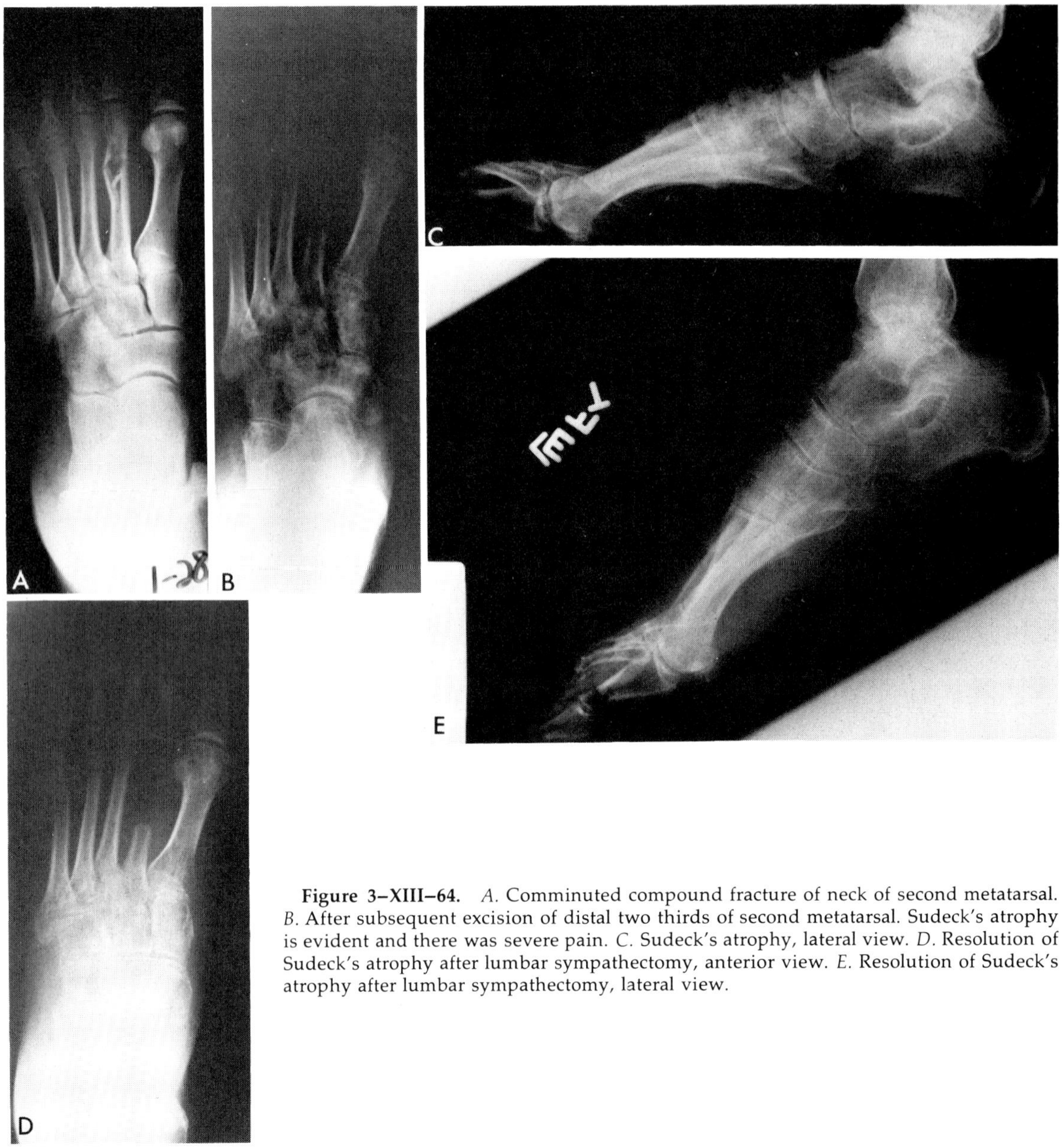

Figure 3–XIII–64. *A.* Comminuted compound fracture of neck of second metatarsal. *B.* After subsequent excision of distal two thirds of second metatarsal. Sudeck's atrophy is evident and there was severe pain. *C.* Sudeck's atrophy, lateral view. *D.* Resolution of Sudeck's atrophy after lumbar sympathectomy, anterior view. *E.* Resolution of Sudeck's atrophy after lumbar sympathectomy, lateral view.

site was disrupted at the time of injury (Fig. 3–XIII–65). It may also occur after surgical intervention for treatment of a closed fracture. Another cause of infection may be hematogenous seeding of organisms in a fracture hematoma from a nidus of infection elsewhere in the body, for instance, carious teeth or the urinary tract. Infection may take the form of either osteomyelitis or infection of a joint space. It may have multiple serious consequences, among which are delayed union, nonunion, joint fusion, chronic osteomyelitis (which may be quiescent for years only to be aggravated and return following relatively minor trauma), synostoses, and multiple systemic manifestations. The systemic complications of infection following a fracture include amyloidosis, distal abscesses from hematologic seeding, and local epidermoid carcinomas around a chronic draining sinus tract. The local treatment of osteomyelitis frequently is saucerization of bone or resection of bone, which is often mutilating. Amputation is often necessary.

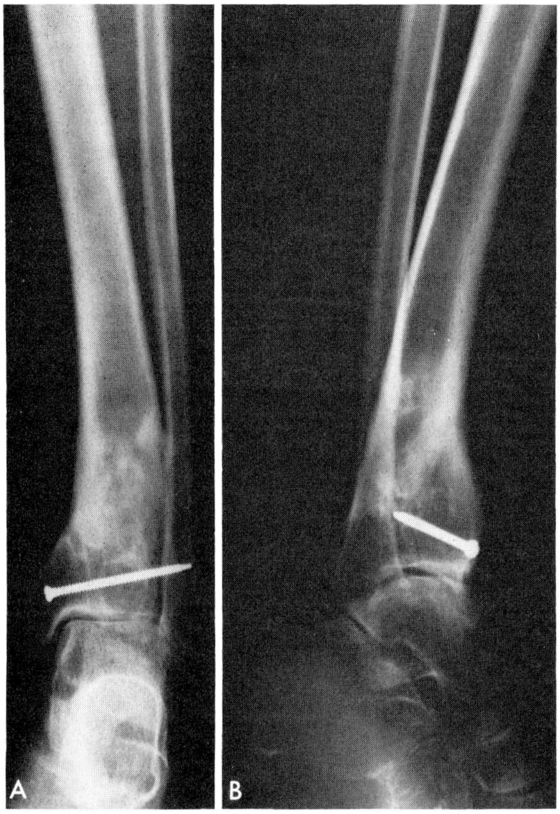

Figure 3–XIII–65. Chronic osteomyelitis of distal tibia after compound fracture. *A.* Anterior view. *B.* Lateral view.

Systemic Effects of Musculoskeletal Injury

Fat Embolism

Fat embolism can follow fracture. It occurs most frequently in patients with multiple fractures of the long bones, pelvis, or ribs. In general, according to Peltier, the amount of embolic fat reaching the lung is proportional to the extent of the bony injury. Hypovolemic shock occurs regularly in patients with multiple fractures because of local blood and fluid loss into the sites of injury. This is particularly true in patients with fractures of the pelvis, in whom retroperitoneal hemorrhage is the most common cause of death. Careless handling of the patient and delay in treatment aggravate this shock. Peltier states that in multiple reports it has been reaffirmed that fat embolism is most apt to occur in patients who have been in severe shock. Fat embolism is a self-limited disease, and if the patient can be supported through the period of respiratory insufficiency, he will recover.[322]

Renal Failure

Acute renal failure can result from severe trauma. In a recent report, Hamburger and associates found the two factors contributing to the development of renal failure to be hypovolemia and infection. It was found that when infection was a factor, the onset of renal failure was significantly later than when hypovolemia alone was present. Vigorous medical management of acute renal failure by control of fluid and electrolytes and protein, and hemodialysis, integrated with aggressive surgical treatment of the infection, resulted in survival and normal renal function in 13 of 15 patients.[323]

Traumatic anuria following muscle ischemia ("crush syndrome") has been repeatedly reported.[324–326] Crushing of a limb induces renal arteriolar constriction and renal ischemia. Myohemoglobin released from damaged muscle is excreted by the glomeruli and produces tubular obstruction, either because it causes physical blockage or because its deposition on the lining epithelium of the tubules interferes with reabsorption of filtrate and leads to an increase of intrarenal pressure (physiologic reabsorption blockage). There is a correlation between the duration of crushing and the morbidity after release. After release of myohemoglobin, escape of fluid into the crushed limb may cause hypotension. Death can occur from renal failure. Damaged muscle, disintegrated red cells, and the electrolytic shift of the catabolic response to injury all contribute to hyperkalemia. In addition to high serum potassium levels, uremia and acidosis follow oliguria. Peritoneal dialysis and hemodialysis have reduced the number of deaths from acute renal failure, but once renal failure has occurred, an appreciable mortality rate still exists.

Vascular Disorders

Thrombosis, thrombophlebitis, and *thromboembolism* occur after musculoskeletal trauma. Bauer stated that thrombosis was 12 times as common among his patients with leg injury as in all the rest of his patients.[327] After orthopedic procedures, the risk involved is fivefold greater in patients aged 40 years or older than in those aged 20 to 30 years.[328] A recent article by Cohen and associates reviewed thrombophlebitis following knee surgery. Of the 35 patients studied, 20 had postoperative venograms that showed fresh venous thrombosis in the lower extremities. Three patients had pulmonary emboli. It was concluded that local factors involved in surgery and postoperative care were responsible for the thromboses.[329] The importance of the study lies in the demonstration of thrombophlebitic complications in numbers far greater than can be appreciated by physical examination, as reported in this and other studies. The recognition of these silent cases of thrombophlebitis is the basis for one of the controversies in orthopedic surgery today. Many physicians have investigated the problem, but as yet there is no clear-cut method of reducing the incidence of silent thrombophlebitis and at the same time avoiding the problems associated with anticoagulant therapy.

PATHOLOGIC FRACTURES

A pathologic fracture is a fracture in a bone already weakened by disease. This may occur without trauma or as the result of a relatively trivial insult. The disorders leading to weakness of the bone may be either a reflection of a general condition or due to a local cause. Some of the general disorders that may lead to pathologic fracture are developmental abnormalities of bone such as osteogenesis imperfecta or osteoporosis; vitamin and nutritional deficiencies such as rickets, scurvy, senile osteoporosis, and disuse osteoporosis; disorders of hormonal balance such as hyperparathyroidism or Cushing's syndrome; and diseases of hematopoietic origin such as multiple myeloma, eosinophilic granuloma, Paget's disease, renal rickets, and polyostotic fibrous dysplasia. Local disorders that may lead to pathologic fracture include cystic diseases of bone such as simple bone cyst or aneurysmal bone cyst; primary benign tumors of bone such as giant cell tumor or hemangiomas; primary malignant bone tumors such as osteogenic sarcomas or fibrosarcomas; metastatic carcinoma and metastatic sarcoma; neurotrophic dystrophies such as syphilis and diabetes; parasitic infections such as hydatid cysts; other infections such as tuberculous osteomyelitis or pyogenic osteomyelitis; and post-irradiation bone changes.

The treatment of these fractures depends upon elucidation of the underlying condition. The increased disability, morbidity, and mortality rates associated with pathologic fractures are in general due to the underlying condition rather than to the fracture itself. A great number of these fractures may be treated successfully in the same fashion as fractures of normal bone. Some of them, however, in which there is a loss of a significant amount of bony substance secondary to the underlying disease process, may present great problems to the orthopedic surgeon. With loss of bone substance, bone-to-bone contact, which is necessary for adequate healing, may be extremely difficult to achieve. The orthopedic surgeon may have to use unusual means of internal fixation such as methyl methacrylate. Harrington and associates point out that when methyl methacrylate is used as an adjunct to internal fixation, there is immediate stabilization of the fracture sufficient to allow full weight-bearing on the extremity as soon as the incisional tenderness allows. This is important because the life expectancy of many of these patients is short, and the aim of fracture management is the immediate restoration of a painless, well-functioning limb.[330]

In general, the treatment of pathologic fractures is dependent upon the treatment of the underlying disease. For example, in an inflammatory disease such as osteomyelitis, the prognosis depends considerably upon which bone is broken, the amount of periosteal reaction, and the amount of local tissue damage. If there is significant bone loss and the fragments become displaced, union may fail to occur and some of the cases will eventually require amputation. In a disease such as rickets, however, the prognosis is good. Since rickets can be cured by a suitable diet with certain supplements added, the fracture should heal as does a fracture in a normal bone.

STRESS FRACTURES (FATIGUE FRACTURES)

Fatigue fractures occur secondary to constant repeated overloading of a bone. These fractures occur chiefly in the lower extremities and may be seen in the metatarsals, fibula, tibia, and femur (Figs. 3–XIII–66 and 3–XIII–67). Indeed, the fatigue fracture of the second metatarsal shaft is so commonly associated with soldiers that it has become known as the "march fracture." Any activity that involves a repeated stress on the lower extremities may result in a fracture. Stress fractures are seen in soldiers, gymnasts, housewives who are on their feet much of the day, policemen, postmen, machine operators, and deck hands. A recent article reported on an unusual fatigue fracture of the tarsal navicular in a long-distance runner.[331] Fatigue fractures have been reported in the clavicle, first rib, and forearm bones, but with less frequency than in the bones of the weight-bearing lower limbs. Watson-Jones records a history of a patient who sustained a fatigue fracture of the ulna after prolonged shoveling of manure.[53]

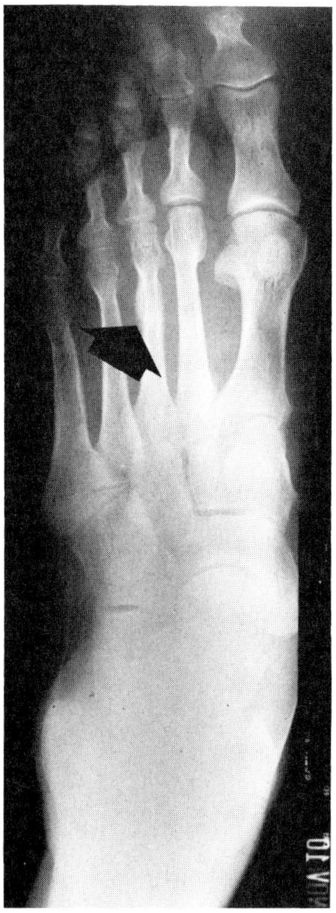

Figure 3–XIII–66. Fatigue fracture (march fracture) of third metatarsal.

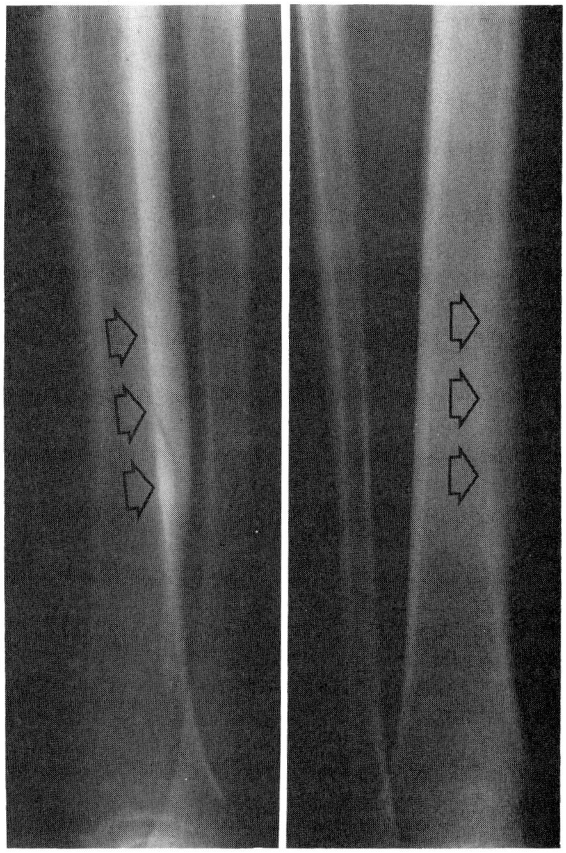

Figure 3–XIII–67. Healed fatigue fracture of distal tibia in cross-country runner.

There are some indications that healing in fatigue fractures takes longer than would otherwise be expected. This may be, in part, because frequently a patient presents with complaints of pain, but x-rays show no fracture line at the time of the initial injury. Follow-up of these patients with x-rays taken serially will show the development of a fracture line. This is especially important in femoral neck fractures in which weight-bearing may lead to displacement and the subsequent problems of nonunion and avascular necrosis. In a recent study of 36 fatigue fractures of the femoral shaft in military recruits, Blickenstaff and Morris pointed out that the most important aspect of treatment was the prevention of displacement. Displacement occurred if diagnosis was delayed too long after the onset of symptoms.[332] Provost and Morris point out that it is extremely important to treat fatigue fractures adequately in the early stages. The extent and severity of the fracture are often impossible to determine or predict initially; therefore patients who complain of pain in the hip after running or marching, who on examination have pain on motion of the hip, should be confined to bed even though roentgenograms of the hips appear entirely normal. Fracture may develop later and may even become displaced while the patient remains in bed.[333]

EXACERBATION OF UNDERLYING CONDITIONS

Many medical conditions are aggravated by trauma. Some of the classic ones are gout, rheumatoid arthritis, other collagen diseases, endocrine disturbances such as Addison's disease, peptic acid disease, asthma, psychiatric disturbances, and metabolic disorders such as hepatic dysfunction. In an acute gouty attack, the deposition of painful uric acid crystals may be precipitated by any one of a number of traumatic factors. Surgical procedures may also produce the acute syndrome in a previously asymptomatic patient. The importance of recognizing the syndrome is emphasized. Patients with underlying rheumatoid arthritis, without previous symptoms, can become symptomatic after trauma. Injury to a particular joint can cause a flare-up of rheumatoid arthritis in that joint, and injury to a lower extremity can cause exacerbation of rheumatoid arthritis symptoms in an upper extremity. The carbohydrate-insulin equilibrium in diabetes is often altered after musculoskeletal trauma or other stresses. Minor trauma in a patient with hemophilia causes consumption of already depleted clotting factors and increases the propensity for hemorrhage in distant sites.

PSYCHIATRIC ASPECTS OF MUSCULOSKELETAL TRAUMA

Psychologic disability plays an important role in the return to work of patients with musculoskeletal injuries. Studies document the importance of psychologic evaluation for optimal rehabilitation effort and suggest that the whole-man concept is a useful, and perhaps necessary, consideration in the rehabilitation of the industrially injured workman.[334] Functional overlay in orthopedic practice can manifest itself by hysteria or a conversion response. Overreaction to organic illness can occur either in previously normal patients or in those who were anxious or depressed prior to their injury. Functional overlay also manifests itself in prolongation of symptoms after the organic disease has subsided. Constitutional and genetic aspects have an important bearing on the fate of people following musculoskeletal injury.[335] Positive motivation to recover from injury results from a combination of instinctual forces and a personality capable of combining hopefulness with realism. Lack of motivation occurs in patients who have had an injury that appears so devastating to them that they lose their will to do well. Injury may be exaggerated or prolonged for monetary gain or for sympathy. Every trauma surgeon can recall countless cases in which patients appear physically healed and show no objective signs of disability, but are unable to return to work because of continuing complaints. A fracture may be completely healed with no functional loss and minimal disfigurement or deformity, but the patient with the injury may refuse to admit his treatment is at an end because there is some slight angulation, bowing, or atrophy. The all too familiar "greenback poultice" applied by an industrial accident board may have greater curative power than the treatment used by a host of attending surgeons. It is often necessary to ask for psychiatric consultation for patients who are refractory to treatment. Even with psychiatric help, it is often difficult to ascertain who is the malingerer and who is the truly functionally disturbed patient. Permanent disability from functional overlay after organic injury can be more severe than the original injury itself.

PRINCIPLES OF DISABILITY EVALUATION

According to McBride, disability

> is a term that implies a transformation of the body structures which results in a depreciation of normal ability to perform the functions of established physical accomplishments.[336]

Physical impairment after an injury will affect an individual's future activities. It is important to take into account that individual's occupation, as disabilities in different parts of the body, depending upon their location and the severity of physical impairment, will affect his ability to perform his previous tasks. A slight permanent disability of an elbow may be of little consequence to a factory worker who runs a machine by means of foot pedals, but the same elbow injury would be severely disabling to a manual worker who sorts out electronic components by performing repetitive maneuvers of pronation and supination. Permanent disability as defined by McBride is a permanent and irreversible state of body impairment that limits the normal capacity of the individual to perform useful work. Permanent total disability implies the impairment of mind or body sufficient to render it impossible to follow a gainful occupation throughout life. Permanent partial disability implies the ability to follow a gainful occupation to a limited degree. Disability is considered temporary when the progress of a patient has not reached its maximum possible degree of improvement. The two principal components in the evaluation of disability are functional deficiency and physical impairment. The loss of function is the result of the physical impairment, but the evaluation of disability involves the proportional weighing of the influences of both components. McBride has suggested seven factors of function that are fundamental: quickness of action, coordination, strength, security, endurance, safety, and prestige of physique for employment. McBride also suggested five factors of physical impairment: anatomical mass damage, clinical manifestations, job restoration restrictions, restrictions of working conditions, and reactionary interferences.[336]

In determining workman's compensation, the goal of treatment is considered to be rehabilitation. The worker is entitled to compensation for disability that ensues from an initial injury sustained while engaging in the duties of his employment. An industrial injury is also compensable if the injury aggravates a preexisting disability. A physician's evaluation of disability is important because judgment is made on the basis of that evaluation. Compensation is awarded to assure that the injured workman and his dependents have adequate means of subsistence during his recovery. In the event of permanent disability or death, adequate means of subsistence is awarded to the injured and his family, according to the evaluation of the examining physician. In establishing disability, one must take into account not only the physical deficit of the patient, but also his age, his educational background and experience, his psychologic strength and weakness, and his capacity for future employment in his previous trade or in a newly learned occupation.

REFERENCES

1. Crenshaw, A. H.: *Campbell's Operative Orthopaedics.* 5th Ed. St. Louis, C. V. Mosby Co., 1971.
2. McLaughlin, H. L.: *Trauma.* Philadelphia, W. B. Saunders Co., 1959.
3. Conwell, H. E., and Reynolds, F. C.: *Key and Conwell's Management of Fractures, Dislocations, and Sprains.* 7th Ed. St. Louis, C. V. Mosby Co., 1961.
4. DePalma, A. F.: *The Management of Fractures and Dislocations: an Atlas.* 2nd Ed. Philadelphia, W. B. Saunders Co., 1970.
5. Charnley, J: *The Closed Treatment of Common Fractures.* 3rd Ed. Baltimore, Williams & Wilkins Co., 1963.
6. Shires, G. T. (Ed.): *Care of the Trauma Patient.* New York, McGraw-Hill Book Co., 1966.
7. Mehrez, M., and el Geneidy, S.: Arthrography of the ankle. J. Bone Joint Surg., *52B*:308, 1970.
8. Gordon, R. B.: Arthrography of the ankle joint. J. Bone Joint Surg., 52A1623, 1970.
9. Nicholas, J. A., Freiberger, R. H., and Killoran, P. J.: Double-contrast arthrography of the knee. J. Bone Joint Surg., *52A*:203, 1970.
10. Fordyce, A. J. W., and Horn, C. V.: Arthrography in recent injuries of the ligaments of the ankle. J. Bone Joint Surg., *54B*:116, 1972.
11. Eisen, A. A.: Electromyography and nerve conduction as a diagnostic aid. Orthop. Clin. North Am., *4*:885, 1973.
12. Kopell, H. P., and Thompson, W. A. L.: *Peripheral Entrapment Neuropathies.* Baltimore, Williams & Wilkins Co., 1963.
13. Omer, G. E.: Evaluation and reconstruction of the forearm and hand after acute traumatic peripheral nerve injuries. J. Bone Joint Surg., *50A*:1454, 1968.
14. Jackson, R. W., and Abe, I.: The role of arthroscopy in the management of disorders of the knee. J. Bone Joint Surg., *54B*:310, 1972.
15. Jackson, R. W.: Arthroscopy of the knee. Current Practice in Orthopedic Surgery, 1973, p. 93.
16. Liebolt, S. L.: *Illustrated Review of Fracture Treatment.* Los Altos, Calif., Lange Medical Publications, 1954.
17. Quigley, T. B., Banks, H. H., and Leach, R. E., et al.: Advances in the management of fractures and dislocations in the past decade. Orthop. Clin. North Am., *3*:793, 1972.
18. Rowe, C. R.: The management of fractures in elderly patients is different. J. Bone Joint Surg., *47A*:1043, 1965.
19. Lam, S. J.: The place of delayed internal fixation in the treatment of fractures of the long bones. J. Bone Joint Surg., *46B*:393, 1964.
20. Smith, J. E. M.: The results of early and delayed internal fixation of fractures of the shaft of the femur. J. Bone Joint Surg., *46B*:28, 1964.
21. McNeur, J. C.: The management of open skeletal trauma with particular reference to internal fixation. J. Bone Joint Surg., *52B*:54, 1970.
22. Flatt, A. E.: *The Care of Minor Hand Injuries.* 2nd Ed. St. Louis, C. V. Mosby Co., 1963.
23. Leffert, R. D.: Brachial plexus injuries. Orthop. Clin. North Am., *1*:399, 1970.
24. Leffert, R. D., and Seddon, H.: Infraclavicular brachial plexus injuries. J. Bone Joint Surg., *47B*:9, 1965.
25. Brown, F. W., and Navigato, W. J.: Rupture of the axillary artery and brachial plexus palsy associated with anterior dislocation of the shoulder. Clin. Orthop., *60*:195, 1968.
26. Bonney, G.: Progress in traction injuries of the brachial plexus. J. Bone Joint Surg., *41B*:4, 1959.
27. Lusskin, R., Campbell, J. B., and Thompson, W. A. L.: Post-traumatic lesions of the brachial plexus. J. Bone Joint Surg., *55A*:1159, 1973.
28. DePalma, A. F.: *Surgery of the Shoulder.* 2nd Ed. Philadelphia, J. B. Lippincott Co., 1973.
29. Bateman, J. E.: *The Shoulder and Neck.* Philadelphia, W. B. Saunders Co., 1972.
30. Moseley, H. F. (Ed.): Surgery of the shoulder region. Surg. Clin. North Am., *43*:6, 1963.
31. Park, J. Y., and Espiniella, J. L.: Rupture of pectoralis major muscle. J. Bone Joint Surg., *52A*:577, 1970.
32. McEntire, J. E., Hess, W. E., and Coleman, S. S.: Rupture of the pectoralis major muscle. J. Bone Joint Surg., *54A*:1040, 1972.
33. Crenshaw, A. H., and Kilgore, W. E.: Surgical treatment of bicipital tenosynovitis. J. Bone Joint Surg., *48A*:1496, 1966.
34. Kernwein, G., Roseberg, B., and Sneed, W. R., Jr.: Arthrographic studies of the shoulder joint. J. Bone Joint Surg., *39A*:1267, 1957.
35. Samilkson, R. L., Raphael, R. L., Post, L., Noonan, C., Siris, E., and Raney, F. L.: Shoulder arthrography. J.A.M.A., *175*:773, 1961.
36. Neviaser, J.: Arthrography of the shoulder joint. J. Bone Joint Surg., *44A*:1321, 1962.
37. Debeyre, J., Patie, D., and Elmelik, E.: Repair of ruptures of the rotator cuff of the shoulder. J. Bone Joint Surg., *47B*:36, 1965.
38. Turek, S. L.: *Orthopaedic Principles and Their Application.* 2nd Ed. Philadelphia, J. B. Lippincott Co., 1967.
39. Russek, A. S.: Scapulo-costal syndrome. J.A.M.A., *150*:25, 1952.
40. Cailliet, R.: *Neck and Arm Pain.* Philadelphia, F. A. Davis Co., 1964.
41. Tyer, H. D. D., Sturrock, W. D. S., and Callow, F. M.: Retrosternal dislocation of the clavicle. J. Bone Joint Surg., *45B*:132, 1963.
42. McKenzie, J. M. M.: Retrosternal dislocation of the clavicle. J. Bone Joint Surg., *45B*:139, 1963.

43. Salvatore, J. E.: Sterno-clavicular joint dislocation. Clin. Orthop., *58*:51, 1968.
44. Allman, F. L., Jr.: Fractures and ligamentous injuries of the clavicle and its articulation. J. Bone Joint Surg., *49A*:775, 1967.
45. Weaver, J. K., and Dunn, H. K.: Treatment of acromioclavicular injuries, especially complete acromioclavicular separation. J. Bone Joint Surg., *54A*:1187, 1972.
46. Jacobs, B., and Wade, P. A.: Acromioclavicular-joint injury. J. Bone Joint Surg., *48A*:275, 1966.
47. Bailey, R. W.: Acute and recurrent dislocation of the shoulder. J. Bone Joint Surg., *49A*:767, 1967.
48. McLaughlin, H. L., and Cavallaro, W. U.: Primary anterior dislocation of shoulder. Am. J. Surg., *80*:615, 1950.
49. Rowe, C.: Prognosis of dislocations of the shoulder. J. Bone Joint Surg., *38A*:957, 1956.
50. Kummel, B. M.: Fractures of the glenoid causing chronic dislocation of the shoulder. Clin. Orthop., *69*:189, 1970.
51. Calvé, J., et al.: Dislocation of the shoulder and vascular lesions. A. Chir., *58*:337, 1941–42.
52. Curr, J. S.: Rupture of the axillary artery complicating dislocation of the shoulder. J. Bone Joint Surg., *52B*:313, 1970.
53. Watson-Jones, R.: *Fractures and Joint Injuries.* 4th Ed. Baltimore, Williams & Wilkins Co., 1960.
54. Bankart, A. S. B.: The pathology and treatment of recurrent dislocation of the shoulder joint. Br. J. Surg., *26*:23, 1938.
55. Chattopadhyaya, P. K.: Posterior fracture-dislocation of the shoulder. J. Bone Joint Surg., *52B*:521, 1970.
56. Pillaman, H. A., and Thompson, R. C.: Bilateral posterior fracture-dislocation of the shoulder. J. Bone Joint Surg., *51A*:1627, 1969.
57. Dorgan, J. A.: Posterior dislocation of the shoulder. Am. J. Surg., *89*:890, 1955.
58. Ralston, E. L.: *Hand Book of Fractures.* St. Louis, C. V. Mosby Co., 1967.
59. Kummel, B. M.: Fractures of the glenoid causing chronic dislocation of the shoulder. Clin. Orthop., *69*:189, 1970.
60. Aston, J. W., and Gregory, C. F.: Dislocation of the shoulder with significant fracture of the glenoid. J. Bone Joint Surg., *55A*:1531, 1973.
61. Neer, C. S.: Displaced proximal humeral fracture. J. Bone Joint Surg., *52A*:1077, 1970.
62. Holstein, A., and Lewis, G. B.: Fractures of the humerus with radial nerve paralysis. J. Bone Joint Surg., *45A*:1383, 1963.
63. Shaw, J. L., and Sakellarides, H.: Radial-nerve paralysis associated with fractures of the humerus. J. Bone Joint Surg., *49A*:899, 1967.
64. Klenerman, L.: Fractures of the shaft of the humerus. J. Bone Joint Surg., *48B*:105, 1966.
65. Sim, F. H., Kelly, P. J., and Henderson, E. D.: Radial nerve palsy complicating fractures of the humeral shaft. J. Bone Joint Surg., *53A*:1023, 1971.
66. Coonrad, R. W., and Hooper, W. R.: Tennis elbow: its course, natural history, conservative and surgical management. J. Bone Joint Surg., *55A*:1177, 1973.
67. Boyd, H. B., and McLeod, A. C.: Tennis elbow. J. Bone Joint Surg., *55A*:1183, 1973.
68. Bosworth, D. M.: The role of the orbicular ligament in tennis elbow. J. Bone Joint Surg., *37A*:527, 1955.
69. Bosworth, D. M.: Surgical treatment of tennis elbow. J. Bone Joint Surg., *47A*:1533, 1965.
70. Roles, N. C., and Maudsley, R. E.: Radial tunnel syndrome. J. Bone Joint Surg., *54B*:499, 1972.
72. Wickstom, J., and Meyer, P. R.: Fractures of the distal humerus in adults. Clin. Orthop., *50*:43, 1967.
73. Miller, W. E.: Comminuted fractures of the distal end of the humerus in the adult. J. Bone Joint Surg., *46A*:644, 1964.
74. Smith, F. M.: *Surgery of the Elbow.* Springfield, Ill., Charles C Thomas, 1954.
75. O'Donoghue, D. H.: *Treatment of Injuries to Athletes.* 3rd Ed. Philadelphia, W. B. Saunders Co., 1976.
76. Radin, E. L., and Riseborough, E. J.: Fractures of the radial head. J. Bone Joint Surg., *48A*:1055, 1966.
77. Bado, J. L.: The Monteggia lesion. Clin. Orthop., *50*:71, 1967.
78. Boyd, H. B., and Boals, J. C.: The Monteggia lesion. Clin. Orthop., *66*:94, 1969.
79. Stein, F., Grabias, S. L., and Deffer, P. A.: Nerve injury complicating Monteggia lesion. J. Bone Joint Surg., *53A*:1432, 1971.
80. Tompkins, D. G.: The anterior Monteggia fracture. J. Bone Joint Surg., *53A*:1109, 1971.
81. McBride, E. D.: *Disability Evaluation and Principles of Treatment of Compensable Injuries.* 6th Ed. Philadelphia, J. B. Lippincott Co., 1963.
82. Tachdjian, M. O.: *Pediatric Orthopedics.* Philadelphia, W. B. Saunders Co., 1972.
83. Flynn, J. E.: *Hand Surgery.* Baltimore, Williams & Wilkins Co., 1966.
84. Sharrard, W. J. W.: *Pediatric Orthopedics and Fractures.* Oxford, Blackwell Scientific Publications, 1971.
85. Herrmann, L. G., and Caldwell, J. A.: Diagnosis and treatment of post-traumatic osteoporosis. Am. J. Surg., *51*:630, 1941.
86. Mazet, R.: Intra-medullary fixation in the arm and the forearm. Clin. Orthop., *2*:75, 1953.
87. Dodge, H. S., and Cady, G. W.: Treatment of fractures of the radius and ulna with compression plates. J. Bone Joint Surg., *54A*:1167, 1972.
88. Smith, J. E. M.: Internal fixation in the treatment of fractures of the shaft of the radius and the ulna in adults. J. Bone Joint Surg., *41B*:122, 1959.
89. Burwell, H. N., and Charnley, A. D.: Treatment of forearm fractures in adults with particular reference to plate fixation. J. Bone Joint Surg., *46B*:404, 1964.
90. Basom, W. C.: Report of two cases of delayed union or non-union treated by prolonged external pin fixation and impaction. Clin. Orthop., *6*:166, 1965.
91. Carroll, R. E., Sinton, W. A., and Garcia, A.: Acute calcium deposits in the hand. J.A.M.A., *157*:422, 1955.
92. Smith, A. M. C. E.: Sprain of the pisiform-triquetral joint. J. Bone Joint Surg., *36B*:618, 1954.
93. Phalen, G.: The carpal-tunnel syndrome. Clin. Orthop., *83*:29, 1972.
94. Langloh, N. D., and Linscheid, R. L.: Recurrent and unrelieved carpal-tunnel syndrome. Clin. Orthop., *83*:41, 1972.
95. Carroll, R. E., and Green, D. D.: The significance of the palmar cutaneous nerve at the wrist. Clin. Orthop., *83*:24, 1972.
96. Shaw, J. C., and Wilson, F. C.: Radial perilunar dislocations. J. Bone Joint Surg., *52A*:556, 1970.
97. Weiss, C., Laskin, R. S., and Spinner, M.: Irreducible radio-carpal dislocations. J. Bone Joint Surg., *52A*:562, 1970.
98. Weiss, C., Laskin, R. S., and Spinner, M.: Irreducible trans-scaphoid perilunate dislocation. J. Bone Joint Surg., *52A*:562, 1970.
99. Stein, F., and Siegel, M. W.: Naviculo-capitate fracture syndrome. J. Bone Joint Surg., *51A*:391, 1969.
100. Siegel, N. W., and Hertzberg, H.: Complete dislocation of the greater multangular (trapezium). J. Bone Joint Surg., *51A*:769, 1969.
101. Hsu, J. D., and Curtis, R. M.: Carpo-metacarpal

dislocations on the ulnar side of the hand. J. Bone Joint Surg., *52A*:92F, 1970.
102. Snook, G. A., Chrisman, O. D., Wilson, T. C., and Wietsma, R. D.: Subluxation of the distal radio-ulnar joint by hyperpronation. J. Bone Joint Surg., *51A*:1315, 1969.
103. Dameron, T. B.: Traumatic dislocation of the distal radio-ulnar joint. Clin. Orthop., *83*:55, 1972.
104. Colles, A.: On the fracture of the carpal extremity of the radius. Edinb. Med. Surg. J., *10*:181, 1814.
105. Pool, C.: Colles' fracture. J. Bone Joint Surg., *55B*:540, 1973.
105a. Böhler, L.: *Treatment of Fractures.* 4th Ed. Baltimore, William Wood & Co. 1929.
105b. Rush, L. U., and Rush, H. L.: Longitudinal pin fixation in Colles' fracture of the wrist. South. Surg., *15*:679, 1949.
106. Cole, J. M., and Obletz, B. E.: Comminuted fractures of the distal end of the radius treated by skeletal transfixion in plaster casts. J. Bone Joint Surg., *48A*:931, 1966.
107. Gartland, J. J., and Werley, C. W.: Evaluation of healed Colles' fractures. J. Bone Joint Surg., *33A*:895, 1951.
108. DePalma, A. F.: Comminuted fractures of the distal end of the radius treated by ulnar pinning. J. Bone Joint Surg., *34A*:651, 1952.
109. Blichert-Toft, M., and Jensen, H. K.: Colles' fracture treated with modified Böhler technic. Acta Orthop. Scand., *42*:45, 1971.
110. Bacorn, R. W., and Kurtzke, J. F.: Colles' fractures. A study of 2,000 cases from The New York State Workmen's Compensation Board. J. Bone Joint Surg., *35A*:643, 1953.
111. Smaill, G. B.: Long-term follow-up of Colles' fractures. J. Bone Joint Surg., *47B*:80, 1965.
112. Ellis, J.: Smith's and Barton's fractures. J. Bone Joint Surg., *47B*:724, 1965.
113. Woodyard, J. E.: A review of Smith's fractures. J. Bone Joint Surg., *51B*:324, 1969.
114. Hunt, D. D.: Dislocation of the extensor pollicis longus tendon in Smith's fracture of the radius. J. Bone Joint Surg., *51A*:991, 1969.
115. De Oliveira, J. C.: Barton's fractures. J. Bone Joint Surg., *55A*:586, 1973.
116. Foéga, H.: Fracture of the lower end of the radius with ulnar nerve palsy. J. Bone Joint Surg., *48B*:514, 1966.
117. Waugh, R. L., and Sullivan, R. F.: Anomalies of the carpus. J. Bone Joint Surg., *32A*:682, 1950.
118. Stewart, M. J.: Fractures of the carpal navicular (scaphoid)—a report of 436 cases. J. Bone Joint Surg., *36A*:998, 1954.
119. Stewart, M. J.: Treatment of fracture of the carpal navicular—conservative versus surgical (with review of 697 cases). J. Bone Joint Surg., *48A*:1025, 1966.
120. Baird, D. B., and Friedenberg, F. B.: Delayed ulnar-nerve palsy following a fracture of the hamate. J. Bone Joint Surg., *50A*:570, 1968.
121. Shea, J. D., and McClain, E. J.: Ulnar-nerve compression syndromes at and below the wrist. J. Bone Joint Surg., *51A*:1095, 1969.
122. Green, J. P.: Proximal avulsion of the iliacus with paralysis of the femoral nerve. J. Bone Joint Surg., *54B*:154, 1972.
123. Epstein, H. C.: Traumatic dislocations of the hip. Clin. Orthop., *92*:116, 1973.
124. Eisenberg, K. S., Sheft, D. J., and Murray, W. R.: Posterior dislocation of the hip producing lumbosacral nerve-root avulsion. J. Bone Joint Surg., *54A*:1083, 1972.
125. Pickett, J. C.: Injuries of the hip. Clin. Orthop., *4*:64, 1954.
126. Kelly, P., and Lipscomb, P.: Primary Vitallium *mold* arthroplasty for posterior dislocation with fracture of the femoral head. J. Bone Joint Surg., *40A*:675, 1968.
127. Henry, A. K., and Bayumi, M.: Fracture of the femur with luxation of the ipsilateral hip. Br. J. Surg., *22*:204, 1934.
128. Dehne, E., and Immerman, E. W.: Dislocation of the hip combined with fracture of the shaft of the femur on the same side. J. Bone Joint Surg., *33A*:71, 1951.
129. Nelson, D. L.: Traumatic recurrent dislocation of the hip. J. Bone Joint Surg., *52A*:128, 1970.
130. Thompson, T. C.: Dislocation of the femoral head into the scrotum. Spectator Correspondence Club Letter, 1948.
131. Epstein, H. C., and Harvey, J. P.: Traumatic anterior dislocations of the hip. Management and results. An analysis of 55 cases. J. Bone Joint Surg., *54A*:1561, 1972.
132. Derian, P. S., and Purser, T.: Intra-articular small-bowel herniation complicating central fracture dislocation of the hip. J. Bone Joint Surg., *49A*:1614, 1966.
133. Larson, C. B.: Fracture dislocations of the hip. Clin. Orthop., *92*:147, 1973.
134. Otto, A. W.: In Pfannenbeckenmisstaltung. Infolge deformierender Osteoarthritis: Neue Seltene Beobachtungen zur Anatomie Physiologie und Pathologie Gehorig. Berlin, Rucker, 1824.
135. Ghormley, R. K., and Dockerty, M. B.: Arthrokatadysis. Surgery, *29*:255, 1951.
136. Friedenberg, Z. B.: Protrusio acetabuli. Am. J. Surg., *85*:764, 1953.
137. Boyd, H. B., and Griffin, L. L.: Classification and treatment of trochanteric fractures. Arch. Surg., *58*:853, 1949.
138. Pauwels, F.: *Der Schenkelhalsbruch Ein Mechanisches Problem.* Stuttgart, Ferdinand Euld, 1935.
139. Garden, R. S.: Low-angle fixation in fractures of the femoral neck. J. Bone Joint Surg., *43B*:647, 1961.
140. Smith, F. B.: Effects of rotatory and valgus malposition in blood supply to the femoral head. J. Bone Joint Surg., *41A*:800, 1959.
141. Banks, H. H.: Factors influencing the results in fractures of the femoral neck. J. Bone Joint Surg., *44A*:931, 1962.
142. Judet, R.: Treatment of femoral fractures with pedicle bone graft. Acta Orthop. Scand., *32*:421, 1962.
143. Meyers, M. H., Harvey, J. P., and Moore, T. M.: Treatment of displaced subcapital and transcervical fractures of femoral neck by muscle pedicle bone graft and internal fixation. J. Bone Joint Surg., *55A*:25F, 1973.
144. Boyd, H. B., and Salvatore, J. E.: Acute fracture of the femoral neck: internal fixation or prosthesis? J. Bone Joint Surg., *46A*:1066, 1964.
145. Hinchey, J. J., and Day, P. L.: Primary prosthetic replacement in fresh femoral-neck fractures. J. Bone Joint Surg., *46A*:223, 1964.
146. Turner, R. H., and Harris, W. H. Personal communication.
147. Crawford, H. B.: Experience with the non-operative treatment of impacted fractures of the neck of the femur. J. Bone Joint Surg., *47A*:830, 1965.

148. Massie, W. K.: Fractures of the hip. J. Bone Joint Surg., *47A*:658, 1964.
149. Boyd, H. B., and Griffin, L. L.: Classification and treatment of trochanteric fractures. Arch Surg., *58*:853, 1949.
150. Evans, E. M.: The treatment of trochanteric fractures of the femur. J. Bone Joint Surg., *31B*:190, 1949.
151. Banks, H. H.: Unstable intertrochanteric fractures. American Academy of Orthopedic Surgeons Instructional Course Lectures. Vol. 19. St. Louis, C. V. Mosby Co., 1970, p. 90.
152. Massie, W. K.: Functional fixation of femoral neck fractures; telescoping nail technique. Clin. Orthop., *13*:230, 1958.
153. Holt, E. P.: Hip fractures in the trochanteric region: treatment with a strong nail and early weight bearing. J. Bone Joint Surg., *45A*:687, 1963.
154. Sarmiento, A.: Intertrochanteric fractures of the femur. J. Bone Joint Surg., *45A*:706, 1963.
155. Dimon, J. H., and Hughston, J. C.: Unstable intertrochanteric fractures of the hip. J. Bone Joint Surg., *49A*:440, 1967.
156. Dimon, J. H., III, and Hughston, J. C.: Unstable intertrochanteric fractures. Part 2. American Academy of Orthopedic Surgeons Instructional Course Lectures. Vol. 19. St. Louis, C. V. Mosby Co., 1970, p. 110.
157. Harrington, K. D., and Johnston, J. O.: The management of comminuted unstable intertrochanteric fractures. J. Bone Joint Surg., *55A*:1367, 1973.
158. Zickel, R. E.: A new fixation device for subtrochanteric fractures of the femur. Clin. Orthop., *54*:115, 1967.
159. Dimon, J. H.: Isolated fractures of the lesser trochanter of the femur. Clin. Orthop., *82*:144, 1972.
160. Zadek, I.: Ossifying hematoma in the thigh. J. Bone Joint Surg., *51A*:386, 1969.
161. Oliver, P.: Myositis ossificans following single trauma. J.A.M.A., *63*:1452, 1914.
162. Holm, C. L., and Embick, R. P.: Traction suspension in fractures of the femur. Northwest Med., *64*:731, 1965.
163. Anderson, R. L.: Conservative treatment of fractures of the femur. J. Bone Joint Surg., *49A*:1371, 1967.
164. Kaufer, H.: Non-operative ambulatory treatment for fracture of the shaft of the femur. Clin. Orthop., *87*:192, 1972.
165. Martyn, J. W., and McGoey, P. F.: Choice of treatment in fractures of the femoral shaft in adults. Can. Med. Assoc. J., *88*:784, 1961.
166. Küntscher, G.: Die Marknagelung von Knochenbrüchen. Arch. Klin. Chir., *200*:443, 1940.
167. Schneider, M.: Part 3, Closed intradeullary nailing of shaft fractures using Küntscher methods. American Academy of Orthopedic Surgeons Instructional Course Lectures. Vol. 22. St. Louis, C. V. Mosby Co., 1973, p. 188.
168. Dencker, H.: Shaft fractures of the femur: comparative study of results of various methods of treatment in 1003 cases. Acta Chir. Scand., *130*:173, 1968.
169. Smith, J. E. M.: The results of early and delayed internal fixation of fractures of the shaft of the femur. J. Bone Joint Surg., *46B*:28, 1964.
170. Gant, G. C., Shaftan, G. W., and Herbsman, H.: Experience with the A.S.I.F. compression plate in the management of femoral shaft fractures. J. Trauma, *10*:458, 1970.
171. Nichols, P. J. R.: Rehabilitation after fractures of the shaft of the femur. J. Bone Joint Surg., *45B*:96, 1963.
172. Kirkup, J. R.: Major arterial injury complicating fracture of the femoral shaft. J. Bone Joint Surg., *45B*:337, 1963.
173. Bonney, G.: Thrombosis of the femoral artery complicating fracture of the femur. Treatment by endarterectomy. J. Bone Joint Surg., *45B*:344, 1963.
174. Wickstrom J., Corban, M. S., and Vise, G. T.: Complications following intramedullary fixation of 324 fractured femurs. Clin. Orthop., *60*:103, 1968.
175. Sarmiento, A.: Functional bracing of tibial and femoral shaft fractures. Clin. Orthop., *82*:2, 1972.
176. Mooney, V., Nickel, V. L., Harvey, J. P., Jr., et al.: Cast-brace treatment for fractures of the distal part of the femur. J. Bone Joint Surg., *52A*:1563, 1970.
177. Mital, M.: Personal communication.
178. Connolly, J. F., and King, P.: Closed reduction and early cast-brace ambulation in the treatment of femoral fractures. J. Bone Joint Surg., *55A*:1559, 1973.
179. Connolly, J. F., Dehne, E., and Lafollette, B.: Closed reduction and early cast-brace ambulation in the treatment of femoral fractures. J. Bone Joint Surg., *55A*:1581, 1973.
180. Neer, C. S., Grantham, S. A., and Shelton, M. L.: Supracondylar fracture of the adult femur. J. Bone Joint Surg., *49A*:591, 1967.
181. Riggins, R. S., Garrick, J. B., and Lipscomb, P. R.: Supracondylar fractures of the femur. Clin. Orthop., *82*:32, 1972.
182. Smillie, I. S.: *Injuries of the Knee Joint.* 3rd Ed. Baltimore, Williams & Wilkins Co., 1962.
183. Ramsey, R. H., and Muller, G. E.: Quadriceps tendon rupture: a diagnostic trap. Clin. Orthop., *70*:161, 1970.
184. Levy, M., Seelenfreund, M., Maor, P., et al.: Bilateral spontaneous and simultaneous rupture of the quadriceps tendons in gout. J. Bone Joint Surg., *53B*:510, 1971.
185. Brooke, R.: The treatment of fractured patella by excision. A study of morphology and function. Br. J. Surg., *24*:733, 1936–37.
186. McMaster, P. E.: Fractures of the patella. Clin. Orthop., *4*:24, 1954.
187. Griswold, A. S.: Fractures of the patella. Clin. Orthop., *4*:44, 1954.
188. O'Donoghue, D. H., Tompkins, F., and Hays, M. B.: Strength of quadriceps function after patellectomy. Western J. Surg., *60*:159, 1952.
189. West, F.: End results of patellectomy. J. Bone Joint Surg., *44A*:1089, 1962.
190. Haliburton, R. A., and Sullivan, C. R.: The patella in degenerative joint disease. A clinico-pathologic study. A.M.A. Arch. Surg., *77*:677, 1958.
191. Wiles, P., Andrews, P. S., and Bremner, R. A.: Chondromalacia of the patella: a study of the later results of excision of the articular cartilage. J. Bone Joint Surg., *42B*:65, 1960.
192. Cave, E. F., and Rowe, C. R.: The patella; its importance in derangements of the knee. J. Bone Joint Surg., *32A*:542, 1950.
193. MacNab, I.: Recurrent dislocation of the patella. J. Bone Joint Surg., *34A*:957, 1952.
194. Gordon, G. C.: Traumatic prepatellar neuralgia. J. Bone Joint Surg., *43B*:41, 1952.
195. Smason, J. B.: Post-traumatic fistula connecting prepatellar bursa with knee joint. J. Bone Joint Surg., *54A*:1553, 1972.
196. Haggart, C. E.: Synovial cyst of the popliteal space: clinical significance and treatment. Ann. Surg., *118*:438, 1943.
197. Burleson, R. J., Bickel, W. H., and Dahlin; D. C.:

Popliteal cyst, a clinico-pathologic survey. J. Bone Joint Surg., *38A*:1265, 1956.
198. Voshell, A. F., and Brantigan, O. C.: Bursitis in the region of the tibial collateral ligament. J. Bone Joint Surg., *26*:793, 1944.
199. Clark, K.: Ganglion of the collateral popliteal nerve. J. Bone Joint Surg., *43B*:778, 1961.
200. Parkes, A.: Intraneural ganglion of the lateral popliteal nerve. J. Bone Joint Surg., *43B*:784, 1961.
201. Towne, L. C., Blazina, M. E., Marmorn, L., and Lawrence, J. F.: Lateral compartment syndrome of the knee. Clin. Orthop., *76*:160, 1971.
202. Collins, H. R.: Reconstruction of the athlete's injured knee. Orthop. Clin. North Am., *2*:207, 1971.
203. O'Donoghue, D. H.: Surgical treatment of fresh injuries to the major ligaments of the knees. J. Bone Joint Surg., *32A*:721, 1950.
204. Clayton, M. L., and Weir, G. J.: Experimental investigation of ligamentous healing. Am. J. Surg., *98*:373, 1959.
205. Feagin, J. A., Abbott, H. G., and Rokous, J. R.: The isolated tear of the anterior cruciate ligament. J. Bone Joint Surg., *54A*:1340, 1972.
206. Trickey, E. L.: Rupture of the posterior cruciate ligament of the knee. J. Bone Joint Surg., *50B*:334, 1968.
207. Nicholas, J. A.: The 5–1 reconstruction for antero or medial instability of the knee. J. Bone Joint Surg., *55A*:899, 1973.
208. Kennedy, J. C.: Complete dislocation of the knee joint. J. Bone Joint Surg., *45A*:889, 1963.
209. Meyers, M. H., and Harvey, J. P.: Traumatic dislocation of the knee joint. J. Bone Joint Surg., *53A*:16, 1971.
210. Connolly, J. F., Whittaker, D., and Williams, E.: Femoral and tibial fractures combined with injuries to the femoral or popliteal artery. J. Bone Joint Surg., *53A*:56, 1971.
211. Kennedy, J. C., Grainger, R. W., and McGraw, R. W.: Osteochondral fractures of the femoral condyles. J. Bone Joint Surg., *48B*:436, 1966.
212. Rosenberg, N. J.: Osteochondral fractures of the lateral femoral condyle. J. Bone Joint Surg., *46A*:1013, 1964.
213. Aichroth, P.: Osteochondral fractures and their relationship to osteochondritis dissecans of the knee. J. Bone Joint Surg., *53B*:448, 1971.
214. Aichroth, P.: Osteochondritis dissecans of the knee. J. Bone Joint Surg., *53B*:440, 1971.
215. Meyers, M. H., and McKeever, F. M.: Fracture of the intercondylar eminence of the tibia. J. Bone Joint Surg., *52A*:1677, 1970.
216. Anderson, R., and Loughlen, I.: Fractures of the tibial plateau: treatment by assured fixation technic. Clin. Orthop., *4*:10, 1954.
217. Porter, B. B.: Crush fractures of the lateral tibial table. J. Bone Joint Surg., *52B*:676, 1970.
218. Roberts, J. M.: Fractures of the condyles of the tibia. J. Bone Joint Surg., *50A*:1505, 1968.
219. Christensen, S.: Dislocation of the upper end of the fibula. Acta Orthop. Scand., *37*:107, 1966.
220. Lyle, H. H. M.: Traumatic luxation of the head of the fibula. Ann. Surg., *82*:635, 1925.
221. Crothers, O. D., and Johnson, J. T. H.: Isolated acute dislocation of the proximal tibio-fibular joint. J. Bone Joint Surg., *55A*:181, 1973.
222. Bateman, J. E.: *Trauma to Nerves in Limbs.* Philadelphia, W. B. Saunders Co., 1962.
223. Devas, M. B.: Shin splints, or stress fractures of the metacarpal bone in horses, and shin soreness, or stress fractures of the tibia, in man. J. Bone Joint Surg., *49B*:310, 1967.
224. Leach, R. E. Hammond, G., and Stryker, W. S.: Anterior tibial compartment syndrome. J. Bone Joint Surg., *49A*:451, 1967.
225. Gillies, H., and Chalmers, J.: Management of fresh ruptures of the tendo Achillis. J. Bone Joint Surg., *52A*:337, 1970.
226. Renne, J. W., and Davis, P. H.: An unusual gastrocnemius muscle syndrome. J. Bone Joint Surg., *55A*:1294, 1973.
227. Judet, R., Mouquin, F., and Patel, A.: Les désinsertions du jumeau interne. Presse Med., *78*:801, 1970.
228. Friedlander, H. L.: Chronic expanding hematoma of the calf. J. Bone Joint Surg., *50A*:1237, 1968.
229. Quigley, T. B., Banks, H. H., Leach, R. E., et al.: Advances in the management of fractures and dislocations in the past decade. Orthop. Clin. North Am., *3*:793, 1972.
230. Nicoll, E. A.: Fractures of the tibial shaft. J. Bone Joint Surg., *46B*:373, 1964.
231. Garrick, J. G., Riggins, R. S., Requa, R. K., et al.: Fracture of the mid-shaft of the tibia and fibula. A survey of treatment. Clin. Orthop., *88*:131, 1972.
232. Sarmiento, A.: A functional below-the-knee *brace* for tibial fractures. J. Bone Joint Surg., *52A*:295, 1970.
233. Sarmiento, A.: A functional below-the-knee *cast* for tibial fractures. J. Bone Joint Surg., *49A*:855, 1967.
234. Müller, M. E., Allgöwer, M., and Willenegger, H.: *Technique of Internal Fixation of Fractures.* New York, Springer Verlag, 1965.
235. Sakellarides, H. T., Freeman, P. A., and Grant, B. D.: Delayed union and non-union of tibial-shaft fractures. J. Bone Joint Surg., *46A*:557, 1964.
236. Wilson, P. D.: *Management of Fractures and Dislocations.* Philadelphia, J. B. Lippincott Co., 1938.
237. Brown, P. W., and Urban, J. G.: Early weight-bearing treatment of open fractures of the tibia. J. Bone Joint Surg., *51A*:59, 1969.
238. Scudese, V. A., Birotte, A., and Gialanella, J.: Tibial shaft fractures: percutaneous multiple pin fixation, short-leg cast and immediate weight bearing. Clin. Orthop., *72*:271, 1970.
239. Owen, R., and Tsimboukis, D.: Ischaemia complicating closed tibial and fibular shaft fractures. J. Bone Joint Surg., *49B*:268, 1967.
240. Elis, H.: Disabilities after tibial shaft fractures. J. Bone Joint Surg., *40B*:190, 1958.
241. MacGowan, W.: Acute ischaemia complicating limb trauma. J. Jone Joint Surg., *50B*:472, 1968.
242. McQuillan, W. M., and Nolan, B.: Ischaemia complicating injury. J. Bone Joint Surg., *50A*:482, 1968.
243. Porter, M. F.: Delayed arterial occlusion in limb injuries. J. Bone Joint Surg., *50B*:472, 1968.
244. Harris, J. D.: A case of arteriovenous fistula following closed fracture of the tibia and fibula. Br. J. Surg., *50*:774, 1963.
245. Evans, T. A., Stone, K. H., and Bailey, D.: Traumatic arteriovenous fistula of the posterior tibial vessels. J. Bone Joint Surg., *49B*:771, 1967.
246. Ghormley, J., and Spear, J.: Anomalies of the posterior tibial tendon, cause of persistent pain about the ankle. Arch. Surg., *66*:512, 1953.
247. DuVries, H. L.: *Surgery of the Foot.* St. Louis, C. V. Mosby Co., 1959.
248. Nava, B. E.: Traumatic dislocation of the tibialis posterior tendon at the ankle. J. Bone Joint Surg., *50B*:150, 1968.
249. Bonnin, J. G.: The hypermobile ankle. Proc. R. Soc. Med., *37*:282, 1944.
250. Bosien, W. R., Staples, O. S., and Russell, S. W.: Residual disability following acute ankle sprains. J. Bone Joint Surg., *37A*:1237, 1955.

251. Smith, M. G. H.: Inferior tibio-fibular diastasis treated by cross screwing. J. Bone Joint Surg., *45B*:737, 1963.
252. Colton, C. L.: Fractures-diastasis of the inferior tibio-fibular joint. J. Bone Joint Surg., *50B*:830, 1968.
253. Mendelsohn, H. A.: Non-union of malleolar fractures of the ankle. Clin. Orthop., *32*:103, 1965.
254. Wilson, F. C., and Skilbred, L. A.: Long-term results in the treatment of displaced bimalleolar fractures. J. Bone Joint Surg., *48A*:1065, 1966.
255. Mukherjee, S. K., and Young, A. B.: Dome fracture of the talus. J. Bone Joint Surg., *55B*:319, 1973.
256. Johnson, E. W., and Ortiz, P. R.: Electro-diagnosis of tarsal tunnel syndrome. Arch. Phys. Med. Rehabil., *4F*:776, 1966.
257. Keck, C.: The tarsal-tunnel syndrome. J. Bone Joint Surg., *44A*:180, 1962.
258. Kopell, H. P., and Thompson, W. A.: Peripheral entrapment neuropathies of the lower extremity. N. Engl. J. Med., *262*:56, 1960.
259. Lam, S. J. S.: A tarsal-tunnel syndrome. Lancet, *2*:1354, 1962.
260. Lam, S. J. S.: Tarsal-tunnel syndrome. J. Bone Joint Surg., *49B*:87, 1967.
261. Edwards, W. G., Lincoln, C. R., Bassett, F. H., III, Goldner, J. L., and Clippinger, F. W.: The tarsal-tunnel syndrome. J. Bone Joint Surg., *51A*:1239, 1969.
262. McGill, D. A.: Tarsal-tunnel syndrome. Proc. R. Soc. Med., *57*:1125, 1964.
263. Skoog, T.: Dupuytren's contraction, with special reference to the aetiology and improved surgical treatment; its occurrence in epileptics; and notes on knuckle-pads. Acta Chir. Scand., (Suppl. 139) *96*:1, 1948.
264. Detenbeck, L. C., and Kelly, P. J.: Total dislocation of the talus. J. Bone Joint Surg., *51A*:283, 1969.
265. Schiller, M. G., and Ray, R. D.: Isolated dislocation of the medial cuneiform bone—a rare injury of the tarsus. J. Bone Joint Surg., *52A*:1632, 1970.
266. Hunt, D. D.: Compression fracture of the anterior articular surface of the calcaneus. J. Bone Joint Surg., *52A*:1637, 1970.
267. Parkes, J. C.: In Giannestras, N. J. (Ed.).: *Foot Disorders: Medical and Surgical Management.* 2nd Ed. Philadelphia, Lea & Febiger, 1973.
268. Coltart, W.: Fractures of the talus. J. Bone Joint Surg., *34B*:545, 1952.
269. Garcia, A., and Parkes, J. C.: Fractures of the foot. In Giannestras, N. J. (Ed.): *Foot Disorders: Medical and Surgical Management.* Philadelphia, Lea & Febiger, 1973.
270. Dunn, A. R., Jacobs, B., and Campbell, R. D., Jr.: Fractures of the talus. J. Trauma, *6*:442, 1966.
271. McKeever, F. M.: Treatment of complications of fractures and dislocations of the talus. Clin. Orthop., *30*:45, 1963.
272. Hawkins, L. G.: Fracture of the lateral process of the talus. J. Bone Joint Surg., *47A*:1170, 1965.
273. Pennal, G.: Fractures of the talus. Clin. Orthop., *30*:53, 1963.
274. Larson, R. L., Sullivan, C. R., and Janes, J. M.: Trauma, surgery, and circulation of the talus—what are the risks of avascular necrosis? J. Trauma, *1*:13, 1961.
275. Mindell, E. R., Cisek, E. E., Kartalian, G., and Dziob, J. M.: Late results of injuries to the talus. J. Bone Joint Surg., *45A*:221, 1963.
276. Kleiger, B.: Fractures of the talus. J. Bone Joint Surg., *30A*:735, 1948.
277. Lance, E. M., Carey, E. J., and Wade, P. A.: Fractures of the os calcis: a follow-up study. J. Trauma, *4*:15, 1964.
278. Carey, E. J., Lance, E. M., and Wade, P. A.: Extra-articular fractures of the os calcis. J. Trauma, *5*:362, 1965.
279. Cave, E.: Fractures of the os calcis, the general problem. Clin. Orthop., *30*:64, 1963.
280. Schottstaedt, E. R: Symposium: treatment of fractures of the calcaneus. J. Bone Joint Surg., *45A*:863, 1963.
281. O'Connell, F., Mital, M. A., and Rowe, C. R.: Evaluation of modern management of fractures of the os calcis. Clin. Orthop., *83*:214, 1972.
282. Lance, E. M., Carey, E. J., and Wade, P. A.: Fractures of the os calcis—treatment by early mobilization. Clin. Orthop., *30*:76, 1963.
283. Thorén, O.: Os calcis fractures. Acta Orthop. Scand., Suppl. 70, 1964.
284. Rowe, C. R., Sakellarides, H. T., Freeman, P. A., et al.: Fractures of the os calcis, a long-term follow-up study of 146 patients. J.A.M.A., *184*:920, 1963.
285. Brav, E. A.: End results of treatment of fractures of the os calcis, an army-wide study. Milit. Med., *130*:23, 1965.
286. Wilson, D. W.: Functional capacity following fractures of the os calcis. Can. Med. Assoc. J., *95*:908, 1966.
287. Nordby, E. J.: Os calcis fractures into the subastragalar joint. Clin. Orthop., *13*:245, 1959.
288. Deyerle, W. M.: Long-term follow-up of fractures of the os calcis. Orthop. Clin. North Am., *4*:213, 1973.
289. Eichenholtz, S. N., and Levine, D. B.: Fractures of the tarsal navicular bone. Clin. Orthop., *34*:142, 1964.
290. Parra, G.: Stress fractures of the sesamoids of the foot. Clin. Orthop., *18*:281, 1960.
291. Giannestras, N. J.: Problems of the forepart of the foot. American Academy of Orthopedic Surgeons Instructional Course Lectures. Vol. 22. St. Louis, C. V. Mosby Co., 1973.
292. Schlonsky, J., and Olix, M. L.: Functional disability following avulsion fracture of the ischial epiphysis. J. Bone Joint Surg., *54A*:641, 1972.
293. Milch, H.: Ischial apophysiolysis—a new syndrome. Clin. Orthop., *2*:184, 1953.
294. Sullivan, C. R.: Fractures of the pelvis. American Academy of Orthopedic Surgeons Instructional Course Lectures. Vol. 17. St. Louis, C. V. Mosby Co., 1961, pp. 92–101.
295. Dunn, A. W., and Morris, H. D.: Fractures and dislocations of the pelvis. J. Bone Joint Surg., *50A*:1639, 1968.
296. MacKinnon, W. B., and Lansdown, E. L.: Total dislocation of the ilium. J. Bone Joint Surg., *54B*:720, 1972.
297. Peltier, L. F.: Complications associated with fractures of the pelvis. J. Bone Joint Surg., *47A*:1060, 1965.
298. Shanmugasundaram, T. K.: Unusual dislocation of symphysis pubis with locking. J. Bone Joint Surg., *52A*:1669, 1970.
299. Levine, J. I., and Crampton, R. S.: Major abdominal injuries associated with pelvic fractures. Surg. Gynecol. Obstet., *116*:223, 1963.
300. Baylis, S., Lansing, E. H., and Glas, W. W.: Traumatic retroperitoneal hematoma. Am. J. Surg., *103*:477, 1962.
301. Braunstein, P. W., Scudder, P. A., McCarroll, J. R., Musolino, A., and Wade, P. A.: Concealed hemorrhage due to pelvic fracture. J. Trauma, *4*:832, 1964.
302. Froman, C., and Stein, A.: Complicated crushing injuries of the pelvis. J. Bone Joint Surg., *49B*:24, 1967.
303. Lawson, L. J., and Wainwright, D.: Massive hemor-

rhage following pelvic fracture. J. Bone Joint Surg., *50B*:380, 1968.
304. Horton, R. E., and Hamilton, S. G. I.: Ligature of the internal iliac artery for massive hemorrhage complicating fracture of the pelvis. J. Bone Joint Surg., *50B*:376, 1968.
305. Mack, H. E., and Tannehill, E. H.: Fractured pelvis complicated by gangrene of extremity–amputation under refrigeration anesthesia. Surg. Gynecol. Obstet., *78*:429, 1944.
306. Wilson, J. N.: Fractures of the pelvis complicated by ischemia of the lower limb. J. Bone Joint Surg., *34B*:68, 1952.
307. Carruthers, F. W., and Logue, R. M.: Treatment of fractures of the pelvis and their complications. American Academy of Orthopedic Surgeons Instructional Course Lectures. Vol. 10. Ann Arbor, J. W. Edwards Co., 1953, p. 50.
308. Harris, W. R., Rathbun, J. B., Worzman, G., and Humphrey, J. G.: Avulsion of lumbar roots complicating fracture of the pelvis. J. Bone Joint Surg., *55A*:1436, 1973.
309. Alker, G. J., Jr., Galsauer, F. E., Zoll, J. G., et al.: Myelographic demonstration of lumbosacral nerve root avulsion. Radiology, *89*:101, 1967.
310. Carlson, D. H., and Hoffman, H. B.: Lumbosacral traumatic meningocele. Neurology (Minneap.), *21*:174, 1971.
311. Goodell, C. L.: Neurological deficits associated with pelvic fractures. J. Neurosurg., *24*:837, 1966.
312. Payne, R. F., and Thompson, J. L.: Myelography in lumbosacral plexus injury. Br. J. Radiol., *42*:840, 1969.
313. Purser, D. W.: Displaced fracture of the sacrum. J. Bone Joint Surg., *51B*:346, 1969.
314. Nicoll, E. A.: Fractures of the dorso-lumbar spine. J. Bone Joint Surg., *31B*:376, 1949.
315. Ray, R. D., Sankaran, B., and Fetrow, K. O.: Delayed union and non-union of fractures. J. Bone Joint Surg., *46A*:627, 1964.
316. Boyd, H. B., Anderson, L. D., and Johnston, D. S.: Changing concepts in the treatment of non-union. Clin. Orthop., *43*:37, 1965.
317. Green, J. P.: Osteochondritis dissecans of the knee. J. Bone Joint Surg., *48B*:82, 1966.
318. Parkash, S., and Kumar, K.: Fibrodysplasia ossificans traumatica. J. Bone Joint Surg., *54A*:1306, 1972.
319. Searle, A. W.: Fibrodysplasia ossificans. J. Bone Joint Surg., *4B*:594, 1966.
320. *Dorland's Illustrated Medical Dictionary.* 25th Ed. Philadelphia, W. B. Saunders Co., 1974.
321. Lord, J. W.: Post-traumatic vascular disorders and upper extremity sympathectomy. Orthop. Clin. North Am., *1*:393, 1970.
322. Peltier, L. F.: Fat embolism. Orthop. Clin. North Am., *1*:13, 1973.
323. Hamburger, R. J., Lindseth, R. E., Kleit, S. A., and Szwed, J. J.: Acute renal failure following trauma. J. Bone Joint Surg., *54A*:1345, 1972.
324. Bentley, G., and Jeffreys, T. E.: The crush syndrome in coal miners. J. Bone Joint Surg., *50B*:588, 1968.
325. Bywaters, E. G. L.: Ischemic muscle necrosis. Crushing injury, traumatic edema, the crush syndrome, traumatic anuria, compression syndrome: a type of injury seen in air raid casualties following burial beneath debris. J.A.M.A., *124*:1103, 1944.
326. Weeks, R. S.: The crush syndrome. Surg. Gynecol. Obstet., *127*:369, 1968.
327. Bauer, G.: Thrombosis following leg injuries. Acta Chir. Scand., *90*:229, 1944.
328. Tubiana, R., and Duparc, J.: Prevention of thromboembolic complications in orthopedic and accident surgery. J. Bone Joint Surg., *43B*:7, 1961.
329. Cohen, S. H., Ehrlich, G. E., Kauffman, M. S., and Cope, C.: Thrombophlebitis following knee surgery. J. Bone Joint Surg., *55A*:106, 1973.
330. Harrington, K. D., Johnston, J. O., Turner, R. H., and Green, D. L.: The use of methylmethacrylate as an adjunct in the internal fixation of malignant neoplastic fractures. J. Bone Joint Surg., *54A*:1665, 1972.
331. Towne, L. C., Blazina, M. E., and Cozen, L. N.: Fatigue fracture of the tarsal navicular. J. Bone Joint Surg., *52A*:376, 1970.
332. Blickenstaff, L. D., and Morris, J. M.: Fatigue fracture of the femoral neck. J. Bone Joint Surg., *48A*:1031, 1966.
333. Provost, R. A., and Morris, J. M.: Fatigue fracture of the femoral shaft. J. Bone Joint Surg., *50A*:1067, 1968.
334. Beals, R. K., and Hickman, N. W.: Industrial injuries of the back and extremities. J. Bone Joint Surg., *54A*:1593, 1972.
335. Yochelson, L.: Psychiatric aspects of orthopedics. In Adams, J. P. (Ed.): *Current Practice in Orthopedic Surgery, 1963.* St. Louis, C. V. Mosby Co., 1963.
336. McBride, E. D.: Disability evaluation and the orthopedic surgeon. Clin. Orthop., *12*:9, 1958.

XIV. Adipose Tissue

by Luke G. Tedeschi

Our knowledge of the response of the fat cell to mechanical trauma is limited to the effects of the extreme degrees of injury, namely those resulting in the death of the cell (*steatonecrosis*) (Fig. 3–XIV–1). Intermediate changes of a minor nature also probably occur; however, the protoplasmic film of the fat cell is so thin that without the application of special methods they cannot be seen and for this reason these likely changes have so far escaped recognition.

THE FEMALE BREAST

Mechanical trauma and pressure are well-known causes of steatonecrosis. The female

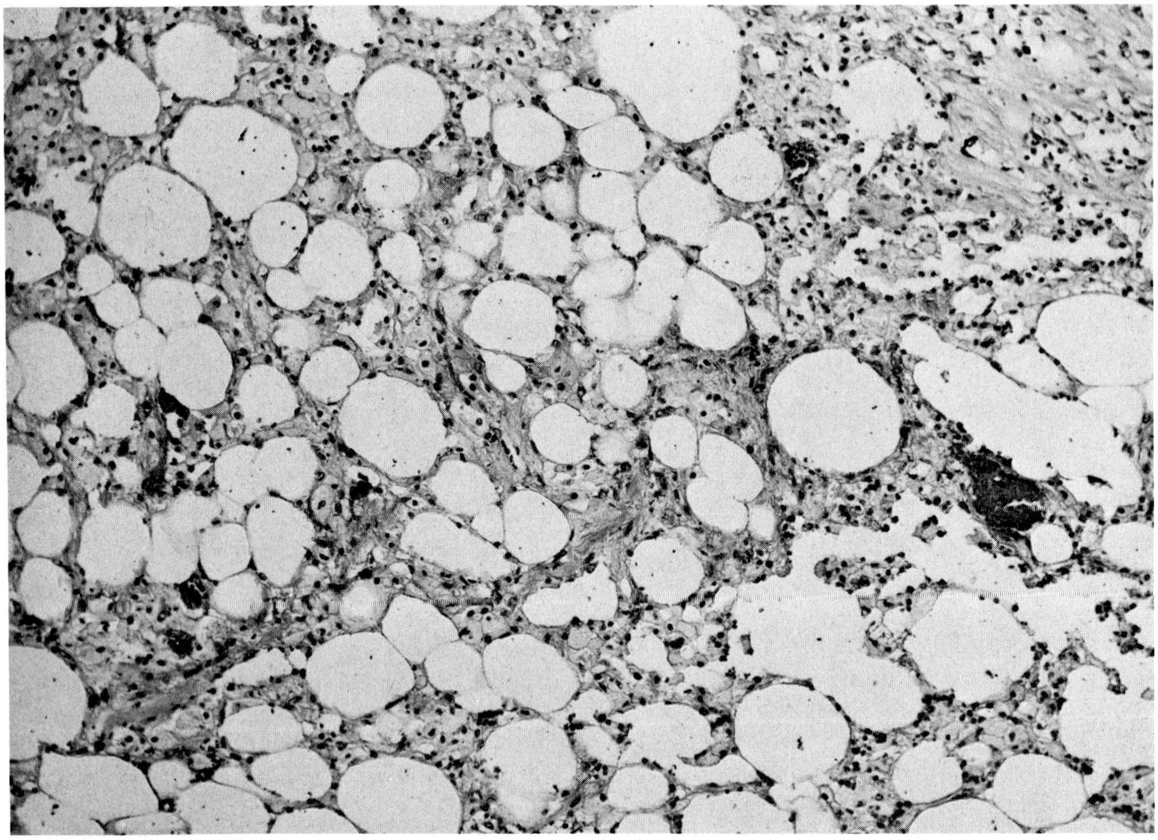

Figure 3–XIV–1. Traumatic steatonecrosis. Notice the lipid-laden macrophages, the incipient fibroblastic tissue proliferation, and the irregularly scattered, bizarre foreign body–type giant cells. From an indurated, painful nodule arising in the breast of a 32-year-old woman subsequent to accidental local trauma.

breast is the organ in which this condition has attracted most attention; the same situation may develop, however, under comparable circumstances, in any area of the body where adipose tissue is present. The process manifests itself as a poorly demarcated area of variable consistency, from hard to rubbery, or elastic, cystic, or soft. Grossly, the lesion is readily recognized by the chalky-white appearance of the fat. The microscopic counterpart is that of a lipophagic granulomatous reaction, which basically does not differ from the same reaction that occurs in the presence of fat necrosis elicited by other causes. Unless there is concurrent bacterial invasion, neutrophils are usually absent in uncomplicated fat necrosis and the inflammatory reaction is predominantly contributed by lymphocytes, mononuclear cells, macrophages, and phagocytic giant cells of the foreign body type. Calcific deposits are likely to occur within the lesion.

Contrary to early reports that large, heavy, pendulous breasts are more inclined to develop fat necrosis, present data indicate that regional or systemic obesity is not as important a factor as previously thought. Whenever a history of trauma can be elicited, as a rule, the traumatic episode is distinctly remembered by the patient as a blow of sufficient severity to produce ecchymosis and pain of variable duration at the site of application of the force. The palpable lump may develop almost immediately, or several years later (up to 17 years according to Adair and Munzer), but in general, within one year of the injury.[1] Attachment of the lump to the skin or less commonly to the deep breast structures, elevation or retraction of the nipple, and not uncommonly enlargement of the axillary lymph nodes—in brief, the classic signs of breast carcinoma—have been described frequently enough in conjunction with fat necrosis to make inescapable the need for careful differentiation between the two conditions.

Trauma, surgical or accidental, is not the only cause of fat necrosis of the breast. In one of the largest reported series of 110 cases (Adair and Munzer), a history of trauma was elicited in only 37 per cent of the cases.[1] A similar incidence (40 per cent) was found by Hadfield in a series of 45 cases.[2] In the remaining cases the cause of the process could not be disclosed.

Periductal mastitis, associated with mammary duct ectasia, is almost regularly accompanied by fat necrosis.[3] An *acute diffuse steatonecrosis limited to the breast*, the cause of which is not known, has also been described.[4, 5]

Thus, the term "steatonecrosis" is used to indicate a quite characteristic pathologic profile rather than a condition necessarily linked to mechanical trauma. Indeed, it has been shown that dietary fat can cause fat necrosis; the same is true for vitamin E deficiency, hypothermia, viruses, and antibiotics (penicillin, actinomycin D).[4, 6, 7] Well known is the association of focal or disseminated fat necrosis, acute pancreatitis, and pancreatic carcinoma. Steatitis, from a whole host of agents, is almost invariably associated with steatonecrosis.[8] Mesenteric lipodystrophy, panniculitis of the mesentery, and retractile mesenteritis (probably different phases of the same condition); pericardial fat necrosis; periureteric liposclerosis; liquefying nodular panniculitis of the buttocks and extremities; the nonsuppurative steatitis of Keil (limited to the anterior abdomen and breast region); poststeroid panniculitis; the panniculitis of Weber-Christian disease; and erythema induratum or erythema nodosum are all examples of conditions in which steatonecrosis is a predominant feature.[4, 9, 10-14]

The fact that a variety of agents, some known and some others still unknown, can produce steatonecrosis should be kept in mind whenever mechanical trauma is being assessed as a presumed cause of the necrosis.

TRAUMATIC FAT NECROSIS OF THE NEWBORN

As the term implies, traumatic fat necrosis of the newborn has been linked to prenatal or perinatal mechanical injury.[15, 18] This concept is well supported by a profuse literature relating the location of the injury to areas of maternal or fetal pressure or to areas of obstetrical manipulation. The mechanical cause of fat necrosis of the newborn is, however, far from being firmly established. Against the assumption that fat necrosis of the newborn is exclusively due to obstetrical manipulation is the occurrence of this disorder in infants delivered by cesarean section. One can go as far as to say that trauma, among other factors, may predispose to the development of this condition. Other theories have been proposed, but none has gone unchallenged; they include exposure to cold; abnormal composition or metabolism of neonatal adipose tissue; asphyxia, with resulting anoxemia; and the effects of lipolytic enzymes, either local or circulating.[19] Other concepts, such as maternal disease (diabetes, syphilis) have been presented but they have not been substantiated by subsequent observations. The not uncommon occurrence of fever and concurrent polymorphonuclear leukocytosis has also led to the speculation that the process could be underlain by an infection.

The condition is inclined to affect full-term, not uncommonly overweight infants born through difficult, prolonged labor. As a rule, the manifestations of the disease make their appearance within the first 10 days of life, less commonly in the second or third week, and the onset is not associated with constitutional symptoms. Rarely the lesions are present at birth. They can be diffuse and affect buttocks, back, shoulders, and the outer aspect of thighs and arms, or localized in the cheeks, limbs, neck, possibly in areas subject to previous pressure. The skin overlying the lesions may be bluish red, red, or of normal color. The lesions may vary in size from nodules several centimeters in diameter to larger plaques, possibly resulting from the confluence of smaller nodules. Nodules and plaques are quite firm and rubbery and do not pit on sustained pressure. The borders of the lesions are ordinarily sharply demarcated and the plaques slightly elevated above the surrounding tissue. By soft tissue radiologic techniques, the affected subcutaneous fat shows a particular areolar appearance.

The lesion persists for several weeks, then gradually disappears spontaneously in three or four months. In the stage of resolution, the skin desquamates and becomes hyperpigmented. Residual atrophy or scarring are uncommon sequelae. Liquefaction of the lesion with formation of pseudocysts may occur, but spontaneous rupture with drainage of oily material is quite rare. Not infrequently the lesion becomes calcified; conversely quite unusual is the occurrence of hemorrhage or abscess within the lesion. Histologically, the process is the nonspecific change associated with steatonecrosis, including deposition of fatty acid crystals and infiltration of macrophages filled with lipid droplets (foam cells) and foreign body giant cells.

A few cases are on record in which the infant died from an intercurrent condition and the visceral fat was found to display changes histologically similar to those in the subcutaneous fat.[20]

Whereas subcutaneous fat necrosis of the newborn typically resolves in a short time, occasionally the process may become more extensive and be complicated by hypercalcemia and its attendant symptoms.

At the present time it does not seem possible to establish a definite relation between idiopathic infantile hypercalcemia and subcutaneous fat necrosis.[21, 24] Subcutaneous fat necrosis can occur without calcification of the lesions, and the calcium level in the serum, as a rule, is not increased in this disorder. By the same token, subcutaneous fat necrosis is not a consistent feature of idiopathic infantile hypercalcemia. It is possible, however, that widespread fat necrosis may alter the calcium metabolism in such a manner as to precipitate the signs and symptoms of a latent hypercalcemia that otherwise might have become manifest at a later age.

Subcutaneous fat necrosis must be differentiated from *sclerema* of the newborn. Grossly the two conditions have similarities. In sclerema, however, the lesion is fairly generalized and, as a rule, only the genitalia, palms, and soles escape involvement. This condition is more likely to develop in debilitated or premature infants, the prognosis is usually grave, and the primary alteration is held to be in the collagen of the tegumental system.[4]

The subcutaneous fat is responsible for the contours of the body and its sex-linked characteristics; thus, the medicolegal implications of steatonecrosis are primarily connected with eventual distortion of body contours resulting from scar formation or contracture, or with pigmentation of overlying skin.

Fat cells do not regenerate or at best they are provided with limited regenerative power. Therefore, from the standpoint of damage compensation, cell death must be considered as a permanent injury. Repair of the lesion can, however, be expected to occur through adipogenic metamorphosis of fat cell precursors as well as by replacement of fatty tissue by fibrous tissue.

REFERENCES

1. Adair, F. E., and Munzer, J. T.: Fat necrosis of the female breast. Report of one hundred ten cases. Am. J. Surg., *74*:117, 1947.
2. Hadfield, G.: Fat necrosis of the breast. Br. J. Surg., *17*:673, 1930.
3. Tedeschi, L. G., Ahari, S., and Byrne, J. J.: Involutional mammary duct ectasia and periductal mastitis. Am. J. Surg., *106*:517, 1963.
4. Tedeschi, C. G.: Pathological anatomy of adipose tissue. In *Handbook of Physiology*. (Edited by A. E. Renold and G. F. Cahill Jr.). Washington, D.C., American Physiological Society, 1965.
5. Fischer, G.: Acute, diffuse steatonecrosis of the breast. Anatomopathologic study of two cases. Ann. Anat. Pathol., *6*:387, 1961.
6. Cox, A. J., Jr., and DeEds, F.: Dietary production of lipogranuloma in rats. Am. J. Pathol., *34*:263, 1958.
7. Herting, D. C., Harris, P. L., and Crain, R. C.: Dietary factors influencing lipogranuloma. Fed. Proc., *18*:529, 1959.
8. MacDonald, A.: Inflammatory diseases of the subcutaneous fat. Geriatrics, *25*:156, 1970.
9. Chester, M. H., and Tully, J. B.: Acute pericardial fat necrosis. J. Thorac. Surg., *38*:62, 1959.
10. Hamburger, J., Richet, C., and Ducrot, H.: A new disease: periureteral liposclerosis. Acq. Medicales Recentes (Paris), *5*:39, 1957.
11. Emmerson, R. W.: Liquefying nodular panniculitis and diabetes. Proc. R. Soc. Med., *59*:252, 1966.
12. Spagnuolo, M., and Taranta, A.: Poststeroid panniculitis. Am. J. Pathol., *20*:783, 1961.
13. MacDonald, A., and Feiwel, M.: A review of the concepts of Weber-Christian panniculitis with a report of five cases. Br. J. Dermatol., *80*:355, 1968.
14. Fountain, R. B.: Lupus erythematosus profundus. Br. J. Dermatol., *80*:571, 1968.
15. Anbari, R.: Subcutaneous fat necrosis of the newborn (adiponecrosis subcutanea neonatorum). Q. Rev. Pediatr., *16*:206, 1961.
16. Browne, K. W., and Burman, D.: Subcutaneous fat necrosis of the newborn. J. Obstet. Gynaecol. Br. Empire, *65*:819, 1958.
17. Holzel, A.: Subcutaneous fat necrosis of the newborn. Arch. Dis. Child., *26*:89, 1955.
18. Weary, P. E., Graham, G. F., and Selden, R. F., Jr.: Subcutaneous fat necrosis of the newborn. South. Med. J., *59*:690, 1966.
19. Noojin, R. O., Pace, B. F., and Davis, H. G.: Subcutaneous fat necrosis of the newborn: Certain etiologic considerations. J. Invest. Dermatol., *12*:331, 1949.
20. Flory, C. M.: Fat necrosis of the newborn. Report of a case with necrosis of the subcutaneous and visceral fat. Arch. Pathol., *45*:278, 1948.
21. Martin, M. M., and Steven, E. M.: Subcutaneous fat necrosis of the newborn with calcification of the tissues. Arch. Dis. Child., *32*:146, 1957.
22. Michael, A. F., Jr., Hong, R., and West, C. D.: Hypercalcemia in infancy, associated with subcutaneous fat necrosis and calcification. Am. J. Dis. Child., *104*:235, 1962.
23. Sharlin, D. N., and Koblenzer, P.: Necrosis of subcutaneous fat with hypercalcemia. A puzzling and multifaceted disease. Clin. Pediatr., *9*:290, 1970.
24. Wilkerson, J. A.: Idiopathic infantile hypercalcemia with subcutaneous fat necrosis. Am. J. Clin. Pathol., *41*:390, 1964.

XV. The Hand

by John J. Byrne

ANATOMY OF THE HAND

Since the hand is an important expediter of the brain, its structure bears close scrutiny.[1] The hand has only five or six general functions that are used in its multitudinous activities. It is the main *sensor* of the body, and in all its activities this is most important. Among its *motor functions* are to pinch, grasp, hook, shovel, and stabilize.

Skin

The skin cover is a fine example of form adapting to function.[2] The dorsal skin is loose to permit the full range of finger motion from the outstretched position to a tightly clenched fist. It is thin and elastic, and possesses hair, sebaceous glands, and sweat glands. If skin loss occurs, it can usually be repaired with local skin flaps or, if more extensive, with split-thickness skin grafts. If there is underlying tendon or bone damage, more extensive skin and subcutaneous tissue grafts are required. Since the dorsal skin is so easily replaced, the dorsum also serves as a donor site for coverage of loss on volar areas of adjacent fingers.

The volar skin is subject to more pressure and, therefore, thicker. Sweat glands are present, but sebaceous glands and hair are missing. Because of the flexion motion of the fingers and thumb, which begin in utero, a series of skin creases develop that are of interest not only to the palmist but also to the surgeon and geneticist. Freely moveable skin on the volar surface would, like a loose glove, slip around when one was grasping or holding objects. Therefore, the digital and palmar creases have a connection with the underlying fibrous tissue that prevents this unstable movement. It is essential for a surgeon to avoid incisions that cross these creases, since they may produce flexion contractures. In the event of injuries that do cross them, the surgeon must minimize the effect by plastic surgical techniques.

Since the hands reflexly protect the body from external violence, there can be many patterns of damage. For example, in flash fires, the hand automatically protects the eyes, leaving the dorsum of the hand prone to burns. The volar surface is the most useful side of the hand and is therefore most prone to damage.

Blood Vessels

The vascular supply, arterial and venous, is extensive. The main *arteries* are the *radial* and *ulnar*, which supply the hand via two arcades in the palm. Injury to one of these channels usually causes no dysfunction, except in the unusual instance in which there is a congenital defect in the arcade systems. Irreparable damage to both vessels usually results in severe ischemic changes in the hand unless the remaining collateral circulation is adequate. In certain operations, vascular injuries may occur, such as damage to the digital vessels in operations on Dupuytren's contracture and damage to the radial artery in volar wrist ganglion removal.

Tendons

The tendons vary on the two sides of the hand. The flexor tendons are strong to enable forceful grasping (Fig. 3–XV–1). Spontaneous rupture is seldom seen unless the tendon is diseased, as in rheumatoid arthritis or severe blunt trauma.

The extensor tendons are flatter and thinner, particularly over the fingers, since great force is not needed for extensor movement (Fig. 3–XV–2). These tendons are more apt to undergo spontaneous rupture. A particularly vulnerable one is the extensor longus of the thumb, which is quite thin and takes a turn around the bony prominence of the radius (Lister's tubercle), where it frays from repeated use and ruptures. Its repair usually involves transfer of an adjacent tendon such as the extensor indicis proprius. The weak extensor tendons over the finger joints are prone to rupture from forced flexion of the joint, giving the characteristic mallet finger of the distal interphalangeal joint and the boutonnière deformity of the proximal interphalangeal joint. The thin extensor tendons over the knuckles are commonly severed when struck against a tooth in fighting.

Tendons have a fibrillar structure, so simple

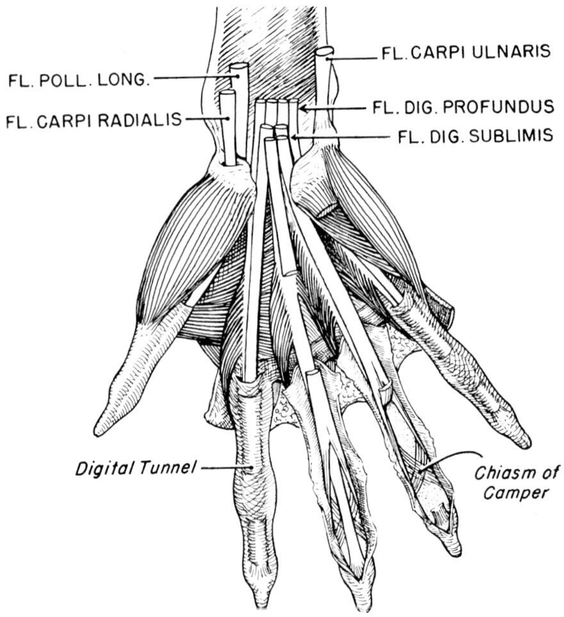

Figure 3–XV–1. The flexor tendons of the hand. The thumb has a single flexor, but each finger has two flexors, a sublimus and a profundus, which glide very closely together in tight fibrous compartments extending from the metacarpophalangeal joints out to the distal portion of the middle phalanx. (From Byrne, J. J.: *The Hand: Its Anatomy and Diseases.* 1959. Courtesy of Charles C Thomas, Publisher, Springfield, Ill.)

suturing is impossible unless the tendon is very flat and can be immobilized and held in place.[3] Numerous techniques have been developed utilizing several principles. One popular suture converts a longitudinal pull into a transverse one by passing the suture in a zigzag fashion back and forth across the tendon, making sure different sets of fibrils are encompassed in each pass (Bunnell technique). The other utilizes the same technique with wire in the proximal tendon, but slides directly through the distal tendon and is passed out through the skin where it is fixed by a button. After healing has taken place, the button is cut off and the wire suture removed proximally by means of another wire loop that was left in place at the time of the original operation (pull-out technique).

Bones and Joints

The bones and joints are well adapted to serve finger and thumb function. The capsules of the digital joints permit flexion and extension but prevent lateral instability. The knuckle joints of the fingers and the carpometacarpal joint of the thumb permit flexion and extension in addition to abduction and adduction so that a circular pattern can be made by each digit. Only the thumb and, to a lesser degree, the fifth finger appear to rotate, but only along an arc, owing to a characteristic saddle-type joint. The latter movement of the thumb permits it to open wide for grasping and to touch its tactile surface to the tacile pads of each finger.

The flexor tendons are intimately adherent to the underside of the finger bones through their tendon sheaths, and malunion of fractures may prevent tendon function.

Fasciae

Where the tendons cross joints they are usually bound down by a *retinacular structure* to prevent bow-stringing with its loss of function. In the wrist, the flexor tendons of the finger and thumb pass under the carpal ligament in company with the median nerve. If the tendons become swollen from overuse or unaccustomed use, they press on the nerve, causing palsy (the entrapment syndromes). As the flexor tendons cross the metacarpophalangeal joints they enter tight synovium-lined fascial tunnels (tendon sheaths). Through overuse or unaccustomed use this sheath may constrict and limit the tendon function (trigger finger or thumb). The same may occur where the abductor pollicis longus and extensor pollicis brevis emerge

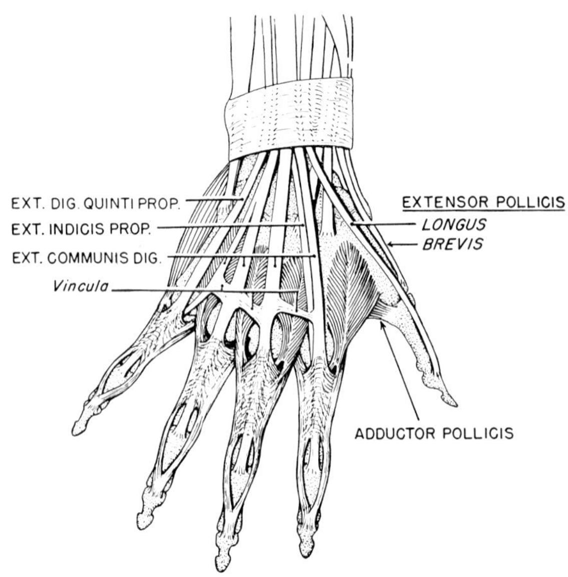

Figure 3–XV–2. The extensors of the hand. Note that the index and fifth fingers have two extensor tendons, while the third and fourth have only one. (From Byrne, J. J.: *The Hand: Its Anatomy and Diseases.* 1959. Courtesy of Charles C Thomas, Publisher, Springfield, Ill.)

from a sheath over the tip of the radius (de Quervain's disease).

The *palmar fascia* is a dense sheet of fibrous tissue arranged in longitudinal bands and held together by transverse bands.[4] It extends in a triangular shape from the base of the palm to the base of the fingers. It serves to ensheath the tendons, nerves, and vessels, holding them in place and protecting them from injury, much like a firm glove. It is subject to nodularity and contracture (Dupuytren's contracture), which is seen more frequently in older persons and may be a reaction to the wear and tear of life's activities. It may also be related to an individual injury.

Muscles

There are muscles that arise and terminate in the hand, the intrinsic muscles (Fig. 3–XV–3). Two sets of three muscles (abductor, flexor, and opponens) form the characteristic balls of the thumb (thenar muscle group) and little finger (hypothenar muscle group). The adductor pollicis (arising from transverse and oblique heads) draws the thumb into the palm and is vital to a strong pinch. The interossei abduct

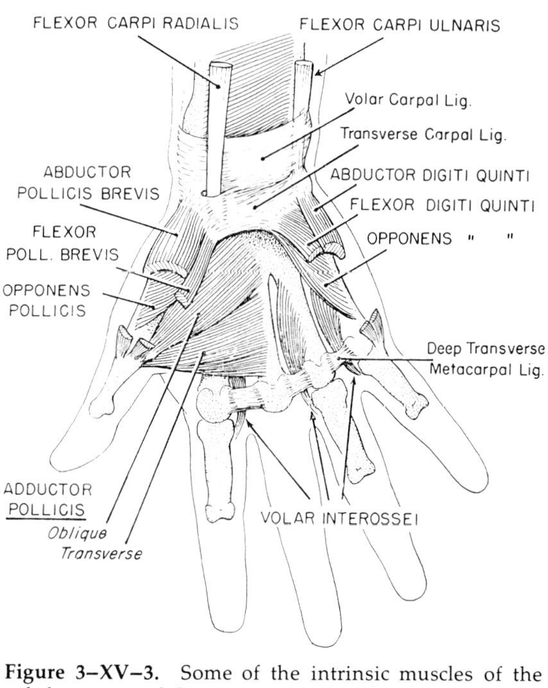

Figure 3–XV–3. Some of the intrinsic muscles of the hand that are vital for its strength and intricate function. The majority of these are supplied by the ulnar nerve; only a few going to the thumb are supplied by the median nerve. (From Byrne, J. J.: *The Hand: Its Anatomy and Diseases.* 1959. Courtesy of Charles C Thomas, Publisher, Springfield, Ill.)

and adduct the fingers. In addition, the interossei in conjunction with the lumbricals perform a unique role: they flex the knuckle (metacarpophalangeal) joint but extend the finger (interphalangeal) joints. Their action gives the hand its strength and most of its complicated function. When these muscles are paralyzed, the hand becomes shrunken and the fingers are held flexed while the knuckle is extended (intrinsic-minus position). Conversely, if these muscles become ischemic, they fibrose and shrink, leaving the finger flexed at the knuckle but extended at the finger joints (intrinsic-plus position), an equally disabling condition.

Synovial Sheaths

The tendons move through the fingers of the hand in their tendon sheaths, which are lined with gliding membranes known as *synovia.* In addition, there is a complicated pattern of synovia that sheathe the tendons as they cross the carpal tunnel. The finger tendons are encompassed in the *ulnar bursa,* which extends from the palm into the wrist and is often connected to one or two of the finger sheaths, usually that of the fifth finger. The tendon sheath of the thumb extends up to the wrist as the *radial bursa.* These tendon sheaths may become inflamed with repeated trauma, giving rise to chronic synovitis. They are subject to other diseases such as tuberculosis and rheumatoid arthritis.

Nerves

The main nerves in the hand are the median and ulnar. The *radial nerve* supplies sensation to the skin on the dorsoradial side of the wrist only. There are no intrinsic muscles in the hand supplied by this nerve. All the extensor muscles are innervated by it, however, and if palsied, they prevent stabilization of the wrist and finger joints, making hand function impossible.

The *median nerve* supplies sensation on the volar surface of the lateral side of the hand, usually including half the ring finger. It also supplies sensation on the dorsum of the thumb and the distal phalanges of the index and middle fingers and the radial side of the ring finger. It supplies the intrinsic muscles associated with the thenar muscle group, which are important for abducting the thumb so that objects can be grasped. Without this action of the thumb, the hand loses the functions of pinching and grasping.

The *ulnar nerve* supplies the ulnar side of the

hand dorsally and ventrally on a line that usually bisects the ring finger. While it is not as important to sensation as is the median, it is all-important to muscle function, since most of the intrinsic muscles of the hand, the seven dorsal interossei, and the adductors as well as the hypothenar eminence are supplied by it. It gives strength to making a fist, and without it the hand is a very weak organ with limited function.

Each nerve consists of neurofibrils arranged in a pattern of interlacing funiculi surrounded by connective tissue perineurium.[5] The numerous funiculi are held together to form a nerve by a connective tissue epineurium. Maps of the funicular pattern have been made by Sunderland.[6]

INFECTIONS

The majority of hand infections are secondary to trauma. Small lacerations not adequately treated may become infected, and puncture wounds drive the bacteria below the skin where deep infections can occur. Persons in certain occupations are more prone to injury than others, e.g., meat cutters, medical workers, glass and metal workers. Wilkes studied a large series of hand infections and found that attempts to prevent them by using protective gloves and improvements in first aid were not effective.[7] It is essential that treatment be early to prevent these infections from becoming more severe.

The majority of infections are caused by staphylococci and streptococci.[8] Culture of specimens from the infected wound should be done immediately to identify the organism and determine its sensitivity to various antibiotics. The choice of antibiotic depends upon the sensitivity of the organism, the cost of the drug, and its safety. Other bacteria may be found and may have a relation to the type of injury or the occupation. The human bite, for instance, inflicted on the knuckles of the hand by teeth during fisticuffs, produces a mixed infection in which anaerobic streptococci are the most significant organisms. Dog and cat bites may result in infections with *Pasteurella multicida.* Anthrax may develop in handlers of sheep, cattle, horses, and swine, or in manufacturers and processors who use their products in factories and canneries. Fish handlers and abattoir workers develop an infection called erysipeloid due probably to an organism called Erysipelothrix. Hand tuberculosis may be seen in people who work with infected cattle.

Localization of Infections in the Hand

There are numerous anatomical compartments in the hand where pus can accumulate. A knowledge of these spaces is essential for correct surgical diagnosis and treatment.

The skin folds around the nail bed may become infected, a condition known as *paronychia.* When incision is needed, the nail matrix should be avoided to prevent permanent damage to the nail. The distal pulp space of each finger forms an isolated pocket to which infection may be confined, since the distal finger crease has a fibrous attachment to the underlying tendon sheath. There are also fibrous septa going from the skin to the periosteum of the distal phalanx, which further compartmentalize this space. Such infections are called *felons,* and they require early incision. Delay may lead to bone sequestration or osteitis with necrosis of skin and fascia, complications that may triple the healing period. Incisions should avoid the volar tactile pad and should be placed as close to the nail bed as possible. Whether to limit the lateral arm of the incision to one side of the finger (hockey-stick incision) or to use both sides (U-shaped incision) depends upon the surgeon's experience. With either incision, the pulp must be opened like a book and the flap packed open for four days.

The *web space* between the fingers contains a fat pad that may become infected from an abrasion in an overlying hand callus. The free border of the web space, which contains the natatory ligament, should not be incised because an adduction contracture of the adjacent fingers could occur. The incision should be placed more proximally on the volar and dorsal boundaries of the space. People dealing with hair or hides may develop lesions in the web spaces from short hairs working into the skin. In the dairy industry these are known as "milkers' granuloma." They are not infrequent in barbers.

There are spaces in the palm of the hand where pus can accumulate in large quantities. If not drained adequately or in time, such collections can result in serious loss of function (Fig. 3–XV–4). These infections are usually caused by direct puncture wounds, but they may be secondary to infections in the finger, which spread proximally along the planes of fascia and tendon, or from infections in the metacarpophalangeal joints. In the *midpalmar* and *pretendinous* spaces infections produce a central palmar fullness and swelling with limitation of motion of some of the fingers (middle, ring, and little). *Ulnar bursa* infections are simi-

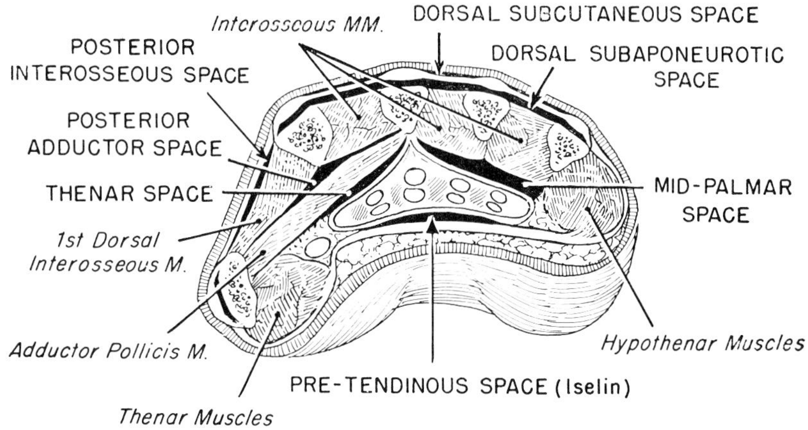

Figure 3–XV–4. The compartments of the palm of the hand in which pus may accumulate and require evacuation. (From Byrne, J. J.: *The Hand: Its Anatomy and Diseases.* 1959. Courtesy of Charles C Thomas, Publisher, Springfield, Ill.)

lar, but in addition may show tenderness and swelling in the volar aspect of the wrist and tenderness along the fifth finger. Incision is made paralleling the palmar crease, and exploration reveals which of these spaces is involved. All such operations require general or regional anesthesia, and a tourniquet is placed on the upper arm so that a bloodless operative field can be obtained. In this way damage to underlying nerves, tendons, and blood vessels will be avoided.

The other palmar space is the *thenar space.* This lies between the ulnar bursa and the adductor pollicis muscle. A collection of pus in this area surrounding the adductor pollicis muscle prevents the thumb from adducting, so that the patient presents with brawny thickening in the web space of the thumb and the thumb held in an abducted position (Fig. 3–XV–5). Incision is made on the dorsal surface

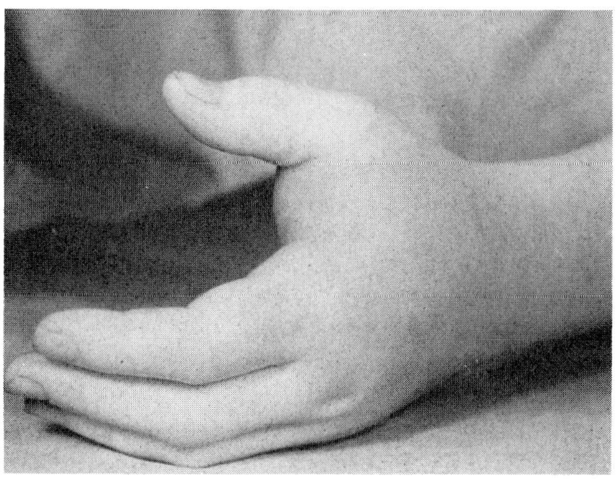

Figure 3–XV–5. A thenar space abscess of the left hand. The thumb is widely abducted from the palm. (From Byrne, J. J.: *The Hand: Its Anatomy and Diseases.* 1959. Courtesy of Charles C Thomas, Publisher, Springfield, Ill.)

of the web space. In this way there is no scarring on the tactile grasping portion of the palm.

The *tendon sheaths* are lined by a synovial membrane that produces a lubricating synovial fluid that enables the tendons to glide easily where they are bound down by fibrous sheaths or ligaments that act as pulleys. The thumb sheath goes up into the wrist as the *radial bursa.* The index, middle, and ring finger sheaths usually stop at the level of the palmar creases. The fifth finger sheath connects usually with the large ulnar bursa, which covers all eight finger tendons as they pass under the carpal ligament. If these isolated sheaths or bursae receive a puncture wound, they may become infected *(acute tenosynovitis).* Treatment is by antibiotics, or by a combination of antibiotics and various methods of drainage if the infection does not respond readily to antibiotic therapy alone. Classically, the sheaths are opened by long incisions suitably placed to avoid undue scarring and flexion contractures. Modifications of the procedure exist in which small incisions are placed proximally and distally, and the involved sheaths are irrigated at varying intervals of time with antibiotic solutions introduced by indwelling catheters.[9] If the infections are not drained soon enough, the end-result is loss of motion in the involved tendons, which may require subsequent reconstructive procedures.

Results of Treatment

There are numerous reasons for poor results after hand infections. Treatment may be inadequate from beginning to end with an improper choice of antibiotics and a lack of incision and drainage when needed. Diabetes mellitus should always be suspected. Sometimes a wrong diagnosis is made; tumors can metastasize to the finger tips and resemble infections, and metabolic disorders such as gout may produce a lesion in the finger that can look like an infection.[10] Improper incisions not only drain the pus poorly so that the infection does not respond readily, but may result in skin contractures and painful scars. Sometimes everything is done properly, but an inappropriate response to the infection results in increased fibrosis in the finger or hand that causes limitation of motion of tendons and joints that may require long periods of physical therapy or reconstructive surgery for improvement.

SKIN INJURIES

The medicolegal aspects of damage to the skin include disfigurement, loss of function, and possible tumor formation. These are usually a result of the initial injury, but they can be made worse by insufficient or injudicious medical therapy.

Disfigurement

This is related to the type of the skin coverage or repair. If the injury is a laceration, repair is by simple suture. Wound healing in the hand is excellent, thanks to its vascularity, and the end-result depends upon the severity of the initial wound. The chief deterrent to good healing is infection. This is usually the result of the initial contamination and the degree of crushing associated with the injury. It may also be connected with the time lag before surgery.

When the skin defect is extensive it is closed by a variety of methods, but generally the dorsum of the hand and fingers can be covered with split-thickness grafts. These may become pigmented in whites or may lose their pigmentation in blacks. The resulting discoloration may be cosmetically disturbing. Full-thickness grafts are needed on the palmar surface and give good cosmetic results even though their failure rate is higher than that of the split-thickness grafts. When extensive tendon or bone repair is needed, the skin defects must be covered by a type of skin flap that includes the subcutaneous fat.[11] The skin flap, usually from a nonhairy portion of the thorax or abdomen, may become quite fatty and resemble a boxing glove if it is on the dorsum of the hand, or a sausage on the fingers.

The degree of disfigurement varies also with the patient's occupation. A defect that might be easily tolerated by a manual worker might cause embarrassment to a person whose hands are constantly in view of his clients, such as a salesperson, a physician, a model, or an entertainment artist.

Some patients, notably blacks, have a tendency to form keloids. These are exuberant overgrowths of fibrous tissue that may be extremely disfiguring.

Loss of Function

This involves pain or limitation of motion. In general, painful scars usually involve nerve injuries (see Painful States). Thin skin coverage on areas subject to constant pressure may also cause pain and require reconstruction.

Skin defects on the dorsal or ventral surfaces of the palm or fingers may produce limitation of motion and prevent flexion or extension.[12] When present in the web spaces, they may prevent abduction or adduction of the fingers and thumb.[13] This may be unavoidable because of the original damage or the inadequacy of initial care. For instance, a simple volar laceration in a finger may have to be lengthened to explore and repair underlying damage proper-

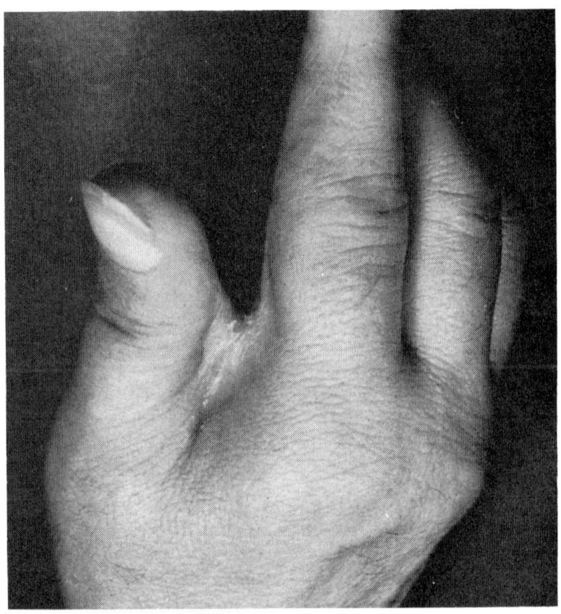

Figure 3–XV–6. A contracture between the index finger and the thumb causing severe disability and requiring a subsequent plastic procedure to restore thumb function. (From Byrne, J. J.: *The Hand: Its Anatomy and Diseases.* 1959. Courtesy of Charles C Thomas, Publisher, Springfield, Ill.)

ly. If the surgeon does this in a longitudinal direction on the volar surface of the finger, he may cause a severe flexion contracture. If, as discussed earlier, a thenar space infection is opened by an incision across the web space of the thumb and index finger, a severe adduction contracture of the thumb may develop (Fig. 3–XV–6). Burns are severe injuries that can result in horrendous deformities, and these may be compounded if skin grafting is not done as soon as feasible.[14]

Most of the finger and hand deformities due to skin contractures can be ameliorated by reconstructive surgery. This should be done as soon as possible to prevent the underlying joint and fascial tissue from becoming irreparably contracted.

Tumor Formation

Thin scars from any cause that are constantly breaking down and rehealing may eventually develop cancer (Marjolin's ulcer). All such scars should be replaced with better skin, or at least observed regularly so that a nonhealing ulcer can be removed for pathologic diagnosis.

TENDON INJURIES

In order to insure proper healing of a lacerated tendon, it is necessary that the two tendon ends be held together for a variable period of time. There is no tension on the distal end, and it can be held in position by proper casting and splinting of the distal phalanges and hand. The proximal end of the tendon, however, is attached to the muscle belly and is therefore subject to varying degrees of tension depending upon the size of the muscle. Because of the fibrillar nature of tendons, ordinary suturing is not possible, since it would easily pull out of the tissue. Usually the suture is placed in a zigzag fashion through the tendon so that the longitudinal pull is partially converted to a transverse pull (Bunnell suture) (Fig. 3–XV–7). These sutures may be left in place or can be so constructed that they can be removed after healing has taken place (pull-out technique

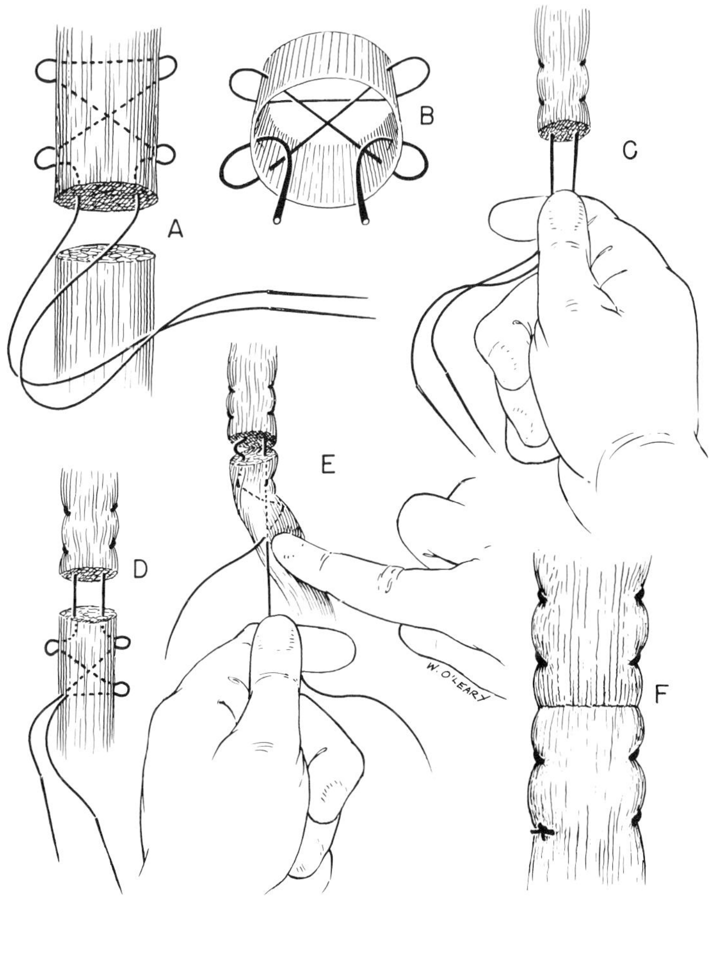

Figure 3–XV–7. The Bunnell suture for restoring tendon continuity. (From Byrne, J. J.: *The Hand: Its Anatomy and Diseases*. 1959. Courtesy of Charles C Thomas, Publisher, Springfield, Ill.)

with wire sutures). For thin flat tendons, mattress sutures are useful. Wherever tendons are grossly disproportionate in size, the smaller end is usually woven through the larger end.

Tendons require three weeks for healing and are immobilized for this period of time in a position that places minimum tension on the junctions and is consistent with restoration of joint mobility. If joints are placed in extreme positions for any length of time, there may be marked limitation of motion. Some tendons are weaker than others and may require protection for a longer time with the hand in a position of function. For instance, the extensor tendons are much thinner and weaker than the flexors, and their junction would be stretched if not protected for the maximum healing period.

The results of tendon suture are good when the tendons are not compressed by tendon sheaths or carpal ligaments, i.e., in the forearm, wrist, palm, back of arm, and hand. When more than one tendon is severed and resutured, the tendons may stick together. If this causes loss of function, reoperation may be necessary to free them (tenolysis). Secondary infection in the wound would also interfere with the tendon gliding motion.

In the finger, because the two flexors pass through a tight tendon sheath, repaired tendons may stick to the sheath and to each other. Many surgeons advocate that initial treatment be confined to cleansing the wound and repairing skin and nerves. In three to four months, a reoperation is done, the severed tendons are removed, and a tendon graft is inserted.[15] The donor tendon is usually from the forearm (the palmaris longus), the leg (plantaris longus), or the foot (extensor longus tendon to the second, third, or fourth toe). In expert hands, the results are excellent to good, but this means two operations. To avoid this, hand surgeons with extensive experience occasionally do a primary repair in incised noncontaminated wounds seen a short time after injury.[16] If there has been extensive scarring of the digit, it may be necessary to form a new tendon sheath by using a temporary silicone rod.[17]

The flexor of the thumb presents its own problems, and secondary repair has been studied by Urbanock and Goldner.[18]

A somewhat similar condition exists when the flexor tendons pass through the carpal canal. When all the tendons are cut, only the profundus tendons and flexor pollicis longus tendon are repaired, since there would not be room for all nine tendon repairs.

Some tendons are so thin that it is difficult to repair them; one such is the extensor tendon of the distal interphalangeal joint. If it is lacerated or ruptured, a characteristic deformity results. The distal interphalangeal joint is held in varying degrees of flexion (mallet finger, baseball finger). In the case of rupture, a splint is applied that immobilizes the distal interphalangeal joint in extension for six to eight weeks, keeping the proximal interphalangeal joint freely moveable.[19] In the case of a laceration or if primary conservative splinting is not successful, repair of the tendon by suturing with occasional reinforcement by tendon grafting may have to be done. The distal interphalangeal joint is held in position for six to eight weeks by either a splint or a small Kirschner wire placed through the joint.

Another such situation arises with injuries (laceration or rupture) of the dorsum of the proximal interphalangeal joint of the fingers. The extensor tendon is torn or stretched and the lateral bands slip volarward, which results in a flexion contracture associated with a hyperextension deformity of the distal interphalangeal joint. This is called a *boutonnière deformity*. For ruptures, conservative splinting of the proximal interphalangeal joint in extension, with attention to active flexion of the distal interphalangeal joint, may give a good result. Reconstructive surgery is difficult, but many operations have been designed.[20]

Spontaneous rupture of tendons seldom occurs unless they are diseased (arthritis) or are small and have an angular range of motion. The extensor pollicis longus is a good example of this. It courses around a small bony tubercle (Lister's) of the radius, where it may fray and rupture in certain occupational movements. This is particularly true if the bony groove becomes irregular from fracture or arthritis.

Repeated or unusual movements of a tendon may lead to inflammatory changes, particularly where it inserts into the bone (traumatic tendonitis). Such areas may become calcified (calcific tendonitis). Examples are the insertions of the extensor carpi radialis longus, the extensor carpi radialis brevis, the flexor carpi radialis, and the flexor carpi ulnaris, and the insertions of the interossei into the proximal phalanges. Treatment is conservative and consists of rest and splinting with or without occasional cortisone injections.

NERVE INJURIES

Trauma to nerves may be caused by laceration by a sharp object, contusion by a blow, inadvertent injury from venous or arterial punctures, ischemia, or compression by another anatomical structure (entrapment syndrome).

Entrapment Syndromes

These are often secondary to encroachment on a nerve by bone or fibrous tissue altered by trauma.[21, 22] The most common is the carpal tunnel syndrome, in which the median nerve is compressed in the narrow carpal canal at the wrist. It may be caused by wrist bones deformed by trauma (usually a Colles' fracture of the radius or ulna), by hemorrhage in the canal from closed or open injuries, or by tendons enlarged by overuse (chronic tendonitis), arthritis, myxedema, or diabetes.

When conservative treatment fails, the carpal ligament should be opened throughout its entire length, thereby widening the carpal canal and taking pressure off the nerve. It is important to operate before paralysis of the nerve results in atrophy of the muscles supplied by it (the muscles at the ball of the thumb), which enable the thumb to open wide (abduction and opposition) in grasping.

Another common entrapment is caused by a fracture of the medial epicondyle of the humerus, which compresses the ulnar nerve as it passes beneath it. Sometimes the ulnar nerve slides from its groove behind the condyle and lies lateral to it where it can be injured by leaning on the elbow on a desk. These conditions may require rerouting of the nerve by a surgical procedure that also fixes the nerve in a more anterior location on the elbow (translocation of the ulnar nerve) or merely neurolysis. There are other causes of entrapment.[22]

Ischemia

Ischemia of a nerve for variable lengths of time (one to three hours) may cause isolated areas of nerve destruction and replacement by fibrous tissue, resulting in complete loss of function. The ischemia may be due to trauma to blood vessels or compression by a tight plaster cast used to immobilize a fracture. Sometimes it is produced by a surgeon who needs a bloodless field in which to operate and applies a tourniquet proximal to the site of injury. My usual precaution is to release the tourniquet at hourly intervals, to permit tissue perfusion for five minutes, and then to reapply the tourniquet if more time is necessary. There is no absolute time limit, however, and other surgeons use different intervals. In general, the shorter the interval of ischemia, the less chance of neurologic complications.[23-25]

If the damage from ischemia is mild, some recovery of function is possible; if it is severe, there is little chance of return of function.

Inadvertent Injection

Chemical neuritis is caused by the injection of medications into a nerve either intentionally to induce anesthesia or inadvertently when giving subcutaneous or intravenous injections.[26]

Laceration

Injuries by a knife or other sharp object can be repaired readily. The usual technique is to try to match up the ends as accurately as possible and sew the outer coat of the nerve ends (epineurium) together with fine interrupted nonabsorbable sutures. The closer the matching of the bundles, the better the end-results. Some surgeons are using microsurgical techniques to sew the funiculi together as well as the outer coat.[27]

In bullet injuries there is greater loss of tissue, and at the time of repair the destroyed nerve has to be resected before good nerve ends can be approximated. If the defects are too extensive, the nerve repair cannot be done. There have been some attempts to use nerve grafts to bridge these defects.

There is some argument about whether nerve injuries should be repaired initially or after a period of time to allow the edema to subside and a better assay of nerve regeneration to be made. In general, American surgeons tend to repair nerve injuries at the time of the initial wound repair.[28]

After the nerves are sutured, a long process of repair takes place in which individual motor and sensory nerve fibrils grow down the distal nerve at a rate of about 1 mm a day. The progress of sensory nerve regeneration can be clinically assayed by tapping the nerve along its course. If new sensory fibrils are present, the patient will feel a "pins and needles" sensation (paresthesia). The most distal point at which the patient feels these "pins-and-needles" when the nerve is tapped is recorded. This test is repeated at monthly intervals to see if this point moves distally down the arm (Tinel's sign). Motor regeneration can be ascertained by nerve conduction tests at an early stage and later by testing for muscle function.

In general, sensory return is usually of fair quality, although two-point discrimination and other fine modalities of sensation do not return. Large muscles usually recover, but small ones, such as the interosseous muscles of the hand, usually atrophy and cannot be reinnervated in time to regain function. Therefore, the degree of function that returns after a nerve injury depends on how far away from the hand the injury occurred.

Little can be done to improve the end-results of sensory return, but numerous tendon transfers are available to improve motor function. If the nerve injury is high in the arm so that a very long (12–18 months) delay is anticipated before nerve recovery, tendon transfers may be done at an early stage to expedite return of function. This is particularly true of radial nerve injuries when the resultant defect renders the hand useless.[29]

If sensation does not return, the numbness results in loss of function, its degree depending on how extensive the loss and its location. For instance, numbness on a nontactile area such as the back of the hand would not have the same significance as numbness on the tactile areas of the thumb or index finger. A new technique has been developed to transfer skin from another tactile area, such as the ulnar side of the finger, with its nerve and vascular bundle intact, to the thumb. In this way some sensation is returned to the digit, albeit an altered one that requires retraining.

Loss of sensory nerve function also involves lack of sympathetic tone, so the skin becomes quite dry and shiny. Shrinkage of soft tissue (atrophy) takes place, and the joints involved become quite stiff (dystrophy).

FRACTURES

The effects of the fracturing forces depend upon the severity of the force, the location of the fracture, and the type of treatment. The force severity will determine if a fracture is simple (either transverse or longitudinal), comminuted, or associated with varying degrees of soft tissue injury that may require amputation.

The location determines the deformity, since various muscles and tendons interplay to pull fragments in various directions.[30] Middle phalanx fractures may angulate dorsally or ventrally depending upon their location in reference to the insertion of the flexor digitorum sublimus: proximal to it there is dorsal angulation; distal to it, volar angulation. Fractures of the middle phalanx may develop a volar angulation owing to the pull of the lumbrical and interosseous muscles, which bow across the fracture site. Fractures of the necks of metacarpals may result in severe volar angulation. Metacarpal shaft fractures tend to cause dorsal angulation because of interosseous muscle contraction. Fractures of the base of the thumb metacarpal produce dorsal angulation owing to the pull of the thenar muscles. If associated with a fracture through the joint so that there is a combined fracture-dislocation (Bennett's fracture), the deformity is very unstable.[31]

Principles of treatment are restoration of normal anatomical relationships, immobilization in a position of function (by means of dressing, plaster cast, Kirschner wires, traction), and early mobilization as soon as there is functional but not necessarily osseous stability.[32]

Fractures may result in deformity, loss of substance, or nonunion. Usually these sequelae are due to the initial trauma and are unavoidable. At times, they can be due to inept treatment. Deformity may result from nonrecognition of the problem, poor reduction of a fracture, or improper immobilization. Loss of substance may be caused by improper debridement of bone fragments. Nonunion may be caused by improper immobilization or failure to recognize the possibility of a fracture, as in those of the navicular bone. Most of these fracture sequelae are remediable by further reconstructive surgery.

The most common sequela of fracture therapy is joint stiffness of all the finger and hand joints. The initial trauma forces play a role in its degree and location. More important are the secondary problems of edema, prolonged immobilization, improper positioning of the joints, ischemia from tight dressings, nonevacuation of hematomas, and infection. In addition, some patients, e.g. those with rheumatoid arthritis and collagen disorders, have a tendency to fibrosis.

The metacarpophalangeal joints usually become fixed in extension, the finger joints in flexion, and the wrist in flexion. Other combinations can occur, however, depending upon the position of immobilization. Their restoration ranges through physical therapy, dynamic splinting, operative capsulotomy, and joint arthroplasty or fusion.

JOINT INJURIES

Types of Injury

Sprains are injuries to the joint apparatus (capsule and ligaments) of varying degrees, including tearing of fibers up to the point of dislocation of the joint. Their treatment involves rest and purposeful splinting in the position of function for 10 to 21 days, depending upon the severity of the sprain. Healing is slow, and there may be prolonged stiffness, pain, and swelling of the involved joint. This delay in healing is worse with increasing age and in patients with a tendency to develop arthritis.

Dislocations are injuries to the joint apparatus (mostly ligaments) of such completeness that the joint becomes angulated or displaced in a dorsal or volar position. These may be reduced to a normal position and have sufficient stability so that they can be treated by splinting for 21 days. After reduction, x-rays are mandatory to be sure there is no associated fracture and that the reduction has maintained itself. When dislocations cannot be reduced or when there is abnormal instability after reduction, surgical repair is needed.

Injuries of Individual Joints

Distal Interphalangeal Joints. These are rarely dislocated and dislocations are usually easily reduced. Ruptures of the extensor tendons resulting in volar angulation have been discussed in the section on injuries to tendons (baseball and mallet finger).

Proximal Interphalangeal Joints. Excellent stability is supplied to this joint by the attachments of the volar plate to the base of the middle phalanx and the two lateral ligament systems (collateral and accessory ligaments). As emphasized by Eaton, dislocation or angulation cannot occur unless there are disruptions of two of these three structures.[33] Dorsal dislocation occurs when the volar plate is torn off its attachment to the middle phalanx and both ligaments are torn longitudinally. It can usually be easily reduced unless there is an associated fracture of the middle phalanx into the joint so that the volar plate is carried with the proximal bone fragment. Such dislocations require open surgery for approximation of the anatomical structures. A volar dislocation of the middle phalanx occurs when the traumatic force drives the head of the proximal phalanx through the extensor mechanism. These usually require surgical repair. Lateral dislocation or angulation occurs with rupture of one collateral ligament (radial much more frequently than ulnar) and the volar plate insertion. They are usually easily reduced and require 21 days of immobilization.

Metacarpophalangeal Joints. These joints are similar to the proximal interphalangeal joints, but there are some anatomical differences that make them less prone to lateral dislocations. The volar plate is attached proximally by a weaker membrane to the palmar fascia, thus hyperextension of this joint is possible. When a dorsal dislocation occurs, the head of the metacarpal pierces this membranous attachment and becomes entrapped by the firm volar plate and adjacent flexor tendons, and often requires surgical intervention. If such injuries are unrecognized, repair is more difficult and some other form of treatment must be attempted, either fusion of the joint or repair with a prosthesis.

Thumb Metacarpophalangeal Joint. This differs from the metacarpophalangeal joints of the fingers in that only flexion and extension can take place. There is limited lateral motion. Dislocations of this joint are most common in the hand, since the thumb is exposed to much trauma. Dorsal dislocation occurs when the forces of injury drive the head of the metacarpal through the proximal volar plate just proximal to the sesamoid bones. The head is trapped between them and the flexor pollicis tendon. Reduction is usually possible; if it is not possible, surgical open reduction must be done (Fig. 3–XV–8). Lateral dislocation or angula-

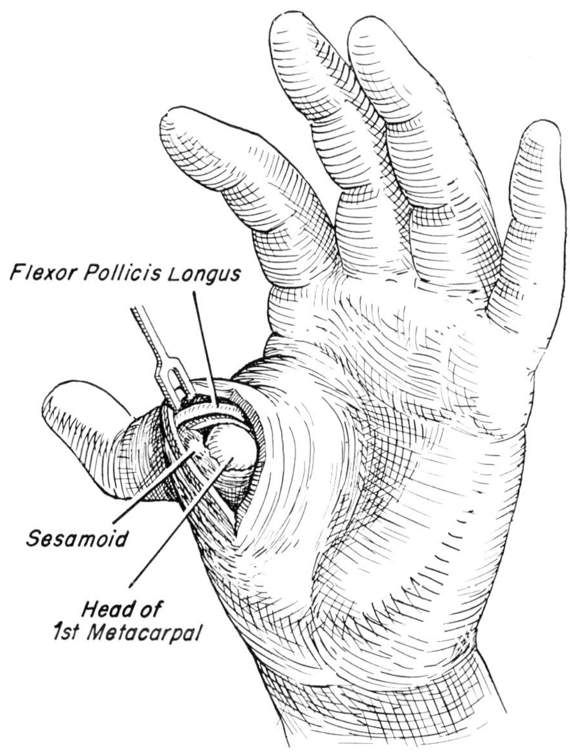

Figure 3–XV–8. Characteristic dislocation of the metacarpophalangeal joint of the thumb that often requires open surgery for reduction. (From Byrne, J. J.: *The Hand: Its Anatomy and Diseases.* 1959. Courtesy of Charles C Thomas, Publisher, Springfield, Ill.)

tion occurs with tears of the collateral ligaments (ulnar 10 times more frequently than radial). If the angulation is severe, even though reducible, such injuries should be explored surgically and the ligaments resutured. Irreducible dislocations, of course, should be repaired surgically. Late cases with significant instability also may need surgical reconstruction.

Thumb Carpometacarpal Joint. Dislocations are rare because of a strong volar attachment to the deep carpal ligaments. Usually, when subject to great stress, the bony beak of the thumb metacarpal stays with the ligament and the remainder of the joint dislocates (Bennett's fracture). When a pure dorsal dislocation occurs, it must be repaired by a reconstructive procedure that anchors the metacarpal in position.

Errors in Diagnosis

Misdiagnosis and consequent inadequate treatment of severe tears of capsular apparatus may result in prolonged or permanent disability of the involved joint. Misdiagnosis or inadequate reduction of a dislocation may similarly result in prolonged or permanent disability.

VASCULAR INJURIES

Vascular injuries are described in another section of this chapter, but there are some that are particularly significant for the hand.

Lacerations

Repair of lacerations of the upper extremity are done by standard surgical procedures. Lacerated radial and ulnar arteries are usually repaired, but if the injuries are to more distal segments (such as metacarpals), there is such good collateral circulation that ligation is done rather than repair. Because the digital vessels are usually too small for general repair, laceration of both vessels usually means that the finger is nonviable. Microsurgical techniques have been developed in some hand centers, however, so that these small digital arteries can be repaired, and even amputated digits are known to have been reimplanted.[34]

Thrombosis

Repeated trauma may result in thrombosis of blood vessels of the hand. Mansfield reported a case of traumatic thrombosis of the ulnar artery in the palm of an engineer who used the palm of his hand to hammer on a chain case during the course of his work.[35] This patient developed tenderness over the base of the hypothenar eminence, and a cordlike structure could be felt. On exploration, this proved to be a thrombosed ulnar artery, which was excised. Zweig and co-workers recently reported 10 such cases.[36] All the patients were male manual laborers who had a definite history of blunt trauma and whose symptoms were sudden pain in the region of the hypothenar eminence. Two categories of symptoms may occur: ulnar nerve irritation and arterial insufficiency. The neurologic symptoms consist of a burning ache or paresthesias on the ulnar side of the hand. The vascular signs are arterial insufficiency in the ring and little fingers. These may be made worse by exposure to cold and may resemble Raynaud's disease. An Allen test will demonstrate that the ulnar artery, not the radial, is diseased. All the patients obtained relief with resection of the thrombosed section of the ulnar artery. The artery is usually damaged in Guyon's canal where, accompanied by the ulnar nerve, it lies in a ligamentous groove between the pisiform bone and a strip of retinaculum coming from the volar carpal ligament to the transverse carpal ligament.

The use of pneumatic tools has resulted in a disease entity quite similar to Raynaud's disease in which the patient manifests cold fingers and the typical color changes of Raynaud's disease. Finger ulcers and gangrene may follow. The cause appears to be the vibration of tools at a rate of between 2,000 and 3,000 revolutions per minute. The basic cause of the vascular change is unknown. There are no histologic changes in the blood vessels, but x-rays reveal multiple obliterative changes. It has been estimated that of 100 men who work with such vibrating tools, 4 per cent show vascular changes in two years, 48 per cent in three years, and approximately 55 per cent between the fourth and fifth years of such use.[37]

Aneurysms

There are various types of traumatic aneurysms that may occur in the hand. In *false aneurysms* there is destruction of the blood vessel wall and formation of a hematoma that becomes a retaining sac of the aneurysm (Fig. 3–XV–9). The most usual trauma to cause this is a puncture wound of the hand. The *true aneurysm* results from a weakening of the arterial wall, and these are usually due to nonpene-

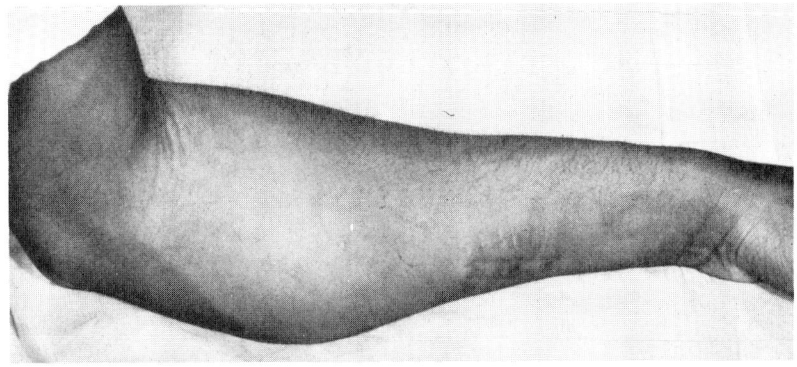

Figure 3–XV–9. A false aneurysm of the forearm produced by a through-and-through gunshot wound. It required subsequent excision and ligation of the ulnar artery.

trating trauma. Such aneurysms are often called *occupational aneurysms*. Excision gives excellent results. Smith demonstrated that most of these occur at sites where the palmar vessels are most superficial and least protected by overlying structures, such as the distal ulnar artery near the hamate bone and the superficial branch of the radial artery at the base of the thenar eminence.[38]

Arteriovenous Fistulae

Traumatic fistulae in the hand are rare civilian injuries. They are usually caused by penetrating trauma. Being of small diameter and a long distance from the heart, they do not produce the serious circulatory problems such as increased pulse pressure, increased heart rate, and increased blood volume with subsequent cardiac failure that can occur with fistulae in other locations. They usually present as small pulsating masses with dilated adjacent veins. A bruit may be heard, and the oxygen content in the involved veins is greater than in normal veins. Simple excision cures the lesions.

Chemical Gangrene

Deliberate arterial injection of gentian violet, ether, and even blood has resulted in gangrene of the hand. Occasionally, arteries are mistaken for veins, especially when the superficial cubital, radial, or ulnar artery is present. Gangrene has also occurred following injections of thiopental, curare, quinine, heavy metals, and antibiotics. Such injuries are becoming more frequent with the increase in narcotic addiction.

General medicinal agents may also produce gangrene. The best-known of these are ergot preparations. In recent years, the use of ergotamine tartrate has resulted in several cases of gangrene of the fingers and lower extremities. The mechanism of increased susceptibility to ergot is probably a combination of excess thyroxin and a damaged liver. Ergot gangrene occurs most often in patients with thyrotoxicosis and jaundice; it almost never follows the use of these alkaloids in the treatment of migraine. Another agent that may produce spasm of blood vessels and cause vascular difficulties is methysergide (Sansert), a serotonin antagonist.

Digital nerve block with anesthetic solution may result in gangrene of the finger, and the author has seen 10 such cases (Fig. 3–XV–10). This can be caused by an admixture of epinephrine in the procaine solution, but secondary factors include the use of a tourniquet and an increased quantity of injected fluid. When forming a digital block, it is recommended that the digital nerve be injected in the palm or certainly in the web space of the finger. Only a small amount of procaine solution should be used and there should be no epinephrine in it.

Ischemic Muscle Contractures

Muscle ischemia may result in the destruction of the muscle and its subsequent fibrosis and contracture. This process may be due to vascular disease, tight compression bandages, or increased volume inside an intermuscular compartment.

Volkmann's contracture involves the muscles of the forearm and usually follows a supracondylar fracture of the humerus or fracture of the bones of the upper forearm. It may, however, occur after any severe trauma to the elbow region. The clinical picture begins with pain in the forearm and hand associated with edema and cyanosis. Hypesthesia and paresthesias develop in the distribution of the median and ulnar nerve. The radial pulse is usually ab-

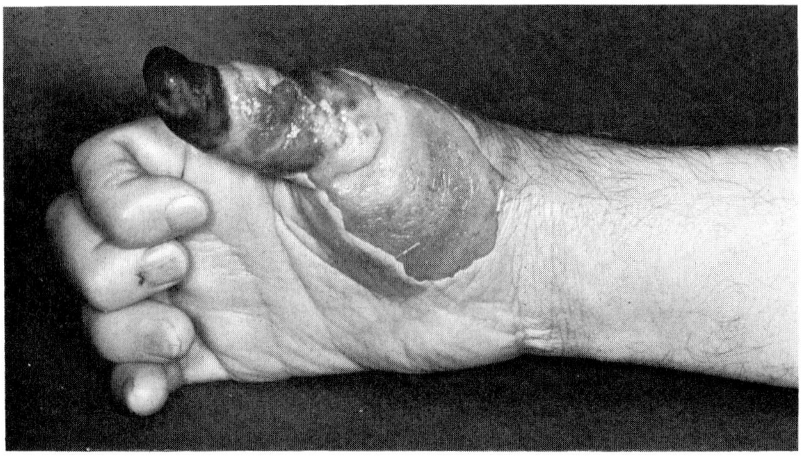

Figure 3–XV–10. Gangrene of the thumb secondary to a digital nerve block.

sent, but this does not have to be so. The fingers are eventually pulled down in flexion, and attempts to extend them are unsuccessful. With time, the muscles become atrophied and contracted, producing severe flexion deformities of the finger as well as persistent neurologic sequelae (Fig. 3–XV–11).

Attention should be given to avoiding this contracture following elbow fractures and, today, also following drug injections. As soon as the pain and cyanosis are evident, the elbow should be extended. If the fractured elbow has been immobilized in a position of acute flexion, the elbow should be extended to see if the radial pulse will return and the pain and edema subside. If they do not, vascular, brachial, and ulnar arteries should be explored, and probably a wide fasciotomy of the anterior compartment of the forearm should be performed.

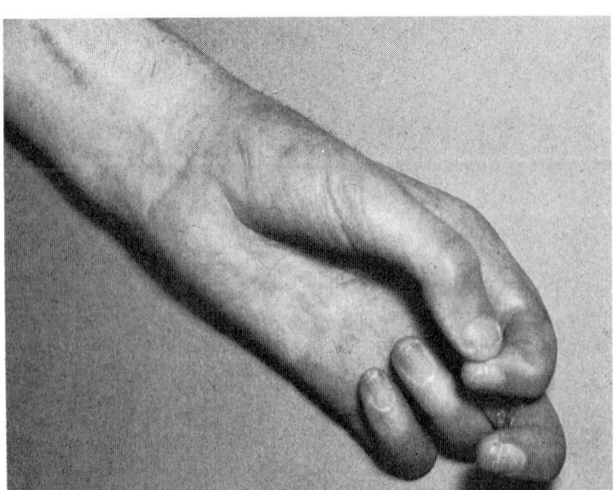

Figure 3–XV–11. Volkmann's contracture with marked clawing of the fingers. (From Byrne, J. J.: *The Hand: Its Anatomy and Diseases.* 1959. Courtesy of Charles C Thomas, Publisher, Springfield, Ill.)

The treatment of an established Volkmann's contracture is complicated and involves various procedures such as tendon lengthening, excision of contracted muscle, and sliding of muscle insertions down along the bone so that extension of the fingers can take place. In addition, one usually has to excise the pronator quadratus and pronator teres muscles in order to prevent locked pronation of the arm.

A similar condition in the intrinsic muscles of the hand is usually caused by a right plaster cast or elastic bandage. This was first described by Bunnell and classified as local ischemic contracture of the hand.[39] As it progresses, the characteristic deformity develops, with the metacarpophalangeal joints held in flexion and the interphalangeal joints in extension. Any attempt to flex the interphalangeal joints with the proximal joint extended is unsuccessful. This is the so-called intrinsic-plus position. It can be prevented by attention to pain; if a patient complains of severe pain after a circular dressing has been applied to the hand, the dressing should be removed to prevent this complication. Particular attention should be given to this type of contracture in any injury associated with metacarpal fractures, pain in the hand, and an intrinsic-plus position of the fingers. In these cases, the interosseous muscle compartment should be incised.[40]

Excessive unaccustomed work may also produce severe swelling of the interosseous muscles so that they shut off their own blood supply inside their tight fascial coverings. The swelling is probably due to fluid retention. This causes severe pain in the involved muscles out of proportion to the swelling, and the required treatment is rapid fasciotomy.[41]

Diagnostic Trauma

The increasing use of diagnostic arteriography and venography has led to a corresponding increase in the number of vascular injuries. The most common is the hematoma, which can usually be prevented and controlled by applying pressure over the puncture site. Large expanding hematomas, however, require exploration and arterial repair.

Thombosis may occur, depending upon preexisting vascular disease, the size of the vessel, the difficulty and duration of injections, and intimal dissection by the catheter. When the thrombosis threatens hand viability or function, exploration and repair are mandatory.[42]

SPECIAL INJURIES

Drug Injuries

A new chapter is being written in hand surgery with the increasing use of hard narcotics by the intravenous route. Toxic or unsterile, or adulterated drugs may be injected inadvertently into the subcutaneous tissue, producing infection and subsequent sloughing of skin and adjacent tendons and joints.

The dorsum of the hand is a common site for these infections, but on adequate drainage, the lesions usually heal without sequelae. Repeated injections also lead to a swelling of the hand from the proximal phalanges to the wrist, which may become permanent (the puffy hand of drug addiction).[43]

McKay and co-workers report that lesions distal to the web space result in more severe disability because the finger skin is less elastic.[44] Injection into the lateral veins of the fingers can produce sloughing that requires skin grafts for coverage.[45] In some patients, flexor tendon sheath infection ensues that necessitates excision of the underlying tendon.

Lesions on the dorsum of the proximal interphalangeal joints can progress to skin slough and extension of the process through the extensor mechanism of the joint. Eventual excision of the necrotic tendon and joint capsule as well as fusion of the joint is necessary.

In addition to local abscesses, cellulitis, and sloughing, injections in the forearm or just below the elbow may cause damage to nerves, arteries, or the contents of the antebrachial space. Nerve injuries are similar to any nerve trauma and may be partial and not require surgical repair. Arterial injuries may result in thrombosis with subsequent gangrene that may require treatment with sympathetic blocks, anticoagulation, and often fasciotomy of the forearm if there is evidence of forearm swelling. Injection into forearm muscles may produce such a severe chemical reaction that they become necrotic and heal with fibrosis resembling Volkmann's contracture of the hand.

Coma induced by an overdose of a narcotic may cause a patient to lie on his arm or lower extremity for an extended period. Such compression of an extremity may result in ischemic necrosis of muscles and nerves manifested by swelling of the muscle compartment. This requires immediate fasciotomy to preserve muscle and nerve function. Muscle necrosis may release large particles of myoglobin, which will appear in the urine (dark color), and this may be associated with renal shutdown.[45]

Occupational Devices

With technologic advances, a multitude of devices have been invented to improve or simplify occupational procedures. All these possess inherent danger if safety precautions are not observed. The list is too long to enumerate completely, but a few examples will suffice.

Grease guns can produce severe injuries if the needlelike ejector comes close to or penetrates the skin when the trigger is on. Grease is then forced into the tissues and spreads along fascial planes all over the finger or hand, depending upon the amount of grease ejected and the ejection pressure. If it cannot be removed, this material causes severe chemical damage, resulting in stiffness of the part and even loss of tissue. In addition, such grease, if left in tissue for long periods of time, may result in a tumorlike growth called an *oleoma*, which may have to be excised.[47, 48] Paint guns produce similar injuries.[49]

In the plastics industry, molten plastics are injected under pressure into various molds. This material may be forced into the hand, producing pain, swelling, and numbness in the involved area as the intensely hot material rapidly solidifies. Severe tendon, bone, and skin damage occurs. The plastic material should be removed and the wound debrided and left open. Reconstructive procedures are then necessary.[49]

Aerosol bombs may leak and cause severe burns of the hand.[50] Tear-gas pens may discharge, penetrate the hand, and produce severe chemical changes in nerves and muscles. In addition, the wad may be injected into the hand and must be carefully looked for at the time of surgical debridement.[9]

Guns for firing nails are now available. The nails have a washer located under the nail head and they also have a plastic collar beneath the washer. The washer drives a piece of skin with it into the deeper tissue, where it may serve as a nidus for a deep infection or even an inclusion cyst at a much later date. Thus, at surgery, not only should the projectile be removed, but a search for the skin fragment should also be made so that it can be removed.[52]

Machines that tear and shred may produce horrible mutilating injuries. The corn picker is a typical example. It produces a devastating wound, usually of the dominant hand. This machine is prone to clogging, and in the attempt to clear the machine, a farmer's hand may be shredded up to the forearm. The wound may consist of lacerations, crushing, and friction burns, which are contaminated with oil, grease, and corn fibers. Treatment includes debridement of nonviable tissue, stabilization of fractures, and primary and delayed skin coverage.[53] A machine for shredding rugs produces a similar injury with the same consequences. I have seen a similar injury recently caused by a frankfurter machine.

Some injuries of the past are of interest since they represent a response of industry to occupational hazards. Faucet handles, once made of porcelain, on twisting would break into sharp pointed edges that lacerated the palm, underlying nerves, and tendons.[54] Beryllium from light bulbs would produce a granulomatous response in the hand lacerated by the glass, which destroyed skin and tendons.[55] Fortunately, these items are no longer manufactured and one finds them only in older houses.

Burns

Burns are the most common of the special injuries. Flame burns occur on the dorsum of the hand when the hand is used to protect the face. Volar burns are usually caused by a hot object.

All serious burns (second- and third-degree) result in severe deformity of the hand, joint stiffness, tight skin, and underlying fibrosis. When underlying tissues (tendons, joints, bones, blood vessels) are damaged, the deformity is more severe and ranges from complete amputation to fixed contractures of digits.

The usual defect is a flexion deformity of the wrist, extension or hyperextension of the metacarpal joints, and flexion of the fingers. It is difficult to prevent this, since adequate splinting is impossible by the usual methods.

Treatment is aimed at resurfacing the injured skin as soon as possible. In intermediate burns, this is done by preventing infection, which would convert the burn to a deeper degree, by using various chemotherapeutic agents (Sulfamylon, silver nitrate). If infection can be prevented, the burn wound will reepithelialize from epithelial remnants in the dermis (sweat and sebaceous glands, hair follicles). In deeper burns (third-degree) the burn eschar should be removed as soon as possible either spontaneously by natural debridement or surgically by excision. The resultant defect is then covered with a split-thickness skin graft.

Much experimental evidence is developing to show that daily dressings with skin grafts from any source (human, porcine, canine) may prevent infection, stimulate epithelialization, and promote eschar removal.[56]

Once the burn wound is covered by skin, physical therapy is begun to develop finger joint and wrist joint function. Subsequent surgical reconstructive procedures may be needed, such as replacement of thin tight skin with thicker skin grafts or even skin flaps. If tendon transfer or grafting is needed, arthrodesis and arthroplasty should be done.

Burn scars have a high potential for cancer development, particularly if they are thin and ulcerate easily. Such scars should be replaced with skin grafts.

Electrical Injuries

These are a major source of trauma. Their severity depends upon the amount of current passing through the tissues. This produces heat that causes intensive local damage to skin, fascia, tendons, blood vessels, and bones. The strength of the current depends upon voltage, duration of exposure, and size and firmness and wetness of contact. Alternating current appears to be worse than direct current. Death may occur from ventricular fibrillation if the current traverses the heart.

The damage is difficult to assess at initial inspection since its effect is progressive owing to widespread vascular injury. The lesions are painless because of nerve destruction. Eventually, inflammatory reaction develops at the periphery of the involved tissue and the area sloughs out very slowly. The forearm and hand may become gangrenous. When the tissues become necrotic they are subject to secondary infection. Repeated hemorrhage from such wounds suggests that hemostatic instruments be kept at the bedside of all such patients.

Initial treatment is conservative, and the affected parts are treated as any other burn. Multiple excisions are required as the necrotic areas become demarcated. Cutaneous homografts may be used after each excision for temporary coverage prior to final autografting. After skin coverage is complete, further reconstructive procedures may be needed such as flap grafts, tendon transfers, joint fusions, or arthroplasties.[57-61]

PAINFUL STATES

Trauma may result in a painful extremity for a variety of reasons. Many of the causes may overlap. In each individual case, these must be searched for, delineated, and treated separately if relief is to be afforded.

Dystrophy of Disuse

Disuse or nonuse of a part from any cause (edema, prolonged immobilization, infection, pain, ischemia) results in joint contracture and atrophy of soft tissue and osteoporosis of bones. This dystrophy is more common with increasing age and in the rheumatoid diathesis. It may respond to resumption of activity with physical therapy after the causes for the disuse or nonuse have been eliminated. Judicious use of an antiinflammatory drug (cortisone injections, phenylbutazone ingestion) may speed up the recovery.

Since there are many causes for the dystrophic stiff hand, every effort should be made for its prevention. Infection should be curtailed by adequate cleansing of the wound, irrigation, and appropriate administration of antibiotics, depending upon the nature of the injury. The edema that precipitates fibrosis should be alleviated by proper compression dressings and postoperative elevation of the extremities. If a sling is used, the hand should be positioned in elevation; improper dependency in a sling produces edema in the hand.[62]

Unnecessary and prolonged immobilization obviously causes stiffness. The immobilization should be restricted to the parts that need it. The position of the hand during the period of immobilization is of utmost importance. The metacarpophalangeal joints are less apt to become stiff when they are kept flexed because of the nature of their anatomy. The proximal interphalangeal joints should be just slightly flexed. This is the position in which all hands that are in prolonged immobilization should be kept whenever possible.

Particular attention should be paid to complaints of pain, especially if a cast has been applied. Pain may indicate pressure sores or ischemia from either vascular damage or a too tight bandage. If the patient's complaints of pain are out of the ordinary for the type of injury he has sustained, the surgeon should remove constricting bandages, which in today's armamentarium usually means Kling, Curlex, and Ace bandages. If there is evidence of interosseous compression, a fasciotomy should be done.

Phantom Limb

Amputation of a part almost always results in some manifestation of the "phantom" limb. This means that at times the patient feels that the amputated part is still present. This is a normal phenomenon, and reassurance by persons caring for the patient will do much to diminish a permanent disability. In a majority of cases, the phantom limb is of no consequence and becomes suppressed. Occasionally, however, if there are emotional or psychiatric problems, such sensations may be aggravated by the central nervous system to a definite painful phenomenon. In addition, some of the localized causes of pain, such as amputation neuromas or reflex sympathetic dystrophy may be present, and correct treatment may relieve the pain from the phantom limb.

Neuromas

Neuromas form at the cut end of an injured nerve, or if the nerve has been partially damaged, they occur along the pathway of the nerve as a neuroma in continuity. When stimulated by pressure, there is exquisite discomfort in the extremity consisting of a "pins-and-needles" sensation or a "shooting" pain radiating from a localized area. The pain may become severe and diffuse, and spread up the entire extremity. This is caused by continued sensation coming from the neuroma, which alters some portion of the spinal cord pathway to the thalamus and makes the pain more severe. It is a difficult problem to understand, and many theories have been brought forth. Some explain it as fiber interaction in injured nerves; others by the fact that the impulses stimulate the internuncial pool or reticular activating system of the spinal cord so that normal impulses reaching the area are interpreted as painful. This same process might also occur in higher regions of the central nervous system. At times, the pain may become permanent, in which case it is almost like a computer in which short-circuiting has occurred and continuous self-sustaining currents are set up.

A neuroma should be carefully searched for by examination of the wound scar with a palpating instrument of small area such as the blunt point of a pencil. The pain can usually be identified at a definite localized spot associated with paresthesias. The neuroma itself may be felt as a discrete mass. Its treatment demands excision of the neuroma, ligation of the nerve end with silk, and replacement of the nerve in an area where it is not subject to contact.

At times, a neuroma may be caught in scar tissue and be aggravated by certain motions of the arm; this type also should be removed, and the nerve end should be relocated distant from the bound area.

Reflex Sympathetic Dystrophy

Some injuries result in a peculiar condition consisting of pain that is often burning in character and aggravated by cold.[63] This may be associated with edema, cyanosis, sweating, and hypesthesia. The resultant motor weakness, atrophy, limitation of joint motion, osteoporosis, or soft tissue atrophy is probably secondary to partial nerve damage and is somewhat akin to the next disease to be mentioned, causalgia. The pain is, however, of a lesser degree, and the vasomotor symptoms are more severe. It may even result in necrosis of the tips of the involved fingers (Fig. 3–XV–12).

Diagnosis should be made early, and these cases should be treated with sympathetic blocks. This usually gives temporary relief, but if repeated attempts with sympathetic blocks are necessary, a sympathectomy may be performed for permanent relief. Other agents of value are vasodilating drugs and, occasionally, drugs such as reserpine (Serpasil). If allowed to progress before treatment is instituted, many of the changes in the hand may become permanent.

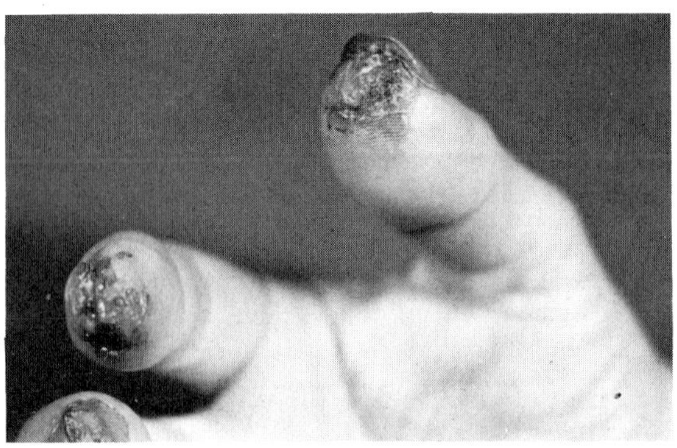

Figure 3–XV–12. Traumatic sympathetic dystrophy with necrosis of the tips of the thumb, index, and middle fingers secondary to minor trauma at the tip of the thumb (From Byrne, J. J. *The Hand: Its Anatomy and Diseases.* 1959. Courtesy of Charles C Thomas, Publisher, Springfield, Ill.)

Causalgia

Causalgia is a definite clinical entity that follows partial injury of a nerve, for instance, the median.[64] There is spontaneous hot, burning pain in the extremity, which is extremely sensitive to touch or even to the suggestion of being touched. Vasomotor manifestations may be present. The cause is basically unknown, but it is felt to be a short-circuiting between the sympathetic and sensory nerves at the site of injury, so that sympathetic discharges are felt as painful sensations. This entity was first described by Weir Mitchell during the Civil War and has been a product of many wars since, but it also may follow civilian trauma. It usually involves partial trauma to a major nerve, such as the median or tibial. Sympathetic blocks give temporary relief and sympathectomy gives permanent relief.

Entrapment of Nerves

This problem has been alluded to earlier. Any injury to bone or soft tissue that results in narrowing of a canal through which a nerve is passing may give rise to painful sensation in the involved nerve. This can occur anywhere from the shoulder outlet to the elbow joint or wrist.

FIBROSES

Dupuytren's Contracture

This is a deformity in the hand produced by contraction of the palmar fascia, which tends to pull the fingers into the palm. The fourth and fifth fingers are most often involved, but all can be. Treatment is by surgical excision of the involved fascia, but there is debate as to how much should be removed and when it should be done. Surgery is not advised unless the finger joints begin to flex. Removal of nodules in the palm is usually not necessary. The extent of surgery depends upon the local anatomical conditions and the age of the patient. The involved bands should be removed (limited fasciectomy), although in very senile patients merely cutting the bands may improve function (fasciotomy). Younger patients with more widespread involvement may require removal of as much palmar fascia as is possible (radical palmar fasciectomy). Some physicians have attempted to destroy the involved fascia with enzyme injections into the fascia followed by forceful extension of the finger to rupture the fascia. The finger is then splinted in extension during the day and protected at night for two weeks. This has been most effective in patients unfit for surgery or as preparation for future surgery.[65]

The cause of this lesion is still obscure, but since it was first clarified by Dupuytren in 1823, it has been thought that trauma plays a major role. Skoog believes the disease originates in small fibrillar ruptures in the aponeurosis.[66] Larsen and co-workers produced tissue resembling Dupuytren's contracture in monkeys by traction on the palmar aponeurosis producing fiber ruptures. Many other conditions have been implicated such as alcoholism, epilepsy, coronary disease. It is more frequent in northern European races, males are affected nine times as often as females, and the disease increases with advancing years. It is probably a response to the wear and tear of everyday existence on that area of the palmar fascia subject to the most stress and use of the hand, the distal palm near the base of the ring finger.[68]

Zachariae reviewed the records of 860 patients with Dupuytren's contracture and found that 54 per cent performed heavy work and the remainder performed light work. Although 782 patients were right-handed, the disease began in the left hand in 43 per cent of the cases.[69] Theisinger reports four cases in which Dupuytren's contracture followed a single trauma.[70] Schroter noticed that it is officially considered an occupational disease in England, the Soviet Union, and Holland, if there is evidence of a long-standing occupational strain on the palmar surface of the hand.[71]

Complications of the operation are not numerous, but involve poor skin healing due to development of very thin skin flaps, hematoma formation, and edema, all of which lead to prolonged immobilization and eventual joint stiffness, particularly in the proximal interphalangeal joints. Hematoma formation is the most common complication, and attempts to prevent it include compression dressing and suction drainage. Some surgeons leave the skin wound open so that blood can be removed immediately during wound healing.[72] Skin necrosis is related to involvement of the skin by the process and the need to develop very thin skin flaps. Digital nerves may be damaged since the disease process incorporates them, particularly in the proximal phalanx. When damaged, they should be repaired; usually there is a good return of function. The blood vessels may also be damaged, and if the blood vessels on both sides of the finger are so destroyed, gangrene of the finger may result.

Stenosing Tenovaginitis

Tendons crossing joints are usually held in place by a fibrous sheath lined with gliding synovial membrane. These may become inflamed and then constricted by fibroplasia, preventing the tendon from gliding smoothly. The most commonly involved sheath is that over the radial stylus containing the abductor pollicis longus and the extensor pollicis brevis (de Quervain's disease); involved nearly as often are the sheath of the flexor pollicis longus and the flexor sheath of the middle and ring fingers.

The basic cause of this process is the repeated motion of the tendons pressing against the sheath. Sperling produced the condition in himself by flexing his little finger 9,000 times in 72 hours.[73] Almost every case involves some occupational motion. It occurs in new workers at an unaccustomed task, old workers out of training for the task, and workers speeding up their jobs. The tasks do not have to be industrial and may be household chores or avocations. It is most common in women whose tendon apparatus may not have been strengthened enough for repeated motions. It may be a first symptom in patients with a tendency to fibroplasia or fibrous inflammation (rheumatoid arthritis).

The process was first described in the tendon sheath of the abductor pollicis longus and extensor pollicis brevis by de Quervain in 1895. This tendon sheath often contains accessory tendons, and some think this increased bulk predisposes the sheath to constriction.[74] There is pain and tenderness over the radial styloid that may be aggravated by the ulnar flexion of the wrist. The thumb motion may be limited in extension and abduction.

The flexor tendon sheaths of the finger and thumb are involved over the metacarpophalangeal joints, where there is tenderness and pain. Tendovaginitis here produces a characteristic snapping or triggerlike action when the involved finger is flexed or extended (trigger finger). Eventually force is applied.

The process may subside with rest and splinting of the involved part with or without the injection of cortisone. If this does not improve the condition, incision of the constricting tendon sheath may be necessary.

REFERENCES

ANATOMY OF THE HAND

1. Littler, J. W.: On the adaptability of man's hand. Hand, 5:187, 1973.
2. Barron, J. N.: The structure and function of the skin of the hand. Hand, 2:93, 1970.
3. Wilson, W. F., and Hueston, J. T.: The intratendinous architecture. Hand, 5:33, 1973.
4. Ritter, M. A.: The anatomy and function of the palmar fascia. Hand, 5:263, 1973.
5. Kuczynski, K.: Functional microanatomy of the peripheral nerve trunks. Hand, *6*:1, 1974.
6. Sunderland, S.: *Nerves and Nerve Injuries.* Edinburgh and London, E. & S. Livingstone, Ltd., 1968.

INFECTIONS

7. Wilkes, R.: Social and occupational study of the causes, cost and prevention of infections of the hand. Br. J. Indust. Med., *11*:269, 1954.
8. Sneddon, J.: Sepsis in hand injuries. Hand, *2*:58, 1970.
9. Pallen, A. G.: Acute infection of the tendon sheaths. Hand, *6*:21, 1974.
10. Graham, W. P, Kilgare, E. S., Williams, E. H., and Gordon, S. L.: Metastatic tumors of the hand. Hand, 5:177, 1973.

SKIN INJURIES

11. Harrison, S. H.: Principles of skin replacement in the hand. Hand, *2*:106, 1970.
12. Bruner, J. M.: Surgical exposure of flexor tendons in the hand. Ann. R. Coll. Surg. Engl., *53*:84, 1973.
13. Mutz, S.: Thumb web contracture. Hand, *4*:236, 1972.
14. Buchan, A. C.: Deep burns—burn contractures. Hand, *3*:90, 1971.

TENDON INJURIES

15. Verdan, C. E.: Half a century of flexor tendon surgery. J. Bone Joint Surg., *54A*:472, 1972.
16. Holms, W.: Primary suture of flexor tendons in the danger zone. Hand, *6*:17, 1974.
17. Hunter, J. M., and Salisbury, R. E.: Flexor-tendon reconstruction in severely damaged hands. J. Bone Joint Surg., *53A*:829, 1971.
18. Urbanick, J. R., and Goldner, J. L.: Laceration of the flexor pollicis longus tendon. J. Bone Joint Surg., *55A*:1123, 1973.
19. Mickic, Z., and Helal, B.: The treatment of the mallet finger by the Oakley splint. Hand, *6*:76, 1974.
20. Suzuki, K.: Reconstruction of post-traumatic boutonniere deformity. Hand, 5:145, 1973.

NERVE INJURIES

21. Phalen, G. S.: The carpal tunnel syndrome. J. Bone Joint Surg., *48A*:211, 1966.
22. Richmond, D. A.: Uncommon causes of nerve compression with hand symptoms. Hand, 5:209, 1973.
23. Wilgis, E. F. S.: Observations on the effects of tourniquet ischemia. J. Bone Joint Surg., *53A*:1343, 1971.
24. Parkes, A.: Ischemic effects of external and internal pressure on the upper limb. Hand, 5:105, 1973.
25. Sanders, R.: The tourniquet, instrument or weapon. Hand, 5:119, 1973.
26. Macon, W. L., and Futrell, J. W.: Median nerve neuropathy after percutaneous puncture of the brachial artery in patients receiving anticoagulants. N. Engl. J. Med., *288*:1396, 1973.
27. Millesi, H.: The microsurgery of peripheral nerves. Hand, 5:157, 1973.
28. Simeone, F. A.: Symposium on operative nerve injuries and their repair. Surg. Clin. North Am., *52*:1097, 1972.
29. Barton, N. J.: Radial nerve lesions. Hand, 5:200, 1973.

FRACTURES

30. Brown, P. W.: The management of phalangeal and metacarpal fractures. Surg. Clin. North Am., *53*:1393, 1973.
31. Hamburg, H. J.: Bennett's fracture. Hand, *4*:224, 1972.
32. Green, D. P., and Anderson, J. R.: Closed reduction and percutaneous pin fixation of fractured phalanges. J. Bone Joint Surg., *55A*:1651, 1973.

JOINT INJURIES

33. Eaton, R. G.: *Joint Injuries of the Hand.* Springfield, Ill., Charles C Thomas, 1971.

VASCULAR INJURIES

34. O'Brien, B. M., and Baxter, R. J.: Experimental digital replantation. Hand, *6*:11, 1974.
35. Mansfield, J. P. J.: Traumatic thrombosis of the ulnar artery in the palm. J. Bone Joint Surg., *36B*:438, 1954.
36. Zweig, J., Lie, K. K., and Posch, J. L.: Thrombosis of the ulnar artery following blunt trauma of the hand. J. Bone Joint Surg., *51A*:1191, 1969.
37. Telforde, D., McCann, M. B., and MacCormack, D. H.: Dead hand in users of vibrating tools. Lancet, *2*:359, 1945.
38. Smith, J. W.: True aneurysms of traumatic origin in the palm. Am. J. Surg., *104*:7, 1962.
39. Bunnell, S.: Ischemic contracture local in the hand. J. Bone Joint Surg., *3A*:88, 1953.
40. Reed, R. L., and Travis, R. T.: Acute necrosis of the second interosseous compartment of the hand. J. Bone Joint Surg., *55A*:1095, 1973.
41. Hughes, J. R.: Ischemic necrosis of the anterior tibial muscles due to fatigue. J. Bone Joint Surg., *30B*:581, 1948.
42. Whelan, T. J., Jr., and Baugh, J. H.: Non-atherosclerotic arterial lesions and their management. Curr. Probl. Surg., 1967.

SPECIAL INJURIES

43. Neviaser, R. J., Butterfield, W. C., and Weicher, D. R.: The puffy hand of drug addiction. J. Bone Joint Surg., *54A*:629, 1972.
44. McKay, D., Pascerelli, E. F., and Eaton, R. G.: Infections and sloughs in the hands of addicts. J. Bone Joint Surg., *55A*:741, 1973.
45. Schreiher, S. N., Liebowitz, M. R., and Bernstein, L. H.: Limb compression and renal impairment (crush syndrome) following narcotic and sedative overdose. J. Bone Joint Surg., *55A*:1683, 1972.
46. Byrne, J. J.: Grease gun injuries. J.A.M.A., *125*:405, 1944.
47. Stark, H. H., Wilson, J. N., and Boyes, J. H.: Grease gun injuries of the hand. J. Bone Joint Surg., *43*:485, 1961.

48. Stark, H. H., Ashworth, C. R., and Boyes, J. H.: Paint gun injuries of the hand. J. Bone Joint Surg., *49A*:637, 1967.
49. Baker, J. M.: Molten plastic injuries of the hand. Plast. Reconstr. Surg., *15*:233, 1955.
50. Metzler, D. F.: Injury resulting from use of aerosol bomb. Public Health Rep., *61*:546, 1946.
51. Adams, J. P., Fee, N., and Kenmore, P. I.: Tear gas injuries. J. Bone Joint Surg., *48*:436, 1966.
52. Braun, R. M.: Nail-gun injury of the hand. J. Bone Joint Surg., *53A*:383, 1971.
53. Melvin, P. M.: Corn picker injuries of the hand. Arch. Surg., *104*:26, 1972.
54. Boyes, J. H., and Melone, F. C.: Injuries of the hand from broken porcelain faucet handles. West. J. Surg., *60*:59, 1952.
55. Flynn, J. E.: Subcutaneous beryllium granulomata of the hand. Ann. Surg., *137*:265, 1953.
56. Rappaport, I., Pepino, A. T., and Dietrick, W.: Early use of xenografts as a biologic dressing in burn trauma. Am. J. Surg., *120*:144, 1970.
57. Mills, W., Switzer, W. E., and Moncrief, J. A. : Electrical injuries. J.A.M.A., *195*:164, 1966.
58. Taylor, P. H., Pugsley, L. E., and Vogel, E. H.: The intriguing electrical burn. J. Trauma, *2*:309, 1962.
59. Lewis, G. K.: Burns from electricity. Ann. Surg., *131*:80, 1950.
60. Brown, J. B., and Fryer, M. P.: Reconstruction of electrical injuries including cranial loss. Ann. Surg., *146*:342, 1957.
61. Kay, N. R. M., and Boswick, J. A.: The management of electrical injuries of the extremities. Surg. Clin. North Am., *53*:1459, 1973.

PAINFUL STATES

62. James, J. I. P.: The assessment and management of the injured hand. Hand, *2*:97, 1970.
63. Boyles, T. B., Judson, W. E., and Potter, T. A.: Reflex sympathetic dystrophy. J.A.M.A., *144*:537, 1950.
64. Mayfield, F. H.: Causalgia. Am. J. Surg., *74*:522, 1947.

FIBROSES

65. Hueston, J. T.: Enzyme fasciotomy. Hand, *3*:38, 1971.
66. Skoog, T.: Dupuytren's contraction. Acta Chir. Scand., Suppl. 139, 1948.
67. Larsen, R. D., Takagishi, H., and Pasch, J. L.: The pathogenesis of Dupuytren's contracture. J. Bone Joint Surg., *42A*:993, 1960.
68. Bruner, J.: The dynamics of Dupuytren's contracture. Hand, *2*:172, 1970.
69. Zachariae, L.: Dupuytren's contracture. Scand. J. Plast. Reconstr. Surg., *5*:116, 1971.
70. Theisinger, W.: Zur Dupuytrenschen Kontractur in der Unfallbegutachtung. Monatsschr. Unfallheilkd., *72*:220, 1969.
71. Schröter, G.: Die Anerkennumg der Dupuytrenschen Kontractur als berufskrankheit. Beitr. Orthop. Traumatol., *18*:78, 1971.
72. McCash, C. R.: The open palm technique in Dupuytren's contracture. Br. J. Plast. Surg., *17*:271, 1964.
73. Sperling, W. P.: Snapping finger. Acta Radiol., *37*:74, 1952.
74. Faithful, D. K., and Lanib, D. W.: DeQuervain's disease—a clinical review. Hand, *3*:23, 1971.

SECTION 1. MECHANICAL INJURY

chapter 4

SYSTEMIC RESPONSE TO TRAUMA

by Herbert B. Hechtman and Luke G. Tedeschi

In the majority of patients who suffer trauma, the restoration of blood volume, blood pressure, and blood flow is readily accomplished and is followed by prompt recovery without residual damage. In a second group of patients, similar resuscitative measures do not lead to rapid improvement. A much more intensive program of care is instituted, extending over days to weeks, and the outcome is not necessarily favorable.[1]

Of the deaths among adult patients who have been severely injured, approximately one third are due to direct involvement of the heart, brain, or kidney by the initial injury or primary disease.[2] About one third result from a process that is primarily septic and involves blood stream infection, usually with gram-negative bacilli or yeasts. Finally, about one third of the fatalities follow progressive respiratory failure, significant gastric bleeding, and myocardial failure despite the absence of direct injury to these organ systems.

Trauma may lead to both direct and indirect injury. Mechanical impact disrupts local tissue and organ architecture, with resultant functional abnormalities. Equally important are the secondary and tertiary reactions that influence multiple body functions far removed from the site of injury. The pathophysiologic mechanisms of these reactions and distant organ injuries are frequently obscure. The occurrence of such phenomena is beyond dispute, however, and is the subject of this chapter.

NEUROHORMONAL RESPONSE

The frequently described fright and flight responses to a threatening situation are mediated via the sympathoadrenal axis. Anxiety, fear, and pain, as well as many subtle emotional factors, can find their common pathway of physical expression both by means of the autonomic nervous system and through sympathetic hormone release. The characteristic pattern of response is an increase in heart rate, blood pressure, and respiratory rate. Redistribution of blood flow results in cooling of the skin, while sweat gland overactivity leads to characteristic sweating. The mouth is dry and the pupils dilated. Young and healthy individuals, such as astronauts or students taking examinations, tolerate these changes induced by stress without incident. Some individuals with preexisting coronary artery disease, which may not be clinically apparent, can exceed the threshold of myocardial work and develop angina or even a myocardial infarction. Other illnesses, such as acute asthma or cerebrovascular accidents, may be triggered by emotional factors.

Another response to fear, for example, the fear of an injection, is a vasovagal reflex that may result in a faint. This common reaction is mediated by the parasympathetic nervous system. Stimulation of this component of the autonomic nervous system leads to sudden thirst due to the functional hypovolemia induced by peripheral vasodilation and tachycardia. If the victim is standing, there is a profound decrease in blood pressure and cardiac output that leads to transient cerebral ischemia and unconsciousness; as he falls to the ground and blood flow is restored to the brain, consciousness is regained and vital signs rapidly return to normal.

An example of an autonomic nervous system response to injury that results in long-term disability is causalgia.[3] It has been observed that major, or even relatively minor, extremity injuries with or without associated fractures may lead to long-term physical and functional impairment. Regional reflex changes with sympathetic overactivity may produce a cool, moist extremity that becomes painful and swollen. This can become an extraordinary handicap. Disuse of the extremity may result in muscle atrophy and frequently osteoporosis. This syndrome has been called Sudek's atrophy or causalgia. It is mentioned as an example of the complexity of the psychologic-neurologic response to trauma.

The long-term emotional response to injury is variable and depends somewhat on the prior mental health of the patient. Physical therapy and occupational retraining are important features for both physical and psychic rehabilitation. The secondary gains of illness must be considered in evaluating the progress or lack of progress in any trauma patient. In general, unsettled suits or compensation tend to perpetuate disability.

In addition to these general neurohormonal and peripheral reflex changes, profound neurohormonal influences may be exerted in a number of organ systems. These include the lungs, brain, heart, alimentary tract, and kidneys.

Increase in the respiratory rate and hyperventilation are usually associated with trauma and may be induced by either a peripheral or central stimulus.[4,5] Fear and pain themselves are adequate causes of hyperventilation. The result of hyperventilation is repiratory alkalosis. It is not uncommon to find the arterial carbon dioxide tension (Pa_{CO_2}) reduced to values in the teens or low twenties (normal $Pa_{CO_2} = 40$). The pH of arterial blood may be 7.5 or 7.6 (normal pH = 7.4). This respiratory alkalosis can occur in minutes and represents a sudden alteration in the internal milieu. Alkalosis may itself produce cerebral vasoconstriction and thereby reduce blood flow to the brain. Anxious individuals can hyperventilate to the point of unconsciousness. Fortunately permanent brain damage is rare. Patients with arteriosclerotic disease of the cerebral vessels, however, may have a critical reduction of blood flow to the brain and suffer irreversible damage.

Alkalosis leads to an abrupt decrease in serum potassium levels. Potassium is taken up into cells while hydrogen and sodium ions enter the serum. Under these circumstances patients, particularly those with heart disease, are more susceptible to cardiac arrhythmias. In addition, the side effects of digitalis become more prominent with hypokalemia.

The normal compensatory response to this alkalosis is the secretion of alkaline urine. This renal mechanism is slow, however, taking hours to days, and is never complete.

In addition to those of the sympathoadrenal axis, other hormones assume regulatory roles in the trauma patient. The metabolically active ones, insulin, glucocorticoids, glucagon, and growth hormone, are discussed later. The mineralocorticoids alter urine composition by increasing potassium and decreasing sodium concentrations.[6] Antidiuretic hormone from the posterior pituitary gland reduces free water clearance from the kidneys. The ultimate importance of many of these hormones is disputed. Frequently, the magnitude of the trauma problem makes many of these fine regulatory mechanisms trivial.[7]

SHOCK

Shock may be defined as a state in which a critical reduction in capillary blood flow causes cellular damage in multiple tissues and organ systems. The magnitude of the damage depends on the discrepancy between tissue needs and supply as well as on the build-up of tissue wastes. This varies from organ to organ. The complexity of the problem of shock is due to the varying rates of organ failure and the interdependence of organ function.

The syndrome of traumatic shock is usually initiated by a loss of circulating blood volume. Major injuries are associated with significant blood or fluid loss, either internally or externally. For example, major external blood loss can result from lacerations of large arteries or veins. Local factors produce vascular constriction and clot formation, which tend to minimize blood loss. Preexisting illness such as arteriosclerosis or clotting defects limit this adaptive response. A patient taking anticoagulant medication such as Coumadin will have an exaggerated blood loss from relatively small wounds.

Internal bleeding is common with both penetrating and blunt thoracic and abdominal injuries. Following blunt trauma to the chest or abdomen, major vessels may be lacerated by shearing forces or by fractured ribs or pelvis. The presence of a fractured rib should alert the physician to possible injuries to the lungs, liver, or spleen. These organs are commonly responsible for internal bleeding.

Hip and pelvic fractures are characteristically associated with the loss of 1 liter or more of blood into tissue spaces of the thigh or retroperitoneum. Blood losses in such circumstances may be massive, but are not always clinically apparent. The general findings of increased pulse and respiratory rates and decreased blood pressure and urine flow must alert the physician to the possibility of blood loss. Occasionally these signs are absent.[8]

Head trauma may also result in internal bleeding either into the brain or into the subdural or epidural spaces. The volume of blood lost is relatively inconsequential. The major significance of the blood is its accumulation within an enclosed space and its displacement of the brain.

Fluid losses other than blood may be significant, and may also be external or internal. Second- and third-degree burns lead to sequestration of plasma or evaporative fluid loss. Such losses are predictable, being based on the size of the burn and the weight of the patient, and may frequently amount to many liters per day.

Internal fluid losses involve sequestration of fluid in cavities or tissues so that the fluid is unavailable to the body. Any traumatized or inflamed area will swell because of fluid accumulation. Inflammatory changes within the abdomen may occur with traumatic pancreatitis and lead to fluid accumulation in the free peritoneal cavity as well as in the walls of the abdominal cavity and intestines. This is similar to an internal burn. Trauma frequently leads to reflex ileus of the gastrointestinal tract, manifest by vomiting and dilatation of the intestine with air and fluid. These fluid shifts may be significant not only in terms of the volume lost but also because of electrolyte shifts.[9] Vomiting or nasogastric suction usually leads to a loss of acid and chloride, resulting in hypochloremic, hypokalemic alkalosis. On the other hand, a traumatic biliary, pancreatic, or duodenal fistula will lead to loss of alkaline secretions. Renal function may be insufficient to reverse these acid-base and electrolyte abnormalities. The kidneys may themselves induce fluid and electrolyte abnormalities. This is often observed during the oliguric as well as the diuretic phases of acute renal failure.

"Hemorrhagic shock," in usual clinical terms, refers to the condition of an anxious patient whose extremities are cool and moist, whose respiratory and pulse rates are increased, and whose blood pressure and urine output are decreased. Such changes in vital signs usually occur after the loss of at least 20 per cent of the blood volume. Elderly patients may be unable to compensate for smaller volume losses because their arteriosclerotic vessels are unable to constrict.

Following hemorrhage, the cardiac output is reduced and redistributed to protect essential organ function. The coronary and cerebral circulation is preferentially maintained while blood flow to the skin and digestive organs is reduced.

In the untreated patient, there is transudation of fluid from the extravascular spaces into the vascular compartment, an attempt by the body to restore blood volume. This process is slow, taking hours, and eventually results in dilution of the red cell mass or a decrease in hematocrit.[10]

Therapy for patients suffering hemorrhage is fluid replacement. There are many conflicting claims in the literature regarding the ideal resuscitation fluid.[11] There is no denial that whole, type-specific blood or low-titer O negative blood is required to maintain oxygen-carrying capacity. The ideal hematocrit or hemoglobin level, however, is disputed. High hematocrits will lead to unacceptable increases in viscosity and will compromise capillary blood flow. It is unlikely, however, that blood viscosity per se (at constant hematocrit) is altered in trauma.[12] Thus, although there is a large literature on fluid therapy, there is little scientific resolution of the problem. Most authors advocate the use of crystalloids, either Ringer's lactate or saline solutions, in combination with blood and albumin.[13]

HYPERDYNAMIC STATE

In 1943 Cournand and co-workers and Richards described the events taking place in hemorrhage that led to a reduction in cardiac output and increased peripheral vascular resistance. The patients studied had suffered both hemorrhage and trauma. These authors concluded that the hemodynamic findings were characteristic of traumatic as well as hemorrhagic shock. Other workers later reported the association of low cardiac output in shock states associated with myocardial infarction and arrhythmias.[16, 17] These several studies resulted in the widely held concept that the combination of low cardiac output and high peripheral vascular resistance was the physiologic basis of shock.

Current observations confirm the presence of low cardiac output in association with hemorrhage and myocardial infarction. Sequential hemodynamic studies after trauma such as blunt abdominal injury and gunshot wounds, however, have repeatedly documented a hyperdynamic state.[18, 19] In patients with trauma alone, the main features are an increased cardiac output, reduced resistance, tachycardia, increased central blood volume, and increased stroke work. These responses occur in the early period after injury, that is, before and during the time of maximal hypotension.[17] The hemodynamic pattern observed in trauma patients who have associated blood loss with moderate or severe hypotension is that of reduced cardiac output, decreased central blood volume, and reduced stroke work. Hemodynamic responses of trauma-hemorrhage patients with mild hypotension closely resemble those of patients with trauma alone.

These hemodynamic events have prognostic significance. Failure of cardiac output to increase and pulmonary and peripheral vascular resistance to decrease are grave signs.[20]

Sepsis is a frequent companion of trauma and may itself lead to shock characterized by hypotension, decreased peripheral vascular resistance, and a normal or increased cardiac output. The hemodynamic picture is very similar to that of pure trauma as just described.[21] The wise clinician who treats trauma is always on the alert for associated sepsis. The diagnosis is often obscure and must always be suspected in patients who fail to show steady improvement.

SEPSIS

Despite recent advances in chemotherapy, infections are frequent following severe trauma, and are often associated with death. Injury upsets the delicate balance between man and his surrounding environment of microorganisms. Antibiotic therapy has now been used for over a quarter of a century. Clinical and laboratory studies have indicated that it has failed to reduce the overall incidence of infection. As Shaw states

> . . . there is at bottom only one genuinely scientific treatment for all diseases and that is to stimulate the phagocytes. Drugs are a delusion.[22]

Many of the pharmacologic agents used in the treatment of trauma have adverse effects on host defense.[23] Some of the commonly used antibiotics are capable of blocking the reticuloendothelial system and suppressing cell-mediated immunity. Almost all the agents used for general anesthesia have been shown to depress lymphocytic function. A single large dose of corticosteroids is capable of diminishing antibody production. Some of the vasoactive agents used in the treatment of shock have deleterious effects of their own on the ability of the host to combat infection. This may in part be due to peripheral vasoconstriction and reduction of blood flow to the injured part, where neutrophilic leukocytes depend on good oxygenation for optimal phagocytosis of microorganisms.

It is probable that despite improvements both in antibiotic therapy and in the general treatment of trauma and shock, substantial reduction in the number of deaths from septic complications will not be achieved until an understanding of the compromised host becomes more complete and specific measures are taken to bolster host defense mechanisms. Like the patient with severe chronic underlying disease, the traumatized patient has lost many host defense mechanisms. This predisposes him to infection with organisms of little virulence.[24] These, after becoming part of the endogenous flora, gain access to the patient through the multiple invasive procedures necessary for his management, such as bladder or tracheal intubation.[25] It is likely that abnormalities of neutrophilic function are the most important variable of immunologic defense relating to the development of opportunistic infections in man.[26, 27]

In addition to circulating neutrophils, there are phagocytic cells in the peritoneum, lungs, liver, and other organs. They have been shown to actively entrap circulating bacteria.[28]

This system, the reticuloendothelial system (RES), is thought to have other significant functions in addition to bacteriostasis. Experimental work has shown that the Kupffer cells in the liver detoxify endotoxin.[29] A number of authors believe that the reticuloendothelial system may be the homeostatic system that serves as the critical common pathway in the pathogenesis of and host adaptation to certain shock states.[30, 31] In animals it has been found that the greater the degree of traumatic shock, the greater are both the magnitude and duration of early phagocytic depression.[32] Such depression may be due to reduced organ blood flow, since histologic and electron microscopic evidence of damage to Kupffer cells of the liver has been demonstrated after hemorrhage.[33, 34]

The following three specific infections relate directly to traumatic wounds. Gas gangrene has been all but eliminated by the military surgeon's emphasis on early and extensive debridement of devascularized muscle.[35] Tetanus is also extremely rare, as prophylaxis is easily administered. Rabies remains somewhat controversial, as current methods of prophylaxis are hazardous and of questionable benefit. In the past 12 years, there have been an estimated two million dog bites per year, with fewer than two cases of rabies per year.[36] These data weigh heavily in support of current therapy, which favors immunization only in cases of known exposure to a rabid animal.

COAGULOPATHY

Under experimental conditions, extensive activation of the hemostatic mechanism produces depletion of platelets and consumable coagulation factors, with a resultant hemorrhagic state.[37] The normal hemostatic mechanism is designed to be activated in vivo by vascular injury. This response involves the interaction of the vascular subendothelium and platelets to form the provisional hemostatic plug through the process of coagulation. Surgical, that is, operative, injury may result in an increase in platelet and fibrinogen consumption, fibrinogen being the final substrate in the coagulation sequence.[38] This type of pathologic consumption is usually referred to as "disseminated intravascular coagulation."[39] Some authors believe this phenomenon is relatively common but often goes unrecognized because platelet and fibrinogen levels in blood (commonly measured coagulation parameters) are normal. These levels may be maintained in the normal range by compensatory increases in production.[38] The mechanism underlying the consumptive process is postulated to involve the release of tissue thromboplastin–like material in response to a cellular injury. This material activates the coagulation process, resulting in the incorporation of platelets in the resulting fibrin plug.

The clinical importance of clotting abnormalities remains controversial. In 12 of 60 patients who had extensive trauma and who required multiple blood transfusions, a diffuse oozing was noted in the postoperative period.[40] Routine clotting profiles showed that a number of these patients had depressed values in all clotting parameters. This may simply have been a function of the dilution of the patients' clotting factors with the large volumes of old banked blood. The alternative postulate is a consumptive coagulopathy. In another study of severe trauma, 13 of 40 patients had markedly abnormal coagulation and fibrinolytic measurements. Three of these thirteen patients developed a diffuse oozing.[41]

Coagulopathy correlated well with the clinical course of trauma patients, serious morbidity being the rule when marked changes in coagulation factors were observed.[41] These correlations still leave unresolved the question of whether disseminated intravascular coagulation causes or results from a deteriorating clinical picture in the shocked patient.

Sepsis may be one of the factors important in inducing clotting defects. Certainly severe alterations in the dynamics of coagulation have been reported in patients in whom systemic sepsis developed after combat wounds.[42] Despite these significant derangements, it is seldom possible to attribute severe intraoperative or postoperative hemorrhage to failure of hemostatic mechanisms.

The practical management of the occasional coagulation disorder following trauma usually involves the giving of fresh blood. Four or five units suffice in most circumstances.[10] Rarely severe bleeding disorders are observed that respond to no known medical therapy. An example of such a problem was a patient treated at University Hospital, Boston. This 28-year-old Nigerian man underwent a hepatectomy involving the left lobe and the posterior segment of the right lobe. The diagnosis was hepatoma. At the conclusion of the operative procedure a diffuse oozing was observed. Clotting study findings were consistent with a coagulopathy. All therapy including massive infusions of fresh blood was without effect and exsanguination ensued.

METABOLISM

The early and delayed effects of trauma on metabolism are just beginning to be unraveled.[43, 44] Fat and carbohydrate are the major metabolic fuels. With a few exceptions, the various tissues of the body can burn either fuel efficiently, but the amounts used tend to vary in reciprocal fashion under different nutritional conditions and with changing demands for energy.

Following trauma, hepatic glycogen stores are converted to glucose at a rate probably faster than in simple starvation. During starvation, these stores are depleted in 36 to 48 hours, and in addition, a series of metabolic adaptations occurs by which energy may be derived from adipose tissue. This results in conservation of protein reserves. The first of these adaptations is glucose exclusion from the majority of tissues, especially those that can readily use free fatty acids as fuel. A second adaptation is the Cori cycle, which shuttles lipid-derived calories, as glucose, to peripheral glycolytic tissues. These tissues, in turn, send the lactate that has been produced back to the liver for resynthesis to glucose. A third and probably the most important adaptation involves the brain, which begins to utilize the ketoacids, β-hydroxybutyrate and acetoacetate, thereby sparing glucose and in turn body protein whose breakdown would be required for glyconeogenesis.

Unfortunately during severe trauma these adaptations either are not adequate or are inoperative. Carbohydrate utilization rate is doubled.[45] The hyperglycemia associated with injury probably results from an increased rate of synthesis from protein or fat or both. In theory, intravenous infusions of amino acids and hypertonic glucose should have a protein-sparing effect. Improvement in cell metabolism has been demonstrated after the infusion of 50 per cent glucose into combat casualties, an effect not explained by the osmotic or volume-expanding action of glucose.[46]

The response of the liver cell, in terms of protein synthesis, to acute stress or injury is rather constant. There is an immediate outpouring of the acute-phase globulins, fibrinogen and haptoglobin, whereas decreased synthesis of albumin and perhaps other proteins such as lipoproteins, transferrin, and prealbumin occurs.[47] The very rapid rate of albumin loss into damaged tissue and the high catabolic rate combine with the decreased rate of synthesis to produce severe hypoalbuminemia. This makes the trauma patient vulnerable to abnormalities in the distribution of water. The distribution of water between plasma and interstitial space is determined in large part by oncotic pressure. A decrease in the plasma oncotic pressure leads to the observed tissue edema and perhaps also to pulmonary edema. Improvement in this water distribution abnormality can be effected by increasing oncotic pressure with liberal albumin therapy, provided there is no capillary damage.[48]

Insulin appears to be the controlling hormone with regard to fuel mobilization and homeostasis during starvation. The precise role it plays following trauma remains to be defined. Certainly growth hormone and adrenal glucocorticoids are of less significance. Glucagon may have important but as yet poorly described activities.

INTRACELLULAR BIOCHEMISTRY

The ultimate understanding of the shock state, and the sequelae of shock in terms of tissue and organ failure, will be accomplished when intracellular derangements have been defined. Damage to one system may in turn affect others. For example, there is considerable evidence that injury to the reticuloendothelial cells occurs in hemorrhagic shock.[49] Instability of lysosomes within these cells and the release of autolytic enzymes may contribute to dysfunction of intracellular biochemical processes. Subsequently, the extracellular leakage of these lysosomal enzymes occurs, causing possible distant damage.

Other studies demonstrate that severe cellular injury, often reversible, occurs in response to both hypovolemic and septic shock. The cellular response is characterized by a reduction of both the active and passive transport mechanisms across the cell membrane.[50] Changes are also documented in the mitochondrial functions of the cells of many organs during shock. Basic regulatory intermediates such as cyclic adenosine monophosphate are thought to function abnormally. The significance of such findings is far-reaching, since such intermediates control hormonal as well as other critical cellular activities.

An example of the importance of intracellular regulatory mechanisms on total body homeostasis may be seen in the effect of 2,3 diphosphoglycerate (DPG) levels in red blood cells. Oxygen delivery to body tissues is a function of blood flow, the oxygen-carrying capacity of blood, and release of oxygen at the tissue level. Pulmonary failure and inadequate respiratory gas exchange limit the oxygen content of arterial blood. This is considered later. For any given alveolar oxygen tension the volume of oxygen contained in blood is primarily related to hemoglobin concentration; the oxygen-hemoglobin dissociation curve describes the relationship of oxygen tension and hemoglobin saturation (Fig. 4–1). Several factors increase the oxygen affinity of hemoglobin and therefore decrease the amount of oxygen released at the tissue level. Elevation of the pH shifts the oxygen-hemoglobin dissociation curve to the left, increasing the affinity of oxygen for hemoglobin. Such a situation is typically found in trauma because of hyperventilation and the associated respiratory alkalosis. The organic phosphate, 2,3 diphosphoglycerate, has also been found to play an important role in oxygen-hemoglobin affinity; low concentrations

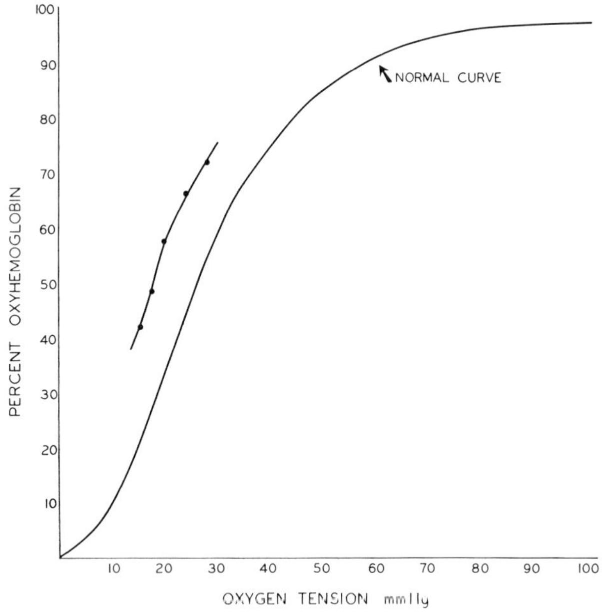

Figure 4–1. The normal oxygen-hemoglobin dissociation curve is sigmoid-shaped. Alkalosis and decrease in red cell 2-3 diphosphoglycerate (2-3 DPG) levels shift the curve to the left. A left-shifted curve makes oxygen unloading from blood to tissues more difficult. Normal venous capillary oxygen tensions are about 35 mm of mercury, at which tension the per cent saturation is 68.5. In order to reduce the per cent saturation to the same level, i.e., supply the same amount of oxygen to tissues, when the curve is shifted as shown, the oxygen tension must be reduced to 25.5 mm of mercury. The body may not be able to accomplish this feat. The abnormal curve that is illustrated (closed circles) resulted from massive transfusions of blood. Stored blood has a low 2-3 diphosphoglycerate level.

lead to significant shifts of the hemoglobin dissociation curve to the left, inhibiting the release of oxygen to tissues.[51, 52]

Patients who have suffered trauma frequently require large infusions of blood. In storage, blood is rapidly depleted of its diphosphoglycerate, acquiring increased hemoglobin affinity for oxygen.[53] Thus, the effect of infusions of stored blood is to shift the oxygen-hemoglobin dissociation curve to the left. Diphosphoglycerate is regenerated following transfusion. The deleterious effect of transfused blood is usually temporary and innocuous except in the acutely ill patient.[54] Acute illness itself may result in a reduction in diphosphoglycerate.[55] Compensation for decrease in oxyhemoglobin levels or for a shift of the dissociation curve to the left in trauma patients is frequently accomplished by a decrease in mixed venous oxygen tension ($P\bar{v}_{O_2}$). If the decrease in $P\bar{v}_{O_2}$ is accomplished by a reduction in oxygen consumption, however, the patient usually will die.[56]

ACUTE RESPIRATORY FAILURE

The association of hypoxemia and hemorrhagic shock was described by Moon over 30 years ago in experimental dogs subjected to hemorrhagic hypotension.[57] The characteristic pathologic findings were pulmonary capillary congestion and patchy areas of atelectasis. In World War II the association of wounding and pulmonary insufficiency was documented. Because of the prominence of edema of the lungs, the term "wet lungs" became a useful clinical term.[58]

In the next two decades several new pathologic and physiologic observations were made. Patients who developed acute respiratory failure (ARF) required higher pressures to inflate their lungs. This decrease in lung compliance (the ratio of tidal volume to peak inspiratory pressure) was termed the "stiff lung" syndrome. Infants who developed acute respiratory failure soon after birth were not only observed to have stiff lungs, but pathologic examination demonstrated hyaline membranes. These same hyaline membranes were soon found in adults dying of acute respiratory failure. The descriptive terms "adult hyaline membrane disease" and "adult respiratory distress syndrome" were coined. The hyaline membranes were composed of proteinaceous materials and cellular debris. Their location within the alveolar air spaces implied the presence of areas of capillary damage through which protein leaked (Figs. 4–2 and 4–3). During the Vietnam war acute respiratory failure was observed to follow shock and trauma.[59] The descriptive phrase "shock lung" became popular as a result of this experience.

In the late 1960's, several authors emphasized the importance of acute respiratory failure in contributing to death.[60] In one series, 9 of 19 patients with severe shock developed respiratory failure, and in 8 of these patients, respiratory failure was a major cause of death.[61] More recent reports substantiate our own expe-

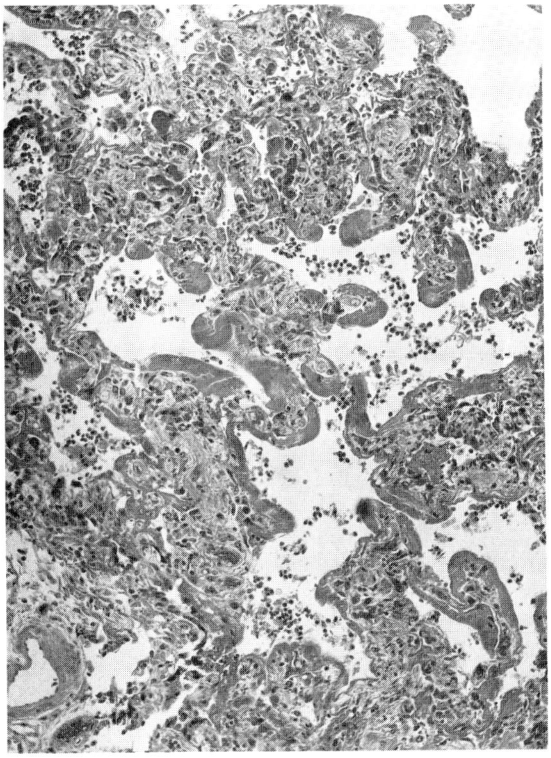

Figure 4–2. Microscopic view of "adult hyaline membrane disease" ("adult respiratory distress syndrome," "shock lung") showing proteinaceous material along the walls of the pulmonary alveoli in a 53-year-old Caucasian man who died in posttraumatic shock.

rience at the Boston University Shock and Trauma Center, where respiratory failure (with an average intrapulmonary shunt of 30 per cent) is seldom a direct cause of death.[62] In only 2 of 25 patients was arterial hypoxemia a sufficient explanation of death.

The etiology of acute respiratory failure is obscure. A clear association between it and trauma frequently cannot be made. Many patients suffering "shock lung" have severe underlying sepsis that may be more directly related to pulmonary problems than the shock itself.[62] Fat embolism is known to lead to respiratory failure and is thought to be a relatively common factor in severe trauma, particularly after long-bone fractures (Fig. 4–4).[63, 64] The syndrome of fat embolism may not only be the result of mechanical blockage of the pulmonary vasculature, but may also relate to the toxicity of lipolytic breakdown products of fat, especially oleic acid.

Other causes of the syndrome include massive transfusions. The considerable debris found in banked blood can pass through standard filters and be picked up by the lungs.[65] The degree of posttraumatic hypoxia has been shown to correlate better with the volume of transfused banked blood than with the degree of trauma or shock per se.[66]

Recent experience has also emphasized the role of aspiration of gastric contents in the evolution of respiratory insufficiency in wounded as well as in other seriously ill or obtunded patients.[67, 68] Other factors such as oxygen toxicity play as yet unknown primary or secondary roles.

The pathophysiology of acute respiratory failure is characteristic, regardless of etiologic factors. The lungs, being rather rudimentary organs, can respond to an insult with a limited repertoire of changes. The major alterations relate to impaired mechanics of ventilation and respiratory gas exchange. The former abnormality may secondarily affect hemodynamics, while the usual gas exchange problem relates to oxygen.

Pulmonary insufficiency characteristically develops one to two days after injury. The patient has an increased respiratory rate, hyperventilates, and may complain of dyspnea. Blood gases demonstrate hypoxia and hypocarbia. Usually the pH is alkaline. The chest x-ray characteristically shows diffuse alveolar collapse and pulmonary edema (Fig. 4–5). The findings by x-ray, however, may not be diagnostic.

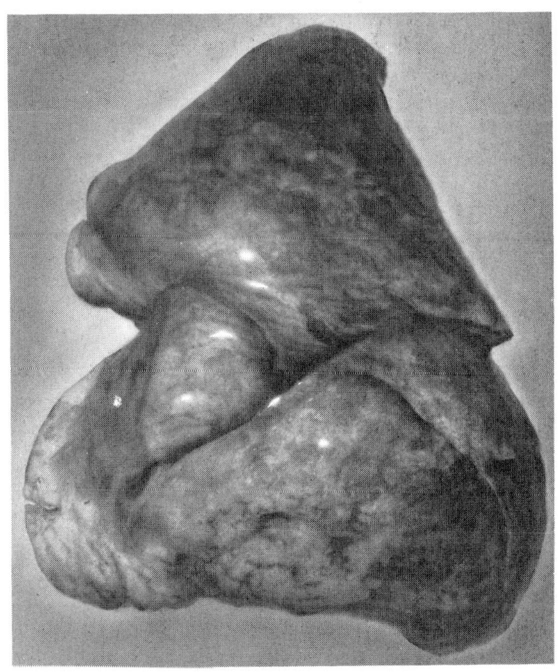

Figure 4–3. Disseminated areas of hemorrhagic pulmonary atelectasis and collapse of large portions of the lung, most prominent in upper and lower lobes, in the same case as Figure 4–2.

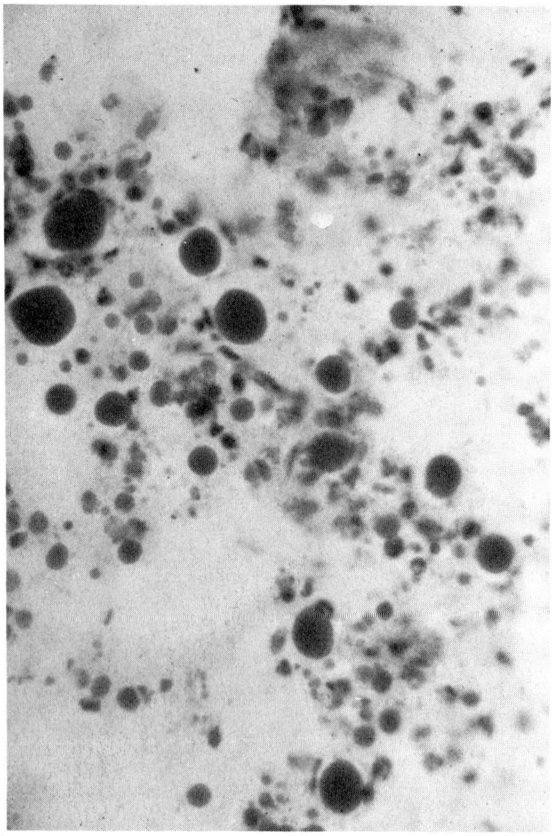

Figure 4–4. Posttraumatic pulmonary fat embolism. Notice the globules of fat both within the lumina of blood capillaries and free in the pulmonary parenchyma. Osmic acid stain. Bilateral fracture of femur following fall from a height.

The pathophysiologic sequence of events leading to respiratory failure is postulated to involve capillary damage and subsequent interstitial edema formation.[62, 69] Edema formation is associated with diminished compliance and therefore leads to increased work of breathing.[70] Although edema per se is not immediately responsible for arterial hypoxemia, it probably will lead to alveolar collapse in the spontaneously breathing patient with low compliance (Fig. 4–6).[71] It is this alveolar collapse, or microatelectasis, that allows the shunting of blood through nonventilated areas, with resultant venous admixture and hypoxemia. These areas of alveolar collapse are diffuse and multiple. Other nonatelectatic regions of the lung are characteristically overventilated and indeed may be ventilated without being perfused, constituting physiologic dead space. Thus, not only are the lungs stiff, but much of the ventilation is wasted, thereby further adding to the work of breathing.

Hypoalbuminemia may potentiate edema formation. It is doubtful, however, that low albumin levels cause the edema seen, and further, left ventricular failure is uncommon in acute respiratory failure.[62, 71] Therefore, elevated hydrostatic pressure is an unlikely cause of edema formation. Despite these considerations, pressure parameters must be measured in the critically ill, especially in those patients who have preexisting cardiac disease.

Surfactant plays a vital role in stabilizing alveoli.[62] Its absence leads to alveolar collapse. Animal work has demonstrated that the biochemical synthesis of surfactant is reduced after hemorrhagic shock.[73] Autopsy specimens of human lungs from patients dying with acute respiratory failure have shown reduced surfactant activity. It is possible that the shock episode leads to an intracellular derangement in the lung, causing failure of the biochemical pathways for the manufacture of this critical material. This postulate remains to be proved in humans.

Head and spinal cord injury frequently leads to respiratory failure, but the mechanism remains disputed. A large clinical study has shown that 50 per cent of patients with central nervous system injuries have arterial oxygen tension (Pa_{O_2}) below 80 mm of mercury, compared with 3 per cent of control patients.[64] Between 10 and 20 per cent of the injured group were severely hypoxemic, with Pa_{O_2} values below 60 mm of mercury. In an analysis of 57 battle casualties in Vietnam, all with head injuries, evidence of pulmonary edema was found in 17 who died soon after wounding, in 11 of 14 who died in less than 24 hours, and in all 15 patients who died between one and seven days after head injury.[75]

Since the observations of Cushing, it has been generally accepted that alterations in intracranial pressure may produce profound changes in cardiovascular hemodynamics.[76] The most frequently cited manifestation of the interrelationship between head injury and circulatory alterations is the association between increased intracranial and systemic arterial pressures. It is postulated that left ventricular failure is induced by the systemic pressure increase, with resultant pulmonary edema. This concept is supported by most animal work, but is not yet substantiated to be the primary causative factor in humans.[77, 78]

Regardless of the etiology of acute respiratory failure, supportive measures usually provide sufficient oxygenation so that death from hypoxemia is rare. The mainstay of treatment is currently the use of volume-cycled respirators. Additional agents such as oxygen, diure-

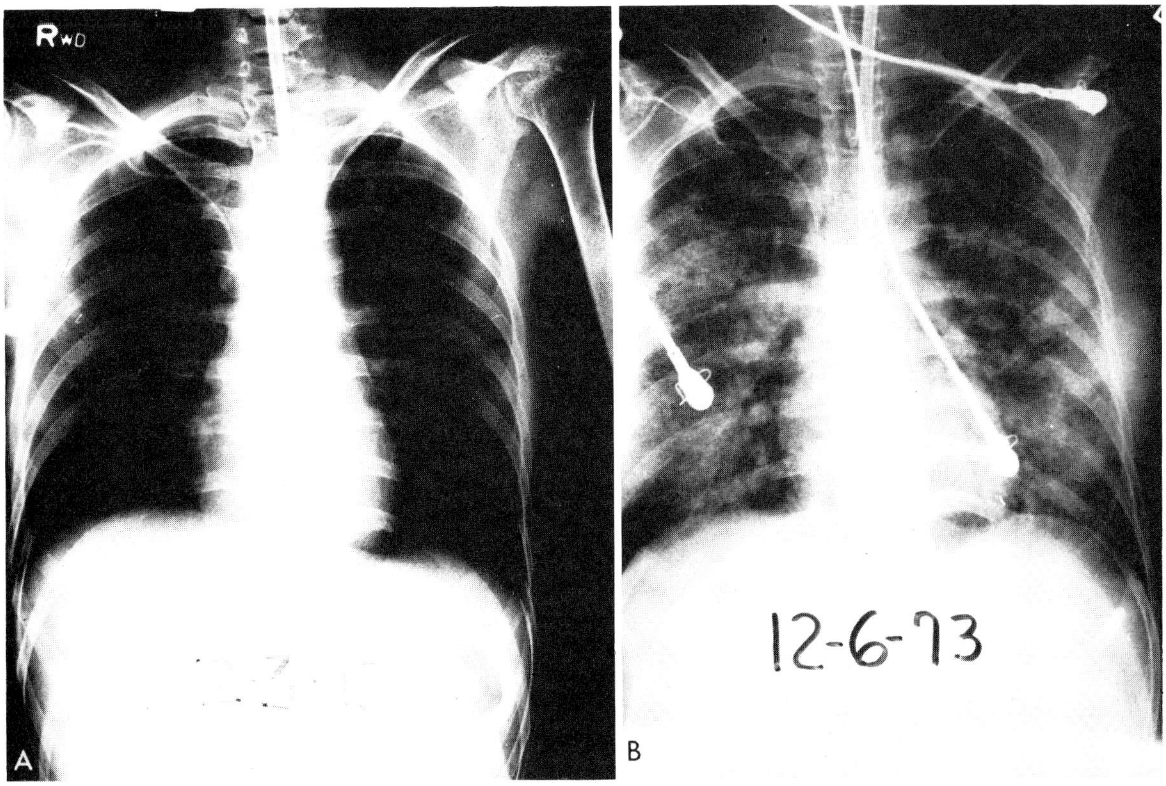

Figure 4–5. This woman suffered blunt injury to her lower abdomen and extremities. She had no known pulmonary disease. Two days following operative repair of a bladder laceration, she became dyspneic. Her arterial oxygen tension on room air was 34 mm of mercury. She had associated respiratory alkalosis. Lung compliance was half of normal. *A*. The chest film demonstrates a normal appearance at admission. *B*. The development of the characteristic fluffy infiltrates associated with acute pulmonary insufficiency.

tics, albumin, and cardiotonic agents are given as required. These agents require careful control, since they may themselves cause pulmonary failure if used improperly.

GASTRODUODENAL ULCERATION

Stress ulceration of the stomach with massive hemorrhage is a frequent companion of trauma. Virtually all patients who have suffered serious trauma or sepsis or both will develop stress ulcers. An excellent clinical study of 42 patients has demonstrated by gastroscopy that within 24 hours of stress, abnormalities appear in the gastric mucosa (Fig. 4–7). Foci of pallor and hyperemia in the proximal part of the body of the stomach were followed by petechiae and shallow erosions, which spread to the entire body of the stomach. The antrum, however, was spared. Diffuse erosions persisted for up to three weeks in some critically ill patients. A number of significant complications developed in this series of 42 patients before clinical bleeding began. These included severe respiratory failure, massive wound sepsis, large intraabdominal abscesses, renal failure, and prolonged ileus. Histologic examinations of the stomach showed focal alterations of surface epithelium, with discontinuities of the limiting membrane and loss of part of the apical cellular region exposing the intracellular contents.[79]

The characteristic pain pattern of chronic duodenal or gastric ulceration is absent with stress ulcers because they are so superficial. Perforation, posterior penetration, and obstruction are extremely unusual.

The incidence rate of significant bleeding from stress ulceration is relatively high. Thirty per cent of severely injured or septic patients require blood transfusions for stress ulcer bleeding. The onset of bleeding is usually several days after the trauma or septic event.

Experimental studies strongly suggest that the basic mechanism producing stress ulceration is an episode of diminished mucosal blood flow.[80] Since most studies have failed to show hypersecretion of acid in these patients, this factor by itself is probably not a critical determinant of ulcer formation. Emphasis is

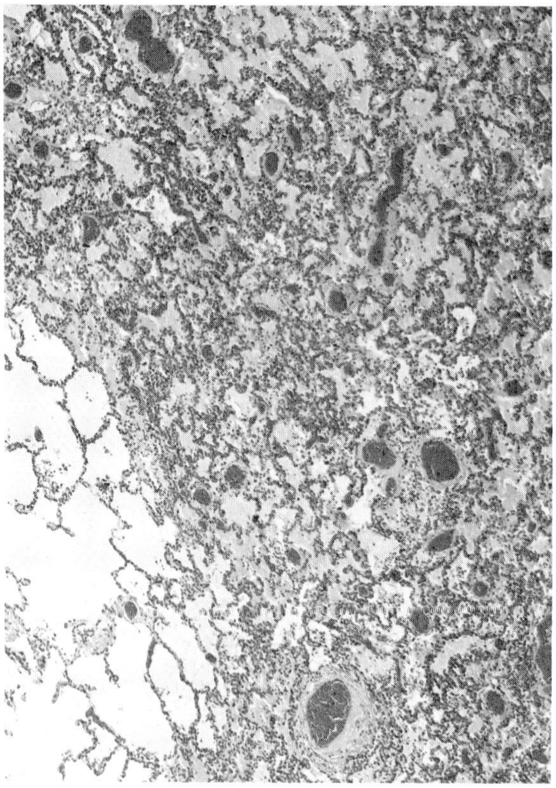

Figure 4–6. Collapse of alveolar walls (microatelectasis) and intraalveolar edema in posttraumatic acute respiratory failure. Notice in the lower right field an area of overventilation (microemphysema). Death occurred two days after a road accident resulting in multiple injuries and acute respiratory failure.

usually placed on ischemia as the most important etiologic factor that must occur in the presence of acid (not necessarily hypersecretion) to result in gastric erosions. Other factors such as reflux of pancreatic juices play unknown roles. It is unlikely that gastric mucus is of much importance in protecting the mucosa against injury.[79]

Two other types of acute ulcerations occur in trauma patients suffering burns or brain injury. This is in addition to chronic ulcer disease. The burn ulcer is generally referred to as a Curling ulcer, in deference to the investigator who first recognized the connection between burn injury and ulcer formation, while the term "Cushing ulcer" is used in homage to the investigator who was first to advance the neurogenic concept of ulcer formation.[81, 82]

Published reports on the incidence of Curling's ulcer have brought forth figures as high as 36.4 per cent in Curling's original series and 21.3 per cent in a recent review.[81, 83] Curling ulcers have been divided into two relatively clear-cut groups.[84] The first type occurs early after burns and has all the characteristics of stress ulcerations already described. The second type occurs later. These are usually duodenal in location and show evidence of chronicity when examined microscopically (Fig. 4–8). These ulcers not only bleed but may also perforate. It is conjectured that they represent acute reactivations of long-standing ulcers.

Cushing ulcers occur in association with intracranial injuries or diseases in which there is increased intracranial pressure.[85, 86] This pressure rise is associated with an outpouring of gastric acid. Various hormones such as adrenal steroids may mediate this response, but the mechanism is poorly understood.[87] It is this hypersecretion that is considered to be the direct cause of the deep ulcerations that are characteristically encountered in the esophagus, stomach, or duodenum. Perforation is not uncommon.

It is doubtful whether neurogenic ulceration in the alimentary tract can progress into a chronic peptic ulcer. In the majority of cases these lesions heal rapidly without leaving a trace. Some observations attest to the contrary, however; the medicolegal implications of the problem are illustrated by the following case in which one of us (L.G.T.) was directly involved.

A 38-year-old construction worker fell from a ladder, from an approximate height of 20 feet, hitting a stone floor. He was brought to the hospital unconscious; there he was found to have a scalp laceration in the occipital area and a horizontal fracture in the occipital bone. About one hour from the time of the accident he regained consciousness, but he remained confused for three to four days and complained of severe headaches. There were no localizing signs of nervous deficits. As the patient was improving, six days after the accident, he suddenly experienced upper abdominal pain and vomited blood. This was interpreted as evidence of acute neurogenic ulceration of the upper alimentary tract. He was treated conservatively with whole blood transfusions and administration of antacids. There was no recurrence of the bleeding episode. Past history failed to indicate signs or symptoms consistent with preexisting chronic gastric or duodenal peptic ulcer, and no evidence of lesions was detected at roentgenologic examination of the upper alimentary tract.

Following discharge from the hospital, the patient was well, except for easy fatigability and occasional headaches, for about one year. Two years after the accident, he consulted his family physician, complaining of severe upper abdominal pain. Roentgenologic examination revealed a lesion in the prepyloric region, along the lesser curvature, that was diagnosed as a peptic ulcer. A medical ulcer regimen was prescribed on which he showed limited

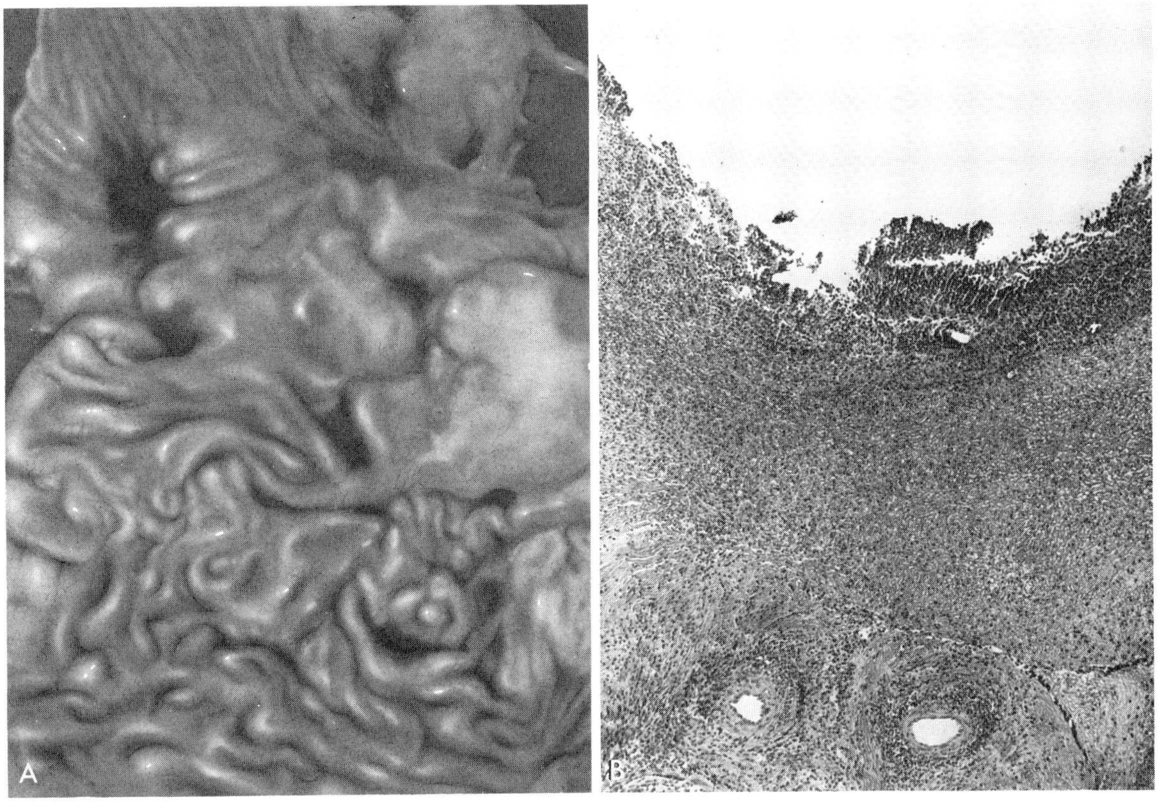

Figure 4–7. *A*. Multiple stress ulcers in the mucosa of the stomach leading to massive gastroenteric hemorrhage in a 48-year-old Caucasian man with severe head trauma. *B*. Microscopic appearance of one of the ulcers shown in *A* displaying absence of surface epithelium, loss of normal mucosal architecture, and leukocytic infiltration.

improvement. One evening, after a heavy meal, he experienced excruciating abdominal pain and vomited blood, both fresh and clotted. Pain and vomiting persisted throughout the night, and early in the morning he was brought to the hospital. While being prepared for surgery, he unexpectedly died.

Postmortem examination revealed a chronic prepyloric peptic ulcer that had perforated the stomach wall. There was blood in the stomach and intestines, and about 1 liter of blood was obtained from the abdominal cavity.

On a decision out of court, the widow received compensation on the assumption that a relationship existed between the fall two years previously and the presumed acute ulcerations in the upper alimentary tract, one of which, according to expert opinion, had progressed to become a chronic peptic ulcer.

Similarly open to controversy is the role of head trauma as a factor aggravating a preexisting chronic peptic ulcer. This situation is illustrated by another case that came under our scrutiny (L.G.T.).

A 58-year old widower fell on his back while carrying a heavy cement bag. He lost consciousness for a few minutes and was brought to the hospital for suturing of a linear laceration in the occipital-parietal region. No other injuries were found, and roentgenologic examination of the skull failed to reveal evidence of fracture. He was kept under observation for the following 24 hours and then discharged. Three days later, he was found dead in his bed by one of his neighbors. There was a bloody discharge from the mouth and nostrils and profuse blood spotting on the pillow and bedclothes.

Postmortem examination showed a chronic peptic ulcer in the duodenum, which had eroded into the superior pancreatic artery. Abundant blood was present in the stomach and duodenum.

History obtained from the only son indicated that the deceased had suffered for years with dyspepsia, for which he had never sought medical advice. Although no request for compensation was made in this case, one wonders whether the head trauma sustained three days prior to death could have been regarded as a precipitating or aggravating factor that led to bleeding of the preexisting ulcer and to the death of the patient.

Therapy for stress ulceration ranges from iced gastric lavage to selective arterial infusion of vasoconstrictor agents, blood replacement, and operation. Regardless of therapy, the prognosis is poor. Once stress ulceration has produced significant hemorrhage, the mortality rate usually exceeds 50 per cent.[79]

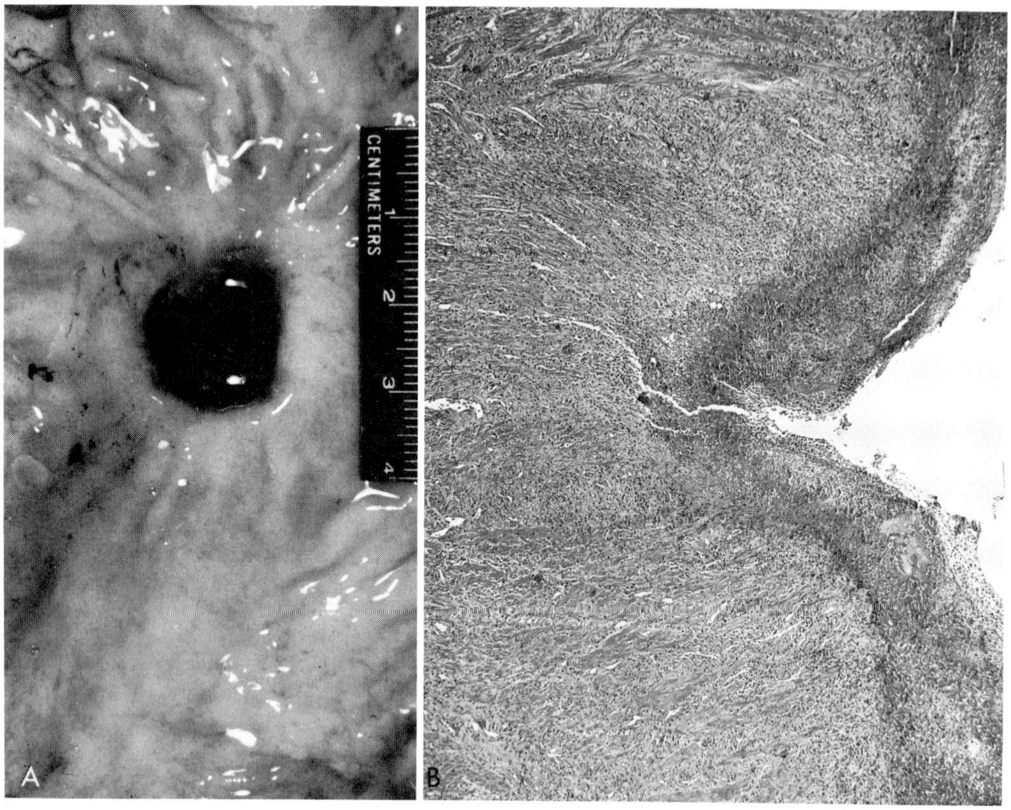

Figure 4–8. *A.* A bleeding Curling ulcer (burn ulcer) in the upper portion of the duodenal mucosa. Death occurred 17 days after extensive body burns sustained in home fire. *B.* Microscopic appearance of the same ulcer shown in *A.* Notice absence of surface epithelium and partial replacement of the mucosa by fibroblastic scar tissue.

MYOCARDIAL DEPRESSION

In the terminal stages of severe trauma, shock, sepsis, or burns, as most clinicians have observed, the patients suffer irreversible left ventricular failure. This is manifest by high left ventricular filling pressure, low cardiac output, and systemic hypotension. This obvious manifestation of cardiac insufficiency is not debated. What is debated is the existence of subclinical forms of myocardial depression that may be manifest soon after trauma, during a time when all vital signs and urine output appear relatively normal.

Cardiac performance may be judged by the relationship of left ventricular filling pressure (pulmonary arterial wedge pressure, left atrial pressure, or left ventricular end-diastolic pressure) to cardiac output—provided cardiac rate, arterial pressure, sympathetic stimulation, and serum catecholamine levels are fixed.[88, 89] As filling pressure is increased, most normal hearts respond by increasing cardiac output. This is true at filling pressures as high as 30 to 35 mm of mercury.[90] In patients with depressed myocardial performance, cardiac output decreases with increasing filling pressures (Fig. 4–9).[2] This phenomenon may not be clinically apparent and has been referred to as subclinical cardiac failure.

In studies conducted in patients who developed sepsis following operative trauma, distinct abnormalities in cardiac function have been observed. Twenty-two patients admitted to the Boston University Shock and Trauma Center were evaluated. Most were found to have a cardiac output that was higher than predicted, averaging 4.3 liters per minute per square meter of body surface. Rapid infusions of colloid solutions were used to raise left ventricular filling pressures. As the filling pressures exceeded 10 mm of mercury, virtually all patients demonstrated reductions in cardiac output, i.e., occult myocardial failure. Since survival was directly related to cardiac output, these patients were treated with fluid infusions to raise their filling pressures just to the point of peak cardiac output.

Other human observations and animal experiments are in accord with the thesis of myocardial depression. There is considerable

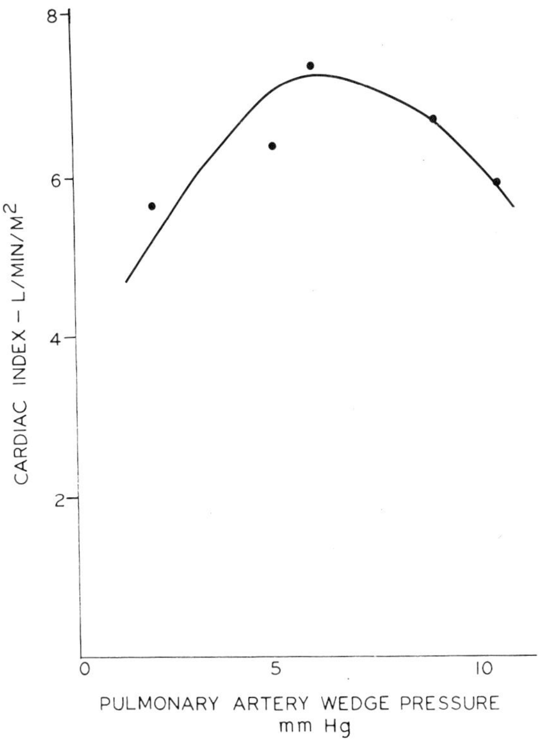

Figure 4–9. A young woman was struck by an automobile as she exited from a street trolley. She suffered multiple long-bone and pelvic fractures and required 7 units of blood in the first 24 hours after the injury. At this time she was hyperdynamic with a cardiac index above 5.5 liters per minute. (Cardiac index = cardiac output/body surface area; the normal cardiac index is 3.5 liters per minute.) The pulmonary arterial wedge pressure, which is equivalent to the filling pressure of the left ventricle, was raised from 2 to 10.5 mm of mercury with a rapid infusion of fluid. The cardiac index rose and then fell. A normal person does not show a decrease in myocardial performance at such filling pressures; the occurrence of such a decrease is evidence of myocardial failure. Optimal fluid therapy should maintain the wedge pressure at 6 mm of mercury.

evidence that a myocardial depressant factor accumulates in the plasma in human shock and in the plasma of animals subjected to hemorrhagic hypotension, mesenteric artery occlusion, or hemorrhagic pancreatitis.[91, 92] Direct in vivo measurement of myocardial performance in animals has confirmed that there is depression following sepsis or severe hemorrhage.[93, 94]

The limitation in myocardial performance is usually set by left ventricular function.[89, 90] Assessment of the functional status of this side of the heart is available through pulmonary arterial catheterization and measure of the pulmonary arterial wedge pressure. Recent experience has demonstrated the ease and safety with which a pulmonary arterial catheter may be positioned in critically ill patients. This catheter has therefore become a valuable adjunct in the guidance of fluid therapy. Since the trauma patient seldom suffers right ventricular failure, the standard central venous pressure readings must be interpreted with great caution.[95]

The etiology of myocardial depression is not certain, and the importance of myocardial depressant factors is debated. In humans dying of severe shock, autopsy evidence of myocardial damage in the form of subendocardial infarcts has been found.[96, 97] It is not certain, however, whether these infarcts are the cause or the effect of myocardial failure.

Other cardiac disorders that attend trauma relate to rhythm disturbances. The alkaline pH and tendency toward hypokalemia make the heart particularly vulnerable to arrhythmias. The most common problem is sinus tachycardia. Preexistent heart disease and the use of digitalis are factors that are associated with a variety of rhythm disturbances that can severely limit cardiac output.

An extensive literature indicates that disorders in rhythm and electrocardiographic changes frequently occur following head injuries.[99, 102] This relationship was first cited by Bramwell in 1934 apropos of the case of a miner, aged 35 years, who, after a blow on the head, developed atrial fibrillation that lasted for four weeks.[98] The most commonly observed changes are: increased Q-T interval, increased voltage of the P wave, increased QRS voltage and raised S-T segments in precordial leads, inverted T waves in precordial leads V_4 to V_6, U waves more than 1 mm in height, sinus arrhythmia with fixed pacemaker, and sinus arrhythmia with pacemaker wandering in the sinoatrial node. As a rule, electrocardiographic abnormalities increase as the level of consciousness deteriorates. Similar disorders have been described during brain operations and pneumoencephalography, and with cerebral tumors, poliomyelitis, and cerebral hemorrhage.[103–108]

Further support of the concept that lesions in the central nervous system may be responsible for the occurrence of cardiac irregularities has come from controlled experiments. Extrasystoles in cats have been induced by stimulation of the posterior hypothalamus.[109] Nodal and ventricular rhythm, multifocal extrasystoles, and shift of the sinoatrial pacemaker have been obtained in cats by stimulating an area between the posterior corpora quadrigemina and the posterior portions of the cerebellum.[110] A variety of rhythm abnormalities have been obtained, also in cats, by stimulation of different subcortical areas.[111] Similarly, Jacobson and Danufsky, in mice submitted to head trauma, have produced electrocardiographic changes that could be prevented by atropine administration; thus their conclusion that the changes were caused by vagal stimulation.[112]

Since postmortem examination of the hearts of humans with rhythm abnormalities following brain damage, as well as the results in experimental animals, has usually failed to show any appreciable cardiac lesion, the concept that neural influences, rather than actual myocardial damage, are responsible for the cardiac abnormalities has gained broad acceptance.[113, 117] The concepts of vagal overactivity, increased sympathetic tone, or excessive release of catecholamines, singly or in variable combinations, have been advocated in support of the neural origin of the cardiac disorders.

In the light of Connor's demonstration that lesions visible under the light microscope can be found in the myocardium of patients with brain trauma, the neural concept must be reconsidered. One of the lesions that Connor has described is referred to as *myocytolysis*. It is characterized by loss of sarcoplasm in small areas of muscle, with retention of the sarcolemma, stroma, muscle nuclei, and lipofuscin granules; coagulative necrosis is absent, and the sarcoplasm seems to have been dissolved. Another type of lesion seen in the early phase of myocardial ischemia, referred to as *fuchsinophilic degeneration*, is characterized by bright eosinophilia in the hematoxylin and eosin stained sections, and by red staining of the transverse striations in the sections stained with cresyl violet–acid fuchsin.[118, 119]

It is of interest that myocardial lesions with similar characteristics in a young epileptic dying with subarachnoid hemorrhage are briefly mentioned by Burch and associates and, in patients dying with insulin shock and poliomyelitis, by Schlesinger and Reiner.[120, 121] Probably the same lesion, in patients dying with head injury, is referred to as "necrosis" by Eichbaum and Bissetti.[122]

Although the cause and significance of these myocardial changes are not clear, their detection in patients with intracranial lesions in 18 of 231 hearts examined in one series (8 per cent) and in 21 of 169 hearts in another series (12 per cent) deserves consideration.[118, 119]

ACUTE RENAL FAILURE

Anyone entrusted with the care of a traumatized patient is well aware of the importance of keeping close records of the quantity and composition of the urine. Important information is provided regarding renal function as well as circulatory dynamics.

Renal failure represents the kidney's inability to excrete the load of metabolic products presented to it. Following trauma, catabolism is increased and greater demands are made upon the kidneys to excrete nitrogenous wastes and potassium. The association of acute renal failure and trauma was recognized during World War I. It was not until World War II, however, that the condition was shown to be associated with shock and especially with the toxic pigments of the crush syndrome. Soon after the war, acute cortical necrosis and acute tubular necrosis or lower nephron nephrosis were described as pathologic entities.[123, 124]

Evidence of some degree of posttraumatic renal insufficiency was noted at autopsy in 39 per cent of 165 Korean battle casualties. Fourteen per cent had been uremic prior to death. However, fewer than 1 per cent of wounded men had evidence of renal failure. In Vietnam War casualties, gross renal function was usually normal. The rarity of flagrant renal failure (approximately 1 in 1,867 casualties) was probably due to rapid evacuation and early treatment of shock. It must be noted, however, that a wide spectrum of renal failure is now recognized. Some patients with overwhelming sepsis following trauma exhibit polyuria with or without azotemia.[126, 127] It is now appreciated that progressive uremia, occurring without a period of oliguria and accompanied by a daily urine volume of more than 1,000 to 1,500 ml, is the most frequent variant of renal failure occurring in association with trauma.

High-output renal failure occurs between 5 and 10 times as frequently as classic oliguric failure, but it occurs in fewer than 1 per cent of victims of severe trauma. The chief complication is hyperkalemia.

The major systemic causes of acute renal failure may be categorized as either inadequate renal perfusion or the effect of toxins. Hypovolemia and low cardiac output are the most frequent causes of inadequate perfusion and oliguria. Mild oliguria is common after trauma. As blood pressure decreases below a systolic pressure of 70 mm of mercury, there is marked oliguria and eventually anuria. In addition to low perfusion pressure, antidiuretic hormone release reduces urine production. Perfusion is shifted away from the cortex to the medulla.[128] This effect may be observed even after restoration of blood volume and blood pressure. These physiologic facts are consistent with morphologic findings in human trauma of large swollen kidneys with pale cortices and medullary congestion (Fig. 4–10).

In the common type of renal failure, the

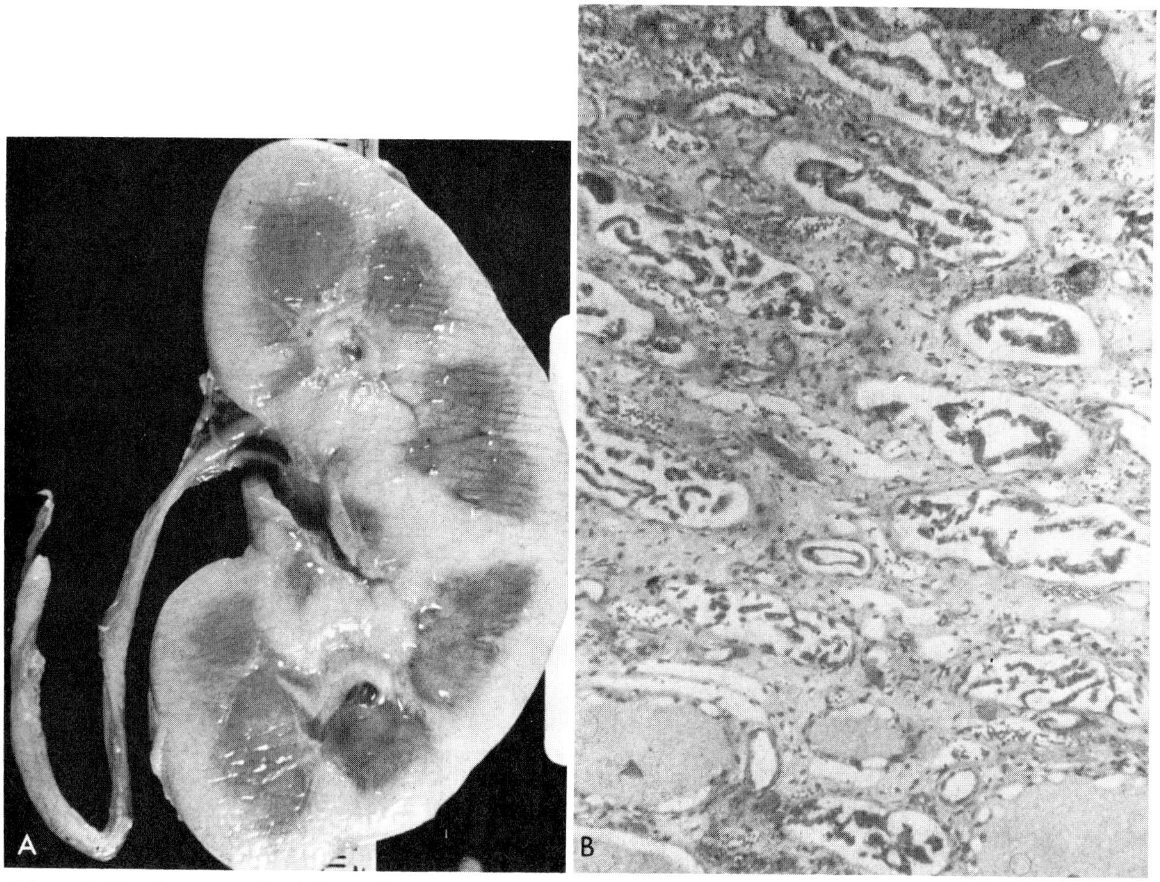

Figure 4–10. Large swollen kidney of "acute tubular necrosis" ("lower nephron nephrosis," "acute cortical necrosis"). Notice the pale cortices and medullary congestion. *B.* Microscopic appearance of the kidney shown in *A*, displaying detachment of tubular epithelium and fragmentation of basement membrane. Death was caused by posttraumatic renal insufficiency.

urine cannot be concentrated, and sodium concentration is characteristically above 60 mEq per liter.[129] Recent micropuncture studies suggest that the primary event in acute renal insufficiency is a decrease in reabsorption of sodium in the proximal tubule. This is a response to either an ischemic or a toxic insult. Stimulation of the renin-angiotensin system then results in a reduction in renal cortical blood flow and glomerular filtration rate.[130]

An extensive literature exists that describes the association of injury, localized to the brain, and impaired renal function. It is of interest to note that the rate of incidence of neurogenic ulcerations of the alimentary tract is high under these circumstances. Albuminuria in cases of brain tumor, grand mal epilepsy, and subarachnoid hemorrhage has been recorded.[131] Transient oliguria has been described in patients with brain tumors and increased intracranial pressure.[132] Impaired tubular function has been reported following cerebral concussion and electroshock therapy; tubular necrosis has been associated with subarachnoid and cerebral hemorrhage.[134–137] Similar findings have been reproduced experimentally, with protection to the kidneys afforded by denervation.[138–140]

The principal toxin associated with acute renal failure is the myoglobulin released from injured or crushed muscle. Other nephrotoxic agents include heme pigments from mismatched blood transfusions. These pigments are probably of little clinical importance unless combined with hypotension. Various iatrogenically introduced toxins must be considered. These are angiographic contrast materials; vasopressor amines such as norepinephrine, phenylephrine hydrochloride (Neo-Synephrine), and metaraminol; the antibiotics kanamycin, gentamicin, amphotericin, polymyxin B, and colistin (Coly-Mycin). Anesthetic agents are rarely nephrotoxic themselves, except for methoxyflurane (Penthrane), providing normal blood volume and pressure are maintained.[141]

Finally, disseminated intravascular coagulation has been implicated in the production of renal failure. This is most commonly seen in association with major sepsis.[142] There is a deposition of fibrin in glomeruli with consequent reduction in glomerular filtration. The pathologic picture is one of cortical necrosis. This lesion, in contrast to acute tubular necrosis, is not reversible.

The critical point upon which hinges the outcome of the lesion, acute tubular necrosis, is the damage done to the basement membrane of the tubule. If the integrity of the basement membrane is preserved, the regenerating epithelial cells will reestablish tubular integrity. In contrast, fragmentation and detachment of the basement membrane prevents reepithelialization and healing of the lesion.[143]

Current therapy for acute renal failure includes the use of ion exchange resins, peritoneal dialysis, and hemodialysis. Each technique has its limitations. Properly selected treatment is usually successful in supporting patients while their renal injury undergoes repair. The required period of support is variable, averaging six days. Occasional patients have recovered renal function after one month. The mortality rate in patients suffering renal failure approximates 20 per cent and in general is related to complications of the injury (usually infection) and not the renal failure.

REFERENCES

NEUROHORMONAL RESPONSE

1. Wilson, R. F., and Krome, R.: Factors affecting prognosis in clinical shock. Ann. Surg., *169*:93, 1969.
2. Moore, F. D., Lyons, J. H., Pierce, E. C., Morgan, A. F., Drinker, P. A., MacArthur, J. D., and Dammin, G. J.: *Post-Traumatic Pulmonary Insufficiency.* Philadelphia, W. B. Saunders Co., 1969.
3. White, J. C., and Sweet, W. H.: *Pain: Its Mechanisms and Neurosurgical Control.* Springfield, Ill., Charles C Thomas, 1955.
4. Shoemaker, W. C., Boyd, D. R., Kim, S. I., Brown, R. S., Dreiling, D. A., and Kark, A. E.: Sequential oxygen transport and acid-base changes after trauma to the unanesthetized patient. Surg. Gynecol. Obstet., *132*:1033, 1971.
5. Baue, A., and Nara, Y.: Regulation of ventilation during hemorrhage and its alterations in response to CO_2. Ann. Surg., *176*:80, 1972.
6. Skillman, J. J., Lauler, D. P., Hickler, R. B., Lyons, J. H., Olson, J. E., Ball, M. R., and Moore, F. D.: Hemorrhage in man: effect on renin, cortisol, aldosterone, and urine composition. Ann. Surg., *166*:865, 1967.
7. Carey, L. C., Cloutier, C. T., and Lowery, B. D.: Growth hormone and adrenal cortical response to shock and trauma in the human. Ann. Surg., *174*:451, 1971.

SHOCK

8. Simmons, R. L., Heisterkamp, C. A., Moseley, R. V., and Doty, D. B.: Postresuscitative blood volumes in combat casualties. Surg. Gynecol. Obstet., *128*:1193, 1969.
9. Moore, F. D.: *Metabolic Care of the Surgical Patient.* Philadelphia, W. B. Saunders Co., 1959.
10. Skillman, J. J., Awwad, H. K., and Moore, F. D.: Plasma protein kinetics of the early transcapillary refill after hemorrhage in man. Surg. Gynecol. Obstet., *125*:983, 1967.
11. Roth, E., Lax, L. C., and Maloney, J. V.: Ringer's lactate solution and extracellular fluid volume in the surgical patient: a critical analysis. Ann. Surg., *169*:149, 1969.
12. McNamara, J. J., Molot, M. D., and Stremple, J. F.: Blood viscosity in combat casualities. Surg. Gynecol. Obstet., *134*:293, 1972.
13. Border, J. R.: Advances and newer concepts in the management of shock. In *Surgery Annual.* Edited by P. Cooper. New York, Appleton-Century-Crofts, 1969, pp. 79–121.

HYPERDYNAMIC STATE

14. Cournand, A., Riley, R. L., Bradley, S. E., Breed, E. S., Noble, R. R., Lauson, H. D., Gregersen, M. I., and Richards, D. W.: Studies of the circulation in clinical shock. Surgery, *13*:964, 1943.
15. Richards, D. W., Jr.: Circulation in traumatic shock in man. Harvey Lect., *39*:217, 1943.
16. Freis, E. D., Schnaper, H. W., Johnson, R. L., and Schreiner, G. E.: Hemodynamic alterations in acute myocardial infarction. J. Clin. Invest., *31*:131, 1952.
17. Gunnar, R. M., Cruz, A., Boswell, J., Co, B. S., Pietras, R. J., and Tobin, J. R.: Myocardial infarction with shock. Hemodynamic studies and results of therapy. Circulation, *33*:753, 1966.
18. Shoemaker, W. C., Printen, K. J., Amato, J. J., Manson, D. O., Carey, J. S., and O'Connor, K.: Hemodynamic patterns after acute anesthetized and unanesthetized trauma; evaluation of the sequence of changes in cardiac output and derived calculations. Arch. Surg., *95*:492, 1967.
19. Shoemaker, W. C., Lim, L., Boyd, D. R., Corley, R. S., Reinhard, J. M., Dreiling, D. A., and Kark, A. E.: Sequential hemodynamic events after trauma to the unanesthetized patient. Surg. Gynecol. Obstet., *132*:651, 1971.
20. Shoemaker, W. C.: Cardiorespiratory patterns of surviving and non-surviving postoperative patients. Surg. Gynecol. Obstet., *134*:810, 1972.
21. Gilbert, R. P., Hinig, K. P., Griffin, J. A., Bicker, R. J., and Adelson, B. H.: Hemodynamics of shock due to infection. Stanford Med. Bull., *13*:239, 1955.

SEPSIS

22. Shaw, G. B.: *The Doctor's Dilemma.* Act I. 1906.
23. Munster, A. M.: The immunology of injury. Surg. Gynecol. Obstet., *136*:666, 1973.
24. Miller, R. M., Polakavetz, S. H., Hornick, R. B., and Cowley, R. A.: Analysis of infections acquired by the severely injured patient. Surg. Gynecol. Obstet., *137*:7, 1973.
25. Bryant, L. R., Trinkle, J. K., and Mobin-Uddin, K.: Bacterial colonization profile with tracheal intubation and mechanical intubation. Arch. Surg., *104*:647, 1972.
26. Alexander, J. W., and Meakins, J. L.: A physiologic basis for the development of opportunistic infections in man. Ann. Surg., *176*:273, 1972.

27. Grogan, J. B., and Miller, R. C.: Impaired function of polymorphonuclear leukocytes in patients with burns and other trauma. Surg. Gynecol. Obstet., *137*:784, 1973.
28. Dorn, B. C., Justice, R. E., McCabe, W. R., and Hechtman, H. B.: A model for bacterial clearance in the lung. Surgery, *71*:414, 1972.
29. Mori, K., Matsumoto, K., and Gans, H.: On the in-vivo clearance and detoxification of endotoxin by lung and liver. Ann. Surg., *177*:159, 1973.
30. Fine, J., Rutenberg, S., and Schweinburg, F. B.: The role of the reticuloendothelial system in hemorrhagic shock. J. Exp. Med., *110*:547, 1959.
31. Zweifach, B. W., Benacerraf, B., and Thomas, L.: Relationship between the vascular manifestations of shock produced by endotoxin, trauma and hemorrhage. II. The possible role of the reticulo-endothelial system in resistance to each type of shock. J. Exp. Med., *106*:403, 1957.
32. Altura, B. M., and Hersey, S. G.: RES phagocytic function in trauma and adaptation to experimental shock. Am. J. Physiol., *215*:1414, 1968.
33. Zweifach, B. W., and Benacerraf, B.: Effect of hemorrhagic shock on the phagocytic function of the Kupffer cells. Circ. Res., *6*:83, 1958.
34. Strawitz, J. G., and Hift, H.: Subcellular changes in hemorrhagic shock. In *Shock and Hypotension*. Edited by L. C. Mills and J. H. Mayer. New York, Grune & Stratton, 1965, pp. 637–642.
35. Neidhardt, J. H., Chadenson, O., and Morin, A.: Gas gangrene of the extremities and the trunk; twenty-two recent observations. Lyon Chir., *68*:191, 1972.
36. Schultz, R. C., and McMaster, W. C.: The treatment of dog bite injuries, especially those of the face. Plast. Reconstr. Surg., *49*:494, 1972.

COAGULOPATHY

37. Monkhouse, F. C., and Milojevic, S.: Changes in fibrinogen level after infusion of thrombin and thromboplastin. Am. J. Physiol., *199*:1165, 1960.
38. Harker, L. A., and Slichter, S. J.: Platelet and fibrinogen consumption in man. N. Engl. J. Med., *287*:999, 1972.
39. McKay, D. G.: *Disseminated Intravascular Coagulation: An Intermediary Mechanism of Disease*. New York, Hoeber Medical Division, Harper & Row, 1965.
40. McNamara, J. J., Burran, E. L., Stremple, J. F., and Molot, M. D.: Coagulopathy after major combat injury: occurrence, management and pathophysiology. Ann. Surg., *176*:243, 1972.
41. String, T., Robinson, A. J., and Blaisdell, F. W.: Massive trauma: effect of intravascular coagulation on prognosis. Arch. Surg., *102*:406, 1971.
42. Hirsch, E. F., Fletcher, J. R., Moquin, R., Dostalek, R., and Lucas, S.: Coagulation changes after combat trauma and sepsis. Surg. Gynecol. Obstet., *133*:393, 1971.

METABOLISM

43. Havel, R. J.: Caloric homeostasis and disorders of fuel transport. N. Engl. J. Med., *287*:1186, 1972.
44. Cahill, G. F.: Starvation in man. N. Engl. J. Med., *282*:668, 1970.
45. Long, C. L., Spencer, J. L., Kenney, J. M., and Geiger, J. W.: Carbohydrate metabolism in man: effect of elective operations and major injury. J. Appl. Physiol., *31*:110, 1971.
46. McNamara, J. J., Molot, M. D., Wissman, D., Collins, C., and Stremple, J. F.: Intravenous hyperalimentation: important adjunct in treatment of combat casualties. Am. J. Surg., *122*:70, 1971.
47. Rothschild, M. A., Oratz, M., and Schreiber, S. S.: Albumin synthesis. N. Engl. J. Med., *286*:816, 1972.
48. Starling, E. H.: *The Fluids of the Body*. Chicago, W. T. Keener & Co., 1909.

INTRACELLULAR BIOCHEMISTRY

49. Bell, M. L., Herman, A. H., Smith, E. E., Egdahl, R. H., and Rutenburg, A. M.: Role of lysosomal instability in development of refractory shock. Surgery, *70*:341, 1971.
50. Shires, G. T., Cunningham, J. N., Baker, C. R. F., Reeder, S. F., Illner, H., Wagner, I. Y., and Maker, J.: Alterations in cellular membrane function during hemorrhagic shock in primates. Ann. Surg., *176*:288, 1972.
51. Benesch, R., and Benesch, R. E.: The effect of organic phosphates from the human erythrocyte on the allosteric properties of hemoglobin. Biochem. Biophys. Res. Commun., *26*:162, 1967.
52. Chanutin, A., and Curnish, R. R.: Effect of organic and inorganic phosphates on the oxygen equilibrium of human erythrocytes. Arch. Biochem. Biophys., *121*:96, 1967.
53. Valtis, D. J., and Kennedy, A. C.: Defective gas-transport function of stored red blood cells. Lancet, *1*:119, 1954.
54. Klocke, R. A.: Oxygen transport and 2,3 diphosphoglycerate (DPG). Chest, *62*:795, 1972.
55. McConn, R., and DelGuercio, L. R. M.: Respiratory function of blood in the acutely ill patient and effect of steroids. Ann. Surg., *174*:436, 1971.
56. Fallon, K. D., Weisel, R. D., and Hechtman, H. B.: P50 determinations: techniques and clinical importance. In *Instrumentation, Methods, and Physiology*. Edited by H. I. Bicher. New York, Plenum Publishing Corp., 1973, pp. 93–97.

ACUTE RESPIRATORY FAILURE

57. Moon, V. H.: *Shock, Its Dynamics, Occurrence and Management*. Philadelphia, Lea & Febiger, 1942.
58. Burford, T. H., and Burbank, B.: Traumatic wet lung: observations in certain physiologic fundamentals of thoracic trauma. J. Thorac. Surg., *14*:415, 1945.
59. Barnes, R. W., and Merendino, K. A.: Post-traumatic pulmonary insufficiency syndrome. Surg. Clin. North Am., *52*:625, 1972.
60. Moore, F. D., Lyons, J. H., Pierce, E. C., Morgan, A. F., Drinker, P. A., MacArthur, J. D., and Dammin, G. J.: *Post-Traumatic Pulmonary Insufficiency*. Philadelphia, W. B. Saunders Co., 1969.
61. Hardaway, R. M., James, P. M., Jr., Anderson, R. W. Bredenberg, C. E., and West, R. L.: Intensive study and treatment of shock in man. J.A.M.A., *199*:779, 1967.
62. Vito, L., Dennis, R., Weisel, R., and Hechtman, H. B.: Sepsis presenting as acute pulmonary insufficiency. Surg. Gynecol. Obstet., *138*:896, 1974.
63. Collins, J. A., Gordon, W. C., Jr., Hudson, T. L., Irvin, R. W., Jr., Kelly, T., and Hardaway, R. M., III: Inapparent hypoxemia in casualties with wounded limbs: pulmonary fat embolism? Ann. Surg., *167*:511, 1968.
64. Collins, J. A., Hudson, T. L., Hamacher, W. R., Rokous, J., Williams, G., and Hardaway, R. M., III: Systemic fat embolism in four combat casualties. Ann. Surg., *167*:493, 1968.

65. Moseley, R. V., and Doty, D. B.: Changes in the filtration characteristics of stored blood. Ann. Surg., *171*:329, 1970.
66. McNamara, J. J., Molot, M. D., and Stremple, J. F.: Screen filtration pressure in combat casualties. Ann. Surg., *172*:334, 1970.
67. Heroy, W. H.: Unrecognized aspiration. Ann. Thorac. Surg., *8*:580, 1969.
68. Moseley, R. V., and Doty, D. B.: Physiologic changes due to aspiration pneumonitis. Ann. Surg., *171*:73, 1970.
69. Robbins, E. D., Cross, C. E., and Zelis, R.: Pulmonary edema. N. Engl. J. Med., *288*:292, 1973.
70. Flemming, W. H., and Bowen, J. C.: The use of diuretics in the treatment of early wet lung syndrome. Ann. Surg., *175*:505, 1972.
71. Hechtman, H. B., Weisel, R. D., Vito, L., Ali, J., and Berger, R. L.: The independence of pulmonary shunting and pulmonary edema. Surgery, *74*:300, 1973.
72. Clements, J. A., Brown, E. J., and Johnson, R. P.: Pulmonary surface tension and the mucous lining of the lungs: some theoretical considerations. J. Appl. Physiol., *12*:262, 1958.
73. Henry, J. N., McArdle, A. H., Scott, H. J., and Gurd, F. N.: A study of the acute and chronic respiratory pathophysiology of hemorrhagic shock. J. Thorac. Cardiovasc. Surg., *54*:666, 1967.
74. Sinha, R. P., Ducker, T. B., and Perot, P. L.: Arterial oxygenation: findings and its significance in central nervous system trauma patients. J.A.M.A., *224*:1258, 1973.
75. Simmons, R. L., Heisterkamp, C. A., Collins, J. A., Bredenburg, C. E., and Martin, A. M., Jr.: Acute pulmonary edema in battle casualties. J. Trauma, *9*:760, 1969.
76. Cushing, H.: Concerning a definite regulatory mechanism of the vasomotor center which controls blood pressure during cerebral compression. Bull. Johns Hopkins Hosp., *12*:290, 1901.
77. Ducker, T. B., and Simmons, R. L.: Increased intracranial pressure and pulmonary edema. II. The hemodynamic response of dogs and monkeys to increased intracranial pressure. J. Neurosurg., *28*:118, 1968.
78. Brown, R. S., Mohr, P. A., Carey, J. S., and Shoemaker, W. C.: Cardiovascular changes after cranial cerebral injury and increased intracranial pressure. Surg. Gynecol. Obstet., *125*:1205, 1967.

GASTRODUODENAL ULCERATION

79. Lucas, C. E., Sugawa, C., Riddle, J., Rector, F., Rosenberg, B., and Walt, A. J.: Natural history and surgical dilemma of "stress" gastric bleeding. Arch. Surg., *102*:266, 1971.
80. Skillman, J. J., Gould, S. A., Chung, R. S. K., and Silen, W.: The gastric mucosal barrier: clinical and experimental studies in critically ill and normal man and in the rabbit. Ann. Surg., *172*:564, 1970.
81. Curling, T. B.: On acute ulceration of the duodenum in cases of burn. Med. Chir. Tr., London, *25*:260, 1842.
82. Cushing, H.: Peptic ulcers and the interbrain. Surg. Gynecol. Obstet., *55*:1, 1932.
83. Moncrief, J. A., Switzer, W. E., and Teplitz, C.: Curling ulcer. J. Trauma, *4*:481, 1964.
84. Sevitt, S.: Duodenal and gastric ulceration after burning. Br. J. Surg., *54*:32, 1967.
85. Dalgaard, J. B.: Brain injury as a cause of esophagogastro-duodenal ulceration. J. Forensic Med., *4*:110, 1957.
86. Dalgaard, J. B.: Cerebral vascular lesions and peptic ulceration. Arch. Pathol., *69*:359, 1960.
87. Tedeschi, C. G.: Gastric mucosal lesions in rats submitted to head trauma. Proc. Soc. Exp. Biol. Med., *57*:268, 1944.

MYOCARDIAL DEPRESSION

88. Guyton, A. C.: *Circulatory Physiology: Cardiac Output and Its Regulation.* Philadelphia, W. B. Saunders Co., 1963.
89. Crexells, C., Chatterjee, K., Forrester, J. S., Dikshit, K., and Swan, H. J. C.: Optimal level of filling pressure in the left side of the heart in acute myocardial infarction. N. Engl. J. Med., *289*:1263, 1973.
90. Hechtman, H. B.: Unpublished observations.
91. Lovett, W. L., Wangenstein, S. L., Glenn, T. M., and Lefer, A. M.: Presence of myocardial depressant factor in patients in circulatory shock. Surgery, *70*:223, 1971.
92. Wangenstein, S. L., Geissinger, W. T., Lovett, W. L., Glenn, T. M., and Lefer, A. M.: Relationship between splanchnic blood flow and a myocardial depressant factor in endotoxin shock. Surgery, *69*:410, 1971.
93. Cann, M., Stevenson, T., Fiallos, E., and Thal, A. P.: Depressed cardiac performance in sepsis. Surg. Gynecol. Obstet., *134*:759, 1972.
94. Crowell, J. W., and Guyton, A. C.: Further evidence favoring a cardiac mechanism in irreversible hemorrhagic shock. Am. J. Physiol., *203*:248, 1962.
95. Gernet, C. F., and Schwartz, S.: Pulmonary artery catheterization. Am. J. Nurs., *73*:1182, 1973.
96. Mallory, T. B.: Systemic pathology of traumatic shock. J. Mount Sinai Hosp., N. Y., *16*:137, 1949.
97. Moon, V. H.: The pathology of secondary shock. Am. J. Pathol., *24*:235, 1948.
98. Bramwell, C.: Can head injury cause auricular fibrillation? Lancet, *1*:8, 1934.
99. Lucke, H.: Über zentral ausgelöste Herzrhythmusstörungen. Dtsch. Arch. Klin. Med., *180*:40, 1937.
100. Doret, J. P., and Ferrero, C.: L'electrocardiogramme dans l'encephalopathie traumatique. Schweiz. Med. Wochenschr., *78*:836, 1948.
101. Nadas, A. S., Alimurung, M. M., and Linenthal, A. J.: Persistent ventricular pacemaker following basal skull fracture; report of case in 5-year old girl. Am. Heart J., *42*:888, 1951.
102. Hersch, C.: Electrocardiographic changes in head injuries. Circulation, *23*:853, 1961.
103. Lepeschkin, E.: *Modern Electrocardiography.* Vol. 1. Baltimore, Williams & Wilkins Co., 1951.
104. Kaunisto, Y.: Electrokardiographische Untersuchungen nach subokzipitaler Luftinsufflation. Acta Chir. Scand., *85*:129, 1941.
105. Giampalmo, V.: Sulle modificanzioni electrocardiografiche nel corso della pneumoencefalografia. Arch. E. Maragliano Patol. Clin., *1*:148, 1946.
106. Paulian, D., Tudor, M., and Constantinesco, G. G.: Les modifications de l'électrocardiogramme dans les tumeurs cérébrales. Arch. Neurol. (Paris), *3*:230, 1939.
107. Gefter, W. I., Leaman, W. G., Luccesi, P. F., Maker, I. E., and Dworin, M.: Heart in acute anterior poliomyelitis. Am. Heart J., *33*:228, 1947.
108. Burch, G. E., Meyers, R., and Abildskov, J. A.: New electrocardiographic pattern observed in cerebrovascular accidents. Circulation, *9*:719, 1954.
109. Beattie, J., Brow, G. R., and Long, C. N. H.: Physiological and anatomical evidence for the existence of nerve tracts connecting hypothalamus with spinal sympathetic centers. Proc. R. Soc. Lond. B, *106B*:253, 1930.

110. Storm van Leeuwen, W.: Arrhythmia cordis door experimentele beschadiging van het centraal zenuwstelsel. Thesis, University of Leyden, 1945.
111. Korteweg, J., Boeles, T. F., and Ten Cate, J.: Influence of stimulation of some subcortical areas on electrocardiogram. J. Neurophysiol., *20*:100, 1957.
112. Jacobson, S. A., and Danufsky, P.: Marked electrocardiographic changes produced by experimental head trauma. J. Neuropathol. Exp. Neurol., *13*:462, 1954.
113. Cropp, G. J., and Manning, G. W.: Electrocardiographic changes simulating myocardial ischemia and infarction associated with spontaneous intracranial hemorrhage. Circulation, *22*:25, 1960.
114. Shuster, S.: The electrocardiogram in subarachnoid haemorrhage. Br. Heart J., *22*:316, 1960.
115. Porter, R. W., Kamikawa, K., and Greenhoot, J. H.: Persistent electrocardiographic abnormalities experimentally induced by stimulation of the brain. Am. Heart J., *64*:815, 1962.
116. Hockman, C. H., Mauck, H. P., Jr., and Hoff, E. C.: ECG changes resulting from cerebral stimulation. II. A spectrum of ventricular arrhythmias of sympathetic origin. Am. Heart J., *71*:695, 1966.
117. Melville, K. I., Blum, B., Shister, H. E., and Silver, M. D.: Cardiac ischemic changes and arrhythmias induced by hypothalamic stimulation. Am. J. Cardiol., *12*:781, 1963.
118. Connor, R. C. R.: Heart damage associated with intracranial lesions. Br. Med. J., *3*:29, 1968.
119. Connor, R. C. R.: Fuchsinophilic degeneration of myocardium in patients with intracranial lesions. Br. Heart J., *32*:81, 1970.
120. Burch, G. E., DePasquale, N., and Malaret, G.: Selected problems in electrocardiography. Ann. Intern. Med., *52*:587, 1960.
121. Schlesinger, M. J., and Reiner, L.: Focal myocytolysis of heart. Am. J. Pathol., *31*:443, 1955.
122. Eichbaum, F. W., and Bissetti, P. C.: Cardiovascular disturbances following acute increase of intracranial pressure. *Proceedings Fifth International Congress of Neuropathology.* International Congress Series No. 100. Amsterdam, Excerpta Medica Foundation, 1966, p. 1016.

ACUTE RENAL FAILURE

123. Trueta, J., Barclay, A. E., Daniel, D. M., Franklin, K. J., and Prichard, M. M. L.: *Studies of the Renal Circulation.* Springfield, Ill., Charles C Thomas, 1947, pp. 112–113.
124. Lucke, B.: Lower nephron nephrosis (renal lesions of the crush syndrome, of burns, transfusions, and other conditions which affect the lower segment of the nephrons). Milit. Surg., *99*:371, 1946.
125. Teschan, P. E., Post, R. S., Smith, L. H., Abernathy, R. S., Davis, J. H., Gray, D. M., Howard, J. M., Johnson, K. E. Klopp, E., Mundy, R. L., O'Meara, M. P., and Rush, B. F., Jr.: In *Battle Casualties in Korea.* Edited by J. M. Howard. Army Medical Service Graduate School. Walter Reed Army Medical Center, Washington, D.C., 1955, Vol. 4, pp. 7–30, 193–233.
126. Rosenberg, I. K., Gupta, S. L., Lucas, C. E., Khan, A. A., and Rosenberg, B. F.: Renal insufficiency after trauma and sepsis: prospective functional and ultrastructural analysis. Arch. Surg., *103*:175, 1971.
127. Shires, G. T., Baxter, C. R., and Zedlitz, W. H.: High output renal failure complicating traumatic injury. J. Trauma, *4*:567, 1964.
128. Carriere, S., Thorburn, G. D., O'Morchoe, C. C. C., and Barger, A. C.: Intrarenal distribution of blood flow in dogs during hemorrhagic hypotension. Circ. Res., *19*:167, 1966.
129. Hopkins, R. W., Sabga, G., Bernerdo, P., Penn, I., and Simeone, R. A.: Significance of post-traumatic and postoperative oliguria. Arch. Surg., *87*:320, 1963.
130. Henry, L. N., Lane, C. E., and Kashgarian, M.: Micropuncture studies of the pathophysiology of acute renal failure in the rat. Lab. Invest., *19*:309, 1968.
131. Guillain, G., and Vincent, C.: Valeur sémeiologique de l'albuminurie dans les hemorrhagies méningées. Semaine Med., *29*:505, 1909.
132. Schmidt, R.: Ueber Hirntumor-Oligurie. Klin. Wochenschr., *12*:105, 1933.
133. Stucke, K., and Carstensen, G.: Nierenfunktionsstörungen nach Commotio cerebri. Dtsch. Med. Wochenschr., *82*:177, 1957.
134. Clute, K. F., and Fitzgerald, G. W.: Anuria following electric shock therapy. Can. Med. Assoc. J., *59*:426, 1948.
135. Goodman, L.: Lower nephron nephrosis following electroconvulsive therapy. Report of two fatalities. J. Nerv. Ment. Dis., *112*:130, 1950.
136. Fishberg, A. M.: Neurogenic nephropathy. Arch. Intern. Med., *99*:129, 1957.
137. Steinmetz, P. R., and Kiley, J. E.: Renal tubular necrosis following lesions of the brain. Am. J. Med., *29*:268, 1960.
138. Green, H. D., and Hoff, E. C.: Effect of faradic stimulation of the cerebral cortex on limb and renal volumes. Am. J. Physiol., *118*:641, 1937.
139. Hoff, E. C., Kell, J. F., Hastings, N., Gray, E. H., and Sholes, D. M.: Acute renal cortical ischemia produced by stimulation of the pressor area of the cerebral cortex. Fed. Proc., *8*:76, 1949.
140. Hoff, E. C., Kell, J. F., Hastings, N., Sholes, D. M., and Gray, E. H.: Vasomotor, cellular and functional changes produced in kidney by brain stimulation. J. Neurophysiol., *14*:317, 1951.
141. Lebowitz, M. H.: Nephrogenic diabetes insipidus following methoxyflurane anesthesia: a report of two cases. Anesth. Analg. (Cleve.), *48*:233, 1969.
142. Fletcher, J. R., Hirsch, E. F., and Lucas, S.: Renal function after sepsis in combat casualties. Surg. Gynecol. Obstet., *133*:237, 1971.
143. Merrill, J. P.: Acute renal failure. In *Diseases of Kidneys.* Edited by M. B. Strauss and L. G. Welt. 2nd Ed. Vol. 1, Chapter 17. Boston, Little, Brown and Co., 1971.

SECTION I. MECHANICAL INJURY

chapter 5

POSTTRAUMATIC EMBOLISM

by Luke G. Tedeschi and Herbert B. Hechtman

The effects of trauma by mechanical force present two major categories of phenomena. On one side are those that are inherent in the anatomical and functional disruption of the bodily structure or structures that are directly affected by the force, and on the other is a broad range of disorders that may occur in conjunction with trauma in general, without direct relation to the location of the injury.

Posttraumatic embolism belongs to the latter category. The term implies the entrance into and transportation in the blood stream of particles of substances that are not normal inhabitants of the blood. Globules of fat or air, tissue cells, fragments of thrombi detached from the intima of an artery (arterial emboli) or a vein (venous emboli), and clusters of bacteria are examples. The ultimate outcome of the phenomenon is the arrest of the circulating particles in the lumina of fine blood vessels in various parts of the body. The vascular occlusion in turn interferes with the blood supply of the area nourished by the obstructed blood vessels, and in the absence of a collateral arterial blood supply the final effect is the death (infarction) of the involved tissue.

Although this sequence of events is a basic feature of embolism, every individual type of foreign circulating particle gives rise to distinctive manifestations that are inherent in the size of the particles, their differences in plasticity, and their particular chemical and biologic properties. Other dissimilarities are linked to the system of channels in which the particles are being transported, whether in the venous or arterial circulation.

THROMBOEMBOLISM

Tissular injury is unavoidably associated with rupture or alterations in the structures of the walls of the blood channels. The exposure of the circulating blood to the endothelial denuded collagen or basement membrane of the injured vessel promotes adhesion of platelets and formation of fibrin, namely, the making of a thrombus.

Intravascular clotting at the site of injury acts as a protective mechanism, preventing or decreasing hemorrhage. This hemostatic plug impairs the blood flow into the involved tissue, however, resulting in local ischemia, an increase in carbon dioxide content, acidosis, and possibly changes in electrical potential, which in turn may disrupt the normal coagulation mechanism.

All tissues contain, in variable concentration, thromboplastin, the material that promotes the formation of thrombin, which is the substance that is essential in the process of clot formation. Upon cellular disintegration, secondary to low-flow states, thromboplastin is released. Whereas at the site of local injury, release of thromboplastin is beneficial in hastening the formation of hemostatic plugs and the clotting of shed blood, its release in excessive concentration into the general circulation can disrupt the overall coagulation mechanism and lead to the formation of disseminated thrombi.

Initially, the local consumption of clotting substances at the site of a massive injury may leave the circulating blood in a hypocoagulable state. There is a decrease in platelets, circulating fibrinogen, prothrombin complex, and factors V, VII, VIII, and X. This depletion is related both to the fact that these substances may be consumed by the process of coagulation at the site of injury and to an outright loss of clotting substance. A rebound period has been described that is characterized by an increase of these substances above normal concentrations. During this period platelets become more adhesive, antithrombin concentrations increase, and there is depletion of fibrin stabilizing factor.[1]

Erythrocyte aggregation also occurs. An experiment in rabbits by Borgstrom and coworkers has shown red blood cell aggregation in the capillary vessels of the bulbar conjunctiva one to three hours after contusion of the muscles of one thigh by repeated light blows.[2]

Systemic hypoxia, shock, and concurrent infection are frequently associated with trauma. Each one, or a combination of these factors, can trigger intravascular coagulation. The adverse effects of systemic hypoxia on coagulation have been reported by Coon and Hodgson in patients with cardiac arrest, and by Crowell and associates in dogs subjected to alternate cardiac arrest and reestablishment of circulation.[3,4]

Shock and the associated lowering of blood pressure are both related to intravascular coagulation.[5,6] Low-flow states and subsequent cell disruption and release of thromboplastin are likely causes of this relationship. This process is postulated to work both ways, with shock leading to intravascular coagulation as well as the reverse.[7] The latter process is debated. The causal relationship of clotting defects in inducing human shock (beyond the production of simple hemorrhage) has yet to be proved (cf. Chapter 4).

Occasionally, the physician is confronted with an injured patient whose bleeding exceeds that explainable by his injury or injuries. Hemostasis results from two major processes: the formation of a primary hemostatic plug of platelets and the generation of thrombin that converts the primary unstable platelet plug into one that is stable. Aberrations of this sequence of events may cause protracted bleeding. Not infrequently this occurrence finds explanation in a preexisting hemostatic defect. This defect may be independent of the systemic disorder in coagulation elicited by the trauma.

Infection is a frequent sequel to injury. Intravascular clumping of platelets and formation of fibrin strands can be evoked by bacterial endotoxins.[8] This phenomenon has been attributed to massive activation of the fibrinolytic enzyme system.

The successful production of disseminated intravascular coagulation in rabbits by intravenous infusion of epinephrine points to the role played by the release of vasomotor substances in the activation of the clotting mechanism.[9] Vasoactive polypeptides are also linked closely to coagulation and the fibrinolytic system.

At the beginning of the century, Cannon presented evidence that adrenal medullary activity hastens blood coagulation, and suggested that the hypercoagulability associated with stress is mediated by the adrenal response.[10,11] This concept implied the existence of a neurohormonal mechanism. Evidence to this effect is now available. Correll has shown that electrical stimulation of the hypothalamus in cats results in an immediate shortening of the clotting time, possibly due to release of an antiheparin factor.[12] Since shortening of the clotting time can be prevented by transection of the midbrain at the level of the inferior colliculus, this may imply that the neurohormonal response is mediated by vagal outflow.[13]

In the past few years disseminated intravascular coagulation (DIC) has been implicated in diverse conditions, such as the "dead fetus syndrome" and allograft rejection.[14,15] Attempts have been made to find mechanisms common to their diverse etiologies. Several systems appear to be operative. These are the plasminogen-plasmin system, the vasomotor system, and the reticuloendothelial system, whose offspring—the macrophage—normally clears and removes fibrin.[16] An additional common pathway for the induction of diffuse intravascular clotting rests on the production of thromboplastin or of some other procoagulant agent capable of activating the "prothrombin converting complex," then thrombin production, and ultimately clot formation.

The localization of the thrombi is dependent upon the condition of the blood vessel wall at the time of the clotting episode. The integrity of the endothelial lining of the microcirculation is a deterrent to the formation of the thrombus.

The same phenomenon that occurs in the microcirculatory system may take place as well in larger blood vessels. Thrombosis is more likely to occur in a vein than in an artery. The formation of a thrombus is favored by the stasis and low velocity of flow characteristic of veins. A venous thrombus may become detached, giving rise to an *embolus* that, following the venous circulation, will be carried to the heart and then to the lungs *(pulmonary thromboembolism)* (Fig. 5–1).

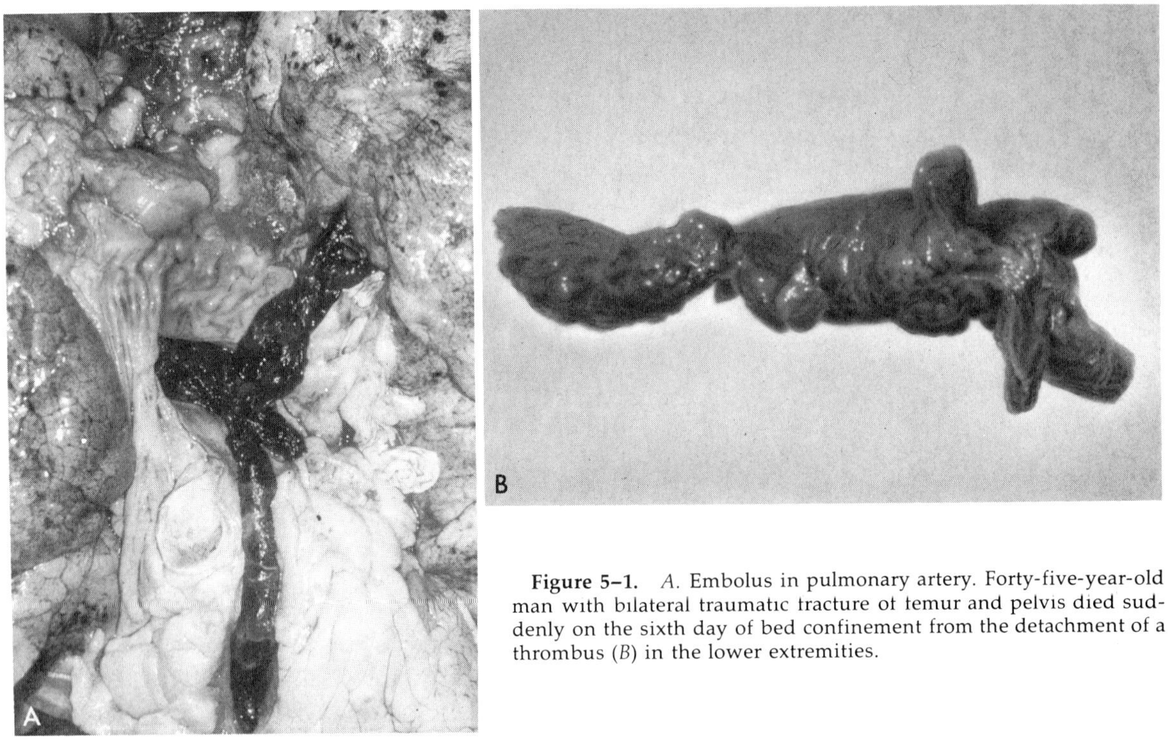

Figure 5–1. *A*. Embolus in pulmonary artery. Forty-five-year-old man with bilateral traumatic fracture of femur and pelvis died suddenly on the sixth day of bed confinement from the detachment of a thrombus (*B*) in the lower extremities.

Saddle embolism is the name given to the life-threatening condition in which the detached thrombus becomes lodged at the bifurcation of the main pulmonary artery, thus interfering with the circulation to both lungs. This occurrence can cause rapid and often fatal right ventricular heart failure. Preexisting heart disease may exaggerate the effect of pulmonary emboli.

Among the *indirect effects* of trauma that are capable of leading to thromboembolism are those resulting from confinement to bed and depressed cardiac function. A thrombus in a vein can develop in the absence of signs and symptoms, and its detachment from the wall of the blood vessel and the ensuing pulmonary thromboembolism may occur days or weeks after the original injury that led to bed rest and immobilization. Virtually all significant venous thromboemboli originate in the veins of the legs or pelvis.

Systemic or *arterial thromboembolism* is much less common and as a rule results from the detachment of a clot from one of the left chambers of the heart. The detached clot travels with the arterial circulation and can lodge in vital organs such as the brain, spleen, kidneys, and intestines. In the absence of active collateral circulation, the end-result of this occurrence will be tissular ischemia followed by infarct necrosis.

The term *septic thrombosis* is used to indicate that a thrombus has become infected. Bacteria are normal inhabitants of every external surface and most of the internal passages of the body. Thus, upon disruption of the barrier provided by the normal continuity of the superficial cell layers (skin, mucosal membranes), bacteria may gain access to the injured tissue and set up a local infection. The dead cells, the outpoured edema fluid and blood elements, the decreased blood supply coincidental to vascular thrombosis and hemorrhage, establish an ideal situation for bacterial growth.

Presence of extraneous material within the wound, such as a bit of glass, a splinter, a projectile, a piece of cloth, and even dead tissue such as a sequestered fragment of bone increase the likelihood of wound infection. Wounds associated with extensive crushing of tissue are more likely to become infected than simple lacerations or puncture wounds.

Often the infection penetrates the vascular walls and extends to involve a concomitant intraluminal blood clot. Microorganisms multiply well in a thrombus. This contributes to the extension of the thrombus as well as to the spread of infection. Septic (infected) thrombi tend to disintegrate more easily than nonseptic thrombi and may serve as a focus of bacteremia or, if they become detached from the vessel wall, can give rise to an abscess wherever they lodge.

Another possible cause of primary wound infection and concurrent septic thrombosis is the trapping in the wound, where resistance is depressed, of bacteria that occasionally circulate in the blood stream even under normal conditions. There is ample evidence to support the concept that pathogenic microorganisms not uncommonly are present in the blood of normal individuals. Under ordinary circumstances these bacteria are quickly removed from the circulation and do not elicit signs or symptoms of disease; however, in coincidence with the reaction to injury and the depressed resistance of the host, the transient bacteria lodge selectively in the wound. They may anchor themselves to an intravascular blood clot, setting up a septic thrombus and a potential septic embolus.

FAT EMBOLISM

According to a definition deeply rooted in the medical literature, fat embolism is a pathologic condition ensuing from the introduction of liquefied fat into the circulation and its transportation by the blood stream to occlude the fine blood vessels in various parts of the body.[17]

In the light of the newer concept that embolic fat may be produced by an alteration in the suspension stability of endogenous serum fat, this definition is no longer entirely adequate.[18, 19]

Under normal conditions fat is present in the blood in the form of glycerides, cholesterol, cholesterol esters, phospholipids, and free fatty acids. The glycerides consist chiefly of triglycerides with long-chain fatty acids that are combined with proteins, resulting in lipoproteins of different density. The amount of glyceride contained in the high-density lipoproteins is relatively small. Low-density lipoproteins in contrast have a relatively large nucleus of triglycerides and cholesterol surrounded by a surface of phospholipids and proteins.

Chylomicrons belong to the latter category. They can be seen in the microscope with darkfield illumination as dancing refractile bodies, from 0.5 to 1.0 μ in diameter.

Chylomicrons do not take fat stains. Conversely fatty particles of apparently analogous composition, but much larger, from 5 to 20 μ in diameter, can be identified with fat stains. Fat embolism has been linked with the presence of fat particles with these characteristics.

Causes of Fat Embolism

Trauma to Bone and Soft Tissue

Trauma to bone is the leading cause of fat embolism. The results of some authoritative series show figures as high as 100 per cent.[20] Fat is mechanically liberated from the bone marrow fat cells and pressed into the veins of the haversian system, which in turn communicates freely with the intramedullary sinusoidal blood channels.

Bone marrow fat is scarce in children, and this explains the rarity of this condition in this age group.[21] A case is on record, however, of posttraumatic fat embolism in a newborn baby.[22]

Direct injury of subcutaneous fat tissue by concussion, contusion, or burns is the second most frequent cause of fat embolism. In this case, the ideal anatomical situation is provided by the dense vascularity of the subcutaneous fat tissue extending to enmesh the individual fat cells in a network of blood capillaries.

Trauma not uncommonly requires surgical or orthopedic procedures. It is worth mentioning that these procedures per se can elicit fat embolism. A profuse literature documents the high incidence rate of fat embolism following orthopedic operations, as well as major and even minor soft-tissue operations.[23-26]

Estimates of the minimal amount of circulating free fat capable of inducing embolic death in man range from 12 to 120 ml.[17] The speed of entry of the fat particles into the circulatory system probably plays a role as important as the amount of fat in determining the outcome of the event.

Nontraumatic Fat Embolism

The notion that fat embolism may occur in conjunction with a broad range of nontraumatic conditions has led to the concept that the phenomenon may be produced by an alteration in the suspension stability of endogenous serum fat resulting in the conversion of chylomicrons into globules of fat emboli.

Fat embolism has been described in man in conjunction with the hyperlipemic stage of diabetic coma, carbon tetrachloride poisoning, pancreatitis, phosphorus poisoning, sodium and ammonium hydroxide intoxications, following excessive alcohol intake, and salvarsan administration.[27-35] It has also been recorded in association with fatty nutritional cirrhosis, and in conjunction with chronic venous congestion and terminal heart failure, an event that has also been linked to fatty liver.[36-40] Additional conditions referred to in the medical literature include a broad range of infectious processes, such as *Clostridium welchii* infection, pneumonia, and bacterial osteomyelitis. It has likewise been mentioned in connection with sickle cell crisis; with total pump-oxygenator perfusion; with extracorporeal circulation in conjunction with cardiopulmonary by-pass; and with prolonged recirculation of plasma in screen, bubble, and disk oxygenators.[44–47] Lymphangiography requires the use of contrast media. Oil embolism has been described in association with this procedure.[48] More recent is the observation of fat embolism in conjunction with arthroplasty utilizing acrylic cement.

The occurrence of fat embolism in affiliation with such a broad spectrum of nontraumatic conditions has led to the search for a common denominator. The search has been rewarding. Evidence is at hand indicating that some of the clinical symptoms ascribed to fat embolism may be caused not as much by the fat emboli as by systemic factors.

In trauma, alterations take place in the physical properties of the blood.[49] With the release of thromboplastin from injured tissue, the red blood cells show a tendency to intravascular aggregation, followed by a decrease in their suspension stability, which is reflected by an elevation of the erythrocyte sedimentation rate.[50] Intravenous injection of thrombin leads to precipitation of fibrin and red blood cells, and also to the formation of intravascular fat.[51]

According to a group of Swedish investigators, the clinical symptoms generally ascribed to fat embolism are caused by impairment of blood flow due to alterations in the physical properties of the blood and coagulation factors. In a series of experiments, Bergentz and coworkers noticed, early in the posttraumatic state (within four hours after surgery), the appearance of platelet aggregates intermingled with abundant chylomicrons and large fat globules; simultaneously the concentration of triglycerides increased in the red blood cells and decreased in the plasma; this was followed (within 24 hours after the injury) by intravascular aggregation of red blood cells concurrent to an increase in fibrinogen and a shift of triglycerides from the red blood cells to the blood plasma. In the subsequent days (from one to seven after the injury) they observed a decrease in the suspension stability of the blood and a rise in the erythrocytic sedimentation rate that they attributed to an increase in lipoproteins, especially fibrinogen and euglobulin.[52–55] Thus, fat embolism is ascribed to decreased blood flow with ensuing acidosis, decreased oxygen consumption, and the "anemia of injury."[57, 58] The premise that the emulsion stability of the blood lipids is closely related to the factors involved in blood coagulation finds additional support in Cammermeyer's report of juxtaembolic thrombosis of fibrin associated with fat embolism.[58]

Along these lines, a fresh outlook on the relationship between trauma and fat embolism has been provided by the suggestion that the biochemical changes occurring in the blood plasma during shock can disrupt the lipid suspension system, resulting in the formation of fatty acids and free fat.[59] Fat embolism and shock are frequently associated in trauma to bone and soft tissues. Under conditions of stress, fats become mobilized as the richest source of stored energy. The hypothesis conceived by David and Musselman that fat mobilized under conditions of stress may act as a trigger mechanism destabilizing fat already present in the blood stream or later mobilized or ingested is gathering support from many sources.[60, 61]

The diagnostic criteria of fat embolism are not clearly defined. This explains why data on the incidence of fat embolism vary considerably, depending on the criteria used to establish the diagnosis. Fat embolism can be classified into three major categories: subclinical, clinically manifest but nonfatal, and fatal forms. In the first category, the amount of embolic fat is so small that no clinical signs or symptoms are elicited. In the second there are definite manifestations, either pulmonary or systemic. The third is self-explanatory.

The challenge to diagnosis is mirrored by the discrepancy in data on the frequency with which this condition occurs. In only 14 of 177 cases of clinically diagnosed fat embolism could the diagnosis be confirmed at autopsy.[62] More recent estimates of the incidence of pulmonary fat embolism range from 0.8 per cent among a thousand battle casualties to 50 per cent in a series of routine hospital autopsies.[63, 64] These differences rest primarily on whether the diagnosis is based on clinical or pathologic criteria.

The Clinical Syndrome

The clinical syndrome commonly ascribed to fat embolism takes two forms: pulmonary and systemic.

Pulmonary embolism can be so mild as to be overlooked. Roentgenograms of the chest may, however, show fine stippling and hazy infiltrations in both lungs, rapidly progressing to the fluffy, dense mottling that is characteristic of pulmonary fat embolism.

When larger emboli are present the overall effect is a severe systemic hypoxemia secondary to microatelectasis (see Chapter 4).[65] The associated symptoms include tachypnea, dyspnea, and in extreme cases cyanosis. Fever is often an added feature.

By means of autoradiographic techniques Fuchsig and co-workers have shown that liberated fat from the depots may not reach the lungs via the blood stream as has been generally assumed, but rather is transported through the lymphatic system to the innominate vein and thence to the lungs.[66, 67]

Systemic embolism takes place when the fat emboli gain access to the systemic circulation. Migration of embolic fat into the systemic circulation is a rather uncommon condition. When this takes place the brain becomes the major target organ. The manifestations of cerebral fat embolism are characterized by signs of generalized brain impairment as well as by evidence of localized neurologic deficit. The former include impairment of consciousness, with varying degrees of somnolence, disorientation, confusional excitement, and stupor gradually deepening into coma; sometimes coma starts suddenly without premonitory symptoms. Decerebrate rigidity of fluctuating intensity and pyramidal signs have also been described. Among the localized neurologic signs, focal seizures, expressive aphasia, hemiparesis, paracentral visual scotomas, conjugate lateral deviation of the eyes, and pupillary inequalities have all been recorded.[68]

The cerebral manifestations of fat embolism mimic so much the manifestations accompanying an intracranial hematoma that a safe distinction between the two can rarely be established without the assistance of cerebral contrast studies and trephination of the skull.

In conjunction with or independently from the cerebral manifestations, oliguria or anuria may develop, reflecting renal involvement. An unusual case of renal fat embolization followed by urostealith formation has been recorded.[69] Whenever the diagnosis of systemic fat embolism is in doubt, a careful search for petechiae may be rewarding. One half to two thirds of the patients with fat embolism show petechiae that fail to blanch on compression. As a rule, they occur on the second or third day after the injury and are most commonly found in the lower palpebral conjunctivae and in the skin of the neck, shoulders, and axillary folds. Biopsy of petechiae can be very helpful in showing sudanophilic material in the lumina of dermal vessels. The same is true of the advocated renal biopsy, a more hazardous procedure.[70, 71]

An equally significant diagnostic sign is the presence of small rosaries of microinfarcts around the maculae of both eyes. In Thomas and Ayyar's series, embolic globules of fat inside the retinal arterioles were identified in 50 per cent of their patients.[68]

Pathology of Fat Embolism

The gross findings at autopsy in systemic fat embolism are not specific. They consist chiefly of petechiae and minute disseminated hemorrhages in the brain and kidneys (Fig. 5–2). The

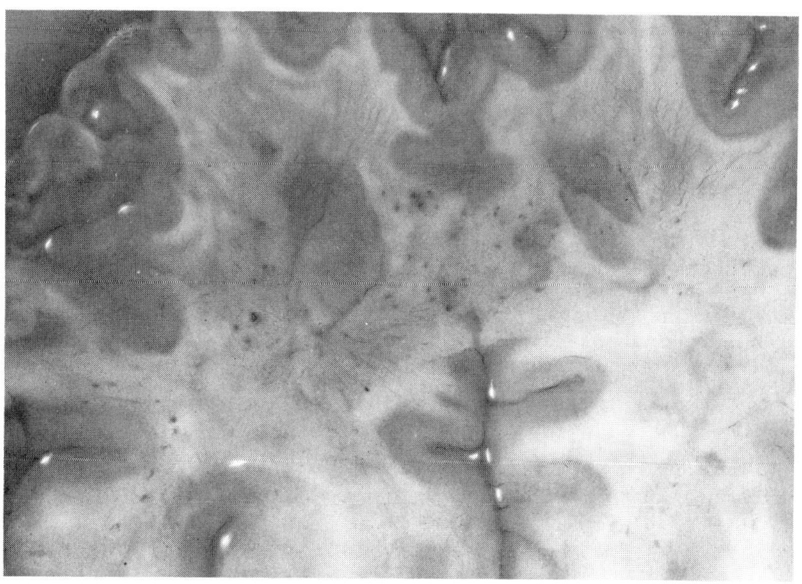

Figure 5–2. Transverse section of cerebral hemispheres showing disseminated petechial hemorrhages at the site of fat emboli. Fifty-nine-year-old truck driver died of systemic fat embolism following multiple bony injuries sustained in a road accident.

diagnosis rests on the identification in the lumina of blood vessels of globules of neutral fat that can be visualized by fat stains (Fig. 5–3). Globules of fat may also be found outside of the walls of blood vessels, either free or phagocytized. An inflammatory response unescapably follows the escape of fat globules in the affected parenchyma, and if the patient survives the immediate impact of the embolism, the tissue involved undergoes the changes associated with interference of blood flow, namely infarct necrosis in the areas of embolic distribution.

Whenever fat embolism results from injury to bone, the presence of bone marrow particles and bony spicules adds validity to the diagnosis.

Red cell aggregates, conglomerates of platelets, and intravascular hyaline microthrombi are not uncommon and probably play an important role in the causation of the microcirculatory disturbances associated with the syndrome of fat embolism.

With increasing interval between trauma and death, the number of emboli found at autopsy is inclined to diminish, and, as a rule, none can be found when the interval is more than four weeks.

Whereas systemic fat embolism is relatively uncommon, minor accumulations of fat globules in the lungs, in the absence of clinical signs and symptoms, are frequently found in patients expiring from various conditions.[72, 73] Frazer, impressed by the frequency of the finding, has suggested that minor degrees of pulmonary fat embolism are a normal accompaniment of digestive lipemia.[74] A similar concept has been expressed by Weld in his study, "Fat Absorption and Lung Oil."

The participation of the lungs in lipid metabolism has been known for a long time.[76] By the same token, well documented is the fact that pulmonary tissue can produce lipase.[77, 78] As a corollary to this demonstration, it has been suggested that release of lipase from the pulmonary tissue may result in hydrolysis of embolic fat and discharge of fatty acids, which in turn can be responsible for at least some of the aspects of the clinical syndrome.[79, 80] Furthermore, the released fatty acids bind calcium as a soap, and the ensuing hypocalcemia may provoke additional effects.

Diagnostic Value of Laboratory Methods

Fat macroglobules can be detected in sputum and blood frequently enough, both in patients with medical disorders and in normal individuals, to deny the finding as valid evidence of fat embolism.[18, 19]

Premortem diagnosis by cryostat frozen sections of clotted blood has been suggested; however, the demonstration of large fat globules in the blood of normal individuals points to the doubtful value of their detection as a diagnostic criterion of fat embolism.[81, 82]

In this connection it is of interest that blood procured by vacuo-collection from human volunteers showed denaturation of plasma proteins and alteration in the suspension stability

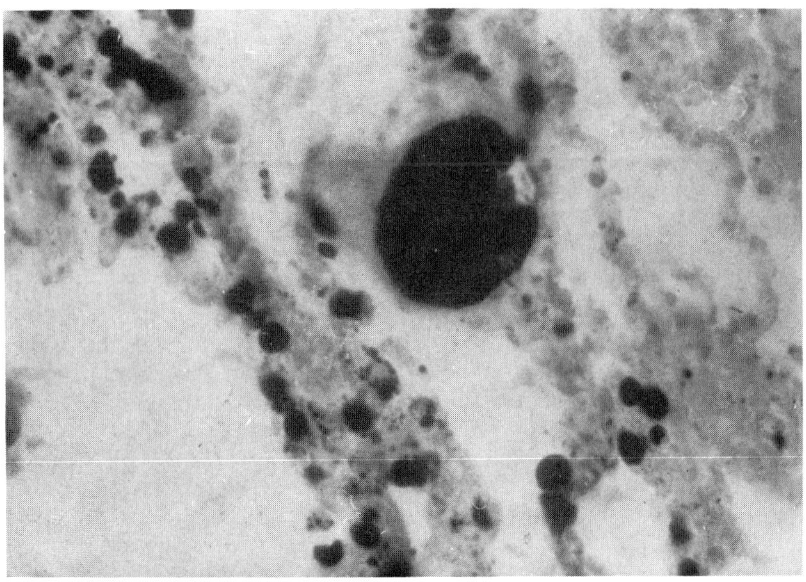

Figure 5–3. Microscopic view of fat globules in the lumina of pulmonary blood capillaries and larger vessels in the same case as Figure 5–2. Osmic acid stain.

of plasma lipids. It has been equally demonstrated that animals autotransfused with vacuo-collected blood may develop fat emboli.[83]

With the expectation of occasional false positive and false negative results, the demonstration of free fat in the urine can strengthen the diagnosis of fat embolism whenever this condition is suspected on the basis of other manifestations. In Thomas and Ayyar's series, lipuria was noted in nearly 50 per cent of the patients.[68]

A few investigators have pointed out a decrease in hemoglobin level to 50 per cent of normal in the absence of external loss of blood, a phenomenon variously attributed to hemolysis or hemodilution or both, from hemorrhage into the lungs or in the traumatized tissue.[68, 84] The platelet count is also worth monitoring inasmuch as it often falls much below normal levels. The underlying cause can be sought in their sequestration in microcirculation. It has been suggested that the petechial rash associated with fat embolism can be a manifestation of thrombocytopenia.[85]

Measurement of serum calcium levels can be of some value. Ross has described a condition of hypocalcemia in fatal cases of fat embolism that he attributed to the affinity of calcium ions for the released free fatty acids as the fat emboli become hydrolyzed.[86]

Examination of spinal fluid specimens in cases of fat embolism has long been neglected. The possibility that fat macroglobules circulating in the blood stream may reach the spinal fluid is substantiated by the observation of Schmidt and of Robb-Smith and associates of sudanophilic fat droplets in the vascular bed of the choroid plexus in patients dying from fat embolism.[87, 88] Sudanophilic fat globules have been shown by Cross in the spinal fluid of a patient with this condition.[89] Nevertheless, the demonstration of fat globules in random spinal fluid specimens seems to parallel their observation in urine, sputum, and circulating blood, showing the presence of free fat in such a variety of conditions, exclusive of trauma, as to invalidate the finding per se as concrete evidence of fat embolism.[90]

Equally uncertain is the value of serum lipase determinations. Evaluations of serum lipase and serum tributyrinase following trauma to bone may show a substantial rise in either or both enzyme levels. The diagnostic value of an increase of either enzyme has been stressed by Peltier and his group; however, it has been shown that morphine, frequently used in traumatized patients, often gives rise to an elevation of serum lipase levels, up to 20 times the normal.[91, 92] Whereas lipuria, as a rule, becomes manifest within 48 hours after the injury, elevation of serum lipase levels occurs later, approximately four days from the time of trauma.

Dines and his group have provided a useful guideline for monitoring the fat embolism syndrome. It includes: (1) determination of arterial blood gases (Pa_{O_2}, Pa_{CO_2}, pH) with the patient breathing room air as a base line, and then one daily determination for three days; (2) examination of cryostat frozen section of clotted blood in every case with Pa_{O_2} of less than 60 mm of mercury for the detection of neutral fat; (3) thoracic roentgenograms on admission and then daily for 72 hours; (4) daily funduscopic examination of 72 hours; and (5) daily determinations of hemoglobin, hematocrit, urinalysis, prothrombin time, platelet count, and serum calcium for 72 hours.[93]

This guideline of laboratory measurements should enable one to detect the subtle manifestations of subclinical fat embolism that are chiefly characterized by coagulation changes (platelet aggregation) and respiratory abnormalities in the absence of the classic signs and symptoms generally ascribed to the fat embolism syndrome.[94]

AIR EMBOLISM

The history of air embolism and that of fat embolism have some points in common. An analysis of underlying causes reveals both to be characterized by: (1) the transport in the circulatory system of foreign particles that are alien to the blood; (2) the ultimate lodging of those particles in the lumina of blood channels with consequent interference with blood flow in the territories affected by the occlusion; and (3) the source of the foreign particles, which can either be aspirated from an external milieu or result from an alteration in the suspension stability of the embolic matter.

For instance the manner in which bone marrow fat gains access to the blood stream in coincidence with a bone fracture is paralleled by the entrance of air through a tear in the wall of a vein or, rarely, an artery. By the same token, the alteration in the suspension stability of endogenous serum fat that results in the conversion of chylomicra into globules of fat is analogous to the liberation of endogenous gaseous nitrogen on exposure to an environmental pressure higher than that at sea level.

Finally, both fat and air embolism not infrequently occur in association. Evidence has been presented that one event (air embolism) can be responsible for the development of the other (fat embolism). Fat embolism resulting from exposure to simulated high altitudes in decompression chambers has been recorded.[95] A not unlikely explanation is that the force of the expanding nitrogen bubbles may tear the walls of the delicate blood channels, both in bone marrow and depot fat, allowing the entrance of free fat into the circulation.

Since fat is the most important reservoir for nitrogen, consideration has been given to the possible role of body build in the occurrence of the phenomenon. Evidence has been presented that during decompression more nitrogen is liberated into the blood stream in obese than in lean subjects.[96]

The subject of gaseous nitrogen embolism is dealt with in the section specifically concerned with the causes and effects of dysbarism or barotrauma (see Chapters 15 and 16). At this point it is sufficient to say that a good deal of similarity exists between the pathophysiologic changes attending the access of gases into the circulatory system and those arising from the liberation of endogenous gaseous nitrogen under conditions of increased or reduced barometric pressure.

The essential environment for normal existence at the cellular level, both in animals and plants, is provided by water and air. Chemical reactions within the cells take place in a water solvent, and air gases gain access to the cells in an aqueous medium.

According to *Henry's laws,* at constant temperature, the amount (by weight) of gas absorbed or dissolved by a given volume of liquid is proportional to the pressure of the gas. Thus, the solubility of gases in blood and tissue fluids is strictly dependent on the external pressure.

Two types of air embolism can occur: venous and arterial.

Prerequisites for the development of venous embolism are: an opened vessel in a state of partial collapse, suction produced by negative intravenous pressure, and the introduction of air under positive pressure.

The air or gas, after entering the blood stream, acts as a foreign particle *(air embolus)* that, following the venous circulation, is carried to the right ventricle, thereby blocking the pulmonary blood flow. If only small amounts of air gain access to the circulation the fine bubbles that are carried from the heart to the pulmonary arteries become disseminated and are absorbed in the lungs, and no harmful effects are elicited. Conversely if large amounts of air reach the heart rapidly, a large air bubble is formed that prevents the blood from flowing from the right ventricle into the pulmonic artery. The resulting churning action is responsible for the loud murmur (audible to anyone in the room), the so called *mill-wheel murmur,* that is diagnostic of air embolism. The resultant right ventricular failure leads to increases in venous pressure with distention of the neck veins, decrease in peripheral arterial blood pressure, a rapid thready pulse, cyanosis, dyspnea, and syncope due to cerebral anoxia. Ultimately cardiac arrest substantiates the diagnosis of venous air embolism.

Diagnosis can be verified at autopsy by in situ clamping of the major blood vessels of the heart, both arteries and veins, and by transferring the heart en bloc with attached blood vessels to a basin filled with water. When the walls of the right side of the heart are incised, the right auricle and ventricle and the pulmonary artery as well are found to be distended by bright red frothy blood, resulting from the thorough mixing of air and blood. Another important finding is a column of bubbles extending from the site of entrance of air to the right chambers of the heart.

Atmospheric oxygen may be demonstrated in the heart up to 72 hours after death. Beyond this time absence of oxygen does not exclude the possibility of air embolism.

Antemortem air embolism must be differentiated from postmortem gas formation in conjunction with invasion of the blood stream by gas-forming bacilli. When this has occurred, bubbles of gas are found throughout the vascular system, arteries and veins as well.

No reliable figures are available on the quantity of air capable of causing death in man. In one case, the patient died after vaginal insufflation of 300 ml.[97] A fatal outcome followed the presacral insufflation of 1000 ml. of oxygen.[98] In the six cases of pneumoperitoneum reported by Burman, one patient receiving 400 ml expired, whereas the others, receiving amounts varying from 300 to 1600 ml, tolerated the procedure well.[99]

Animal experiments have given equally variable results. In a study in dogs, 7.5 ml of air per kilogram of body weight, injected in five seconds or less, produced death in all tested animals.[100] This would be equivalent to 525 ml in a 70-kg man. Obviously, the speed with which the air gains access to the circulation plays a very important role in determining the outcome of the event. An experiment by Richardson and co-workers indicates that one dog was able to tolerate 1377 ml of air in 460 minutes before dying.[101]

With reference to the amount of air, the situation arising in conjunction with arterial embolism is of an entirely different nature. The access of a few milliliters of air in the arterial circulation can be lethal if the bubble becomes impacted in the inflow vessel to a vital organ. Myocardial infarction has been recorded in concurrence with air embolism in one of the coronary arteries coincidental to artificial pneumothorax.[102, 103]

Injuries in the neck, involving the carotid artery or the jugular veins or both, are most likely to give rise to arterial air embolism. If the air enters the carotid artery it is carried directly to the brain; if instead it gains access to one of the jugular veins, the embolus is carried to the left chambers of the heart and then into the systemic circulation.

Coincidental to cerebral embolism, a broad spectrum of neurologic manifestations may develop, including sudden aphasia, blindness, hemiplegia, and convulsions. Ophthalmoscopic examination may reveal air bubbles in the retinal arteries. The diagnosis of air embolism may be further substantiated by the unexpected appearance of a marbled discoloration of the skin, usually in the upper parts of the body. A small incision in the skin so affected may show that the blood contains air bubbles. This phenomenon, known as "air bleeding," is definite proof that arterial embolism has taken place.[104]

When a patient dies, the head should be examined first and the calvaria removed with caution to avoid aspiration of air into the cerebral vessels. As in fat embolism, the demonstration of the emboli in the vascular bed of the choroid plexus provides convincing evidence of air embolism. The presence in the brain of disseminated areas of ischemic necrosis further substantiates the diagnosis. It is not clear why the infarcts attending air embolism are as a rule ischemic, in contrast with the infarcts associated with solid bodies, which in general are of the hemorrhagic type.

Air embolism produces two independent vascular effects that in reality do not differ from the response elicited by any other kind of embolic foreign body: one is mechanical obstruction, and the other is of the nature of a neurovascular spasm.[105]

An experiment in animals by Moore and Braselton indicates that the minimum lethal dose of oxygen is 10 per cent greater than that of air. Comparing the effects of carbon dioxide and air, these investigators noticed that 0.25 ml of air per pound of body weight was ineffectual, whereas over 0.5 ml per pound was consistently lethal. In contrast, carbon dioxide, up to 3 ml per pound, had no ill effects. This would correspond to 37.5 ml in a 150-lb man.[106]

Harkins and Harmon, comparing the effects of air and oxygen introduced into the peripheral circulation, found that the minimal lethal dose of both gases was the same – 8 ml per kilogram.[107] In a similar investigation in dogs, Goodwin and Harmel noticed that helium and oxygen had comparable effects and that intraarterial administration of the gas was better tolerated than the intravascular inoculation by the venous route.[108]

The greater safety of carbon dioxide probably is due to its twentyfold greater solubility in blood as compared to air and to its ability to combine with the alkaline buffer systems of the blood. It would seem that oxygen is intermediate in its embolic potential, and that the effects of helium and nitrogen parallel those of air.

Devices are available to trap, quantitate, and analyze in an airtight system gases obtained from the heart or blood vessels. Erben and Nádvorník's apparatus, which basically consists of an aspirometer and oxygenometer, allows the simultaneous determination of air and putrefactive gases.[109]

Air embolism can occur under a wide variety of circumstances, including therapeutic error or carelessness.

Wounds in the neck are apt to involve large veins and arteries, and because of this, can be rapidly fatal. Penetrating wounds of the lungs can equally lead to aspiration of air into the pulmonary veins and from there into the general circulation, ultimately resulting in cerebral air embolism.

Two cases are on record of suicidal attempts by injection of air; in one case 60 ml of air was self-injected into an antecubital vein, and in the other 20 ml was injected on two different occasions. In both cases the attempt failed and there were no adverse effects.[110] Most unusual is the case reported by Cooke of self-induced death, either accidental or deliberate, following injection of air in the urethra with an atomizer bulb.[111] Equally unusual was the self-inflicted death of a transvestite following injection of air in the scrotal sac with a bicycle pump.[112]

Any operative procedure about the head or neck affords the possibility of air entering a vein. Death has occurred during tracheostomy, thyroidectomy, lavage of the nasal sinuses, and neurosurgical procedures, particularly when the patient was in Fowler's or sitting position.[116, 117]

The use of gases as contrast media for the radiologic visualization of portions of the human body are not so popular today as formerly, just because of the hazards connected with the procedure.

Death has been reported following injection of air into the knee joint, presacral insufflation of air, ventriculography, and pneumoencephalography.[118-122] Injection of air into the male urethra coincidental to urethrocystography has also been responsible for embolic death.[123] The recent advent of open heart surgery with extracorporeal circulation has provided another avenue for the entrance of air into the pulmonary artery.[124]

Transfusion of blood under pressure probably accounts for more deaths by air embolism than any other procedure. While the use of collapsible plastic blood containers has reduced the hazards connected with the method, the container is only one part involved in the system and there is no way to deliver blood under pressure without the potential risk of producing venous air embolism and death. Indeed, any needle placed in the venous system carries the risk of causing air embolism.[125]

With the advent of chemotherapy and antibiotic administration for the treatment of tuberculosis, pneumothorax and pneumoperitoneum have been abandoned. When these therapeutic procedures were fashionable, many deaths from air embolism were recorded. Just to cite a single large series, 74 deaths from air embolism were reported by Dasher and associates in 1954 among 127 patients subjected to pneumoperitoneum.[126]

The majority of conditions predisposing to air embolism are found in the areas of gynecology and obstetrics. The presence of large venous sinuses in both the gravid and the nongravid uterus combined with a source of air such as that provided by vaginal insufflation and douching, tubal insufflation, presacral pneumography, and attempted self-abortion set an ideal stage for air embolism. According to Haynes, more than 100 cases of fatal air embolism following attempts at abortion had been reported up to 1956.[127] Death by air embolism has even occurred during normal labor, without any injection of air.[128-130] This situation belongs to the unusual. Equally unusual, but well-documented, is air embolism from aspiration of air into the lower genital tract during knee-chest exercises shortly after childbirth, in concurrence with ruptured uterus, and following postpartum surgical sterilization.[130-133]

From the study of Cockett, Mangelson, and Kado it would appear that prompt parasympathetic blockage by intravenous atropine may significantly improve the ultimate outcome for patients who develop oxygen embolism while undergoing a variety of procedures.[134]

EMBOLISM FROM TISSUE COMPONENTS

Pulmonary embolism from tissue or tissue components is a well-recognized and far from uncommon phenomenon. Pulmonary embolism involving chorionic tissue takes place in about 50 per cent of women in the course of normal gestation, and to some extent it can be considered a physiologic event. Chorionic emboli usually degenerate and disappear; however, maternal death from right-sided heart failure has been reported in both normal and abnormal gestation following massive embolism of chorionic elements.[135, 136] In the loosely analogous situation of patients with chorionic tumors, dissemination of the neoplastic trophoblast into the systemic circulation has been recorded with equal frequency. Park and Lees, in their analysis of the common sites of metastases in 123 patients dying of choriocarcinoma, state that about one third of the patients had involvement of brain, liver, and kidney, and about one fifth had involvement of spleen and intestines.[137] Also in the field of obstetrics, and equally well documented, is embolism by amniotic fluid.[138]

Injury by mechanical trauma is regularly associated with disarrangement of tissue structure and tearing of the walls of small blood channels. This combination provides an ideal situation for the entrance into circulation of fragments of tissue or tissue components.

Pulmonary embolism by liver cells in coincidence with hepatic trauma and bone marrow embolism in concurrence with fracture of long bones are of common knowledge.[139] A report in the medical literature describes skin embolism from a venipuncture site; and another case is on record of embolism from transitional epithelium, presumably arising at the site of a severe ulcerative urethritis.[140, 141]

Brain components must be included among the tissues capable of embolizing following disruption of normal structure. With 15 cases on record up to 1967, and, as far as we could ascertain, no additional cases reported thereafter, pulmonary embolism by brain tissue, without a doubt, is a rare phenomenon.[144-152] McMillan's 4 cases, the largest individual series so far reported, drawn from 213 cases of severe head injury, give to the phenomenon an incidence of approximately 2 per cent.[149]

The dimensions of the embolism may vary from a single microscopic embolus of brain tissue, accidentally found in the lung of a 23-month-old child who died following a head injury, to massive embolization of cortical tissue in a patient who underwent a decompression operation for skull fracture (in this case, fragments of brain tissue were visible grossly in the major pulmonary arteries).[145, 147]

In 11 of the recorded cases, the embolism could be linked to head trauma of one type or another, resulting in skull fracture and severe laceration of the brain. The remaining four cases were in infants who presumably suffered trauma at delivery.[142, 143, 152]

The contrast between the relative frequency of head injury, either during delivery or incident to trauma in postnatal life, and the rarity of pulmonary brain embolism, suggest that certain uncommon predisposing factors must be present to determine the occurrence of the phenomenon. The nature and types of these factors have not been clarified yet.

Pulmonary brain embolism is an event entirely distinct from heterotopia of neural tissue in the lung parenchyma. The differentiation rests primarily on the fact that in the heterotopias the neural tissue is embedded within the pulmonary tissue, whereas in posttraumatic embolism, the neural tissue is found within branches of the pulmonary vessels. This does not rule out that the heterotopias also may have their remote origin in some traumatic experience early in gestation, with resultant embolization of neural tissue to the lungs.

Since mature cells, once detached from their milieu, usually degenerate and, given time, disappear, the deleterious effects evoked by emboli from normal tissue components by and large do not differ from those elicited by a blood embolus or an air bubble.

A situation of an entirely different nature attends the embolization by tumor cells (Fig. 5–4). The potentiality of a malignant tumor to produce *metastases* is one of the major features of a cancerous growth. In keeping with their invasive characteristics, tumor cells enter the blood or lymph stream, or both, become seeded in distant organs, and under favorable conditions, multiply, giving rise to a tumor, which to a considerable extent possesses the same characteristics as the tumor from which they have originated. Tumor cells in transit (so-called neoplastic emboli) can frequently be retrieved from the blood of cancer patients, primarily from the venous blood draining the tumor.

Rather uncommon is the situation of major arterial obstruction, distal vascular insufficiency, and gangrene of the affected tissue from detached fragments of a tumor, mostly a cardiac myxoma or a vascular endothelial tumor.[153-157]

Similarly unusual is the occurrence of fibrin (hyaline) thrombi in conjunction with tumor cell embolus from mucinous adenocarcinoma.[158]

The concepts of growth, rate of growth, and tumor metastases are inherent in the natural history of cancer. This being the case, the question whether mechanical trauma, single or repeated, can hasten the course of the disease by

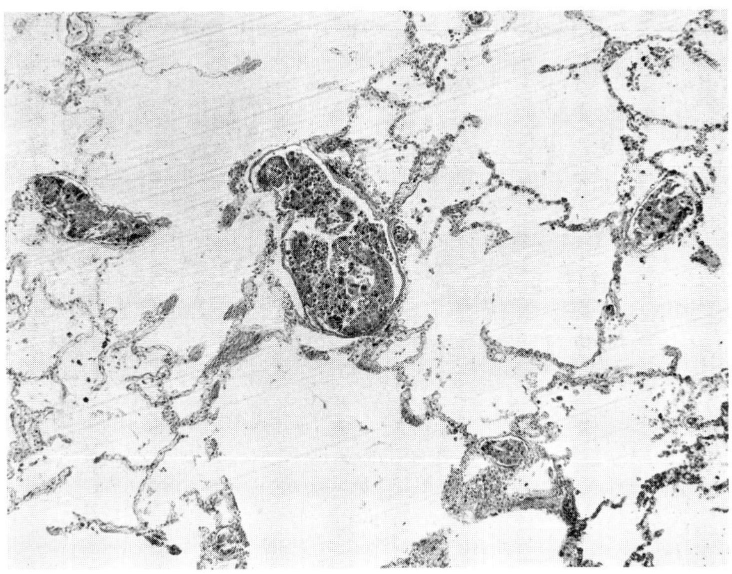

Figure 5–4. Emboli of tumor cells (hepatocellular carcinoma) in pulmonary blood vessels.

inducing tumor metastases or influencing their localization provides a complex challenge in compensation courts.[159-162]

The idea that a single mechanical injury can stimulate the occurrence of tumor metastasis lacks scientific substantiation. Occasional reports, however, bring forth some evidence in support of a causal relation between trauma and localization of tumor particles circulating in the blood or lymph stream. By the same token, it has been stated that repeated rubbing or squeezing of a tumor can produce tissue disruption and thus favor the development of metastasis.

Since the cause of cancer is unknown, and equally poorly understood is the intimate life history of the process, it can hardly be expected that a fair opinion be rendered by a court of law on the causal relationships between uncomplicated trauma and cancer formation and any of its manifestations.

FOREIGN BODY EMBOLIZATION

The first report of embolization by a foreign body, according to Straus, is attributed to Davis (1834). The embolus consisted of a large wooden fragment that, from the right anterior aspect of the chest, entered the superior vena cava to be carried to the heart, ultimately lodging in the right ventricle. The patient survived 37 days and presumably died of sepsis.[163]

A relatively extensive literature thereafter records venous embolization to the heart of foreign bodies of the most extravagant nature, including pins, thorns, bones, bullets, and iatrogenically introduced objects such as hypodermic and radium needles, intravenous catheters, and cotton fiber during angiography.[164–169]

Among the embolizing objects, bullets rank first in Padula and co-workers' survey: 27 of the 43 embolized objects were bullets. In about half the cases, the bullet migrated to the heart immediately after entering the venous circulation, whereas in the other half a delay of two days to 13 months intervened between wounding and embolization.[170]

Most unusual is Hiebert's case, reported by *Time* magazine, of a bullet entering the skull, penetrating the transverse sinus, and migrating to the right ventricle of the heart.[171] Similarly astonishing are the circumstances related to a case described by Padula and associates of a bullet embolized from the abdomen to the right ventricle and removed 14 years later because of severe cardiac neurosis.[170]

Foreign bodies within the heart chambers are generally well tolerated. Although the majority of foreign objects in most locations within the heart may remain dormant and produce no serious difficulties, irreversible or fatal complications may arise when the foreign body is of relatively large dimensions or impinges upon papillary muscles, chordae tendinae, or valve leaflets. Infection from contaminated objects is another major threat.

With the relative safety of cardiac surgery today, the prevailing opinion is that intracardiac foreign bodies should be removed.[172, 173] Surgical intervention and removal of the foreign body are primarily indicated to prevent the embolus from mobilizing and proceeding further, to reduce the danger of detachment of the frequently associated thrombus, and to diminish the incidence of bacterial endocarditis and recurrent pericardial effusions.

The psychologic morbidity arising in concurrence with intracardiac foreign bodies is another element not to be overlooked. Cardiac neurosis is a frequent complication associated with an intracardiac foreign body. Bland and Beebe, in their 20-year follow-up study of World War II veterans with missiles in the heart, stress the cardiac neurosis factor that can reach such serious proportions as to incapacitate the patient entirely, even in the absence of any cardiac functional disorder.[174]

Peripheral embolization from an intracavitary bullet wound is uncommon but its occurrence has been recorded.[175] Most frequently peripheral embolization is caused by a gunshot wound of the chest involving the thoracic aorta.[176] Expectedly the left iliac and femoral arterial system are the most frequent sites of embolization because of the lesser angle at the point of origin of the artery at the aortic bifurcation. Of 36 patients in which this occurrence was assessed, in 17 the bullet had migrated to the left iliac artery or lower, and in the other 9 the embolus had lodged in the aorta or had entered upper extremity vessels.[177] Clot formation and propagation are frequent complications of distant bullet embolism.

REFERENCES

THROMBOEMBOLISM

1. McKay, D. G.: Trauma and disseminated intravascular coagulation. J. Trauma, *9*:646, [Aug.] 1969.
2. Borgstrom, S., Gelin, L. E., and Zederfeldt, B.: The formation of vein thrombi following tissue injury: an experimental study in rabbits. Acta Chir. Scand. Suppl., *247*:1, 1959.
3. Coon, W. W., and Hodgson, P. E.: Fibrinolysis in surgery patients. I. Possible relationship to a hemorrhagic diathesis. Surg. Gynecol. Obstet., *95*:717, 1952.

4. Crowell, J. W., Sharpe, G. P., Lambright, R. L., and Read, W. L.: The mechanism of death after resuscitation following acute circulatory failure. Surgery, *38*:696, 1955.
5. Hardaway, R. M.: *Syndromes of Disseminated Intravascular Coagulation.* Springfield, Ill., Charles C Thomas, 1966.
6. Crowell, J. W., and Read, W. L.: In vivo coagulation: a probable cause of irreversible shock. Am. J. Physiol., *183*:565, 1955.
7. Whitaker, A. N., and McKay, D. G.: Induction of hypotension in rhesus monkeys and rabbits by intravenous thrombin infusion. Lab. Invest., *20*:79, 1969.
8. McKay, D. G., Margaretten, W., and Csavossy, I.: An electron microscope study of endotoxin shock in rhesus monkeys. Surg. Gynecol. Obstet., *125*:825, 1967.
9. Whitaker, A. N., and McKay, D. G.: Disseminated intravascular coagulation in rabbits by intravenous infusion of epinephrine. Fed. Proc., *27*:569, 1968.
10. Cannon, W. B., and Gray, H.: Factors affecting the coagulation time of blood. II. The hastening or retarding of coagulation by adrenalin injection. Am. J. Physiol., *34*:232, 1914.
11. Cannon, W. B., and Mendenhall, W. L.: Factors affecting the coagulation time of blood. IV. The hastening of coagulation in pain and emotional excitement. Am. J. Physiol., *34*:251, 1914.
12. Correll, J. W.: Central neural structure and pathways important for control of blood clotting: evidence for release of anti-heparin factor. International Conference on Microcirculation. Abstract. 1968, p. 36, Gothenburg.
13. Attar, S., Boyd, D., Layne, E., McLaughlin, J., Mansberger, A. R., and Cowley, R. A.: Alterations in coagulation and fibrinolytic mechanisms in acute trauma. J. Trauma, *9*:939, [Nov.] 1969.
14. Hodgkinson, C. P., Thompson, R. J., Hodari, A. A.: Dead fetus syndrome. Clin. Obstet. Gynecol., *7*:349, 1967.
15. Myburgh, J. A., Williams, G. M., Hume, D. M., Hudson, R. P., Jr., Morris, R. J., Kano, K., and Milgram, F.: Hyperacute rejection in human kidney allografts. Shwartzman or Arthus? N. Engl. J. Med., *281*:131, 1969.
16. Lee, L., Prose, P. H., and Cohen, M. H.: The role of the reticuloendothelial system in diffuse, low grade intravascular coagulation. Thromb. Diath. Haemorrh. Suppl., *20*:97, 1966.

FAT EMBOLISM

17. Tedeschi, C. G.: Pathologic anatomy of adipose tissue. In *Handbook of Physiology.* Section 5. Chapter 14. Edited by A. E. Renold and G. F. Cahill, Jr. Washington, D.C., American Physiological Society, 1965, pp. 141–168.
18. Tedeschi, C. G., Castelli, W., Kropp, G., and Tedeschi, L. G.: Fat macroglobulinemia and fat embolism. Surg. Gynecol. Obstet., 126:83, 1968.
19. Tedeschi, C. G., Walter, C. E., and Tedeschi, L. G.: Shock and fat embolism: an appraisal. Surg. Clin. North Am., *48*:431, 1968.
20. Grant, R. T., and Reeve, E. B.: *Observations on the General Effects of Injury in Man.* Medical Research Council, Special Report Series 277. London, His Majesty's Stationary Office, 1951.
21. Speed, K.: *Fractures and Dislocation.* Philadelphia, J. B. Lippincott Co., 1916.
22. Nicod, J. L.: Fat embolism in the newborn. Schweiz. Med. Wochenschr., *19*:845, 1938.
23. Bissell, W. W.: Pulmonary fat embolism: a frequent cause of post-operative surgical shock. Surg. Gynecol. Obstet., *25*:8, 1917.
24. Carter, B. N., Christainsen, J. N., and Prior, J. A.: Fat embolism as a post-operative complication of extrapleural thoracoplasty. J. Thorac. Surg., *10*:641, 1941.
25. Ferguson, H. F.: Fat embolism following incision of female breast for diffuse suppuration. Br. Med. J., *1*:584, 1895.
26. Robinson, J. R.: Fat embolism following abdominal surgery. Am. J. Surg., *78*:401, 1949.
27. Kent, S. P.: Fat embolism in diabetic patients without physical trauma. Am. J. Pathol., *31*:399, 1955.
28. Warren, S.: Fat embolism. Am. J. Pathol., *22*:69, 1946.
29. Zon, L., and Warren, S.: The chylomicron count in diabetes mellitus. Proc. Soc. Exp. Biol. Med., *33*:236, 1935–1936.
30. MacMahon, H. E., and Weiss, S.: Carbon tetrachloride poisoning with macroscopic fat in the pulmonary artery. Am. J. Pathol., *5*:623, 1929.
31. Lynch, M. J.: Nephrosis and fat embolism in acute haemorrhagic pancreatitis. A.M.A. Arch. Intern. Med., *94*:709, 1954.
32. Carrara, M.: Ueber die Fettembolie der Lungen in ihren Beziehungen zur gerichtlichen Medicin. Fried Bl. Gerichtl. Med. Sanitätspol., *49*:241, 1898.
33. Fazekas, I. G.: Fettembolien bei experimenteller Natriumhydroxyd-und Ammoniumhydroxyd-Vergiftung. Frankfurt Z. Pathol., *51*:524, 1938.
34. Lynch, M. J. G., Raphael, S. S., and Dixon, T. P.: Fat embolism in chronic alcoholism. A.M.A. Arch. Pathol., *67*:68, 1959.
35. Burns, E. L., and Bromberg, L.: Fatal multiple fat embolism in a patient given salvarsan. Am. J. Syph., *14*:43, 1930.
36. Case Record No. 48-1962, Massachusetts General Hospital. N. Engl. J. Med., *267*:200, 1962.
37. Owens, G., and Sokal, J. E.: Liver lipid as a source of embolic fat. J. Appl. Physiol., *16*:1100, 1961.
38. Owens, G., and Northington, B. A.: Liver lipid as a source of post-traumatic embolic fat. J. Surg. Res., *2*:283, 1962.
39. Raphael, S. S., and Lynch, M. J. G.: Kimmelstiel-Wilson glomerulo-nephropathy: its occurrence in diseases other than diabetes mellitus. A.M.A. Arch. Pathol., *65*:420, 1958.
40. Whiteley, H. J.: Relation between tissue injury and the manifestations of pulmonary fat embolism. J. Pathol. Bacteriol., *67*:521, 1954.
41. Cooke, W. T., et al.: Clostridial infections in war wounds. Lancet, *1*:487, 1945.
42. Catsaras, J.: Embolies graisseuses pulmonaires dans la bronchopneumonie grippale. Presse Méd., *28*:618, 1920.
43. Hedri, A.: Wann and wie soll die Osteomyelitis im akuten Stadium operiert werden? Langenbecks Arch. Klin. Chir., *138*:596, 1925.
44. Graber, S.: Fat embolization associated with sickle-cell crisis. South. Med. J., *54*:1395, 1961.
45. Miller, J. A., Fonkalsrud, W. W., Latta, H. L., and Maloney, J. V.: Fat embolism associated with extracorporeal circulation and blood transfusion. Surgery, *51*:448, 1962.
46. Owens, G., Adams, J. E., and Scott, H. W.: Embolic fat as a measure of adequacy of various oxygenators. J. Appl. Physiol., *15*:999, 1960.
47. Lee, W. H., Krumharr, D., Fonkalsrud, E., Schjeide, O. A., and Maloney, J. V.: Denaturation of plasma proteins as a cause of morbidity and death after intracardiac operations. Surgery, *50*:29, 1961.

48. Bron, K. M., Baum, S., and Abrams, H. L.: Oil embolism in lymphangiography; incidence, manifestations and mechanism. Radiology, *80*:194, 1963.
49. Gelin, L. E.: Disturbances of the flow properties of blood in surgery. Acta Chir. Scand., *122*:287, 1961.
50. Borgstrom, S., Gelin, L. E., and Zederfeldt, B.: Formation of vein thrombi following tissue injury. Acta Chir. Scand. (Suppl.), *247*:1, 1959.
51. Adkins, R. B., Foster, J. H., and O'Salle, D.: Experimental study of the genesis of fat embolism. Ann. Surg., *156*:515, 1962.
52. Bergentz, S. E., Gelin, L. E., and Rudenstam, C. M.: Intravascular aggregation of blood cells following intravenous infusion of fat emulsions. Acta Chir. Scand., *120*:115, 1960.
53. Bergentz, S. E.: Studies on the genesis of post-traumatic fat embolism. Acta Chir. Scand., (Suppl.) *282*:1, 1961.
54. Bergentz, S. E., Gelin, L. E., and Rudenstam, C. M.: Fats and thrombus formation. Thromb. Diath. Haemorrh., *264*:474, 1961.
55. Bergentz, S. E., Gelin, L. E., Hallgren, B., Rudenstam, C. M., and Svanborg, A.: Influence of trauma on the lipids in blood and lung tissue. Acta Chir. Scand., *124*:377, 1962.
56. Löfström, B.: Intravascular aggregation and oxygen consumption. Aggregation of red cells produced by high molecular weight dextran or by hypothermia. Acta Anaesthesiol. Scand., *2*:41, 1959.
57. Gelin, L. E.: Studies in anemia of injury. Acta Chir. Scand., (Suppl.) *210*:130, 1956.
58. Cammermeyer, J.: Subacute cerebral fat embolism complicated by juxtaembolic thrombosis of fibrin. A.M.A. Arch. Pathol., *56*:254, 1953.
59. Fuchsig, P., Brücke, P., Blümel, G., et al.: A new clinical and experimental concept of fat embolism. N. Engl. J. Med., *276*:1192, 1967.
60. Davis, H. L., and Musselman, M. M.: Blood particle agglomeration and fat embolism. Int. Rec. Med., *167*:439, 1954.
61. Brücke, P., Bümel, G., and Gottlob, R.: Über die Fettresorption bei Volumenmangel: Ein experimenteller Beitrag zur Pathogenese der Fettembolie. Arch. Klin. Chir., *313*:1049, 1965.
62. Scriba, J.: Untersuchungen über die Fettembolie, Dtsch. Z. Chir., *12*:118, 1880.
63. Wilson, J. V., and Salisbury, C. V.: Fat embolism in war surgery. Br. J. Surg., *31*:384, 1943.
64. Lehman, E. P., and McNattin, R. F.: Fat embolism. III. Incidence at postmortem. Arch. Surg., *17*:179, 1928.
65. Wiener, L., and Forsyth, D.: Pulmonary pathophysiology of fat embolism. Am. Rev. Resp. Dis., *92*:113, 1965.
66. Fuchsig, P.: Neue Erkentnisse in Pathogenese and Therapie der Fettembole. Arch. Klin. Chir., *316*:243, 1966.
67. Fuchsig, P., Brücke, P., Blümel, G., and Gottlob, R.: A new clinical and experimental concept of fat embolism. N. Engl. J. Med., *276*:1192, 1967.
68. Thomas, J. E., and Ayyar, D. R.: Systemic fat embolism. Arch. Neurol., *26*:517, 1972.
69. Wagman, E., Barbara, A., Marquis, J., Chirls, M., and Falla, A.: Renal fat embolization and urostealith formation complicating femoral fracture. J.A.M.A., *198*:721, 1966.
70. Sevitt, S.: Significance and classification of fat embolism. Lancet, *2*:825, 1960.
71. Stephens, J. H., and Fred, H. L.: Petechiae associated with systemic fat embolism. Arch. Dermatol., *84*:515, 1962.
72. Scully, R. E.: Fat embolism in Korean Battle casualties; its incidence, clinical significance and pathologic aspects. Am. J. Pathol., *32*:379, 1956.
73. Tedeschi, C. G., Walter, C. E., and Tedeschi, L. G.: Shock and fat embolism: an appraisal. Surg. Clin. North Am., *48*:431, 1968.
74. Frazer, A. C.: Comment. Proc. R. Soc. Med., *34*:651, 1941.
75. Weld, C. B.: Fat absorption and lung oil. Can. J. Res., E., *26*:274, 1948.
76. Sieber, N.: Splitting of fats by lung tissue. Hoppe Seylers Z. Physiol. Chem., *55*:177, 1908.
77. Rona, P., and Reinicke, D.: On the study of toxicity. Biochem. Z., *118*:213, 1921.
78. Gomori, G.: Distribution of lipase in the tissues under normal and pathological conditions. Arch. Pathol., *41*:121, 1946.
79. Peltier, L. F., Adler, F., and Lai, S.: Fat embolism: the significance of an elevated serum lipase after trauma to bone. Am. J. Surg., *99*:821, 1960.
80. Scuderi, C. S.: Fat embolism. A clinical and experimental study. Surg. Gynecol. Obstet., *72*:732, 1941.
81. Huaman, A., Nice, W., and Young, I.: Fat embolism syndrome: premortem diagnosis by cryostat frozen section. J. Kans. Med. Soc., *70*:487, 1969.
82. Tedeschi, L. G., Castelli, W. P., and Tedeschi, C. G.: Fat particles in plasma. The macroglobule: its relevance to the concept of fat embolism. Hum. Pathol., *2*:165, 1971.
83. Fadali, A. M. A., and Walstad, P. M.: In vacuo blood collection: a possible cause of fat emboli. Surgery, *71*:738, 1972.
84. Fischer, J. E., Turner, R. H., Herndon, J. H., et al.: Massive steroid therapy in severe fat embolism. Surg. Gynecol. Obstet., *132*:667, 1971.
85. Wertzberger, J. J., and Peltier, L. F.: Fat embolism: the importance of arterial hypoxia. Surgery, *63*:626, 1968.
86. Ross, A. P.: The fat embolism syndrome: with special reference to the importance of hypoxia in the syndrome. Ann. R. Coll. Surg. Engl., *46*:159, 1970.
87. Schmidt, O. (Breslau): Zum Nachweis cerebralen Fett- und Luftembolie. Dtsch. Z. Gesamte Gerichtl. Med., *13*:231, 1929.
88. Robb-Smith, A. H. T., Hung, A. H., Russell, D., and Greenfield, J. G.: Discussion on fat embolism and brain. Proc. R. Soc. Med., *34*:639, 1941.
89. Cross, H. E.: Examination of cerebrospinal fluid in fat embolism: report of a case. Arch. Intern. Med., *115*:470, 1965.
90. Tedeschi, C. G., Walter, C. E., Lepore, T., and Tedeschi, L. G.: An assessment of the cerebrospinal fluid and choroid plexus in relation to systemic fat embolism. Neurology (Minneap.), *19*:586, 1969.
91. Peltier, L. F., Adler, F., and Lai, S. P.: Fat embolism: the significance of an elevated serum lipase after trauma to bone. Am. J. Surg., *99*:821, 1960.
92. Wapshaw, H.: The pancreatic side effects of morphine. Br. Med. J., *1*:373, 1953.
93. Dines, D. E., Linscheid, R. L., and Didier, E. P.: Fat embolism syndrome. Mayo Clin. Proc., *47*:237, 1972.
94. McCarthy, B., Mammen, E., Leblanc, L. P., and Wilson, R. F.: Subclinical fat embolism: A prospective study of 50 patients with extremity fractures. J. Trauma, *13*:9, 1973.

AIR EMBOLISM

95. Haymaker, W., and Davison, C.: Fatalities resulting from exposure to simulated high altitudes in decompression chambers: A clinicopathological study

of five cases. J. Neuropathol. Exp. Neurol., *9*:29, 1950.
96. Armstrong, H. G.: *Principles and Practice of Aviation Medicine*. 2nd Ed. Baltimore, Williams & Wilkins Co., 1943.
97. Martland, H. S.: Air embolism: fatal air embolism due to powder insufflators used in gynecologic treatments. Am. J. Surg., *68*:164, 1945.
98. Ransom, C. L., Londes, R. R., and McLelland, R.: Air embolism following retroperitoneal pneumography. J. Urol., *76*:664, 1956.
99. Burman, D.: Air embolism during pneumoperitoneum treatment. Thorax, *11*:49, 1956.
100. Oppenheimer, M. J., Durant, T. M., and Lynch, P.: Body position in relation to venous air embolism and the associated cardiovascular-respiratory changes. Am. J. Med. Sci., *225*:362, 1937.
101. Richardson, H. F., Coles, B. C., and Hall, G. E.: Experimental gas embolism. Can. Med. Assoc. J., *36*:584, 1937.
102. Durant, T. M.: The occurrence of coronary air embolism in artificial pneumothorax. Ann. Intern. Med., *8*:1625, 1935.
103. Pollak, M.: Air embolus. Am. Rev. Tuberc., *28*:187, 1933.
104. Cohen, A. C., Glinsky, G. C., Martin, G. E., and Fetterhoff, K. I.: Air embolism. Ann. Intern. Med., *35*:779, 1951.
105. Chase, W. H.: Anatomical and experimental observations on air embolism. Surg. Gynecol. Obstet., *54*:569, 1934.
106. Moore, R. M., and Braselton, C. W., Jr.: Injections of air and of carbon dioxide into pulmonary vein. Ann. Surg., *112*:212, 1940.
107. Harkins, H. M., and Harmon, P. H.: Embolism by air and oxygen: comparative studies. Proc. Soc. Exp. Biol. Med., *32*:178, 1934.
108. Goodwin, W. E., and Harmel, M. H.: Intravascular administration of oxygen and helium. Experiments on intravascular administration of oxygen and helium. Curr. Res. Anesth. Analg., *28*:255, 1949.
109. Erben, J., and Nádvorník, F.: The quantitative demonstration of air embolism. J. Forensic Med., *10*:45, 1963.
110. Nitsche, H. G., quoted by Buxton, C. L.: Death from air embolus. Report of case following tubal insufflation. Am. J. Obstet. Gynecol., *74*:430, 1957.
111. Cooke, R. T.: Self-induced air embolism in a man. Br. Med. J., *2*:1197, 1961.
112. Adelson, L.: Fatal air embolism following intrascrotal injection in a transvestite. J. Forensic Sci., *2*:291, 1957.
113. Asherton, N.: Tracheostomy: sudden death from air embolism. J. Laryngol., *72*:743, 1958.
114. Larson, L. M., and Nordland, M.: Air embolism complicating thyroidectomy. Am. Surg., *99*:112, 1934.
115. Thomson, K. F.: Air embolism following antral lavage. J. Laryngol., *69*:829, 1955.
116. Emery, E. R.: Air embolism. A report of two cases. Anaesthesia, *17*:455, 1962.
117. Hunter, A. R.: Air embolism in the sitting position. Anaesthesia, *17*:467, 1962.
118. Kleinberg, S.: Pulmonary embolism following oxygen injection of a knee. J.A.M.A., *89*:172, 1927.
119. Russ, F. H., Glenn, D. L., and Gianturco, C.: Gas embolism during extraperitoneal insufflation. Radiology, *61*:637, 1953.
120. Glassman, I., Chapiro, R., and Robinson, F.: Air embolism during presacral pneumography. J. Urol., *75*:569, 1956.
121. Meppner, F.: Air embolism eight hours after ventriculography. Acta Radiol., *38*:291, 1952.
122. Jacoby, J., Jones, J. R., Ziegler, J., Classen, L., and Garvin, J. P.: Pneumoencephalography and air embolism; simulated anesthetic death. Anesthesiology, *20*:336, 1953.
123. Forbes, K. A., and Cordonnier, J. J.: Circulatory collapse following urethrocystography. J. Urol., *70*:975, 1953.
124. Milnes, R. F., Vander Wonde, R., Morris, J. D., and Sloan, H.: Problems related to a bubble oxygenator system. Surgery, *42*:986, 1958.
125. Gottlieb, J. D., Ericsson, J. A., Sweet, R. B.: Venous air embolism: a review. Anesth. Analg. (Cleve.), *44*:773, 1965.
126. Dasher, W. A., Black, J. P. M., Weiss, W., and Bogen, E.: Air embolism complicating pneumoperitoneum: a review. Am. Rev. Tuberc., *69*:396, 1954.
127. Haynes, D. M.: Cerebral hypoxia from air embolus following attempted abortions. Am. J. Obstet. Gynecol., *71*:1111, 1956.
128. Brodsky, J. D., and Greenstein, L.: Air embolism associated with pregnancy and the puerperium. Ill. Med. J., *112*:1, 1957.
129. Mylks, G. W., Brown, A. B., and Robinson, C. N.: Air embolism during labor. Can. Med. Assoc. J., *56*:427, 1947.
130. McCullough, K. M., and Morales, E.: Air embolism following post-partum surgical sterilization. Md. State Med. J., *4*:273, 1955.
131. Redfield, R. L., and Bodine, H. R.: Air-embolism per vaginam. J.A.M.A., *113*:671, 1939.
132. Stroh, J. E., and Olinger, M. T.: Air embolism. Am. J. Obstet. Gynecol., *35*:711, 1938.
133. Scrimgeour, J. W. F., and Carrick, M. E.: Fatal air-embolism associated with ruptured uterus. Lancet, *1*:485, 1955.
134. Cockett, A. T. K., Mangelson, N. L., and Kado, R. T.: Pathophysiology of aeroembolism following intravenous injection of oxygen. Aerosp. Med., *39*:407, 1968.

EMBOLISM FROM TISSUE COMPONENTS

135. Toy, B. L., and Tedeschi, L. G.: Embolic trophoblast in peripheral circulation during pregnancy. Proc. Soc. Exp. Biol. Med., *106*:865, 1961.
136. Tedeschi, L. G., and Toy, B. L.: Experimental transpulmonary migration of trophoblast. Obstet. Gynecol., *21*:55, 1963.
137. Park, W. W., and Lees, J. C.: Choriocarcinoma. A general review with an analysis of five hundred and sixteen cases. A.M.A. Arch. Pathol., *49*:205, 1950.
138. Sznejder, M. A.: Maternal death from rupture of the uterus and amniotic fluid embolism. Am. J. Obstet. Gynecol., *84*:249, 1962.
139. Dunhill, M. S.: The pathology of pulmonary embolism. Br. J. Surg., *55*:790, 1968.
140. Nosanchuk, J. S., and Littler, E. R.: Skin embolus to lung. Arch. Pathol., *87*:542, 1969.
141. Wilson, T., and Becker, S. N.: Postoperative death from pulmonary and paradoxic emboli containing transitional epithelium. Obstet. Gynecol., *39*:286, 1972.
142. Gardiner, W. R.: Massive pulmonary embolization of cerebral cortical tissue: an unusual fetal birth injury. Stanford Med. Bull., *14*:226, 1956.
143. Tryfus, H.: Massive pulmonary embolism of cerebellar tissue in a newborn. Arch. Dis. Child., *38*:292, 1963.
144. Merkel, H.: Observations on intra-vital and post-mortem displacement of brain substance within the

vascular system. Dtsch. Z. Gesamte Gerichtl. Med., *7*:217, 1926.
145. Krakower, C.: Pulmonary embolism containing cerebral tissue. Arch. Pathol., *22*:113, 1936.
146. Walcher, K.: Vital reactions. Ergbn. Allg. Pathol., *35*:209, 1940.
147. Oppenheimer, E. H.: Massive embolization by cerebral cortical tissue. Bull. Johns Hopkins Hosp., *94*:86, 1954.
148. Nunes, M. A.: Embolism of cerebral tissue. Gaz. Méd. Port., *8*:247, 1955.
149. McMillan, J. B.: Emboli of cerebral tissue in lungs following severe head injury. Am. J. Pathol., *32*:405, 1956.
150. Pisch, W.: Demonstration on the theme, sudden death: cerebral tissue embolism into the lungs as a result of head crushing. Acta Med. Leg. Soc. (Liege), *17*:95, 1964.
151. Tackett, L. R.: Brain tissue pulmonary emboli. Arch. Pathol., *78*:292, 1964.
152. Valdes-Dapena, M. A., and Arey, J. B.: Pulmonary emboli of cerebral origin in the newborn. A report of two cases. Arch. Pathol., *84*:643, 1967.
153. Light, H. G.: A tumor embolus causing infarction of small bowel. Pa. Med., *73*:37, 1970.
154. Balas, P., Katsaras, E., and Zoitopoulos, M.: Peripheral arterial embolism by malignant tumor. Vasc. Surg., *5*:27, 1971.
155. Mandel, M. M., and Strimel, W. H., Jr.: Ventricular myxoma associated with cerebral embolism. J.A.M.A., *214*:2154, 1970.
156. Sladden, R. A.: Neoplasia of aortic intima. J. Clin. Pathol., *17*:602, 1964.
157. Windelmann, R. K., Van Heerden, J. A., and Bernatz, P. E.: Malignant vascular endothelial tumor with distal embolization. A new entity. Am. J. Med., *51*:692, 1971.
158. Cohan, M., Pittman, G., and Hoffman, G. C.: Hemolytic anemia, tumor cell emboli, and intravascular coagulation. Arch. Pathol., *93*:305, 1972.
159. Adelson, L.: Injury and cancer. Western Reserve Law Rev., 5:150, 1954.
160. Behan, R. J.: *The Relation of Trauma to New Growths.* Baltimore, Williams & Wilkins Co., 1939.
161. Ellenbogen, L. S.: Traumatic cancer. J. Med. Soc. N.J., *51*:276, 1954.
162. Hueper, W. C.: Medicolegal aspects of cancer. Am. J. Clin. Pathol., *25*:116, 1955.

FOREIGN BODY EMBOLIZATION

163. Straus, R.: Pulmonary embolism caused by a lead bullet following a gunshot wound of the abdomen. Arch. Pathol., *33*:63, 1942.
164. McRae, A. T., Medalle, V. M., Pate, J. W., and Richardson, R. L.: Polyethylene catheter embolus. Am. Surg., *39*:57, 1973.
165. Blair, E., Hunziker, R., and Flanagan: Catheter embolism. Surgery, *39*:57, 1973.
166. Dolring, R. B., Stemmer, E. Z., and Connolly, J. E.: Complications of indwelling venous catheters with particular reference to catheter embolus. Am. J. Surg., *114*:259, 1967.
167. Ross, A. M.: Polyethylene emboli: how many more? Chest, *57*:307, 1970.
168. Wellmann, K. F., Reinhard, A., and Salazar, E. P.: Polyethylene catheter embolism. Review of the literature and report of a case with associated fatal tricuspid and systemic candidiasis. Circulation, *37*:380, 1968.
169. Kay, J. M., and Wilkins, R. A.: Cotton fibre embolism during angiography. Clin. Radiol., *20*:410, 1969.
170. Padula, R. T., Sandler, S. C., and Camishion, R. C.: Delayed bullet embolization to the heart following abdominal gunshot wound. Am. Surg., *169*:599, 1969.
171. The Wandering Bullet. Time, p. 52, December 25, 1964.
172. Harken, D. E., and Zoll, P. M.: Foreign bodies in and in relation to the thoracic blood vessels and heart. III. Indication for the removal of intracardiac foreign bodies and the behavior of the heart during manipulation. Am. Heart J., *32*:1, 1946.
173. Morton, J. R., Reul, G. J., Arbegast, N. R., Okies, J. E., and Beall, A. C., Jr.: Bullet embolus to the right ventricle. Am. J. Surg., *122*:584, 1971.
174. Bland, E. F., and Beebe, G. W.: Missiles in the heart: a 20 year follow-up report of World War II cases. N. Engl. J. Med., *274*:1039, 1966.
175. Lewis, R. J., and Kunderman, P. J.: Bullet embolus of the heart. Chest., *62*:627, 1972.
176. Keeley, J. L.: A bullet embolus to the left femoral artery following a thoracic gunshot wound. J. Thorac. Surg., *21*:608, 1951.
177. Painter, M. W., and Britt, L. G.: Distal bullet embolism after gunshot wound of the chest: a case report. Am. Surg., *37*:106, 1971.

SECTION 1. MECHANICAL INJURY

chapter 6

TRAUMA AND PREGNANCY

by Warren M. Crosby

In spite of the generally accepted feeling that pregnancy is a "delicate" state, modern women do not reduce the level of their activity while pregnant. Indeed, the reverse seems to be the case: rooms are made ready for the baby, or the whole family moves to a new home. Pregnancy increases the number of visits from family and friends, and this entails an obligatory increase in the amount of cleaning and straightening of the home in preparation for guests. In early pregnancy, patients become tired easily and fainting spells are not uncommon. Hyperventilation and altered emotional states render the pregnant woman more vulnerable then than at other times in her life. In later pregnancy, loosening of pelvic joints and alteration in the center of gravity owing to the protuberant abdomen produce unsteadiness. Minor accidental injury is more common during pregnancy than at perhaps any other time in adult life.[1] Nor do pregnant women refrain from travel. Because of increased activity, they may actually travel more during pregnancy. In California, automobile accidents caused 13.9 per cent of all maternal deaths; in Minnesota, the automobile was the most frequent nonobstetrical cause of death.[2,3] The protuberant abdomen of late pregnancy is the target for violence directed at the pregnant woman. The fetus and uterus are the recipients of beatings, stabbings, and gunshot wounds.[4,5] The state of pregnancy imposes physiologic changes on nearly all organ systems, and these changes must be taken into account when treating the pregnant trauma victim. Physicians who are not obstetricians generally lack familiarity with the state of pregnancy and the physiologic changes that accompany it. They also are keenly aware of potential litigation when the trauma victim is pregnant. Possibly because of this, there is a general unwillingness to operate on a pregnant woman that does not exist when the victim is not pregnant. This arises from the fear of stimulating labor or, more frequently, the fear of being blamed for premature labor or abortion that might have occurred anyway. Because of this fear, the physician may ignore the unfamiliar pregnancy and train his attention on superficial wounds, which, though dramatic, may be of lesser importance than internal injuries that may involve the pregnant uterus.

This chapter provides a reference for the physician and the attorney regarding the effects of automotive and other trauma on pregnancy.

TRAVEL DURING PREGNANCY

Obstetricians generally recommend that travel be kept to a minimum during pregnancy, and for good reasons: waves of nausea or periods of syncope are not uncommon at this time, and if the pregnant woman is driving by herself and suffers one of these episodes, the risks of accidental trauma are increased. In early pregnancy, 15 to 20 per cent of patients undergo spontaneous abortion. This process is accompanied by pain and hemorrhage, and may be suddenly incapacitating. For this to occur in a strange community or completely away from medical services subjects the woman to a decided risk that she would not have suffered had she stayed at home. In later pregnancy, the onset of labor may occur away from home, which is undesirable because the woman may then be attended by a physician who is not familiar with her case and does not have access to her previous records, and she will be liable to the increased anxiety attendant upon such an unfamiliar setting at such a vulnerable time. Alterations in blood coagulability and venous hemodynamics in late pregnancy also contribute to the development of thrombophlebitis among traveling pregnant women.

But travel itself does not apparently affect pregnancy adversely. Several controlled studies, comparing women who traveled during pregnancy with women who did not, have concluded that travel is not harmful to the majority of pregnant women. For instance, Beach questioned over 700 recently delivered women and compared the outcome of pregnancy of those who had traveled for substantial distances with that of those who had not. There was a slightly greater number of perinatal deaths among those mothers who had not traveled, although this was not a statistically significant difference.[6] Diddle studied travel during pregnancy and its relationship to pregnancy interruption and stated

> It may be concluded that travel in modern conveyances seldom if ever initiates interruption of pregnancy, unless intrinsic and extrinsic factors are already in action.[7]

Guilbeau studied nearly 2,000 women who had traveled during pregnancy and, in this detailed analysis, found no relationship between the length of the journey and the incidence of pregnancy loss.[8] Additional reports have presented similar conclusions regarding travel by air and other conveyances.[9–11]

AUTOMOTIVE TRAUMA

Maternal Injuries

The incidence of injury to victims of automobile collisions varies considerably because of many factors, including the physical severity of the damage to the vehicle, the seating position of the victim, the type of collision, the size and weight of the vehicle and its construction, and the use of occupant restraint systems, to name but a few of the better understood ones.[12, 13] In their study of pregnant victims of automobile collisions, Crosby and Costiloe found that 53 per cent of the collisions inflicted minor damage to the vehicles and that in these only three victims were injured and none died. It is clear that unless there is severe damage to the modern automobile, the likelihood of major or life-threatening injury to the pregnant occupant is small. This study revealed that pregnant drivers were less frequently ejected from the vehicle than passengers in the right, front, or rear seats, a fact that may account for the lower mortality rate enjoyed by drivers. The total injury rate, however, was similar regardless of seating position because drivers, while they died less frequently, had correspondingly more nonfatal injuries. Being the driver thus does not decrease the chance of being hurt in a severe collision, it just lessens the chance of dying from the injury. There was also a significantly lower rate of ejection from the vehicle among pregnant passengers who were wearing lap belts. Because of this and the attendant increase in survival, the authors recommended that pregnant as well as nonpregnant passengers use lap belt restraint.

Of the 15 pregnant women who died as the result of automobile collisions, as reported by Crosby and Costiloe, 7 died of head injuries and 6 from exsanguinating hemorrhage associated either with rupture of major blood vessels or with pelvic fracture. It may be important that those victims sustaining injuries to the upper half of the body died primarily of head injuries sparing the abdominal viscera, while those who died from hemorrhage had sparing of the head. Nonfatal but life-threatening injuries also included pelvic fractures and internal injuries to the liver and spleen, but did not include serious head injury.

The uterus was ruptured in two of the fatally injured victims, and the uterine rupture was only one of several injuries, each of which would have been fatal in itself. Woodhull reported 42 cases of traumatic uterine rupture that had resulted from falls and beatings and accidents involving horse-drawn vehicles. He was apparently the first to report a uterine rupture due to an automobile collision.[15] Several other cases of automobile collisions in which uterine rupture occurred have been reported.[16–22, 24] Uterine rupture has been reported as early as at three months' gestation, and in that instance, the blow that purportedly caused the rupture of the uterus was considered by the authors to be insignificant. One report concerns a mother who was struck down and then run over by a heavy bus. The fetus was extruded from the uterus by the tremendous force and was removed from the subcutaneous tissue of the mother's thigh. It is of some interest that the physician was able to repair the uterine defect after removing the fetus, and the patient survived.[16] An unusual situation was reported in the *Detroit Free Press* in March 1971. A serious collision occurred on a freeway, and early arrivals at the scene found the body of a woman with a very large laceration in her abdomen. In a search through the debris somewhat later, a baby was found alive and crying 85 feet from the body of the mother. It was apparent that the mother had been ejected through the windshield of the automobile and that a piece of the broken windshield had opened her abdomen and uterus without injury to the baby.[23]

Rubovits first demonstrated that uterine rupture might occur with lap belt restraint. He felt that compression of the lower abdomen of the mother by the lap belt resulted in an increase in pressure, causing uterine rupture.[26] Crosby and Costiloe found no uterine ruptures among 28 belted victims of severe automotive collisions, while there were two among the 180 unrestrained victims.[12] I have collected three additional cases of uterine ruptures in belted victims of automobile collisions. In each of these cases and in that of Rubovits, the mother survived following hysterectomy. None of the fetuses survived, however. These case reports show that the pregnant uterus can be ruptured with or without the presence of a lap belt. The presence of the lap belt may focus some of the force of deceleration on the pelvic structures when the forward flexion of the mother's body compresses the uterus between the lap belt and her thigh. This may also occur in the unbelted mother when her unrestrained body crashes against various parts of the interior of the car. A centrally located belt buckle would tend to increase the pressure over the narrow area of the buckle. It has also been reported that previous uterine surgery may increase the risk of rupture during sudden increases of uterine pressure.[27]

The pregnant uterus, by acting as a hydraulic shock absorber for forces directed at the anterior abdominal wall and dissipating them in its elasticity, provides protection for the remainder of the abdominal organs. The larger the uterus, the greater the protection offered. In nonpregnant victims, automotive collisions injure the spleen, kidney, liver, and intestines with about equal frequency. Injury to the abdominal wall, mesentery, pancreas, and diaphragm are unusual, and retroperitoneal bleeding is uncommon.[28] Farrell noted, however, that closed abdominal trauma as the sole injury was the exception rather than the rule and pointed out that while the physician's attention was diverted from severe closed abdominal injury, the patient might die from unrecognized retroperitoneal hemorrhage.[29] When the automotive collision victim is pregnant, hemorrhage plays a considerably larger role in morbidity and death. Elliott reported 38 pregnant women who were seriously injured. The primary cause of death in each of the eight fatal cases was uncontrollable hemorrhage into the retroperitoneal space or the intraperitoneal space, or from premature separation of the placenta. The author felt that the increased vascularity of the pelvic organs during pregnancy resulted in a larger number of deaths due to hemorrhage.[30] Sparkman reported 16 traumatic ruptures of the spleen during pregnancy. Only 2 were associated with automobile accidents. In 10, the trauma was "apparently trivial." Because of this relatively minor degree of trauma required to rupture the spleen in pregnant women, Sparkman concluded that pregnancy predisposed to splenic rupture. In comparison with the frequency of reported cases of spontaneous rupture of the spleen in other diseases, its frequency in pregnancy is second only to that in malaria.[31]

Fracture of the pelvic ring in the trauma victim presents even greater problems when the victim is pregnant.[32,33] The increased vascularity of the pelvis during pregnancy increases the risk of death from retroperitoneal hemorrhage associated with pelvic fracture. It has been estimated that the retroperitoneal space has a capacity of 4,000 ml at the pressure normally found in pelvic veins.[34] With this large capacity for concealed hemorrhage and the enhanced likelihood of bleeding during pregnancy, pelvic fracture is a more serious injury in the pregnant than in the nonpregnant individual.

Deformity of the pelvis great enough to interfere with the process of healing of a pelvic fracture during pregnancy is unusual, and delivery through a recently fractured pelvis is not attended by serious complications.[4,35,36] Injury to the bladder and urethra has, however, been reported following delivery through a recently fractured pelvis.[37]

Fetal Injury

The leading single cause of fetal death in accidents is death of the mother. Minor injury to the mother is infrequently accompanied by fetal loss. In the study reported by Crosby and Costiloe, there were four pregnancy losses among the victims of 233 minor collisions and in only two of these was the fetal loss related temporally to the collision.[12] Fort and Harlin reported 210 instances of minor trauma during pregnancy. Only 27 involved automotive collisions. There were two patients in whom the pregnancy terminated within 48 hours of the trauma, and both fetuses survived. In each instance in which the baby died, the pregnancy had progressed normally for several weeks following the traumatic episode. The incidence rates for abortion, stillbirth, and neonatal death were not statistically different from those of controls.[1]

Premature Separation of the Placenta

The cause of fetal loss is not always apparent. Premature separation of the placenta can be produced by trauma and may result in fetal loss. During a collision or any incident in which force is directed at the uterus, the uterine wall changes shape in accordance with the laws of fluid mechanics. Since the uterine wall is elastic, the uterus may elongate or shorten, and attendant stress is placed on the attachment to the placenta. The placenta, in contrast to the uterine wall, is nonelastic and cannot contract or expand to the same extent as the uterine wall to which it is attached. Thus placental attachments may be sheared during the impact and its aftermath. Premature separation of the placenta is therefore an expected result of severe abdominal trauma in late pregnancy. It occurred to a clinically recognizable degree, however, in less than 6 per cent of pregnant victims of severe automotive collisions.[12]

Following the shearing of the placental attachment, bleeding into the decidua from the arterioles and veins draining the intervillous space occurs. The blood may clot and the hematoma become self-limited. If the clot remains limited and there is no external bleeding, the hematoma may become organized, producing a depression in the maternal surface of the placenta that is later replaced by fibrous tissue, a placental infarct. Placental infarcts are common, but it is not known how frequently they are due to placental separations of a small degree. Small placental infarcts are of little clinical significance. In 80 per cent of cases of premature separation of the placenta, there is external bleeding, and in 20 per cent the bleeding is concealed behind the placenta.[38] The severity of clinical symptoms and the outcome for the fetus both depend on the area of the placental surface involved. In the near-term pregnancy, when less than 25 per cent of the placental surface is separated, external bleeding and premature labor ordinarily occur, but the fetus can be expected to survive. Conversely, when more than 50 per cent of the placenta is involved in the separation, it is unlikely that the fetus will survive, and there is usually maternal shock, tetany, and uterine tenderness. This syndrome may be followed by disseminated intravascular coagulation.[39] Among patients with clinically recognizable premature separation of the placenta, the maternal mortality rate is 1 per cent or less, and the fetal mortality rate ranges between 30 and 68 per cent depending upon the criteria for establishing the diagnosis.[40]

How frequently trauma produces placental separation is difficult to establish with accuracy, but trauma is universally considered one of the many causes of premature separation of the placenta.[41,42] Pritchard reported a 1 per cent incidence of trauma as the cause of premature separation of the placenta severe enough to cause fetal death in utero. One of the two cases reported was the victim of a head-on automobile collision and the other suffered a beating from her husband.[43] Kimbrough reported one premature separation of the placenta due to trauma among 383 cases of all grades of severity.[44] Paintin reported 213 cases, of which only 3 were felt to be in any way related to trauma. Automotive collisions were not mentioned by this author.[45] Dyer and Barclay reported two cases of premature separation of the placenta among 30 victims of automotive collisions admitted to the Charity Hospital of Louisiana. One was found in conjunction with other internal injuries at the autopsy of a fatally injured mother. The other was that of a woman who had been injured by the steering wheel during a head-on automotive collision. The fetal death occurred, as evidenced by the cessation of fetal movement, the day of the collision. Labor, however, did not ensue for nine weeks following the accident. The macerated stillborn baby was accompanied by a fibrotic placenta with a central depression. The authors felt that the collision produced a central placental hematoma, which killed the fetus but did not result in delivery for nine weeks.[4]

It is possible for trauma to produce a small area of separation or decidual hemorrhage that clots and later becomes organized and produces a small infarct. This could be associated with a limited amount of external bleeding following trauma, but such small infarcts are unlikely to result in death of the fetus. In the series reviewed and my own experience there has not been a case of premature separation of the placenta produced by trauma that did not terminate the pregnancy within 48 hours of the traumatic episode. In the single case reported by Dyer and Barclay, in which the dead fetus was retained for over two months, it was clear that the fetus died the day of the collision. In addition, Peyser and Toaff reported a case in which the fetal surface of the placenta was torn during an automobile collision. The fetus died immediately from exsanguination into the amniotic fluid, but was not delivered for five days.[46] This does not represent a premature separation of the placenta with bleeding into the decidua, but actually a laceration of the placenta. In the absence of bleeding into the decidua, the stimulus for labor would not be so strong. The implication is that if the area of separation is large enough to kill the fetus, labor or fetal death will occur shortly. If these do not occur, harm to the fetus from placental separation is unlikely, if it ever occurs.

Maternal Shock

Another factor that has been identified as producing fetal death is maternal shock. Hypotension in the mother is dealt with by the usual physiologic mechanisms of vasospasm and increase in heart rate, so that the vital organs of the mother may be protected. Unfortunately, the uterus is not considered a vital organ in the mother's vascular economy and thus the fetus may frequently be sacrificed in the interest of making what blood volume there is available for the mother. As a result, the maternal organism can survive shock for a considerably longer time than can the fetus. A similar stress response mechanism may account for fetal distress in the absence of recognized maternal shock. Catecholamines that may be released during the acute stress of injury may produce a marked reduction in uterine blood flow, even though the maternal blood pressure may never be recorded at a low level. The reduction in blood flow to the pregnant uterus may be severe enough to result in fetal death. This hypothesis is supported by experimental evidence reported by Romney and associates, by Greiss, and by Boba and others.[48–50]

Direct Trauma

Direct trauma to the fetus has been reported as a cause of fetal death following trauma to the mother. Brinton, in a largely anecdotal review in 1884, reported 53 cases of in utero fetal injury from trauma. The majority of these babies survived.[51] Smith accepted only 32 of Brinton's cases as representing true in utero traumatic fractures and added 12 more cases in which the criteria for inclusion were more stringent than Brinton's. In Smith's series, the bone most frequently fractured was the clavicle, followed by the skull, those of the extremities, and the scapula.[52] More recently, injuries to the fetus have been reported involving the cervical spine,[18] the jaw,[53] the clavicle,[25] and the ribs,[54, 55] and intracranial hemorrhage without fracture.[4, 56]

The most commonly reported fetal injury that remains apparent at birth is skull fracture.[57–61] In each of these situations, the mother sustained a fracture of the pelvis and the fetus was near term and was in cephalic presentation. It was concluded that the fetal skull was crushed by the pelvic fracture and dislocation of the pelvic bones. Intracranial hemorrhage may accompany fetal skull fracture even though the skull fracture itself may not be extensive.[62, 63] The lap belt may also cause injury to the fetal skull in the absence of maternal pelvic fracture. In one of the author's cases, flexion of the mother's body over a lap belt crushed the fetal skull between the belt (or the buckle) and the sacral promontory.[25] Overall, it may be stated that fetal injury may be produced by trauma with either fatal or nonfatal results for the fetus, depending upon the extent of the injury and its location. Fetal soft-tissue injury may heal more slowly than similar lesions after birth.[37]

Premature Labor

Premature labor may be an indirect cause of death of the baby following trauma to the pregnant mother. Many patients report contractions of the uterus ("false labor") following trauma or emotional shock of almost any kind. If the baby is then born prematurely at any time following such an incident, the incident is frequently blamed for the premature delivery of the baby and its subsequent impairment or death. There are very few data regarding the frequency of true premature labor following trauma. Crosby and Costiloe reported 363 mothers between 13 and 36 weeks of gestation at the time of the automotive collision. Thirty-five of these pregnancies terminated prematurely. In 17 cases, the mother sustained severe injuries, including placental separation, head injury, uterine rupture, internal injuries, and multiple fractures. In each case, the fetus was stillborn within a few days of the collision. In addition, there were eight premature stillbirths within a week of the accident in uninjured mothers. Thus, in 25 of 35 premature deliveries, there was at least a temporal relationship between the collision and the premature delivery. It is significant that none of these fetuses survived. In the 10 remaining cases, premature delivery occurred between 2 and 16 weeks following the collision. Two of the ten fetuses were stillborn. In one case, the mother sustained a basilar skull fracture during the collision and delivered the macerated fetus four weeks later. In another, the mother had fibroid tumors of the uterus and a congenital uterine deformity, either of which might have been responsible for the premature birth in the absence of trauma.[12] Since the cause or causes for the normal onset of labor are poorly understood at present, it is not possible to say with authority whether any additional factors might be related to any individual labor. With this fact in mind it seems apparent that for a direct causal relationship to be presumed between trauma and the onset of premature labor, there must be some identifiable lesion that is related both to trauma and to the onset of premature labor, such as premature separation of the placenta, maternal shock, or death of the fetus with or without fetal injury. The medicolegal aspects of this relationship are further discussed later.

Abortion

Abortion may follow injury to the mother, but it is often difficult to establish a causal relationship between the two, because any abortion that occurs within a few days of the traumatic episode may have already been in progress at the time the injury occurred. Conversely, embryonic injury caused by trauma may not result in an abortion for several weeks or even months following the incident.[64] Spontaneous abortion due to defective development of the embryo and placenta terminates between 10 and 20 per cent of pregnancies before the twentieth week of gestation.[65] Approximately one third of spontaneously aborted fetuses are normally developed, and other than abnormal development may be involved. Uterine abnormalities and maternal diseases may account for some of these abortions, but the majority result from unknown causes. Many studies have shown that travel in the absence of trauma does not increase the incidence of abortion.[6, 8, 66, 67] Javert studied 2,000 spontaneous abortion specimens. Seven of the patients gave a history of antecedent trauma. In each of these seven, there was bleeding within a few hours of the trauma, and two patients aborted within the next 24 hours. This might suggest that trauma caused the abortion, but degeneration of the decidua and villi were already advanced beyond the stage that would have been possible in such a short period of time. In five, the abortion occurred from three days to one month following the trauma, "making it virtually impossible to correlate the abortion with the trauma."[68] Fort and Harlin, and Crosby and Costiloe found that the abortion rate following trauma did not differ significantly from that expected in the normal population.[1, 12] That abortion following trauma can be related to the trauma has, however, been suggested by Hertig and Sheldon. Of 1,000 consecutive abortion specimens that they studied, 9 had a history of antecedent trauma. In each case, embryonic or placental defects were present that would have led to abortion irrespective of the trauma. These authors did report two cases, however, in which an automobile collision was followed soon afterward by bleeding and subsequent passage of a normal fetus and placenta. They suggested that these latter two were instances in which there was a causative relationship between collision and the abortion. They suggested that in order to establish such a causative relationship, the trauma must be followed within hours by a sequence of events that leads to the expulsion of a normally developed fetus.[64] These two cases may be the only ones documented in which there is sufficient evidence to substantiate such a causative relationship between the traumatic event and the subsequent abortion.

Prevention of Automotive Injury During Pregnancy

Injury to occupants of automobiles occurs as a result of collision between the occupant and the vehicle. The most common maternal injuries involve the head and the extremities, and the impact of these parts against the interior of the vehicle dissipates some of the force of the collision. Unless directly struck, the uterus and placenta are spared the effect of force absorbed by other parts of the mother's body. When the victim wears a lap belt, the decelerative force is directed toward the pelvis by the restraining action of the belt. The belt thus reduces maternal injury by preventing ejection and by limiting secondary impacts within the interior of the vehicle. But the amount of force directed toward the pregnant uterus when the body of the mother jackknifes over the belt may exceed that occurring in unrestrained mothers. The fetus of the belted mother thus may be subjected to a part of the force in every severe collision, whereas in unrestrained pregnant victims, the major part of that force is only occasionally directed against the pregnant uterus. The overall benefit that should thus accrue to the pregnant victim by lap belt restraint may be offset by the increase in fetal injury brought about by folding the mother's body over the lap belt. Ejection from the vehicle is substantially reduced or eliminated by lap belt restraint, however, and thus reduces the risk for the accident victim herself. Crosby and Costiloe, in weighing these two divergent effects of lap belt restraint, showed that prevention of ejection improves both maternal and fetal death rates.[12] These studies provided no evidence that lap belt restraint increased the mortality rate for mother or fetus regardless of the physical severity of the collision. They recommended lap belt restraint for pregnant travelers. The addition of a shoulder harness to the lap belt is now standard on automobiles manufactured in the United States. This three-point restraint system should reduce even further the frequency of maternal and fetal injury by distributing the decelerative force more evenly and by preventing forward flexion. While data are lacking as to the beneficial effects of this newer system in pregnant humans, Crosby and associates have shown a statistically significant improvement in fetal survival among pregnant baboons using three-point restraint when compared with animals restrained by lap belt alone.[69] A complete review of the problem of occupant restraint for maximum protection has recently been published by Snyder.[70]

NONAUTOMOTIVE INJURY

In view of the incidence of violence in our society, there are surprisingly few gunshot or stab wounds reported involving pregnant women. Dyer and Barclay reported eight cases of penetrating wounds of the pregnant uterus in their review of 25 years' experience at the Charity Hospital of Louisiana.[4] Badia and Charlton reported a knife wound of the pregnant uterus in a case in which both the mother and the fetus survived, the fetus being delivered three months following surgical repair of the uterine perforation.[71] Similar cases with fetal survival have been reported.[72, 73] McNabney and Smith reported a uterine stab wound in which the fetus was also injured. Both fetus and mother underwent exploratory laparotomy and both survived.[5] Frequently, however, the fetal outcome is poor.[74-76] Dyer and Barclay reported one case in which the umbilical cord was severed by the knife and another in which the fetus died, apparently of maternal shock. In the latter case, hysterotomy was performed to achieve hemostasis.[4]

Gunshot wounds apparently are more frequent than stab wounds. Koback and Hurwitz reported 31 cases prior to 1964. The maternal mortality rate in their series was 9 per cent with no deaths of mothers treated since 1912. The fetal mortality rate in pregnancies advanced to seven months or more, however, was 55 per cent. Buchsbaum reported 16 cases with no maternal deaths. The fetal mortality rate in this series was 75 per cent.[37] Since then, several reports have appeared with essentially the same results.[4, 5, 73, 76, 78-82] Dyer and Barclay have stressed that penetrating wounds of the abdomen during pregnancy invariably involve the gravid uterus.[4] A recent case reported by Kaufer and co-workers is the exception that proves the rule: In this bizarre case, the patient fell three stories from a building and landed upright on an auto jack, which perforated the rectum, liver, and right lung without involving the pregnant uterus.[83]

MEDICOLEGAL CONSIDERATIONS

One of the more difficult problems faced by physicians is to be asked by legal counsel for one of their patients whether a traumatic event—an auto collision, a fall, a beating—"caused" something to happen to her pregnancy—abortion, fetal death, premature labor, or premature separation of the placenta. There is little experience upon which to base an opinion. The problem is that pregnancy is a precarious state: Abortion or premature labor may occur, the fetus may die, or the placenta separate, all without any known "cause." The vast majority of such complications occur in the absence of trauma of any kind. In addition, traumatic events, even those that seriously injure the mother, are infrequently followed by pregnancy loss. With these inconsistencies in mind, the physician often will side with the claims made by his patient. This may serve his patient's interests, but may not serve justice. The following discussion is intended to help the attorney and the physician establish guidelines with which to establish or rule out a probable relationship between a traumatic event and a pregnancy loss.

The law has difficulty in dealing with the fetus, as evidenced by a recent United States Supreme Court decision concerning abortion. In that decision, the court stated:

> . . . we need not resolve the difficult question of when life begins. When those trained in the respective disciplines of medicine, philosophy and theology are unable to arrive at any con-

sensus, the judiciary, at this point in the development of man's knowledge, is not in a position to speculate as to the answer.

It should be sufficient to note briefly the wide divergence of thinking on this most sensitive and difficult question. There has always been strong support for the view that life does not begin until live birth. This was the belief of the Stoics. It appears to be the predominant, though not the unanimous, attitude of the Jewish faith. It may be taken to represent also the position of a large segment of the Protestant community, insofar as that can be ascertained; organized groups that have taken a formal position on the abortion issue have generally regarded abortion as a matter for the conscience of the individual and her family. As we have noted, the common law found greater significance in quickening. Physicians and their scientific colleagues have regarded that event with less interest and have tended to focus either upon conception or upon live birth or upon the interim point at which the fetus becomes "viable," that is, potentially able to live outside the mother's womb albeit with artificial aid. Viability is usually placed at about seven months (28 weeks) but may occur earlier, even at 24 weeks. The Aristotelian theory of "mediate animation," that held sway throughout the Middle Ages and the Renaissance in Europe, continued to be official Roman Catholic dogma until the 19th century, despite opposition to this "ensoulment" theory from those in the Church who would recognize the existence of a life from the moment of conception. The latter is now, of course, the official belief of the Catholic Church. As one of the briefs *amicus* discloses, this is a view strongly held by many non-Catholics as well, and by many physicians. Substantial problems for precise definition of this view are posed, however, by new embryological data that purport to indicate that conception is a "process" over time, rather than an event, and by new medical techniques such as menstrual extraction, the "morning-after" pill, implantation of embryos, artificial insemination, and even artificial wombs.[84]

The law appears to deal with the fetus in two separate ways. In the first instance, an abortion that was caused by the action of another person may be compensable by the defendant but in a limited way: The mother or the family that was deprived of the joys anticipated by completion of the pregnancy may be compensated for their mental anguish but not for the productivity of the aborted fetus as if it were a potential wage earner and citizen. Indeed it is said:

> A pregnant woman who, by reason of injuries negligently or wrongfully inflicted, suffers a miscarriage, is entitled to recover such damages as will fairly compensate her for the mental and physical pain and suffering and any impairment of her health occasioned by the miscarriage. Some courts hold that only the increased pain and suffering caused by the miscarriage, over what would naturally have ensued, are to be considered by the juries; but the more general, and apparently more reasonable, rule is that the pain and suffering which would naturally have come to the mother cannot be deducted from that occasioned by the miscarriage.
>
> Insofar as it is a part of the mother's personal injuries, mental anguish concerning the loss or birth of her child is a proper element of damages, and she is entitled to recover for her mental distress due to her fear or apprehension before the birth of the child that it will be deformed in consequence of such negligence, as well as for her disappointment at the birth of the deformed child. . . .
>
> Furthermore, it is generally held that in an action for personal injuries resulting in a miscarriage, recovery cannot be had for the injury to, or death of, the unborn child, or for the loss of its prospective earnings.[84]

In a series of medical-legal abstracts that have appeared in the *Journal of the American Medical Association*, the editors have observed the development of this concept.[86-89]

Wrongful death statutes generally provide that an action may only be maintained for the death caused wrongfully by a third party if the party who died was a "person." It is therefore important whether the fetus was actually a person, or viable, at the time of the accident. Jurisdictions are split as to the propriety of such an action even if the fetus is viable. The laws of most states in which a wrongful death action may be maintained hold that a "viable" child is a "person" within the meaning of the statute and that

> . . . "viable fetus" means the child has reached such a state of development that it can presently live outside the female body as well as in it. A fetus generally becomes a viable child between the sixth and seventh month of its existence. . . .[90]

Cases holding to the contrary state that

> . . .an unborn child is a part of the mother until birth and, as such, has no juridical existence.[91, 92]

Abortion

Abortion is defined as the termination of pregnancy prior to the attainment of fetal viability. Between 10 and 20 per cent of recognized pregnancies terminate in abortion. Hertig and Sheldon reported that 61.7 per cent of abortions were associated with ovular defects (absence or defects of embryos, placental abnormalities).[64] Such a defective pregnancy will always abort, regardless of what happens to the mother. Abortion of a defective ovum, therefore, should not be grounds for compensation, even if the abortion closely follows a traumatic event.

There is no general rule governing what facts permit recovery for traumatic abortions. Each case must stand on its own merit. In the case of *Finks* v. *Gillum*, the state Supreme Court allowed a jury verdict to stand that found that Mrs. Gillum's miscarriage was caused by the collision in which she was involved. The miscarriage occurred three days after the accident and, although there was evidence that the collision did not proximately cause the miscarriage, the court found evidence supporting the jury's verdict, and, therefore, allowed the award to be affirmed.[93]

Similarly in *Smith* v. *Philip Morris Company*, tried without a jury, the judge allowed the plaintiff mother to recover for her miscarriage occurring two to three weeks following the accident.[94]

On the other hand, in *Abend* v. *Sieber*, the appellate court reversed a judgment in favor of the mother, stating there was no causal connection between the accident and the miscarriage although an operation five weeks after the accident revealed an abdominal pregnancy with the fetus outside both the uterus and the fallopian tubes. Following the accident there were bruises on the body and a discharge of vaginal blood.[95]

In response to a letter to the editor regarding abortion following trauma, the *Journal of the American Medical Association* suggested several factors that should be determined in establishing a causal relationship between trauma and abortion: There should not be an abnormality of the fetus that might cause abortion but could not have resulted from trauma to the mother; there should not be constitutional factors in the mother predisposing to abortion, such as dietary or vitamin deficiency or a history of previous abortion; there should not be the existence of local infections that are sometimes held responsible for abortion; pelvic abnormalities such as myomas, cysts, cervicitis, severe lacerations, pelvic inflammatory disease, and retroversion should also not be present; nor should systemic diseases such as syphilis, tuberculosis, or toxemia of pregnancy; there should be an absence of exposure to toxic agents such as lead, irradiation, or "too much alcohol or nicotine"; there should not have been previous operative procedures such as trachelorraphy; nor should intercourse have taken place immediately prior to abortion; and finally, there should not be vigorous douching with either cold or hot water.[96] The editor who was the author of this comment in our opinion overstated the case, since there is no convincing evidence that drinking alcohol or smoking cigarettes or having intercourse has ever caused an abortion that would not have occurred otherwise. In fact, the two cases reported by Hertig and Sheldon may be the only ones documented in recent literature in which there is sufficient evidence to substantiate a causative relationship between trauma and abortion.

From the foregoing it is apparent that trauma may cause termination of pregnancy prior to the development of fetal viability, i.e., an abortion, although this is rare. The following criteria suggest that a probable causative relationship exists between a traumatic event and a subsequent abortion: (1) The traumatic event was followed within 24 hours by a process that led ultimately to abortion. (2) The fetus and placenta were studied pathologically and found to have been normal. (3) The appearance of the fetus and placenta were compatible with the stage of gestation at which the traumatic event occurred. (4) There is an absence of factors that are known to cause abortion, such as abnormalities of the uterus (including congenital defects of uterine development, leiomyomas, endometrial polyps, and incompetent cervical os), a history of repeated abortion in the absence of any known cause, chronic infections in the mothers (syphilis, tuberculosis, or toxoplasmosis involving the uterus), and a history of exposure to abortifacients (x-ray, lead, folic acid antagonists) or a physical attempt to induce abortion. These criteria are consistent with recognized legal requirements.[97]

It is clear that it is difficult to establish a probable relationship between an abortion and a traumatic event. This is as it should be. In the first place, traumatic events are not very often followed by abortion. When they are, the pregnancy usually proves to have been defective. The author agrees with Hertig and Sheldon, and with the Louisiana Court, that evidence to prove a causal relationship should be subjected to the strictest examination and that the burden of proof that a causative relationship exists between the trauma and a subsequent abortion should rest with the person who alleges that such a relationship exists.[64, 87] If these criteria are met, it is unlikely that a traumatically induced abortion would go unrecognized. Similarly, it is unlikely that an abortion that would have occurred in the absence of trauma will be compensated. It is recognized that on rare occasion a missed abortion that was in fact due to a traumatic event, such as that reported by Dyer and Barclay, or the Breus' mole noted by Hertig and Sheldon, will go uncompensated.[4, 64] The latter cases are extremely rare and are not ordinarily associated with great maternal distress or medical difficulty.

Premature Labor

Premature labor occurs spontaneously, the rate of incidence being between 6.69 and 14.18 per cent, depending upon socioeconomic status and race.[98] Etiologic factors can be ascertained in less than 40 per cent of premature labors, although trauma has long been considered a possible cause. In some cases, rupture of membranes or premature separation of the placenta has been attributed directly to trauma. If trauma can be established as the cause of either of these two events, premature labor that results therefrom can clearly be related to the trauma itself. A case of the author's is an example. A 28-year-old mother of three was in her fourth pregnancy. She was the right front seat passenger in an automobile that struck a large truck at approximately 3 to 5 miles per hour. She was thrown abruptly against the dashboard, but did not sustain any visible injuries. She became quite upset during the discussion that followed between the police, the driver of the truck, and the driver of the automobile in which she was riding, and she walked two blocks to her home, where she noted that fluid was leaking uncontrollably from the vagina. The following day, she reported to her obstetrician, who confirmed the diagnosis of premature rupture of the membranes. Five days later, she delivered a 1-lb 13-oz premature baby. The child is hopelessly mentally retarded following severe and prolonged anoxia as a result of inadequate pulmonary maturation. It would appear that the temporal sequence of events confirmed the traumatic cause of the premature rupture of the membranes. In the first place, the mother had had three normal term deliveries without premature rupture of the membranes preceding the present pregnancy. There was no history of factors known to cause premature labor. Membrane rupture occurred within 30 minutes of the traumatic event.

The elements of proof suggesting premature birth are:

History of earlier pregnancy to full term.
Evidence of live fetus in normal position.
Absence of physiological evidence of conditions within the mother that would produce premature delivery.
Shock accompanying injury.
Rupture of amniotic sac as evidenced by escape of amniotic fluid at time of or immediately after accident.
Beginning of labor pains soon after accident, pains continuing until delivery of a premature infant.
Weight of infant not in excess of 2,500 grams at birth, regardless of period of gestation.[99]

Premature separation of the placenta is not often caused by trauma. In a recent study of 201 cases of premature separation of the placenta severe enough to kill the fetus, trauma was the cause of the placental separation in only two.[43] Among 213 cases, Paintin was unable to find any patients whose premature separation of the placenta was caused by a fall, a beating, or an automobile collision. He did report, however, that 1.3 per cent of the cases were related to "trauma," which consisted of external cephalic version under anesthesia, coitus, or sudden escape of amniotic fluid in conjunction with polyhydramnios.[45] From the standpoint of patients with severe injuries, however, premature separation of the placenta is considerably more frequent than was previously recognized. For instance, at the Charity Hospital of Louisiana, Dyer and McCaughey reviewed a 10-year experience and found 214 cases of abruptio placentae occurring in 39,076 deliveries. None were felt to be due to trauma.[42] Conversely, when reporting accidental trauma complicating pregnancy at the same institution, Dyer and Barclay cited two instances of traumatic separation of the placenta among 30 seriously injured pregnant victims of automobile collisions, an incidence rate of 6.6 per cent.[4] Crosby and Costiloe reported 41 seriously injured victims of automobile collisions. Twelve developed premature separation of the placenta (29.2 per cent).[12] Thus, it appears that the range of incidence of premature separation of the placenta among seriously injured victims of automobile collisions is between 6 and 30 per cent. In 13 of the 14 cases just reported, pregnancy terminated within 48 hours of the traumatic episode. In the single case reported by Dyer, the dead fetus was retained within the uterus for over two months. It is thus clear that trauma does not often cause premature separation of the placenta, but there is little question that it does sometimes. Trauma-induced placental separation that does not kill the fetus or produce labor within 48 hours is extremely uncommon if it occurs at all.

On the basis of the studies just cited, if one is to postulate that a traumatic event caused premature separation of the placenta, the following criteria should be satisfied: (1) The pregnancy should have been advancing normally until the traumatic event. (2) There should be no evidence of factors known to predispose to premature separation of the placenta: previous vaginal bleeding, hypertension, toxemia of pregnancy, or abnormalities of the uterus, including leiomyoma or congenital septa. (3) The signs and symptoms of placental separation, including vaginal bleeding, uterine tetany, fetal death, and uterine tenderness should begin within 48 hours of the traumatic event and terminate the pregnancy shortly thereafter. (4) The diagnosis should be confirmed by an adherent clot or a depression of the placental surface.

While it is possible for a placental separation to result in fetal death without immediate delivery (as in the case reported by Dyer and Barclay), for a causal relationship to exist there should be evidence of fetal life shortly before the accident and its absence shortly thereafter, with evidence of placental separation whose degree of organization when studied pathologically after delivery is compatible with the length of time passed since the traumatic event.

Fetal Injury

Trauma may cause fetal injury or death. The most commonly reported fetal injury that remains apparent at birth is skull fracture. The mechanism of injury is dislocation of the pelvic bones of the mother, which crushes the fetal skull by compression.

If fetal death does occur in the absence of significant uterine or placental injuries, maceration may mask the fetal injury, and it may go unrecognized. Fetal injury need not necessarily result in fetal death. Soft-tissue injury may be repaired in utero and be unidentifiable at birth, but fractures may be identified by x-ray, and the progress of the normal healing processes may reveal the length of time since the fracture occurred. If that time coincides with the traumatic event, a cause and effect relationship may be established. Except in cases of osteogenesis imperfecta congenita, in utero fractures of fetal bones prior to labor are extremely uncommon. There have been at least 14 cases reported following trauma in which the appearance of the fractures on x-ray coincided with the time lapse since the traumatic event.

In the law relative to prenatal injury the "viable-nonviable" dichotomy arises again. The more recent cases have allowed recovery of damages for prenatal injuries regardless of the viability at the time of the accident, if the child is subsequently born alive. Some courts, however, have limited recovery to those instances in which the fetus was viable at the time of the accident, and at least one jurisdiction disallows recovery in any instance.[100]

Some states by statute disallow the child his own cause of action for negligently inflicted prenatal injuries, while case law allows such a right of action in other states. Most states do not allow the parents an independent cause of action for prenatal injuries of children.[101]

For there to be a cause and effect relationship between a traumatic event and an apparent fetal injury in utero, the following criteria should be satisfied: (1) The pregnancy should be advancing normally at the time the accident occurred. (2) The appearance of the injury should be consistent with the lapse of time since the traumatic event. In the case of fractures, the healing process can be accurately dated by roentgenologic appearance. Depressed skull fractures can occur during the birth process, as can fractures of the long bones or the clavicles, and strict attention must be paid to the roentgenologic appearance of these lesions to differentiate birth trauma from accidental trauma preceding birth as the true cause of the injury.

SUMMARY

Trauma is rarely followed by interruption of pregnancy in the absence of serious or life-threatening injury to the mother. In the latter situation, the pregnancy is not always involved. This communication has, it is hoped, developed criteria to aid in establishing or disproving a causative relationship between a traumatic event and subsequent pregnancy injury.

Acknowledgments: The author acknowledges the invaluable help of Robert S. Baker, esquire, who researched the legal literature and offered advice on the finished manuscript.

REFERENCES

1. Fort, A. J., and Harlin, R. S.: Pregnancy outcome after non-catastrophic maternal trauma during pregnancy. Obstet. Gynecol., 35:912, 1970.
2. Montgomery, T. A., Lewis, A., and Hammersly, M.:

Maternal deaths in California, 1957–1962. Calif. Med., *100*:412, 1964.
3. Barno, A., Freeman, D. W., and Baker, M. P., Jr.: Minnesota mortality study. Minn. Med., *45*:847, 947, 1962.
4. Dyer, I., and Barclay, D. L.: Accidental trauma complicating pregnancy and delivery. Am. J. Obstet. Gynecol., *83*:907, 1962.
5. McNabney, W. K., and Smith, E. I.: Penetrating wounds of the gravid uterus. J. Trauma, *12*:1024, 1972.
6. Beach, W. B.: Travel in pregnancy. Am. J. Obstet. Gynecol., *54*:1054, 1947.
7. Diddle, A. W.: Trauma and interruption of pregnancy. Texas State J. Med., *44*:520, 1948.
8. Guilbeau, J. A.: Effect of travel on interruption of pregnancy. Am. J. Obstet. Gynceol., *66*:1224, 1953.
9. McFarland, R. A.: *Human Factors in Air Transportation.* New York, McGraw-Hill Book Co., 1953. p. 758.
10. Shillito, F. H.: Medical considerations of the air traveler. N.Y. State J. Med., *47*:2201, 1947.
11. Whittingham, H. E.: Air transport of pregnant women. Practitioner, *166*:156, 1951.
12. Crosby, W. M., and Costiloe, J. P.: Safety of lap belt restraint for pregnant victims of automobile collisions. N. Engl. J. Med., *284*:632, 1971.
13. Schwimmer, J., and Wolf, R. A.: Leading causes of injury in automobile accidents. Automotive Crash Injury Research of Cornell University, N.Y. (June), 1962.
14. Huelke, D. F., and Gikas, P. W.: Causes of deaths in automobile accidents. J.A.M.A., *203*:1100, 1968.
15. Woodhull, R. B.: Traumatic rupture of the pregnant uterus resulting from an automobile accident. Surgery, *12*:615, 1942.
16. Coutts, D.: Fetus removed from mother's thigh following rupture of the uterus. Proc. R. Soc. Med., *29*:308, 1936.
17. Eastman, N. J.: Editorial comment. Obstet. Gynecol. Survey, *13*:69, 1958.
18. Elias, M.: Rupture of the uterus by external violence. Lancet, *2*:253, 1950.
19. McCarty, V., and Risely, D. R.: Traumatic rupture of the uterus in early pregnancy. J. Int. Coll. Surg., *26*:228, 1956.
20. Snidow, F. A.: Spontaneous rupture of the uterus at sixth month of pregnancy. Am. J. Obstet. Gynecol., *29*:751, 1935.
21. Stapleton, G.: Rupture of the pregnant uterus from indirect injury. Br. Med. J., *2*:367, 1937.
22. Parkinson, C. E.: Traumatic rupture of the gravid uterus. Am. J. Roentgenol., *80*:684, 1958.
23. *Detroit Free Press.* March 23, 1971.
24. Morrison, J. H., and Douglass, L. H.: Rupture of the uterus. Am. J. Obstet. Gynecol., *50*:330, 1945.
25. Crosby, W. M.: Pathology of obstetric injuries in pregnant automobile accident victims. In *Accident Pathology.* Edited by K. M. Brinkhous. Washington, D.C., U.S. Government Printing Office, 1970, p. 204.
26. Rubovits, F. E.: Traumatic rupture of the pregnant uterus from "seat belt" injury. Am. J. Obstet. Gynecol., *90*:828, 1964.
27. Crosby, W. M., Snyder, R. G., Snow, C. C., et al.: Impact injuries in pregnancy I: Experimental studies. Am. J. Obstet. Gynecol., *101*:100, 1968.
28. Griswold, R. A., and Collier, H. S.: Blunt abdominal trauma. Int. Abstr. Surg., *112*:309, 1961.
29. Farrell, J. J.: Nonpenetrating abdominal trauma. J. Fla. Med. Assoc., *43*:1104, 1957.
30. Elliott, M.: Vehicular accidents and pregnancy. Aust. N.Z. J. Obstet. Gynaecol., *6*:279, 1966.
31. Sparkman, R. S.: Rupture of the spleen in pregnancy. Am. J. Obstet. Gynecol., *76*:587, 1958.
32. Schumann, W.: Fractured pelvis in obstetrics. Am. J. Obstet. Gynecol., *23*:103, 1932.
33. Eliason, E., and Johnson, J.: Fractures of the pelvis. Surg. Clin. North Am., *17*:1571, 1937.
34. Gomcyekow, G. E., cited by Baylis, S. M., Lensing, E. H., and Glas, W. W.: Traumatic retroperitoneal hematoma. Am. J. Surg., *103*:477, 1962.
35. Mulla, N.: Fracture of the pelvis in pregnancy. Am. J. Obstet. Gynecol., *74*:246, 1957.
36. Voegelin, A. W., and McCall, M. C.: Some acquired bony abnormalities influencing the conduct of labor. Am. J. Obstet. Gynecol., *48*:361, 1944.
37. Buchsbaum, H. J.: Accidental injury complicating pregnancy. Am. J. Obstet. Gynecol., *102*:752, 1968.
38. Hellman, L. M., and Pritchard, J. A.: *Williams Obstetrics.* 14th Ed. New York, Appleton-Century-Crofts, 1971, p. 624.
39. Page, E. W., King, E. B., and Merrill, J. A.: Abruptio placentae: dangers of delay in delivery. Obstet. Gynecol., *3*:385, 1954.
40. Hellman, L. M., and Pritchard, J. A.: *Williams Obstetrics.* 14th Ed. New York, Appleton-Century-Crofts, 1971, p. 635.
41. Levi, A. A.: The pregnant uterus—external trauma and its consequences: annotated bibliography. Obstet. Gynecol., *21*:755, 1963.
42. Dyer, I., and McCaughey, E. V.: Abruptio placentae: a ten year survey. Am. J. Obstet. Gynecol., *77*:1176, 1959.
43. Pritchard, J. A.: Genesis of severe placental abruption. Am. J. Obstet. Gynecol., *108*:22, 1970.
44. Kimbrough, R. A.: Antepartum hemorrhage. Am. J. Obstet. Gynecol., *78*:1161, 1959.
45. Paintin, D. B.: The epidemiology of antepartum hemorrhage. J. Obstet. Gynaecol. Br. Common., *69*:614, 1962.
46. Peyser, M. R., and Toaff, R.: Traumatic rupture of the uterus. Obstet. Gynecol., *34*:561, 1969.
47. Dilts, P. V., Brinkman, C. R., III, Kirshbaum, T. H., and Assali, N. S.: Uterine and systemic hemodynamic interrelationships and their response to hypoxia. Am. J. Obstet. Gynecol., *103*:138, 1969.
48. Romney, S. L., Gabel, P. V., and Takada, Y.: Experimental hemorrhage in late pregnancy. Am. J. Obstet. Gynecol., *87*:636, 1963.
49. Greiss, F. C.: Uterine vascular response to hemorrhage during pregnancy. Obstet. Gynecol., *27*:549, 1966.
50. Boba, A., Plotz, E. J., and Linkie, D. M.: Effect of atropine on fetal bradycardia and arterial oxygenation: experimental study in the dog during graded hemorrhage and following vasopressor administration. Surgery, *58*:267, 1965.
51. Brinton, J. H.: Report of two cases of intrauterine fracture. Trans. Am. Surg. Assoc., *2*:425, 1884.
52. Smith, R. S.: Intrauterine fracture. Surg. Gynecol. Obstet., *17*:346, 1913.
53. Broadbent, T. R., and Hochstrasser, A.: Fracture of the mandibular condyle in the newborn. Plast. Reconstruct. Surg., *20*:171, 1957.
54. Shrove, R. S., Gee, P. J., and Cross, A. P.: Schizophrenia during pregnancy associated with injury to foetus *in utero.* Br. Med. J., *1*:686, 1968.
55. Musselli, N. G.: Uterine, fetal and placental injuries due to a motor car accident. J. Obstet. Gynaecol. Br. Common., *79*:379, 1972.
56. Raney, E. H.: Fetal death secondary to non-penetrating trauma of the gravid uterus. Paper presented before District VI meeting of American College of

Obstetricians and Gynecologists. Omaha, Neb., Oct. 12–15, 1966.
57. Jones, G. F., and O'Nan, W. L.: Intrauterine skull fracture. J. Ky. Med. Assoc., *38*:273, 1940.
58. Seear, T., and Woeppel, C. J.: Traumatic fetal death resulting from fractured pelvis. Am. J. Obstet. Gynecol., *65*:450, 1953.
59. Theurer, D. E., and Kaiser, I. H.: Traumatic fetal death without uterine injury: report of a case. Obstet. Gynecol., *21*:477, 1963.
60. Pike, J. B.: *In utero* depressed fracture of the fetal skull. Med. Times, *86*:869, 1958.
61. Alexander, E., Jr., and Davis, C. H., Jr.: Intrauterine fracture of the infant's skull. J. Neurosurg., *30*:446, 1969.
62. Parkinson, E. B.: Prenatal loss due to external trauma to the uterus. Am. J. Obstet. Gynecol., *90*:30, 1964.
63. Poulson, A. M., Jr., and Gabert, H. A.: Fetal death secondary to nonpenetrating trauma to the gravid uterus. Am. J. Obstet. Gynecol., *116*:280, 1973.
64. Hertig, A. T., and Sheldon, W. H.: Minimal criteria required to prove *prima facie* case of abortion. Ann. Surg., *117*:596, 1943.
65. Hellman, L. M., and Pritchard, J. A.: *Williams Obstetrics.* 14th Ed. New York, Appleton-Century-Crofts, 1971. p. 496.
66. Diddle, A. W.: Effect of travel on the incidence of abortion. Am. J. Obstet. Gynecol., *48*:354, 1944.
67. Webb, C. F., and Harvey, H. B.: Travel during pregnancy. Obstet. Gynecol., *4*:222, 1954.
68. Javert, C. T.: Role of the patient's activities in the occurrence of spontaneous abortion. Fertil. Steril., *11*:550, 1960.
69. Crosby, W. M., King, A. I., and Stout, L. C.: Fetal survival following impact: improvement with shoulder harness restraint. Am. J. Obstet. Gynecol., *112*:1101, 1972.
70. Snyder, R. G.: Human impact tolerance. In *Proceedings; International Automobile Safety Conference.* New York, Society of Automotive Engineers, 1970, pp. 712–756.
71. Badia, P. D., and Charlton, A.: Stab wound of a seven-month pregnant uterus. N.Y. State J. Med., *40*:1797, 1940.
72. Wright, C. H., Posner, A. C., and Gilchrist, J.: Penetrating wounds of the gravid uterus. Am. J. Obstet. Gynecol., *67*:1085, 1954.
73. Quast, D. C., and Jordan, G. L., Jr.: Traumatic wounds of the female reproductive organs. J. Trauma, *4*:839, 1964.
74. Moss, L. K., Schmidt, F. E., and Creech, O.: Analysis of 550 stab wounds of the abdomen. Am. Surg., *28*:483, 1962.
75. Gordon, P. R. G.: Antenatal uterine and foetal injuries by stabbing; maternal survival, foetal death. J. Obstet. Gynaecol. Br. Emp., *73*:155, 1966.
76. Bochner, K.: Traumatic perforation of the pregnant uterus. Obstet. Gynecol., *17*:520, 1961.
77. Koback, A. J., and Hurwitz, C. H.: Gunshot wounds of the pregnant uterus. Obstet. Gynecol., *4*:383, 1954.
78. White, W. H., Jr.: Gunshot wound of the gravid uterus. J. S.C. Med. Assoc., *58*:82, 1962.
79. Geggie, N. S.: Gunshot wound of the pregnant uterus with survival of the fetus. Can. Med. Assoc. J., *84*:489, 1961.
80. Bost, T. C.: Gunshot wounds of the pregnant uterus. South. Med. J., *34*:1040, 1941.
81. Beattie, J. F., and Daly, R. F.: Gunshot wound of the pregnant uterus. Am. J. Obstet. Gynecol., *80*:772, 1954.
82. Bryant, J. F., and Moore, M. D.: Gunshot wound of the gravid uterus with simultaneous exploration of mother and fetus. Am. Surg., *30*:207, 1964.
83. Kaufer, N., Shein, S., and Levowitz, B. S.: Impalement injury of the rectum: an unusual case. Dis. Colon Rectum, *10*:394, 1967.
84. *Wade* v. *Roe*, 93 S.Ct. 705 (1973).
85. 22 Am. Jur. 2d, Damages, S125:
86. J.A.M.A., *144*:785 (Oct. 28), 1950.
87. J.A.M.A., *146*:1527 (Aug. 18), 1951.
88. J.A.M.A., *149*:1673 (Aug. 30), 1952.
89. J.A.M.A., *150*:1337 (Nov. 29), 1952.
90. *Mitchell* v. *Couch*, Ky., 185 S.W.2d.
91. *Holloway* v. *Davis*, Okl., 261 P2d 217 [1953].
92. *Dradbels* v. *Skelly Oil Company*, 50 N.W. 2d 229 [Neb., 1951].
93. *Finks* v. *Gillum*, 273 S.W.2d 722 (Tenn., 1954).
94. *Smith* v. *Philip Morris Company*, 107 Cal.App.2d 361, 237 P2d 295 (1951).
95. *Abend* v. *Sieber*, 161 Md. 645, 158 Atl. 63 (1932).
96. Editorial: Trauma and abortion. J.A.M.A., *107*:2152, 1936.
97. 1 Am. Jur. Proof of Facts 16.
98. Hellman, L. M., and Pritchard, J. A.: *Williams Obstetrics.* 14th Ed. New York, Appleton-Century-Crofts, 1971, p. 529.
99. 2 Am. Jur. Proof of Facts, 530.
100. Eaton, E. J., and Danziger, R. F.: Traumatic disruption of pregnancy. Obstet. Gynecol., *30*:16, 1967.
101. 40 ALR3d 1222, *Liability for Prenatal Injuries.*

SECTION 1. MECHANICAL INJURY

chapter 7

TRAUMA IN PREGNANCY – INJURY TO THE FETUS AND NEWBORN

by Abraham Towbin

"Birth injury," as the term is generally used, indicates organic damage present in the newborn, and generally implies brain damage suffered by the infant during delivery. Despite its frequency, the processes of neonatal organic damage, its causes, and its sequelae remain poorly understood clinically. Misconceptions are deeply rooted in medical and lay literature. "Birth injury" is often pictured as mechanical trauma resulting from artless, forceful application of obstetrical forceps. Medical texts still present diagrams showing forceps crushing the head of the half-delivered fetus, depicting this as a major cause of mental retardation and cerebral palsy.

The investigation of perinatal complications and their sequelae not only involves many medical specialties – obstetrics, pathology, neurology, psychiatry – but also engages the efforts of many paramedical workers and concerned laymen. These problems, related to diseases of pregnancy and birth as complications leading to mental retardation and cerebral palsy, are of natural interest to the general public and increasingly occupy the attention of social, educational, and philanthropic agencies, and currently, the news media. Legal authorities are expressly concerned; recent years have seen an incongruous number of lawsuits involving obstetricians and other doctors in cases of "birth injury." Present estimates indicate there are over 4 million children and adults in the United States with organic mental retardation and other crippling nervous system disorders stemming from gestation and birth.

Despite the need for broader information clinically, the study of fetal-neonatal disease, the investigation of perinatal brain damage and its sequelae, remains one of the most fertile and least explored fields in medicine. In an effort to bridge this hiatus, the National Institutes of Health in 1959 formulated the Collaborative Perinatal Project (Collaborative Study of Cerebral Palsy, Mental Retardation, and Other Neurologic and Sensory Disorders of Infancy and Childhood), a study of 50,000 pregnant women and their offspring, with 15 medical centers across the country participating.[1] Clinically, the Collaborative Perinatal Project has been a source of information correlating perinatal data with follow-up pediatric neurologic studies extending from birth through childhood. Pathology studies carried out in the project's postmortem investigation of neonatal deaths have provided fundamental information defining the nature of organic damage present at birth. Detailed neuropathologic studies were carried out in which, in over 600 cases, whole-brain histologic sections were prepared and stored in the Warren Anatomical Museum, Harvard University Medical School.

Further clinicopathologic data have been obtained in studies carried on in the Norwood Perinatal Project, an ongoing interdisciplinary investigation conducted by the Department of Pathology and the Department of Obstetrics and Gynecology, Norwood Hospital, Norwood, Massachusetts, to analyze patterns of organic damage in newborn infants in a circumscribed (suburban American) population.[2]

From the Collaborative project and the Norwood Project, and from other current studies of fetal-neonatal disease, two basic concepts have emerged: (1) Most organic damage present in the newborn is of prenatal occurrence, due to prenatal factors, and often the damage is incurred hours, days, or weeks before birth. This applies especially to central nervous system damage. (2) Two main causal processes–mechanical trauma and, more often, hypoxia–are the cause of most organic damage present in the newborn.

A host of varied other pathologic processes–genetic anomalies, infectious disease, metabolic defects–occur in the newborn, but are comparatively uncommon. In recent times, the terms "congenital defects" and "birth defects," pointing to hereditary processes, are commonly used in close association with mental retardation, implying that genetic factors are the basic, important cause of nervous system crippling stemming from birth. Genetic disorders, although accounting for but a small proportion of neonatal mortality and morbidity, continue to consume vast, often dominant, research attention, while the common processes of perinatal hypoxia and mechanical injury are overlooked and often misinterpreted.

OBSTETRICAL CULPABILITY

In obstetrics, as in all clinical medicine, of imminent concern today is the prevailing inflation of malpractice suits confronting the physician. As pointed out in the lay media, the obstetrician is a particularly prime target.[3] There is need for more clinical awareness of iatrogenic (and apparent iatrogenic) mechanisms of obstetrical injury, processes defined in past and recent literature and indicated here.

At autopsy of the individual newborn with organic damage, in determining the causal factors–nature of onset, symptoms, latency–the interpretation of some problematical cases is difficult because there is no clear-cut information recorded regarding perinatal disturbances or delivery room complications. The clinical obstetrical history available often offers no clue to the time of origin of the damage evident postnatally; a vexing incongruity often exists between the extent of organic damage present at autopsy and the paucity of symptoms noted in the clinical record.

In appraising culpability for organic damage present at birth, it is necessary, clinically and medicolegally, to consider three aspects of the injury: its origin, the temporal factors, and the degree of latency.

The *origin*, the primary initiating cause of the fetal-neonatal injury, like that of other pathologic processes, may be endogenous, stemming from intrinsic defects in the biologic system, or may be exogenous, arising from external forces in the environment, from extrinsic agents. *Endogenous perinatal disorders* are complications that develop internally in the maternal-placental-fetal organization–eclampsia, toxemia, structural defects of the uterus, defective placentation, umbilical cord compression, or fetal malposition. *Exogenous mechanisms of perinatal damage* include physical trauma to the mother and conceptus, infectious disease, and of increasing concern, toxic drugs and other substances that affect the fetus. Likewise to be considered with exogenous processes is iatrogenic injury, damage to the fetus resulting from external obstetrical measures, such as spinal injury due to excessive traction applied in assisted delivery.

The *temporal factor*, the chronologic pattern, the time of onset and course of development of the perinatal complication, sharply determines the ultimate form and severity of injury present in the newborn. Thus the occurrence of placental detachment or umbilical cord compression in the prenatal period commonly proves fatal, whereas the same complication developing intranatally is more readily recognized and controlled. The degree of *latency*, the presence or absence of symptoms of the intrauterine complication, is likewise of immediate significance in determining the outcome of hypoxic and mechanical perinatal injury.

Obstetrical Responsibility with Reference to Clinical Patterns of Perinatal Complications

Based on the causal factors just defined–the origin of the pathologic process, the temporal factor, and latency–perinatal complications affecting the fetus emerge in four distinctive clinical patterns, each pattern reflecting a corresponding level of obstetrical responsibility.

Pattern 1. Prenatal Latent Complications with Immediate Damaging Effects on the Fetus

Precipitous silent complications that compromise the maternal-placental-fetal unit, the unheralded development of a tight umbilical cord knot, or sudden massive abruptio placentae–conditions with rapid consequent hypoxic damage in the fetus, often fatal–remain unpreventable, inculpable problems in obstetrical practice.

Pattern 2. Prenatal Latent Complications with Progressive, Subacute Attrition of the Fetus

Complications developing prenatally, such as progressive infarction of the placenta or the slow accumulation of an occult retroplacental hematoma, gradually compromise placental function and, if they occur early and develop by degrees, may exert damaging effects over a long period. In the fetus, protracted deprivation of nutrition and oxygen results in corresponding proliferation of cerebral and other visceral damage. Such cases, with placental insufficiency and hypoxia, are often marked clinically by decreased fetal activity.[4, 5] This often enigmatic loss of intrauterine activity, this apparent state of fetal unconsciousness, has been characterized as the "fetus-in-coma." The impoverished fetus may quietly perish in utero or, enfeebled, may succumb during the stress of parturition or soon after, or the infant may survive with organic damage of varying severity, often with cerebral disability—the familiar story of placental insufficiency, low birth weight, dysmaturity. In cases in which the prenatal course is outwardly symptomless and the process of intrauterine attrition clinically latent, cases in which the pregnant mother received all indicated standard prenatal care, the rescue of the compromised fetus and salvage of an unblemished neonate, appear beyond the province of the clinician.

Pattern 3. Prenatal Complications with Delayed Effects

With this type of complication, defects in the maternal-placental-fetal organization become established early in the prenatal period, remain latent, do not exercise their effects, and do not cause trouble for the fetus until labor begins. This kind of diphasic pathologic mechanism, such as placenta or vasa previa, is like a time bomb—poised, threatening the still healthy fetus. With this pattern of gestational-parturitional complication, obstetrical responsibility lies in a gray zone, varying from case to case, depending on the nature of the complication and, more directly, on an early diagnosis. The early detection of fetal jeopardy and the prevention of damage to the fetus are in turn dependent upon adequate prenatal care and appropriate monitoring after labor begins. In most instances in which the complication is recognized before labor becomes advanced, with active obstetrical intercession, a favorable outcome is to be expected.

Pattern 4. Complications Originating During Delivery

With complications that originate intranatally, fetal damage is commonly due to hypoxia, as occurs with sudden placental detachment or umbilical cord prolapse, or to mechanical processes, as occurs with rupture of the liver in prematures or spinal injury in breech deliveries. Damage of this order, the pathologic process having its genesis after the onset of labor, in a sense may be viewed as "birth injury." Complications arising during parturition often are precipitous, the manifestations immediately evident. The adequate management of such intranatal emergencies is the direct responsibility of the attending obstetrician, who must anticipate and diagnose the complication early by timely monitoring, and prevent far-advanced fetal damage by expeditious intervention.

DIAGNOSIS OF FETAL-NEONATAL DAMAGE

Fetal-neonatal organic damage, particularly in the central nervous system, has in the past often been diagnosed in a vague, equivocal way. Diagnoses such as biologic immaturity, dysmaturity, asphyxia neonatorum, sepsis, oversedation, parturitional shock, placental insufficiency, thrombosis of cord vessels, thymic death, and fetal atelectesis are often applied ambiguously, often without organic basis, often in error. The terms "birth injury," "cerebral trauma," and "brain-damaged infant," at once implying mechanical and hypoxic injury, are used variously to indicate nervous system damage in the newborn. Likewise at autopsy examination of the brain, diagnoses of "intracranial hemorrhage," "anoxic damage," and "encephalomalacia," often applied, are pathologically inconclusive and plainly circumvent the question of etiology.

In the following consideration of basic patterns of fetal-neonatal injury, priority is given to the most commonly occurring processes. Central nervous system damage is emphasized here because of its dominant incidence in the newborn and is of clinical concern in two major aspects: neonatal mortality and neonatal morbidity. First, it is increasingly evident in clinicopathologic investigations that central nervous system damage is the most important factor contributing to fetal-neonatal death. Second, the most important cause of neuropsychiatric disorders in infancy and child-

TABLE 7-1. CENTRAL NERVOUS SYSTEM DAMAGE IN THE NEWBORN

MECHANICAL INJURY
Spinal cord and brain stem injury
Subdural hemorrhage due to dural-venous laceration
HYPOXIC INJURY
Deep cerebral venous infarctional damage in premature infants
Cortical cerebral venous infarctional damage in term infants

hood—cerebral palsy, epilepsy, mental retardation, and related psychopathy—stems from organic injury in the fetal-neonatal period.[6–13]

Studies in the Collaborative Perinatal Project and in the Norwood Perinatal Project indicate that the effects of mechanical trauma and hypoxia, the major causes of central nervous system damage in newborn infants, take four basic forms (Table 7-1). *Mechanical injury* leads to two main types of damage, spinal injury and subdural hemorrhage. *Hypoxia* results in brain damage of two different forms, affecting the deep cerebral structures in the premature and the cortical cerebral elements in infants at term.

Patently, damage to the nervous system, in the fetus as in the adult, even in minor degree, is inherently more serious than most visceral injury. Small focal lesions affecting vital centers in the brain stem prove lethal. In the nervous system, even in the fetus, regeneration of tissue does not occur; loss of structure is permanent, resulting in crippling of function or death. Comparable damage, even major destruction, occurring in other parenchymal structures and organs that have a substantial margin of safety, may be reversible through regeneration and repair, and cause no lasting functional loss.

MECHANICAL INJURY IN THE FETUS AND NEWBORN

Mechanical injury to the fetus, present in the newborn, may result from intrinsic mechanisms or from extrinsic agents. Intrinsic processes of injury stem from fetal malposition, prematurity, precipitous labor, or prolonged labor due to dystocia. Extrinsic mechanisms, often iatrogenic, are commonly associated with forceful obstetrical manipulation in extracting the fetus. External causes of fetal injury include direct trauma to the abdomen of the pregnant mother, especially in automobile collisions, resulting in cranial injury or spinal injury in the fetus.[14–16] Severe injury to the mother at times causes, secondarily, fetal hypoxia due to maternal shock or traumatic placental detachment. In a reflection of the violence of our society, the fetus is at times the victim of penetrating wounds of the abdomen of the mother, gunshot wounds being apparently more frequent than stab wounds.[17]

In ordinary clinical circumstances, as viewed in the delivery room, most of the many varied forms of injury present at birth are superficial, of no lasting significance clinically; these minor injuries are not dealt with here.

In the case material of the Collaborative and Norwood projects there were three main types of mechanical injuries of serious consequences. Central nervous system damage, as noted, was by far the predominant form of fetal-neonatal injury. Noteworthy, also, were the unanticipated incidence of liver injury with rupture and, as is discussed later, the occurrence of pneumothorax.[1, 2]

Rupture of the Liver

Compression injuries of the abdomen, especially rupture of the liver, are common in the newborn, are often lethal, and are often undiagnosed.[18–20] Traumatic lesions of the liver occurring during parturition vary in severity from small superficial blisterlike subcapsular hematomas to deep, mangling lacerations involving an entire lobe of the organ (Figs. 7-1 and 7-2). Exsanguination into the peritoneal cavity, fatal hemoperitoneum, commonly results and may occur following rupture of a small or large subcapsular hematoma, as well as from a deep laceration.

The cause of such liver injury in the fetus and newborn is usually intrinsic, but at times may be related to force applied in delivery. Most injuries of the liver result from crushing of the abdomen during parturition, during descent, in a manner analogous to intracranial damage consequent to excessive molding compression of the head during delivery. The stress of lateral compression to which the fetus is subjected in its descent through the birth canal may in some cases of cephalic delivery cause intracranial damage, while in other instances, with breech delivery, the same lateral compression, exerted against the abdomen, results in rupture of the liver. With breech presentation, with the lower extremities flexed and pressing into the abdomen of the fetus, crushing injury of the bulky soft liver is likely to occur, especially if expulsion of the fetus is forceful and precipitous. In some cases trauma to the liver is thought to be due to external obstetrical manipulation, forceful grasping of the trunk of the half-delivered fetus during extraction of the aftercoming head.

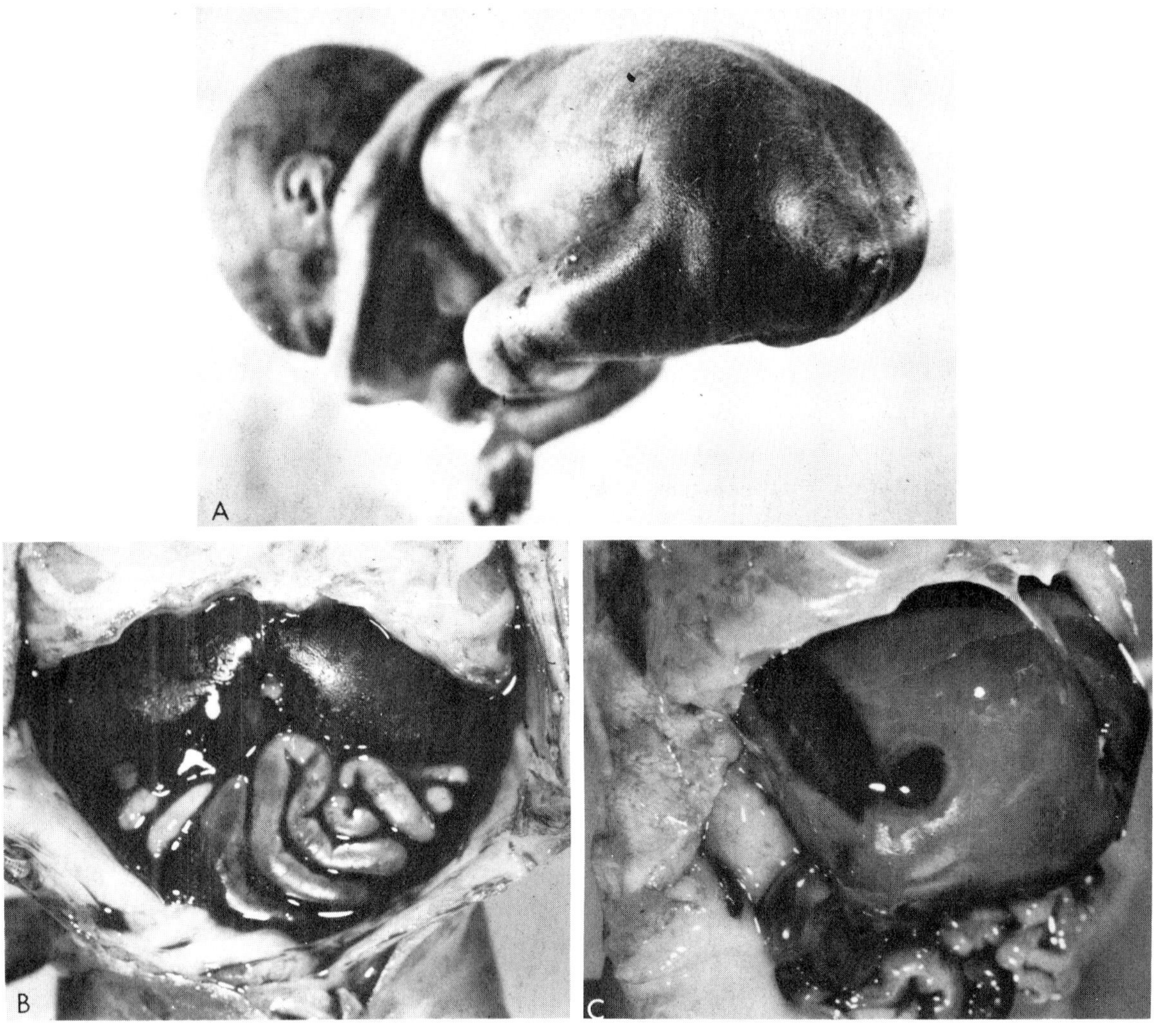

Figure 7–1. *A.* Premature infant delivered by breech (note edema and hemorrhage of buttocks) with flexed lower extremities forced against the body, compressing the abdomen and chest and causing crush injury; death during delivery. *B.* At autopsy, primary incision revealed massive hemoperitoneum. *C.* Liver showed contusion with bleblike subcapsular hematomas leaking blood into the abdomen. Right oblique view of the body with the liver drawn downward and forward to expose the hematomas on the upper anterior surface (C–10).

Newborn infants with liver injury tend to be either very small or very large. Prematurity is an obvious contributing factor; lethal liver rupture is especially common in small fetuses (500- to 1,500-g stillbirths), but generally goes unrecognized, since these small fetuses are not usually subjected to autopsy in most hospitals. Also in very large postmature fetuses, liver rupture is apt to occur, especially with a difficult breech presentation.

The frequency of perinatal rupture of the liver is not generally realized by obstetricians and pediatricians. Well-documented studies of consecutive neonatal autopsies reveal the occurrence of hepatic hemorrhage in from 3.6 to 5.0 per cent of stillbirths and neonatal deaths.[19] Affected infants present a characteristic picture: most commonly, a spindly pale premature without cyanosis and with a soft distended abdomen. The appearance is in distinct contrast to the edematous suffusion and cyanosis associated with asphyxia.

In most cases, liver rupture is rapidly fatal, with death occurring during the course of parturition. The effects of the injury may be delayed; Potter reported 40 cases of babies born alive with liver rupture.[21] In cases of latent liver injury, with a subcapsular hematoma gradually expanding, rupture and massive fatal hemoperitoneum may occur hours or days after birth—clinically, a neonate in apparently good health suddenly developing pallor and rapid irreversible shock.

Mechanical injury of other abdominal organs—rupture of the spleen or subcapsular hemorrhage of the kidney—are reported to

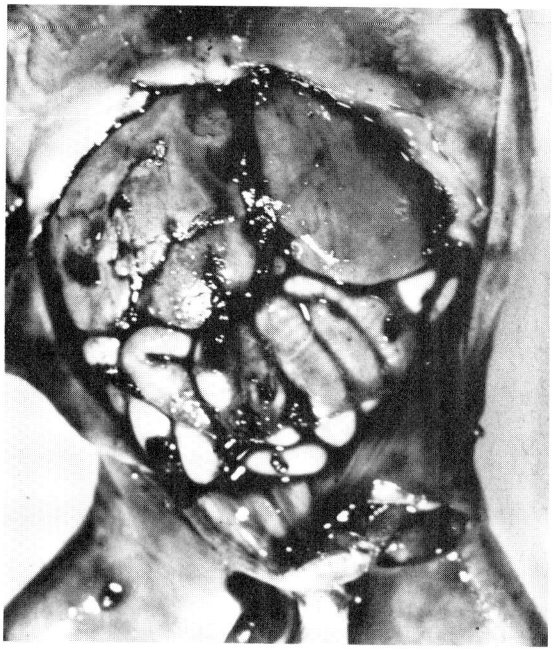

Figure 7–2. Rupture of liver with hemoperitoneum. Premature labor; breech extraction. At autopsy, abdomen was distended; clotted and fluid blood spread throughout the abdomen, between loops of intestines and other viscera and about the surface. Right lobe of liver showed deep, jagged lacerations. Severe spinal injury was also present in this case (N–1888).

occur, but are rare compared to liver rupture. Fetuses with hepatomegaly and splenomegaly, as in erythroblastosis and with maternal diabetes, are highly susceptible to liver and spleen injury.

Central Nervous System Mechanical Injury

The two most important forms of fetal-neonatal central nervous system damage resulting from mechanical trauma, spinal injury and subdural hemorrhage, have a wide range of effects, often sublethal, at times leading to lasting crippling injury. Perinatal mechanical trauma, although significant, is less important than hypoxia as a cause of chronic central nervous system disability. Mechanical injury, however, very often has immediate severe effects and, as such, is a major cause of stillbirth and early neonatal death.

Spinal Cord and Brain Stem Injury

Many clinicians are unaware that spinal injury, varying in severity, is of frequent occurrence in the fetus and newborn (Table 7-2). Such injury is often latent and at times de-

TABLE 7–2. SPINAL CORD AND BRAIN STEM INJURY IN THE FETUS AND NEWBORN

STRUCTURE	TYPE OF LESION
Meninges	Epidural hemorrhage Subdural hemorrhage Arachnoidal congestion and subarachnoid hemorrhage
Cord	Laceration Malacia Edema and congestion Hemorrhage
Brain Stem	Laceration Cerebellar contusion and abrasion Hemorrhage
Spinal and Cranial Nerves	Avulsion of roots Tears and hemorrhage
Musculoskeletal system	Spinal muscle laceration and hemorrhage Vertebral fracture-dislocation

velops prenatally through endogenous mechanisms. More often, neonatal spinal injury is the result of exogenous force, traction applied in delivery. The symptoms of spinal injury in the newborn often go unrecognized clinically, and the damage, even when severe, frequently escapes detection at autopsy.[22, 23]

The significance of spinal and brain stem injury in the adult is well known; the lesions, occurring after hyperextension or hyperflexion, vary from scattered petechiae to frank laceration and hemorrhage in the cord, brain stem, and meninges; death often is precipitous, at times following ostensibly minor trauma, often with incongruously minimal pathologic findings at autopsy.[24-26] Spinal injury of this nature, with epidural hemorrhage, is known to occur frequently in infants two to six months old in the syndrome of sudden infant death.[27, 28]

Clinical observers in the past were well aware of the problem of spinal injury in the newborn. Over a hundred years ago, in England, Kennedy called attention to spinal injury at birth and described "spinal apoplexy" as a cause of neonatal death.[29] Autopsy investigations in the past in which the spinal structures were examined in detail indicated the occurrence of spinal injuries in 10 to 33 per cent of deaths of newborn infants.[18, 22, 30–33]

In the newborn, as in the adult, elementary biologic processes are maintained and regulated, not by the cerebrum, but by the brain stem. Neonates with severe damage in the cerebrum often survive; anencephalics may live for prolonged periods. Survival of the newborn depends on the integrity and function of vital centers in the brain stem and upper spinal cord. It has been emphasized clinically that most signs of neonatal injury observed in the delivery room are neurologic, that the Apgar score, appraising respiratory action, cardiac function, reflex irritability, and other elementary signs in the newborn, is in essence an assessment of the presence or absence of damage in the brain stem and spinal cord.

In the case material studied by the author in conjunction with the national Collaborative Perinatal Project, of 170 cases in which adequate specimens of the spinal cord were available with the brain specimens, 16 showed extensive spinal cord lesions of traumatic nature; less severe lesions were present in 14 additional cases.[1] Brain stem injury of an extensive degree was evident in 6 of 430 brains studied; lesions of less pronounced extent were present in 7 other brains.[32]

The most frequent spinal injury was epidural hemorrhage (Figs. 7–3 and 7–4). This lesion, known to follow mechanical trauma in adults as well as in infants, is often overlooked, its importance underestimated.[25] Kennedy, in his pioneer studies of injury at birth, in describing neonatal "spinal apoplexy," pointed out the frequent presence of spinal epidural hemorrhage in newborn infants examined postmortem.[29] In affected infants, the hemorrhage may be limited to the loose areolar tissue surrounding the dura in the spinal canal, but at times, the damage accompanying the epidural hemorrhage is extensive, involving the cord and penetrating outward into the intervertebral structures and beyond into the soft tissues surrounding the spinal column. In itself, spinal epidural hemorrhage is not a killing lesion; its presence, however, reflects significant trauma: the force of injury causing the epidural lesion, extending its effects and impairing the function of the cord and medulla, leads to "spinal shock," with suppression of respiration and other vital functions.

In cases of spinal injury, in addition to epidural hemorrhage, damage of varying severity may occur in structures within the spinal canal—dural laceration with intramural and subdural hemorrhage, avulsion of nerve roots,

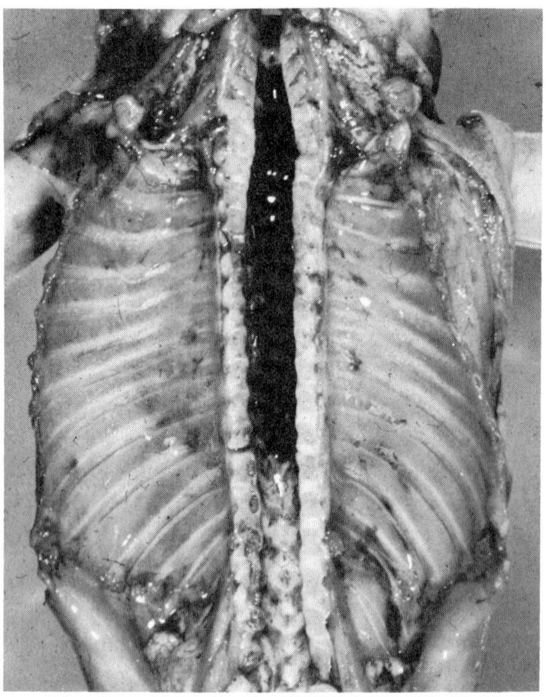

Figure 7–3. Spinal injury in a premature. Precipitous delivery in a primipara. Infant was apneic at birth, survived four hours. Autopsy revealed spinal epidural hemorrhage, thoracocervical portion of vertebral canal coated with a gelatinous hemorrhagic extravasate lying extradurally (M–54). (From A. Towbin: Central nervous system damage in the human fetus and newborn infant. Am. J. Dis. Child., *119*:529, June, 1970. Copyright 1970, American Medical Association. Reprinted by permission.)

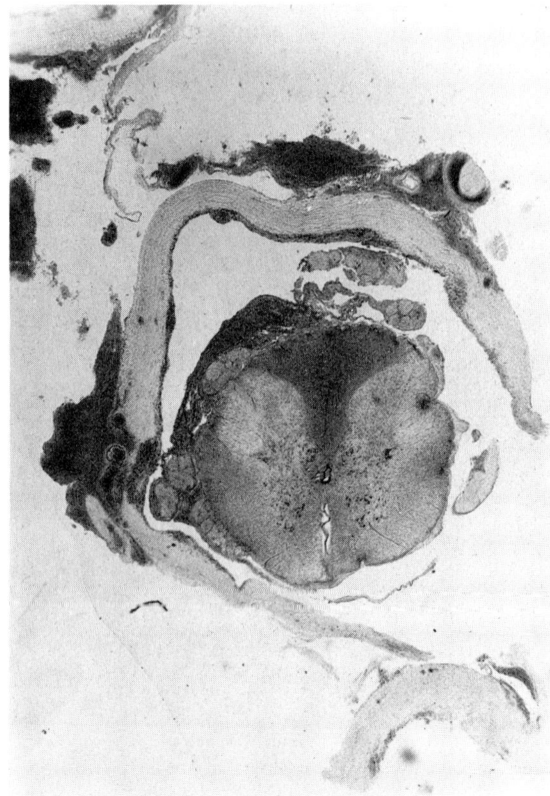

Figure 7–4. Spinal epidural hemorrhage; hemorrhagic extravasation about the spinal nerve at the point of exit through the dura. Premature delivery; Apgar score 4 at five minutes; hypotonia and respiratory depression; infant died 16 hours after delivery (W–107). (From A. Towbin: Central nervous system damage in the human fetus and newborn infant. Am. J. Dis. Child., *119*:529, June, 1970. Copyright 1970, American Medical Association. Reprinted by permission.

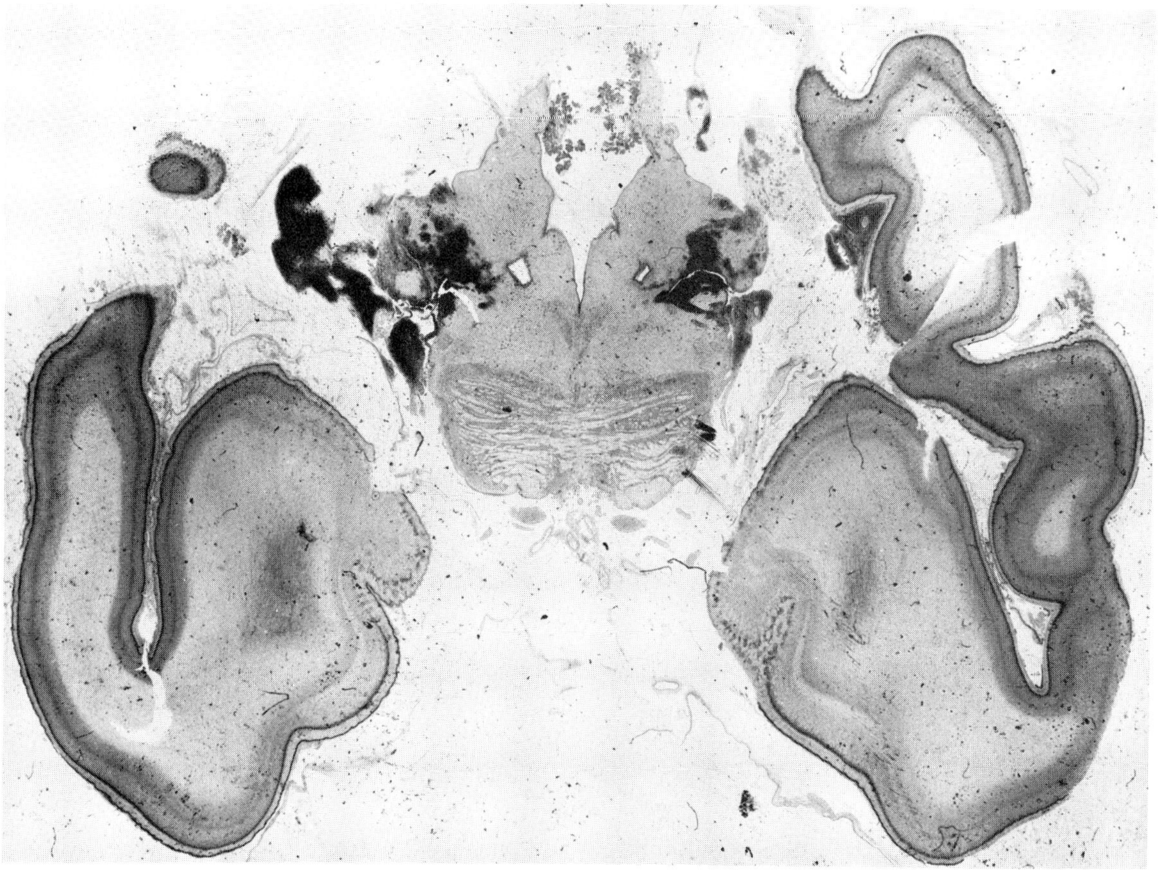

Figure 7–5. Brain stem injury incurred at delivery. Stretch injury with laceration and hemorrhage involving cerebellar peduncles and other structures about the fourth ventricle. Clinically, a complicated breech extraction with difficulty in delivering the arms and aftercoming head. Infant in poor condition after birth, pale, hypotonic, cyanotic, and with feeble respirations. Death occurred after 24 hours. Postmortem examination revealed a major spinal injury as well as the stretch injury of the brain stem (W–39). (From A. Towbin: Spinal cord and brain stem injury at birth. Arch. Pathol., 77:620, June, 1964. Copyright 1964, American Medical Association. Reprinted by permission.)

and when injury is more severe, softening, laceration, and hematoma formation in the substance of the cord. Similar injuries occur in the brain stem (Figure 7–5). Transectional lesions of the cord and brain stem with frank fracture-dislocation of the spine, as shown in Figure 7–6, or traction decapitation, as described in the past, occur infrequently today.

In the past, spinal injury in the newborn was generally attributed to exogenous force, to excessive traction applied at delivery. Recent studies, however, have focused attention on endogenous spinal injury, damage incurred by the fetus prior to labor or early in parturition. Clinically and pathologically, analysis of the underlying pathogenesis with regard to the temporal factor reveals conclusively that perinatal spinal injury may occur (1) during intrauterine life because of malposition, (2) during midlabor, as the fetus is forced down the birth canal, and (3) during the final extraction of the fetus.

Exogenous Causes of Spinal Cord and Brain Stem Injury. Forceful longitudinal traction—particularly when combined with flexion, hyperextension, or torsion of the spinal axis—has been considered the most important cause of neonatal spinal and brain stem injury.[22, 30, 34, 35] Two basic mechanical components are involved: stretch injury and compression injury. Stretch injury occurs when excessive traction is applied on the trunk to obtain the after-coming head in breech delivery (Fig. 7–7). It also may occur with forceps traction in cephalic presentation. With traction there is stretching and tearing of soft structures, of blood vessels, meninges, and nerve roots, and tearing and hemorrhage within the substance of the cord and brain stem (see Fig. 7–5). The effect of forceful obstetrical traction, stretch injury, was studied experimentally by Duncan, who tested the tensile strength of the spinal column in the fresh mature fetus. He found that in some instances with traction of 90 lb the vertebral column yielded; decapitation occurred with 120 lb of force. Duncan commented, "This is probably far from being what most obstetricians would regard as great force."[36]

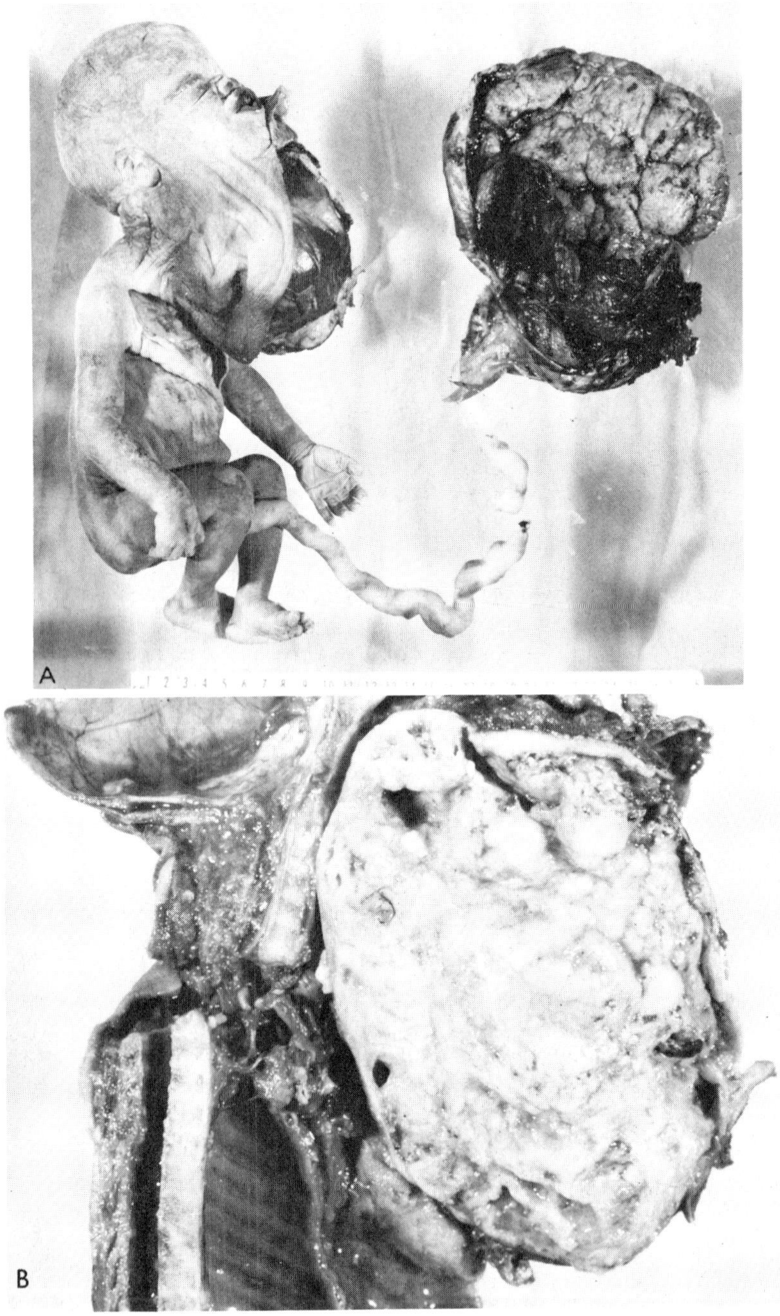

Figure 7–6. Parturitional fracture-dislocation of cervical spine. Premature labor in primipara; vaginal delivery. Footling presentation with extreme difficulty in delivering the aftercoming cervical-cephalic mass. *A.* Fetus, 4 lb 6 oz, with massive submaxillary teratoma. *B.* Sagittal view showing teratomatous mass and fracture-dislocation of spine (N–2).

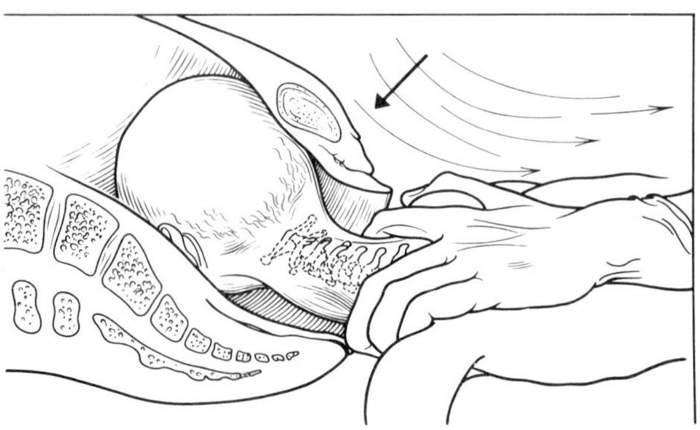

Figure 7–7. Trauma to cervical spinal structures by traction, torsion, and lateral flexion during extraction of the aftercoming head in breech delivery. (From A. Towbin: Neonatal damage of the central nervous system. In *Neuropathology: Methods and Diagnosis.* Edited by C. G. Tedeschi. Boston, Little, Brown and Co., 1970. Reprinted by permission.)

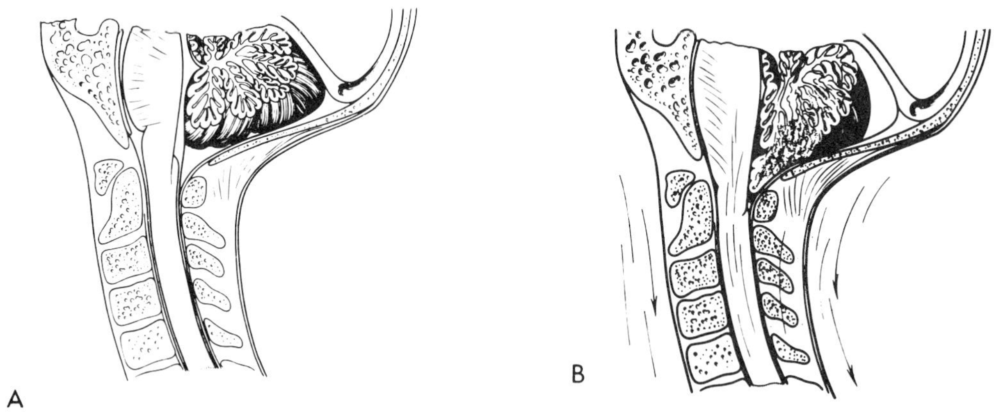

Figure 7–8. *A.* Normal relationship of brain stem and cord to base of skull and foramen magnum. *B.* Damage to brain stem due to traction; forceful traction leads to herniation of brain stem into the foramen magnum, with stretch injury of the brain stem and compression and erosion of cerebellar structures. (From A. Towbin: Neonatal damage of the central nervous system. In *Neuropathology: Methods and Diagnosis.* Edited by C. G. Tedeschi. Boston, Little, Brown and Co., 1970. Reprinted by permission.)

Brain stem damage is at times found in conjunction with stretch injury of the spinal cord. Forceful traction tends to produce compression injury of the brain stem, the medulla being drawn down and herniated into the foramen magnum (Figs. 7–8 and 7–9). The lower brain stem, throttled in the foramen, suffers surface injury as well as compression. The cerebellum, lying posteriorly, impaled on the edge of the foramen magnum, may be severely damaged as the surface structures grind against the base of the skull and are torn.

In a similar manner, the brain stem may be displaced downward by compression of the

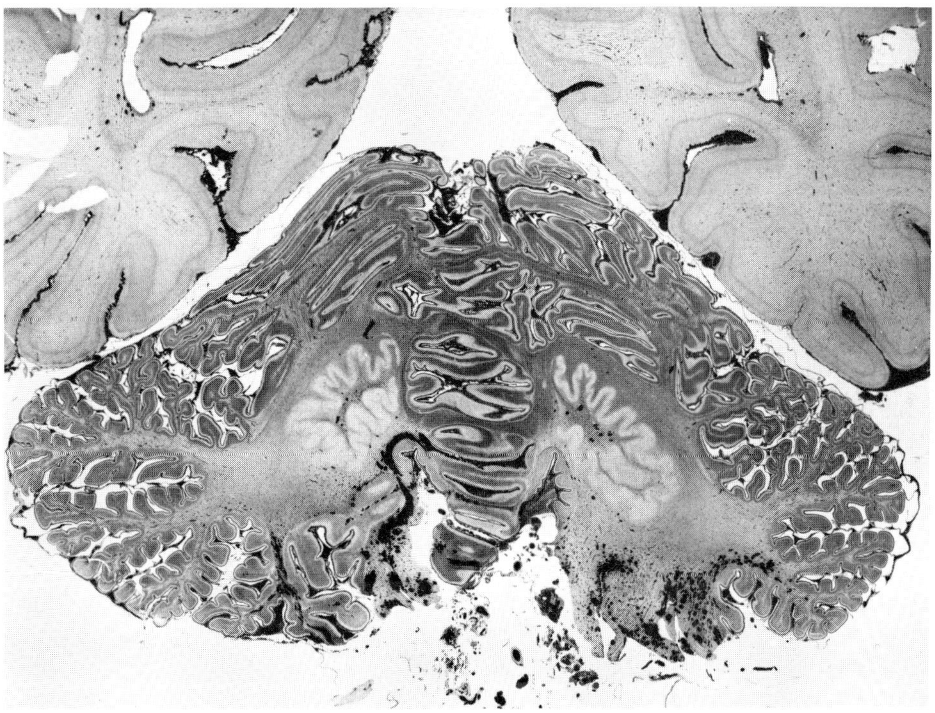

Figure 7–9. Cerebellar herniation damage incurred at birth. Surface contusion and fragmentation, the effects of traction herniation. Damaged midposterior portion of cerebellum positionally related to the margins of the foramen magnum. Term infant, cephalic delivery with forceps extraction. At birth, prolonged apnea, with spontaneous respiration delayed for 23 minutes; death occurred after four hours. Autopsy revealed spinal injury as well as cerebellar damage (W--55). (From A. Towbin: Spinal cord and brain stem injury at birth. Arch. Pathol., 77:620, June, 1964. Copyright 1964, American Medical Association. Reprinted by permission.)

head, produced obstetrically when manual pressure is applied to the suprapubic region of the mother to hasten delivery of the after-coming head in breech delivery.

Endogenous Perinatal Spinal Injury. The process of birth, even under controlled conditions, whether assisted or spontaneous, is potentially a higher traumatic event for the fetus. The fetus may suffer injury prior to manifest labor or early in labor. Significantly, spinal injury has been observed in infants delivered by cesarean section. Malposition, causing hyperextension or hyperflexion of the fetus, is the major factor in endogenous spinal injury (Fig. 7-10). In some cases of unrelieved abnormal cephalic presentation and at times in breech or transverse presentation, with persisting hyperextension or hyperflexion, the resulting narrowing of the spinal canal and compression of the cord, especially at the foramen magnum, reduces the cord segment to frank mush. Hellström and Sallmander and others have reported cases of sublethal spinal injury of this type; in the cases described, x-rays prior to delivery had shown fetal malposition with severe hyperextension; the infants at birth were paraplegic and, by x-ray and at surgery, showed traumatic cervical cord lesions.[37] Endogenous spinal injury due to unrelieved face or brow presentation commonly proves lethal, with death often occurring intranatally, as in the following case.

The mother, admitted far advanced in active labor, indicated there had been a loss of fetal activity. The heart tone, heard momentarily, disappeared. Examination revealed a face presentation.

At postmortem examination there was a severe "caput" over the face; the cervical spine showed a fracture-dislocation of the vertebrae and compression necrosis of the upper cervical cord.

In breech deliveries endogenous spinal injury is relatively frequent. Damage is commonly present in the lower thoracic, lumbar, and sacral segments and is attributable to hyperflexion of the spine during descent of the fetus. In other cases of breech delivery, spinal injury may be of exogenous obstetrical origin, due to traction or manipulation in extracting the aftercoming head. Former obstetrical techniques, the common application of version and extraction, frequently resulted in iatrogenic cervical cord injury.

When causes of fetal-neonatal injury are analyzed, it is manifestly evident that *duration of labor* is a most significant factor, contributing to mechanical damage—spinal injury as well as subdural hemorrhage—and also to hypoxic damage in the fetus. The extremes—prolonged labor and precipitous labor—both are associated with high incidence of neonatal morbidity and mortality. (It is evident that the safest vaginal delivery is that of moderate duration.)

Prolonged labor connotes the existence of obstetrical complications, impediments to parturition that produce fetal trauma and hypoxia. After long, difficult parturition, frequently in cases of fetal-pelvic disproportion, spinal injury is present—at times endogenous, at times exogenous, at times both. In the primipara with prolonged labor, especially the elderly primipara, neonatal spinal injury occurs commonly.

Precipitous delivery, of the premature as well as the mature fetus, in which the unmolded head traverses an inadequately relaxed birth canal, fosters both intracranial and spinal injury; such injury is at times iatrogenic, following the use of oxytocin (Pitocin).

Prematurity, especially when associated with precipitous delivery, is a basic intrinsic factor in the pathogenesis of mechanical injury in the

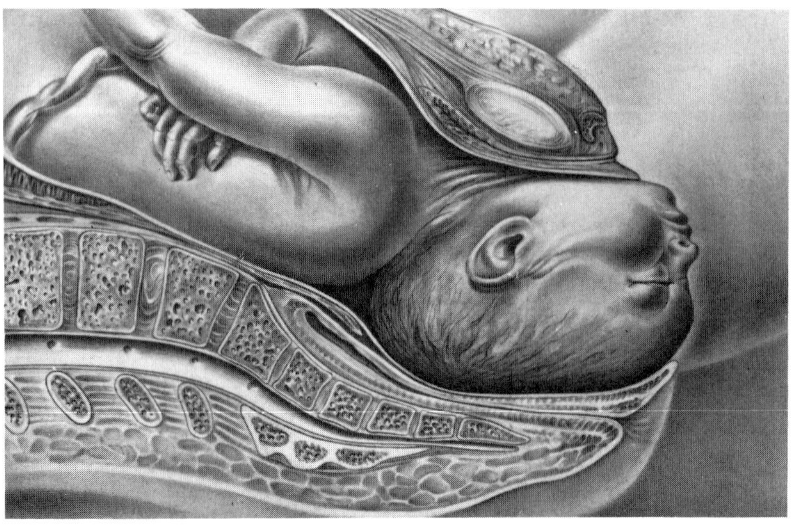

Figure 7–10. Hyperextension of the cervical spine in cephalic delivery. (From A. Towbin: Neonatal damage of the central nervous system. In *Neuropathology: Methods and Diagnosis.* Edited by C. G. Tedeschi. Boston, Little, Brown and Co., 1970. Reprinted by permission.)

fetus. In premature infants, especially in very early, small prematures, spinal injury is frequent and at times directly responsible for death (cf. Figs. 7–3 and 7–4). In many instances spinal injury occurs when premature delivery is spontaneous and unattended. The common supposition that the body of a very small premature fetus will pass through the birth canal easily and unhurt is wrong. The premature fetus, fragile and unfinished, suddenly forced through a rigid cervical opening and an unrelaxed birth canal, readily incurs spinal and brain stem injury.

Susceptibility to spinal injury, the innate constitutional vulnerability of the fetus to such injury, varies from case to case, as is evident clinically and pathologically. Exposure to mechanical stress during parturition may have no apparent effects in one case, while similar stress may prove lethal in another. Even standard orthodox obstetrical procedures may prove intolerable to the fetus. Thus in one instance of a difficult assisted delivery, no evidence of injury is present in the newborn infant, while in another instance, an "easy delivery" of a baby that "just wouldn't breathe," the autopsy may reveal extensive spinal injury.

The pathologic processes described here focus attention on the inadvisability, the wrongness, of the traditional upside-down spanking of the newborn infant in the delivery room to stimulate breathing—and equally, the danger of the nurse's insistent, well-intended massage of the back of the apneic neonate, apneic often because of spinal injury.

Effects of Spinal and Brain Stem Injury. Apnea is the prime symptom of spinal cord and brain stem injury. The clinical pattern of neonatal spinal injury as characterized in the old German literature pictured the newborn infant "mit Hertzschlag aber nicht Atmen," with heartbeat but not breathing. As previously pointed out, the inititation of respiration, sustained cardiac function, muscle tone, irritability, and other elementary signs related to the Apgar score are dependent on an intact brain stem and cervical cord.

The direct effects of neonatal spinal cord and brain stem injury appear in three main clinical groups. In the first group, death occurs rapidly during labor or soon after birth, the consequence of intolerable injury to vital regulatory centers in the brain stem or upper cord. In infants who survive initially, central respiratory depression, punctuated by periods of apnea, is often complicated terminally by superimposed peripheral pulmonary respiratory distress due to hyaline membrane disease or pneumonia. The second group comprises infants who survive for long periods, often years, with crippling neurologic defects directly due to spinal injury present at birth. Disability may range from the transient and mild to permanent paraplegia.[37] As Ford has pointed out, there must exist a large number of instances of perinatal injury of mild degree, with minimal neurologic symptoms, in children who are awkward or spastic, that are relegated to the category of cerebral palsy.[38] In cases of spinal injury at birth in which damage to the cord and nerve roots occurs clinically there may result corresponding neurologic defects affecting limbs, diaphragm, or other parts.[31] Damage to cranial nerve nuclei or nerve roots associated with brain stem trauma at birth may be a causal factor in congenital facial diplegia, extraocular muscle imbalance, and other cranial nerve deficits in children.[39] The third group of cases comprises newborn infants with spinal injury who, secondarily, suffer cerebral hypoxic damage. Respiratory depression and systemic hypoxia imposed at birth by spinal injury may result in widespread hypoxic devastation of the cerebrum. The effects of the superimposed cerebral damage may prove far more crippling than those of the primary spinal injury; infants so blighted may ultimately manifest symptoms of mental retardation, cerebral palsy, epilepsy, and other neurologic disorders.[7]

The overall incidence of neonatal spinal injury is not known. It is likely that a small but significant percentage of the general population bear latent sequelae stemming from perinatal spinal and brain stem injury.[38, 39] From data in past and current investigations, it is estimated that yearly in the United States over 10,000 neonatal deaths occur because of spinal and brain stem injury. Neonatal injury of this nature merits wider attention so that preventive measures may be pursued, iatrogenic injury may be averted, and in affected newborn infants early consideration may be given to this form of injury and this neurologic diagnosis.

Subdural Hemorrhage and Related Cranial Trauma

Subdural hemorrhage in the newborn, resulting from dural-venous laceration, as well as spinal and brain stem injury, is closely associated with four other related pathologic processes that affect the cranial structures, traumatic processes of greater or less importance: caput succedaneum, cephalhematoma, skull fracture, and molding of the head. The occurrence of these four forms of cranial injury, when they are severe, is significant in that they visibly reflect excessive parturitional stress, often heralding the presence of more severe damage intracranially, brain stem injury or subdural hemorrhage.

Caput Succedaneum. This is an area of boggy swelling that forms in the scalp over the presenting part of the head in cephalic presentations. The elevated, rounded area of the caput succedaneum corresponds to the portion of the scalp surface that is exposed within the opening of the dilated cervix during labor. Pathologically, the scalp in the area of the caput is swollen to three to four times its normal thickness and is suffused by edematous fluid (Fig. 7–11). The circumscribed area of edema and congestion is due to local interferences with venous return produced by the close embrace of the rigid cervical ring; this local swelling and edema of the scalp is similar to that which occurs distal to a tourniquet on a limb.

The location of the caput succedaneum is such that it adds to the elongation-distortion that develops with the process of parturitional cranial molding. Most commonly, the caput occurs asymmetrically over the crown of the head, in the parietal region, in association with vertex presentations. With breech presentations, analogous swelling and hemorrhagic discoloration occur over the buttocks and scrotum or labia (Fig. 7–12). With brow presentation, the swelling occurs over the frontal area and forehead, and in face presentation the eyelids, cheek, and nose are edematous and reddened.

Postnatally the caput succedaneum gradually diminishes, often disappearing during the first day after birth. The presence of a large caput, consequent to a protracted labor with strong uterine contractions, although not of direct bearing neurologically, does signify that injury to dural and other intracranial structures may be anticipated.

Cephalhematoma. This is a localized accumulation of blood deep to the scalp, between the periosteum and bone surface (Fig. 7–13). Unlike the variably located caput succedaneum, the hematoma is confined to the periosteal sheath of a single bone, commonly the right parietal bone, and never crosses a suture line. Cephalhematoma is rare, occurring in less than 1 per cent of newborns, and varies in size from a centimeter to golf ball proportions.

Cephalhematoma is generally considered to be due to mechanical trauma; during labor, with the cyclic uterine contractions, the presenting surface of the fetal head is subjected to forward and backward movements and compression against the sides of the birth canal. The friction of this repeated tangential traction and recoil, it is thought, causes loosening and avulsion of the periosteum, tearing blood ves-

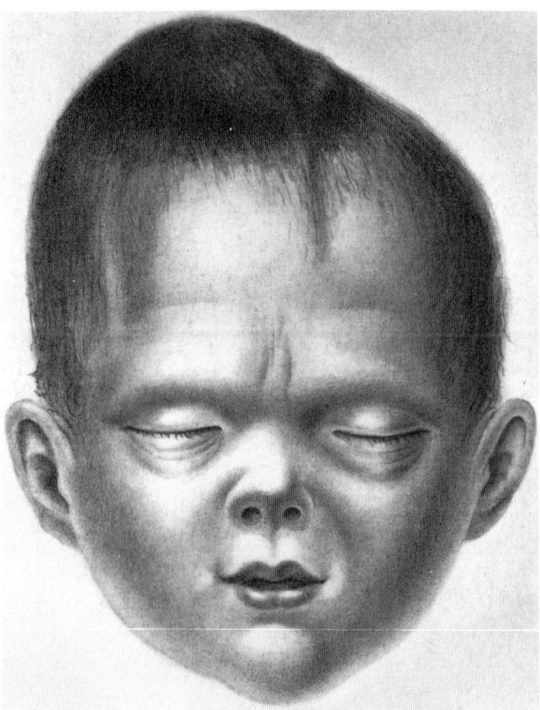

A

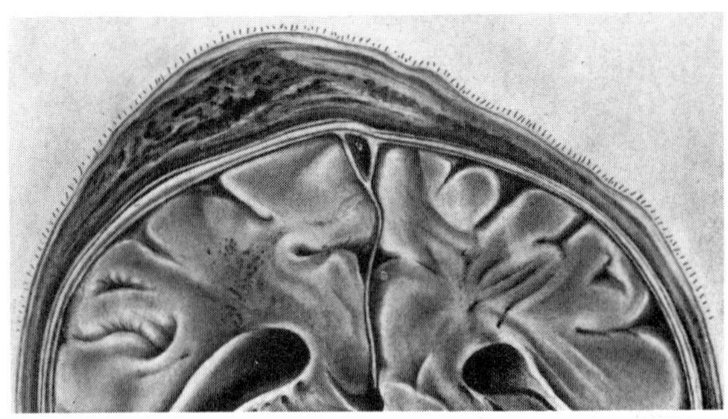

B

Figure 7–11. *A.* Caput succedaneum, an area of boggy swelling forming in the scalp, corresponding to the presenting part of the fetus. *B.* Frontal section through the involved region of the head; edema and hemorrhage in the scalp, in the layer between the galea and the periostium. (From A. Towbin: Neonatal damage of the central nervous system. In *Neuropathology: Methods and Diagnosis.* Edited by C. G. Tedeschi. Boston, Little, Brown and Co., 1970. Reprinted by permission.)

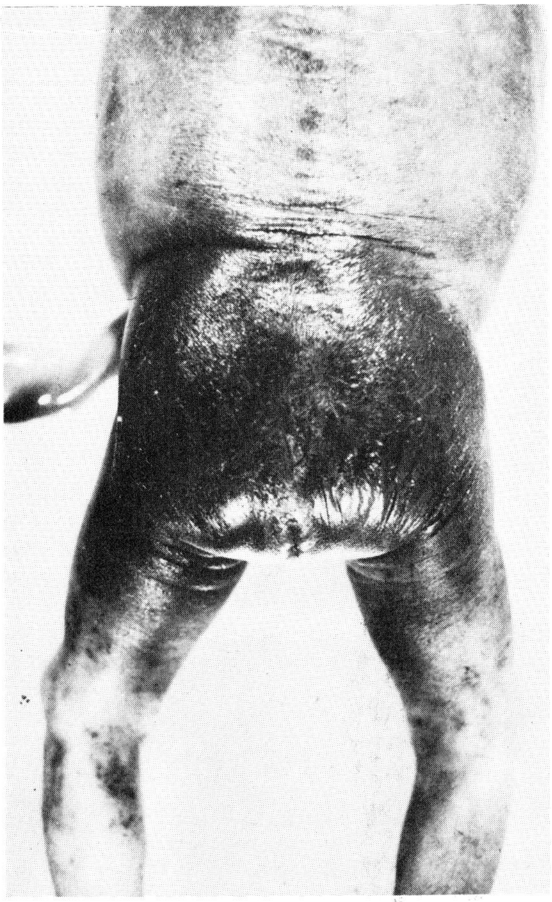

Figure 7–12. Hemorrhagic discoloration and edema of buttocks in breech presentation, analogous to caput succedaneum with cephalic presentation. (Same case as in Figure 7–1.)

sels and leading to hematoma formation. Linear fractures of the parietal bone subjacent to the hematoma may contribute to the subperiosteal bleeding; such fractures are reported to occur in 25 per cent of cephalhematomas.[40]

Cephalhematoma is a more serious lesion than caput succedaneum. The hematoma swelling often tends to increase during the first day or two after birth, as more and more blood accumulates, but gradually recedes in subsequent weeks as the blood is absorbed. At times the hematoma becomes infected through a small excoriation of the overlying skin, leading to protracted suppuration. Occasionally the outer wall of the hematoma develops a crackling calcified crust, and rarely, the entire hematoma is converted to an exostosis.

Although exerting no direct effect on the underlying brain, cephalhematoma, like caput succedaneum, reflects a difficult parturition, and at times its presence is immediately overshadowed by concomitant major intracranial hypoxic or mechanical injury.

Damage to the scalp during delivery may take the form of bruises or lacerations. Forceps may produce damage of varying pattern and severity in the scalp; if used to rotate the head, the tip or edge of the blade may cut the skin and injure the underlying bone. Misapplication and slipping of forceps may produce bony damage as well as severe soft-tissue injury. Injury to the scalp may be incurred during other obstetrical procedures; the medicolegal literature cites cases in which the scalp was incised

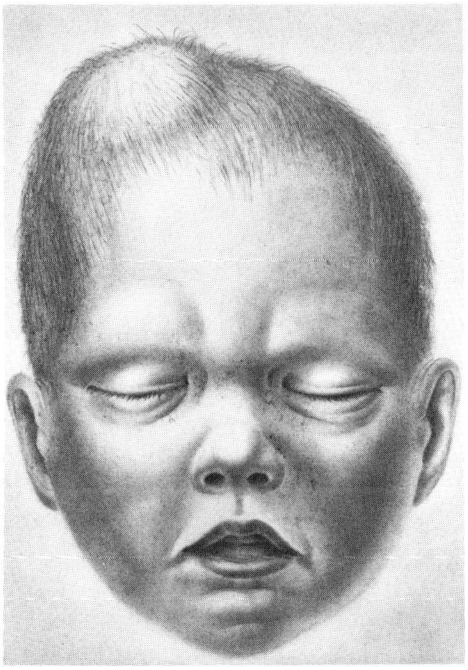

A

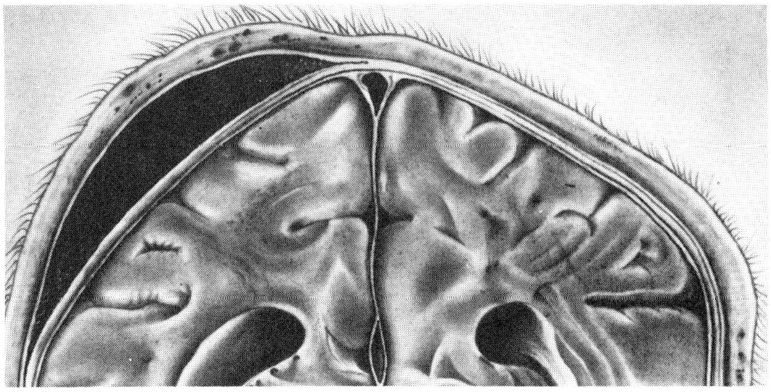

B

Figure 7–13. Cephalhematoma over the right parietal bone. *B.* Frontal section through the involved region of the head, through the hematoma over the right parietal bone; the extravasation of blood is confined to the subperiosteal stratum. (From A. Towbin: Neonatal damage of the central nervous system. In *Neuropathology: Methods and Diagnosis.* Edited by C. G. Tedeschi. Boston, Little, Brown and Co., 1970. Reprinted by permission.)

accidentally when a prominent caput succedaneum was mistaken for bulging membranes.

Fractures of the Skull. Extensive fractures of the skull incurred during delivery of the fetus—crushing of the head by obstetrical forceps, still commonly pictured in medical and lay texts—are rare in present-day obstetrical practice. Injury to the head of the fetus, with skull fracture, does occur at times in cases of severe accident injury to the mother during pregnancy. Fracture of the maternal pelvis with dislocation of the bones may result in crushing of the fetal head.[41] In some automobile accidents, fracture of the skull may result from compression of the fetus' head by the seat belt worn by the mother.[15]

The infrequency of skull injury in the fetus and newborn is largely due to the elasticity and compressibility of the soft cranial bones, to the ease with which they can override one another at their broad, loose sutures The most common traumatic lesion of the skull, the so-called "depressed fracture," is usually not a fracture at all, but merely an indentation of the wall of the calvarium, appearing as a depression in the cranium, usually 3 to 4 cm wide (Fig. 7–14). Indentations are the result of flicking inward of the flexible resilient plate of bone, like depressing the side of a ping-pong ball. Most commonly the deformity is produced as the head is pulled under the protruding promontory of the pelvis during a breech or forceps extraction. The deformity of the skull in most cases is easily corrected, and the lesion is usually without complications.

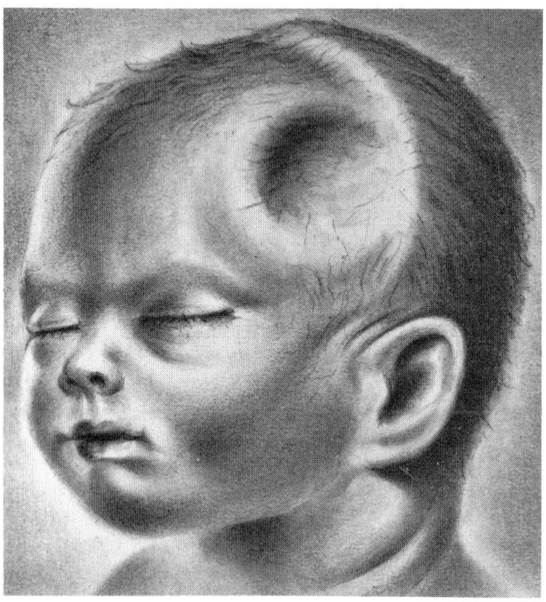

Figure 7–14. Indentation of the calvarium ("depressed fracture" of the frontal bone). Note the associated persisting downward displacement of the frontal bone and the overriding of the parietal bone. (From A. Towbin: Neonatal damage of the central nervous system. In *Neuropathology: Methods and Diagnosis.* Edited by C. G. Tedeschi. Boston, Little, Brown and Co., 1970. Reprinted by permission.)

True fractures, though uncommon, appear in many forms, varying from linear cracks, so-called fissures, to bizarre fragmentation of the bones with displacement and damage to underlying structures, at times with laceration of dural venous sinuses and subsequent subdural hemorrhage. Most serious fractures are the consequences of forceful termination of delivery. Severe fractures are, however, known to make their appearance after ostensibly easy routine delivery.

Of medicolegal importance is the differentiation of the parturitional skull fracture from that of infanticide. It is generally regarded as unlikely that skull fractures will result from precipitate, unattended birth, even when the neonate falls to the floor. Skull injuries inflicted in infanticide can usually be positively differentiated from delivery trauma; homicidal fractures usually are deeply depressed, multiple, and irregularly distributed and often the overlying skin exhibits the impression of the murder tool.

Molding of the Head. Plastic changes in the shape of the head during parturition, when extensive, often portend corresponding distortion and injury to structures intracranially. Molding occurs during labor as a consequence of the lateral compression exerted on the fetus in its passage through the birth canal. This parturitional compression converts the head from a rounded ball to an elongated cylindrical structure (Fig. 7–15). Molding of some degree occurs regularly in cephalic delivery, the oversized fetal head—positioned as the forward element—penetrating, dilating, overcoming the circumferential resistance of the birth canal. The plastic changes of the head in molding are possible because of the softness of the bone and because the broad, loose sutural connections permit displacement and overlapping or overriding of the individual skull bones (Fig. 7–16). Overriding is usually most conspicuous over the parietal region, one parietal bone being tucked under the other, but also commonly involves the parietal bones in conjunction with the frontal or occipital bones. Molding may be initiated at the time of the engagement of the fetal head in the pelvis, a week or more before term, or may be delayed until the onset of active labor. In the newly born infant, the elongation of the head caused by molding usually is

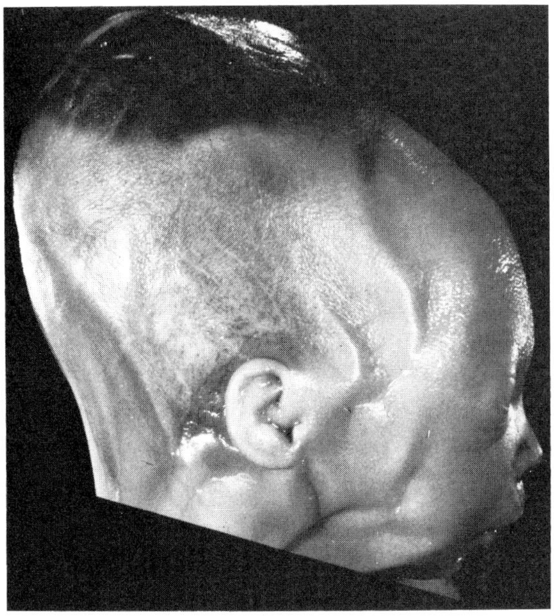

Figure 7–15. Molding of the head following vertex presentation and vaginal delivery. Elongation of the cranium due to protrusion of the parietal bone over the frontal and occipital bones at the sutural margins was further exaggerated by the presence of the bulging and discolored yarmulke-like caput succedaneum.

further increased and exaggerated by the presence of a caput succedaneum.

The shape of the molded head, the pattern of the distortion and the direction of the elongation, is determined primarily by the position of the fetal head as it becomes engaged and traverses the birth canal (Fig. 7–17). Vertical

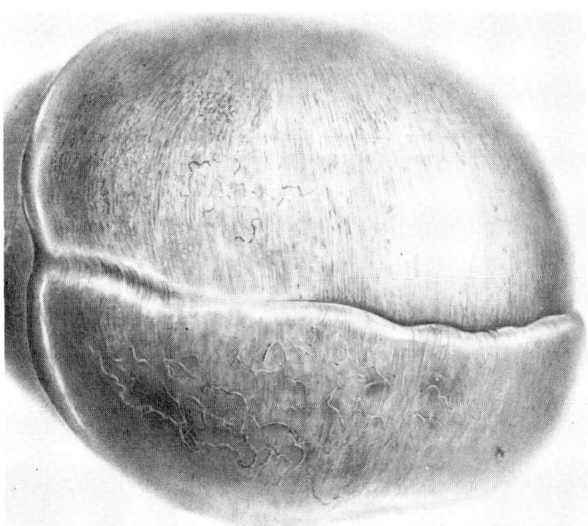

Figure 7–16. Molding distortion of the head, upper anterior view with scalp reflected. Overriding of the skull bones, with the right parietal tucked under the left along the interparietal fissure, and the frontal bone depressed under the parietals anteriorly. (From A. Towbin: Neonatal damage of the central nervous system. In *Neuropathology: Methods and Diagnosis.* Edited by C. G. Tedeschi. Boston, Little, Brown and Co., 1970. Reprinted by permission.)

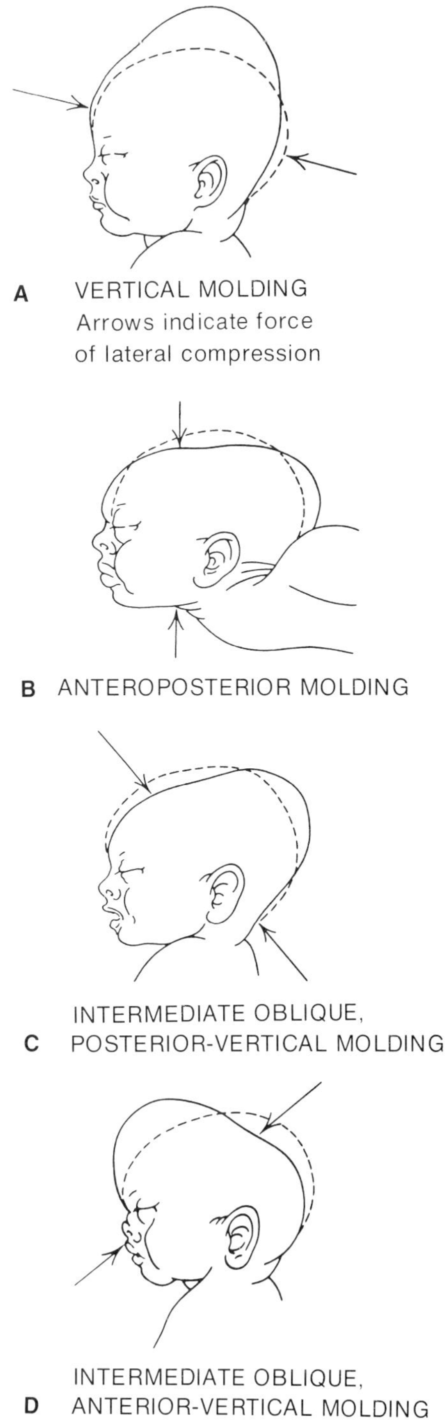

Figure 7–17. Patterns of cranial molding during parturition. *A.* Vertical elongation, resulting from compression in the anteroposterior diameter, commonly occurs in vertex presentations. *B.* Anteroposterior elongation, consequent to compression between the base of the skull and the vault, commonly occurs in face presentation and with breech delivery. *C.* Intermediate pattern of molding, with prominence of the parietooccipital region, as occurs with contracted pelvis. *D.* Intermediate pattern of molding, with prominence of the frontal region, as occurs in brow presentation. (From A. Towbin: Neonatal damage of the central nervous system. In *Neuropathology: Methods and Diagnosis.* Edited by C. G. Tedeschi. Boston, Little, Brown and Co., 1970. Reprinted by permission.)

elongation of the head, the most common form of molding, occurs with vertex presentations; the face and forehead are compressed and flattened; the vault of the head is arched sharply along the sagittal suture. The squame of the occipital bone is bent inward and under the parietal bones; the frontal bone also tends to be inserted under the parietals. The parietal bone that lies against the promontory during delivery is usually depressed and overlapped by the other parietal.

In the young fetus, even though the head is small, severe molding distortion may develop as the head is pressed through the narrow unrelaxed birth canal prematurely. The popular impression that the skull cannot be molded in the postmature is incorrect. Molding of the head may be apparent after breech delivery; with labor lasting a long time after the membranes rupture, the head, pressed down by the fundus, becomes elongated and distorted.

Molding is often viewed as a physiologic part of the process of parturition, a mechanism that allows delivery of the relatively oversized head through the tight pelvic conduit. Pathologically, it is of concern because the forces that bring it about may also produce intolerable stress and damage to intracranial structures. There is no doubt that severe parturitional distortion of the fetal head, excessive molding, imposes strain on the dural structures, and that the resulting stretching and tearing of the dura and its venous channels leads to subdural hemorrhage.

Dural-Venous Laceration with Subdural Hemorrhage. Of the pathologic processes that affect the central nervous system of the newborn infant, subdural hemorrhage is the most familiar clinically. Although common, subdural hemorrhage has generally been overdiagnosed in newborn infants, the diagnosis being applied much more frequently than the condition actually occurs. Clinically, in the past, in infants with neurologic symptoms after birth, this diagnosis was applied empirically, almost automatically, routinely, and generally in error, as ultimately shown at autopsy. In recent years there has been increasing cognizance of the predominance of hypoxic brain damage, rather than subdural hemorrhage, as the main cause of postnatal neurologic disability.

Likewise there has long existed the misconception that severe intracranial damage, tentorial tears and subdural hemorrhage, is mostly caused by obstetrical forceps compressing the infant's head during delivery. No doubt the hasty or faulty application of forceps may cause direct cranial damage. As previously discussed, however, the forceful employment of forceps combined with excessive traction usually causes damage, not directly to the cranium, but indirectly to the spinal structures and brain stem.

Etiologically, dural-venous laceration is mainly endogenous in origin, in most cases occurring intranatally during active labor in the descent through the birth canal. The immediate causal mechanism, as previously indicated, is directly related to parturitional molding of the fetal head. In the fetus and newborn, the dura, which lines the cranial cavity and also forms tight partition sheets (the falx cerebri between the cerebral hemispheres and the tentorium posteriorly between the cerebrum and cerebellum), is of special significance pathologically (Fig. 7–18). Incorporated within the dural sheets, intramurally, are numerous venous sinuses, large thin-walled blood vessels superficially located and highly vulnerable to injury. The dural sinuses lying at the edges of the tentorium and falx receive the venous drainage of the cerebrum through the vein of Galen and other bridging veins. During delivery with molding, the taut tentorium and falx, tightly attached to the cranial bones, are forced to adjust to the altered, elongated shape of the head; in the fetus, the dural sheets, stretching across the cranial cavity like guy wires, resist excessive change in the shape of the head. If molding is

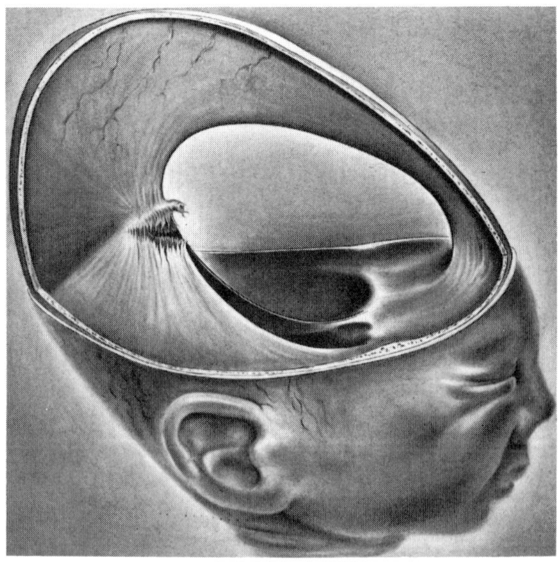

Figure 7–18. Laceration of the tentorium. View of intracranial dural structures, the falx cerebri above and the tentorium spreading downward. Stretch injury consequent to vertical molding elongation distortion of the head; characteristic laceration of the tentorium at its attachment to the falx, penetrating the straight sinus, with tearing away of the attached end of the vein of Galen. (From A. Towbin: Neonatal damage of the central nervous system. In *Neuropathology: Methods and Diagnosis.* Edited by C. G. Tedeschi. Boston, Little, Brown and Co., 1970. Reprinted by permission.)

protracted and severe, or if it is applied suddenly, the fibrous dural septa, subjected to intolerable tension and strain, give way, split, and tear as shown in Figure 7–18. Stretch tearing of the tentorium and other dural structures results in rupture of the venous sinuses within the dura and avulsion of the attached bridging veins from the brain—with consequent subdural hemorrhage.

Contributing causes are both endogenous and exogenous. The most important factor obstetrically in the pathogenesis of dural-venous laceration is the duration of labor. Prolonged labor and precipitous labor are both associated with a high rate of incidence of subdural hemorrhage in the newborn.

In prolonged cephalic delivery in the presence of cephalopelvic disproportion, with the head receiving the brunt, the repeated direct thrust of each uterine contraction through a long labor, mechanical injury of some degree is inevitable. In the newly delivered infant, the external physical marks of prolonged labor—a large caput succedaneum and excessive molding—often indicate concomitant intracranial injury, laceration of dural and venous structures, and subdural hemorrhage.

Precipitous delivery proves as dangerous as, or more dangerous than, prolonged labor. Ordinarily, with cephalic presentation, when the process of parturition advances at a balanced pace and the compressive forces mount slowly, permitting gradual molding of the head, the strain on the cranium and dural structures generally is tolerated without significant injury. When the process advances rapidly, however, when the rounded, unmolded head is pressed quickly through the resisting, incompletely relaxed ligamentous birth canal and cranial compression is applied suddenly, the dural structures are unable to adapt. Tears and hemorrhage result.

Of special concern are two exogenous causes of neonatal subdural hemorrhage that are iatrogenic, stemming from obstetrical procedures and precipitate delivery: (1) the use of oxytocin (Pitocin), in some instances resulting in sudden powerful uterine contractions and rapid expulsion of the fetus; and (2) the sudden forceful application of obstetrical forceps during a threatening intranatal complication, may cause catastrophic injury to the skull and intracranial structures. Such sudden compression of the head, especially in the premature, results in distortion of the cranium conducive to stretching and tearing of dural structures. Forceps that grip the head obliquely or in the fronto-occipital diameter are especially likely to cause such damage.

Fetal presentation is a primary factor in the pathogenesis of subdural hemorrhage. Cephalic delivery, with the head exposed foremost to lateral compression during descent, provides anatomical conditions obviously conducive to injurious molding with consequent dural-venous laceration and hemorrhage. Breech delivery, however, does not entirely safeguard the fetus from such head injury; intracranial damage may occur in utero, in middelivery, because of direct compression of the head by the uterine fundus, or more often, when difficulty is encountered in extracting the after-coming head. Even when cesarean section is resorted to, after failure of trial labor or with the development of other parturitional problems, there are cases in which the infant, traumatized in utero prior to the section, is born with subdural hematoma.

The size of the fetus, patently, is a direct factor in the occurrence of subdural hemorrhage. While even very small premature infants may show extensive subdural hemorrhage, the injury is more frequent in the mature and postmature. The frequency and severity of subdural hemorrhage vary directly with the size, the weight, and the gestational age of the infant.

In addition to fetal-pelvic disproportion, varied other obstetrical conditions that offer resistance to parturition influence the occurrence of subdural hemorrhage—pelvic malformations, uterine leiomyomas, abnormal fetal presentations, and primiparity, especially in older mothers. In rare instances, intracranial bleeding from dural-venous laceration may be exaggerated by hemorrhagic diatheses in the newborn.

The prenatal occurrence of subdural hemorrhage, developing prior to active labor, has been observed. It is apparent that the fetus may suffer substantial intracranial injury during the last weeks of gestation, when lightening takes place, when the fetus descends and settles into the pelvis, with engagement, with the beginning molding of the head. The clinical picture at this time is often clouded by the occurrence of latent labor, or so-called false labor, as observed in the following case.

Uterine contractions occurred intermittently two weeks prior to term, subsided, and were considered to be false labor pains. The mother, after leaving the hospital, reported an apparent loss of fetal activity. Later, on examination, the fetal heart was not audible. Active labor then developed; the stillborn infant showed a large caput succedaneum and a massive subdural hemorrhage.

Significantly, subdural hemorrhage may make its appearance after easy, ostensibly uncomplicated, spontaneous labor of moderate duration. Extensive lacerations of the tentorium and other dural structures are at times present in such circumstances. It is apparent that the force of one or more strong expulsive labor pains, especially if the fetus is constitutionally weak and susceptible, is sufficient to cause intracranial injury.

As Gröntoft has pointed out, dural laceration can occur after death of the fetus, and its presence by itself, without substantial hemorrhage, in stillbirths is not always conclusive indication of the cause of death.[42] In the presence of concomitant evidence of mechanical injury, histopathologic study of the dural lesion may permit a definitive diagnosis.

Pathologically, dural lacerations in the newborn are of varied form and severity. The mildest traumatic alteration in the tentorium and falx are not lacerations but consist of purpuric spots of hemorrhagic discoloration on the dural surfaces, observed almost universally in neonatal autopsies. Tentorial lacerations characteristically appear as broad shredded zones of disintegration, rarely as sharp-edged tears. Bits of clotted blood adhere to the frayed, stringy edges of the laceration, or blood oozes from torn vessels.

Each basic form of cephalic molding, vertical or anteroposterior, tends to produce dural tears in specific locations intracranially (Table 7–3). In the newborn, dural-venous laceration occurs at five main sites, at each giving rise to subdural hemorrhage at corresponding specific sites: (1) laceration of the tentorium, particularly at its junction with the falx; (2) tears of the falx; (3) tears of the vein of Galen near its junction with the straight sinus; (4) direct injury to the circumferential dural sinuses in association with fractures, displacement, and overriding of cranial bones; and (5) tearing of the superficial cerebral bridging veins at their attachment to the superior sagittal sinus.

Of the main forms of dural and venous injury indicated here, the most serious is laceration of the tentorium, with the tear extending medially to the straight sinus and to the point of attachment of the vein of Galen (Fig. 7–18). Regardless of the pattern of molding, whether the head is elongated in the vertical or horizontal diameter, the tentorium in this area at its junction with the falx cerebri, despite its protection by reinforcing fibers, proves extremely vulnerable. Tears in this triangular area, extending and opening major blood channels such as the straight sinus and the vein of Galen, result

TABLE 7–3. NEONATAL SUBDURAL HEMORRHAGE DUE TO DURAL-VENOUS LACERATION

Dural-Venous Lesion	Causal Factors	Location of Hemorrhage	Effects	Occurrence
Tentorial tear at junction of tentorium and falx	Vertex presentation with excessive vertical molding; forceps application in in anteroposterior diameter Face and brow presentation producing anteroposterior elongation of head	Basal cerebral hemorrhage with "incomplete" tentorial tears Posterior fossa hemorrhage due to tears extending to straight sinus and vein of Galen	Supratentorial hemorrhage usually tolerated Posterior fossa hemorrhage rapidly fatal	More common in term than in premature infants
Falx tears	Face and brow presentation producing anteroposterior elongation	Longitudinal cerebral fissure, over corpus callosum	Usually incidental finding at autopsy	Rare
Vein of Galen tear	Vertical and anteroposterior elongation	Commonly posterior fossa Also combined with basal cerebral hemorrhage	Posterior fossa hemorrhage produces rapid lethal compression of brain stem	Term and premature infants
Circumferential dural sinus injury	Fractures Occipital bone diastasis with laceration of lateral sinus Overriding of parietal bones with laceration of superior sagittal sinus	Region of sinus injury	Rapid accumulation of blood Precipitous death with lateral sinus laceration and posterior fossa hemorrhage	Rare
Superior superficial cerebral veins (bridging veins), stretch tears	All forms of cephalic molding, especially vertical Overlapping of interparietal fissure	Usually thinly spread over superior surface of cerebrum (subarachnoid bleeding often also occurs) Localized hematoma, frontoparietal, at times	Usually well tolerated when dispersed over hemisphere Cerebral compression with localized hematoma	Rare in premature infants Common at term in minimal form Large hematomas rare

in rapidly fatal subdural hemorrhage into the posterior cranial fossa.

Subdural bleeding from other torn dural-venous structures varies in extent and distribution and correspondingly varies in importance pathologically. In neonates, two patterns of subdural hemorrhage, regionally located, are commonly of concern (cf. Table 7–3).

The *cerebral form*, with blood over the convexity of the hemispheres, occurs mainly at term and, although common, is usually mild. With molding of the head during labor, the bridging veins between the medial superior aspect of the cerebrum and the superior sagittal sinus become stretched and may tear. Bleeding in this area is usually limited to a thin film of blood forming over the cerebrum (Fig. 7–19). Contrary to the general clinical impression, large subdural hematomas over the cerebral hemispheres are uncommon in the newborn. In prematures, especially in very small infants, the superficial veins over the cerebrum are still underdeveloped, and in these infants subdural hemorrhage about the cerebrum is rare.

Posterior fossa subdural hemorrhage occurs in both premature and term infants and, as previously indicated, is almost always fatal. The accumulation of blood in the posterior fossa, usually the consequence of a tear at the junction of the falx and tentorium near the attachment of the vein of Galen, results in lethal compression of the brain stem (Fig. 7–20).

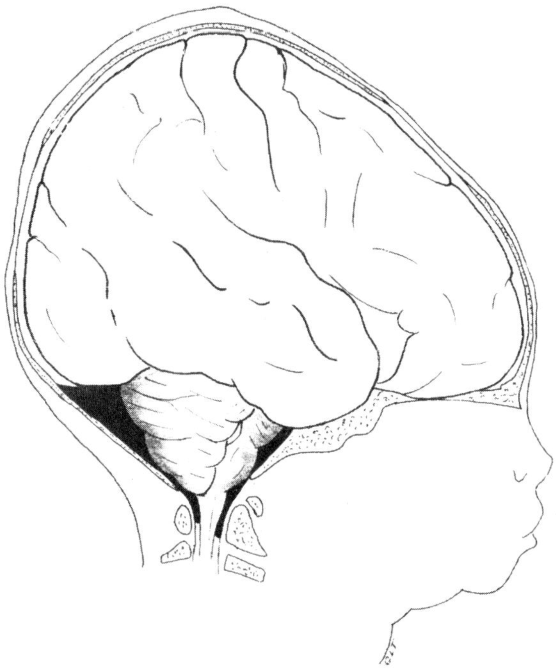

Figure 7–20. Posterior fossa subdural hemorrhage, commonly the consequence of tentorial laceration. The accumulation of blood leads to rapidly fatal compression of the brain stem.

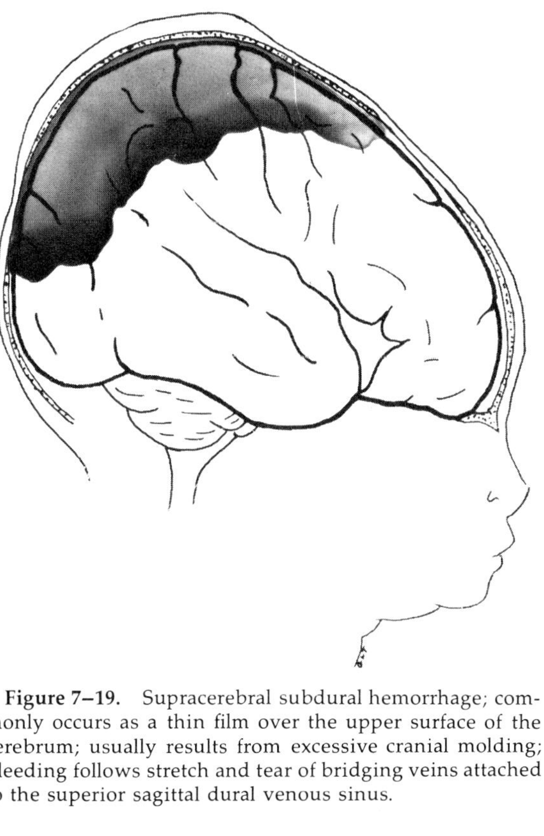

Figure 7–19. Supracerebral subdural hemorrhage; commonly occurs as a thin film over the upper surface of the cerebrum; usually results from excessive cranial molding; bleeding follows stretch and tear of bridging veins attached to the superior sagittal dural venous sinus.

The axiom is well conceived that subdural hemorrhage in the neonate exerts an all-or-none effect. As is evident, the clinical consequence of subdural bleeding in the newborn depends on its location. Cerebral (supracerebral) extravasation, in the majority of instances, is asymptomatic and innocuous, usually being lightly dispersed over the hemispheres. This type of bleeding is thought by some to occur, in minor degree, almost universally in term deliveries. It is not unusual to find evidence of old subdural bleeding, traces of hemosiderin, or even latent encysted subdural hematomas over the cerebral convexity in infants who survive for a period and die of other systemic diseases. In contrast, with hemorrhage into the posterior fossa, a small confined chamber where the trapped blood causes compression and injury of vital regulatory centers in the brain stem, death usually takes place at once. Manifestly, in the neonate, the process of subdural hemorrhage, because of the extremes of its effects—harmless or lethal—leaves few cases with chronic crippling neurologic sequelae. Accordingly, while subdural hemorrhage is of major concern as a factor in neonatal mortality, it is the cause of relatively few cases of mental retardation, cerebral palsy, or other lasting cerebral disability.

In the newborn infant, injuries to the nervous system are often multiple, incorporating both mechanical injury and hypoxic damage, one type of injury overlapping and exacerbating another. In infants with dural-venous laceration, the process of hemorrhage may be intensified by hypoxia; in infants born cyanotic and moribund, in hypoxic circulatory failure, the subdural bleeding is reinforced by mounting systemic venous congestion. As stated earlier, in infants with spinal cord and brain stem injury, respiration becomes depressed, causing superimposed hypoxic cerebral damage of varying severity. In the newborn, after complicated deliveries, it is not uncommon to find subdural hemorrhage, spinal injury, and hypoxic infarctional cerebral damage, all present in the same case.

HYPOXIC PROCESSES OF INJURY IN THE FETUS AND NEWBORN

Organic injury present at birth, poorly understood in the past, was commonly thought to be due mainly to mechanical obstetrical trauma. Current investigations provide increasing evidence that hypoxic complications are far more important than mechanical trauma as a cause of fetal and neonatal injury and death. Furthermore, it is evident that in a majority of cases, hypoxic damage has its origin prenatally and in most instances results from endogenous, intrinsic complications; less often, it is due to extrinsic obstetrical factors. Hypoxia is the most important cause of neonatal mortality and morbidity—the most important pathologic process contributing to stillbirth and death of the newborn and the main cause of chronic neurologic disability stemming from the perinatal period. Plainly it is the responsibility of the obstetrician, for clinical, academic, and medicolegal reasons, to distinguish between endogenous and exogenous processes leading to hypoxic injury. It is likewise of primary importance to the clinician that hemorrhage and other organic processes due to hypoxia in the newborn be recognized as such and not be attributed to mechanical trauma.

Systemic and Local Effects of Hypoxia

All the visceral and somatic structures of the body are susceptible to injury by hypoxia. In the fetus, as in the adult, hypoxia causes injury of varying severity to tissues, damage to parenchyma and stroma that may or may not be reversible. The tubular necrosis that occurs in the kidney and the fatty changes in the liver cells are reversible, and destroyed elements may be regenerated. Likewise, compensatory changes tend to occur in the heart and other organs. In the brain, however, the more highly specialized cellular elements, the nerve cells, are readily affected by oxygen deprivation and, once destroyed, are not replaced.

The processes that, during fetal and neonatal life, lead to hypoxic brain damage are analogous to the pathologic mechanisms that occur

TABLE 7–4. PATHOGENESIS OF PERINATAL HYPOXIC ORGANIC DAMAGE

(1) THE HYPOXIC ONSET

In the Fetus	In the Newborn
Hypoxic intrauterine complications: premature placental detachment, placental infarction, placenta previa; umbilical cord knots, compression, and other conditions disrupting the maternal-placental-fetal organization	Hypoxia due to central respiratory failure following parturitional spinal cord or brain stem damage, or due to postnatal peripheral pulmonary complications (pneumonia, hyaline membrane disease, pneumothorax)

↓

(2) CONGESTIVE HEART FAILURE

Hypoxia, affecting the myocardium, leads to cardiac decompensation with systemic circulatory congestion (backward failure), to generalized bodily venous engorgement in the fetus and newborn

↓

(3) LOCAL VISCERAL VENOUS STASIS-THROMBOSIS

↓

Infarction (hemorrhagic)

↓

Local hemorrhage

in the adult in the respiratory brain death syndrome and, in other circumstances, often in the aged, in conditions in which congestive heart failure leads to intracranial venous stasis with thrombosis and ultimately to infarctional damage in the brain.[43, 44]

The pathogenesis of hypoxic injury in the fetus and newborn, damage to the brain and other organs, evolves through a consistent series of clinicopathologic processes, through three consecutive stages, each stage precipitating the next. The onset, the hypoxic gestational complication, leads to congestive heart failure, systemic circulatory congestion in the fetus, which in turn results in visceral (cerebral) venous infarctional damage and hemorrhage (Table 7–4).[8]

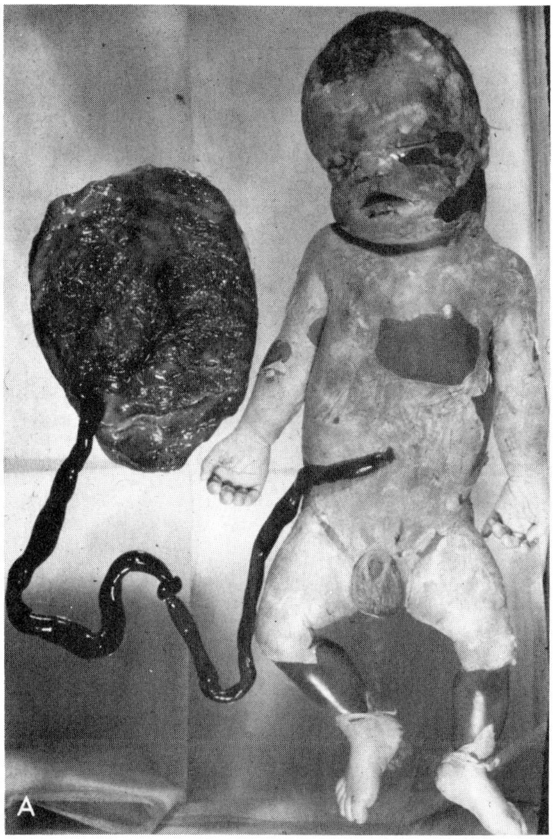

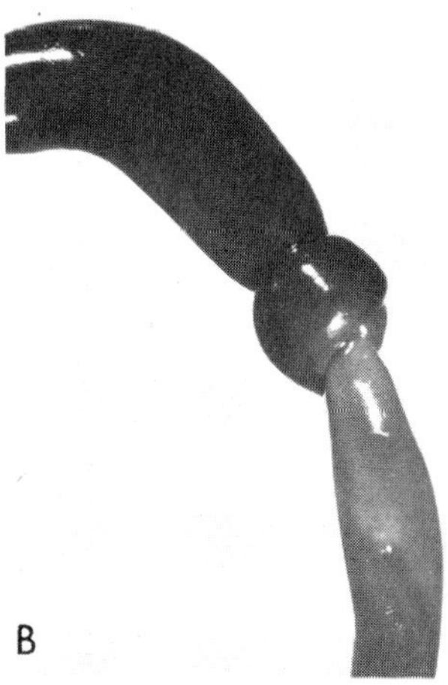

Figure 7–21. *A.* Hypoxic intrauterine death due to umbilical cord knot. Near-term pregnancy. Maternal history of decreasing fetal activity (fetus-in-coma) developing gradually in a period of 10 days prior to labor. Fetus shows early maceration, is edematous and cyanotic (M–38). *B.* Tight true cord knot.

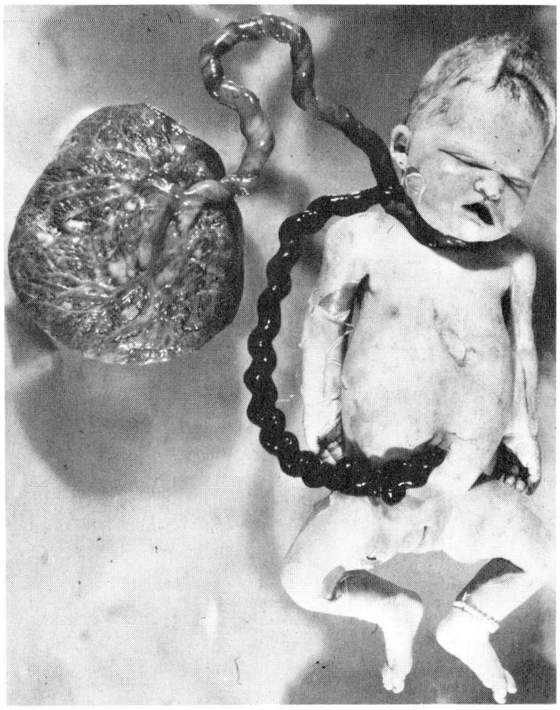

Figure 7–22. Fetal hypoxia due to entangled loop of cord around the neck. Gradual loss of fetal activity (fetus-in-coma) prior to delivery. Congenital long cord; note proximal segment of cord, attached to fetus, is swollen and discolored, in contrast to the distal placental segment. Fetus edematous, in congestive heart failure (N–1544).

The systemic and visceral changes that take place in these three stages follow basic pathologic patterns.

Stages of Hypoxic Injury

The Onset. The hypoxia-producing complication may have its onset prenatally, intranatally, or postnatally, and may have its origin in any of the components of the maternal-placental-fetal organization.

Various maternal complications, particularly eclampsia, toxemia, hypertension, and isoimmunization, as well as infections, anemia, and diabetes mellitus, exert their hypoxic effects on the fetus. Physical injury, often automobile accidents, in which the pregnant mother suffers severe trauma with shock results in intrauterine hypoxia.[14-16] Fetal hypoxic damage at times results from accidental or suicidal maternal

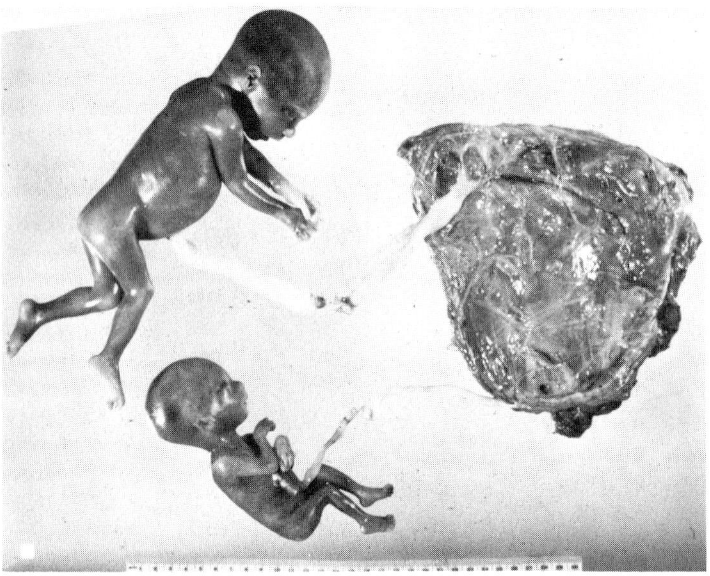

Figure 7–23. Chronic fetal hypoxia associated with placental vascular shunts (intrauterine transfusion syndrome). Monochorionic twins; 20 weeks' gestation. In this placental disorder, vascular shunts result in unequal distribution of blood to the twins, leading to chronic hypoxia and other nutritional deprivation and stunting of growth of one twin, the other twin becoming functionally dominant and organically hypertrophied and plethoric. As in this case, hydramnios commonly develops with premature birth, with superimposed acute parturitional hypoxia (L–22). (From A. Towbin: Central nervous system damage in the human fetus and newborn infant. Am. J. Dis. Child., *119*:529, June, 1970. Copyright 1970, American Medical Association. Reprinted by permission.)

asphyxia.[11, 45–47] During gestation and delivery, the occurrence of a tight umbilical cord knot, nuchal cord, and other forms of cord entanglement and compression are familiar causes of hypoxia (Figs. 7–21 and 7–22). Frequently fetal hypoxia is due to placental complications, especially infarction and retroplacental hemorrhage, clinically often signaled by the occurrence of vaginal bleeding and false labor (Figs. 7–23 through 7–26). Varying from case to case, hypoxia resulting from placental disorders such as retroplacental hemorrhage, placenta previa, or infarction may be sudden and lethal, or may be protracted, latent.

Frequently in cases of placental disease the acute hypoxic state initiated during intrauterine life, present at birth, is extended postnatally; in such cases, as is discussed later, the affected newborn, especially the premature, commonly develops hyaline membrane disease, meconium aspiration pneumonia, pneumothorax, or other peripheral pulmonary complications, further aggravating the systemic hypoxia.

Systemic Circulatory Failure. This develops regularly after protracted hypoxia in the fetus and newborn (cf. Table 7–4).[42, 48–52] During parturition, as hypoxic complications occur, monitoring very soon registers the altered, weakened cardiac function of the affected fetus. In the delivery room the effects of hypoxia are plainly evident; the newly born infant is cyanotic, bloated, limp, and comatose, and usually rates an Apgar score of less than 5.

Hypoxia produces essentially the same systemic clinical and pathologic effects in the human fetus and newborn as in the adult. As evident in the monitored fetus, hypoxia immediately manifests its first crippling effects directly on the heart, on the myocardium; ventricular contraction is weakened; resulting cardiac decompensation leads to systemic circulatory congestion (backward failure) and to generalized bodily venous engorgement. In perinatal deaths after protracted terminal hypoxia, postmortem examination consistently reveals the characteristic picture of congestive heart failure—cyanosis, peripheral edema, ascites, hydrothorax, hydropericardium, cardiac dilatation, distention of the venae cavae, and enlargement and engorgement of the liver, spleen, and other viscera; the brain is very soft, swollen, and congested.

Local Visceral Venous Infarction. This is the end event in the sequence of organic processes that develop in the hypoxic fetus and newborn. With increasing hypoxic circulatory failure and local stagnation of venous blood flow, stasis-thrombosis occurs, especially in peripheral veins, very often intracranially.[18, 48, 50, 53–58] In the parts of the body involved, this results in hemorrhagic infarction (cf. Table 7–4). Venous thrombosis with infarction occurs at times in the kidney, adrenal, thymus, and other organs; the cerebrum, however, is the most frequent site of venous infarction in the fetal-neonatal period.[58] Infarctional damage varies in pattern and extent. In the affected organs, in the wake of the infarctional damage, bleeding develops, often progressing to massive hemorrhage.

The significance and frequency of venous infarction and its role as a cause of hemorrhage, especially intracranial hemorrhage, are not generally realized clinically. In analyzing the processes of infarction and hemorrhage, often elementary principles of pathology are passed over. Basically, infarction in an organ

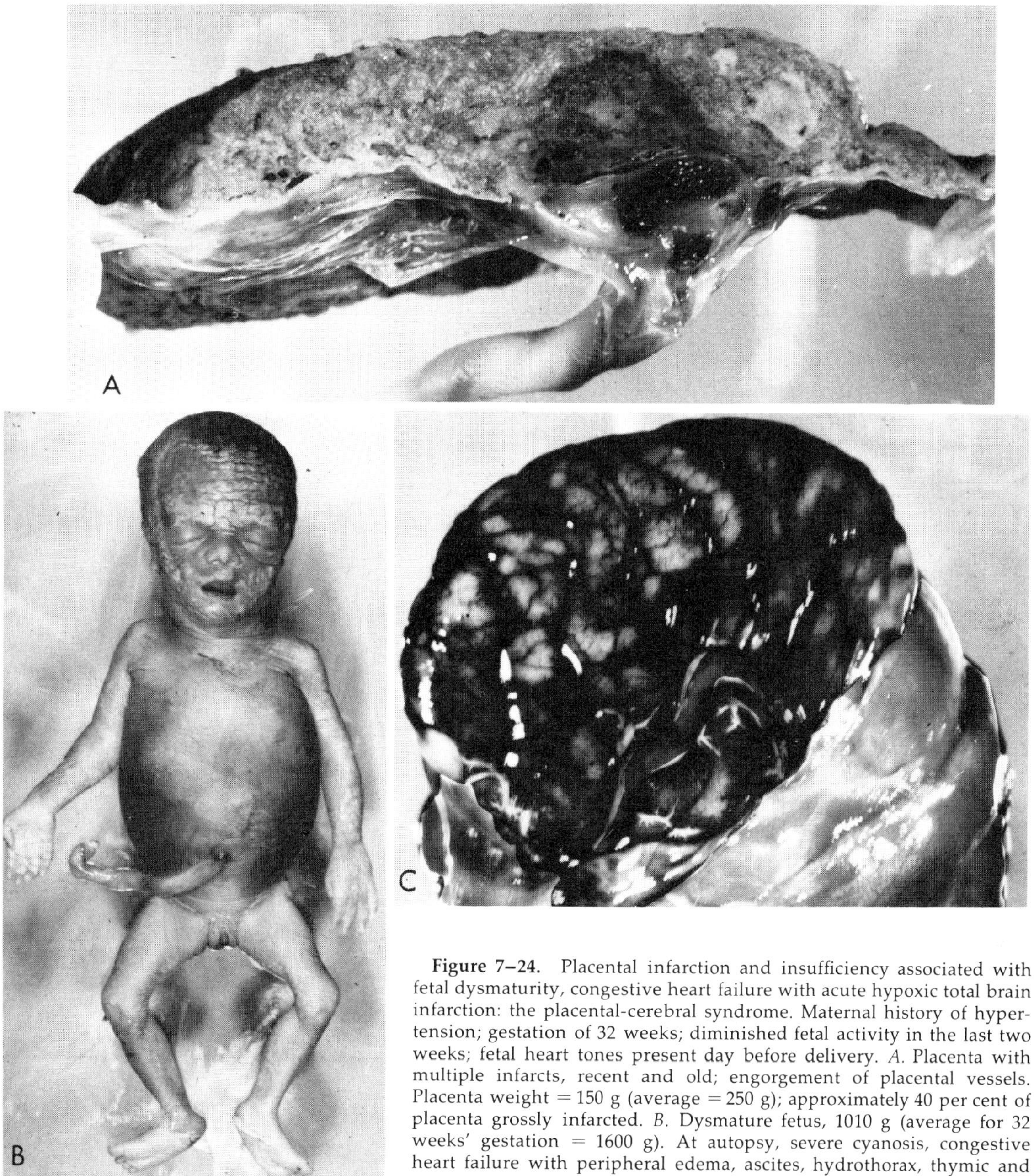

Figure 7–24. Placental infarction and insufficiency associated with fetal dysmaturity, congestive heart failure with acute hypoxic total brain infarction: the placental-cerebral syndrome. Maternal history of hypertension; gestation of 32 weeks; diminished fetal activity in the last two weeks; fetal heart tones present day before delivery. *A.* Placenta with multiple infarcts, recent and old; engorgement of placental vessels. Placenta weight = 150 g (average = 250 g); approximately 40 per cent of placenta grossly infarcted. *B.* Dysmature fetus, 1010 g (average for 32 weeks' gestation = 1600 g). At autopsy, severe cyanosis, congestive heart failure with peripheral edema, ascites, hydrothorax, thymic and adrenal atrophy. *C.* Brain exposed at autopsy; venous stasis with diffuse cerebral infarction. Brain weight and cerebral convolutional differentiation commensurate with 32 weeks' gestation (W–133).

develops because of interference with local circulation, the suppression of either arterial inflow or venous outflow. Although both mechanisms are known to occur, the process of *arterial* infarction is more familiar, much better known medically. In practice, with clinicians and pathologists, an infarct found in an organ is most often presumed to be due to arterial occlusion, infarction due to venous thrombosis generally escaping consideration.

Venous infarcts occur mainly in organs with great circulatory exchange, commonly the brain, kidney, and intestine; characteristically the venous lesions are hemorrhagic, in contrast to arterial infarcts, which are usually pale and dry. The process of venous infarction is gradual. In affected areas, with slowing of local blood flow, with or without thrombosis, attritional changes occur in the tissue—histologic damage leading to necrosis. Breakdown of tissue is evident, not only in the parenchymal cells but also in the stromal elements, especially in the thin-

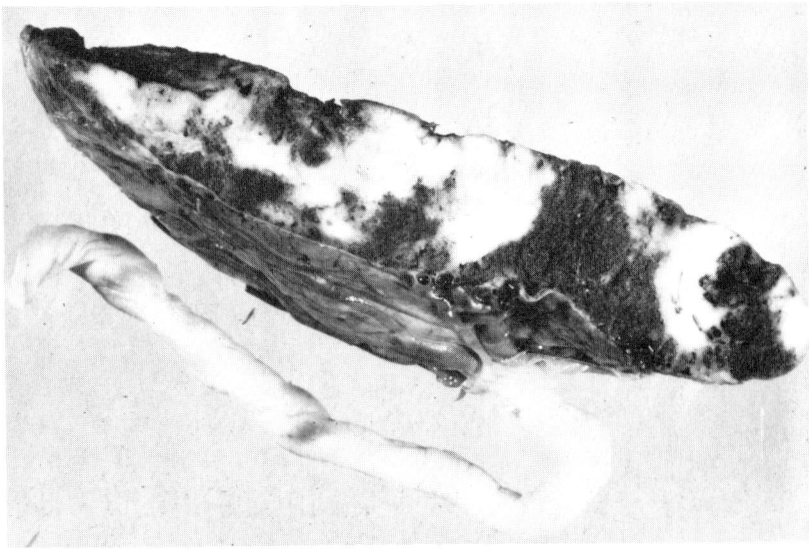

Figure 7–25. Placental infarction and insufficiency, fetal dysmaturity. Mother of average body build; prenatal course essentially uncomplicated; examinations during the last trimester, however, indicated an apparent decrease in fetal growth. Gestation of 40 weeks. Placenta weighed 400 g, was estimated 50 per cent infarcted. Newborn, weight 2200 g, in fair clinical condition postnatally but with physical characteristics of dysmaturity (N–1467).

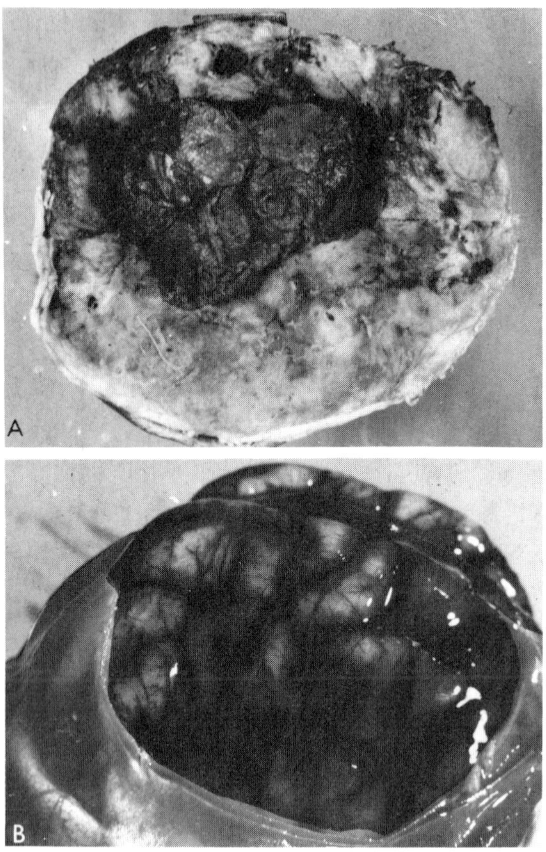

Figure 7–26. *A.* Retroplacental hematoma, old and recent. Prenatal vaginal bleeding. Gestation of 30 weeks. Gradual loss of fetal activity two days before delivery. Placental weight, 175 g (average = 210 g). Stillborn; weight, 1250 g (average = 1400 g). Autopsy revealed slight maceration, cyanosis, congestive heart failure with ascites, hydrothorax, and visceral congestion. *B.* Brain exposed at autopsy. Diffuse venous stasis-thrombosis with massive bilateral cerebral infarction. Placental-cerebral syndrome (N–49).

walled veins. As a result, early in the course of venous infarction minute bleeding points, small focal hemorrhages, make their appearance in the tissues affected. Thus in the intestine with mesenteric vein thrombosis, beginning infarction signals its presence first by the appearance of minute hemorrhages in the mucosa and, soon thereafter, with bleeding into the lumen of the organ. Similarly, with renal vein thrombosis and early infarction, hematuria results—in the newborn as in the adult. In the same way, in the hypoxic fetus and newborn, with infarction developing in the brain, very soon focal hemorrhages appear in the cerebral walls, and blood escapes into the ventricles and subarachnoid space. Hemorrhage, with blood escaping from disintegrating veins and suffusing through the necrotic tissue, is thus the ultimate manifestation of venous infarction.

In general, hemorrhage, in the fetus and newborn as in the adult, may be of venous or arterial origin; hemorrhage may be due to defects or injury of vessel walls, may be associated with intravascular hypertension, and at times may be due to defective blood coagulation. Arterial hemorrhage and arterial thrombosis are relatively rare in the newborn. In studies in the past, observers have in some instances incorrectly interpreted the common hemorrhagic cerebral infarctions in the newborn as the consequence of arterial occlusion.[59, 60] In another view also, neonatal bleeding was commonly thought to be due mainly to vitamin K deficiency. Current studies indicate that although other etiologic processes occur, hypoxia with consequent venous infarction is the most common cause of neonatal cerebral and other visceral hemorrhage.

Kidney, Adrenal, and Other Visceral Damage Due to Hypoxia

In the fetus and newborn, hypoxic damage of varying pattern and extent occurs commonly in the kidney, the adrenal, and other organs, especially the brain. The degree and distribution of the damage is generally related to the severity of the hypoxic exposure. Three main patterns of organic hypoxic damage appear. (1) Diffuse damage to essential parenchymal cells may be more or less evenly spread through the organ; in a given case, widespread neuronal damage may be present in the cerebrum, together with tubular necrosis in the kidneys and fatty metamorphosis in liver cells and in myocardial fibers.[18, 51, 58] (2) Focal hemorrhagic infarcts frequently appear as small scattered lesions, minute infarcts, hemorrhagic extravasates in the form of petechiae, on the pericardium and other serosal surfaces and in the thymus and other viscera (Figs. 7–27 and 7–28). With extension of the infarctional process,

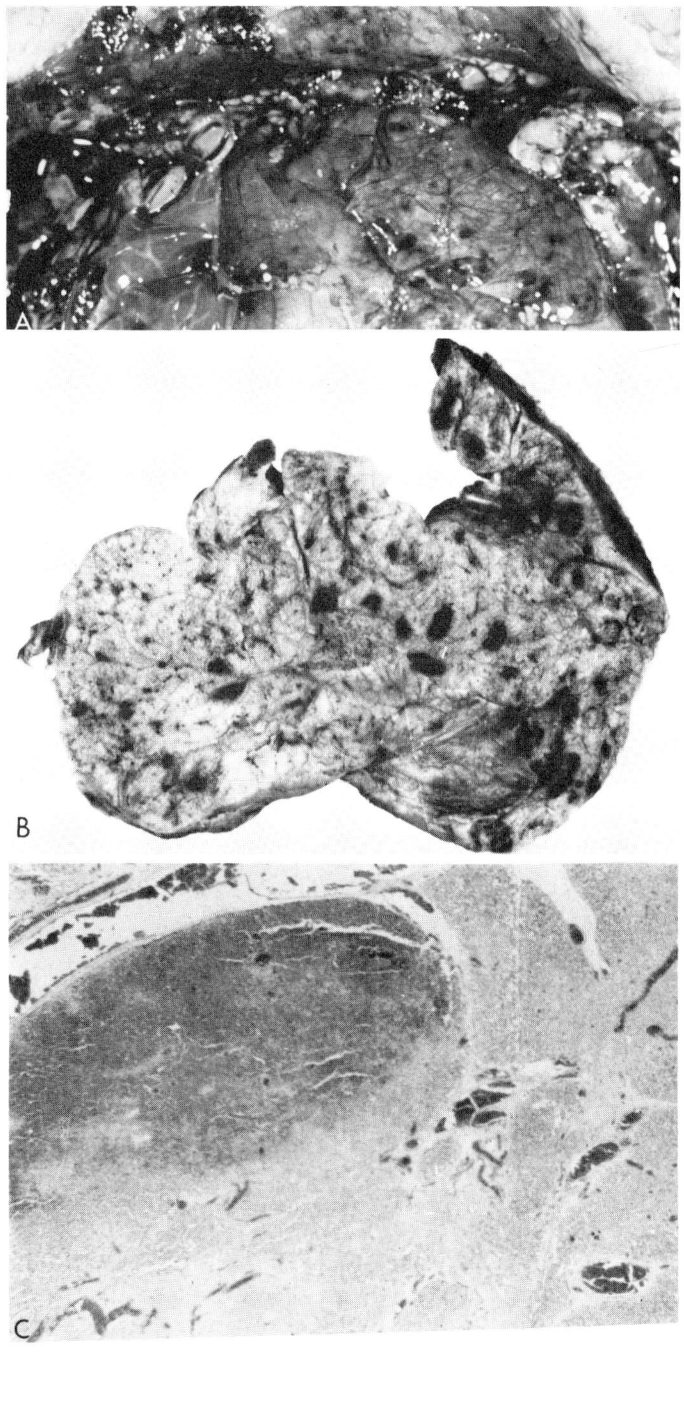

Figure 7–27. Hypoxic focal hemorrhagic infarcts (petechiae) of thymus. Term pregnancy; decreased fetal movements day before delivery (fetus-in-coma). Evidence of fetal distress during labor; cesarean section revealed umbilical cord compression, meconium staining; stillbirth. At autopsy, congestive hepatosplenomegaly, hydrothorax, aspiration of amniotic fluid. *A.* Autopsy dissection exposing thymus and other structures in upper thorax; small focal hemorrhagic lesions evident on the external surface of the thymus. *B.* Corresponding hemorrhagic lesions in the transected surface of the thymus. *C.* Histologically these prove to be microinfarcts; the area of hemorrhagic necrosis in the upper left portion of the section is associated with engorged small venous channels (M–9).

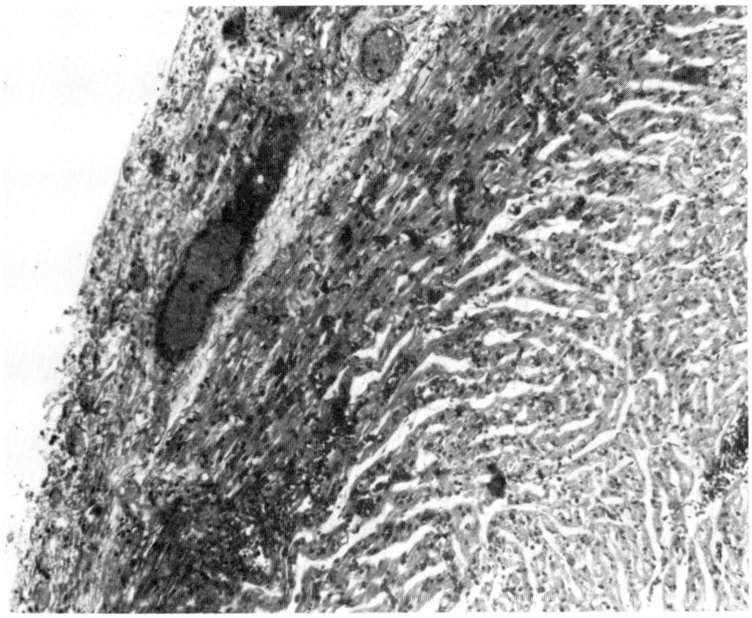

Figure 7–28. Focal myocardial hemorrhagic infarction, grossly appearing as pericardial petechia. Prolonged fetal-neonatal hypoxia in premature (M–52).

the focal areas of necrosis may become confluent, forming larger infarcts, occupying major portions of the organ. (3) The hypoxic damage may extend to total organ infarction.

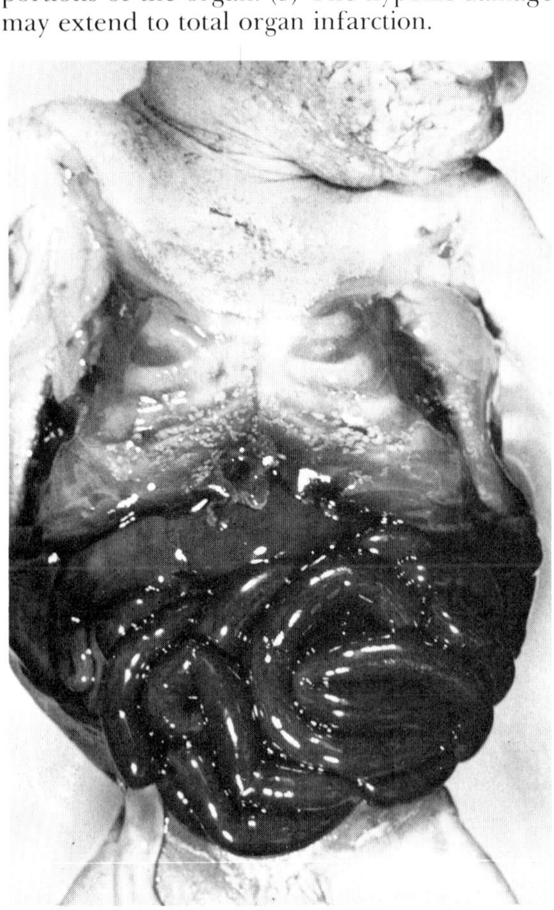

Figure 7–29. Intestinal infarction in newborn. Massive placental infarction and cerebral infarction (same case as in Figure 7–24; W–133).

The kidney, adrenal, testis, thymus, and intestinal tract often are severely involved, at times showing total organ infarction (Figs. 7–29 through 7–33).[48, 61-64] Renal vein thrombosis with diffuse infarction of the kidney appears second only in frequency to infarction of the brain. Morison described 17 cases of renal vein thrombosis and infarction occurring in newborn infants.[61] Neonatal renal vein thrombosis has been attributed to asphyxia with concomitant vascular congestion. Venous infarction of the kidney has been described following delivery after abruptio placentae. At autopsy in some instances renal vein thrombosis has been found in association with cerebral venous thrombosis.

Cerebral Hypoxic Damage

Patterns and Pathogenesis

In the central nervous system, as in other structures of the newborn, hemorrhage is the most common indication of injury, resulting as it does both from mechanical trauma and from hypoxia. In analyzing neonatal injuries that present extensive hemorrhage, especially in the central nervous system, it is of elementary importance to identify the causal mechanism, to distinguish mechanical injury from hypoxic damage. Clinically and pathologically, in the differential diagnosis of neonatal hemorrhagic processes, the cause is often left vague and equivocal. Patently, *hemorrhage* is not a clinical or pathologic entity. As applied in the central nervous system, the diagnosis "intra-

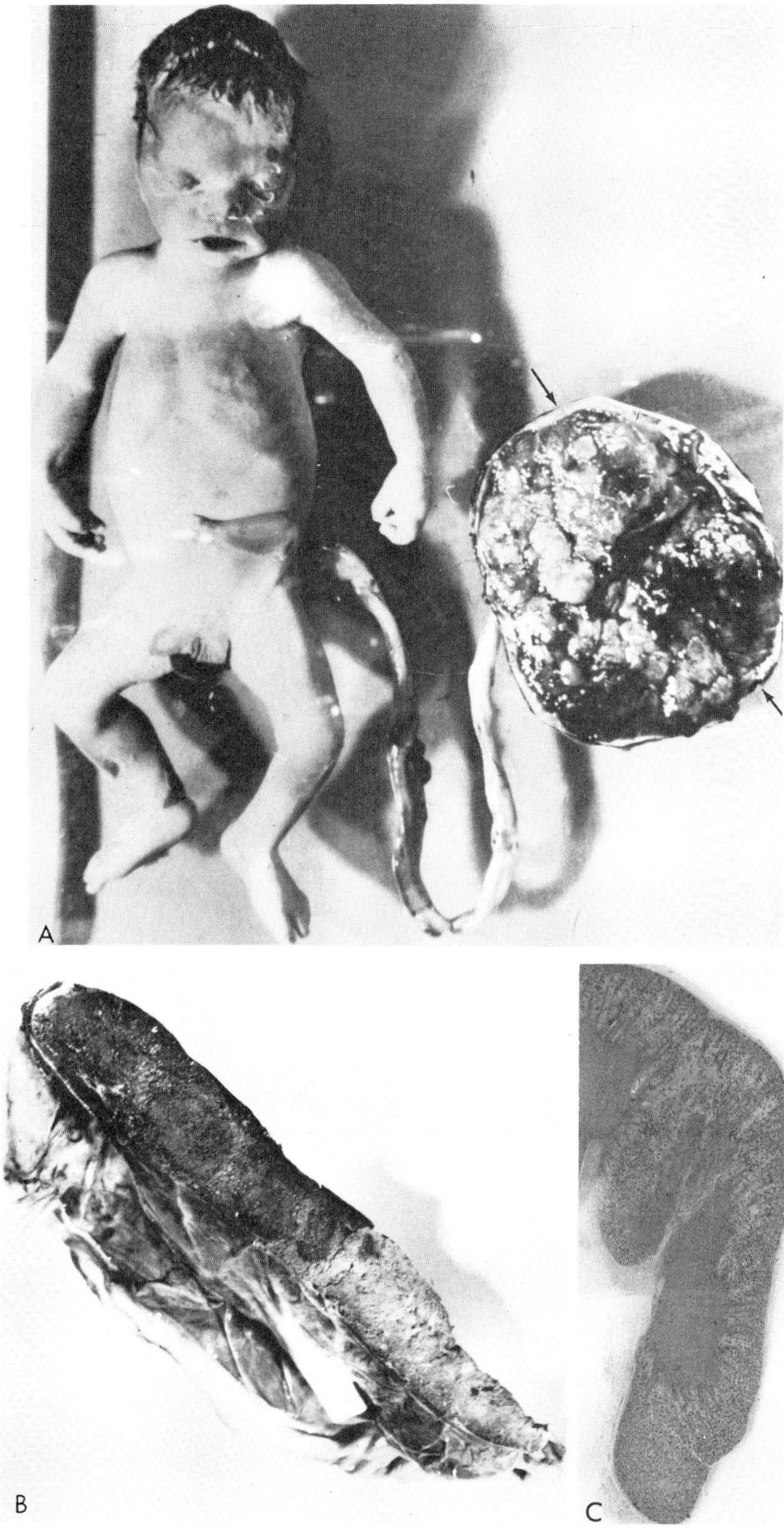

Figure 7–30. Placental infarction with associated kidney infarction. *A.* Fetus, near term, stillborn; cyanotic; autopsy findings of congestive heart failure. Upper arrow indicates swollen acutely infarcted portion of placenta. Placenta transected along line between arrows. *B.* Cut surface of placenta; upper left portion swollen, with confluent areas of indurated reddened infarction; lower portion relatively intact, pink, soft. *C.* Kidney with acute hemorrhagic cortical infarction in upper portion; lower portion relatively unaffected (C–78).

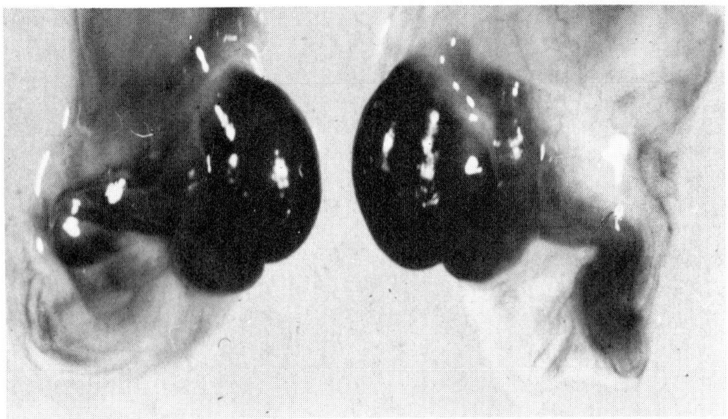

Figure 7–31. Infarction of testes. Premature infant; breech extraction. Infant cyanotic edematous; survived one hour (N–79).

cranial hemorrhage" is ambiguous, not meaningful, unless consideration is given to the underlying pathogenesis. In the past there has been a tendency to lump together all forms of neonatal intracranial hemorrhage, subdural as well as intracerebral, and to consider them summarily as being due to "trauma."

Studies carried out in the Collaborative Perinatal Project defined four main types of neonatal central nervous system hemorrhage (Table 7–5).[1, 58] Two of these pathologic processes, hemorrhage due to spinal and brain stem injury, and subdural hemorrhage, have already been discussed here. The other two major forms of intracranial hemorrhage, processes in the cerebrum consequent to hypoxia, are reviewed in the sections following.

The direct study of perinatal brain damage is important not only in defining the acute, immediate processes, but also in elaborating the pathologic study of the brain. The location and age of the damage in the brain, correlated with obstetrical data, provides basic information for determining the time when the damage occurred—distinguishing prenatal damage from intranatal or postnatal damage—and for defining underlying gestational-parturitional causal mechanisms. Further, with regard to chronic nervous system sequelae, the temporal organic relationships so defined are of importance diagnostically to the pediatrician, neurologist, and psychiatrist in the study of children who survive after perinatal hypoxia. The gestational age at the time of the hypoxic injury consistently governs the location of the cerebral structural damage and hence may also determine the sequelant clinical pattern of cerebral functional disability.

In the fetus and newborn with developing systemic congestive heart failure with local venous stasis-thrombosis consequent to hypoxia, the resulting hemorrhagic infarcts in the brain are of consistent, specific pattern. As defined in Collaborative Perinatal Project studies, the in-

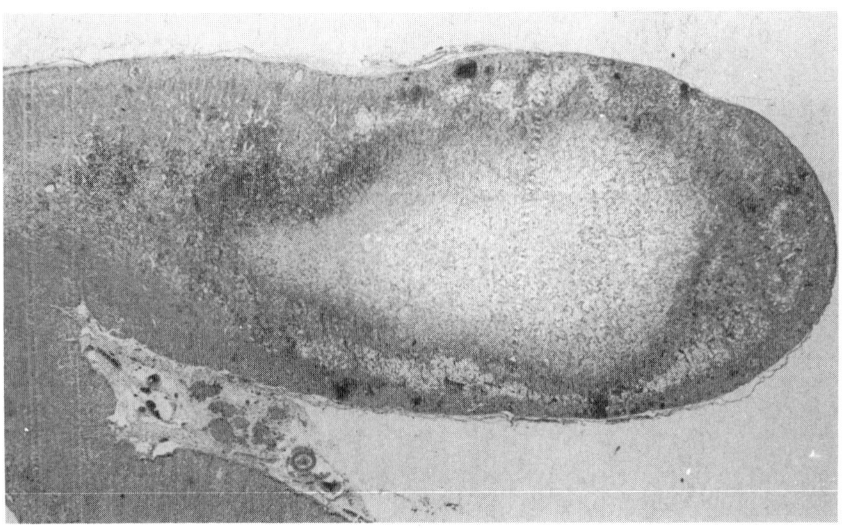

Figure 7–32. Adrenal infarct. Premature infant lived three days. Autopsy revealed severe congestive heart failure—visceral engorgement, hydrothorax, hydropericardium, and ascites; infarctional damage also present in the gastric mucosa and in the cerebrum (M–6).

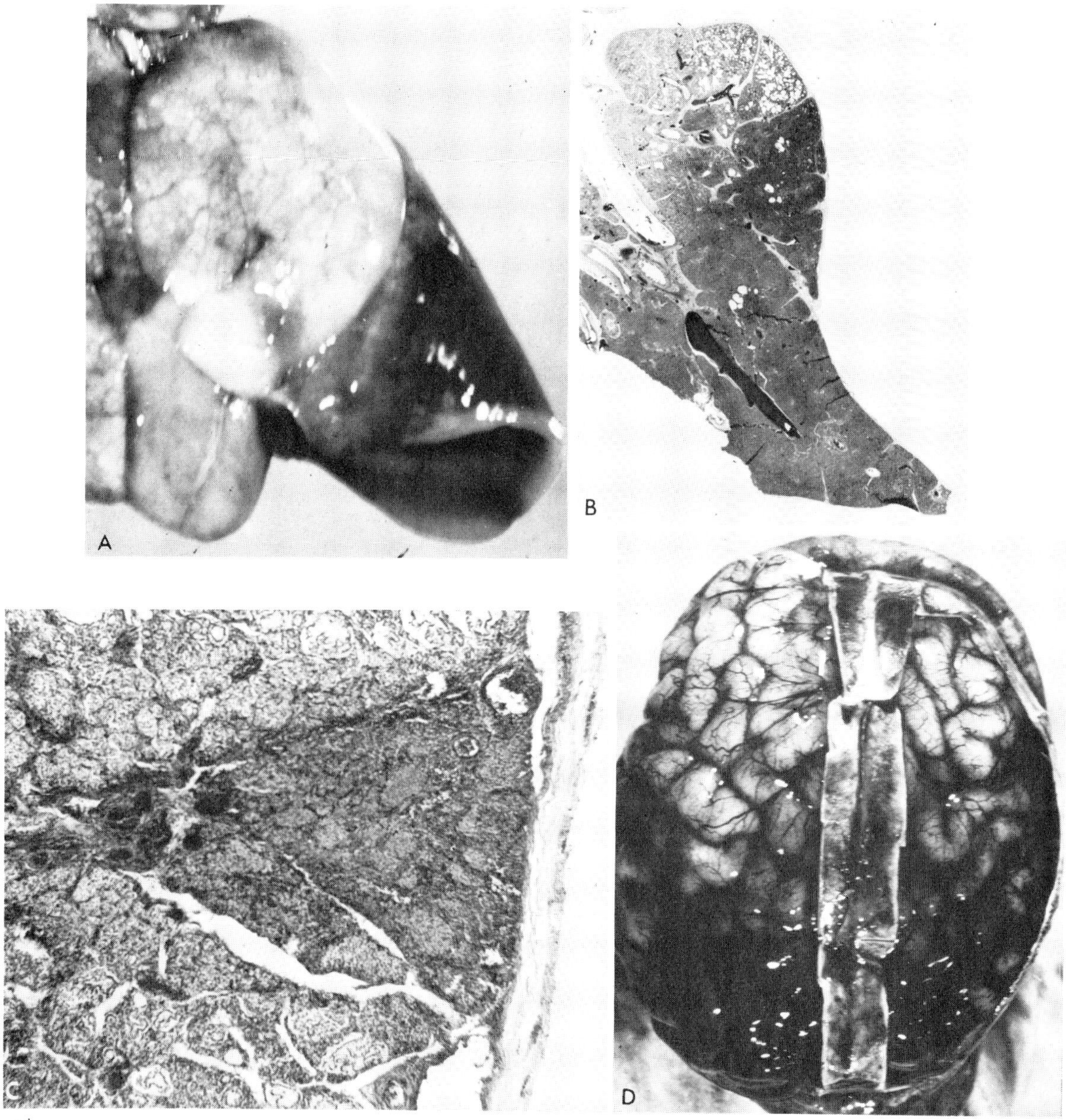

Figure 7–33. Multiple visceral infarcts in premature infant, 35 weeks' gestation; retroplacental hemorrhage; infant lived three days. Severe congestive heart failure. *A.* Pulmonary infarction evident at autopsy. *B.* Corresponding longitudinal section of lung showing thrombosis of large vein and infarction of lower lobe. *C.* Focal infarct in thyroid; thrombosis of small veins at the left is associated with wedge-shaped infarct at the margin. *D.* Massive infarction of posterior portion of the cerebral hemispheres and associated thrombosis of dural venous sinuses (N–15).

TABLE 7–5. INTRACRANIAL HEMORRHAGE IN THE NEWBORN INFANT

Type	Occurrence	Cause	Pathogenesis	Patterns	Pathologic Significance	Clinical Effects
Subdural	Supratentorial in term infants mainly Subtentorial in premature and term	Trauma	Molding and other forceful cranial distortion; tearing of dural venous structures	Supratentorial bleeding (slight) common Subtentorial (posterior fossa)	Supratentorial form usually latent Posterior fossa hemorrhage leads to brain stem compression	Supratentorial forms usually tolerated Subtentorial form usually rapidly fatal
Brain stem (spinal cord)	Premature and term infants	Trauma	Excessive traction, torsion, and flexion during delivery leading to stretch injury and pressure injury in upper cord and brain stem	Spinal epidural hemorrhage most common lesion observed grossly Posterior fossa hemorrhage consequent to brain stem lacerations	Spinal epidural hemorrhage indicates trauma to cord structures. Traction with cerebellar herniation, leads to erosion and deep brain stem laceration	Hemorrhage usually of secondary importance; mortality, morbidity due to associated injury to vital centers and consequent depression of respiration
Intraventricular due to periventricular venous infarction	Premature infants	Hypoxia	Fetal-neonatal hypoxic systemic circulatory failure, deep cerebral venous stasis; infarction of subependymal germinal matrix	Bleeding varies from slight oozing to massive intraventricular hemorrhage with extension to subarachnoid space of posterior fossa	Mild forms often latent; massive hemorrhage in posterior fossa leads to compression of vital medullary structures	Mild forms tolerated; neurologic deficits in surviving infants Massive hemorrhage precipitates death
Subarachnoid due to cortical venous infarction	Term infants	Hypoxia	Fetal-neonatal hypoxic systemic circulatory failure; stasis of superficial cerebral venous circulation	Cerebral subarachnoid bleeding usually focal and of minor degree	Lesions localized or diffuse; usually not lethal	Hemorrhage usually tolerated neonatally; chronic neurological deficits in surviving infants due to underlying cortical damage

farctional lesions occur in two basic forms, characterized by their location in the cerebrum: *deep* cerebral damage and *cortical* cerebral damage (Fig. 7–34).[65] The pattern of the damage, the distribution of the infarcts, is related to the gestational age at the time of the hypoxic event. In the premature fetus and newborn, at 25 to 35 weeks' gestation, the hypoxic damage consistently is located in the deep cerebral strata, mainly in the periventricular tissues. In the mature fetus and newborn, acute damage in this deep location is infrequent; acute cerebral damage incurred at or near term generally affects the surface elements, the cortex becoming the primary target of hypoxic injury.[8, 11, 65–67]

*In the Premature: Deep Cerebral Infarction**

Acute Stage. The specificity in location of acute hypoxic damage in the fetus and newborn, the predilection for deep cerebral struc-

*See References 12, 18, 54–57, 68–70.

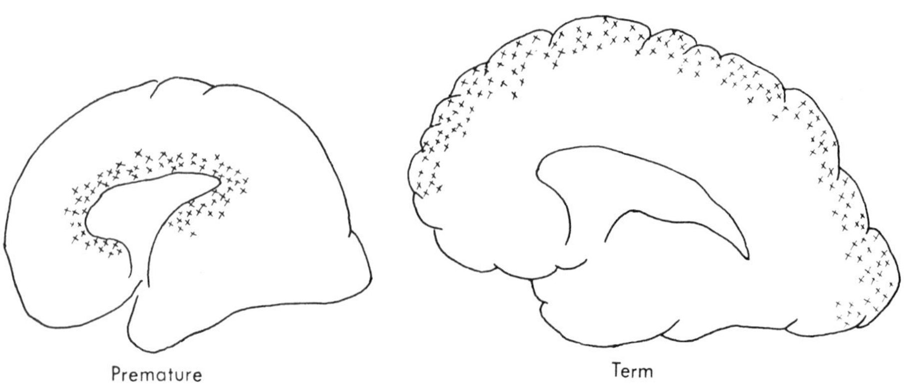

Figure 7–34. Two basic patterns of hypoxic cerebral infarctional damage related to the gestational age. In the premature, hemorrhagic infarction of the periventricular germinal matrix tissue and adjoining deep structures predominates; at term, the cortex with the subjacent white matter is the predominant site of hypoxic infarctional damage.

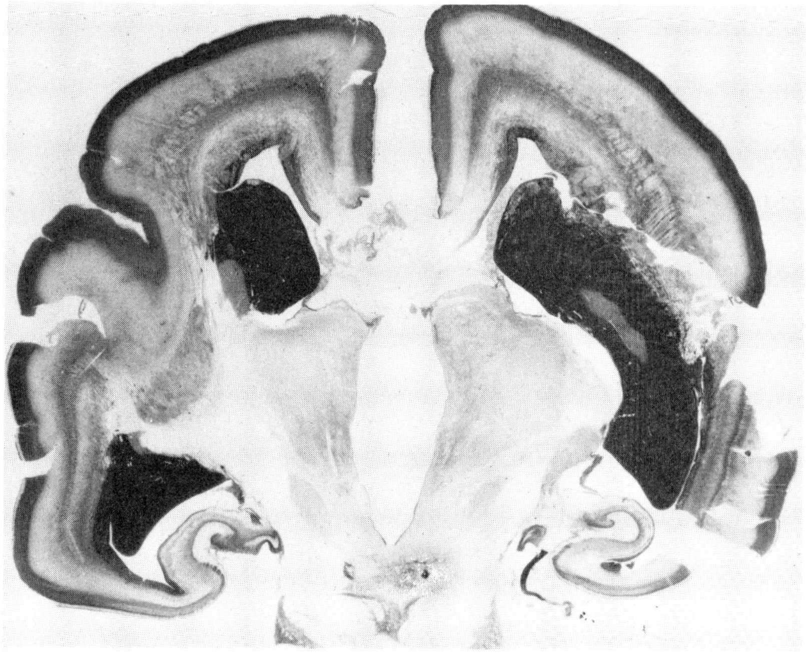

Figure 7–35. Germinal matrix tissue deposits in subependymal zones of lateral ventricles. Germinal matrix deposits appear as polypoid sheets of compact deeply staining tissue projecting from ependymal surface into lateral ventricles; most prominent during midfetal life, diminishing toward term. Stillborn, 19-week gestation, frontal section of brain (W–52).

tures in the premature and for the cortex at term, is not a random occurrence but is influenced by three biologic factors, all related to gestational age: the presence or absence of germinal matrix tissue, the momentum of local organogenesis, and the level of development of local intracranial vascular elements.[8]

Germinal tissue in large deposits remains present in the brain of the premature, in the deep strata of the cerebrum—thick deeply staining compact cellular subependymal masses bulging into the lateral ventricles, especially prominent at each side of the groove between the caudate nucleus and the thalamus (Fig. 7–35). The germinal matrix tissue is gradually used up as the brain matures and is almost gone in the mature fetus. The healthy growth and development of the fetal brain requires that the germinal matrix tissue be adequate and maintained undamaged. Structural development of the brain in the premature is most active at the center of the cerebrum, in the periventricular tissues, where elaboration of cerebral components from germinal matrix is highly visible. These deposits of spongioblastic matrix cells, representing depots of anlage elements, are required for the ultimate formation of the basal ganglia and other deep neuronal assemblies and contribute to the formation of the cerebral cortex. The large periventricular deposits of germinal matrix, swollen bulging pads of soft, friable tissue, are highly vulnerable to hypoxia, readily undergoing disintegration.

Vascular structures at the core of the cerebrum become differentiated early in the premature brain, the deep veins of Galen standing out prominently in close association with the periventricular germinal matrix deposits. In contrast to the structural activity in the deep tissues, development of the surface structures of the premature cerebrum is delayed; the cerebral cortex remains smooth, a rudimentary inert thin dense ribbon, with its vascular elements, the surface veins and dural sinuses, appearing inconspicuous until near term.

With the premature fetus and newborn exposed to hypoxia, with systemic congestive failure mounting and circulatory stasis in the cerebrum reflected upstream, the vein of Galen and its deep tributaries become dilated and engorged, often undergoing thrombosis.[8, 55, 56, 69, 71] At the core of the cerebrum, as the process of venous congestion and thrombosis manifests its infarctional effects, the surrounding deep deposits of germinal matrix and neighboring periventricular tissues undergo necrosis with hemorrhage (Fig. 7–36). The process of hemorrhagic infarction may utilimately extend deeply into the cerebral wall as occurred in the following case.

Premature labor developed at 27 weeks of gestation; extraction of the fetus was impeded by a complex presentation. The fetus died during the delivery. The placenta showed extensive recent retroplacental and retromembranous hemorrhage.

Severe spinal injury was evident at postmortem examination in addition to massive hemorrhagic infarction of the left cerebral hemisphere. Serial whole-brain histologic sections demonstrated thrombosis

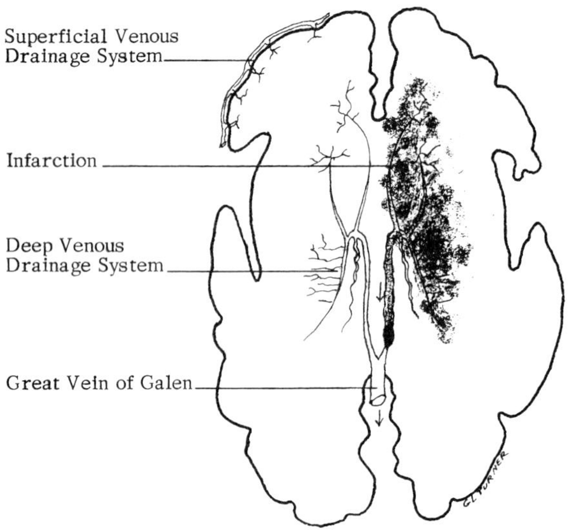

Figure 7–36. Mechanism of deep cerebral venous infarction in premature infant. On the right, the deep cerebral vein showing dilatation and stasis-thrombosis, corresponding infarction of the deep cerebral structures, and hemorrhagic extravasation through the infarct. Deep cerebral veins are prominently developed, in contrast to rudimentary superficial cerebral veins. (From A. Towbin: Central nervous system damage in the human fetus and newborn infant. Am. J. Dis. Child., *119*:529, June, 1970. Copyright 1970, American Medical Association. Reprinted by permission.)

of the corresponding deep cerebral vein at the foramen of Monro on the left. On the other side of the brain, infarctional damage was less advanced and, as evident in Figure 7–37, the terminal vein in the cerebral subependymal germinal matrix was distended, occupied by an organizing thrombus.

With less severe hypoxic exposure, the infarctional damage in the premature brain, the periventricular destruction, is less penetrating, less extensive, as in the case demonstrated in Figure 7–38.

The infant was born at 35 weeks' gestation, weighed 2,390 g. The gestational course had been uneventful until premature rupture of membranes and spontaneous labor occurred. The mother had controlled mild diabetes. The infant at birth was cyanotic and edematous; respiratory distress developed. Toward the end of the first day the infant showed sudden neurologic deterioration, became unresponsive, and died 23 hours after birth.

Autopsy revealed acute passive congestion of the liver, spleen, and other viscera; hyaline membrane disease and bronchopneumonia were present. Significantly, in the histologic sections of the brain in this case, the zone of necrosis in the cerebral wall was more extensive than the area of hemorrhage, indicating that the primary nature of the lesion was infarctional and that the hemorrhagic suffusion was secondary. With breakdown of the hemorrhagic infarct, leakage of blood occurred into the lateral ventricles. Within the hemorrhagic debris lining the ventricle, dilated veins and thromboses were evident.

Hypoxic cerebral infarctional damage is of course not an all-or-none process. While the

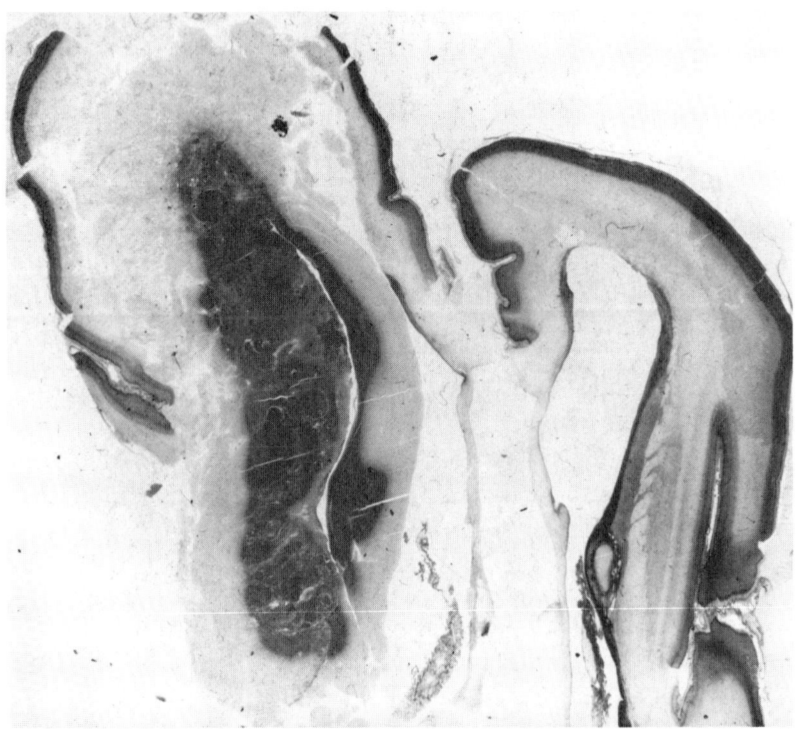

Figure 7–37. Massive hemorrhagic venous infarction of the left cerebral hemisphere, extending from the deep periventricular tissues outward. Also, on the right side, the deep cerebral vein, lying in the lateral periventricular tissues, is distended, occupied by an organizing thrombosis. Gestation of 27 weeks; intranatal death; placenta with massive retroplacental and retromembranous hemorrhage (B–265). (From A. Towbin: Cerebral intraventricular hemorrhage and subependymal matrix infarction in the fetus and premature newborn. Am. J. Pathol., *52*:121, 1968. Reprinted by permission.)

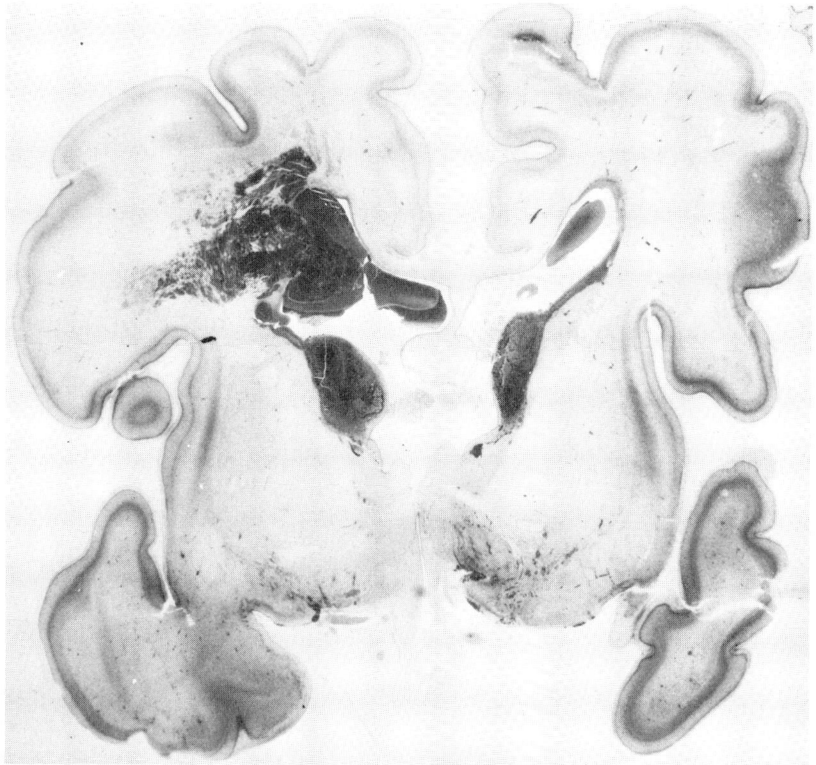

Figure 7–38. Infarction of cerebral subependymal matrix tissue and adjoining periventricular white matter; hemorrhagic suffusion of infarcted cerebral substance; thrombosis of periventricular veins; intraventricular hemorrhage. Premature rupture of membranes with delivery at 35 weeks' gestation; infant showed progressive neurologic deterioration and respiratory distress; death at 23 hours. Autopsy showed hyaline membrane disease and congestive heart failure with the cerebral infarction (W–59). (From A. Towbin: Cerebral intraventricular hemorrhage and subependymal matrix infarction in the fetus and premature newborn. Am. J. Pathol., *52*:121, 1968. Reprinted by permission.)

hemorrhagic devastation at times is massive, as illustrated, more often the lesions are small, focal, of minimal extent, and often present in the brain in premature infants dying of other systemic disorders.

Minimal hypoxic cerebral damage characteristic of the premature is demonstrated in Figure 7–39.

The infant was born prematurely, at 32 weeks' gestation, and lived two days. The mother had had

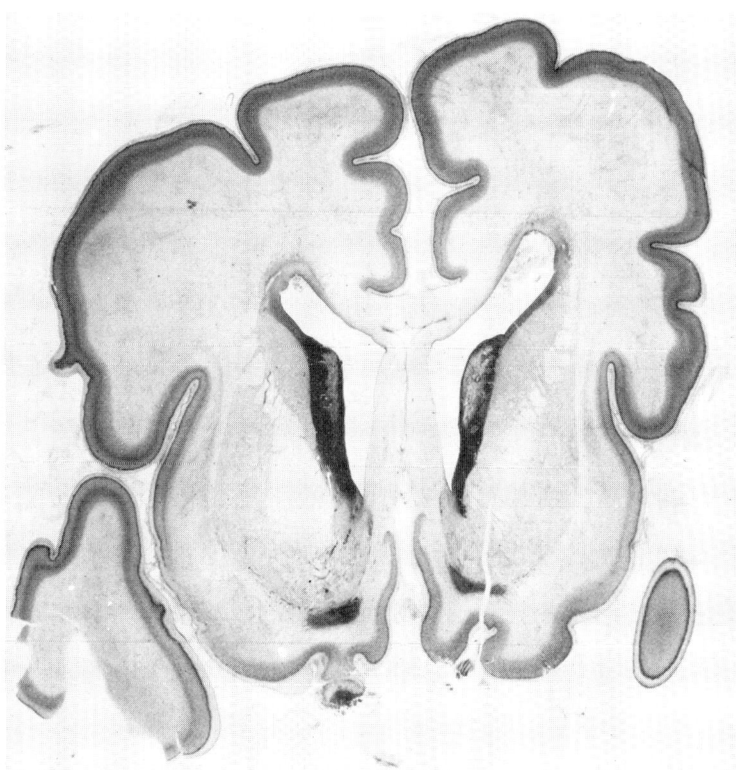

Figure 7–39. Minimal hypoxic infarctional damage of cerebral germinal matrix. Frontal section of brain shows deeply staining deposits of periventricular matrix tissue at the lower lateral aspects of the ventricles, with irregular patches of infarctional devastation; thromboses of small veins in the matrix. Premature delivery at 32 weeks following abruptio placentae. Infant lived two days, showing central and peripheral respiratory complications with increasing apnea. Autopsy showed, in addition to hyaline membrane disease and the cerebral matrix infarctions, multiple visceral venous thromboses, intestinal infarction, and pulmonary embolism (W–73). (From A. Towbin: Cerebral intraventricular hemorrhage and subependymal matrix infarction in the fetus and premature newborn. Am. J. Pathol., *52*:121, 1968. Reprinted by permission.)

moderate hypertension. She was admitted in active labor; moderate hydramnios was evident. With the cervix dilated at 6 cm, amniotomy was performed; bright red blood escaped, indicative of abruptio placentae. The infant, delivered from a vertex presentation, appeared in good condition and cried spontaneously. Weight was 3 lb 4 oz. The placenta showed evidence of premature separation. The infant developed respiratory complications, both of central and peripheral nature; repeated episodes of apnea occurred.

Autopsy revealed multiple visceral thrombotic and embolic vascular occlusions; the portal vein contained a thrombus; the entire small intestine was infarcted. Pulmonary embolism was present. Hyaline membrane disease was evident histologically. In the examination of the brain, in the histologic section through the frontal region of the cerebrum shown in Figure 7–39 there is a persisting heavy deposit of germinal matrix, a thick mound of deeply staining tissue at the lower lateral aspect of each lateral ventricle. Within the matrix are patches of pale necrotic tissue, areas of infarction, portions of which are hemorrhagic. The matrix veins are distended with conglutinated blood. Posteriorly in the cerebrum the periventricular lesions were enlarged and, related to this, there was extravasation of blood into the ventricles.

Minimal lesions occur not only in the germinal matrix deposits but also in the surrounding white matter, small areas of necrosis of the nature of microinfarcts, lesions known as "periventricular leukomalacia" (Fig. 7–40).[12, 72] These small focal lesions in the periventricular white matter are intimately associated with the presence of venous stasis, with thromboses, and as pointed out by Banker, are usually in the distribution of the deep venous drainage system of the cerebrum.[72]

Deep cerebral infarctional damage is the most frequent, most significant pathologic process observed in perinatal autopsies. The periventricular hemorrhagic lesions are present in some degree almost universally in premature infants examined postmortem.[8, 18] In studies in the Collaborative Perinatal Project, in a series of 140 premature newborn infants studied at autopsy, deep infarctional damage of severe to moderate degree was present in 48 per cent of the cases; significantly, in the other 52 per cent of cases, acute hypoxic lesions of minimal type were present, often scattered diffusely through the germinal tissue.[9] Intraventricular hemorrhage, often massive exsanguination into the ventricles, was commonly present and usually consequent to large periventricular hemorrhagic infarction, but at times resulted from minor focal subependymal matrix lesions.

Thrombosis of deep cerebral veins with destruction of periventricular germinal tissue and subsequent shedding of cellular debris and blood into the ventricular cavities in some cases leads to blocking of the aqueduct and foramina of Luschka and Magendie, and ultimately to noncommunicating hydrocephalus in surviving infants.[71]

The ultimate fate of the acute hypoxic infarctional lesions in the brain depends on the severity of the process and the length of survival after the hypoxic episode. Massive hemorrhagic cerebral infarction with rapid intraventricular exsanguination is lethal. When the process is less severe, not fatal, the local lesions evolve through an intermediate *subacute* stage, with the necrotic hemorrhagic debris becoming phagocytized and the area of de-

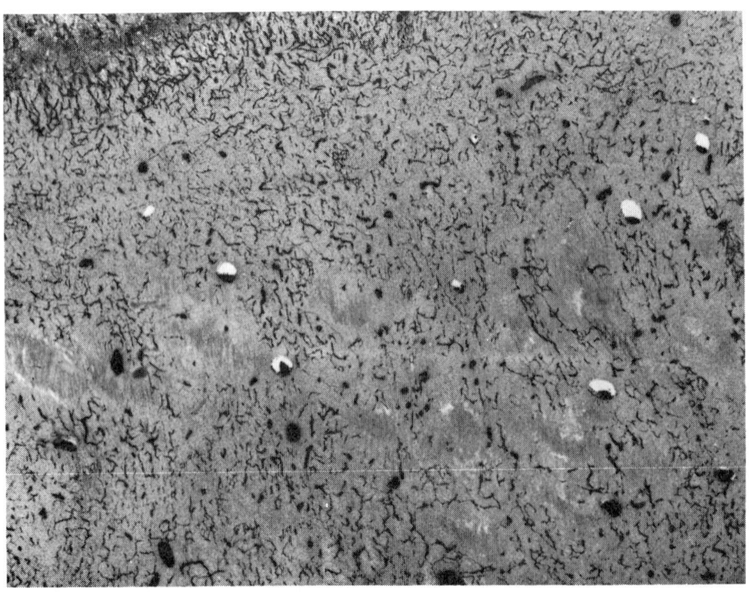

Figure 7–40. White matter microinfarcts in periventricular tissue of cerebrum ("periventricular leucomalacia"), commonly present in prematures, associated with systemic hypoxia and local venous stasis. Section shows cloud-like islands of infarctional necrosis surrounded by network of engorged capillaries; small veins with thromboses.

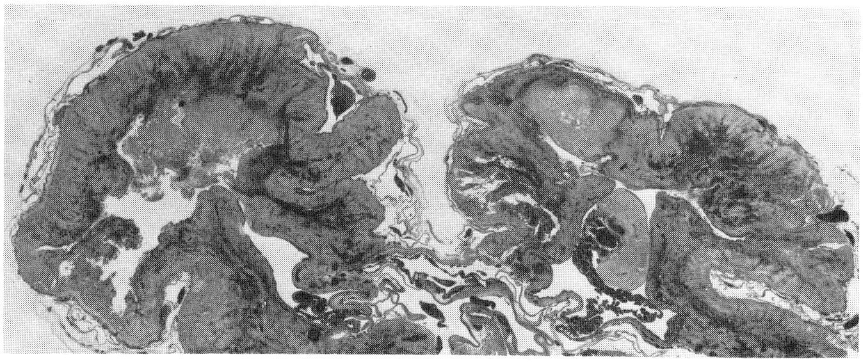

Figure 7–41. Subacute periventricular cerebral venous infarction; deep areas of advanced infarction undergoing organization with formation of granulation tissue and scarring. Prenatal history of severe maternal illness with vaginal bleeding two months before delivery at term (T–1). (Compare with pattern of acute infarctional damage as occurs in the premature, Figure 7–38). (From A. Towbin: Central nervous system damage in the human fetus and newborn infant. Am. J. Dis. Child., *119*:529, June, 1970. Copyright 1970, American Medical Association. Reprinted by permission.)

struction becoming organized by ingrowth of vascular elements and glia. If the infant then survives for months or years, the lesion becomes *chronic*, forming dense scars and irregular cavitations.[9-13, 55, 70, 73, 74]

Subacute Stage.† Perinatal cerebral hypoxic damage in the form of subacute infarcts, studied in newborn infants, provides an indispensable pathologic link relating the processes of acute neonatal cerebral damage to the chronic lesions found in mental retardation and cerebral palsy. These transitional subacute lesions vary in extent, appearing in the brain as areas of gelatinous tan discoloration with hyperemic margins. An example of this subacute transitional pattern of damage is illustrated in the following case.

Two months before term the mother became acutely ill with a respiratory infection; she developed

†See References 9, 11, 55, 69.

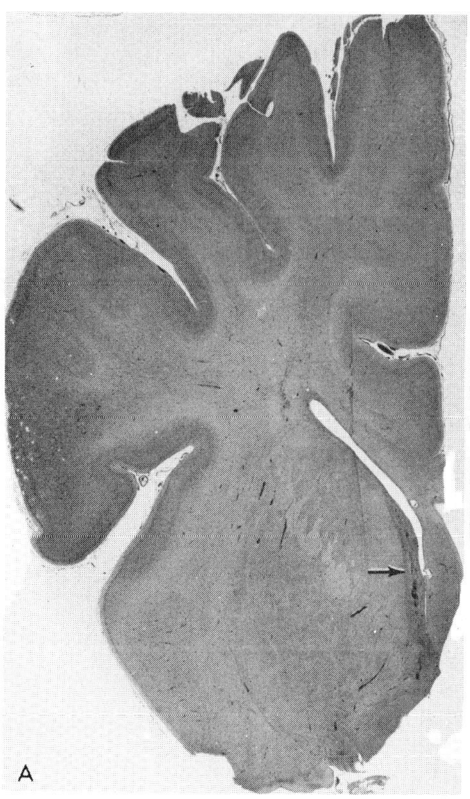

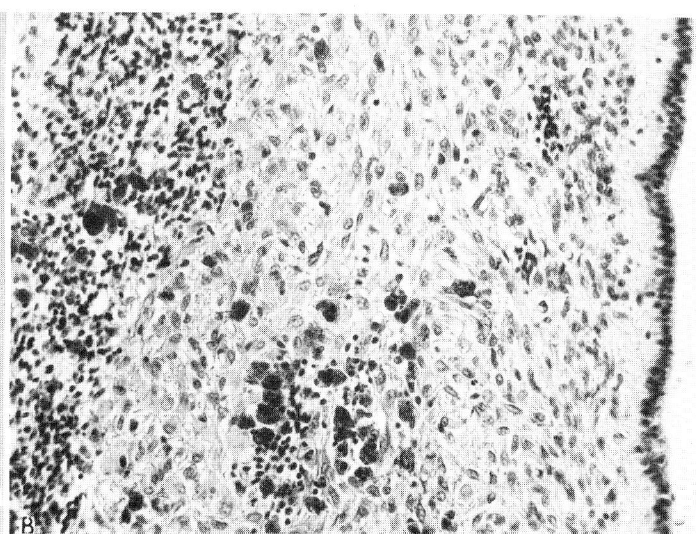

Figure 7–42. *A.* Subacute minimal infarctional lesion in the periventricular germinal matrix tissue in the premature; infant with congenital heart disease with protracted hypoxia, survived 16 days. The gross specimen of the brain showed a small focus of brown discoloration in the subependymal tissue of the cerebrum in the caudothalamic area. Corresponding histologic section showed glial-hemosiderin scar in this area (arrow), site previously occupied by germinal matrix tissue (T–131). *B.* Higher magnification of area indicated by arrow. Ependymal lining at the right; subependymal strata show heavy proliferation of plump glial cells, with clusters of large, deeply staining hemosiderin-laden phagocytes. At the left, clusters of small dark cells, the residue of germinal matrix tissue. (From A. Towbin: Organic causes of minimal brain dysfunction. J.A.M.A., *217*:1207, August 30, 1971. Copyright 1971, American Medical Association. Reprinted by permission.)

vaginal bleeding and was hospitalized. The pregnancy was maintained. The infant, delivered at term, weighed 2,770 g and lived 18 hours. Externally the infant appeared well formed; the head was of proportionate size.

At autopsy the brain was found to be very small, weighing 130 g (average, 360 g). The miniature cerebrum, occupying the depths of the cranial cavity, showed well-defined convolutions, giving the specimen the appearance of a collapsed loaf of braided bread. The histologic sections of the cerebrum indicated clearly the mechanism of damage; the vein of Galen and its deep cerebral tributaries contained well-established thromboses, and the periventricular layers of the cerebrum were destroyed by multiple confluent infarcts undergoing organization and scarring (Fig. 7–41). The cerebrum appeared reamed out by the infarction, the hemispheres remaining as irregular thin-walled sacs covered with cortical tissue.

Minimal lesions of subacute form are commonly observed in hypoxic premature infants who live for a period of weeks or months. The subacute lesions, corresponding in location to the fresh infarcts seen in the newborn premature, occur deep in the cerebrum, in the region of the periventricular germinal matrix deposits at the caudothalamic groove (Fig. 7–42). Varying in size, the subacute lesions grossly appear as focal areas of tan softening and histologically show glial scarring and persisting clusters of hemosiderin, the residues of previous hemorrhagic infarction. In the course of time, in infants who survive, the infarcted soft tan areas become contracted and scarred, at times cystic, as the lesions become chronic in nature.

Chronic Forms.‡ In premature infants who survive for protracted periods through the subacute "healing" stage, the deep cerebral infarctional damage present at birth ultimately becomes transformed into deep areas of scarring and cavitation. Following fetal-neonatal hypoxia in the premature, residual chronic lesions are found located in the basal ganglia and other periventricular structures. The damaged regions of the cerebrum become distorted, scarred, loculated, locally reduced in substance. The leathery indurated cystic lesions microscopically show gliosis and rarefaction, often with hemosiderin phagocytosis, changes characteristic of old hemorrhagic infarction. Figures 7–43 and 7–44 show the common pattern of chronic cerebral lesions, with deep scarring and necrosis, found in children and adults with a history of perinatal hypoxia and clinical cerebral palsy, mental retardation, epilepsy, and other major nervous system disabilities.

The clinical-pathologic relationship between early prenatal hypoxia and subsequent deep cerebral lesions—the effect of hypoxia on the premature fetus—is demonstrated in past reports by Neuburger and Hallervorden, and recently by Bankl and Jellinger and Csermely.[11, 45–47] In the cases described, the fetuses were subjected to hypoxia months before birth during maternal attempts at suicide by asphyxia. In the offspring, clinically, there were manifestations of severe mental retardation, motor disturbances, and other major neurologic disabilities. Postmortem studies in these cases revealed extensive cerebral destruction, with scarring and cavity formation in the deep white matter and basal ganglia.

Prematurely born infants who survived for extended periods after severe perinatal hy-

‡See References 9, 11, 55, 69.

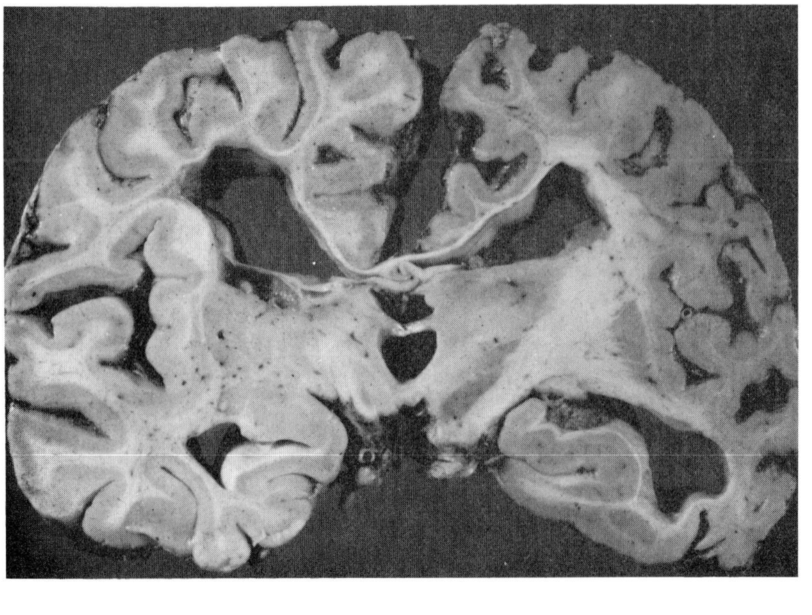

Figure 7–43. Chronic cerebral lesion characteristic of cerebral palsy and mental retardation; common periventricular location, involving the basal ganglia, thalamus, and deep white matter. Cystic areas of necrosis and scarring, residues of perinatal infarction. Eight-year-old girl with mental retardation and spastic quadriplegia (CSS–10762). (Compare with acute infarctional lesion shown in Figure 7–38.) (From A. Towbin: Pathology of cerebral palsy; cerebral palsy due to encephaloclastic processes. A.M.A. Arch. Pathol., *59*:529, May, 1955. Copyright 1955, American Medical Association. Reprinted by permission.)

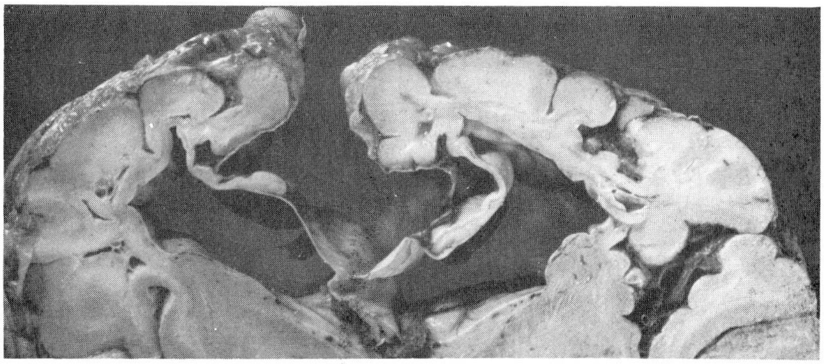

Figure 7–44. Chronic cerebral lesions, cystic necrosis and scarring, stemming from birth, in seven-year-old with cerebral palsy and mental retardation. The pattern of chronic lesions is analogous to subacute cerebral infarctional damage present in Figure 7–41 (CSS 5064). (From A. Towbin: Pathology of cerebral palsy; cerebral palsy due to encephaloclastic processes. A.M.A. Arch. Pathol., *59*:529, May, 1955. Copyright 1955, American Medical Association. Reprinted by permission.)

poxia, the sequelant clinical manifestations, and the residual chronic cerebral lesions have been described by Brand and Bignami. In one case, an eight-week-old infant born at 34 weeks' gestation following abruptio placentae, the cerebrum showed softening and cavitation of the periventricular white matter. In another infant, born at 30 weeks' gestation, the cerebrum showed severe gliosis of the white matter around the lateral ventricles. In contrast to this pattern of chronic damage—deep cerebral lesions that develop in hypoxic prematures—is the process of damage that occurs at term, affecting mainly the cortex.

At Term: Cortical Cerebral Infarctional Damage

Hypoxic cerebral damage occurring at term generally affects the cortex. The process of cortical damage, basically of venous infarctional nature, is analogous pathologically to the deep hypoxic damage that takes place in the premature, and in surviving infants, the lesions evolve through the same patterns of acute, subacute, and chronic tissue changes.[10, 11, 13] The cortical hypoxic lesions incurred at term are essentially of the same pattern as occur in the brain in adults after hypoxia.

The difference in localization of perinatal cerebral hypoxic lesions, deep in the premature and cortical in the mature, as shown in Figure 7–34, is of broad significance pathologically and clinically, providing an organic basis for the interpretation of chronic lesions such as occur in mental retardation and for distinguishing lesions incurred prenatally from intranatal and postnatal damage.

Acute Stage.§ Fetal-neonatal hypoxia at term stems essentially from the same complications that affect the premature, disturbances in the maternal-placental-fetal organization, very often of an acute, precipitous nature. At term, as in the premature, the sequence of pathologic processes is initiated by hypoxic complications beginning just prior to labor, during delivery, or after birth, leading to fetal-neonatal heart failure and ultimately to local venous stasis-thrombosis and hemorrhagic infarction (cf. Table 7–4). The local pathologic process, the pattern of hypoxic brain damage, for which the target is the cerebral cortex, is governed by factors tangential to advancing gestational age. As the fetus ages and approaches term, in the cerebrum the germinal matrix deposits become exhausted, used up in the formation of the basal ganglia and other maturing nuclear structures. The momentum of local structural activity shifts from the core of the cerebrum to the surface, where the convolutional pattern becomes demarcated and more and more complicated. Histologically, in the cortex the laminar pattern becomes differentiated. The surface vasculature, the superficial cerebral veins and dural sinuses, becomes clearly determined. At term, with this surge of biologic activity at the cerebral surface, the cortex proves increasingly vulnerable to hypoxia, and becomes the main site of hypoxic infarctional damage.

Depending on the severity of the hypoxic gestational-parturitional complication at term, the extent of damage to the cortex and subjacent tissue varies. In the most severe form, autopsy reveals well-established thromboses in dural sinuses and superficial veins, and associated broad hemorrhagic infarcts extending through portions or entire lobes and at times encompassing the entire cerebrum—whole-brain infarction. Massive cerebral infarctional damage occurred in the case illustrated in Figure 7–45.

In the fetus late in gestation and in the newborn near term, hypoxic damage in the cere brum tends to be located intermediately—not in the cortex nor in the periventricular tissues, but in the middle strata of the hemispheric wall, as occurred in the following case.

§See References 11, 65, 66, 76.

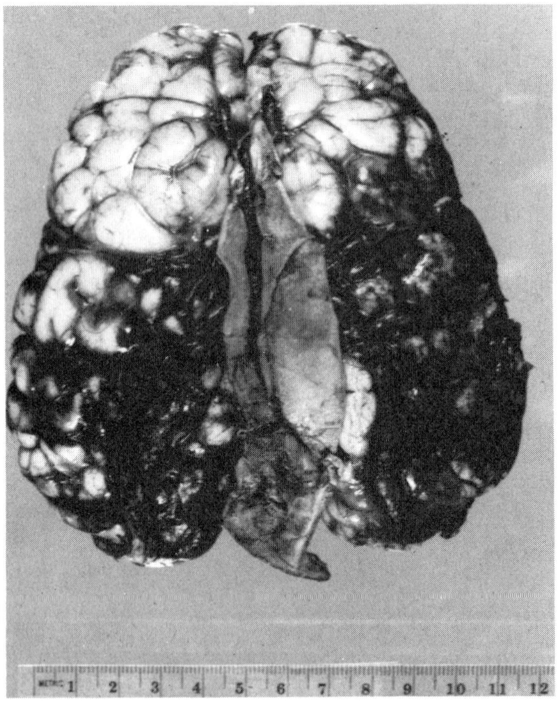

Figure 7–45. Acute cortical cerebral infarction in mature newborn; thromboses present in superior longitudinal dural venous sinus. Infant with multiple malformations, including cardiac defects, showed progressive neurologic deterioration and increasing congestive circulatory failure after birth; death after three weeks (C–93).

The fetus was the smaller of male twins, with manifestations of the intrauterine transfusion syndrome evident. The larger twin, biologically dominant and providing the main circulatory impulse, survived; the smaller member, dependent and stunted, died during delivery. The imbalance in the fetal circulation was related to a demonstrated vascular shunt. The larger twin, delivered first, was active and alert, but plethoric. (Ultimately, at the age of two years, he showed manifestations of cerebral palsy, reflecting perinatal brain damage.) Examination during labor had indicated both fetuses were alive; heart tones were heard eight minutes prior to the delivery of the first twin. Death of the second twin occurred during parturition; the stillborn infant, delivered eight minutes after the first, was small, cyanotic, about half the size of the surviving twin, crown-rump length being 260 mm compared to 320 mm in the surviving twin. Gestational age was estimated to be near 36 weeks.

At autopsy the smaller twin showed generalized effects of congestive heart failure, with engorgement of viscera; the brain was swollen, edematous, and congested. Thrombosis of superficial cerebral veins and subcortical veins was present. On both sides of the cerebrum the occipital lobe showed a large hemorrhagic infarction occupying the central white matter (Fig. 7–46). Histologic study of the lesions indicated the infarctional process was of prenatal origin, several days old.

Less severe hypoxia in the fetus near term produces a correspondingly less severe pattern of cerebral convolutional damage that takes the form of laminar necrosis of the cortex, as in the following case example.

The mother had several episodes of false labor and vaginal bleeding in the days prior to delivery. The infant was stillborn at term. The placenta showed extensive retroplacental hematomas, varying in age.

At autopsy there was diffuse visceral congestion, with the brain engorged and edematous. Histologic sections of the cerebral convolutions showed widespread patchy cortical devastation, broad areas of laminar cortical necrosis (Fig. 7–47).

The minimal form of hypoxic cerebral cortical damage occurring at term is commonly neuronal, with varying numbers of individual cells injured and eliminated. Histologically the cortex becomes punctuated by shrunken, deeply staining neurons that appear singly or in clusters, as demonstrated in Figure 7–48, a section of cerebral cortex from a postmature infant who

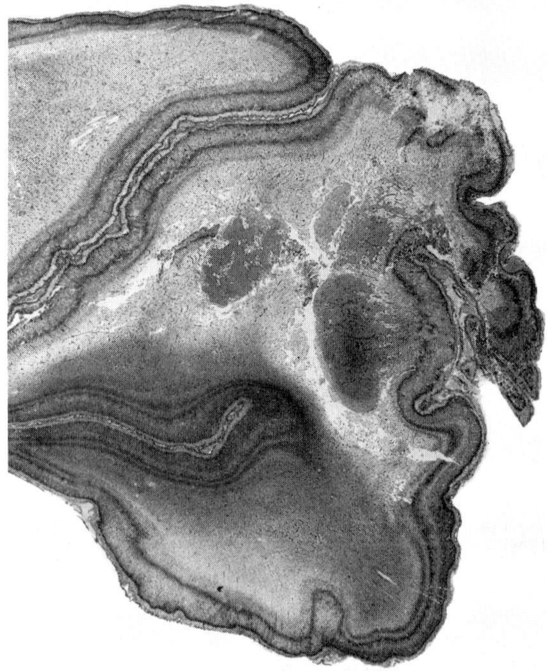

Figure 7–46. Cerebral venous infarction involving central white matter. Intrauterine transfusion syndrome associated with twin pregnancy and placental vascular shunt. Smaller of twins; gestation estimated to be 36 weeks; fetal death occurred during delivery. At autopsy, congestive heart failure; brain swollen, stasis-thrombosis of superficial and deep cerebral veins; infarctional processes in brain were histologically several days old, of prenatal origin (W–36). (From A. Towbin: Neonatal damage of the central nervous system. In *Neuropathology: Methods and Diagnosis*. Edited by C. G. Tedeschi. Boston, Little, Brown and Co., 1970. Reprinted by permission.)

lived one day. Some of the affected elements that are more labile become shriveled and necrotic ("ischemic neuronal necrosis"), and are quickly wiped out by the oxygen deprivation. Neighboring cells of similar form, having a higher threshold and proving more durable, appear unchanged and survive. In the newborn infant, as in the adult after hypoxic exposure, such devastation may spread over broad areas of the cerebrum.

The late effects of acute hypoxic cortical cerebral damage incurred at term, the evolution of the lesions through the subacute and chronic phases, are illustrated in the cases that follow.

Subacute Stage. Surface destruction extending over wide lobar regions of the cerebrum, of subacute nature pathologically, was present at birth in a mature infant in the case shown in Figure 7–49.

The mother had developed infectious hepatitis late in the last trimester; the pregnancy was maintained to term. At delivery the mother was still seriously ill, still jaundiced. The infant was stillborn.

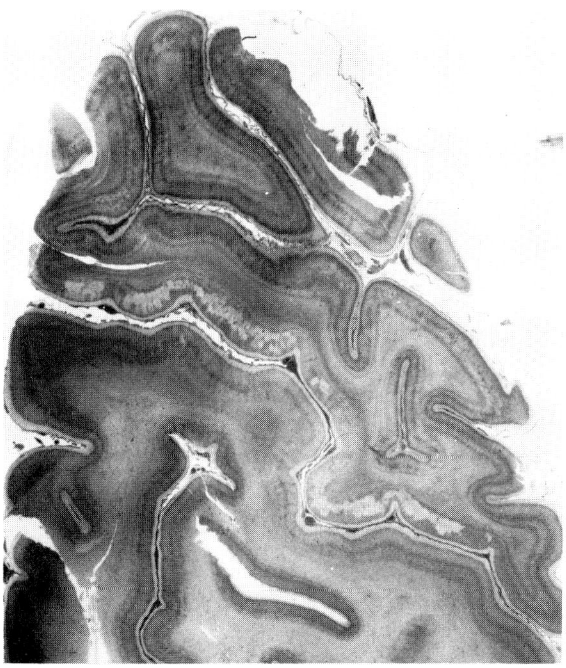

Figure 7–47. Cortical cerebral infarctional damage occuring at term. Intrauterine hypoxia due to premature partial detachment of placenta; maternal history of prenatal bleeding. Placenta showed old and recent retroplacental hematomas. Mature infant stillborn; autopsy revealed severe systemic venous congestion; brain edematous and congested, histologically showing cortical cerebral laminar pattern of necrosis, convolutions with patchy acute devastation, pale "moth-eaten" areas in the cortex, diffusely scattered over the cerebral hemispheres, damage of prenatal origin (W–18). (From A. Towbin: Organic causes of minimal brain dysfunction. J.A.M.A., *217*:1207, August 30, 1971. Copyright 1971, American Medical Association. Reprinted by permission.)

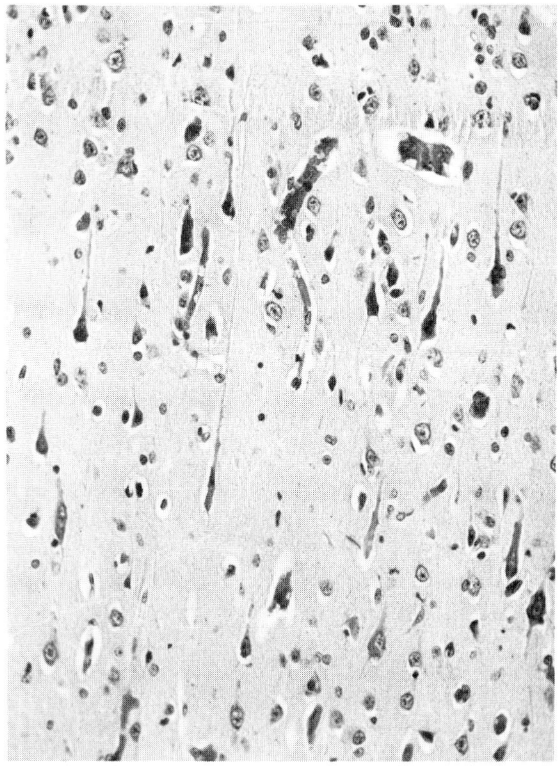

Figure 7–48. Minimal cortical neuronal hypoxic cerebral damage; postmature infant lived one day. Section of motor cortex; damaged Betz cells shrunken, elongated, deeply staining; surviving neurons, biologically more durable, appear with large clear-staining nuclei and central nucleoli. History of complicated, prolonged parturition. Autopsy revealed spinal epidural hemorrhage, severe systemic venous congestion, focal myocardial infarcts, meconium aspiration pneumonia (M–47). (From A. Towbin: Organic causes of minimal brain dysfunction. J.A.M.A., *217*:1207, August 30, 1971. Copyright 1971, American Medical Association. Reprinted by permission.)

At autopsy, the brain was small and showed broad lobar areas of cerebral devastation, the convolutions effaced and flattened, and the cortex replaced by rubbery yellow tissue. Histologically, the damaged hemispheric wall showed the pattern of progressive venous infarction, varying from acute hemorrhagic necrosis in some areas to subacute reaction in other parts. Most of the destruction was far advanced, with structural obliteration and scarring.

Chronic Lesions.‖ The late organic cerebral effects of hypoxia at term—cortical neuronal depletion, at times focal or diffuse convolutional scarring—are observed in cases of mental retardation and cerebral palsy. Likewise, experimentally in animals, cortical cerebral devastation, convolutional destruction, and atrophy occur in monkeys that survive for prolonged periods after hypoxia at term.[67, 70]

‖See References 6, 7, 10–13, 74.

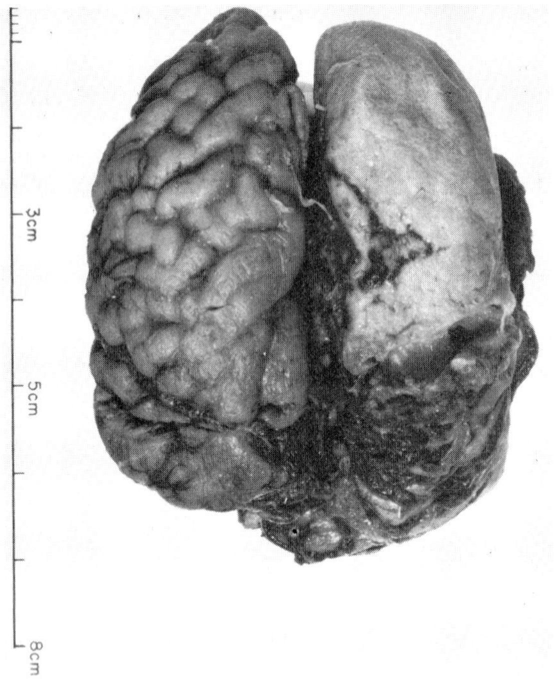

Figure 7–49. Subacute cortical cerebral infarctional damage. Maternal hepatitis during last weeks of gestation; pregnancy maintained to term. Infant stillborn. The brain at autopsy, disproportionately small in the cranial vault, appeared loosely suspended from the dura by strands of thick veins; the frontoparietal portion of the right cerebrum, with arachnoid removed, was of smooth rubbery texture; surrounding superficial cerebral veins dilated, filled with thromboses. Left temporal lobe (not shown in illustration) also with similar infarction. The process of cerebral infarction, pathologically several weeks old, reflects the duration of maternal illness in the prenatal period (T–2).

The chronic sequelae of perinatal hypoxia at term are evident in the following case, an adult psychiatric patient with a history of complicated term birth.

At the time of delivery, after prolonged labor, with vaginal parturition unsuccessful, a cesarean section was resorted to. The infant was described as a "good baby" by the obstetrician. During infancy and childhood, however, emotional problems developed; she was described as a "nervous child" and was withdrawn from regular school. She had difficulty in learning to read, and was considered to be moderately retarded mentally. As she grew older, increasing personality changes appeared, and she was institutionalized at 18 years of age with the diagnosis of schizophrenia. Significantly, physical examination at this time revealed slight spasticity of the left extremities, with hyperactive deep reflexes, ankle clonus, and positive Babinski response on this side. She remained institutionalized. Death occurred at 42 years.

Postmortem study of the brain showed fibrotic occlusion of the anterior portion of the superior sagittal sinus and obliteration of adjoining surface veins. In the right frontal lobe, on the cerebral surface at the side of the occluded dural venous sinus, there was a circumscribed, old contracted infarction of the cortex, involving the precentral and adjoining frontal convolutions (Fig. 7–50).

In this case, with a history of complications at birth, the cortical lesion provided the organic basis for the development of neurologic and behavioral disturbances, ultimately elaborated in adulthood.

The "Fetus-in-Coma" Syndrome

With the occurrence of intrauterine hypoxia, manifestations of fetal brain damage are often evident early, often before changes in the fetal heart action. In many instances there occurs a consistent sequence of clinical changes, the syndromic pattern of "fetus-in-coma," reflecting impairment of vital cerebral function in the fetus.

Traditionally fetal death is thought of as occurring catastrophically, suddenly, in minutes. This concept is basically in error. In most cir-

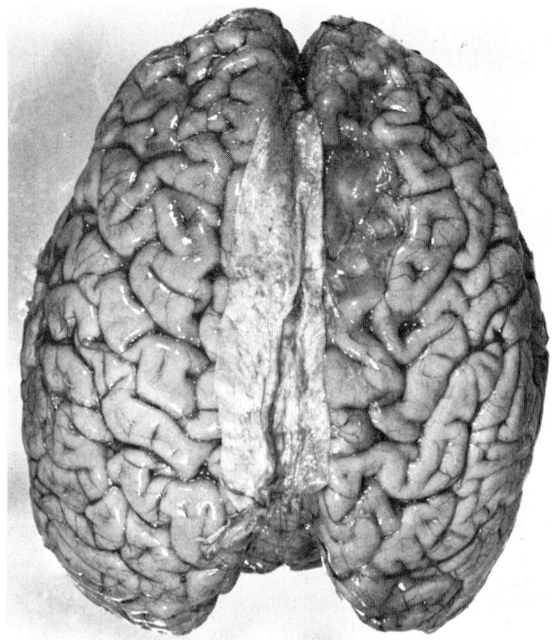

Figure 7–50. Focal cortical cerebral scarring, area of remote infarction; thrombotic occlusion of adjacent anterior portion of superior sagittal dural venous sinus. Forty-two-year-old woman; left-sided spasticity. History of complicated cesarean birth, behavioral disturbances during childhood, and learning disability; institutionalized at 18 years with diagnosis of schizophrenia. Cerebral lesion found at autopsy consistent with venous infarction stemming from birth (D–59). (From A. Towbin: Organic causes of minimal brain dysfunction. J.A.M.A., *217*:1207, August 30, 1971. Copyright 1971, American Medical Association. Reprinted by permission.)

cumstances of asphyxia, in the fetus as in the adult, death occurs gradually in stages. This is not generally fully taken into account in obstetrical management. Clinically correlated autopsy studies provide substantial evidence that in many cases the fetus's death is preceded by a protracted agonal period, extending for hours or days. This terminal period is marked clinically by a decline in fetal activity, the "fetus-in-coma." Clinical studies in such cases indicate that the loss of fetal activity is usually the consequence of hypoxia, often due to placental insufficiency.[4,5]

Characteristically in this syndrome, the mother reports a recent decrease or loss of fetal movement. Early examination of the mother, however, often reveals a good heart tone. Some degree of labor may occur—variable uterine contractions, often latent, unrecognized by the mother or dismissed as false labor.

These clinical events, translated organically, echo the following intrauterine pathologic processes: The primary intrauterine disturbance, commonly a partial abruption or other placental disorder, renders the fetus hypoxic and, secondly, may precipitate premature contractions. As in the adult with unrelieved asphyxia, neuromuscular function of the fetus weakens, leading to manifest paralysis and coma and ultimately to loss of vital function. At autopsy in such cases the brain shows advanced hypoxic infarctional damage, accounting for the progressive fetal paralysis evident prenatally in the syndrome of the fetus-in-coma.

The following case (T-443) is illustrative.

The mother, a 23-year-old primipara near term, reported a loss of fetal movements; however, immediate examination revealed fetal heart tones of good quality. Active labor ensued six days later; considerable fetal-pelvic disproportion was manifest; the mother delivered a slightly macerated stillborn infant. The placenta showed a large subacute infarction and an associated circumscribed retroplacental hematoma.

The infant at autopsy presented a thick, well demarcated caput succedaneum and in the upper spinal canal a heavy epidural hemorrhage. Far-advanced cerebral hypoxic damage was evident.

In correlating the clinical and pathologic findings in this case, it was apparent that with the development of the placental abruption, an initial episode of unrecognized latent labor occurred, days before the ultimate parturition, resulting in the early formation of the thick caput and the spinal injury—compounding the hypoxic injury already incurred by the still-living but comatose fetus. Although the clinical course had extended over a period of a week, marked by loss of fetal movements, it was evident from the limited degree of maceration found at autopsy that death of the fetus was relatively recent.

The occurrence of this clinical state, the so-called "fetus-in-coma," merits more serious consideration as a monitoring measure. The importance of this syndrome lies in recognizing that in the beginning, with early hypoxic brain damage occurring, the loss of fetal activity represents a period of fetal unconsciousness, not death—a period during which immediate cesarean intervention may save the infant. As summarized by Sandovsky and associates, "Fetal kicking may be a better indicator of fetal health than the heart beat."[5] Pathologically, this syndrome focuses attention again on the occurrence and significance of latent prenatal brain damage.

Postnatal Hypoxic Processes

Hypoxia beginning during fetal life is often increased by related complications developing after birth. Meconium aspiration pneumonia, pneumothorax, and hyaline membrane disease are significant examples, being related to perinatal hypoxia both in cause and in effects.

Meconium Aspiration (Intrauterine) Pneumonia

Aspiration of amniotic fluid occurs commonly in utero, especially with the occurrence of hypoxic gestational and parturitional complications. The fetus, under the stress of mounting hypoxia, frequently evacuates meconium into the amniotic fluid. Meconium, containing bile elements and intestinal enzymes, is an irritant substance. Subsequently, with fetal distress increasing, respiratory movements are initiated in utero and meconium-contaminated amniotic fluid, loaded with desquamated debris and enzymes, is deposited in the lung. After delivery, a chemical and foreign-body type of pneumonia develops, further impairing the oxygenating mechanism of the often neurologically crippled neonate (Fig. 7–51).

Pneumothorax

Postnatal pneumothorax is common, said to be present in 1 to 2 per cent of all newborn. A minor degree of pneumothorax may occur spontaneously in neonates and is often without symptoms, evident radiologically in infants who required no resuscitation at delivery.[77,78] Pneu-

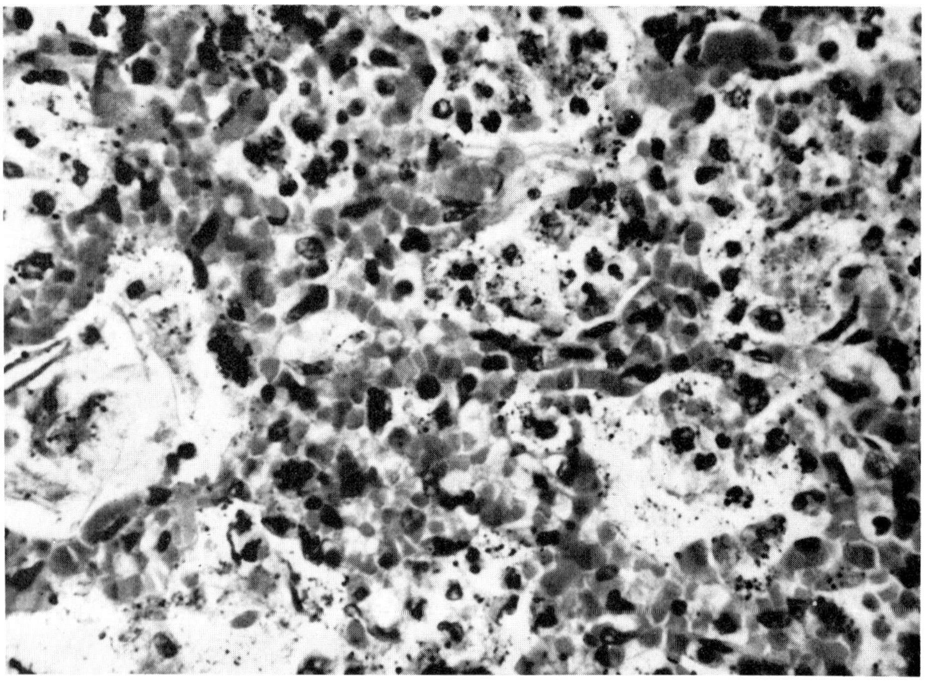

Figure 7–51. Meconium aspiration penumonia in newborn. Complicated delivery; prolonged (13-hour) labor; amniotic fluid thick, heavily stained with meconium. Postmature infant; 10 lb; Apgar score 4 at one minute, 6 at five minutes. Central and peripheral respiratory complications; lived one day. Autopsy revealed spinal epidural hemorrhage, congestive heart failure with hypoxic damage in myocardium and cerebrum (see Fig. 7–48). Lungs large with firm ropy texture and mottled gray pink, dark red, and purple; microscopically, alveoli with many macrophages containing bile pigment, numerous aspirated squames, and many acute inflammatory cells (M–47).

mothorax of severe form usually is the consequence of injudicious use of resuscitation measures; the incidence of injury of this type increased especially after the introduction of positive pressure resuscitation methods. Hyperdistention of alveoli leads to rupture of alveolar septa, with consequent development of pulmonary interstitial emphysema and exten-

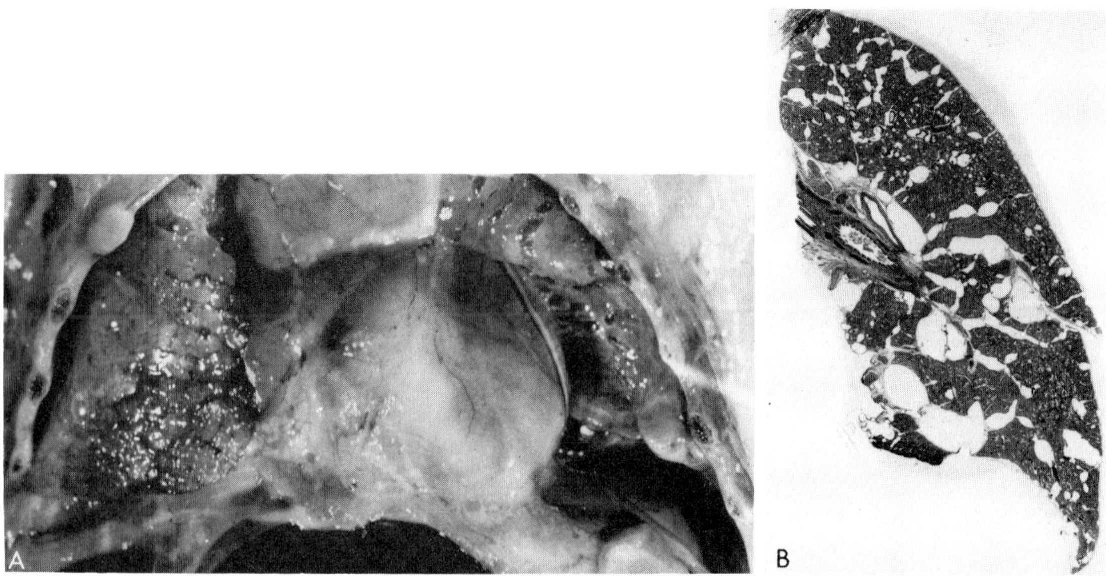

Figure 7–52. Pneumothorax, interstitial emphysema, in newborn. Spontaneous occurrence in premature infant, in good condition at birth; developed labored respiration and, terminally, increasing periods of apnea. Presence of numerous small clear cysts, pockets of trapped gas in the interstitial tissue, evident on the pleural surfaces in *A*, and distributed through the lung substance in *B*. Rupture of surface gas cysts resulted in pneumothorax, with compression atelectasis of the left lung, evident in *A*. Death was attributable to cerebral periventricular infarction, with intraventricular and subarachnoidal hemorrhage, evident at autopsy, in addition to the pneumothorax (N–82).

sion of air into subpleural and interlobular connective tissue and into the mediastinum (pneumomediastinum). Extension of the air dissection through the tissues results in subcutaneous emphysema and at times pneumopericardium; more often, the interstitial emphysema leads to progressive bilateral pneumothorax (Fig. 7–52). If unrelieved, this complication, usually occurring tangential to other hypoxic perinatal complications, is commonly the terminal mechanism of injury superimposed on the newborn, frequently an infant already in distress with central respiratory depression due to antecedent hypoxic or mechanical injury to the brain or spinal cord, or at times with meconium aspiration pneumonia.

Respiratory Distress Syndrome

Premature infants with central nervous system damage frequently develop hyaline membrane disease.[12, 79, 80] The nervous system injury causes central respiratory depression; the resulting hypoxia leads to cardiac failure with systemic visceral venous congestion (cf. Table 7–4). Investigators in the past have pointed out the importance of local hypoxia, exercising its effects on the lung tissue, as a major facet of the pathogenesis of hyaline membrane disease.[12, 80] When the lung is examined microscopically, it is evident that the areas with the most severe venous congestion also have the thickest hyaline membrane deposits (Fig. 7–53). In this syndrome, with the premature infant surviving for days and the pathologic changes in the lung advancing, the clinical manifestations of secondary peripheral respiratory failure increase. Essentially, the mounting systemic hypoxia leads to further cerebral damage. Ultimately, if the process is unrelieved, the accrued central and peripheral respiratory disability and nervous system damage prove fatal.

CONCLUSIONS

Sequelae of Perinatal Injury

A majority of children in "State Schools," children with *mental retardation, cerebral palsy,* and *epilepsy* are there as a consequence of

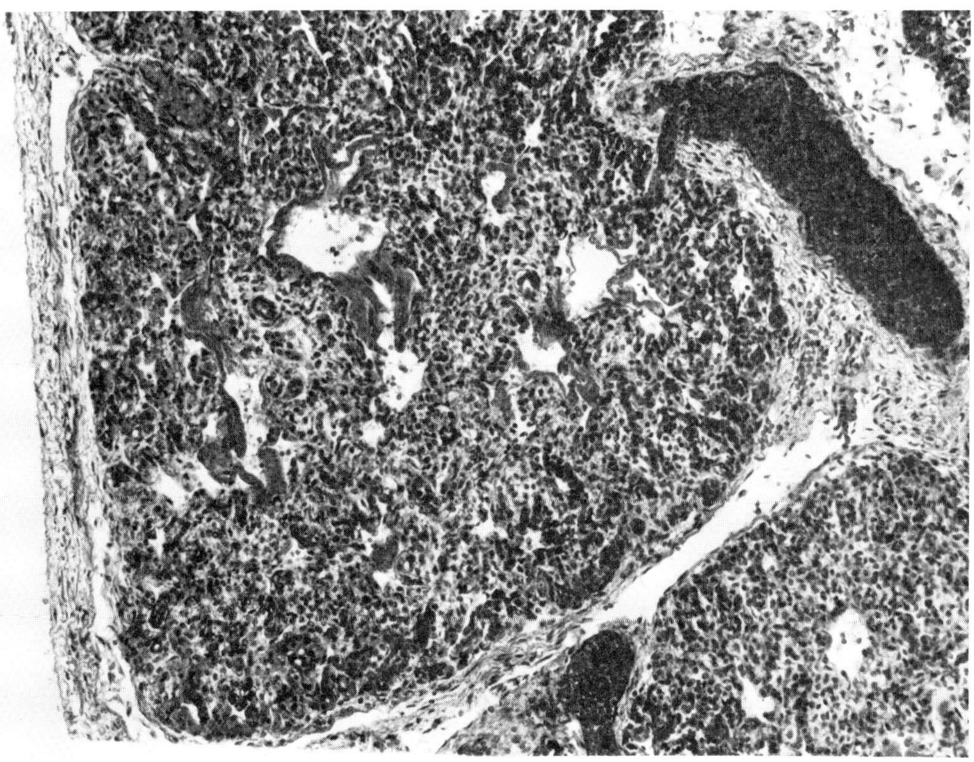

Figure 7–53. Hyaline membrane disease; premature delivery, abruptio placentae; approximately 32 weeks' gestation; lived 21 hours. Developed central and peripheral respiratory complications, with periods of apnea and periods of labored respiration. Autopsy showed infarctional damage of brain and myocardium (cf. Fig. 7–28); lungs mottled gray and red, rubbery, aerated centrally, firm peripherally. Microscopic section shows irregular despoits of "hyaline" material about the lining of alveoli and small bronchioles; mainly in the peripheral portions of the lung, present in association with local dilatation and engorgement of neighboring venous channels (M–52).

perinatal cerebral damage. This causal relationship was pointed out by Little over a hunded years ago, emphasized by Freud in his detailed clinical-neuropathologic studies of cerebral palsy, and has been confirmed in numerous other clinical and pathologic studies through the years.[7, 9, 10, 13, 76, 81-85] Linked to the triad of mental retardation, cerebral palsy, and epilepsy, a fourth segment of chronic postperinatal cerebral disability has now become increasingly recognized, the occurrence of *psychiatric disorders*. Psychoses in children and adults, childhood schizophrenia, manic conditions, and other forms, a major group of cases, are associated with gestational-parturitional etiopathologic factors.[86-90] Minor forms of neuropsychiatric disability, e.g., the syndrome of minimal brain dysfunction, likewise in a large portion of cases, are recognized to be of organic nature, stemming from perinatal cerebral damage.[74, 91-93]

With both major and minor forms of chronic nervous system sequelae, it is increasingly evident that the underlying organic damage is largely incurred *prenatally* and, closely related to this factor, is the large incidence of prematurity recorded in these cases.

Prenatal Injury

Correlation of recent and past studies of perinatal organic damage reviewed here provides essential evidence that most cerebral damage leading to mental retardation and other related neuropsychiatric disability has its origin prior to delivery.[12, 23, 42, 50, 68, 86-88, 94, 95]

In times past, the clinical-pathologic analysis of case material such as that illustrated in Figures 7–43, 7–44, and 7–50, the study of chronic cerebral lesions stemming from the fetal-neonatal period, generally yielded meager information. Efforts to distinguish lesions of prenatal occurrence from those of intranatal and postnatal origin by studying the end picture, the chronic lesions, years after the injury occurred and usually with little or no clinical information about the perinatal period, met with limited success. The interpretation of causal mechanisms—analyses of the chronic lesions without recourse to studies of antecedent acute forms of brain damage in the newborn—often led to misconceptions. Resolution of the problem defining underlying processes of pathogenesis was significantly advanced in the last decade in the Collaborative Perinatal Project studies and other current investigations. Facets of key information acquired in the Collaborative Project provide a basis for the transitional correlation of acute and subacute perinatal brain damage with patterns of chronic cerebral lesions found in mental retardation, cerebral palsy, and related neuropsychopathy.

In earlier studies by Malamud and coworkers and by other past observers, it was shown that in cerebral palsy and mental retardation there were two basic patterns of chronic cerebral lesions: *deep cerebral damage* with destruction in the basal ganglia and other periventricular tissues (this was the common form); and *cortical damage* the other chronic form, with lesions primarily in the surface tissues of the cerebral convolutions (this pattern, with focal and diffuse cortical scarring, was relatively infrequent in the chronic case material).[6, 7, 55, 59, 83, 85]

A significant connection emerges between Malamud's past studies of the *chronic* lesions and the recent studies of acute perinatal cerebral damage carried out in the Collaborative Perinatal Project, linking perinatal events with childhood and adult nervous system crippling. The close organic tie is evident when one compares the fresh perinatal lesions in Figure 7–38 and with the subacute pattern of damage in Figure 7–41 and then with the common deep form of late chronic residual lesions in cerebral palsy and mental retardation in Figures 7–43 and 7–44. The cerebral lesions in the newborn and the chronic lesions in the cases of cerebral palsy and mental retardation are of the same nature pathologically—both are infarctional—differing only in age, one being acute, the other chronic.

Further, when the acute and chronic case material is compared, there is evident an important relationship in the location and incidence of the cerebral lesions. In both the acute and chronic cases, the incidence of *deep* cerebral lesions is much greater than that of *cortical* damage. Primary cortical cerebral damage proves relatively infrequent both in the newborn acute cases and in the chronic cases with mental retardation and cerebral palsy.

This clinical-pathologic correlation, linking acute and chronic patterns of damage, provides a formula for interpreting retrospectively the time of incurrence of chronic cerebral lesions in cases of cerebral palsy and mental retardation. Lesions located in the deep periventricular cerebral structures reflect damage incurred at 22 to 35 weeks' gestation or earlier; destruction involving mainly cortical elements indicates damage incurred later in the fetal-neonatal period, near or at term, or postnatally.

The predominance of deep cerebral lesions found in cerebral palsy and mental retardation indicates that in most cases the original acute damage was incurred by the fetus prenatally, or by the premature newborn, a significant length of time prior to term.

It merits emphasis that in newborn infants with cerebral hypoxic damage, the pattern of the lesion, its deep or cortical localization, depends on the gestational age at the time of the hypoxic complication, not on the gestational age at birth. In instances of term gestation such as that illustrated in Figure 7–41, in which the fetus incurred cerebral damage prenatally, the result of sublethal hypoxic exposure weeks or months before birth, the cerebral lesion present in the mature newborn is of subacute form, located in the deep cerebral structures.

Acute and subacute cerebral lesions incurred during fetal life may be inapparent clinically in the newborn infant. At times the prenatal intrauterine hypoxic complication, although causing major fetal cerebral damage, is transient, the process remaining clinically silent and asymptomatic during the entire period of gestation; at term, the gestation and delivery are recorded as essentially uncomplicated. The mature newborn infant may show no noticeable immediate manifestations of the latent damage already imprinted in the cerebrum. Regrettably, in most instances the manifestations of cerebral crippling are only postponed. This syndromic pattern is frequently the basis for the common enigmatic occurrence of cerebral palsy and organic mental retardation in patients with a history of uncomplicated, noncyanotic term delivery. The development of such organic central nervous system crippling in infants with no apparent prenatal or parturitional complications, in "good babies" with Apgar score of 10/10, is often the result of latent intrauterine hypoxia in which infarctional cerebral lesions were imprinted-days, weeks, or months before delivery.

"Minimal" Brain Damage¶

The occurrence of latent perinatal brain damage merits wider consideration. Minute deep cerebral matrix infarcts and minimal cortical lesions are usually inconspicuous anatomically, and their importance often is underestimated clinically—the newborn infant with latent damage of this nature often being without noticeable symptoms in the delivery room. The late sequelae of such lesions, however, often surfacing in childhood or adolescence as "minimal brain dysfunction," pose a problem increasingly recognized, of concern clinically and pathologically.[74, 89, 91–93]

¶See References 12, 72, 74, 76.

Clinically the severity of acute and late sequelae of cerebral hypoxia, in the newborn as in the adult, corresponds basically to the amount of damage incurred in the brain. It is well established that in infants who survive after extensive hypoxic infarctional perinatal cerebral damage, the lesions become subacute and, after years, form large scars and cavitations, with consequent related clinical manifestations of mental retardation, cerebral palsy, and other nervous system crippling. Plainly, since hypoxic cerebral damage is not an all-or-none process, the conclusion is inescapable that smaller cerebral lesions incurred in the perinatal period are correspondingly responsible for residual small chronic lesions and, clinically, for the consequent appearance of related minimal patterns of nervous system disability. Hypoxic damage in the germinal matrix and deep white matter, even though the lesions appear minute, imposes an irrevocable loss of anlage tissue, a loss of maturing neuronal elements, creating a lasting handicap. Pathologically, in autopsy material from cases of mental retardation and cerebral palsy and in other case material from neuropsychiatric institutions, in children and adults, there are often present in the cerebrum corresponding small subependymal cavities and pigmented scars at the caudothalamic groove. These small chronic lesions, generally overlooked or dismissed as incidental, may in some instances represent residues of periventricular infarctions dating from the fetal-neonatal period, contributing to varied nervous system disabilities.

Cortical damage of minor degree, as shown in Figure 7–50, likewise may lead to varying chronic neuropsychiatric disability. Also of particular significance are the late effects of diffuse, widely scattered cortical neuronal destruction that may occur at term with hypoxia. In experimental studies with pregnant monkeys near term subjected to asphyxia, the surviving offspring showed pronounced reduction in spontaneous activity and dexterity; examined after 10 years' survival, the brains of the animals showed substantial depletion of nerve cells in the cerebrum, most clearly evident in the precentral motor cortex.[67]

It is likely that the cerebral cellular loss resulting from hypoxia is, in a significant measure, qualitative in nature. As in any population subjected to a noxious environment, it is likely that with exposure to hypoxia, the most highly specialized members, the most differentiated cells, the prime neuronal elements, succumb first.

With hypoxia, the ultimate decrease in neurons that occurs may be so lightly distributed as to escape detection microscopically. A depletion of cells up to 30 per cent may go unrecognized even by experienced neuropathologists. Pathologically, cases of such posthypoxic mental retardation with no discernible decrease in nerve cells in the brain have been characterized as "subanatomical" forms.[7, 76] Scholz has emphasized that neuronal loss such as this, diffusely distributed through the brain, although inconspicuous anatomically, may ultimately lead to significant disability, manifestations of minimal brain dysfunction, or more serious neurologic crippling.[96]

Minimal organic damage to the brain is common in the perinatal period, and it can be concluded that some degree of damage, minimal or more, is present in every newborn infant. Preceding the stresses of birth are the effects of intrauterine environmental deprivation—organic attrition resulting from sublethal perinatal disturbances. The hazards confronting the fetus mount during the hours of labor the process of birth being the most endangering experience to which most individuals are exposed. The perinatal period has a death rate greater than any other time of life. Parturition, even under optimal controlled conditions, is a traumatic, potentially crippling event for the fetus. Compressed and forced through the birth canal, it is subjected to rapid, often turbulent alterations in environment and is required to make complicated changes in circulation, respiration, and other system functions. Often, the borderline between what is physiologic and what is pathologic is not distinct. Although all the structures of the body are vulnerable to hypoxia and mechanical injury during birth, the most sensitive target is the brain. For the fetus, premature or at term, during its tenuous existence in utero and as it is forced down the birth canal and separated, some measure of hypoxic and mechanical injury to the central nervous system is inescapable.

Prematurity

Basic to the problem of perinatal brain damage and of concern clinically, is the large incidence of neuropsychiatric disorders in children and adults with history of premature birth.[23, 68, 87, 88, 97, 99-101] The scope of this problem is reflected in the fact that, in the general population, 5 to 10 per cent of persons are born prematurely. It is not the province of this report to deal broadly with the pathogenesis of premature labor. In obstetrical practice, however, one group of premature cases has come under increasing scrutiny: iatrogenic prematurity—the ready inclination to induce labor a week or two after the calculated date has passed with the result, commonly, that the newborn is obviously two or three weeks premature instead of postmature. Today, with all the diagnostic aids available, this is essentially avoidable. The infants in this induced group, constituting an increasingly major portion of prematures, are subject to all the hazards of premature birth and its sequelae.

Children with cerebral palsy have a history of premature delivery in over 25 per cent of cases.[7] In prematurely born children with organic mental retardation, the occurrence and severity of the cerebral impairment is essentially proportional to the degree of prematurity. Studies in the Collaborative Perinatal Project reveal that in premature infants with birth weight under 2,500 g, the incidence of mental retardation (IQ less than 70) is over 10 per cent, almost twice that in infants born at term. Very small prematures, infants with birth weight of 1,500 g or less, who survive into childhood have IQ scores 10 to 12 points lower than children born at term. In this group of very small prematures, 25 per cent have an IQ of 80 or less.[100] Behavioral disorders—minimal brain dysfunction, delinquency, and psychopathy—in children born prematurely have received increasing consideration in recent years.[99, 101-103]

In the past the persisting handicaps of the prematurely born were believed to be due largely to organic "immaturity," a lasting impairment in structural and functional differentiation and growth. That this concept is basically in error is indicated in current clinical and pathologic investigations. It is increasingly evident that, in children prematurely born, the persisting manifest disturbances in development and function are attributable, not to an enduring biologic "immaturity," but essentially to organic injury sustained prenatally and during the processes of premature delivery. With premature labor, injury of varying severity, hypoxic as well as mechanical, is an imminent threat to the fragile and unready fetus. In its descent through the vaginal canal the premature fetus is repeatedly subject to recurrent hypoxic-mechanical-hypoxic injury. First, with the onset of the prenatal complication, there is usually an accompanying initial period of hypoxia; the intrauterine disturbance, commonly of placental origin—abruption, infarction, placenta previa, or other placental disorder—while precipitating premature labor, at the same time causes hypoxia in the fetus. Second, with active labor developing, the fragile hypoxic fetus is forced through a rigid physiologically unprepared, unrelaxed birth canal, frequently suffering superimposed mechanical trauma—spinal injury, tentorial laceration with subdural hemorrhage, compression-laceration of the liver, or other physical injury. Finally, surviving vaginal parturition, the small hypoxic traumatized premature infant is vulnerable to another hypoxia-producing complication, the development of pulmonary hyaline membrane disease—the respiratory distress syndrome—with the consequence that more hypoxic cerebral damage is added to that already accrued during fetal life.

Experience demonstrates that in many cases of prenatal vaginal bleeding and related complications, the accompanying hypoxic process in the fetus and the resulting intracranial damage are far advanced by the time the moribund infant is delivered. The traditional obstetrical practice in such cases—watchful waiting, delaying until evidence of fetal distress is established—deserves rethinking. Today, the surgical risk to the mother in a cesarean section is indeed minor compared to the predictable dangers to which the premature fetus is subjected by a conservative course of prolonged waiting and vaginal birth. The fact, frequently pointed out, that many prematures seemingly escape injury in vaginal delivery does not mitigate the problem. From autopsy studies of infants of 32 weeks' gestation and older, there is convincing evidence that death of most small prematures is due to injury, hypoxic and mechanical; that such deaths cannot be validly attributed to "immaturity" or other "natural causes"; and that prior to the effects of the delayed vaginal birth, the fetus was viable.

In the light of these clinical and pathologic considerations, it is conclusive that, to resolve the dilemma of premature parturition, early cesarean section is necessary in order to obtain, as nearly as possible, an unblemished neonate. Far better that the neonatal pediatrician be presented with an intact and healthy small premature than with a hypoxic, mechanically traumatized newborn of slightly older gestational age. With some reasonableness it is said, "The premature is born too early and too late."

Corollary to this consideration, and of current concern is the matter of elective legal abortion performed by hysterotomy late in pregnancy, at 20 to 24 weeks' gestation. The traditional view that such small fetuses and newborns are "not viable" is based upon opinion derived from experience with vaginal delivery of traumatized fetuses. The conclusion is inescapable that a fetus of this age, alive before hysterotomy and having avoided the trauma of premature vaginal delivery, will be born alive, and given special care, the newborn may survive.

Implicit in the problem of prematurity is the need, in general, for more direct attention to the clinical condition of the fetus. In practice the obstetrician is preoccupied with the well-being of the mother, only secondarily with the health of the fetus. The pediatrician, in turn, is usually keyed to the needs mainly of older infants and children, and often is disinclined to incorporate into his practice critically distressed, debilitated newborns. Concern for the future well-being of the newborn should begin, not in the delivery room at the moment of birth, but months earlier. In this vein, the emerging concept of "prenatal pediatrics," as expressed by Batstone and co-workers, reflects the need for more comprehensive handling of fetal-neonatal disease.[104] The organically injured newborn, especially the premature, requires intensive emergency care, treatment by a trained neonatologist—a clinician who is not an obstetrician, not a pediatrician, but a specialist with a foot in each of these two disciplines. It is mandatory that the clinician responsible for the health of the newborn be knowledgeably involved in the case during the prenatal period as well as postnatally, especially in the event of a gestational complication in which the gestation terminates prematurely.

Viewed broadly, parturitional injury to the premature, and concern with its processes, and prevention of its occurrence bear upon three facets of obstetrical discipline: adequate monitoring of the fetus, in conjunction with the neonatologist; early cesarean section; and detailed pathologic examination of placentas.

Placental Examination

A clear understanding of the pathologic processes leading to hypoxic damage during fetal life, in the premature and mature, depends in large measure on information derived from study of the placenta. Biologically, the maternal-placental-fetus relationship is delicately balanced. The placenta has a narrow margin of safety. Maternal disease, as well as placental disorders and other intrauterine disturbances, immediately affects the fetus. The importance of the placenta pathologically, the role of this organ in the genesis of fetal disability, especially cerebral damage, is increasingly clear. Current correlated clinical-pathologic studies in the Collaborative and Norwood perinatal projects have focused attention on processes of hypoxic damage in the fetus, especially in the brain, resulting from placental disorders. This organic pathologic pattern, the frequency with which disease of the placenta leads to hypoxic damage in the fetal brain, defines a consistent cause-and-effect relationship: the placental-cerebral syndrome. In preliminary studies in the Norwood Perinatal Project, in the routine laboratory examination of placentas from consecutive deliveries, significant pathologic changes were evident in a major portion of the specimens. Clinically, in deliveries in which significant placental disease was present, the Apgar score, reflecting nervous system involvement, was decreased correspondingly in most cases. Of the neonatal deaths that occurred, a majority of the cases had extensive cerebral hypoxic damage; the close link between the cerebral damage and the placental disease was repeatedly demonstrated at autopsy.

The necessity, clinically and medicolegally, for a careful examination of each placenta cannot be overemphasized. In many instances, in obstetrical cases in which there is hypoxic fetal damage, basic information bearing on the etiopathogenesis can be obtained only from detailed study of the placenta. To obtain a substantial definition of the cause of a perinatal death, laboratory study of the placenta, correlated with a competently performed autopsy, is mandatory. If the placenta is not submitted to the laboratory for examination, is discarded in the delivery room as is the common practice, essential information is lost and, in many instances, the cause of the fetal-neonatal injury remains enigmatic. Consequently, with organic injury present at birth, the causal mechanism uncertain, and the underlying pathologic process overlooked, responsibility for the infant's disability or death is often misinterpreted.

REFERENCES

1. Collaborative Perinatal Project: Research Profile No. 11. Public Health Service Publication No. 1370. Bethesda, Md., National Institute of Neurological Disease and Blindness, National Institutes of Health, 1965.
2. Norwood Perinatal Project. Profile of Research Program. Department of Pathology and Department of Obstetrics and Gynecology, Norwood Hospital, Norwood, Mass. Project Protocol Publication No. 2. 1970.
3. Editorial comment: Suing the doctor. Time, July 15, 1974, p. 78.
4. Matthews, D. D.: Fetal movements and fetal wellbeing. Lancet, *1*:1315, 1973.
5. Sandovsky, E., Yaffe, H., and Polishuk, W. Z.: Fetal movement monitoring in normal and pathologic pregnancy. Int. J. Gynecol. Obstet., *12*:75, 1974.
6. Norman, R. M.: Atrophic sclerosis of the cortex associated with birth injury. Arch. Dis. Child., *19*:111, 1944.
7. Towbin, A.: *The Pathology of Cerebral Palsy.* Springfield, Ill., Charles C Thomas, 1960.
8. Towbin, A.: Cerebral intraventricular hemorrhage and subependymal matrix infarction in the fetus and premature newborn. Am. J. Pathol., *52*:121, 1968.
9. Towbin, A.: Mental retardation due to germinal matrix infarction. Science, *164*:156, 1969.
10. Towbin, A.: Cerebral palsy. In *The Pathology of the Nervous System.* Edited by J. Minckler. Vol II. New York, McGraw-Hill Book Co., Inc., 1971.
11. Csermely, H.: Perinatal anoxic changes of the central nervous system. Acta Paediatr. Acad. Sci. Hung., *13*:283, 1972.
12. Schwartz, P., and Anderson, G. W.: Birth lesions of the nervous system. In *Pathology of the Nervous System.* Edited by J. Minckler. Vol III. New York, McGraw-Hill Book Co., 1972.
13. Towbin, A.: Mental retardation. In *Pathology of the Nervous System.* Edited by J. Minckler. Vol III. New York, McGraw-Hill Book Co., Inc., 1972.
14. Dyer, I., and Barclay, D. L.: Accidental trauma complicating pregnancy and delivery. Am. J. Obstet. Gynecol., *83*:907, 1962.
15. Crosby, W. M.: Pathology of obstetric injuries in pregnant automobile-accident victims. In *Accident Pathology.* Edited by K. M. Brinkhous. Washington, D.C., U. S. Government Printing Office, 1970.
16. Crosby, W. M., and Costiloe, J. P.: Safety of lap belt restraint for pregnant victims of automobile collisions. N. Engl. J. Med., *284*:632, 1971.
17. Kobak, A. J., and Hurwitz, C. H.: Gunshot wounds of the pregnant uterus. Obstet. Gynecol., *4*:383, 1954.
18. Yllpö, A.: Pathologisch-anatomische Studien bei Frühgeborenen. Z. Kinderheilkd., *20*:212, 1919.
19. Henderson, J. L.: Hepatic hemorrhage in stillborn and newborn infants. J. Obstet. Gynaecol. Br. Emp., *48*:377, 1941.
20. Gruenwald, P.: Rupture of liver and spleen in the newborn infant. J. Pediatr., *33*:195, 1948.
21. Potter, E. L.: Quoted by Schaffer, A. J., in *Diseases of the Newborn,* Ed. 1. Philadelphia, W. B. Saunders Co. 1960, p. 515.
22. Stoltzenburg, F.: Zerreissungen der intervertebralen Gelenkkapseln der Halswirbelsäule, eine typische Geburtsverletzung. Berl. Klin. Wochenschr., *48*:1741, 1911.
23. Towbin, A.: Latent spinal cord and brain stem injury in newborn infants. Dev. Med. Child Neurol., *11*:54, 1969.
24. Marburg, O.: Die traumatischen Erkrankungen des Gehirns und Rückenmarks. In *Handbuch der Neurologie.* Vol. 2. Edited by O. Bumke, and O. Foerster. Berlin, Springer Verlag, 1936.
25. Wilson, S. A. K.: Spinal haemorrhage. In *Neurology.* Edited by A. N. Bruce. Vol. 3. London, Butterworth and Co. Ltd., 1955.
26. Lindenberg, R., and Freytag, E.: The brainstem lesions characteristic of traumatic hyperextension of the head. Arch. Pathol., *90*:509, 1970.
27. Towbin, A.: Spinal injury related to the syndrome of sudden death in infants (crib-death). Am. J. Clin. Pathol., *49*:562, 1968.
28. Harris, L. S., and Adelson, L.: "Spinal injury" and sudden infant death. A second look. Am. J. Clin. Pathol., *52*:289, 1969.
29. Kennedy, E.: Cerebral and spinal apoplexy in newborn. Dublin J. Med. Sci., *10*:419, 1836.
30. Litzmann, C. C. T.: Ein Beitrag zur Kenntnis der

spinalen Lähmung bei Neugeboren. Arch. Gynaecol., *16*:87, 1880.
31. Crothers, B., and Putnam, M. C.: Cord birth injuries. In *Birth Injuries of the Central Nervous System.* Edited by F. R. Ford, B. Crother, and M. C. Putnam. Medicine Monographs, No. 11. Baltimore, Williams & Wilkins Co., 1927.
32. Towbin, A.: Spinal cord and brain stem injury at birth. Arch. Pathol., *77*:620, 1964.
33. Walter, C. E., and Tedeschi, L. G.: Spinal injury and neonatal death. Am. J. Obstet. Gynecol., *106*:272, 1970.
34. Ehrenfest, H.: *Birth Injuries of the Child.* New York, Appleton-Century-Crofts, 1931.
35. Föderl, V.: Die Halsmarkquetschung eine Unterart der geburtstraumatischen Schädigung des Zentralnervensystems. Arch. Gynaekol., *143*:598, 1931.
36. Duncan, J. M.: Laboratory note: on the tensile strength of the fresh adult foetus. Brit. Med. J., *2*:763, 1874.
37. Hellström, B., and Sallmander, U.: Prevention of cord injury in hyperextension of the fetal head. J.A.M.A., *202*:1041, 1968.
38. Ford, F. R.: *Diseases of the Nervous System in Infancy, Childhood, and Adolescence.* 4th Ed. Springfield, Ill., Charles C Thomas, 1960.
39. Yates, P. O.: Birth trauma to vertebral arteries. Arch. Dis. Child., *34*:436, 1959.
40. Kendall, N., and Woloshin, H.: Cephalhematoma associated with fracture of the skull. J. Pediatr., *41*:125, 1952.
41. Alexander, E., Jr., and Davis, C. H., Jr.: Intrauterine fracture of the infant's skull. J. Neurosurg., *30*:446, 1969.
42. Gröntoft, O.: Intracerebral and meningeal haemorrhages in perinatally deceased infants. Acta Obstet. Gynecol. Scand., *3*:308, 1953.
43. Towbin, A.: The respirator brain death syndrome. Hum. Pathol., *4*:583, 1973.
44. Towbin, A.: The syndrome of latent cerebral venous thrombosis: its frequency and relation to age and congestive heart failure. Stroke, *4*:419, 1973.
45. Neuburger, F.: Fall einer intrauterinen Hirnschädigung nach einer Leuchtgasvergiftung der Mutter. Beitr. Z. Gerichtl. Med., *13*:85, 1935.
46. Hallervorden, J.: Über eine CO-Veriftung im Fetalleben mit Entwicklungsstörung der Hirnrinde. Allg. Z. Psychiatr., *124*:289, 1949.
47. Bankl, H., and Jellinger, K.: Zentralnervöse Schäden nach fetaler Kohlenoxydvergiftung. Beitr. Pathol. Anat., *135*:350, 1967.
48. Cruikshank, J. N.: Child Life Investigations: The Causes of Neonatal Death. Privy Council, Medical Research Council, Special Report Series No. 145. London, His Majesty's Stationery Office, 1930, p. 47.
49. Clifford, S. H.: The effects of asphyxia on the newborn infant. J. Pediatr., *18*:567, 1941.
50. Macgregor, A. R.: The pathology of still-birth and neonatal death. Br. Med. Bull., *4*:176, 1946.
51. Gruenwald, P.: Axphyxia, trauma and shock at birth. Arch. Pediatr., *67*:103, 1950.
52. Burnard, E. D., and James, L. S.: Failure of the heart after undue asphyxia at birth. Pediatrics, *28*:545, 1961.
53. Hutinel, V.: *Contribution a l'etude des trouble de la circulation veineuse chez l'enfant et en particulie chez le nouveau-né.* Paris, V. Adrien Delahaye et Cie, 1877.
54. Courville, C. B.: Venous channel thrombosis as a possible cause of cerebral paralysis of early life. Arch. Pediatr., *76*:129, 1959.
55. Young, E. F., and Courville, C. B.: Central softening of the cerebral hemispheres in the newborn. Clin. Pediatr., *1*:95, 1962.
56. Kalbag, R. M., and Woolf, A. L.: *Cerebral Venous Thrombosis.* London, Oxford University Press, 1967.
57. Takashima, S.: Studies on vascular architecture and cerebral vascular diseases of the newborn infants. Fukuoko Acta Med., *61*:376, 1970.
58. Towbin, A.: Neonatal damage of the central nervous system. In *Neuropathology: Methods and Diagnosis.* Edited by C. G. Tedeschi, Boston, Little, Brown and Co., 1970.
59. Hallervorden, J., and Meyer, J. E.: Cerebrale Kinderlähmung. In *Handbuch der speziellen Pathologischen Anatomie und Histologie. Nervensystem.* Edited by F. Henke, O. Lubarsch, and R. Rössle. Vol. 13, part 4. Berlin, Springer-Verlag, 1956, pp. 194–282.
60. DeReuck, J., Chattha, A. S., and Richardson, E. P., Jr.: Pathogenesis and evolution of periventricular leukomalacia in infancy. Arch. Neurol., *27*:229, 1972.
61. Morison, J. E.: Renal venous thrombosis and infarction in the newborn. Arch. Dis. Child., *20*:129, 1945.
62. Zuelzer, W. W., Kurnetz, R., and Fallon, R. L.: Circulatory diseases of the kidneys in infancy and childhood. Thrombosis of renal veins. Am. J. Dis. Child., *81*:27, 1951.
63. Avery, M. E., Oppenheimer, E. H., and Gordon, H. H.: Renal-vein thrombosis in newborn infants of diabetic mothers. N. Engl. J. Med., *256*:1134, 1954.
64. Servida, E., and Tropeano, L.: Infarcimento emorragico renale nel neonato. Folia Hered. Pathol., *7*:77, 1959.
65. Towbin, A.: Cerebral hypoxic damage in fetus and newborn. Arch Neurol., *20*:35, 1969.
66. Larroche, J. C.: Nécrose cérébrale massive chez le nouveau-né. Biol. Neonat., *13*:340, 1968.
67. Windle, W. F.: Brain damage at birth. J.A.M.A., *206*:1967, 1968.
68. Towbin, A.: Central nervous damage in the premature related to the occurrence of mental retardation. In *Physical Trauma as an Etiological Agent in Mental Retardation. Proceedings of a Conference on the Etiology of Mental Retardation.* Bethesda, Md., National Institute of Neurological Diseases and Stroke, 1970.
69. Schwartz, P.: Birth injuries. In *Pathology of the Nervous System.* Vol. II. Edited by J. Minckler. New York, McGraw-Hill Book Co., Inc., 1971.
70. Meyers, R. E.: Two patterns of perinatal brain damage and their conditions of occurrence. Am. J. Obstet. Gynecol., *112*:246, 1972.
71. Larroche, J. C.: Post-haemorrhagic hydrocephalus in infancy. Anatomical study. Biol. Neonatc, *20*:287, 1972.
72. Banker, B. Q.: Cerebral vascular disease in infancy and childhood. J. Neuropathol. Exp. Neurol., *20*:127, 1961.
73. Rydberg, E.: Cerebral injury in newborn children consequent on birth trauma; with an inquiry into the normal and pathological anatomy of the neuroglia. Acta Pathol. Microbiol. Scand. Suppl., *10*:247, 1932.
74. Towbin, A.: Organic causes of minimal brain dysfunction. Perinatal origin of minimal cerebral lesions. J.A.M.A., *217*:1207, 1971.
75. Brand, M. M., and Bignami, A.: The effects of chronic hypoxia on the neonatal and infantile brain. Brain, *92*:233, 1969.
76. Courville, C. B.: *Birth and Brain Damage.* Pasadena, Cal., Margaret Farnsworth Courville, Publ., 1971.

77. Bargh, W.: Pneumothorax in the neonate. Br. J. Anaesth., *36*:456, 1964.
78. Chernick, V., and Avery, M. E.: Spontaneous alveolar rupture at birth. Pediatrics, *32*:816, 1965.
79. Neubuerger, K. T., and Schneck, S. A.: Lesions of the brain in hyaline membrane disease of infants. In *Proceedings of the IV International Congress of Neuropathology.* Stuttgart, Thieme, 1962.
80. Towbin, A.: Nervous-system damage related to hyaline-membrane disease. Lancet, *1*:890, 1969.
81. Little, W. J.: On the influence of abnormal parturition, difficult labor, premature birth, and asphyxia neonatorum, on mental and physical condition of the child, especially in relation to deformities. Lancet, *2*:378, 1861.
82. Freud, S.: Die infantile Cerebrällahmung. In Nothnagels *Handbuch der speziellen Pathologie und Therapie.* Vol. 9, pt. 3. Vienna, A. Hölder, 1897.
83. Benda, C. E.: *Developmental Disorders of Mentation and Cerebral Palsies.* New York, Grune & Stratton, 1952.
84. Masland, R. L., Sarason, S. B., and Gladwin, T.: *Mental Subnormality.* New York, Basic Books, 1958.
85. Malamud, N., Itabasi, H. H., Castor, J., and Messinger, H. B.: An etiologic and diagnostic study of cerebral palsy. J. Pediatr., *65*:270, 1964.
86. Taft, L. T., and Goldfarb, W.: Prenatal and perinatal factors in childhood schizophrenia. Dev. Med. Child. Neurol., *6*:32, 1964.
87. Dalen, P.: Family history, the electroencephalogram and perinatal factors in manic conditions. Acta Psychiatr. Scand., *41*:527, 1965.
88. Mednick, S. A.: Breakdown in individuals at high risk for schizophrenia: possible predispositional perinatal factors. Ment. Hyg., *54*:50, 1970.
89. Goldfarb, W., and Yahraes, H.: The causes and treatment of childhood schizophrenia. In *The Mental Health of the Child.* Public Health Service Publication No. 2168. Rockville, Md., 1973, p. 293.
90. Garmazy, N., and Streitman, S.: Children at risk: the search for the antecedents of schizophrenia. Pregnancy and birth complications. Schizophrenia Bull., *8*:28, 1974.
91. Pasamanick, B., and Lilienfeld, A. M.: Association of maternal and fetal factors with development of mental deficiency. 1. Abnormalities in the prenatal and paranatal periods. J.A.M.A., *159*:155, 1955.
92. Clements, S. D.: *Minimal Brain Dysfunction in Children.* NINDBH Monograph 3. Public Health Service Publication 1415, 1966.
93. Connors, C. K.: The syndrome of minimal brain dysfunction: psychological aspects. Pediatr. Clin. North Am., *14*:749, 1967.
94. Toverud, K. U.: Etiological factors in neonatal mortality, with special reference to cerebral hemorrhage. Acta Paediatr. Scand., *18*:249, 1936.
95. Pasamanick, B., Rogers, M. E., and Lilienfeld, A. M.: Pregnancy experience and the development of behavior disorder in children. Am. J. Psychol., *112*:613, 1956.
96. Scholz, W.: Die nicht zu Erweichung führenden unvollständigen Gewebsnekrosen (Elektive Parenchymnekrose). In *Handbuch der Speziellen Pathologischen Anatomie und Histologie: Nervensystem.* Edited by F. Henke, O. Lubarsh, and R. Rössle. Vol. 13, part 1. Berlin, Springer-Verlag, 1956, pp. 1285–1325.
97. Benton, A. L.: Mental development of prematurely born children. Am. J. Orthopsychiatry, *10*:719, 1940.
98. Churchill, J. A.: The relationship of Little's disease to premature birth. Am. J. Dis. Child., *96*:32, 1958.
99. Harper, P. A., and Wiener, G.: Sequelae of low birth weight. Annu. Rev. Med., *16*:405, 1965.
100. Berendes, H.: Quoted in Medical Tribune, *9*:20, 1968.
101. Drillien, C. M.: Aetiology and outcome in low-birthweight infants. Dev. Med. Child Neurol., *14*:563, 1972.
102. Denhoff, E.: Bridges to burn and build. Dev. Med. Child. Neurol., *7*:3, 1965.
103. Rosen, E. J.: Behavioral and emotional disturbances associated with cerebral dysfunction. Appl. Ther., *11*:531, 1969.
104. Batstone, G. F., Blair, A. W., and Slater, J. M.: *A Handbook of Pre-natal Paediatrics.* Philadelphia, J. B. Lippincott Co., 1971.

SECTION 1. MECHANICAL INJURY

chapter 8

THE LAW OF PRENATAL AND PERINATAL INJURIES

by Lee S. Goldsmith and Ira A. Cohen

This chapter deals with the historical and legal development in the United States of the causes of action for prenatal and perinatal injuries. It delves into the liability for damaging in utero a fetus that is subsequently born alive with a disability, for producing a trauma causing the fetus to be born alive and, subsequently, to die, or for causing the fetus to be stillborn. The effects that the recent Supreme Court decisions concerning abortion have had on these fetal wrongful death actions are analyzed.

Finally, the very difficult problems posed by the so-called "wrongful life" lawsuits are discussed, as are the reasons for which the judges have approached these cases with trepidation and why this author feels that plaintiffs will meet with increasing success with them.

HISTORICAL DEVELOPMENT OF CAUSE OF ACTION FOR PRENATAL INJURY

Under the common law, there was no recognized cause of action for prenatal injury. Justice Holmes, in *Dietrich* v. *Northampton*, laid down the reasoning that would be followed in American courts for years to come.[1,2] This reasoning, maintaining that a fetus has no existence independent from its mother, stated that it had no right to bring a cause of action for trauma inflicted on the mother while she was pregnant.

During this period, the state of Louisiana allowed an action for prenatal injuries, but that was a situation peculiar to their civil law system.[3]

The first common law state to allow recovery was California. Their decision, however, was grounded in a section of their civil code that was at the time peculiar to their state. California Civil Code 29 provided that

> . . .[a] child conceived, but not yet born, is to be deemed an existing person, so far as may be necessary for its interests in the event of its subsequent birth.[4]

Obviously, with this statutory provision in effect, it would be impossible to deny recovery to a child who, as a result of a trauma suffered en ventre sa mere, was born alive with a disability.

It was not until 1949 that a case in which recovery was permitted for a prenatal injury was decided solely on its merits. *Bonbrest* v. *Kotz* was a case of obstetrical malpractice involving a child who was injured while being removed from its mother.[5] *Bonbrest* rejected the old, commonly held theory that a fetus was part of its mother and that a trauma to the mother injuring the fetus could result in a cause of action for the mother only, and not for the subsequently born child.

Bonbrest v. *Kotz* was able to break the hold of *Dietrich* v. *Northampton* and its progeny by rejecting the "entity" theory, and stating that the mother and fetus were distinct and independent beings. "Medicine is replete with cases," said the court, "of living children being taken from dead mothers."

This was, of course, a compelling case with which to make new law. How could the court have reasoned that the mother and fetus are a single entity when the fetus was in the process of being born and when the trauma was, in fact, directly to the fetus!

The "entity" theory was not the only grounds used to reject the cause of action for prenatal injury in the early cases. The avowed difficulty of proving that the trauma to the mother was the proximate cause of the injury to the fetus gave courts a second ground for dismissal. Two important cases, however, put an end to this argument. *Woods* and *Damasiewicz* both held that a person cannot be barred from instituting a cause of action merely because it would be difficult to prove the case.[6]

PRENATAL TRAUMA RESULTING IN INJURY TO FETUS BORN ALIVE

Almost every American jurisdiction that has considered the question has now allowed recovery to a child, born alive, who suffered a disability as a result of prenatal trauma.

> States that have allowed such actions when the question has been presented to the court are: Alabama, California, (a case based on a peculiar California statute), Connecticut, Delaware, District of Columbia, Georgia, Illinois, Iowa, Kansas, Kentucky, Louisiana, Maryland, Massachusetts, Michigan, Minnesota, Mississippi, Missouri, Nevada, New Hampshire, New Jersey, New York, North Carolina, Ohio, Oregon, Pennsylvania, Rhode Island (plaintiff born with physical defects because of doctor's failure to prescribe gamma globulin for mother exposed to German measles), South Carolina, Tennessee, Texas, Washington (negligent failure to treat an anemic condition of the mother during delivery caused anoxia of the mother, and the child was, as a result, born with athetoid quadriplegia; $89,000 verdict for the plaintiff), West Virginia, and Wisconsin.[7] Recovery has also been allowed under the Federal Tort Claims Action, when $260,000 damages were awarded to a child unable to see, speak, use his limbs, or control his muscles as a result of trauma suffered by the mother in an automobile accident during the sixth month of pregnancy.[7a]

Because *Bonbrest* v. *Kotz* was based in large part upon the reasoning that a fetus could exist independently of its mother, this independence—or fetal viability—has remained an important element in prenatal injury cases. In other words, to recover in many jurisdictions, the fetus must have sustained the injury as a result of trauma that occurred at a period of gestation when the fetus was viable.

Many jurisdictions allowing recovery for fetal injuries caused by trauma suffered when the fetus is not viable, base their decisions upon the grounds that the fetus becomes a separate entity at the moment of conception. *Kelly* v. *Gregory* was the first case to reject the viability rule as a standard. Here, a child was born severely handicapped after its mother was hit by an automobile during her third month of pregnancy.[8] Other jurisdictions merely ignore the viability rule, stating that it is a completely arbitrary standard.[9]

Proving that the fetus was viable at the instant of trauma—in jurisdictions where this is required—could in some cases be a difficult proposition.

Some legal commentators have theorized that the Supreme Court, in its recent landmark decisions legalizing abortion, has solved the problem. It is maintained that by allowing the states to regulate or proscribe abortion during the third trimester, the court must have determined that the legal standard of viability would begin at the seventh month.[10-12]

The *Roe* v. *Wade* "standard," however, has not been accepted as the standard of fetal viability. More likely the courts will require viability to be established by sound medical testimony. The medical definition of viability is the ability of the fetus to remain alive, separate and independent from its mother. There are several standards against which this can be measured. First, the fetal lungs and central nervous system must be sufficiently developed to be able to sustain respiration. Second, the fetus must have reached a sufficient size. The World Health Organization has set 1.1 lb as the standard of viability. Most medical authorities, on the other hand, have stated that a fetus would have to weigh 2.2 lb to have a reasonable chance to live. Actually, the lightest child on record to be born alive weighed only 396 g (under 14 oz). Finally, gestational age is a standard commonly applied to determine viability. The World Health Organization standard of viability is 20 weeks. Most medical authorities, however, maintain that the fetus would have to have reached between 24 and 28 weeks of gestation to have a chance of survival. The records reveal that one baby was actually born during the eighteenth week of pregnancy and survived.

Obviously, the standards of viability vary, and proof will have to be determined by a multiplicity of factors skillfully presented.

PRENATAL TRAUMA RESULTING IN DEATH OF THE FETUS

Where a state's wrongful death statute allows recovery for the wrongful death of a child, almost all jurisdictions that permit actions for prenatal injury generally also allow recovery when a child born alive subsequently dies as a result of trauma suffered while in utero. (See, e.g., *Wendt* v. *Lillo, Shousa* v. *Matthews Driveurself Serv. Inc., Callahan* v. *Slevsky, Leal* v. *C. C. Pitts Sand & Gravel, Inc.*, [a case in which the fetus lived for two days following birth]; *City of Louisville* v. *Stuckenberg* [in which the mother fell on the sidewalk, causing the child to be born five weeks prematurely; the child was born alive and subsequently died]; and *Huskey* v. *Smith*.)[13]

Recovery for wrongful death of a stillborn fetus, however, is a concept the courts have had far more difficulty with. To understand why, one must keep in mind the fact that the cause of action for prenatal injury is a relatively recent phenomenon. Further, the cause of action for wrongful death in the United States has been almost entirely a statutory development.

At common law, there was no cause of action for wrongful death.[14] This common law principle was accepted in the United States in the 1848 case of *Carey* v. *Berkshire R.R.* and was eventually followed in almost every American jurisdiction.[15]

Eventually, every state except Hawaii (which has a common law action for wrongful death) passed a statute allowing a cause of action for wrongful death. These statutes were, for the most part, based on Lord Campbell's Act, which stated that

> whensoever the death of a person shall be caused by a wrongful act, neglect or default, and the act, neglect or default is such as would, if death had not ensued, have entitled the injured to maintain an action and recover damages in respect thereof, then and in every such case, the person who would have been liable if death had not ensued shall be liable to an action for damages, not-withstanding the death of the party injured, and although the death shall have been caused under such circumstances as amount in law to a felony.[16]

The problem the courts have had with applying this to the wrongful death of a stillborn infant has stemmed from their reluctance to interpret the word "person" contained within these statutes as including a fetus.

Of course, the common law has always recognized the property rights of an unborn child when that child is subsequently born alive and when such recognition is to the child's benefit.[17] An Oklahoma court in 1912 recognized the right of an unborn child subsequently born alive to take as a beneficiary of the proceeds of his father's wrongful death action.[18]

Of course, this concept is one that applies to the law of estates and property. It recognizes that there are inchoate rights that will vest upon the happening of an event at an unspecified future date (e.g., the birth of an unconceived or unborn child). These rights could not vest unless and until the child was born, however, because under the law, an unborn child could not pass on property rights.

If the law of property and succession recognized that a fetus had no rights of its own until it was born alive, the criminal abortion statutes expressed a different philosophy. Under the criminal law, it had always been a misdemeanor to kill a viable child, and it eventually became a crime to kill any unborn child.[19]

It is maintained by some commentators that the abortion statutes existed primarily for the protection of the mother, with the right to life of the fetus subordinated to the health and welfare of the mother. To support this position, it is pointed out that abortion was generally allowed to save the life of the mother or protect her mental well-being.[20] It is more likely that the prohibition against abortion was primarily designed to protect the unborn child. It squares more with the property law concept that the property rights of a child would be recognized where it was to his benefit, and it is more in keeping with the then current concepts of morality. Allowing abortion under limited circumstances to avoid the death or severe mental breakdown of the already living was a reflection of the balancing of interests that the law always finds itself exercising.

In order to overcome the major block against allowing recovery for a stillborn fetus, the courts had to recognize the fetus as a "person" under the wrongful death statutes. To do so, it had first to reject the "entity" theory expressed in *Dietrich* v. *Northampton*, supra, that the mother and the fetus were one. Justice Boggs's dissent in *Allaire* v. *St. Luke's Hospital* was the first major voice raised against Justice Holmes's theory and the first eloquent expression of the idea that a fetus had an independent existence in the law.

The first cases of prenatal wrongful death in which recovery was allowed all involved obstetrical malpractice in which the doctor's or hospital's negligence caused the death of the fetus while in the process of delivery.[21] These were ideal cases to change the law in this country because they dramatized the arbitrariness of requiring a live birth before a right to recover would vest.

The rejection of the "entity" theory becomes especially important in states that deny a cause of action for prenatal wrongful death while still allowing recovery for postnatal death resulting from prenatal injury. The rejection of the action for prenatal wrongful death in these states is often based on the theory that the tort is not complete until the harm occurs, and the harm occurs when the fetus dies and not when the trauma occurs. The fetus, if it has no separate existence from the mother, cannot suffer a harm, and if it is never born alive, the tort is never complete. If, on the other hand, the fetus enjoys a legal existence independent from the mother, the harm will occur when the trauma occurs. The tort will thus be complete at the point of trauma, and if this trauma causes death in utero, the fetus's right to a cause of action for wrongful death will vest.[22]

This approach, coupled with a rejection of the viability test previously alluded to, would allow recovery for the wrongful death of a fetus no matter when the trauma occurred. Very few states, however, allow recovery for wrongful death of a stillborn fetus when the trauma occurs prior to viability.[23]

Most jurisdictions that do not allow a cause of action for prenatal wrongful death base their decision on the ground that the word "person" does not include a fetus within the meaning of their wrongful death statute.

Some jurisdictions, especially those whose statutes use pecuniary loss as the measure of damages in a wrongful death action, use as a basis for rejection of the fetal wrongful death action the ground that damages would be remote, speculative, and difficult to ascertain.[24] Such statutes would not consider the loss of the prospective child, along with the companionship, society, and services it would have provided had it lived, a measurable loss in pecuniary terms.

Endresz v. *Friedberg*, supra, perhaps best sums up the arguments used for denying recovery for fetal death. Judge Fuld held in that case that the law had never considered the fetus as having a legal existence separate from its mother unless it was necessary to protect the child's own rights. He stated that while justice required that there be a right of action for an infant injured en ventre sa mere and subsequently born alive with some handicaps, it was not so compelling

> . . . where the foetus, deprived of life while yet unborn, is never faced with the prospect of impaired mental or physical health.

Judge Fuld went on to say that

> . . . there is but a "conditional prospective liability created when an unborn child . . . is injured" through the wrongful act of the defendant, and such liability attaches only upon the fulfillment of the condition that the child be born alive.[25]

The courts' ability to recognize the cause of action for fetal wrongful death will be greatly enhanced by a recognition of the concept that recovery in such suits (as well as recovery in all suits involving the death of young children) serves primarily to vindicate the rights of the parents rather than the rights of the unborn fetus. In reality, this is similar to the objectives of *all* wrongful death actions—that is, to benefit the living (as recovery for the death of a wage earner is designed to permit the decedent's family to enjoy the continued benefits of the decedent's existence).

Currently, 20 states have decided cases allowing recovery for the wrongful death of a stillborn fetus:

Alabama, Connecticut (difficulty of proving causation should not bar the right to a cause of action), Delaware, District of Columbia (mother died in childbirth at full term, and doctor negligently failed to deliver the baby alive), Georgia (no necessity for the fetus to be viable at the time of the injury), Illinois, Indiana, Kansas, Kentucky, Louisiana, Maryland, Michigan, Minnesota (state has pecuniary loss statute), Mississippi, Nevada (state has pecuniary loss statute; court said that the loss to the survivors is the same as it would have been had the child been born alive and subsequently died; court further held that the difficulty in proving damages is not a bar to a cause of action), New Hampshire, Ohio (state has pecuniary loss statute), South Carolina (difficulty of ascertaining amount of damages does not bar a cause of action), West Virginia (state's statute allows automatic injury award of $10,000, without reference to pecuniary loss, and allows recovery for pecuniary loss where same can be reasonably proved), and Wisconsin (state has pecuniary loss statute).[26]

There are 12 states that have decided cases denying recovery for fetal wrongful death:

California (fetus not a "person" within meaning of the wrongful death statute), Florida, Iowa (unborn fetus not a "person" within the meaning of the survival statute), Massachusetts, Nebraska, New Jersey (unborn child's pecuniary value is not ascertainable), New York (in one case, no measurable damages until birth; in another, court would not issue letters of administration for the purpose of instituting a wrongful death action for a fatal injury to a fetus), North Carolina (pecuniary value of unborn fetus is not ascertainable),

Oklahoma, Pennsylvania (damages too speculative), Tennessee, and Virginia.[27]

Finally, there are two states that have denied recovery in such lawsuits, but under circumstances that leave the basic question of recovery open:

> Alaska (case based upon nonviable fetus) and Missouri (state has a pecuniary loss statute, and court ruled that aunts and uncles suing as plaintiffs in this case could not show pecuniary loss).[28]

It should be noted, however, that most jurisdictions rejecting recovery for the wrongful death of the unborn child do allow recovery for the pain, suffering, and emotional distress suffered by the mother as a result of the loss, and for the husband's loss of his wife's services and consortium.[29]

Because the United States Supreme Court in its recent landmark decision on abortion stated that "the word 'person,' as used in the Fourteenth Amendment, does not include the unborn," it has been asked whether the court has sounded the death knell for the wrongful death action of the stillborn fetus.[30] *

If a fetus does not have a constitutionally protected right to life, does the admonition in *Endresz* v. *Friedberg*, supra, that a fetus has "but a conditional prospective right to recovery which attaches only when the child is born alive" become the law throughout the United States?

The answer to this question can be found in three sources. First, the law has always recognized conflicting theories of law as it has suited the purposes of the law of torts, estates, future interests, and abortion. Second, recovery for wrongful death of a stillborn fetus, especially in states with pecuniary loss statutes in effect, really serves as vindication of the rights of the parents rather than those of the unborn child. This recognition is the only way the courts can

> . . . be consistent with the historical purposes of wrongful death statutes and at the same time avoid conflict with *Roe* v. *Wade*'s declaration that "due process" legal personality is not acquired until the instant of birth.[32]

Finally, the language of *Roe* v. *Wade* itself provides us with a solution. Justice Blackmun stated in dictum that the ruling of the case was not inconsistent with the policy of some states to permit parents of a stillborn child to maintain an action for wrongful death due to prenatal injuries. Blackmun's reasoning was that it is really the *parents'* rights that are being vindicated in such actions, and that such a cause of action for the *parents* would not be inconsistent with the view that the fetus represents a mere potentiality of life.[33]

THE CAUSE OF ACTION FOR "WRONGFUL LIFE"

A so-called "wrongful life" case involves a lawsuit instituted as a result of an act of negligence that causes the birth of a child either unplanned by the parents or unwanted or both. A basic respect for human life and a great reluctance on the part of the courts to acknowledge that an unplanned or unwanted or handicapped child is an undesirable and compensable alternative to the absence of the child have resulted in a general lack of success of these cases.

For the most part, and with very few exceptions, courts allowing recovery in wrongful birth cases have done so in cases involving the negligent performance of a sterilization operation and the resultant birth of an unplanned child.[34] † Some of these cases have been grounded on a breach of contract theory.[35]

In the *Doerr* case, a sterilization operation was performed on a man. His wife subsequently became pregnant and gave birth to a retarded child. The wife brought an action against the surgeons for breach of an oral contract to make her husband sterile. Damages were assessed by the court for all medical expenses and for the costs necessary for the special care and attention required by this child.

Whether a case is based on negligence or on breach of contract, it is easy to understand the courts' occasional willingness to award damages in these cases. The plaintiffs here sought treatment specifically to prevent the birth of a child. The physician's negligent performance of the surgery not only caused it to fail to achieve its purpose but caused the plaintiffs to fail to use other means of birth control and thus produce a child. The cause and effect, and damages

*An excellent discussion of the effects of *Roe* v. *Wade* on this area of law appears in the case note, "Wrongful Death and the Unborn: An Examination of Recovery After *Roe* v. *Wade*," in the *Journal of Family Law*.[31]

†See, e.g., *West* v. *Underwood*, *Shaheen* v. *Knight*, *Doerr* v. *Villate*, *Bishop* v. *Byrne*, *Custodia* v. *Bauer*, *Coleman* v. *Garrison*.

flowing therefrom, are clear and easily assessable.

An action whose theoretical basis is closely related to the preceding cases is *Troppi* v. *Scarf*. In this case, a pharmacist negligently filled a prescription for birth control pills and erroneously sold a woman tranquilizers instead. The woman became pregnant, gave birth to a normal child, and sued the pharmacist for the costs of rearing the child. The court based its decision for the plaintiff on five grounds: First, the court held the pharmacist to a high standard of care in filling a prescription, which standard was not met in this case. Second, the pharmacist's negligence was a direct cause of the pregnancy, and the pregnancy was a foreseeable result of that breach. Third, it does not violate public policy to allow this recovery, since it is within the public's interest to foster family planning. Fourth, the court rejected the defendant's argument that the benefits of parenthood outweighed the costs of rearing a child. They held, instead, that this weighing process is a question of fact that must be left to the discretion of the jury. Finally, the court rejected the defendant's contention that damages were unascertainable, holding instead that difficulty in assessing damages cannot be a bar to a cause of action.[36]

In *Troppi*, as in the sterilization cases, the breach was a direct cause of the birth, and the court's resistance to allowing recovery in wrongful birth cases generally was met by the compelling nature of the facts.

In all other classes of wrongful birth cases the courts have found the facts far less compelling.

There have been several unsuccessful lawsuits brought for illegitimate birth. In *Zepeda* v. *Zepeda*, an illegitimate child sued his father for the damages resulting from the stigma of being born a bastard.[37] While the court recognized that the plaintiff had in fact suffered damages, they dismissed the complaint on the ground that to allow such an action to succeed would open the doors of litigation to all persons born under a social handicap.[38]

In *Williams* v. *State*, a woman was a patient in a state mental institution, where she was assaulted and raped by a male inmate. This attack resulted in the birth of a boy. The infant subsequently sued the state of New York on the grounds that he was born

> . . . deprived of property rights,. . . of a normal childhood and home life,. . .of proper parental care, support and rearing,. . . [and bearing] the stigma of illegitimacy.[39]

The court, while recognizing both the state's negligence in the operation of the hospital and the damage suffered by the child, denied that the plaintiff had a cause of action:

> [T]he law knows no cure or compensation for [being born out of wedlock], and the policy and social reasons against providing such compensation are at least as strong as those which might be thought to favor it. Being born under one set of circumstances rather than another or to one pair of parents rather than another is not a suable wrong that is recognizable in court.[39]

The cases that have posed the greatest philosophical difficulty for the courts have been those in which an alleged act of negligence resulting neither in an injury or deformity to a child, nor in the birth of a child, has, rather, resulted in the failure of the mother to obtain an abortion. For the most part, a cause of action has generally not been recognized in this class of cases.

The first important case in this area was *Gleitman* v. *Cosgrove*.[40] In *Gleitman*, a woman developed German measles during her first month of pregnancy. The physician she consulted informed her that the measles would have no effect on the fetus, although in fact, there was a generally recognized 20 to 50 per cent risk that the child would be born deformed. The child was born with severe birth defects involving sight, hearing, and speech. The parents claimed that, had they known of this, they would have sought further medical advice about the performance of an abortion.

Of course, the physician's negligent medical treatment did not in this case cause the child's birth defects. Rather, it was the cause of his birth, and if he were to have a cause of action, it would have to be for being born. The court, citing previous decisions for *illegitimate* birth, stated that it would be impossible to measure the difference between life with defects and no life at all.

The parents' cause of action was decided on analogous grounds—that one cannot measure the difference between the denial of the benefits of parenthood against the emotional and financial injuries suffered as a result of the birth of this deformed child. Citing the public's interest in protecting human life, the court stated further that the right to life of the child is greater than the parents' right to be spared the emotional and financial trauma of the birth.

Three years after *Gleitman*, the New York court, in *Stewart* v. *Long Island College Hospital*, faced a similar situation.[41] Mrs. Stewart also developed German measles during pregnancy.

She, however, specifically requested a therapeutic abortion. The hospital, following a 2 to 2 vote of their abortion committee, refused to perform the abortion. Mrs. Stewart's physician failed to notify her that an abortion might be obtained elsewhere and advised her against seeking other avenues for securing this abortion.

Though the Stewart child was born with severely disabling deformities, the court denied recovery, basing their denial on *Zepeda, Williams*, and *Gleitman*. In dismissing the child's cause of action, the court held that

> . . . there is no remedy for having been born under a handicap . . . when the alternative . . . is not to have been born at all.[41]

The parents' cause of action for physical pain and mental anguish was dismissed on the basis that

> . . . it would be virtually impossible to evaluate, as compensatory damages, the anguish to the parents of rearing a malformed child as against the denial to them of the benefits of parenthood.[41]

A recent case in New York serves as a striking contrast to *Gleitman* and *Stewart*.[42] In *Ziemba* a physician negligently failed to diagnose a pregnancy. The mother consulted a second doctor, whose diagnosis was that she was four and a half months pregnant. The mother did not want to be pregnant, and alleged that if she had been told earlier, she would have obtained an abortion (which at this point was perfectly legal). At four and a half months, however, abortion is not totally safe, and the mother chose to have the child rather than undergo the risks of abortion. A normal child was subsequently born, and the parents brought an action against the doctor, asking damages for pain and suffering, loss of consortium, and the potential educational and medical expenses of the child.

The defendant physician brought a motion to dismiss the action, citing the speculativeness of the damages and the mother's failure to obtain an abortion—which was available. The court denied the defendant's motion, thus allowing the case to go to trial. The court's decision was based on the opinion that all the matters raised in the defendant's motion were questions that were within the competence of a jury to decide. Difficulty in weighing damages cannot bar a cause of action, and if the alleged damages flow naturally from the physician's breach, then the task of measuring elements of damage must be left to the jury's discretion. Furthermore, the mother's failure to obtain an abortion cannot bar her cause of action as a matter of law, since that refusal could have been based on sound medical grounds, which would be jury questions at trial. *Stewart* was significant because when *Stewart* was decided, abortion was illegal. *Ziemba's* significance, if it serves as a basis for future decisions, should lie in its leaving to the jury questions of damage.

Gleitman and *Stewart* in effect refused *as a matter of law* to consider certain types of damage compensable. This is a position that is difficult to maintain on both logical and historical grounds. Is it not within the discretion of the jury—and therefore a question of fact—whether or not a person has suffered damages? The better judicial reasoning has always been that difficulty in determining or measuring damages cannot bar a cause of action. Rather, the real question should be whether the alleged acts of negligence caused the claimed injuries. If causation is thus proved, then the jury must decide whether the plaintiff has suffered an injury and what that injury is worth. (Is not the question of whether the anguish and expense of rearing a malformed or unwanted child is worse than the benefits of parenthood a question of *fact*, and therefore within the sole province of the jury?)

CONCLUSION

History in the law of prenatal torts will be made in the future with the development of the cause of action for wrongful birth.

Consider the following:

That both *Gleitman* and *Stewart* were based on an assumed interest of the state in protecting the right of the unborn fetus over that of the parents.

That when these cases were decided, abortion was either illegal or considerably proscribed.

That the courts based many of their decisions on their inability to assume that the expense and anguish of rearing an unwanted, unplanned, or deformed child is worse than parenthood.

That the courts held as a matter of law that the damages just enumerated were not compensable, even if they flowed naturally from the alleged breach of duty, and even if they in fact constituted damages.

Consider further that *Roe* v. *Wade* held that a fetus has no constitutionally protected right to life, that abortion is generally legal and within the discretion of the mother, that historically the courts have held that difficulty in assessing damages could not bar a cause of action, and that the weighing of the scales of benefit versus burden in a damage action has traditionally been the jury's privilege.

These considerations should weigh heavily on the minds of judges pondering the fates of plaintiffs in wrongful birth suits brought in the future, and their compelling nature should cause many courts to reevaluate their prior reluctance to consider these matters worthy of jury consideration.

REFERENCES

1. Dietrich v. Northampton, 138 Mass. 14 (1884).
2. Lipps v. Milwaukee Elec. Ry. & Light Co., 159 N.W. 916 (Wisc. 1916); Stanford v. St. Louis–S. F. Ry., 108 So. 566 (Ala. 1926); Drobners v. Peters, 232 N.Y. 220; Magnolia Coca-Cola Bottling Co. v. Jordan, 78 S.W. 2d 944 (Tex. 1935); Newman v. City of Detroit, 274 N.W. 710 (Mich. 1937).
3. Cooper v. Blanck, 39 So. 2d 352 (La. 1923).
4. Scott v. McPheeters, 92 P. 2d 678 (Calif. 1939).
5. Bonbrest v. Kotz, 65 F. Supp. 138 (D.D.C. 1946).
6. Woods v. Lancet, 102 N.E. 2d 691 (N.Y. 1951); Damasiewicz v. Gorsuch, 79 A. 2d 550 (Md. 1951).
7. Alabama–Wolf v. Isbell, 280 So. 2d 758 (Ala. 1973).
   California–Scott v. McPheeters, supra.
   Connecticut–Tursi v. New England Windsor Co., 111 A. 2d 14 (Ct. 1955).
   Delaware–Worgan v. Greggo & Ferrara, Inc., 128 A. 2d 557 (Del. 1956).
   District of Columbia–Bonbrest v. Kotz, supra.
   Georgia–Tucker v. Howard L. Carmichael & Sons, Inc., 65 S.E. 2d 909 (Ga. 1951); Fallow v. Hobbs, 147 S.E. 2d 517 (Ga. 1966).
   Illinois–Amann v. Faidy, 114 N.E. 2d 412 (Ill. 1953); Rodriguez v. Patti, 114 N.E. 2d 721 (Ill. 1953).
   Iowa–Wendt v. Lillo, 182 F. Supp. 56 (D.C. Iowa 1960).
   Kansas–Hale v. Manion, 368 P. 2d 1 (Ka. 1962).
   Kentucky–Mitchell v. Couch, 285 S.W. 2d 901 (Ky. 1955).
   Louisiana–Cooper v. Blanck, 39 So. 2d 352 (La. 1923).
   Maryland–Damasiewicz v. Gorsuch, supra.
   Massachusetts–Keyes v. Construction Service, Inc., 165 N.E. 2d 912 (Mass. 1960).
   Michigan–Womack v. Buchhorn, 187 N.W. 2d 218 (Mich. 1971).
   Minnesota–Verkennes v. Corniea, 38 N.W. 2d 838 (Minn. 1949).
   Mississippi–Rainey v. Horn, 72 So. 2d 434 (Miss. 1954).
   Missouri–Steggal v. Morris, 258 S.W. 2d 577 (Mo. 1953).
   Nevada–White v. Yup, 458 P. 2d 617 (Nev. 1969).
   New Hampshire–Poliquin v. McDonald, 135 A. 2d 249 (N.H. 1957).
   New Jersey–Smith v. Brennan, 157 A. 2d 497 (N.J. 1960); Knutson v. Brown, 226 A. 2d 460 (N.J. 1966).
   New York–Woods v. Lancet, supra; Kelly v. Gregory, 125 N.Y. S. 2d 696 (1953).
   North Carolina–Stetson v. Easterling, 161 S.E. 2d 531 (N.C. 1968) (dicta).
   Ohio–Williams v. Marion Rapid Transit, Inc., 87 N.E. 2d 334 (Ohio 1949).
   Oregon–Mallison v. Pomeroy, 291 P. 2d 225 (Ore. 1955).
   Pennsylvania–Sinkler v. Kneale, 164 A. 2d 93 (Pa. 1960).
   Rhode Island–Sylvia v. Gobeille, 220 A. 2d 222 (R.I. 1966).
   South Carolina–Hall v. Murphy, 113 S.E. 2d 790 (S.C. 1960).
   Tennessee–Shousa v. Matthews Driveurself Serv., Inc., 358 S.W. 2d 471 (Tenn. 1962).
   Texas–Leal v. C. C. Pitts Sand & Gravel, Inc., 419 S.W. 2d 820 (Tex. 1967); Yandell v. Delgado, 471 S.W. 2d 569 (Tex. 1971).
   Washington–Seattle-First National Bank v. Rankin, 367 P. 2d 835 (Wash. 1962).
   West Virginia–Panagopoulous v. Martin, 295 F. Supp. 220 (D.C.W. Va. 1969).
   Wisconsin–Kwaterski v. State Farm Mutual Insurance Company, 148 N.W. 2d 107 (Wisc. 1967).

7a. Under the Federal Tort Claims Act–Sox v. United States, 187 F. Supp. 465 (E.D.S.C. 1960).

8. Kelly v. Gregory, 125 N.Y. S. 2d 696 (1953).
9. Bennett v. Hymers, 147 A. 2d 108 (N.H. 1958); Sinkler v. Kneale, 164 A. 2d 93 (Pa. 1960). Other cases rejecting the viability standard: Hornbuckle v. Plantation Pipe Line Co., 93 S.E. 2d 727 (Ga. 1956) (trauma during third month of pregnancy); Puhl v. Milwaukee Auto. Ins. Co., 99 N.W. 2d 163 (Wisc. 1959) (dicta); Smith v. Brennan, 157 A. 2d 497 (N.J. 1960) (viability-nonviability distinction abolished); Daley v. Meier, 178 N.E. 2d 691 (Ill. 1961); Sylvia v. Gobeille, 220 A. 2d 222 (R.I. 1966) (causation, and not viability, is the sole test); Torigian v. Watertown News. Co., 225 N.E. 2d 926 (Mass. 1967); Delgado v. Yandell, 468 S.W. 2d 475 (Tex. 1971); Womack v. Buchhorn, 187 N.W. 2d 218 (Mich. 1971); Wolf v. Isbell, supra (trauma at sixth month of pregnancy).
10. Case Note: Damages for the wrongful death of a fetus–proof of fetal viability. 51 Chicago–Kent Law Rev. 227 (Summer, 1974).
11. Roe v. Wade, 410 U.S. 113 (1973).
12. 51 Chicago–Kent Law Rev. 227, 239.
13. Wendt v. Lillo, 182 F. Supp. 56 (N.D. Iowa 1960); Shousa v. Matthews Driveurself Serv. Inc., 358 S.W. 2d 471 (Tenn. 1962); Callahan v. Slevsky, 385 P. 2d 674 (Colo. 1963); Leal v. C. C. Pitts Sand & Gravel, Inc., 419 S.W. 2d 820 (Tex. 1967); City of Louisville v. Stuckenberg, 438 S.W. 2d, 94 (Ky. 1968); Huskey v. Smith, 265 So. 2d 596 (Ala. 1972).
14. Baker v. Bolton, 1 Campb. 493, 170 Eng. Rep. 1033 (K. B. 1803).
15. Carey v. Berkshire R. R., 55 Mass. 475 (1848).
16. Lord Campbell's Acts, 9 & 10 Vict., C. 93 (1846).
17. 1 *Blackstone's Commentaries* §175; Marsellis v. Thalhimer, 2 Paige 35 (N.Y. 1830); Hall v. Hancock, 32 Mass. 255 (1834); McLain v. Howald, 79 N.W. 182 (Mich. 1899); Wehrman v. Farmers' & Merchants' Savings Bank, 259 N.W. 564 (Iowa 1935).
18. Herndon v. St. Louis & S.F.R. Co., 128 P. 2d 727 (Okla. 1912).
19. Commonwealth v. Parker, 50 Mass. 263 (1845); Mitchell v. Commonwealth, 78 Ky. 204 (1879).
20. Case Note: Torts–Wrongful death–unborn child–the estate of an unborn child has a cause of action for wrongful death. 70 Mich. Law Rev. 729 (March 1972).
21. Verkennes v. Corniea, 38 N.W. 2d 38 (Minn. 1949); Rainey v. Horn, 72 So. 2d 434 (Miss. 1954).
22. State ex rel Odham v. Sherman, 198 A. 2d 71 (Md. 1964).
23. Poliquin v. MacDonald, 135 A. 2d 249 (N.H. 1957); West v. McCoy, 105 S.E. 2d 88 (S.C. 1958); Mace v. Jung, 210 F. Supp. 706 (D. Alas. 1962) (fetus 4-

4½ months old); Rapp v. Hiemenz, 246 N.E. 2d 77 (Ill. 1969); O'Neill v. Morse, 188 N.W. 2d 785 (Mich. 1971).

24. Endresz v. Friedberg, 248 N.E. 2d 901 (N.Y., 1969); In re Bradley's Estate, 269 N.Y. S. 2d 657 (1967); Gay v. Thompson, 146 S.E. 2d 425 (N.C. 1966); Graf v. Taggert, 204 A. 2d 140 (N.J. 1964).
25. Endresz v. Friedberg, 248 N.E. 2d 901, 903.
26. Alabama—Wolf v. Isbell, supra.
Connecticut—Hatala v. Markiewicz, 224 A. 2d 406 (Ct. 1966).
Delaware—Worgan v. Greggo & Ferrara, Inc., supra.
District of Columbia—Simmons v. Howard University, 323 F. Supp. 256 (D.D.C. 1971).
Georgia—Porter v. Lassiter, 87 S.E. 2d 100 (Ga. 1955).
Illinois—Chrisafogeorgis v. Brandenburg, 304 N.E. 2d 88 (1973).
Indiana—Britt v. Sears, 277 N.E. 2d 20 (Ind. Ct. App. 1971).
Kansas—Hale v. Manion, 368 P. 2d 1 (Kan. 1962).
Kentucky—Mitchell v. Couch, 285 S.W. 2d 901 (Ky. 1955); Rice v. Rizk, 453 S.W. 2d 732 (Ky. 1970).
Louisiana—Valence v. Louisiana Power & Light Co., 50 So. 2d 847 (La. Ct. App. 1951).
Maryland—State ex rel. Odham v. Sherman, supra.
Michigan—O'Neill v. Morse, supra.
Minnesota—Verkennes v. Corniea, supra.
Mississippi—Rainey v. Horn, supra.
Nevada—White v. Yup, supra.
New Hampshire—Poliquin v. MacDonald, supra.
Ohio—Stidam v. Ashmore, 167 N.E. 2d 106 (Ohio 1959).
South Carolina—Fowler v. Woodward, 138 S.E. 2d 42 (S.C. 1964).
West Virginia—Baldwin v. Butcher, 184 S.E. 2d 42 (W. Va. 1971); Panagopoulous v. Martin, supra.
Wisconsin—Kwaterski v. State Farm Mutual Auto. Ins. Co., supra.
27. California—Norman v. Murphy, 268 P. 2d 178 (Calif. 1954); Bayer v. Suttle, 23 Cal. App. 3d 361, 100 Cal. Rptr. 213 (1972).
Florida—Stokes v. Liberty Mutual Ins. Co., 213 So. 2d 695 (Fla. 1968).
Iowa—McKillip v. Zimmerman, 191 N.W. 2d 706 (Iowa 1971).
Massachusetts—Leccese v. McDonough, 279 N.E. 2d 339 (Mass. 1971).
Nebraska—Drabbels v. Skelly Oil Co., 50 N.W. 2d 229 (Neb. 1951).
New Jersey—Graf v. Taggert, 204 A. 2d 140 (N.J. 1964).
New York—Endresz v. Friedberg, supra; In re Bradley's Estate, supra.
North Carolina—Gay v. Thompson, 146 S.E. 2d 425 (N.C. 1966); Stetson v. Easterling, 161 S.E. 2d 531 (N.C. 1968).
Oklahoma—Padillo v. Zirod, 426 P. 2d 16 (Okla. 1967).
Pennsylvania—Caroll v. Skloff, 202 A 2d 9 (Pa. 1964); Marko v. Philadelphia Transp. Co., 216 A. 2d 502 (Pa. 1966).
Tennessee—Durrett v. Owens, 371 S.W. 2d 433 (Tenn. 1963).
Virginia—Lawrence v. Craven Tire Co., 169 S.E. 2d 440 (Va. 1969).
28. Alaska—Mace v. Jung, 210 F. Supp. 706 (D.C. Alas. 1962).
Missouri—Acton v. Shields, 386 S.W. 2d 363 (Mo. 1965).
29. Tunnicliffe v. Bay Cities Consol. Ry., 61 N.W. 11 (Mich. 1894); Malone v. Monongahela Valley Traction Co., 140 S.E. 340 (W. Va. 1927); Fehely v. Senders, 135 P. 2d 283 (Ore. 1943); Stafford v. Roadway Transit Co., 70 F. Supp. 555 (W.D. Pa. 1947); Duncan v. Martins Restaurant, Inc., 106 N.E. 2d 731 (Ill. 1952).
30. Roe v. Wade, 410 U.S. 113, 158 (1973).
31. Case Note: Wrongful death and the unborn: an examination of recovery after *Roe* v. *Wade*. 13 J. Family Law 99 (1973–74).
32. 13 J. Family Law 99, 105; 410 U.S. 113, 162.
33. 410 U.S. 113, 162.
34. West v. Underwood, 40 A. 2d 610 (N.J. 1945); Shaheen v. Knight, 11 Pa. D. & C. 2d 41 (1957); Doerr v. Villate, 220 N.E. 2d 767 (Ill. 1966); Bishop v. Byrne, 265 F. Supp. 46 (D.C. W. Va. 1967); Custodia v. Bauer, 261 Cal. App. 2d 303, 59 Cal. Rptr. 463 (1967); Coleman v. Garrison, 281 A. 2d 616 (Del. Super. 1971).
35. Shaheen v. Knight; Doerr v. Villate, supra.
36. Troppi v. Scarf, 187 N.W. 2d 511 (Mich. 1971).
37. Zepeda v. Zepeda, 190 N.E. 2d 849 (Ill. 1963), cert denied 379 U.S. 945 (1964).
38. Pinkney v. Pinkney, 198 So. 2d 52 (Fla. 1967).
39. Williams v. State, 223 N.E. 2d 343 (N.Y. 1966).
40. Gleitman v. Cosgrove, 227 A. 2d 689 (N.J. 1967).
41. Stewart v. Long Island College Hospital, 313 N.Y. S. 2d 502 (App. Div., 2d Dept. 1969) affd. 332 N.Y. S. 2d 640, 283 N.E. 2d 616 (1970).
42. Ziemba v. Sternberg, 357 N.Y. S. 2d 265 (App. Div. 1974).

SELECTED READINGS

43. Note: Torts—wrongful death—unborn child—the estate of an unborn child has a cause of action for wrongful death. 70 Mich. Law Rev. 729 (March, 1972).
44. Note: The law and the unborn child: the legal and logical inconsistencies. 46 Notre Dame Lawyer 349 (Winter, 1971).
45. Note: Negligence and the unborn child: a time for change. 18 S. D. Law Rev. 204 (Winter, 1973).
46. Comment: Wrongful death and the unborn: an examination of recovery after *Roe* v. *Wade*. 13 J. Family Law 99 (1973–74).
47. Note: Damages for the wrongful death of a fetus—proof of fetal viability. 51 Chicago—Kent Law Rev. 227 (Summer, 1974).
48. Dachs, N. H.: Liability for wrongful harm to the unborn—past, present and future. 158 N.Y. Law J., (August 2, 3 and 4, 1971).
49. *Prosser on Torts* 354 (3d ed. 1974).
50. Gordon: The unborn plaintiff. 63 Mich. Law Rev., 579 (1965).
51. Culiner: Trauma to the unborn "child." Trauma, *5*:5, 1963.

SECTION 1. MECHANICAL INJURY

chapter 9

SELF-INFLICTED WOUNDS

by William G. Eckert

Bodily harm that is self-induced may take the form of localized mutilative injury or injury that may have systemic effects. Malingering and psychiatric disorders are the most frequent underlying factors.

Historically, mutilation, self-induced or done by others with the consent of the injured party, was practiced by the Amazons. Indeed, the term "Amazon" means "without breast," and presumably the procedure was carried out by the warrior women to feel more free during combat. The subject has been thoroughly discussed by Schechter.[1]

In self-mutilation, the skin is the most frequent target and the fingernail is the primary tool of injury. Halprin classified three categories of tegumental self-inflicted wounds: *neurotic excoriations*, *delusions of parasitosis*, and *factitial dermatitis*.[2]

Patients within the first two categories readily admit causing the lesions. The latter are irregularly shaped and are usually found on the chest, the lateral aspects of the thighs, and the arms and face. Healing is associated with scarring with or without pigmentation. Left-sided lesions are more prominent in right-handed individuals, and right-sided lesions in left-handed individuals. Fresh lesions and scars alternate irregularly, and as a rule, the general health of the person is not impaired (Fig. 9–1).

Patients with delusions of *parasitosis* are convinced their skin harbors parasites and they attack them with caustics, sharp instruments, and fingernails. The distribution of the lesions is similar to that seen in neurotic excoriations. Paranoid tendencies are usually pronounced, and these delusions are used to maintain some contact with reality.

Factitial dermatitis is associated with denial of any knowledge of the cause of the lesions. The patient describes a burrowing or crawling sensation in the skin followed in one or two days by lesions of bizarre configuration. The lesions are not symmetrical, appear singly or in crops, and heal readily with scar formation. Biopsy indicates an injury that lacks characterization. The injury is produced most frequently by lighted cigarettes or caustic agents; cutting instruments and injection of toxic or irritant materials are less frequently used.[3] Rubbing of skin cuts with ink may produce a tattoo effect.

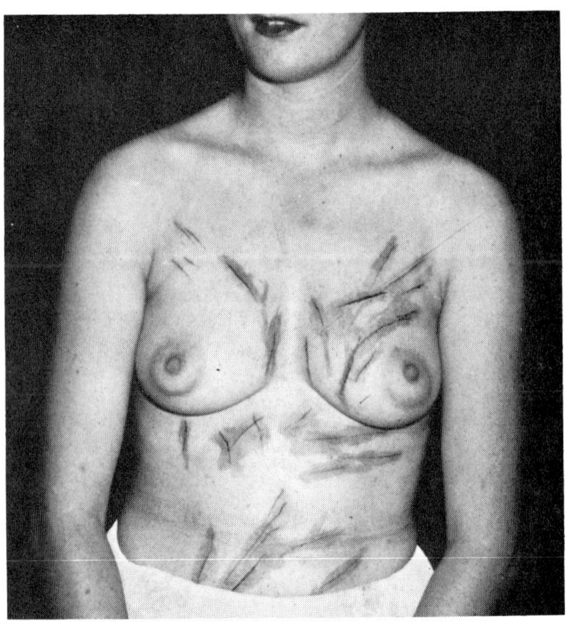

Figure 9–1. Self-inflicted injuries made in an effort to gain attention.

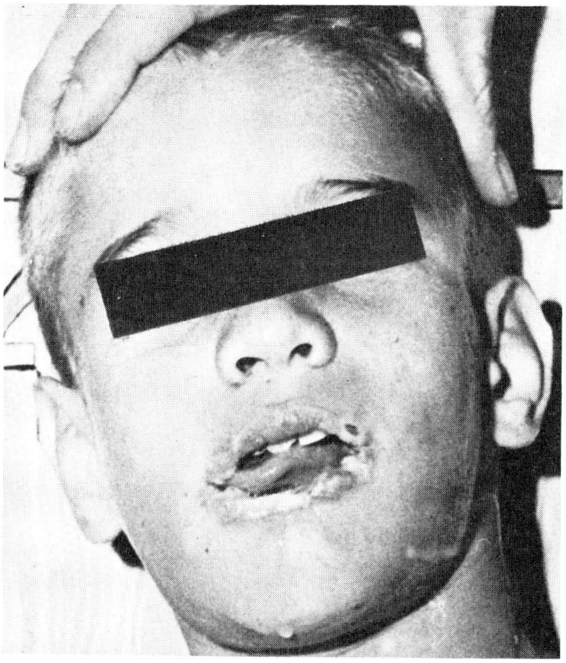

Figure 9–2. Biting of the lips in a mentally retarded male child (Lesch-Nyhan syndrome).

Onychophagia (nail-biting), leading to maceration of the skin and infection, may be considered another form of self-mutilation. The habit may extend to biting of fingers, hands, and forearms, and if the joints are lax, of ankles, feet, and genitalia. Scaling, pigmentation, and hypertrichosis may develop at the site of the bites. Lip biting, in extreme cases, may lead to leukoplakia, and cheek biting may cause stimulation of fibroblastic tissue simulating tumor, as seen in epilepsy in conjunction with phenytoin (Dilantin) treatment.

Self-destructive biting is part of the Lesch-Nyhan syndrome, a familial disorder of uric acid metabolism associated with mental retardation, which occurs in different racial groups (Fig. 9–2).[4]

Head banging or bumping occurs in 10 to 20 per cent of full term babies; sometimes the habit persists in childhood in overactive or mentally disturbed children, causing subcutaneous hematomas as well as injuries to the distal phalanges and subungual hemorrhages.

Grinding of the teeth *(bruxism)* is frequently seen in the mentally retarded and it can lead to abnormal tooth wear, bilateral hypertrophy of the masseter muscles, and pain on chewing. In the same group of individuals, lip licking may be noticed; this results in the enlargement of the tongue, excessive salivation, and maceration of the lips.

Picking of acne eruptions is also common and may finally lead to severe disfigurement.

Pressure on the subcutaneous tissue by a tightly tied cord, belt, or similar item wrapped around a part of the body, often the waist, may lead to atrophy. Tribal customs of some natives of Africa may include the wrapping of metal bands about the neck or legs to the extent that permanent disfigurement occurs.

Pulling of body hair *(trichotillomania)* may be considered another form of self-mutilation. The same is true for the pulling of the labia or nipples, tips of the fingers or toenails, ears or nose, all of which result in lesions of the affected parts as seen in repeated mechanical trauma. The cauliflower ear, as it occurs in boxers, can be self-inflicted as well.

Thermophilia is another aspect of self-destruction. In this case the abnormal behavior leads to exposure of parts of the body to heat radiating from open fires, radiators, or protective grills over radiators.

"Benign" self-mutilation or "goldbricking," as defined by Waisman, is the exacerbation of a skin disorder by self-induced excoriation prior to an appearance before a Veterans Administration pension reexamination board or a hearing before a Workmen's Compensation Court. This is done deliberately to magnify the extent of an existing dermatitis.

Self-inflicted injury may occur in people who are not psychotic but who wish to escape a condition of stress. Thus during wartime, shooting or cutting off a finger or a toe may get a soldier removed from the front line, or counterfeited lesions may get a prisoner under sentence of hard labor admitted to the hospital where he will receive more food and rest.

Self-inflicted injuries may equally be employed to create a new identity by tattooing or scarring, or to destroy a recorded identity by obliterating fingerprints with acids or by cutting or burning. The attempt can go as far as to require the expertise of a plastic surgeon to change the facial conformation.

Self-mutilation, as psychotic behavior, may go much beyond superficial tegumental injuries. Self-inflicted enucleation of the eye, tongue severance, severance of fingers and toes and of the Achilles tendon, and even autocannibalism, have all been recorded. Cases have also been described in which self-inflicted dislocation was claimed to be the result of being bumped by a car and the "victim" threatened to call the police in order to receive a quick payoff. Even bony fractures have been simulated by introducing threads into the subcutaneous tissue, possibly with the assistance of medical or paramedical personnel.

The list of misdemeanors is endless indeed. The skull has been penetrated with nails or spikes, the chest wall and the lungs with splinters of wood, and the urinary bladder with lead pencils or hairpins through the female urethra.

Self-mutilation of the genitalia in the non-pregnant woman is rather uncommon. The opposite is true, however, if one considers self-induced abortion in the category of self-mutilation.[6] Sepsis, shock, peritonitis, vaginal ulceration, and placental as well as uterine necrosis are well-known sequelae of chemical (e.g., potassium permanganate, soap, turpentine) or instrumental abortifacients. Even stabbing or gunshot wounds of the pregnant uterus have been used in an attempt to kill the embryo. A case is on record in which an auto–cesarean section was performed. Vedrine reports the severance of a prolapsed uterus with a kitchen knife by a 70-year-old woman, and Krzyzowski reports an attempt to interrupt pregnancy by the intraabdominal injection of ether.[7, 8]

Male self-mutilation includes castration as a self-destructive mechanism.[9] The act is often precipitated by depression and may be followed by death caused by hemorrhage and shock. The author was directly involved in a case in which a hippie was found floating in a sandpit. The left testis had been amputated. Slashes, resembling hesitation cuts, were present in the skin of the left inguinal region. Investigation of this case revealed that the deceased was a drug user who, assumedly, had died as a result of hemorrhage and shock before completely submerging in the water.

Lesions do not have to be self-inflicted or counterfeited by traumatic methods. The case has been reported of a factitial Weber-Christian syndrome (a disease of adipose tissue) self-induced by the injection of milk in the subcutaneous tissue.[10] Injection of air mimicking subcutaneous emphysema has been reported also, as has self-injection of fecal material with resultant abscess formation.[11]

A puzzling entity is the factitious anemia described by Daily. It can be caused by instrumentally induced bleeding from the vagina or the anus or both. In an even more complex case, a laboratory technologist attempted to produce hemolytic anemia by lysing red cells that she had drawn from her own vein. She used sterile water to do this, and then she reinjected the lysed blood into her own vein.[12] Factitious proteinuria is on record following the introduction of egg white by catheter into the urinary bladder. The list of methods devised to simulate disease is indeed endless; among these one should mention chronic ingestion of arsenic-containing preparations to cause anemia and ingestion of coumarin to induce a hemorrhagic diathesis.

Mention of the condition that Asher and associates have called the "Münchausen syndrome" is pertinent at this point. This syndrome is exemplified by the case of the patient who presents himself at the doctor's office or the hospital emergency room with an entirely fabricated medical history often supported by clinical manifestations of a congenital or long-standing, and not uncommonly self-induced, condition. Fruitless clinical investigation often leads to surgical explorations, which also fail to establish a diagnosis. The patient leaves the hospital without authorization, to be admitted to another hospital where the same performance is repeated—over and over.[13]

These patients are psychopaths who are expert at deceiving even the most astute observer. According to the main presenting features, Asher has proposed the following classifications:

1. Patients with acute abdominal symptoms (laparotomaphilia migrans).
2. Patients with bleeding from a bodily orifice (haemorrhagia histrionica).
3. Patients with acute neurologic manifestations, such as coma, blackouts, and headaches (neurologia diabolica).[13]

To simulate a condition affecting the upper alimentary tract, the patient may injure his nasopharynx with a sharp instrument, swallow the blood, and regurgitate it in front of the examining physician to mimic hematemesis. A skillful puncturing of the anal or vaginal mucosa may produce a realistic bleeding episode, sufficient to convince the examining physician of the authenticity of the problem. A search of the patient's belongings may reveal clothing from other hospitals, broken thermometers, pins or other sharp instruments, and possibly medical literature from which ideas are obtained.

The excessive intake of digitalis preparations to simulate a heart condition can be listed among the methods employed to self-induce factitial syndromes, primarily with the objective of fraudulently receiving disability payments.

Carotinemia, simulating jaundice, was an easy way out of the trenches in World War I—just by eating carrots in great amounts.[14]

REFERENCES

1. Schechter, I.: Breast mutilation in Amazons. Surgery, *51*:554, 1962.

2. Halprin, K.. The art of self mutilation. J.A.M.A., *198*:777, *198*:1207, 1966; *199*:119, 1967.
3. Butterworth, T., and Strean, L. P.: Behaviour disorders of interest to the dermatologists. Arch. Dermatol., *88*:859, 1963.
4. Lesch, R., and Nyhan, W. L.: A familial disorder of uric acid metabolism and central nervous system function. Am. J. Med., *36*:561, 1964.
5. Waisman, M.: Pickers, pluckers and imposters. Postgrad. Med., *38*:620, 1965.
6. Reish, L. H., and Weber, T.: Female genital self-mutilation. Obstet. Gynecol., *41*:239, 1973.
7. Vedrine, J.: Voluntary genital mutilation in women. Med. Leg. Domm. Corpor., *2*:165, 1969.
8. Krzyzowski, J.: Attempt at interrupting pregnancy by means of self mutilation. Psychiatr. Pol., *1*:607, 1967.
9. Chanulal, R.: An unusual method of suicide. Forensic Sci., *2*:379, 1973.
10. Ackerman, A. B.: Factitial Weber-Christian syndrome. J.A.M.A., *198*:7, 1966.
11. Gershwin, M.: Factitious subcutaneous emphysema. Ann. Intern. Med., *75*:585, 1971.
12. Daily, W. J., Coles, J. M., and Creger, W. P.: Factitious anemia. Ann. Intern. Med., *58*:533, 1963.
13. Asher, R.: Münchausen's syndrome. Lancet, *1*.339, 1951.
14. Tedeschi, C. G.: Sulla carotinemia. Arch. Stud. Fisiopatol. Ricambio, *2*:1, 1934.

SECTION 1. MECHANICAL INJURY

chapter 10

THE BATTERED CHILD

by Bernard Knight

The "battered child" refers to the infant—usually under three years of age—who suffers repeated nonaccidental injuries, sometimes fatal, caused through episodes of violence by a parent or guardian.

The syndrome was virtually unrecognized until the early 1960's, since when it has received almost explosive publicity in both the medical and the lay press. This has led to long-overdue recognition of a problem of vital concern to pediatricians, sociologists, medicolegists and law enforcement authorities.

HISTORICAL BACKGROUND

In 1946, an American radiologist, J. Caffey, described a puzzling association of brain membrane hemorrhages and multiple limb fractures occurring in infants. In six babies, no less than 23 fractures had appeared, most of them at intervals after the subdural hematoma. At that time, Caffey could offer no explanation for the lesions.[1]

A second paper by Caffey, in 1957, described similar lesions, and he suggested that parental violence might be a more likely cause than some obscure disease process.[2] Even before this date, Wooley and Evans (1955) and Silverman (1953) had published cases and offered the opinion that parental violence was involved.[3, 4] New reports followed rapidly: Griffiths and Moynihan (1963), Fairburn and Hunt (1964), Parker (1965), Cameron, Johnson and Camps (1966), and Kempe and associates (1962) were among the many in the vanguard, and these and many more recent papers have placed the "battered child" or "battered baby" syndrome in the position of a newly-recognized clinical and pathologic entity.[5-9] The National Society for Prevention of Cruelty to Children (NSPCC) in Britain established a special Battered Child Research Unit, and several useful publications have emanated from it, especially that of Skinner and Castle in 1969.[10]

Thus after an unknown period—possibly many decades or even centuries—in which nonaccidental parental injuries to small children had gone undetected and unsuspected by members of the medical profession, the term "battered child" was recognized within a few short years by every doctor and by a large section of the general public.

THE BATTERED CHILD SYNDROME

Age of the Child

Almost all battered infants are below the age of three years, though occasionally older children may be so victimized. In Cameron's survey in London, 55 per cent of the victims were under one year old and 79 per cent were less than two years old, the mean age being 14 months. Similarly, Scott's series of fatal London cases showed an average age of 15 months. In the NSPCC survey of Skinner and Castle, 56 per cent of the infants were less than a year old. It should be noted that many published surveys include only fatal cases, and these are not necessarily entirely representative of the syndrome as a whole, the fatally injured victims frequently being younger than the victims in the "clinical" instances.

Sex Variation

Though, as in the sudden infant death syndrome, there appears to be a slight weighting against male infants, this does not seem significant and appears to bear no relationship to causation or type or severity of injuries. As with so many disease processes and traumatic conditions throughout the whole span of life, the male appears slightly more vulnerable.

Position in Family

Reports vary somewhat, it being suggested by some surveys that one child of a family, almost invariably the youngest, may be the "scapegoat," receiving most of the battering while his siblings escape. Skinner and Castle do not confirm this, however, though their series strongly indicates that children born subsequent to the first battered child are very much at risk. In general terms, it does seem that there can be a marked disparity between the treatment meted out to different children in the same family, and the tendency for the youngest child to be battered has even led to the term "Cinderella syndrome" sometimes being used.

Racial Incidence

Results from various surveys differ according to the locale in which they were carried out, but in Britain ethnic factors have been studied in two London series. Scott's series of fatal cases indicated that 90 per cent were white and 10 per cent were colored, though he does not relate this to the racial proportions in London at the time. He does note that a large proportion of Irish adults were involved.[11] In the series of Cameron and co-workers, 21 per cent were colored children, which he says is a disproportionately high figure in comparison with their numbers in the population as a whole.[8]

Nature of Injuries

One of the noticeable features of battering is that it tends to be "noninstrumental," i.e., the assaults are usually carried out by the unaided hands of the adult without the intervention of instruments that is commonly seen in adult homicide. There are, of course many exceptions to this, and feeding bottles, pokers, shovels, and similar implements have been described as causing injury—but the general rule remains that direct manual violence is the most common method of injury.

Though the spectrum of injuries is very wide, certain recurrent features are of great diagnostic value.

Bruises, Abrasions, and Lacerations

Soft-tissue injuries are almost universal, several series reporting an incidence between 80 and 100 per cent (Figs. 10–1 and 10–2). The head, face, and neck are most commonly affected, with bruises, abrasions, and lacerations as frequent features. Bruising of the scalp and forehead is naturally associated with the common underlying skull and brain injuries, and bruising of the external ear, cheeks, and especially lips is extremely common. Bruising in the scalp may not be overtly apparent, but in a search above the hairline and, in postmortem

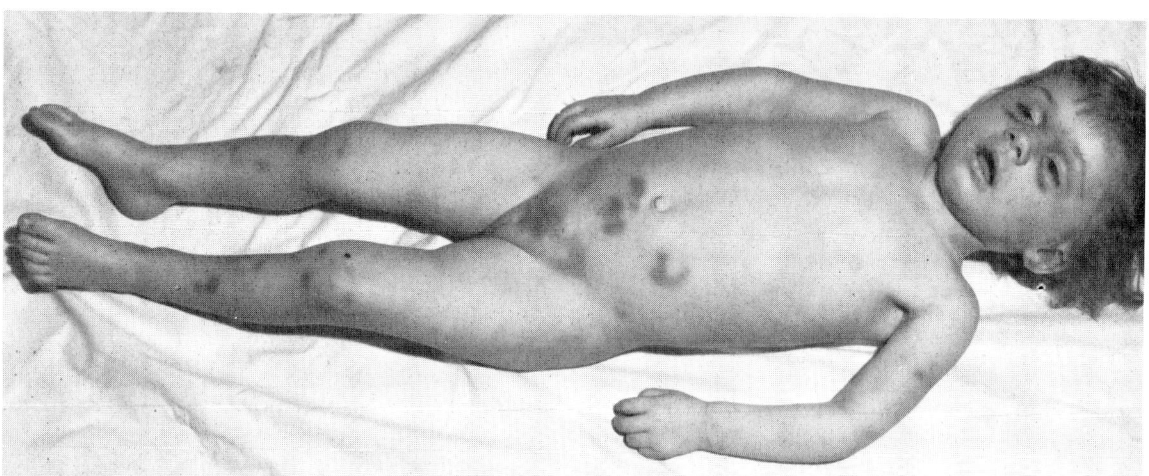

Figure 10–1. Widespread bruising in typical sites—on the abdomen, legs, around the eyes and mouth—inflicted by male consort of mother. Alleged to have "slipped while bathing."

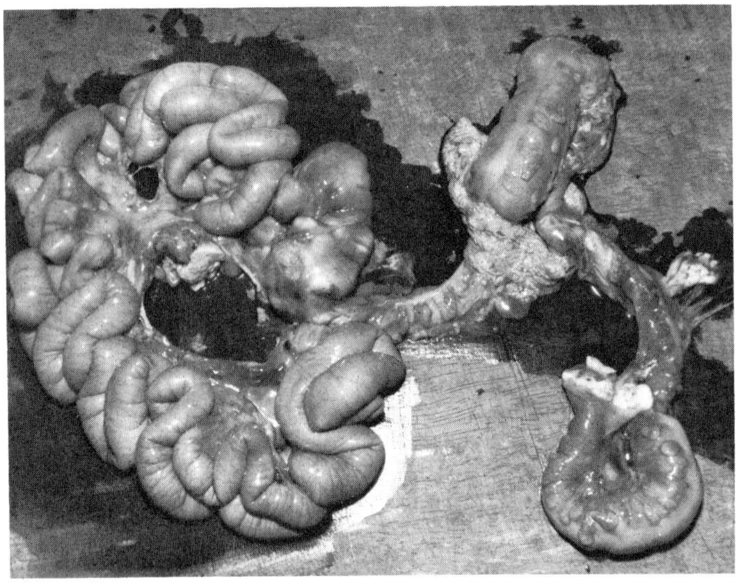

Figure 10–2. Intestines of child shown in Figure 10–1, showing multiple lacerations of mesentery leading to fatal peritoneal bleeding. The child lay dead overnight before medical help was sought.

examinations, on reflection of the scalp, extensive bruising may be obvious in this area.

A particular lesion of diagnostic significance is bruising of the lips, especially the upper lip, commonly with lacerations of the inner aspect (Fig. 10–3). The frenulum (the band of tissue connecting the center of the upper lip to the gum) is often ruptured, and detachment of the inner surface of the lip from the gum margin is a noticeable feature, suggesting slapping or punching of the mouth region. Bruising of the cheeks and ears is also due to slapping with the adult hand.

Bruising of the neck and sides of the chest may sometimes reveal finger-tip pressure marks. The neck may be held on each side in turn to immobilize the face while it is assaulted with the other hand, and this may leave symmetrical bruises beneath the angle of the jaw. A common method of assault, especially of smaller babies, is to grip the child forcefully on each side of the thorax while shaking him violently. This tends to leave bruises on the skin of the armpits and lower ribs, often in association with multiple fractures of the posterior parts of the ribs from

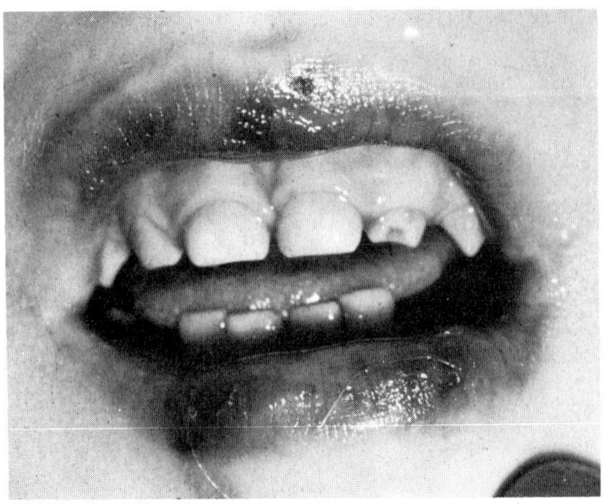

Figure 10–3. Extensive bruising of lips and a small laceration of the upper lip due to slapping by a parent.

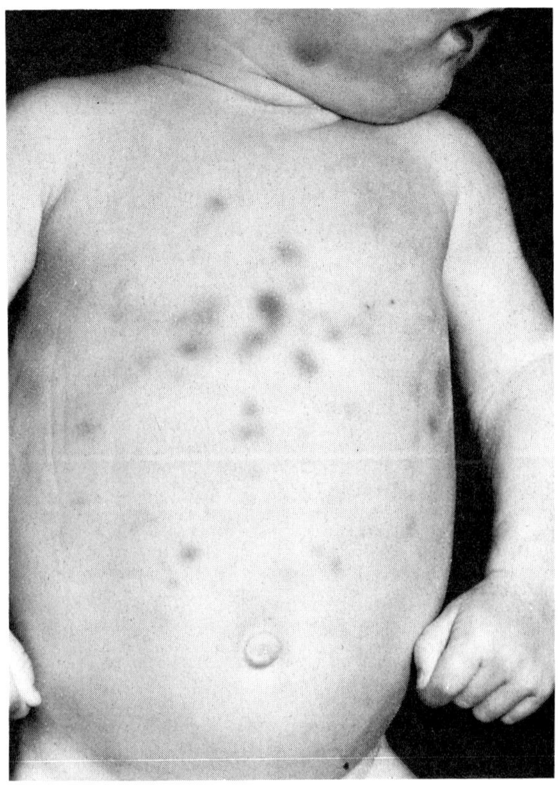

Figure 10–4. Multiple bruising of chest and abdomen, with further lesions on face, was due to forcible prodding by finger tips of male consort of mother in an attempt to stop child's crying.

compression of the chest between the squeezing adult hands.

Bruising of the abdomen is very common (Fig. 10–4). After head injuries, ruptures of abdominal organs are the commonest fatal lesions, and the external signs may be finger-tip or larger bruises (often called "sixpenny-piece" bruises) extending from the breast bone to the pubis (Fig. 10–5). Though these are common, it must be noted that gross internal injuries may still be present even though there are few external signs such as those just described.

The limbs may also show multiple bruising, especially the forearms, upper arms, and legs, often in a bilateral fashion. These areas form convenient "handles" for the irate parent to grasp the child.

Bites are a well-known phenomenon in the battered child syndrome and seem to be almost solely the prerogative of the mother (Fig. 10–6). They must be carefully differentiated from bites caused by other children, and the expert advice of and examination by a dentist experienced in forensic matters is to be recommended, to confirm or confound the parental explanation that they were caused by a sibling.

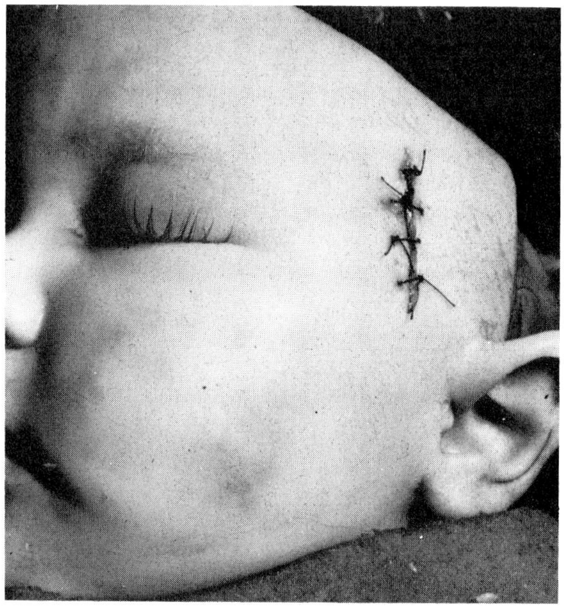

Figure 10–6. Two semicircular marks on the cheek of a child dying from a fractured skull. These were bite marks consistent with the size of the mother's dental arches.

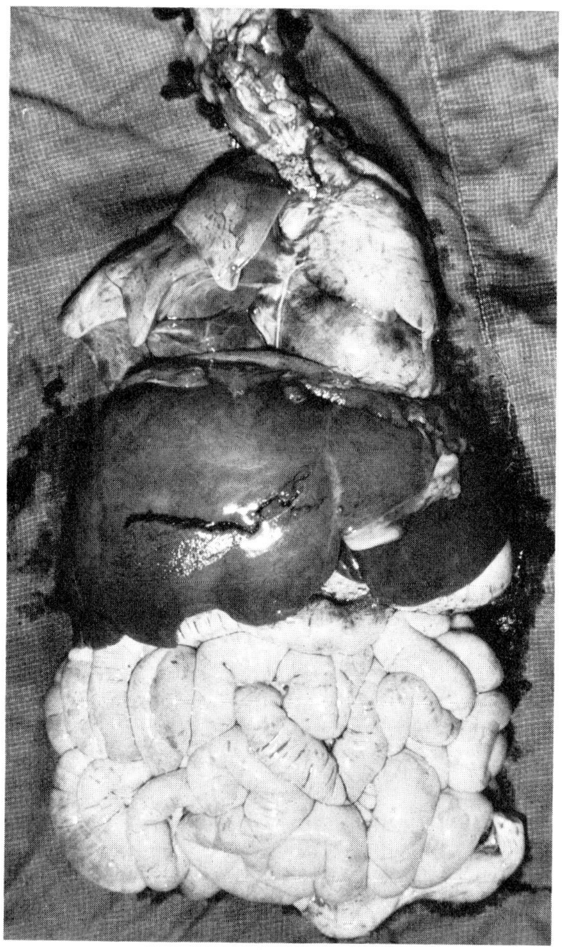

Figure 10–5. Abdominal contents of child shown in Figure 10–4. A laceration of the liver completely traverses the organ.

Eye Injuries

Injuries to the eye have only recently been described in detail in the battered child syndrome. Retinal separation, lens displacement, retinal hemorrhages, subconjunctival hemorrhages, and subhyaloid hemorrhages have all been described. Because of this, the assistance of the ophthalmologist should be sought as well as that of the radiologist and the dentist.[12, 13]

Head Injuries

Head injuries are common, and fractured skull and brain damage form the most frequent cause of death.

External scalp injuries have already been mentioned. Subdural hematoma, the lesion that first came to the attention of radiologists in this syndrome, is common. Deeper brain damage accounts for the high rate of incidence of permanent cerebral dysfunction that is such a distressing feature of many cases. Of Cameron's series of fatal cases, no less than 69 per cent had a fractured skull; in Scott's more recent London series of deaths, 69 per cent had a subdural hematoma with or without a fractured skull, and in Skinner and Castle's series of nonfatal cases, 28 per cent had this lesion.[8, 10, 11]

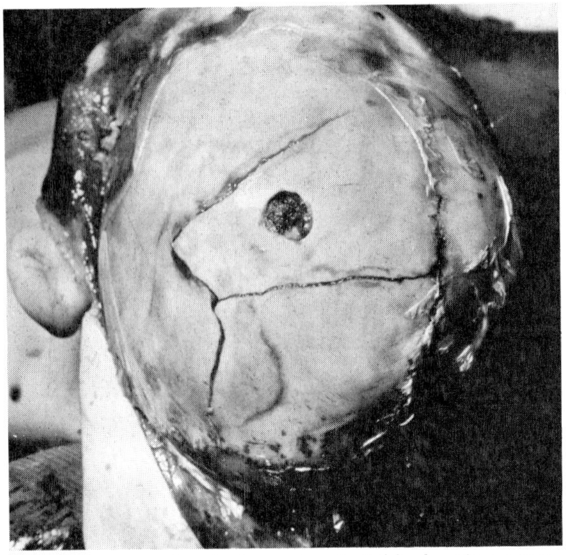

Figure 10–7. Skull of a battered child, showing extensive fissured fractures. There was a large subdural hemorrhage, which aspiration through the burr hole failed to relieve. There were other skeletal injuries of varying ages, all allegedly due to a simple fall from the father's arms.

The usual type of skull fracture is a fissured, sometimes fragmented, break in the parietal area caused by the impact of the head against a solid object rather than by a direct blow against a fixed head (Fig. 10–7). Apart from frank subdural hematomas and cerebral contusions, scattered patches of bleeding in the membranes of the brain are frequently seen.

Visceral Injuries

Visceral injuries are the next most common cause of death. Ruptures of liver, intestine, or mesentery account for most of the fatalities and are due to blows on the front of the abdominal wall. The most gross internal injuries may be present with minimal external signs, though many cases exhibit the multiple bruising described earlier. A through-and-through penetration of the liver and complete severing of the third part of the duodenum across the front of the spinal column has been seen in infants with few external signs of injury. Lacerations of the liver—often on the under surface—may be associated with gross intraperitoneal bleeding, which may also occur from tears in the mesentery of the small bowel where it is stretched across the prominence of the lumbar spine. Such injuries may be falsely attributed by parents to a simple fall or to an innocent accident, such as a "swing banging against his little tummy."

Skeletal Lesions and Radiologic Appearances

In both fatal and nonfatal cases, radiography is *all-important* in the battered child syndrome. In every suspect fatal case, whole-body x-ray *must* be performed before formal autopsy. In live infants, any substantial degree of suspicion should call for similar treatment, the minimal risk of radiation exposure being far outweighed by the danger of missing a true battered child. Radiography may provide two useful kinds of information: first, about general skeletal damage, especially of differing times of infliction; and second, about characteristic bony lesions.

Lesions of different ages are demonstrable by the stage of the healing process in older fractures as compared with fractures of recent origin. Callus formation is important in this respect in identifying and approximately dating old healing fractures.

Characteristic radiographic lesions include separation of epiphyses, especially around the elbow and the knee joints, although any limb joint may be involved; and shearing and elevation of the periostium, which is not firmly attached in infants. This leads to subperiostial calcification in periostial hemorrhages, a characteristic radiographic feature of the battered child. Fractures of the ribs, which were mentioned earlier, are commonly multiple and seen as a line running down near the posterior angles of the ribs, revealing themselves radiographically as a "beading" effect when callus formation has had time to occur. These are due to fracturing from lateral compression of the chest. Fractures of the clavicle are also common and may be seen in the same anteroposterior film.

Chipping of the corners of epiphyses at the large joints of the limbs is again a characteristic feature and was described in one of the early papers on the battered baby; Astley, describing cases in Birmingham, mentioned "metaphyseal fracture-like defects"—translucent zones on radiographs, which divided off peripheral parts of the metaphyses at the ends of long bones—"cutting a corner off the ends." Many of these lesions are due to the shaking and rotating strains imposed upon the limbs by the forceful application of adult hands. Metaphyseal fragmentation is another common finding. Fractures of the shafts of the long bones may result from direct blows either from a fist or from the child hitting a fixed object. Fractures of spine and pelvis are uncommon in the battered child syndrome. The fractured skull lesions have already been described.

Burns

A relatively common and most distressing lesion in the battered child syndrome is the burn inflicted on the infant victim by various

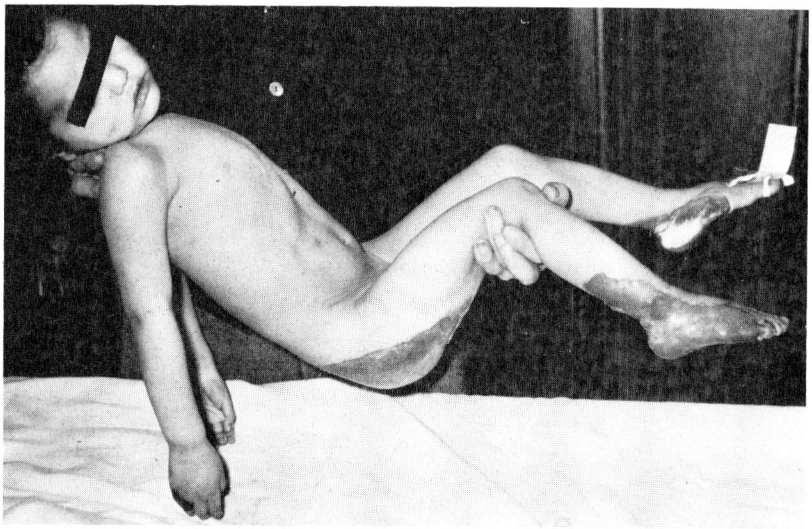

Figure 10–8. Scalds on a child's buttocks and feet, showing a horizontal level and indicating the method of immersion. The child was locked out of the house and persistently complained of being cold. She was dipped into very hot water by a female adult relative to "teach her a lesson." (Photograph kindly provided by Dr. W. R. L. James.)

means. Punctate burns, often accompanied by older scars, may indicate deliberate stubbing of cigarette ends upon the child's skin. Instances of the child being seated upon a hot stove or electric radiator as a punishment for continual soiling of napkins or the like have been reported frequently. Dipping in very hot fluids is another sadistic punishment; the accompanying photograph shows the distinct "fluid level" passing across the buttocks onto the heels, indicating the method by which the child was dipped into very hot water (Fig. 10–8). Often the localized and well-demarcated nature of the burns may suggest the unusual circumstances and possibly the deliberate etiology.

Delay in Seeking Medical Advice

Another highly significant feature is the frequently long interval between injury and seeking of medical advice. Though in genuine accidents it is the natural impulse to seek the aid of a doctor as soon as possible, the parents of the battered child often wait an inexplicably long time before bringing the child to the attention of a medical attendant. In Cameron's large London series, there was a mean period of over 20 hours before medical aid was provided for the child.[8] Even in fatal cases, an unusual delay may occur before a doctor is called. Guilt and the hope that the child may eventually recover seem to outweigh the normal parental impulse to summon medical assistance. In Scott's series, the most constant feature of the action taken by the guilty father was "unnecessary delay in seeking help."[11]

Discrepancy Between History and Findings

Apart from delay in seeking medical advice, another characteristic feature is the frequent inconsistency of the parent's explanation with the extent and chronology of the injury. Though genuine accidents to children are quite common, the histories offered by the battering parents do not account for the multiplicity of bruises or the spacing of multiple fractures in different stages of healing. The parents—especially the father—are characteristically "glib" and in the past have easily convinced unsuspecting doctors of the genuine nature of the "accident."

An explanation is put forward that is quite consistent with *one* of the injuries, but when widespread lesions are found or the features of the injuries indicate that they have been inflicted over a period of time, the offered excuses become unacceptable.

Frequent parental explanations—which may change several times on repetition—include "fell out of my arms while feeding," "fell from the perambulator," "punched by his older brother," "knocked himself against the furniture," "hit in the stomach with a swing," and so on—with almost infinite variations. However, the presence of a dozen abdominal bruises, bilateral parietal bruising, old fractures of the ribs, and a recent fracture of the skull would be obviously inconsistent with any such simple explanation. This inconsistency is one of the most important diagnostic features when genuine accidents are being sifted from potential batterings.

Another significant pointer is the tendency of guilty parents to take the child to a different doctor or to a different accident center at each episode of injury. This obvious precaution tends to defeat the arousal of medical suspicion, as communication between doctors and hospital casualty departments may be dependent upon the parent's own cooperation, which is naturally suppressed in the presence of guilt.

Thus the repetitive nature of injuries may be concealed for some time and may only be recognized in retrospect when definite battering is diagnosed.

This is a syndrome in which the physician is entirely dependent upon a vicarious history from the parents, as the child is usually unable to divulge the true course of events. This is one reason why whole-body x-ray is so important because, as Cameron so graphically stated, "the skin and bones tell a story which the child is too young or too frightened to tell."[8]

The Family and the Parents

This aspect of the syndrome has attracted most discussion, speculation, and research. A detailed discussion is out of place in a textbook of traumatology, but the main points may be touched upon. Sociology, psychiatry, and penology converge to try to explain what exactly are "battering parents," what made them so, and what may be done about it. Opinions vary, especially on the two sides of the Atlantic, but certain factors pertaining to the family appear to be fairly consistent:

1. All social classes may batter their children, but there is a definite loading toward the lower end of the social spectrum. In Scott's series, the largest group among the battering fathers were semiskilled workers, and this appears to be a valid impression for many of the remainder of cases. No social class is exempt, however.

2. The age of the parents tends to be in the early twenties, sometimes with the mother considerably younger. In the three series of Cameron, Johnson, and Camps, of Skinner and Castle, and of Scott, the average age of the father was 28, 24, and 25 years respectively, and that of the mother 24, 22, and 23 years respectively.[8, 10, 11]

3. A frequent finding is that the family is isolated, i.e., cut off from normal family relationships with grandparents and often removed geographically from its origins. The itinerant factory worker is a typical example, though general shiftlessness and unemployment seem uncommonly prevalent among the fathers.

4. Discord between the parents is almost a constant finding, and the marriage may be unstable. Very often the "father" is not the child's biologic father but a later consort of the mother.

5. Very often, the child is unwanted, either being a later undesired addition to the existing family or the result of a failed abortion, a failure of contraception, or sometimes of real or suspected adultery. This may account for the cases in which the battered child is the scapegoat of the family, the other children – usually older – escaping injury.

6. The physical provision for the family is usually good, and the battered child obviously belongs in quite a separate category from the dirty, wasted, neglected child. The overt standard of mothering may be good, and the nutrition and physical well-being of the children excellent.

7. The intelligence of the parents may be quite normal, especially that of the father, who frequently is a quick-thinking, smooth-talking person who thus can more easily project a reasonable story to the doctor to account for the injuries. Immaturity and aggressiveness were reported by Scott in most of the fathers of fatal cases in London, but there seems little evidence in Britain of marked moral or psychologic insufficiency in the majority of parents, which is somewhat at variance with some reported series in the United States. The defect appears to lie in character rather than in IQ. Often a general impression of a dominant, aggressive father or consort and a less intelligent, dominated, and overstressed mother appears to characterize the typical picture of the battering family. Many of the fathers have been reported to have had criminal records as well as being frequently unemployed; in Scott's series 65 per cent had previous convictions for criminal offenses.

8. Lack of stability of the family in the geographical sense is common, and in Britain a disproportionate number of cases appear to occur among caravan dwellers. This appears to be related to their general social isolation and unwillingness or inability to form social links, which might help to ease intrafamily tensions.

9. It appears that a considerable number of battering parents were themselves battered children. This was confirmed by Scott's series in which 19 of 29 indicted fathers came from "punitive backgrounds," 12 of these remembering parental violence.[11]

10. There is a striking absence of suicide attempts among parents after infliction of fatal batterings on children; this contrasts markedly with other types of filicide, in which attempts at self-destruction from remorse are frequently seen. This trait appears to underline the dissociation that parents can produce after battering, and helps to explain the frequent delay in seeking help, the frequent absence of any action whatsoever following severe battering, and

in some cases, the apparent unconcern over the whole episode.

11. An almost constant feature is the precipitation of violence by actions of the child itself. Crying, refusal to be quiet, persistent soiling of napkins, or the like invariably acts as the precipitating stimulus to an episode of violence. It has been pointed out more than once that these stimuli are those that affect most parents to the point of exasperation but that, in the battering parents, arouse a reaction that is abnormally violent and repetitive. Again, a defect of behavior rather than an outright psychotic state is detectable in the offending parent.

MORTALITY, MORBIDITY, AND RECURRENCE RATES

The cases of the battered child that come to light are those in which attempts at concealment failed. It is thus obvious that concealment is successful in a number of other cases, and this number is a matter for conjecture. As Simpson says, "we might only be seeing the tip of the iceberg."[15] No accurate estimate of the incidence can be made, but it is clear that on both sides of the Atlantic, the amount of morbidity and the number of deaths are appreciable.

Kempe and co-workers, in a 12-month survey, collected 302 cases from 71 hospitals: 33 of these children died and 85 had permanent brain damage. Over the same period, he received reports of 447 cases from 77 district attorneys; 45 per cent of these children died.

Both American and British surveys indicate that of children recognized as being battered on one occasion, 60 per cent will return with further parentally inflicted injuries and 10 per cent will eventually receive fatal injuries.

Skinner and Castle further offer the rather pessimistic statement that the rebattering rate among battering families known to a protective agency does not compare favorably with their estimate that, in the absence of any such intervention, 25 to 50 per cent are rebattered. They go on to say that the findings suggest that multiplicity of workers and overfrequent observation of battering families can increase family stress, and a type of supervision of a family that is limited to an anxious watchfulness without specific treatment goals is not in the child's interest.

In some families there was a favorable response to social case work, but the study highlights the need for greater skill by all workers who, for the purpose of child protection, intervene in crisis situations.

When, in a family with more than one child, the first-born was battered, records show that there was a 13 to 1 chance that the subsequent child would be injured. This observation, again by Skinner and Castle from the NSPCC records in Britain, revealed the risk that exists to children born into families in which the first-born has been battered, and, as mentioned, it questioned the reliability of previous suggestions that a particular child in a family is often singled out for battering. The latter appears to occur when the battering attitude of the parents develops later in the course of family evolution, the older child escaping if the family stresses are delayed until the birth of a later child.

DIAGNOSIS OF CHILD BATTERING

Much of the delay in recognition of this syndrome has been due to the attitude of the medical profession. By selection and training, doctors tended to be sympathetic and relatively unsuspicious; this has led to either genuine unawareness of the parental responsibility for the injuries or even a subconscious rejection of such suspicions.

Much of the early evolution of the recognition of the syndrome was clouded by enthusiastic seeking after genuine pathologic conditions affecting bones, skin, and blood vessels that might account for the lesions in a nontraumatic way. Thus the early literature is filled with discussion of such entities as osteogenesis imperfecta, hemorrhagic diatheses, and subclinical scurvy, which, although they must not be ignored in differential diagnosis, have not yet been fully relegated to their proper and somewhat insignificant place in the list of probabilities.

It is as important not to brand the innocent parent as a "batterer," however, as it is to miss a true battered child. Accidents to small children are frequent and careful evaluation is necessary to distinguish the one from the other.

Certain pointers may be of use, but the doctor's "suspicion threshold" must remain low. When any doubt exists, either watchful supervision or discreet reporting to a protective agency is advisable and can do no harm.

The suggestive pointers to true battering are:

1. Variations and inconsistencies in the parental explanation, even though the variations themselves may sound convincing when taken individually. A changing story, even over a few hours or days and especially when different versions are given to different investigators, is suspicious.

2. Delay in seeking medical advice or treatment.

3. Inconsistency of the injuries contrasted with the explanation. The inconsistency may be in the number of lesions or in the time factor involved, i.e., a simple fall cannot give rise to multiple bruises in different areas of the body, and similarly, injuries in different stages of healing, such as bruises and fractures, cannot have been caused by a single traumatic event.

4. Classic lesions such as torn upper lip frenulum; multiple bruises on the face, thorax, or abdomen and around the larger limb joints; bite marks and unusual burns; fractures in different stages of healing; multiple bruises with different color spectrum of age.

5. Evidence of repeated visits to different doctors or different medical centers, especially when these facts may not have been volunteered or are even actively concealed from the attending physician.

6. A general, almost intuitive feeling about the family—the rather glib father, perhaps a dominated wife, and a social pattern consistent with the foregoing descriptions in this chapter.

All these factors must be taken in combination, not isolation. When there is doubt, the opinions of a colleague, especially an experienced pediatrician, and also of members of child protection agencies are of great help.

Even if the current episode cannot be definitely attributed to battering, but suspicion remains, it is vital that treatment not be limited to that of the acute injury and that the child not be returned to a possibly hostile environment without any follow-up. The organizations such as the NSPCC in Britain can be depended upon to exercise a tactful supervision of any suspect families, which is vital if the tragic sequelae of further injury, frequent brain damage, and a 10 per cent mortality rate are to be avoided.

REFERENCES

1. Caffey, J.: Multiple fractures of long bones in infants suffering from subdural hematoma. Am. J. Roentgenol., *56*:163, 1946.
2. Caffey, J.: Some traumatic lesions in growing bones other than fractures and dislocations: clinical and radiological fractures. Br. J. Radiol., *30*:225, 1957.
3. Wooley, P. V., and Evans, W. A.: Significance of skeletal lesions in infants resembling those of traumatic origin. J.A.M.A., *158*:539, 1955.
4. Silverman, F. N.: Roentgen manifestations of unrecognized skeletal trauma in young infants. Am. J. Roentgenol., *69*:413, 1953.
5. Griffiths, D. L., and Moynihan, F. J.: Multiple epiphyseal injuries in babies. Br. Med. J., *2*:1558, 1963.
6. Fairburn, A. C., and Hunt, A. C.: Caffey's third syndrome—a critical evaluation. Med. Sci. Law, *4*:123, 1964.
7. Parker, G. E.: The battered child syndrome. Med. Sci. Law, *8*:160, 1965.
8. Cameron, J. M., Johnson, H. R. M., and Camps, F. E.: The battered child syndrome. Med. Sci. Law, *6*:2, 1966.
9. Kempe, C. H., Silverman, F. N., Steele, B. F., Droegmuller, W., and Silver, H. K.: Battered child syndrome. J.A.M.A., *158*:539, 1962.
10. Skinner, A. E., and Castle, R. L.: *78 Battered Children: a Retrospective Study.* London, National Association for Prevention of Cruelty to Children, Sept. 1969.
11. Scott, P. D.: Fatal battered baby cases. Med. Sci. Law, *13*:197, 1973.
12. Mushin, A. S.: Ocular injuries in the battered baby syndrome. Brit. J. Ophthal., *55*:343, 1971.
13. Mushin, A. S.: Ocular damage in the battered baby syndrome. Br. Med. J., *3*:402, 1971.
14. Astley, R.: Multiple metaphyseal fractures in small children. Br. J. Radiol., *26*:577, 1953.
15. Simpson, C. K.: Battered babies: conviction for murder. Br. Med. J., *1*:393, 1965.

SELECTED READINGS

16. Adelson, L.: Slaughter of the innocents. N. Engl. J. Med., *26*:1345, 1961.
17. Altman, D. H., and Smith, R. L.: Unrecognized trauma in infants and children. J. Bone Joint Surg., *42A*:407, 1960.
18. Barabas, A. P.: Heterogenicity of the Ehlers-Danlos syndrome. Br. Med. J., *1*:612, 1967.
19. Bodian, M.: Transient loss of vision following head trauma. N.Y. State J. Med., *64*:916, 1964.
20. Bryant, H. D., et al.: Physical Abuse of Children: an Agency Study. Child Welfare, *42*:125, 1963.
21. Castle, R. L., and Kerr, A. M.: A Registry of Suspected Abuse Cases. London, National Association for Prevention of Cruelty to Children, 1972.
22. Central Health Services Council: The Battered Baby: a Memorandum. London, Department of Health and Social Security, 1970.
23. Fontana, V. J., Donovan, D., and Wong, R. J.: The maltreatment syndrome in children. N. Engl. J. Med., *269*:1389, 1963.
24. Defrancis, V.: Child Abuse. Denver, American Humane Association, Children's Division, 1963.
25. Gibbens, T. C., and Walker, N.: Cruel Parents. London, Institute for Study and Treatment of Delinquency, 1956.
26. Gil, D. G.: Nationwide survey of legally reported physical abuse of children. Unpublished paper, Brandeis University, 1968.
27. Gilkes, M. J., and Mann, T. P.: Fundi of battered babies. Lancet, *2*:468, 1967.
28. Griffith, J. F., and Dodge, P. R.: Transient blindness following head injury in children. N. Engl. J. Med., *278*:648, 1968.
29. Gwinn, J. L., Lewin, K. W., and Paterson, H. G.: Roentgenographic manifestations of unsuspected trauma in infancy. J.A.M.A., *176*:926, 1961.
30. Harcourt, B., and Hopkins, D.: Ophthalmic manifestations of the battered baby syndrome. Br. Med. J., *3*:398, 1971.
31. Helfer, R. E., and Kempe, C. H.: *The Battered Child.* Chicago, University of Chicago Press, 1968.
32. Holzel, A., and Tobin, J.: Fundi of battered babies. Lancet, *2*:723, 1967.

33. Kempe, C. H.: Pediatric implications of the battered baby syndrome. Arch. Dis. Child., *46*:28, 1971.
34. Kempe, C. H., and Helfer, R. E. (Eds.): *Helping the Battered Child and his Family*. Philadelphia and Toronto, J. B. Lippincott Co., 1972.
35. Merrill, Kaufman, Dodge and Schoepfer: Protecting the Battered Child. Denver, American Humane Association, Children's Division, 1961.
36. Nurse, S. M.: Familial patterns of parents who abuse their children. Smith Coll. Stud. Soc. Wk., *35*:11, 1964.
37. Oppe, T. E.: Battered babies. Health Trends. London, Dept. of Health and Social Security, 1972.
38. Rae, L. J.: Chapter 8 in *Recent Advances in Forensic Pathology*. Edited by F. E. Camps. London, J. & A. Churchill Ltd., 1968.
39. Simons, B.: Child Abuse Survey. Denver, American Humane Association, Children's Division, 1966.
40. Simpson, K.: Child abuse—the battered baby. In *Modern Trends in Forensic Medicine*. 3rd Ed. Edited by A. K. Mant. London, Butterworth & Co., 1973.
41. Tate, R. J.: Facial injuries associated with the battered baby syndrome. Br. J. Oral Surg., *9*:41, 1971.
42. Turner, E.: Battered baby syndrome (letter). Br. Med. J., *1*:308, 1964.
43. Turner, J. W. A.: Indirect injuries of the optic nerve. Brain, *68*:40, 1943.
44. Young, L.: *Wednesday's Children: a Study of Neglect and Abuse*. New York, McGraw-Hill Book Co., 1964.

SECTION 2. INJURY BY FIREARMS, BOMBS, AND EXPLOSIVES

chapter 11
FIREARM INJURIES

by Bernard Knight

Owing to the frequency of firearm injuries in both civilian medicolegal practice and in military medicine, an extensive literature exists on the subject. In addition, there is an even greater volume of literature concerning the weapons that cause these injuries. Though it is true that no real understanding or interpretation of gunshot wounds can be made without some knowledge of the construction and functioning of weapons, some medical authors provide such an enthusiastically detailed treatise on the "hardware," that one suspects that they are themselves caught up in the common fascination with firearms that is all too frequently a tragic feature of accidental shootings.

In order to avoid an excessive overlap of the medical aspects of firearm wounds with the purely technical forensic science discipline of firearms examination (or "ballistics"), a discussion of the laboratory and its capabilities and some pertinent manufacturer's data concerning cartridge specifications, bullet types, and rifling lands are presented in Chapter 12.

The medical examination of firearm wounds would, however, be meaningless without a certain basic knowledge of the types of weapon that could have inflicted the injury. Much of this knowledge must already be possessed by every graduate of a medical school, and the remainder can be learned in an hour's reading. It is the application of this basic technical knowledge to the findings in the autopsy room that requires meticulous observation, common sense, and above all, experience.

PERTINENT FACTS ABOUT WEAPONS

Gun Types

The gun barrels through which projectiles are emitted may be smooth internally or may be rifled, i.e., have a number of shallow spiral grooves. The smooth-walled weapons, or shotguns, which are by far the most frequent wound inflictors seen in Britain, are sporting guns that almost invariably fire a large number of small lead pellets. These diverge as they leave the end of the barrel, their path tracing out a long narrow cone that spreads *very approximately* at the rate of 1 inch (2.5 cm) width per yard (90 cm) distance from the muzzle.

Rifled weapons comprise pistols or handguns (revolvers and automatic pistols) and long-barreled weapons such as rifles and military self-loading or automatic weapons.

The diameter of the barrel of a smooth-bore shotgun is described either by the internal diameter in inches or metric units, or more commonly in English-speaking countries by the rather archaic "bore" or "gauge" system, which refers to the number of spheres of pure lead totaling 1 lb in weight, that would exactly fit the interior of the barrel. In the first nomenclature, a common size is the .410-inch caliber, and in the second system the most common is a larger weapon the "12-bore" of gauge .738 inches. In the United States, the description

"12-gauge" is usually used in place of the European term "12-bore."

Rifled weapons are almost invariably described by their internal barrel diameter expressed in inches or metric units. For instance, many revolvers have a caliber of .45, .38, or .32 inches. Automatic weapons may have similar calibers, but many of European origin such as the Mauser, Beretta, or Luger are calibrated in millimeters, commonly 7.65 mm and 9 mm. Outside these ranges of size, another very common caliber is the 0.22-inch weapon, either a handgun or a rifle.

Rifles and self-loading or automatic weapons with long barrels are either hunting or military weapons, and the diversity of types is extremely great. When the need arises, such specifications as might be useful in interpretation of wounds may be obtained from appropriate nonmedical sources, preferably via the crime laboratory firearms expert. In countries with sophisticated law enforcement facilities, the days of the "do-it-yourself" firearms pathologist have long since passed.

Ammunition

More important than the details of the weapon, as far as the doctor is concerned, is the nature of the projectile and of the components of the propellant. Any or all parts of the ammunition may contribute to the wounds upon the victim.

The following constituents emerge from a shotgun discharge and may be present in or around the injury:

Gas. The detonation of 1 grain weight of propellant produces between 200 and 900 ml of gas, according to whether black powder or a nitrocellulose-type propellant is used. This gas consists of carbon dioxide, carbon monoxide, nitrogen, hydrogen sulfide, hydrogen, methane, and other substances, all at a very high temperature.

Shot. Up to several hundred small lead spheres, the number depending upon the size of the load and the size of the individual pellet, constitute the shot. The permutations of number and size can vary enormously with different manufacturers, as well as with home-made or modified cartridges. Exceptionally, one single large projectile, such as the Foster rifled slug, may be loaded into a shotgun. In even more exceptional circumstances—as by terrorists during the Malayan emergency—bolts, metal fragments, wood screws, and the like may be used in lieu of shot.

Propellant. Unburned, burning, or partially burned propellant is frequently emitted from the muzzle, though this is much less common with the modern "clean" smokeless nitro-based type than with the old black gunpowder.

Wads. These are fitted into shotgun cartridges distal to the propellant. Usually there is a thin cardboard disk immediately on top of the propellant, followed by a thick felt wad, then another thin cardboard disk. The shot comes next, and the upper end of the cartridge is closed by another cardboard or plastic disk, over which the edges of the cartridge cylinder walls are crimped. With modern ammunition, plastic is being used more and more, so that some of these older constituents are no longer seen.

Exceptionally, some parts of the cartridge case itself may be emitted from the muzzle, for instance, fragmented cardboard, plastic, and fragments of primer.

With rifled weapons, gas, propellant, and primer fragments may emerge as with the shotgun discharge. In addition there may be grease, wax, copper, or cadmium coating the bullet and functioning as a lubricant. In all types of weapon, there may be fragments of metal torn from the inside of the barrel by the passage of the bullet, especially if, for example, the cylinder chamber of a poorly made or damaged revolver is not correctly aligned with the axis of the barrel. All these elements may contribute to the appearance of the wound.

CHARACTERISTICS OF FIREARM WOUNDS

Because of the numerous permutations of type and size of weapons, together with factors such as range and direction, descriptions and interpretations of firearm wounds can become very confusing. In an attempt to create an intelligible scheme of interpretation, their various characteristics of importance are described first and later correlated.

Entrance or "In-Shot" Wounds

Site and Size

A homicidal firearm wound may be in any part of the body consistent with a mortal result. Suicidal and accidental wounds tend to occupy certain sites, though this factor alone can rarely be relied upon to indicate the nature of the incident. This topic is discussed further later.

The size of the entrance wound gives no direct measurement of the size of the weapon of infliction, save that a shotgun wound, especially with peripheral pellet marks, is obviously recognizable at sight. Factors such as range and gas penetration greatly modify the size of the wound; even so, the experienced eye can often differentiate between, say, a .22 and a .38 bullet hole, though naturally this inspired guessing is no substitute for later meticulous confirmation. The reason for the noncoincidence of skin puncture and missile size is that the projectile *indents* the skin before puncturing it, so that the perforation is made with the skin under tension. After the bullet passes through, the skin returns to its former size and the edges of the wound contract. Offset against this, of course, is the enlargement of the hole caused by gas pressure when the range is short, as is discussed later.

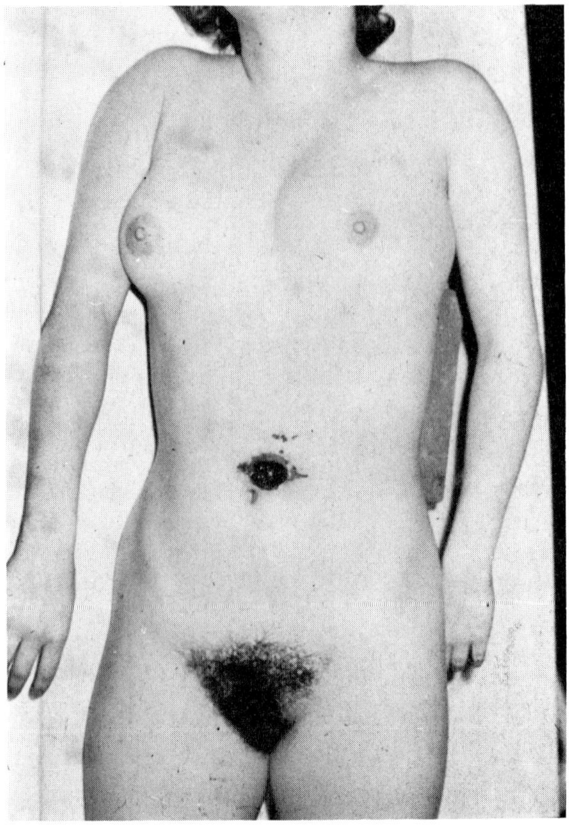

Figure 11–1. Near-contact entrance wound from a 12-bore shotgun (homicide). Interposition of clothing has prevented soiling of the skin by powder and smoke. There is peripheral bruising and a few adjacent marks from stray fragments of cartridge contents. (Courtesy of Dr. W. R. L. James.)

Skin Damage and Soiling

Splitting of Skin. Often gross splitting of the skin may be seen in the case of a contact or near-contact wound. Gas under high pressure from the muzzle is forced into the wound and greatly distends the subcutaneous tissues. This is much more marked where there is a hard structure immediately beneath the skin, such as skull or sternum. This prevents the gases from dispersing, and the back pressure causes a ragged tear in the region of the wound. Over soft areas such as abdominal wall or fatty tissue, this tearing of the wound may be absent, as the elasticity of the tissues allows the gas pressure to disperse less violently.

The wounds may be stellate, cruciate, triform, or rarely, linear in nature. The surrounding skin and underlying tissues may be distinctly pink in color owing to absorption of carbon monoxide by the hemoglobin and myoglobin. Even if not visible, it may be detectable by chemical or physical means; in cases in which there has been doubt as to which was the entrance and which the exit wound, this examination has occasionally proved useful, though in the case of shotgun wounds, monoxide may be present throughout the length of the track.

Abrasion and Bruising. There may be abrasions or even bruising at the site of entry, from two causes.

First, around the margin of the entry wound, there is almost invariably a ring of skin damage due to the longitudinal and rotatory movement of the missile (Fig. 11–1). This is called the "abrasion collar" or the "marginal abrasion"; it may not be visible in contact wounds over firm tissue. This abrasion collar, especially after some postmortem interval, is of a reddish brown color, sometimes reminiscent of the "parchment appearance" seen on any abrasion or ligature mark where the epidermis has been rubbed off. This coloration, however, may be obscured by grease marks, smoke, or powder deposition. If the bullet has entered perpendicularly to the skin surface, the abrasion ring is circular and uniform, but if the bullet has entered obliquely, it presents a more elliptical shape, the longer axis pointing in the direction of approach of the missile (Figs. 11–2 and 11–3). If the projectile approaches at a very small angle to the skin, there may be a furrow ploughed through the epidermis before complete entry occurs. Occasionally a bullet may strike the body tangentially and never actually enter, so that an elongated furrow is left; sometimes this may be so deep as to cause exposure of the underlying tissues and muscle (Figs. 11–4 and 11–5).

Apart from an abrasion collar, there may sometimes be a wider zone of bruising around

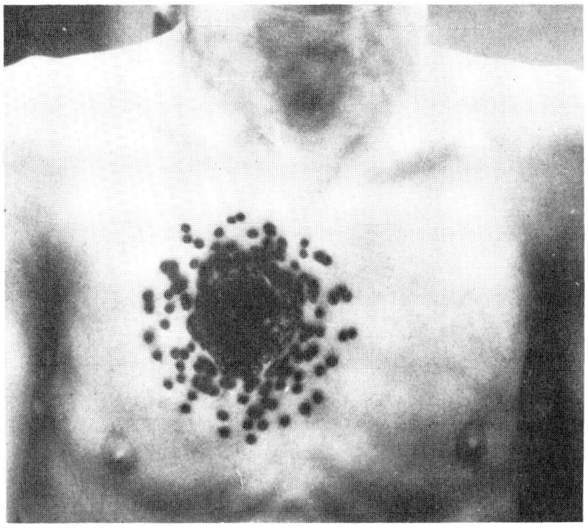

Figure 11–2. Shotgun discharge (12-bore) at about 5 yards (homicide). The symmetrical, circular wound indicates a firing position directly in front of the body. (Courtesy of Dr. W. R. L. James.)

the entrance wound owing to general tissue trauma in the area. Sometimes this may be seen as petechial stippling, but these lesions are frequently absent.

The other cause of a skin lesion in the region of an entrance wound is not the projectile itself, but the muzzle of the weapon in a contact discharge. Where the end of the barrel is in contact with the skin at the time of firing, the body surface may be "ballooned" by the entry of gases. This forces the surface against the muzzle, and the skin may take a bruised imprint of the face of the weapon. This is sometimes erroneously said to be due to "recoil" of the weapon, but this cannot be so, as recoil tends to move the weapon *away* from the skin. In fact, probably many muzzle impressions fail to be recorded because of the rapid removal of the weapon by recoil. In any event, the mark left on the skin may be an incomplete, indistinct bruise or occasionally may be a perfect imprint of the end of the weapon. Apart from the actual tip of the muzzle, the rib of a revolver barrel may produce a linear mark above the wound of entrance. Similarly, the retractor spring rod of some automatic pistols may produce a small circular abrasion below the entrance wound. Similar patterns may sometimes be discovered on clothing, especially when viewed by special techniques such as infrared photography. The interposition of clothing may, of course, prevent any distinct skin mark being made in a contact wound, though this is not invariably the case.

Grease Ring. In addition to the abrasion, a coating of foreign material may often be found around the margin of the entrance wound. It is due to removal of substances from the bullet as it passes through: bullet lubrication, gun oil from the interior of the barrel, lead from the surface of the bullet, barrel debris, and the like. With jacketed bullets of hard metal, such soiling is less common.

Flame Effects. Though modern propellants produce far less smoke and flame than the old black powder, contact and very close discharges may still cause appreciable heat effects, which may leave their own marks upon the body. The flame from the muzzle reaches a few inches in the case of a revolver, up to a foot from a shotgun. Where no clothing is interposed, the surface hairs, if present, may be either completely removed by burning down to skin level or may be shriveled, blackened, and clubbed

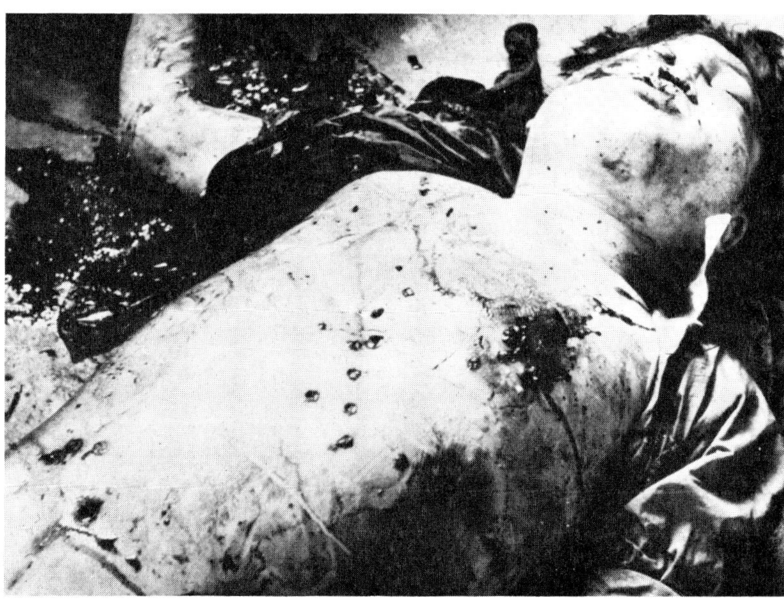

Figure 11–3. Multiple entrance wounds from a military automatic weapon (Sten gun during Malayan terrorist emergency). The large wound on the left breast is due to closely grouped wounds.

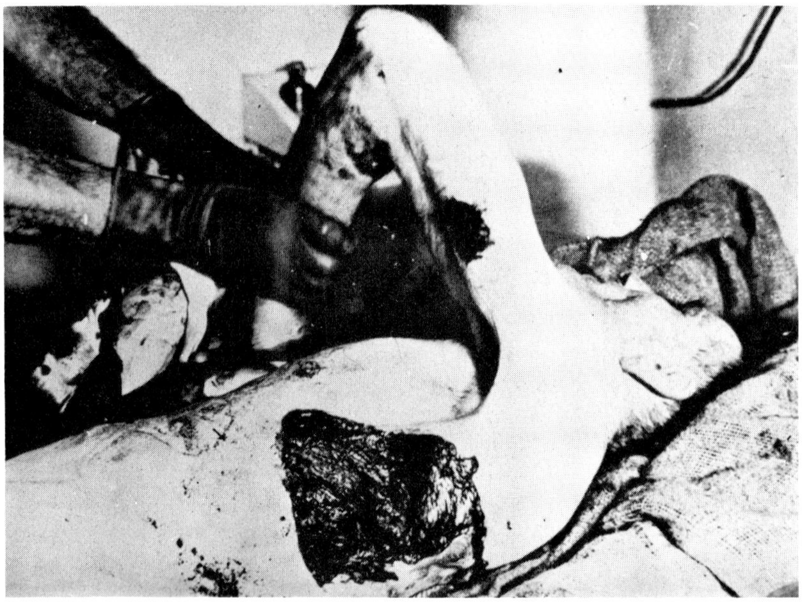

Figure 11–4. Superficial wounds due to a shotgun blast passing tangentially across the chest wall without deep penetration. There are opposing wounds on the arm. (Courtesy of Dr. W. R. L. James.)

owing to burning and melting of the keratin. The skin itself may show all the characteristics of burning from any cause, with scorching of the epidermis, a reddish brown flare, and if the victim survives for any length of time, reactive hyperemia, swelling, and possibly blistering as with other types of burn.

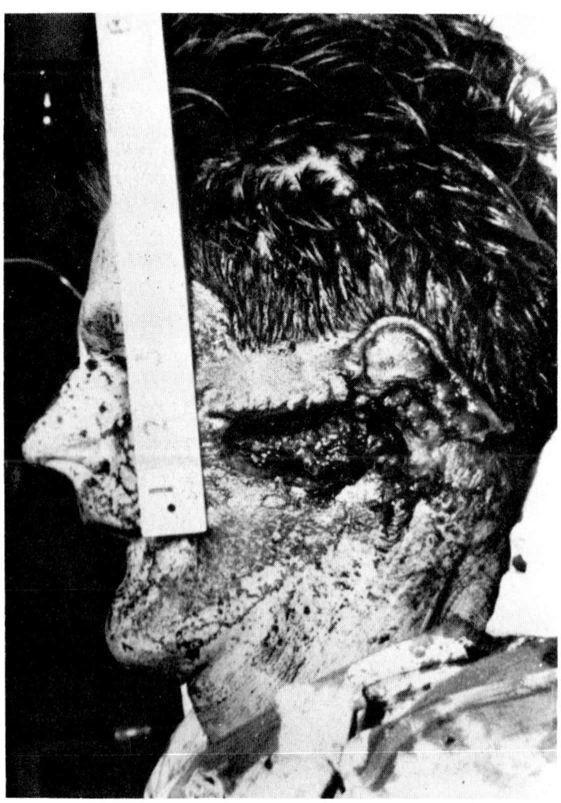

Figure 11–5. Tangential wound from 12-bore shotgun at about 2-yard range, furrowing the face and ear (homicide).

Smoke Blackening. This is alternatively called "smudging," "fouling," or "blackening," and like other characteristics, is far more marked with black powder than with the modern nitrocellulose-type propellants that are now far more commonly encountered. Along with the flame from the barrel, black powder produces a jet of carbon-containing gas, which at contact and near-contact ranges, may be deposited upon clothing or skin. Apart from considerations of range, this smoke mark may be useful in demonstrating the direction of impact, as the circular deposition typical with a perpendicular wound will be progressively lengthened and become elliptical as the angle to the skin decreases (Fig. 11–6).

Powder Tattooing. Also referred to as "stippling" or "peppering," these marks are due to unburned and partially burned powder and are, again, far more common with black powder discharges than with modern propellants. They may range from a millimeter size downward to minute specks, either black or red in color. If large grains were still burning, there may be a halo of skin burn around them when they are viewed with a lens. With modern propellants, this black stippling may be absent, though small flakes and threads of a gelatin-like substance may be visible on close examination. The presence and extent of powder tattooing, and also of smoke effects, can be more readily demonstrated by infrared photography on both skin and clothing.

The Wound Itself

This varies greatly according to such factors as the location in the body, the range, and the type of weapon.

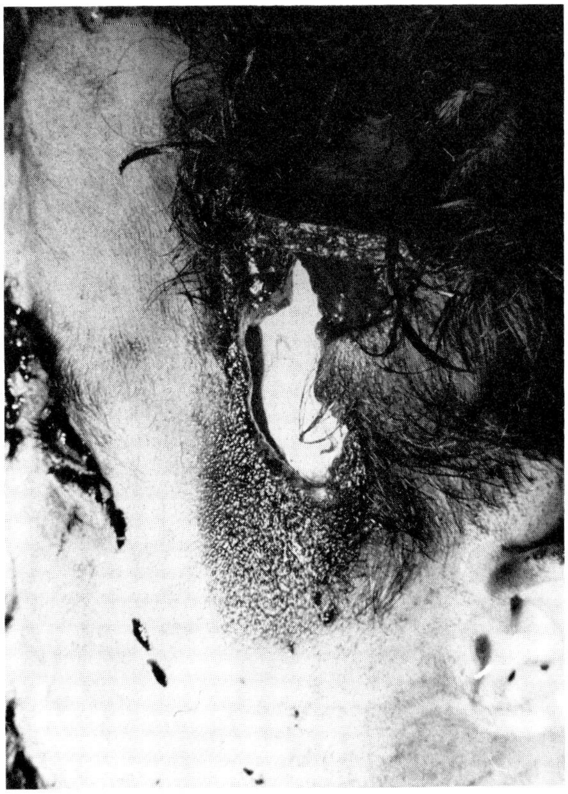

Figure 11–6. Suicidal shotgun wound of the temple, almost contact. The elliptical shape of the powder blackening below the entrance wound indicates that the muzzle was held at a marked angle to the skin surface.

An intermediate-range rifled-weapon injury would typically show a clean-cut circular hole with inverted edges. This has been described as similar to "poking a lead pencil through the skin." Toward the extreme range of a weapon, a single projectile striking the body may cause a larger, jagged entry wound because the steady gyroscopic spin of the bullet, maintained by the initial velocity, is being lost. The bullet may then begin to pursue an erratic course with marked "tail-wag" and even "tumbling," turning head-over-heels along its path. In this situation, it may cause a most irregular wound, which may be misinterpreted either as an exit wound or as a contact wound unless other criteria are carefully evaluated. Such a bullet may not have sufficient momentum at the end of its flight to traverse the body, and there may thus be no exit wound.

The "tail-wag" referred to may also occur at close ranges before the bullet has had time to settle down into a steady gyroscopic progression. The tip of the bullet may follow the axis of the trajectory, but the tail of the bullet may describe a circle (or rather *spiral*) around the line of flight. If the bullet strikes the body during this phase, the entrance wound may be much larger than if the bullet had been fired from an intermediate distance. This again accentuates the dangers of making a snap judgment about the caliber of the weapon from the size of the entrance wound.

As smooth-bore shotguns cause by far the majority of firearm wounds in Britain, the shotgun lesion has particular relevance there. Except at contact or short range, the shotgun wound can hardly be confused with that from the single projectile fired from a rifled weapon, as at any range beyond a few feet, there will be multiple entrance wounds in all but the most unusual circumstances. The lead pellets of a shotgun cartridge emerge from the muzzle of the gun as a single mass, but soon begin to diverge into a long narrow cone. Thus at the muzzle they will cause a single large wound, but as the distance increases this wound will be progressively smaller. The central mass of packed shot becomes smaller, owing to divergence of peripheral pellets, which will then make their own individual marks in a circular fashion around the diminishing central core. At a certain distance—which varies greatly according to circumstances—there will be no central hole, only a diffuse peppering with shot, and this state of affairs will continue (with increasing distance between the individual shot holes) until the maximum penetrating range of the weapon is reached. A formula hallowed by long usage is that the diameter of the spread of the shot pattern on the skin in inches is roughly equal to the distance from the muzzle in yards. Unfortunately the word "roughly" is the most important feature of this rule of thumb, and it is imperative that test firings of such weapons be carried out with similar ammunition in order to arrive at a more trustworthy estimate of range.

Many factors modify the spread of the pellet pattern in a shotgun discharge: first, the configuration of the gun barrel is very important. A parallel-sided barrel is referred to as the "cylinder" and a barrel that tapers slightly toward the muzzle is known as a "choke" barrel. The degree of taper varies with the manufacturer and model of the weapon, and there are intermediate degrees such as "modified choke," "improved cylinder," and "half choke." Frequently a double-barrel shotgun has a cylinder on the right and a choke barrel on the left. Some weapons are equipped with a facility for removing one particular type of barrel so that it may be replaced with a different degree of choke. In addition, modern accessories can convert a cylinder to a choke barrel—for example, variable chokes such as the Poly-Choke, Kutts Compensator, and Weaver-Choke are available. These technical matters are for the firearms examiner to investigate, but naturally his findings must be correlated with the interpretation of the physical wound found at autopsy.

Another complication with shotguns is the increased modern tendency to fire a single projectile through the smooth bore. This has been done for many years in the form of a solid round "pumpkin ball" or the Brenneke rifled slug, but more recent types include the Foster rifled slug and the French Blondeau, which is dumbbell-shaped.

Other modern modifications of shotguns include the increased use of plastic, especially to replace traditional wads. Some of these—such as the "Power-Piston"—have the shot contained inside a polythene cup, which may itself be involved in the wounding process. In some modern cartridges, plastic granules may be used as a filler between the lead pellets, and this highly colored material may also be found within wounds or upon the skin.

Shotgun wounds at close or contact range may cause far more destruction of tissue than rifled weapons because the amount of gas produced is far greater, owing to the larger amount of propellant employed. Gross tearing and laceration of tissues is a common feature of shotgun wounds, especially those contact wounds of the head frequently seen in suicides.

Estimates of range of discharge of the shotgun may be further complicated by the fact that even one particular weapon may produce totally different divergence patterns when different cartridges are fired. This may be due not only to differences in type and manufacture of the ammunition; aging, deterioration due to storage, and deliberate tampering with ammunition may radically alter the discharge properties. For example, tampering with the cartridge contents may include removing the top closure card and fusing the shot together with melted paraffin wax or even pitch in order to prevent dispersion. The cartridge case may also be partially cut through at the level of the plunger wad so that the top half becomes detached on firing and acts as a receptacle for the shot, the whole upper part of the cartridge sometimes entering the body.

The components of a shotgun cartridge, being so different from revolver or automatic loads, are important in the autopsy examination of firearm wounds. Apart from the shot and propellant described earlier, the wads of cardboard or felt or plastic may also be found within the wound or may cause separate wounds of their own. The latter are usually limited to superficial bruising or abrasion, but on occasion the wads can actually cause laceration and penetration. Their presence in a wound is important in the estimation of range.

Exit Wounds

Like entrance wounds, there may be great variation in the appearance of the exit or "outshoot" wound from a firearm. In many cases, of course, there will be no exit wound because the projectile or projectiles remain within the body. This is a common occurrence, either because the bullet from a rifled weapon is fired from an extreme range so that its momentum is insufficient to traverse the body completely and exit on the other side, or because it strikes a hard body structure that fragments it or dissipates its energy. Similarly, it is the exception rather than the rule for shotgun pellets to emerge on the farther side of the body, unless this is in a narrow area such as the head, neck, or limbs.

Taking first the single projectile from a rifled weapon, the exit wound commonly presents a

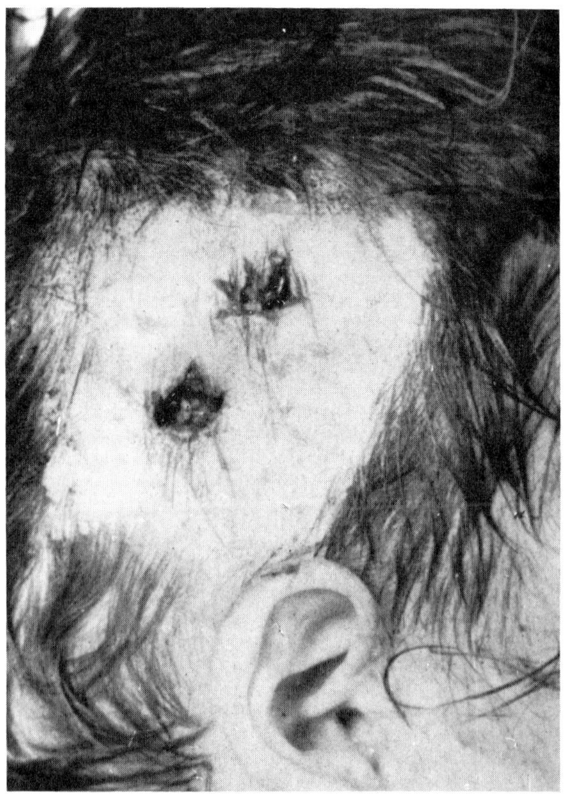

Figure 11–7. Two exit wounds from a 0.22 rifle on the scalp of a child (homicide). The absence of soiling, hair burning, and the like indicates that the stellate shape was not due to contact entrance.

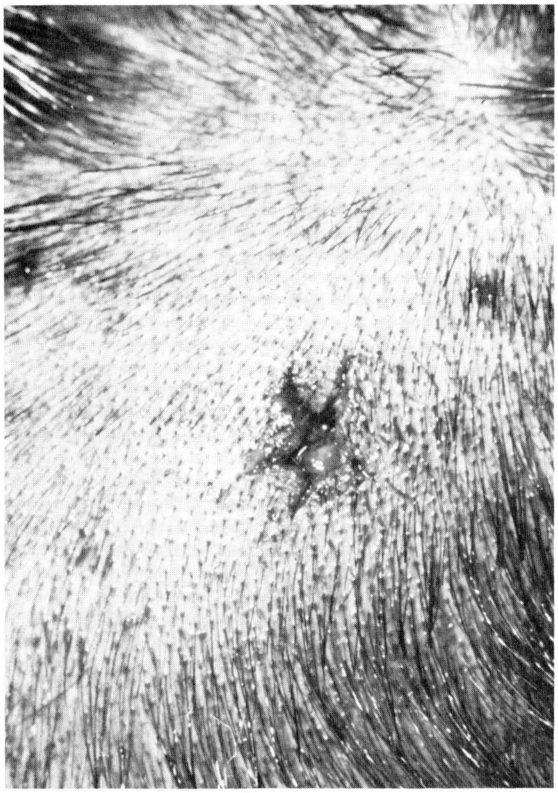

Figure 11–8. Exit wound of a 9-mm automatic rifle bullet on the scalp. The stellate wound cannot have been caused by contact entrance, because other signs on the surrounding skin and hairs are lacking. (Courtesy of Dr. W. R. L. James.)

larger and more ragged appearance than the corresponding entrance wound, though exceptions are numerous (Figs. 11–7 and 11–8).

A bullet that hits the body from intermediate range may cause a very small entrance wound because of its steady trajectory and the elasticity of the skin. On leaving the body on the farther side, it tends to produce an *everted* wound, as opposed to the *inverted* entrance wound, and there may well be enlargement and tearing of the margins due to disturbance of the steady gyroscopic path that exists before impact. Because the unsupported skin is struck from within, the wound tends to burst outward, and frequently fragments and tags of subcutaneous tissue are seen either at the margins or actually extruded. An important exception to this is the exit of a bullet at a point that is well supported, either by tight clothing such as a waistband or corset or where the victim was pressed against a firm surface such as a wooden or plasterboard wall, car upholstery, or the like. Here the pressure of the external substance tends to hold the skin surface rigid, causing the exit wound to be a clean puncture, sometimes indistinguishable from the entrance wound except for the absence of inversion, grease, and other soiling.

Another cause of a large ragged exit wound is the tumbling of the bullet due to resistance against the body tissues, which therefore smashes its way out of the body in a more irregular fashion. Even more severe tissue destruction is caused when the bullet strikes a hard body component such as bone or a solid organ such as the liver, heart, or kidney. In this case, the trajectory will be greatly distorted and the bullet may fragment, some of the fragments exiting in separate places. Another cause of extensive damage may be that the energy of the bullet is transmitted to fragments of bone, which then themselves become projectiles. These may cause severe and sometimes multiple exit lacerations that can be mistaken for other types of wound (Fig. 11–9).

When the energy of the missile is spent before exit occurs, the projectile may come to rest immediately beneath the skin, which is second only to bone and cartilage in its resistance to penetration. Shotgun pellets are frequently found in this position and may be palpated under the skin.

Difficulties in distinguishing entrance from exit wounds may be accentuated if the body is

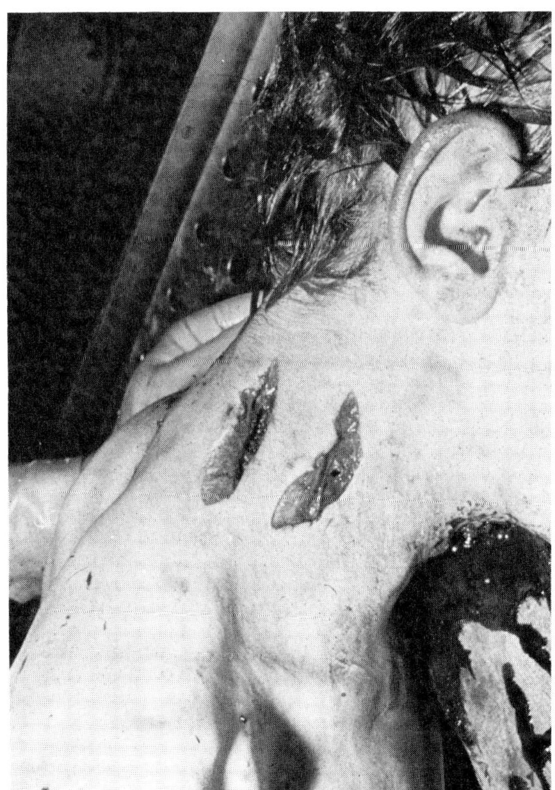

Figure 11–9. Accidental shotgun wound of the neck, showing two exit wounds caused by bone fragments displaced from the spine. These were initially suspected by the police to be knife wounds.

decomposed, especially after maceration due to immersion in water. Sometimes fragments of clothing and other foreign material may be found in the track between the two wounds, and their orientation may assist in differentiating the two lesions. Carbon monoxide is usually confined to contact or close-range entrance wounds, though the amount generated by large shotgun cartridges may be sufficient to produce chemically detectable monoxide right through the track, even around the exit wound.

Wounds in Particular Sites

Head Wounds

Gunshot wounds of the head are frequent in both suicidal and homicidal shootings. One of the elective sites of the suicide is in the mouth and the other is in the temple, both with either smoothbore or rifled weapons. The effects can be extremely destructive, especially with shotguns, which may completely explode the cranium.

A well-known aspect of bullet wounds is the differentiation between entrance and exit wounds through the skull tables. This can easily be determined in almost every case, because the passage of the bullet leaves a clean-cut hole on the approach side and a beveled crater on the exit side. This applies to both traverses of a "through-and-through" wound of the cranium, so that the beveling occurs on the *inside* of the skull at the *entrance* wound and on the *outside* at the *exit* wound. The crater effect is produced when the unsupported diploë everts and fragments on the side where the bullet leaves, this in contrast to the approach side where the rim of the defect is supported by the underlying bone. The differences are well shown in Figure 11–10.

Associated linear fractures are common, radiating out from the bullet holes. As in skin wounds, bullet holes in the skull can leave an excellent record of the angle and direction of the shot, seen in the asymmetry of the bony defect, which becomes more elliptical as the angle decreases. The direction along the axis of the ellipse from which the bullet came is obvious on inspection, from the undercutting effect. Not infrequently, the bullet expends most of its momentum in penetrating the skull at one point and cannot escape on the opposite side. It may be able to traverse the soft brain tissue, but may be arrested by the tough dura on the opposite side. In children, this is possible in the absence of explosive-propelled weapons; in two cases seen in the Cardiff department, the thin temporal bones of the children were penetrated by the small lead slugs of 0.177-inch air rifles. Each slug caused a wide track of destruction across the brain and came to rest against the opposite cranial wall (Fig. 11–11).

Bullets may enter the cranial cavity and, though they have insufficient energy remaining to exit on the opposite side, may ricochet from the inside of the skull and cause secondary tracks of damage or even skid around the inside of the skull in a circumferential manner.

High-velocity projectiles, especially those

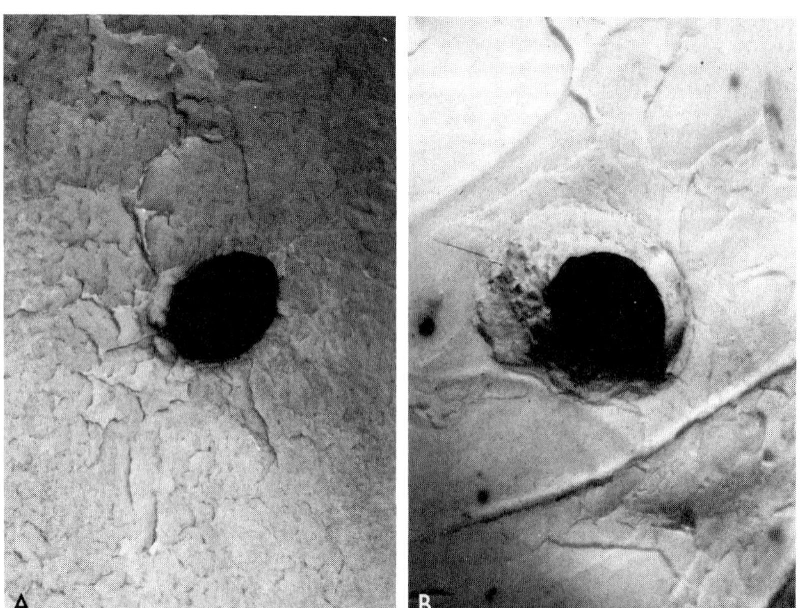

Figure 11–10. Passage of a 0.22 bullet through the skull. *A.* The clean-cut outer aspect. *B.* The beveled appearance on the inner table. This bullet passed right through the head, causing the reverse of these appearances on the opposite side of the skull vault.

from military weapons, may cause gross damage to the head by virtue of the total release of their extremely high kinetic energy. The effects may be so destructive as to cause virtual decapitation, and the injuries may sometimes be confused with those due to high explosive rather than to a simple projectile (Fig. 11–12).

Wounds of Chest and Abdomen

The most frequent sites for fatal firearm wounds are the chest and abdomen, partly because of the sites chosen in suicides and partly because of the larger target area presented in accidents and homicides.

In the chest, the wounds may be complicated by the interposition of the bony thoracic cage, the entrance wound being supported in some instances by underlying sternum or rib. Rib or spine may interfere with the passage of the bullet, and there may be extensive exit wound damage from bone fragments. Vital organs such as heart, lungs, and great vessels are frequently damaged, and these injuries are usually the immediate cause of death from tissue destruction and gross hemorrhage. With shotgun injuries of the chest, the pellets may be widely distributed within the lungs and behind the parietal pleura, within the costal spaces, and beneath the skin of the opposite side of the thorax.

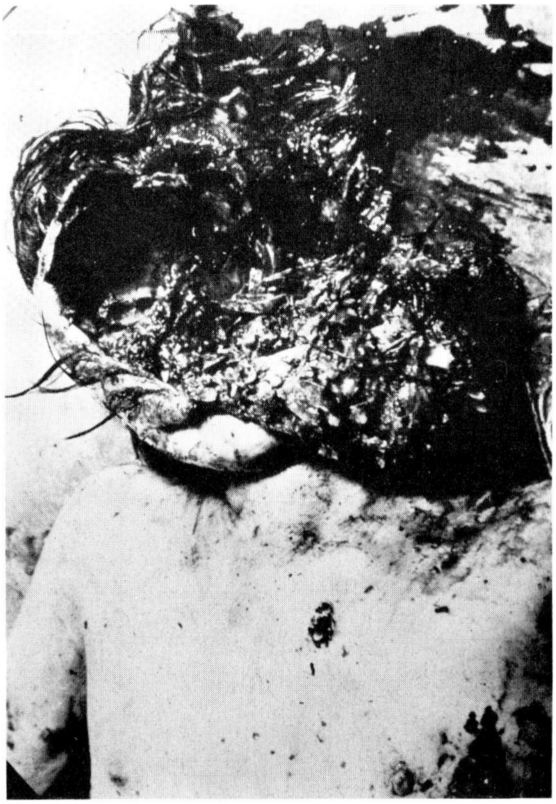

Figure 11–12. The head of a female Malayan terrorist, hit in the left auditory meatus by a single bullet. Owing to the exceptionally high muzzle velocity of the weapon (a military Belgian Fabrique Nationale rifle), the head has exploded because of the violent deceleration of the missile in the dense bone at the base of the skull.

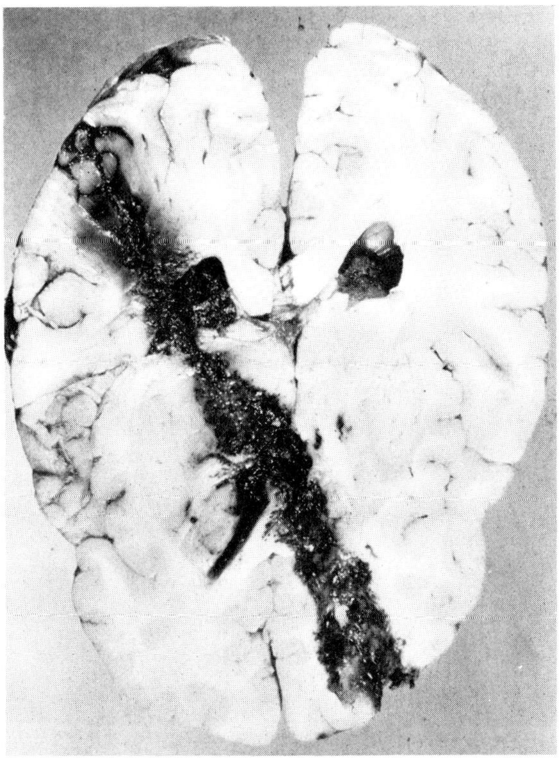

Figure 11–11. The brain of a child, showing the passage of a 0.177-inch air gun slug, which can just be seen in the occipital cortex. Even with such a relatively low-velocity missile, the width of the track of destruction can be seen to be many times the size of the slug. (Courtesy of Dr. W. R. L. James.)

All permutations of organ damage may be seen, and it would be profitless to describe the many varieties, as careful examination and dissection will reveal the extent of the lesions in each case. It is worth remembering that in bullet wounds, the track of damage, especially through the lung, is far wider than the diameter of the projectile itself. In close discharges, especially from shotguns, the destructive effect of gases must be added to the effects of the projectiles.

Wounds of the abdomen may cause all manner of organ destruction and damage as well as bony lesions in the lumbar spine, sacrum, and pelvis. In shotgun wounds, coils of small bowel may lie outside the abdomen, their extrusion probably being aided by entry of gas into the peritoneal cavity in a contact or near-contact discharge (Fig. 11–13). Internally, the cause of death is usually massive hemorrhage directly

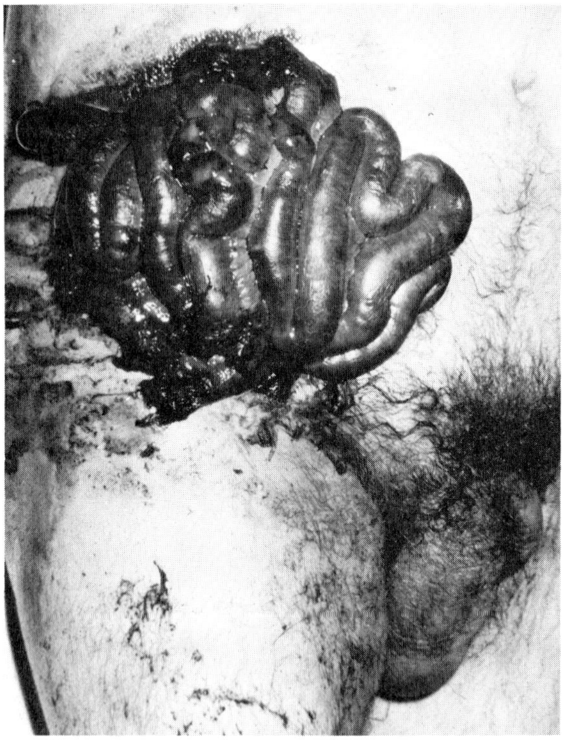

Figure 11–13. Extrusion of coils of intestine through abdominal shotgun wound. The size of the close-discharge wound and the abdominal muscle spasm have forced the gut through the defect. (Courtesy of Dr. W. R. L. James.)

from aorta, vena cava, or vascular organs such as the mesentery and liver, as well as from shock from tissue destruction and bowel perforation.

Estimation of Range

The several factors discussed in the first part of this chapter may be employed to give some estimate of range, though it cannot be overemphasized that a definitive opinion depends on collaboration with a criminalistics firearms expert after any suspect weapon has been tested.

Shotgun Wounds

The *contact wound* is a large wound, often ragged because of gas tearing. Underlying destruction of tissue is great. There is smoke soiling of surrounding skin, though if contact is firm, this may be slight. Wads are found within the wound. In the head or neck, a large exit wound or complete destruction is frequent. When the shot was fired into the mouth, the whole head may be exploded, with only the lower face intact.

Near-contact wounds, up to about 1 foot, appear similar to contact wounds though there is more extensive smoke soiling and powder tattooing owing to the opportunity for emission between the muzzle and the skin. Wads are found in the wound, and wound margins show laceration by gas, though not invariably. Up to about 1 yard, the wound is likely to be single, depending on the weapon characteristics. Beyond this, satellite pellet holes begin to appear around the main wound margins. Wads are still present in the wound. There is extensive singeing of hair, if unprotected by clothing. Carbon monoxide is found in tissues around the entry, possibly through the whole track.

At *moderate range*, between 1 and 5 yards, the wound will begin to spread and the approximate formula of "total diameter in inches equals range in yards" may be very loosely applied. Smoke soiling will be absent and powder tattooing will be less evident or may be invisible to the naked eye, though powder grains may be visible on magnification or by infrared photography. Wads are still present in the wound up to a variable distance, usually up to 6 feet and occasionally as far as 20 feet.

At *more distant range*, beyond 5 yards, the spread of pellets becomes greater according to the choke of the barrel and other factors until the central hole vanishes at around 8 to 12 yards, to be replaced by a uniform "peppering" of shot marks. At longer ranges these begin to fail to penetrate the skin, leaving small abrasions with occasional pellets embedded in the dermis. There are no tattooing or smoke marks. No wads are found in wounds at ranges over 5 to 6 yards. Death from the direct effects of shot is rare beyond 30 yards, unless some vital structure such as the eye is penetrated or there is associated cardiovascular disease in which cardiac arrest might be precipitated by the pain and shock.

Rifled Weapons

Contact wounds show tearing of tissue in a cruciate or stellate manner if underlying tissues are firm, e.g., skull or sternum. Bruising of surrounding skin by impact onto muzzle is frequent, as are marginal abrasion, grease ring, and localized peripheral burning and flame effects. The latter may be absent or minimal in firm contact wounds. Smoke blackening is possible if the muzzle is not tight against the skin. Carbon monoxide is found in tissues, and there is frequently an exit wound unless bone is struck within the body. The wound is almost always larger than the bullet, except over soft tissue.

Near-contact wounds are small; there is less likelihood of ripping of margins unless the muzzle is very nearly in contact with skin supported by bone. Extensive blackening and powder tattooing are present if black powder propellant is used; alternatively, fragments of nitro compounds are found. Abrasion collar and grease ring are present, as are flame effects with singeing of hair and carbon monoxide in tissues.

At *close range*, up to 1 to 2 feet, there are decreasing heat effects, smoke soiling, and powder tattooing. Singeing of hairs is unlikely. The wound is small, and no gas effects in tissues (with modern propellants) or macroscopic skin effects are likely.

At *intermediate range*, from 2 feet up to the effective range of the weapon, the entrance wound is small with regular margins, grease ring, and abrasion collar. There are no macroscopic or chemically detectable residues on skin and no burning or singeing.

Extreme range entrance wounds may be irregular owing to tumbling of the bullet and may be indistinguishable from typical exit wounds. No help in estimation of range is offered by the appearance of the entrance wound in the intermediate distance between a few feet and toward the extreme effective range of the weapon.

Accident, Suicide, or Murder?

The medical evidence can sometimes confirm or exclude certain of the possible motives for the shooting, but in the majority of cases, collateral evidence from witnesses and investigating officers provides most of the data upon which a decision is made. The doctor must be sure that in his examination he does not ignore the conclusions that can be drawn from circumstantial evidence; it must always be borne in mind that the most extraordinary events occur in medicolegal practice and that a careful evaluation must always be made to ensure that dogmatic statements by medical witnesses do not mislead the investigating authorities. For example, a fatal shooting occurred in England in which there was an entrance wound on the chest of the victim and an exit wound on the back. There was another entrance wound on the back, and inside the thorax was a deformed revolver bullet. The natural assumption was that the victim had been shot twice from two different directions, but this was inconsistent with the circumstances, and on careful investigation it was discovered that the deceased had been standing against a brick wall. A single projectile had entered the front of the chest, passed through the back, ricocheted from the wall, and reentered the back. Other experienced forensic pathologists doubtless have far more bizarre examples, all of which illustrate the fact that experience, common sense, and a willingness to consider other possibilities are as essential in the practice of legal medicine as the possession of a compendious store of theoretical knowledge.

With these reservations in mind, there are certain patterns of injury in gunshot wounds that either indicate, suggest, or are consistent with certain methods of causation.

Suicide

In almost every case, the weapon is present at the scene. Rarely, an exception is found in which the suicide has survived long enough to remove himself from the vicinity of the shooting. There are numerous cases on record in which even the most gross injuries, including partial destruction of the brain, have been consistent with survival and mobility for some time after the shooting.

There are well-recognized sites of election for a suicidal gunshot wound. Most suicides shoot themselves in either the temple, the chest, or through the mouth or front of the neck. The commonly made statement that right-handed people shoot themselves in the right temple and vice versa is by no means accurate, and no firm conclusions can be drawn from evidence of a contralateral discharge when the "handedness" of the deceased was known. Apart from these major sites of election, occasional wounds in other parts of the body may be seen in undoubted suicides, but such cases must be treated with more than usual care. A useful observation is that suicides rarely shoot themselves through their clothing, but usually pull it aside to bare the skin.

If the wound is in an obviously inaccessible site such as the back of the neck or the back of the thorax or abdomen, then murder or accident must be suspected until excluded by other factors. It is rare for suicides to shoot themselves through the eye or through the abdomen. It is also very unusual—at least in Britain—for a woman to shoot herself, a fact in line with the general rule that women usually destroy themselves by less violent methods than men.

The presence of more than two bullets or evidence of two discharges is obviously a strong pointer toward homicide rather than suicide or accident. There are, however, many instances on record of a suicide being able to fire two or more shots into himself, each apparently potentially and immediately lethal.

In spite of these exceptions, the presence of two mortal gunshot wounds must be accepted as evidence of homicide until proved to the contrary.

Naturally, this presumption must be modified if an automatic (not self-loading) weapon is involved with which continuous pressure on the trigger results in repetitive discharges.

The range of the discharge is naturally all-important. For obvious reasons the vast majority of suicidal gunshot wounds are either contact or near-contact in nature. Thus all the characteristics of near-discharges become important in the examination.

When short firearms such as revolvers and automatic pistols are used, the usual sites of election may be found. When long-barreled weapons such as rifles or shotguns are used, then the sites of election are limited by the necessity for the person to be able to reach the trigger. Thus shotgun wounds in the mouth, front of the head, and front of the thorax are common. When a long-barreled gun is used, a device may be used to actuate the trigger that is out of reach of the fingers. Strings, sticks, and even more complicated mechanical apparatus may be found. In fact, some suicides have been reported in which quite sophisticated mechanical apparatus has been devised, some of which even discharged the weapon from a distance that would have aroused suspicion of murder if the machinery had not been visible. In these cases there seems to be some element of the bizarre, an almost masochistic pleasure, in devising such apparatus. In most cases, however, the presence of the weapon and the presence of a contact or near-contact wound are consistent with a diagnosis of suicide, though naturally this needs corroboration.

Exceptions do occur, a classic example being the political murder of King Ananda of Thailand in 1946, in which the rigged "suicide" failed because the site of election was wrong. The entrance hole was over the center of the eyebrow, an unusual position. There was a revolver on the bed where death occurred, but although of the correct caliber, it was not the one that fired the fatal shot.

Accidents

It is impossible to differentiate accident from homicide merely on examination of the firearm wound. Both conditions may involve close or distant discharges, and in both the wound may be in almost any part of the body, there being less tendency for a limited number of sites of election than in suicide. Here again, investigation and collateral evidence are all-important.

Some pointers may be useful, however. Like suicide by shooting, accidental gunshot wounds are very rare in women because of the almost complete prerogative of men for the handling of, and fascination with, firearms. Many accidental shootings occur in young men or youths who appear to have a compulsive need to handle firearms. Elements of "brinkmanship" and almost a death wish have been seen in numerous cases of accidental firearm wounds. The typical situation is seen where a young man is alone in his room with a weapon, which he is dismantling, cleaning, and generally toying with in an almost loving manner. These deaths are sometimes hard to differentiate from suicides, except there is no evidence of external circumstances that might have led to the victim taking his own life. Some accidents do genuinely occur during the manipulation of guns, though the absolute foolhardiness of manipulating a loaded weapon often suggests that the victim was indulging in some activity other than purely utilitarian maintenance and cleaning. In these cases the fatal wound is often on the front of the upper part of the body, especially through the chest, neck, or head.

Other more obviously genuine accidents with shotguns are frequently seen among sportsmen and farmers. The latter often seem to possess ancient weapons that are very unsafe, and testing of these firearms may reveal that the trigger mechanism is so worn that a slight impact causes the gun to discharge. Many countrymen seem to be incredibly indifferent to the potential dangers of their weapons. Instances have been seen in which fatal discharges occurred when the owner was using the gun as a walking stick or using it to push aside bushes in a hedgerow.

Other accidents occur when weapons are discharged at a distance without any thought of the possibility of human injury being present in the mind of the firer. Such accidents have occurred when a hunter fired at some movement in undergrowth, but the "animal" turned out to be human. From the medical examiner's point of view, there is nothing about the wound in such cases that will differentiate an accident from a deliberate homicide. As with the differentiation from suicides, the presence of two bullets or of two discharges strongly suggests homicide, but there are many exceptions to this assumption.

Homicide

When a distant discharge has occurred, when no weapon is present at the scene, or when the site of election is inconsistent with suicide, the differentiation between accident and homicide depends upon the circumstances and the results of inquiries. The proportion of such events that are eventually apportioned to one classification or the other depends to a considerable extent on the geographical situation. In Britain, owing to the very strict regulations concerning possession of firearms, the majority of such tragedies are accidental, but in the United States, by far the greater majority are homicidal.

A pointer suggesting homicide, as opposed to accident, includes repetitive discharges, especially when there are several bullets in the body and an automatic weapon is not involved. The caution mentioned earlier in respect to suicides must be repeated, however, because cases are on record in which a suicide has been able to fire the weapon several times even when the first discharge might well have been expected to be immediately fatal.

Sites of election for homicidal gunshot wounds are not so clearly demarcated as in suicide, but they are frequently seen in the back of the head, back of the neck, sides of the trunk, abdomen, and proximal parts of the limbs, all sites that are shunned by suicides. Gonzales, Vance, Helpern, and Umberger reviewed 274 homicidal shootings in New York City and reported that in 70 per cent the wounds resulted from a single bullet penetrating a vital portion of the body: 25 per cent involved the abdomen, 23 per cent the chest, 10 per cent the head, 7 per cent the spine, 3 per cent the neck, and 2 per cent the extremities. In the remaining 30 per cent of the total, wounds by more than one bullet were encountered.

Wounds in inaccessible places such as the back of the head, neck, or thorax obviously raise the suspicion of homicide, especially if they are contact or near-discharge wounds, less likely to be accidental. Probably the most single useful factor in suggesting that firearm wounds are homicidal is the multiplicity of discharges. Naturally if other evidence such as attempted disposal of the body, tying of the limbs, or other evidence of suspicious activities is combined with a fatal gunshot wound, the possibility of homicide is greatly strengthened.

Survival Time and Activity After Shooting

A matter that is not infrequently raised in inquests and criminal trials is the possibility of the fatally injured person being able to move or survive following the gunshot wound. In a number of authenticated cases, the duration of such survival and activity seems incompatible with the anatomical damage, but in the face of absolute evidence, it must be admitted that it is highly unsafe to be dogmatic about the limitation of such activity.

In one case reported by Glaister, the man shot himself with a .45-caliber pistol beneath the chin. The bullet entered the cranium and pulped the frontal and temporal lobes of the brain before making its exit through a $1\frac{1}{2}$-inch diameter defect in the skull. Following this injury the man walked from a garden shelter (where the shooting had occurred and where later pieces of skull and brain were found on the ceiling), walked around some gardens for at least 165 yards, returned to the shelter for some time, then walked home to his house, where he arrived at least one hour after the shooting. He spoke in an apparently normal fashion to the maid who admitted him, hung up his overcoat and umbrella, and walked upstairs to his room. Death did not take place until at least four hours after the shooting.

Faced with a case like this, it is risky to be dogmatic about the length of survival time, especially when cerebral injuries are involved. Of course, when there has been gross cardiovascular damage with copious blood loss, the medical expert is on firmer ground when he offers an opinion that death must have occurred within a short time, but surprises never cease to occur.

Postmortem Examination Technique in Shooting Fatalities

Autopsies on victims of firearm wounds present special problems over and above those of the usual medicolegal postmortem examination. In all cases a very careful and detailed autopsy must be performed, with particular attention to retention of certain trace evidence for the forensic science laboratory.

The clothing must be handled with particular care because of possible projectiles, powder residues, metallic traces, and similar material that may be around the entrance wound and that can be partly lost by mishandling. The advice of the forensic scientist, who is usually present at the autopsy or at the scene, should be respected, and full access should be granted to him to inspect and deal with such trace evidence in the manner that he thinks best. If no laboratory assistance is available at the time of autopsy, the clothing should be carefully retained in clean brown paper or plastic bags, care being taken to observe the chain of continuity of evidence with investigating officers. Before removal of the clothes, the exact position of the gunshot defects in the clothing should be measured so that they can later be compared with the position of the wounds in the body. This may be done by photography and also by measuring the position of the clothing defects from certain fixed points, such as heel level to give distance above the ground, from the center line of the body, and from some anatomical landmark such as the jugular notch of the manubrium sterni. Further specialized techniques of examination of the clothing, such as infrared photography, chemical and physical examination of powder residues, and even more sophisticated techniques, are now the province of the crime laboratory; the role of the pathologist is confined to correlating the position of the clothing defect with the wound in the body and in ensuring that no trace evidence is lost. He also naturally incorporates the initial naked-eye evidence of close-discharge powder soiling and burning and the like with later scientific evidence offered by the laboratory in coming to his final conclusion about the range and direction of the discharge.

Once the clothing has been removed or if the gunshot is in an unclothed area of skin, the pathologist's next duty is to inspect carefully and record the nature of the external wounds and to decide which is the entrance and which the exit if both are present. He should stoutly resist any misguided attempts of inexperienced mortuary attendants to wash the body surface. He must give investigating authorities full access for photography, and supplement it by his own photography if he thinks it necessary. Again he should give full access to the crime laboratory personnel should they wish to take samples from around the wound by swabbing or any other means, though this should not take place until he has satisfied himself that he has examined and recorded all the aspects of the wound that he deems necessary.

The next move depends partly upon the facilities available: if radiographic equipment is available in the mortuary, films of the body should be taken prior to internal examination to demonstrate the position of any bullets or metallic fragments. Should the autopsy have to be performed where such facilities are not available, the pathologist must decide from the factors in the particular case whether he wishes to proceed "blind" or whether the body should be removed to a place where they are available. Sometimes this decision has to be made after the postmortem examination has been started because of difficulties in locating bullets or fragments. If the case is one of homicide, it is better to suspend operations until radiography is available than to press on blindly, possibly encountering the bullet unexpectedly with instruments and damaging characteristic rifling and other marks.

The bullets, fragments, or lead shot must be recovered as complete and intact as possible and preserved in a condition in which they will not deteriorate before the crime laboratory can run its tests. For example, a soft lead revolver bullet should not be dropped into a glass bottle for transport to the laboratory, as prolonged rattling about inside the hard container may well blur the fine recognition marks, which may be vital in the case. The bullet should be packed in a soft material such as gauze or cotton wool and preferably handed at the scene of the autopsy to a crime laboratory scientist or to a responsible investigating officer for dispatch, once again ensuring that the continuity of the chain of evidence is preserved.

Similarly, fragmented bullets, cards, and wads from shotgun cartridges should be carefully retained. The number of lead pellets in a shotgun injury may present a tedious job of recovery, but as full a clearance as possible should be made so that the laboratory can have the chance to identify the type of ammunition used by measuring the total load of shot. Again, radiography may greatly assist, as pellets may lodge in the most unlikely and distant places, often not visible in the bloody conditions of an autopsy.

After the autopsy is completed and the damage to internal structures evaluated, several questions need to be answered.

The cause of death is usually a relatively straightforward matter; its determination, being based on the pathologist's previous experience of postmortem examinations, is normally a matter of considering the total amount of tissue damage, vascular damage, and hemorrhage. At this point some estimate of the rapidity of death might be hazarded, with the reservations mentioned previously.

The type of weapon used, i.e., rifled or smoothbore, and if possible, the caliber.

The number of discharges that have impinged upon the body. This is also usually a straightforward matter, but in cases in which two wounds have been superimposed upon one another, difficulties may certainly arise. This is why the total amount of metallic material and associated objects—such as wads and cards—must be recovered as fully as possible from the body.

The range at which the discharge took place, which has already been discussed at length.

The direction from which the shot was fired relative to the body, both in the horizontal and vertical planes. This must be assessed by: (1)

the appearance of the entrance wound, taking account of any departure from a circular pattern of either the skin defect or associated powder blackening and smoke fouling, and any undercutting of the margin at one side; and (2) by the anatomical direction of the track between entrance and exit wound or between entrance and internal damage. Caution must be used where internal structures have been struck by the missile, which may produce distortion of the direction of the track. In shotgun wounds with multiple pellets, diffusion of shot may sometimes render an accurate estimation of direction difficult. The apparent direction within the body of a bullet track is naturally not necessarily the same as its orientation relative to ground level or other fixed structures at the scene of the incident. The direction of the track depends upon the posture of the body at the time of impact. Dogmatic statements about the position of a weapon must be tempered with caution, as it is unsafe to assume that the body was in the normal upright position.

The height from heel level, i.e., from ground level, of the entrance wound and exit wound, must be measured as it may well have some relevance in reconstructing the incident.

When there have been internal thoracic or abdominal injuries, *the volume of blood* in the pleural, pericardial, or peritoneal cavities should be measured, as this may sometimes be of some help in estimating the likely survival time after the injury—or at least indicating that death was not immediate, if there has been time for a large volume to collect. When large vessels such as the aorta, pulmonary veins, or vena cava have been lacerated, this estimation is of little value, as extensive postmortem leakage can occur.

Width of the Bullet Track

Where a projectile, especially one emitted from a weapon with a high muzzle velocity such as an automatic pistol or rifle, passes through tissues, the most noticeable appearance is that the track of damage is far wider than the diameter of the projectile. High-speed cinephotography has revealed that the most extraordinary deformation occurs in a semisolid medium used to simulate brain, lung, liver, or other such organ. When the missile enters the tissue, cinephotography at 8,000 frames per second shows, its passage is followed by an extensive transient cavitation due to lateral transfer of energy, a large semivacuum forming behind the bullet for a width many times the diameter of the projectile. The tissue around this cavity then collapses and pulsates with decreasing amplitude for a few milliseconds, coming to rest with a wide track of destruction of a diameter intermediate between that of the original cavity and that of the projectile.

This effect is best seen with a single projectile from a rifled weapon; the pattern is complicated by the divergent paths of the numerous pellets in a shotgun discharge, though undoubtedly the same effect occurs for each individual pellet, leading to a summation of their effect in the tissues in a more diffuse manner.

Blank Cartridge Injuries

Cartridges filled only with a propellant load and no metallic projectiles can still cause severe injuries. Such ammunition may be used in practice weapons, starting guns, theatrical work, and the like. A paper or plastic cover holds the charge in place in the absence of a missile or pellets.

Wounds can be caused from either the discharge of gases or from the occluding device in the end of the cartridge. When the gun is fired at contact or very close range, the disruption caused by the gases may be as severe as that seen in a wound caused by conventional ammunition. Gonzales, Vance, Helpern, and Umberger reported the death of a boy of 14 years who fired a .32 blank cartridge in contact with the skin of his chest, blowing a hole through the skin, into the costal muscles, pericardium, and right ventricle.

Clothing may be disrupted and carried into the wound, and there is the danger of infection, including tetanus.

A number of cases have been reported in which paper wadding used on top of a blank cartridge caused fatal injuries when discharged at a distance of a few feet. In one classic old case, a member of the audience in a theater, sitting in the gallery, had part of his hand blown away by a piece of greased newspaper that had been discharged from a small cannon on the stage. It is obvious, from the many cases reported over the years, that the severity of injury can be much greater than expected; it depends upon the amount and compression of the wadding, together with the total propellant charge of the cartridge.

Wounds from Veterinary "Humane" Killers

A number of injuries, some fatal, have been described as the result of the use of slaughtering guns employed in abattoirs and by veterinary surgeons. These are of two main types: one resembles a handgun, but instead of a free projectile, a steel "captive bolt" emerges through the muzzle, propelled by a blank cartridge behind. The other type consists of a metal bell a few inches in diameter, the face shaped to fit the head of a large animal, behind which is a metal tube. A bullet-containing cartridge is fitted into the end of this tube, the bell applied to the animal, and the end of the rod struck a blow, which detonates the cartridge, sending the bullet down the tube and into the animal's head.

Both these weapons have been used by suicides, and accidental discharges have caused human injuries and fatalities. Polson, and Hunt and Kon have described injuries from these instruments.

Weapons that fire a free bullet are usually of about 0.32 caliber; the captive bolt extends from the muzzle for a distance of about 5 cm. The face surface of the bell of one type of weapon often has a pattern of concentric circles, presumably intended to stop slipping, and these may be imprinted upon the human skin after discharge.

Weapons of a similar nature are used in the building industry for driving fixing devices into masonry. These are variously known as "masonry guns," "nail guns," or "stud guns" and fire a hardened steel pin into concrete or similar material by means of a blank cartridge. A number of wounds have been reported, caused either by direct impact on the human body or by ricochet from the masonry surface. Exceptionally, a pin has penetrated a thin partition and wounded workmen on the other side.

SELECTED READINGS

GENERAL SOURCES

1. Glaister, J., and Rentoul, E.: *Medical Jurisprudence and Toxicology*. 12th Edition. Edinburgh, E. & S. Livingstone, 1966.
2. Gonzales, T. A., Vance, M., Helpern, M., and Umberger, C. J.: *Legal Medicine*. 2nd Edition. New York, Appleton-Century-Crofts Inc., 1954.
3. Knight, B.: *Legal Aspects of Medical Practice*. London, Churchill-Livingstone, 1972.
4. Picton, B.: *Murder, Suicide or Accident*. London, John Hale & Co. [New York, St. Martin's Press], 1971.
5. Polson, C. J.: *Essentials of Forensic Medicine*. 2nd Edition. Oxford, Pergamon Press, 1965.
6. Simpson, C. K. (Ed.): *Taylor's Principles and Practice of Medical Jurisprudence*. 12th Edition. London, J & A Churchill Ltd., 1965.
7. Sturner, W. Q., and Petty, C. S.: in *Modern Trends in Forensic Medicine*. 3rd Series. Edited by A. K. Mant. London, Butterworth & Co., 1973.

USEFUL ARTICLES

8. Adelson, L.: A microscopic study of dermal gunshot wounds. Am. J. Clin. Pathol., *35*:393, 1961.
9. Black, A. M., Burns, B. D., and Zuckerman, S.: Wounding mechanism of high velocity missiles. In *War Medicine*, Edited by W. S. Pugh. New York, F. Hubner & Co., 1942.
10. Breitenecker, R.: Shotgun wound patterns. Am. J. Clin. Pathol., *52*:258, 1969.
11. Breitenecker, R.: Shotgun patterns. An experimental study on the influence of intermediate targets. J. Forensic Sci., *12*:193, 1967.
12. Callender, G. R.: Wound ballistics: mechanism of production of wounds by small bullets and shell fragments. War Med., *3*:337, 1943.
13. De Muth, W. E., Jr.: Bullet velocity and design as determinants of wounding capability. An experimental study. J. Trauma, *6*:222, 1966.
14. De Muth, W. E., Jr.: The mechanisms of gunshot wounds. J. Trauma, *11*:219, 1971.
15. Di Maio, V. J., and Spitz, W. V.: Injury by birdshot. J. Forensic Sci., *15*:396, 1970.
16. Diamond, F. C., Jr., and Rich, N. M.: M-16 rifle wounds in Vietnam. J. Trauma, *7*:619, 1967.
17. Gonzales, T. A.: Wounds by firearms in civil life. Am. J. Surg., *26*:43, 1934.
18. Graham, J. W., Petty, C. S., Flohr, D. M., and Peterson, W. E.: Forensic aspects of frangible bullets. J. Forensic Sci., *11*:507, 1966.
19. Harvey, E. N., McMillen, S. H., and Puckett, W. O.: Mechanism of wounding. War Med., *8*:91, 1945.
20. Helpern, M., and Hickam, J. B.: Wounding effect of high energy missiles. J. Aviation Med., *17*:504, 1946.
21. Hunt, A. C., and Kon, V. M.: The patterns of injury from humane killers. Med. Sci. Law, *2*:197, 1962.
22. Mant, A. K.: An unusual gunshot injury. Med. Sci. Law, *8*:256, 1968.
23. Mason, M. F., Rose, E., and Alexander, F.: Four nonlethal head wounds resulting from improper revolver ammunition. J. Forensic Sci., *12*:205, 1968.
24. Mattoo, B. N.: Shot penetration from ballistic data. J. Forensic Sci., *14*:521, 1969.
25. Mattoo, B. N., and Nabar, B. S.: Evaluations of effective shot dispersion in buckshot patterns. J. Forensic Sci., *14*:263, 1969.
26. Mattoo, B. N., and Wani, A. K.: Casualty criteria for firearm wounds with special reference to shot penetration. J. Forensic Sci., *14*:120, 1969.
27. Petty, C. S.: Firearms injury research. The role of the practicing pathologist. Am. J. Clin. Pathol., *52*:277, 1969.
28. Petty, C. S.: Advanced Ballistics Workshop for Medical Examiners, South-Western Institute of Forensic Sciences, Dallas, Texas, April 4–6, 1970.
29. Petty, C. S.: In *Medical Jurisprudence*, Edited by J. R. Waltz and F. E. Inbau. New York, Macmillan, 1971, p. 329.
30. Petty, C. S.: Firearms and the Forensic Pathologist. American Society of Clinical Pathologists Commission on Continuing Education, 1966.
31. Petty, C. S., and Hauser, J.: Rifled shotgun slugs: woundings and forensic ballistics. J. Forensic Sci., *13*:144, 1968.
32. Petty, C. S., David, J., and Howard, L.: Factors Modifying Firearms Wounds. American Society of Clinical Pathologists Commision of Continuing Education, Forensic Pathology Seminar, Atlanta, Georgia, September 14, 1970.
33. Smith, S., and Glaister, J.: In *Recent Advances in Forensic Medicine*. 2nd Edition. London, J. & A. Churchill, 1939.
34. Spitz, L.: Air rifle injuries in children. S. Afr. Med. J., *43*:557, 1969.
35. Spitz, W. U., and Wilhelm, R. M.: Stud gun injuries. J. Forensic Med., *17*:5, 1970.
36. Stahl, C. J.: Forensic aspects of tear-gas pen guns. J. Forensic Sci., *13*:442, 1968.
37. Stahl, C. J., and Davis, J. H.: Missile wounds caused by tear-gas pen guns. Am. J. Clin. Pathol., *52*:270, 1969.
38. Vance, B. M.: Bullet wounds of the heart. Am. J. Sci., *168*:872, 1925.

SECTION 2. INJURY BY FIREARMS, BOMBS, AND EXPLOSIVES

chapter 12

THE FORENSIC BALLISTICS LABORATORY

by Stanton O. Berg

This discussion of the forensic ballistics laboratory and its capabilities is intended to provide the pathologist with a ready reference to turn to when confronted with a firearms problem. While a comprehensive treatment of the field of firearms and forensic ballistics is not possible, the fundamentals of firearms, ammunition, and forensic ballistics are broadly and carefully outlined and explored to give him sufficient knowledge and understanding of the subject to appreciate the use, value, limitations, and implications of the firearms evidence that he will encounter in his day-to-day professional work and of the boundaries to the assistance that can reasonably be expected from a forensic ballistics laboratory.

THE SCIENCE OF BALLISTICS

As with most technical subjects, the basic definitions and associated terms are important to a proper understanding. Accordingly a discussion of the essential terms follows.

Types of Ballistics

Interior Ballistics. Interior ballistics (internal ballistics) is that branch of the science of ballistics that deals with what happens to a cartridge and its bullet from the time the trigger of the gun is pulled until the bullet exits from the gun barrel—those things that happen in the interior of the gun barrel and chamber. It deals with primers, primer ignition, gunpowders, burn rate, rifling, rate of rifling twist, chamber and barrel dimensions, breech pressure, and velocity.

Exterior Ballistics. Exterior ballistics (external ballistics) is the branch of the science of ballistics that deals with what happens to a bullet or projectile from the moment it leaves the gun barrel to the moment of impact on a target or object. Essentially, exterior ballistics is concerned with the flight of the bullet and the bullet trajectory. It deals with air resistance, bullet drop and gravity, bullet drift, and bullet stability.

Terminal Ballistics. Terminal ballistics is concerned with the effect of the bullet on the target at impact and until it comes to rest. The bullet penetration and the release of bullet energy are some of the factors considered.

Wound Ballistics. Wound ballistics is a part of terminal ballistics. As its name implys, it relates to the bullet effects resulting in wounds to persons or animals. Penetration, severity, and appearance of the wound are some of the factors considered.

Forensic Ballistics. Also known as firearms identification, this is one of the departments of the forensic sciences. Forensic ballistics deals with the examination of fired bullets and cartridge cases and their identification as having been fired in a particular gun to the exclusion of all others. It also relates to distance determinations made from an examination of shot pellet patterns and firearms combustion residue patterns. In a broad sense it may be considered as any scientific investigation of firearms evidence in a criminal or civil matter of litigation. The term was coined by Col. Calvin H. Goddard, the American pioneer in this field. There is some controversy among firearms examiners whether "forensic ballistics" or "firearms identification" is the proper designation for the science. In any event, it seems beyond dispute that the term "forensic ballistics" has caught both the public and the story writers' fancy, and it is unlikely that it will give way to the rather ambiguous term of "firearms identification."

Physics Basic to Ballistics

Velocity

In physics, velocity has two components. It has speed or rate of motion and it has direction of motion. As commonly used in the field of firearms, velocity refers simply to the speed of the bullet or projectile at a predetermined point in its flight. The cartridge manufacturers usually publish ballistics tables in which they show the approximate bullet velocity of the particular cartridge at the muzzle of the gun. In the case of centerfire rifles, the remaining velocity also is usually shown at distances of 100, 200, and 300 yd, and the corresponding energy figures are also given for the same points of distance. Velocity is commonly expressed in feet per second (fps); for example, a .38 special cartridge with a 158-grain bullet may have a muzzle velocity of 855 fps.

Energy

There are two basic types of energy: *static* or *potential energy*, and *motion* or *kinetic energy*. In firearms and ballistics the term "energy" has reference to kinetic energy or energy due to motion. Energy, the capacity for doing work, is expressed in foot-pounds (ft-lb). This unit has reference to the work (or force) resulting when a weight of 1 lb is dropped from a height of 1 ft. For example, the aforementioned .38 special 158-grain bullet at a velocity of 855 fps would have an energy of 256 ft-lb. The formula for kinetic energy is:

$$E_k = \frac{MV^2}{2}$$

Inertia

Inertia is defined by Newton's first law of motion, which basically states that a body at rest will tend to remain at rest and a body in motion will tend to remain in motion unless acted on by outside forces. A bullet that has been shot out of a gun barrel tends to continue to move forward, but its path (trajectory) and its velocity are changed by the outside forces of air resistance and gravity.

Gravity and Trajectory

Gravity is the force of attraction exerted by a celestial body such as the earth. It is the force that causes all unsupported objects, including bullets, to fall to the earth. As soon as a bullet leaves the gun barrel, gravity begins to act upon it, drawing it toward the earth. Inasmuch as the bullet is also moving outward at the same time as it is being drawn to the earth, the motion follows a curved path called its trajectory. This curve is usually very slight over short distances, and the trajectory may almost appear to be a straight line. Over larger distances, the curved path of the bullet becomes more apparent (Fig. 12–1).

Because of the action of gravity, a bullet must be projected above the line of sight in order to compensate for the gravity drop. The downward acceleration of an object owing to gravity is approximately 32 fps. The higher its velocity, the greater the distance a bullet can travel outward before being drawn to the ground, and consequently the less the compensation for drop that must be made over a given distance. One might describe it as a race of the bullet to move forward or outward as far as possible before being grounded by gravity.

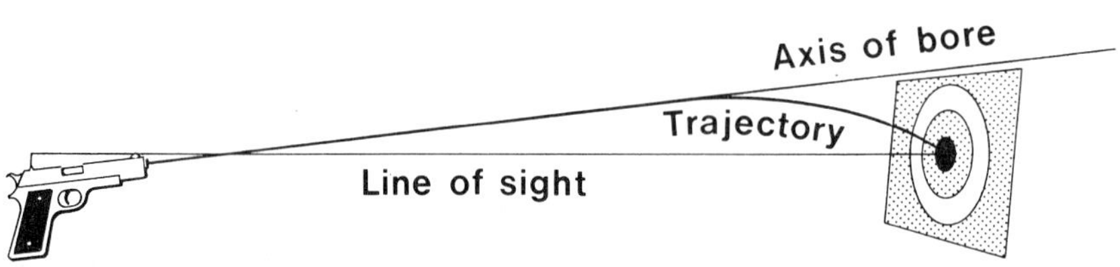

Figure 12–1. Diagram of a bullet's trajectory (exaggerated for clarity).

Ballistics Coefficient

This is a technical term (abbreviated as C) used to describe the ability of a bullet to maintain its velocity against air resistance. Mathematically it is calculated from a formula ($C = \frac{M}{id^2}$ in which M is mass, i is a form factor, and d is diameter) in which the sectional density (weight in relation to cross-section) of a bullet is divided by a form factor (shape of the bullet). The larger the coefficient, the more efficient the bullet or projectile. Air resistance and gravity are the two most significant forces acting upon a bullet during its flight prior to impact on a target. An example of the effect of air resistance can be seen by examining the resulting velocity loss during flight of a .22 long rifle rimfire 40-grain (weight) bullet. Its velocity of 1335 fps at the muzzle drops to 1045 fps at 100 yd because of air resistance. This represents a loss of approximately 22 per cent of the initial velocity. The better the ballistics coefficient of a bullet, the less velocity loss it will suffer over a given distance.

Rifling

Rifling is the name given to the series of spirally cut grooves in the interior of the bores of handguns and rifles. The higher or raised portions of the barrel interior remaining after the grooves have been cut are called the lands. The spiral barrel rifling, composed of an equal number of lands and grooves, may rotate either to the right (clockwise) or to the left (counterclockwise), depending on the preference of the manufacturer. The number of lands and grooves may vary from 2 to more then 20; however, 6 is the most common (Fig. 12–2). The purpose of rifling is to impart a spin to the bullet to stabilize it during its flight (gyroscopic action). One might compare a bullet fired from a rifled barrel to a properly thrown football.

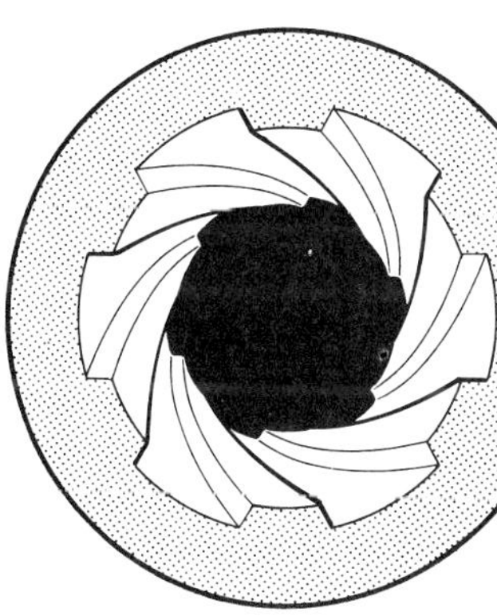

Figure 12–2. Diagram of rifling the bore of a gun barrel.

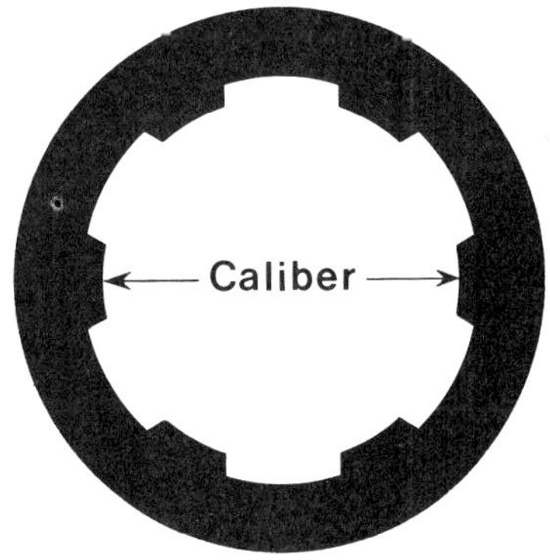

Figure 12–3. Diagram of caliber determination in a gun barrel.

Caliber or Gauge

The caliber of a rifle or handgun is the bore diameter of the rifled barrel, the distance between the two opposite lands (Fig. 12–3). In the United States and England, caliber is measured in decimal fractions of an inch. In Europe the caliber is measured in millimeters. The United States military establishment is converting to the metric system of caliber designation. Cartridge designations unfortunately are not always the same as caliber designations. The classic example is the .38 special cartridge, which is actually .35-caliber in bullet diameter.

In shotguns the bore size is referred to as gauge. The term "gauge" had its origin many years ago when the bore size was designated by the number of round lead balls (to the pound) that would fit the bore. The 12-gauge shotgun, then, would require 12 balls of its bore diameter to make a pound. The exception to this system is the .410 gauge, more properly called the .410 bore, which refers to the bore diameter and has no relation to the number of lead balls to a pound.

THE LABORATORY

Most firearms laboratories handling evidence in criminal cases are operated by a branch of the government, whether it be at federal, state, county, or municipal level. Where such laboratories are located within, or are a part of the police department, they are usually staffed by members of that particular police department. State crime laboratories (and their firearms sections) are usually staffed by civilians, except perhaps where such laboratories are a branch, or unit, of a state police organization. Laboratories of this type are usually equipped to handle most examinations of firearms and related evidence of a criminal nature. They provide laboratory services to law enforcement and governmental investigative agencies within their particular jurisdictional limits. Normally they do not provide services in connection with purely civil matters. The laboratory may, however, be involved in investigating the criminal aspects of a case that later may be the subject of civil litigation. Purely civil cases (firearms accidents) are handled by an independent laboratory or an independent firearms examiner. In contrast to the number of crime laboratories, there are very few independent arms laboratories or examiners available, and overall, the volume of firearms work available to them is somewhat limited. Because of the relatively large number of governmental police laboratories, the prosecution in a criminal case rarely utilizes the services of an independent firearms examiner. It has also been infrequent in the past that an independent was utilized by the defense attorney. At least in part, this is due to the high professional and ethical standards maintained by government laboratory personnel. Frequently, when an independent is employed by the defense in a criminal case, it is to interpret and analyze firearms evidence for an attorney who has little or no knowledge of firearms. Such usage can be expected to become more common in the future because of the influence of the many criminal law seminars and institutes on both state and local levels that are at present being sponsored by the universities and bar associations. The bulk of the independent examiner's work at the present time is therefore in the civil litigation field (e.g., hunting and shooting accidents, product failures, and questionable suicide or accident cases involving insurance). The ethical standards of most of our law enforcement laboratories do not permit members of their staffs to handle private or civil case work. While the volume of civil firearms cases has not been great in the past, it is expected that this area will show significant growth in the future because of the virtual legal revolution that has occurred in the products liability field, with movement away from the old legal concept of warranty-privity of contract and negligence to doctrines of strict and absolute liability. This is currently reinforced by a greater concentration of legal effort and education in products work.

Functions and Capabilities of a Firearms or Ballistics Laboratory

The services rendered by most governmental firearms laboratories generally consist of (but are not restricted to): (1) examination of evidence fired bullets or evidence fired cartridge cases and a particular firearm to determine if the bullet or cartridge case was fired from that firearm; (2) examination of two or more evidence fired bullets or cartridge cases to determine whether they were all fired from the same gun; (3) examination of fired bullets and cartridge cases for possible determination of the make and model of the gun from which they were fired; (4) examination of cartridges, bullets, cartridge cases, and other ammunition components to determine the identity of the manufacturer; (5) test firing for powder and combustion residue patterns for possible determination of the distance between the gun muzzle and the victim or the target at the time the shot was fired; (6) test firing for shot patterns for possible distance determination; and (7) tests of firearm trigger pulls and general function or safety (important from the standpoint of possible accidental discharges).

The laboratory of the independent firearms examiner, in addition to the foregoing, also determines and analyzes the causes of cartridge or firearms failures (of a burst or blown up gun and cartridge, or of accidental discharges), analyzes design and operational features (for example, measuring velocity and pressure), and performs similar related services.

Instrumentation

Although the instrumentation of a ballistics or firearms laboratory is somewhat dependent on the services offered, there is some very basic equipment that is found in the majority of laboratories.

The workhorse of almost every laboratory is a *stereomicroscope* (Fig. 12–4). Such a microscope permits long working distances and a wide field of view, the images are right side up and three-dimensional, and a wide range of examinations can be carried out. It can be used to examine bullets, cartridges, gunpowder and other cartridge components, and bullet holes and surfaces around such holes, as well as surfaces of firearms or firearms parts. It is an extremely useful instrument.

The basic instrument for bullet and cartridge identification (the matching of a particular bullet or cartridge case to a specific gun) is the *comparison microscope* (Fig. 12–5). It is basically two microscopes joined together by a comparison bridge and eyepiece, and permits the viewing of a portion (usually half) of the field of view from each microscope side by side in the eyepiece, which may be of either the monocular of binocular type. The examiner can view a portion of two different bullets or cartridge cases simultaneously in a single microscopic field and determine points of similarity or difference between them. Further discussion of the actual comparison techniques follows later.

Many times a standard laboratory microscope is equipped with a filar micrometer eyepiece and a mechanical stage with a bullet holder for making measurements of rifling marks on a bullet. Such a microscope may be used for any measurements requiring the precision of a thousandth of an inch.

The laboratory also has photographic equipment permitting photography through the various microscopes as well as of guns, cartridges, their components, and other related evidence.

In addition, numerous miscellaneous instruments are used, such as a micrometer and vernier calipers and gauges, barrel interior inspecting devices, scales, and balances. A bullet recovery box or tank should also be available to recover test-fired bullets in an undamaged condition.

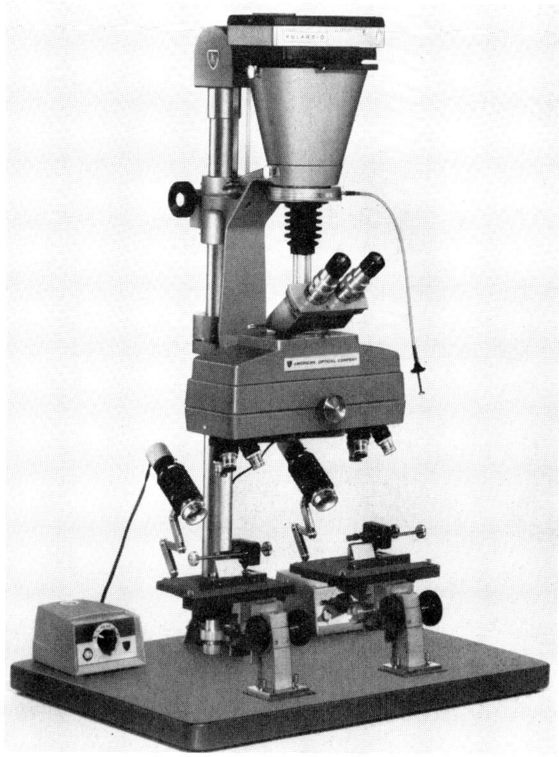

Figure 12–5. American Optical forensic comparison microscope. (Courtesy of the American Optical Corporation.)

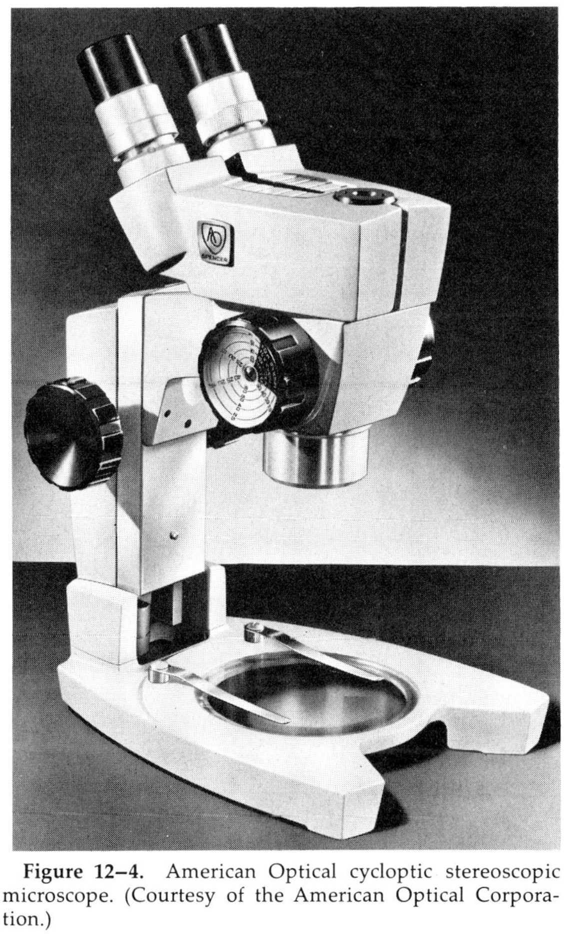

Figure 12–4. American Optical cycloptic stereoscopic microscope. (Courtesy of the American Optical Corporation.)

The independent laboratory, in addition to the foregoing, would have such instruments as are needed for products liability investigations: velocity chronographs, pressure barrels, metal hardness testers, and reloading equipment.

Reference Collections

Every firearms laboratory has a critical need for an abundance of reference material. The reference collections are a constant source of information, and a laboratory functioning without them would be operating under a definite handicap. They include:

Reference Library. A good library of books, published articles, photographs, and color slides covering the many ramifications of firearms, cartridges, firearms investigation and identification, and firearms wounds is essential to an efficient operation.

Reference Collections of Firearms and Materials. Such collections comprise a cartridge collection (illustrated in Figure 12–6), a gunpowder collection, bullet and shot size collections, specimens of fired bullets and car-

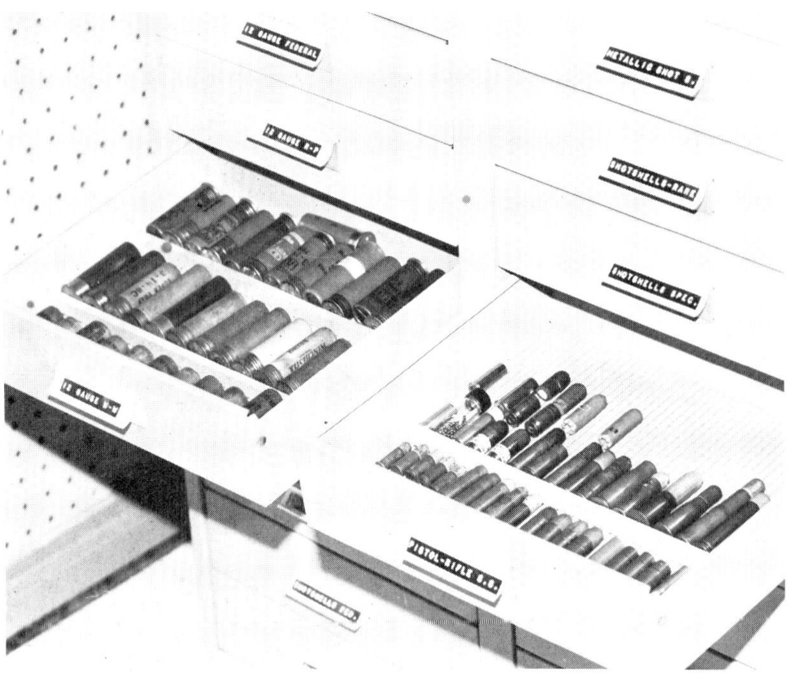

Figure 12–6. Shotshell portion of the author's cartridge collection showing general arrangement.

tridge cases from as many different guns as possible, firearms of basic types and makes, and shot and powder residue pattern collections for varying distances.

To keep such reference collections and materials up to date, they must constantly be added to. Most laboratories subscribe to the pertinent professional journals and firearms publications and maintain membership in professional societies and organizations.

The Report of Examination

The report of the findings of the firearms laboratory examination tends to vary greatly between laboratories and individual examiners; no standard form is utilized in reporting on an examination. The reports of most government laboratories tend to be very brief and are usually confined to a list of the items of evidence received by the laboratory for examination and a short statement of the conclusions reached as a result of such examinations (Fig. 12–7). Usually, the procedures followed and the findings that resulted in the conclusions are not covered in the report. Photographs and diagrams are usually not attached, but the laboratories are prepared to make up special court exhibits when these are requested or needed.

The reports of independent examiners and laboratories also tend to vary, but in general are more detailed and go into some depth on the basis for the findings and conclusions. They are frequently supported by diagrams and photographs, and the results of experiments and tests are usually covered in detail. They may be form reports, with detailed comments, or may be of a narrative type. Such detail is usually not needed in the initial reports of the crime laboratories' findings, but the greater detail in the independent reports is necessary because they are concerned with matters of civil litigation, are directed to the attorneys representing the parties, and may constitute almost the entire basis for either defending or pressing a claim for damage. The reports may be used for preparation of or for negotiation and settlement of the cases. In criminal cases, however, many times the firearms evidence makes up only a single facet of the overall evidence. Figure 12–8 is an example of the author's report of findings in an examination for safety function.

HISTORICAL BACKGROUND

Forensic Ballistics (Firearms Identification)

In looking back to find the roots of our present-day science of forensic ballistics or firearms identification we must go back to the mid 1800's when some very basic and elementary principles were applied to simple forms of

Text continued on page 536

CONFIDENTIAL REPORT OF LABORATORY FINDINGS
DJ-LE-103 (Rev. 4/73)

STATE OF WISCONSIN / DEPARTMENT OF JUSTICE
Division of Law Enforcement Services
CRIME LABORATORY BUREAU
4706 University Avenue
Madison, Wisconsin 53705

District Attorney:

Date: January 1, 1974

Submitting Agency:

Case No.: 74-000

Other Agencies:

Agency No.:

Case Name: Doe, John (V) - Shooting Investigation, City, County, State

Laboratory Analyst:

I do hereby certify this document, consisting of 1 page(s), to be a true and correct report of the findings of the Crime Laboratory Bureau on the items examined as shown by this report.

ADMINISTRATOR
TITLE

SIGNATURE

The Smith and Wesson Model 10 Military and Police .38 Special caliber double action revolver, serial number 000000, item A, was examined, test fired and found to be mechanically functional.

Trigger pull determinations revealed that a pull of approximately 3-1/2 and 8-3/4 pounds was required to fire the revolver single and double action, respectively.

Comparison microscope examinations were made involving the submitted .38 caliber fired bullets, items B, C, and D and test fired bullets from the above revolver. Based on the marked similarity of rifling class and individual characteristics observed common to the test fired bullets and items B, C, and D it is the opinion of the examiner that the bullets, items B, C, and D, were fired from the above described revolver, item A.

Similar comparison microscope examinations were made involving the submitted Remington-Peters .38 Special caliber fired cartridge cases, items E, F, and G, and cartridge cases test fired in the above revolver. Based on the marked similarity of class and individual characteristics observed common to the firing pin and breech face impressions on items E, F, and G and the test fired cartridge cases, it is the opininon of the examiner that the cartridge cases, items E, F, and G, had been fired in the previously described revolver, item A.

DISTRIBUTION: White - Laboratory
Canary - District Attorney
Blue - District Attorney
Pink - Submitting Agency
Green - Extra

Figure 12–7. Example of a state crime laboratory report of examination of firearms evidence. (Courtesy of The Crime Laboratory Bureau of the State of Wisconsin.)

STANTON O. BERG

Firearms Examiner

6025 GARDENA LANE N. E. MINNEAPOLIS, MINN. 55432

788 - 7132

Date: 22 February 1973

FIREARMS EXAMINATION REPORT

1. **IDENTIFICATION. Source:** Received from Jim Jones of Jones, Jones, Jones & Jones, 815 Cargill Bldg., Northstar Center, Minneapolis, Minn. on 10 Feb. 1973.

Make: Suinimra **Caliber:** .38 Special

Model: M W 38 **Type:** Revolver **Action:** Double Action

Magazine: 6 chamber cylinder **Serial No.:** 402115

Special Markings: Left Upper front of frame: Stamping of a "Head". Under the "Head" is the markings: "M W 38" On the left lower front of the frame: Three German proof marks. Also proof mark on left side of barrel. Above the grip on the left side is a black and gold medallion of a "Head" with the wording" "Suinimra". On right lower side of frame: "Made in Germany". Serial No. on right front side of frame.

2. **PRELIMINARY DATA. Case or Holster:** Received in a holster.

Description: Black leather holster with strap. Marked "Federal Man" B450. It appears that a bullet has been fired through the end of the holster. Perforation with sooty interior.

Position of Safety: None **Loaded or unloaded:** Unloaded

See comments on next page concerning safety feature.

Barrel or Cylinder residues: The barrel and cylinder has light amount of combustion residues.

NOTE: Gun and holster were tagged as follows: "Jones, Jones, Jones & Jones, 815 Cargill Bldg., Northstar Center, Minneapolis, Minn.

3. **CONDITION. Grips or stocks:** Two piece molded brown plastic grips. Small nicks, scratches and abrasions on the surface.

Metal Parts: Blued finish is largely intact. All metal parts have a few nicks, scratches and abrasions. **Screw Heads:** Good - slightly burred.

Missing or altered parts: Ordinary stove bolt used to hold grips to frame.

4. **Barrel Rifling:** Right Twist-10 grooves. **Condition:** Good.

Barrel Length: Approx. 4 inches.

Sights: Ramp style - Flat top front sight. Rear sight is milled slot in frame.

Figure 12–8. Example of the author's firearms examination in a civil case.

Illustration continued on opposite page

FIREARMS EXAMINATION REPORT CONT. -2- **Date:** 22 February 1973
Suinimra Model MW 38, No. 402115

Weight: Approx. 31 ounces. (unloaded) **Trigger Pull:** Double Action: 17 lbs. Single Action: Approx. 5½ lbs.

Breech Face: Horizontal tool marks. Firing pin has circular tool marks. Pushing on rear of hammer will permit the firing pin to protrude approx. .010" from the breech face surface.

5. **SAFETY:** The firing pin is separate spring loaded rebounding type contained within the recoil shield. When the trigger is held to the rear the hammer in falling is free to strike the rear of the firing pin. A safety block is provided to prevent the hammer from contacting the rear of the firing pin except when the trigger is held fully to the rear. As pointed out above, the hammer is permitted to contact the rear of the firing pin slightly. This is sufficient to move the firing pin out of the firing pin hole beyond the breech face surface approx. .010". To this extent the safety block is partially ineffective. If the hammer did not make contact, the firing pin spring would hold the firing pin

6. **TEST FIRING. Ammunition:** REMINGTON .38 Special Police (continued below)

Service. 158 grain lead bullet. Index 5138. 25 rounds.

Ejection: Hand ejection - Without malfunction.

Mechanical Operation: Cylinder rotates to the right. After firing the 1st and 2nd rounds the gun cocks hard for the 3rd thru 6th rounds. This was due to the fired cases dragging against the breech face as the cylinder is rotated. Cylinder crane is loose and wobbly due to loose screw or bolt running through crane.

Malfunctions: Firing, extraction and ejection without malfunction. Examination of the test fired and recovered bullets would indicate improper cylinder to barrel alignment.

NOTE: SEE EXPERIMENTS BELOW, CONDUCTED WITH UNLOADED BUT PRIMED CARTRIDGE CASES.

7. **ADDITIONAL NOTES AND COMMENTS:** 5. Cont. in a retracted position within the firing pin hole. This does result in a safety hazard in that without the trigger being depressed the hammer can bring the firing pin into contact with the primer on a cartridge case. I experimented with primed cartridges in which the bullet and powder had been removed. I lifted the hammer a short distance and let it drop(with no trigger pressure) The primer fired. I tried the same experiment with the gun in the holster and the strap across the back of the hammer. There is enough play between the strap and the hammer to permit the hammer to be lifted approx. .3". Again the primer fired. Further experiments were conducted with primed cases in which the rear of the hammer was struck a blow. A rubber hammer was used to simulate a sudden blow by a firm part of the body such as the forearm etc. Although significant primer indentation was achieved each time this was tried, only one out of four primed cartridge cases fired in this manner. However if a steel hammer was used, only a light tap was needed to fire the primed cases. Three out of three fired in this manner.
The Gun is defective in that the safety block does not prevent the hammer from contacting and moving the firing pin forward.

STANTON O. BERG

(SB 5/69)
(-10/72)

Figure 12–8 *continued.*

identification. These principles were later gradually expanded and built upon until, in the early portion of this century, a science evolved.

Early Beginnings

1835—London. A policeman, Henry Goddard, secured the conviction of a murderer by matching a bullet with a flaw to a bullet mold that produced exactly the same flaw in all bullets cast from it. The mold had in it a gouge that produced a ridge on the bullet.

1863—United States: The Civil War. A bullet was identified by caliber and shape. Confederate General Stonewall Jackson was fatally wounded on the evening of May 2 at Chancellorsville, Virginia, under unusual circumstances. An examination of the bullet removed from his wound revealed it to be a round ball of .67 caliber. It then became apparent that the wound had been accidentally inflicted by one of his own men. The ball was of the type used in an obsolete musket common to Hill's division of the Confederate Army, while the bullet in common use in the Union Army was a cylindroconoidal-shaped .58-caliber minié ball.

1879—Minnesota. The case of *Minnesota* vs. *Edward Lawlor* involved simple identification by rifling marks on a bullet. This is a rather colorful case that arose in the city of Winona and involved a bordello operator known as French Lou. Three gentlemen got into an altercation over Lou's affections, with the result that one was shot to death. The question then arose of which of the remaining two had done the shooting. One was armed with a .32-caliber Smith and Wesson revolver, and the other with a .32-caliber Hood revolver. At the trial, a gunsmith was permitted to testify that the Smith and Wesson had a rifled barrel, whereas the Hood did not, except for some false rifling grooves at the muzzle. The gunsmith's testimony concluded that from their appearance, the bullets taken from the decedent's body could not have come from the Smith and Wesson, but might well have come from the Hood revolver.

1900—Buffalo, New York. The first significant literature on bullet identification by rifling marks, an article entitled "The Missile and the Weapon," by Dr. Albert L. Hall, appeared in the June 1900 *Buffalo Medical Journal*. The article covered in detail how measurements of land and groove markings as well as measurements of bullet diameter are made. It also called attention to the variations in bullet shape and style between manufacturers.

Advent as a Science—The Early Pioneers

In the early 1900's, the science had progressed to the point that bullets and cartridge cases could be linked and identified to a particular gun.

1907—The Brownsville, Texas, Riot. In 1907 some soldiers from a United States Infantry regiment were involved in a riot in the town of Brownsville. After the riot, 39 cartridge cases from .30-caliber rifles were recovered, as well as some bullets. This evidence, along with the suspected rifles, was sent to the staff at Frankford Arsenal for examination. The staff at the Arsenal studied the evidence and determined that the fired cartridge cases could be identified with the guns that fired them by matching the breech face markings on the cases; 33 of the fired cartridge cases were identified with four of the suspected rifles. The other six fired cases could not be linked to any of the guns submitted. No conclusions were drawn about the fired bullets.

1909–1923—Paris, France. During this period, V. Balthazard, a professor of legal medicine at the University of Paris, published a number of papers on his method of identifying bullets to a particular gun by taking a series of photographs of rifling marks around the bullets' circumference. Such photographs of test and evidence bullets were then enlarged and compared. Balthazard also made cartridge case identification through photographs based on the firing pin, extractor, ejector, and breech face markings and their comparison. During the same period of time, work was being done in Great Britain by Sir Sydney Smith, Hugh Pollard, and A. Lucas.

1925–New York. This was a most significant year. Four gentlemen joined their talents together and became known as the Bureau of Forensic Ballistics. These gentlemen were Mr. C. E. Waite, a special investigator of the New York attorney general's department, Mr. Philip O. Gravelle, a microscopist and photographer, Mr. John H. Fisher, a tool designer and authority on precision measurements, and Lt. Col. Calvin H. Goddard, an Ordnance Reserve officer. This association resulted in a number of significant events. The *comparison microscope* was adapted to bullet and cartridge identification at the suggestion of Mr. Gravelle. Although the microscope had been used in other fields for the comparison of similar substances, this is its first known application to firearms evidence. Microscopic examination and comparison has remained the standard method of bullet and cartridge identification. The Bureau of Forensic Ballistics, through Fisher's initiative, also developed the helixometer to measure the twist of rifling and to examine the interior of a gun barrel. This instrument's practical use is limited to the needs of the advanced researcher. The term "forensic ballistics" was also coined by Goddard at that time. The term has proved popular with the public and with writers, although many firearms examiners do not consider it properly descriptive of the science and prefer "firearms identification" instead. Goddard produced a number of articles on the subject during this period, the first of which appeared in *Army Ordnance* magazine of November-December 1925 under the title "Forensic Ballistics." He later moved his laboratory to Chicago and established the Scientific Crime Detection Laboratory at Northwestern University in 1930.

The Refinements

The comparison microscope has remained the basic instrument for cartridge and bullet comparison and identification for over 50 years. The instruments are now much improved and more convenient to use. Binocular eyepieces are used now rather than the original monocular eyepiece, the field of view can be varied from one side to the other, and bullet and cartridge holders are improved, as is the lighting and the associated photographic equipment.

The science has built up its own body of literature, including several textbooks. The earliest English language text was the one by Burrard, originally published in 1934 in London under the title *The Identification of Firearms and Forensic Ballistics*. This was followed by Hatcher's textbook published in the United States in 1935, *Textbook of Firearms Investigation, Identification and Evidence*. The same year saw *The Identification of Firearms* published by Gunther and Gunther in New York. The Hatcher text was completely rewritten and updated in 1957 by Jury and Weller. In 1958, Davis published his book, *An Introduction to Tool Marks, Firearms and the Striagraph,* in which he presented a new method of firearms identification. Davis adapted the Timken Roller Bearing Company's profilograph to bullet identification and called it the Striagraph. The device records surface irregularities on a graph. Identification is based on a comparison of the graphs of bullet surface irregularities. The most monumental work in the field was produced by Dr. J. H. Mathews, of the University of Wisconsin. This work, *Firearms Identification,* was originally published as two volumes in 1962, with a third volume being added in 1973.

All sciences eventually form their own professional organizations. In 1969, in Chicago, a professional association of firearms and toolmark examiners was formed and called the Association of Firearm and Toolmark Examiners.

Development of Arms and Ammunition

This brief history is intended to give only a bird's-eye view of the development of arms and ammunition and to list some of the more prominent milestones along the way. No in-depth treatment is intended; there are many textbooks that cover the area in great detail for those readers who care to pursue the subject further.

Gunpowder

It is not known for sure who actually discovered gunpowder or when the discovery took place—one of the many events that are lost in the mists of antiquity. For many years, the Chinese have been credited with the discovery of gunpowder sometime in the thirteenth century. This myth persists, although no present-day authority or firearms scholar will credit the Chinese with the discovery and recent research tends to completely discredit the idea. Although Marco Polo crisscrossed China (1254–1324), he did not report seeing as much as one Chinese firecracker. The Mohammedans of Moorish Spain were working with combustible powder in the twelfth century, and it is thought that the Mohammedan traders introduced gunpowder to China via a land route through North Africa. The first record of gunpowder in China is somewhat later.

The use of gunpowder as a propellant for projectiles occurred in the early 1300's. It was first used only in cannons and was later developed for use in crude portable hand firearms called hand cannons. These devices were fired by a burning stick, a lighted match, a hot iron, or a live cinder. The early form of gunpowder, called black powder, was a mixture of sulfur, charcoal, and saltpeter (potassium nitrate). On firing, it produced considerable smoke and combustion residue. In 1885, smokeless powder was developed by Vieille in France. This new propellant lacked the extensive smoke-producing properties of black powder, was cleaner burning, and was more powerful. Gunpowders of the smokeless type were essentially of two kinds. The single-base powder as developed by Vieille in France and the double-base powder developed a little later in 1889 by Abel and Dewar in England. In the single-base powders nitrocellulose was the base. In double base powders, both nitrocellulose and nitroglycerine were the main ingredients. Present day commercial ammunition is all loaded with smokeless powder. Black powder, however, is still available to the "black powder enthusiasts" who enjoy the shooting and use of the old style weapons designed for this particular type of propellant.

Ignition Systems

The development of ignition systems is illustrated in Figure 12–9.

1450—Matchlock System. This is the ap-

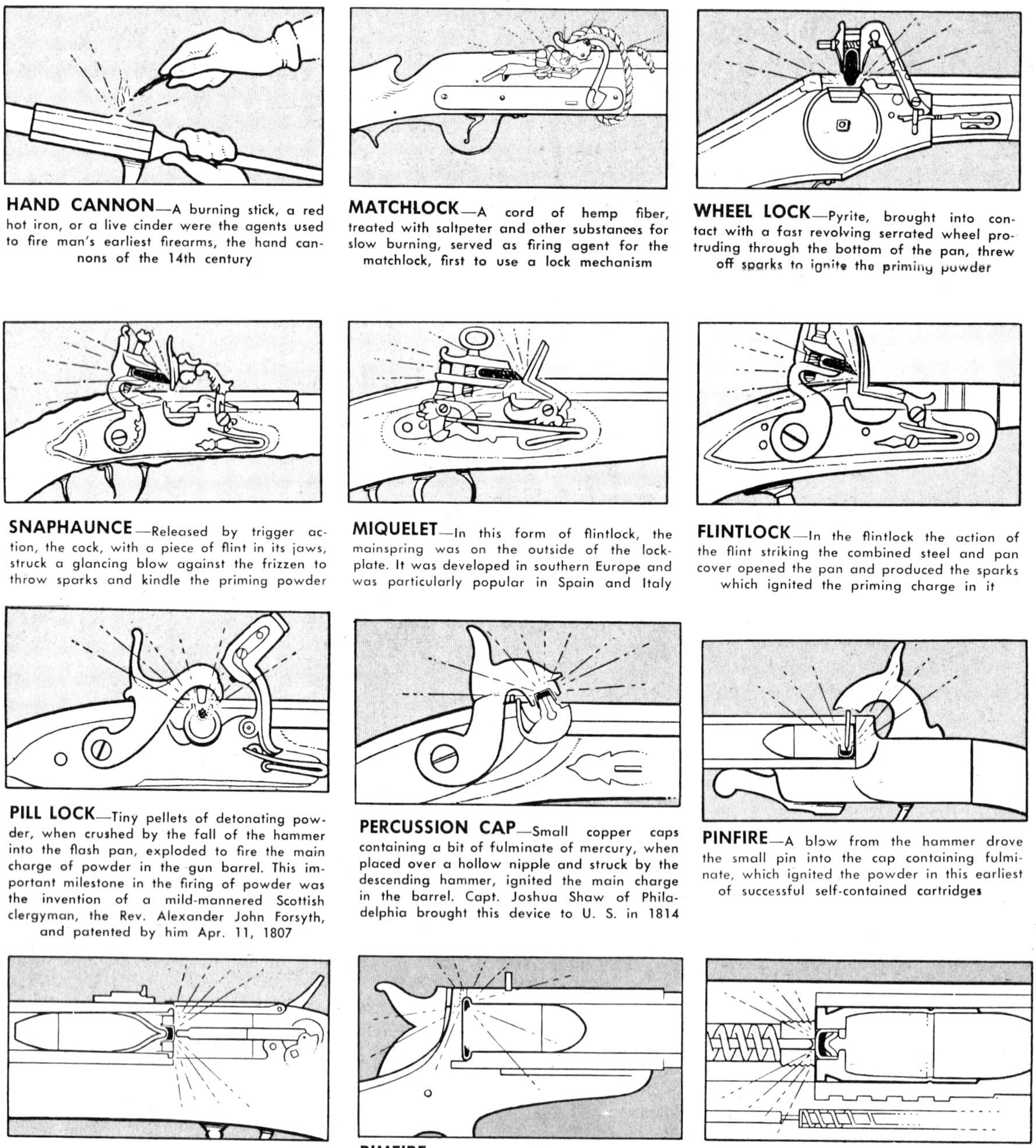

HAND CANNON—A burning stick, a red hot iron, or a live cinder were the agents used to fire man's earliest firearms, the hand cannons of the 14th century

MATCHLOCK—A cord of hemp fiber, treated with saltpeter and other substances for slow burning, served as firing agent for the matchlock, first to use a lock mechanism

WHEEL LOCK—Pyrite, brought into contact with a fast revolving serrated wheel protruding through the bottom of the pan, threw off sparks to ignite the priming powder

SNAPHAUNCE—Released by trigger action, the cock, with a piece of flint in its jaws, struck a glancing blow against the frizzen to throw sparks and kindle the priming powder

MIQUELET—In this form of flintlock, the mainspring was on the outside of the lock-plate. It was developed in southern Europe and was particularly popular in Spain and Italy

FLINTLOCK—In the flintlock the action of the flint striking the combined steel and pan cover opened the pan and produced the sparks which ignited the priming charge in it

PILL LOCK—Tiny pellets of detonating powder, when crushed by the fall of the hammer into the flash pan, exploded to fire the main charge of powder in the gun barrel. This important milestone in the firing of powder was the invention of a mild-mannered Scottish clergyman, the Rev. Alexander John Forsyth, and patented by him Apr. 11, 1807

PERCUSSION CAP—Small copper caps containing a bit of fulminate of mercury, when placed over a hollow nipple and struck by the descending hammer, ignited the main charge in the barrel. Capt. Joshua Shaw of Philadelphia brought this device to U. S. in 1814

PINFIRE—A blow from the hammer drove the small pin into the cap containing fulminate, which ignited the powder in this earliest of successful self-contained cartridges

MORSE—A percussion cap was exploded when crushed against the heavy wire anvil attached to the inside of the case of this early metallic cartridge patented in 1858

RIMFIRE—Containing fulminate in its rim, this cartridge has undergone but little change in outward appearance since it was developed by Smith & Wesson nearly a century ago

RIMLESS—Utilizing a modern primer embodying the action of both explosive compound and anvil, the present-day center-fire cartridges are the result of centuries of development

Figure 12–9. Firearms ignition systems. (Courtesy of the National Rifle Association of America.)

proximate date that the matchlock system of ignition of propellants in firearms was developed. This was a decided improvement over the ignition system for the hand cannon described earlier. A device was attached to the gun to hold a lighted, specially treated cord and to bring it into contact with the powder charge in the gun.

1517—Wheel Lock System. In this system, invented by a German by the name of Johan Kiefuss, pyrite was brought into contact with a fast-moving serrated wheel (spring action previously hand wound), which threw sparks into a pan of priming powder. It was a swifter, surer, and more convenient form of ignition.

1575—First Cartridge. This early form of cartridge has very little in common with present-day cartridges. Essentially, it was a paper package containing the projectile and a premeasured amount of powder. Its advantage was in the speed of loading and avoidance of the inconvenience of carrying loose powder.

1550–1615—Flintlock Firearm. This firearm was developed in stages, the Snaphounce, the earliest version, coming out in 1550 in Scandinavia. The ignition system utilized the striking action of a cock and flint against a battery, or frizzen, to produce a shower of sparks into a primed pan. This was followed in 1600 by the miquelet lock (Spanish and Italian) and the English dog lock. These versions combined the battery and the priming pan cover into one unit. Finally, in 1615, the refined flintlock came into being in France. It had the foregoing refinements, but the significant difference was an internal lock mechanism in place of the exposed mechanisms used in the earlier versions.

1776—Breech-Loading Firearm. This year saw the introduction of a breech-loading firearm in place of the previous muzzle-loading arms. The Ferguson breech-loading rifles were placed in use in the British Army at this time.

1807—Percussion System. This system was developed by the Scottish clergyman Alexander J. Forsyth, who determined that certain compounds could be detonated by a blow and could be used to ignite powder charges in a firearm. These compounds were formed into tiny pellets and used in a gun with a hammer to strike and detonate them. Such firearms were called pill locks.

1814—Percussion Cap. Joshua Shaw, from Philadelphia, developed a percussion cap using the Forsyth principles. This cap contained a detonating compound and became the most commonly used primer for the muzzle-loading firearm.

1835—Revolver. Samuel Colt patented his revolver in this year. The first practical revolver, it contained a cylinder with a number of drilled-through chambers. The cocking of the hammer rotated the cylinder to bring a fresh chamber and cartridge in line with the barrel.

1836—Pin-Fire Cartridge. In this cartridge, developed by LeFaucheux in France, a protruding pin was struck by the hammer and driven into the interior of the cartridge and into a cap of priming mixture. It is considered to be the first self-contained cartridge to come into general use. By "self-contained cartridge" we mean the bullet, the powder, and the primer all together in one unit with the cartridge case.

1845—Rimfire Cartridge. Flobert, in France, developed the first rimfire cartridge, which he called the "bullet breech." In this cartridge the priming compound is contained in a hollow cartridge rim. The gun's firing pin, or hammer, strikes the cartridge rim, crushing it and detonating the priming compound.

1858—Centerfire Cartridge. This cartridge, developed by Morse and containing a percussion cap in the center of the head of the cartridge, was introduced at this time. The event marked the beginning of a series of rapid developments in centerfired cartridges. The basic centerfire and rimfire methods of ignition are the standards for modern ammunition.

1884—Machine Gun. Hiram Maxim, in the United States, designed the first fully automatic firearm in which the recoil of the weapon served to load and fire the gun as long as the trigger was depressed and ammunition remained. It had a profound effect on warfare.

1892—Automatic Pistol. These pistols are more properly called semiautomatic, or self-loading, because they require a separate pull on the trigger to fire each shot. The first practical pistol of this type was designed by Schonberger and manufactured in Austria. There is some dispute as to who produced the first successful automatic pistol, but it is generally conceded that the first *commercially* successful one was designed by an American, Borchardt, in 1893.

Rifling

The first references to rifling are found between the years 1450 and 1500 and seem to have originated in Germany and Austria. It was, however, many years after this that rifling came into general use. Rifling is, as described and illustrated earlier, the helical grooving that runs lengthwise along the inside of the barrel. Rifling methods and types have taken many forms over the years.

MODERN FIREARMS

This discussion is intended to give the working doctor and pathologist only general information about the more common types of guns that he will encounter in his day-to-day work so that he will be able to differentiate between them. Most modern firearms are equipped with a safety device that may either lock the trigger or block and lock the sear mechanism. The sear mechanism is simply a lever arrangement between the trigger and the hammer or the firing pin. Safeties cannot be relied upon because during the lifetime of a gun they may become worn and defective.

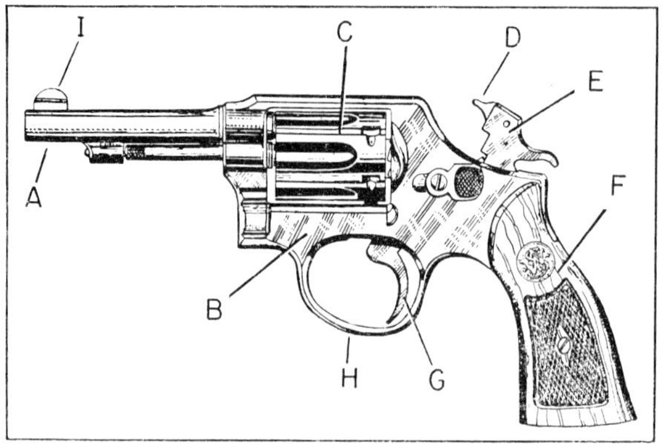

Figure 12–10. A typical revolver. A, Barrel; B, frame; C, cylinder; D, firing pin; E, hammer; F, grips; G, trigger; H, trigger guard; I, front sight. (Courtesy of the Institute of Applied Science.)

Handguns

This is the class of guns that is most commonly encountered in police investigations. A handgun is intended to be held and fired from one hand. Most modern ones have barrels with spirally cut rifling grooves down the length of the barrel.

There are a great many handgun manufacturers, both domestic and foreign. A few of the better-known American manufacturers are Smith & Wesson, Colt, Harrington & Richardson, Iver Johnson, High Standard, and Ruger. Generally, handguns are of three distinct types.

The simplest form of handgun is the *single-shot pistol.* This gun has no magazine or cylinder, or similar device, to hold additional cartridges in readiness for firing. The single shot chamber is loaded with a single cartidge, and hence the name. After the single cartidge has been fired, the empty cartridge case must be extracted or ejected from the chamber and replaced with a live cartidge before the gun can again be fired. The barrel frequently tips up or pivots at the chamber to permit loading. Derringer pistols are usually single-shot pistols. Special target pistols are also frequently of the single-shot type. Unfortunately, there is also a type of handgun called the zip gun, which is a crudely hand-fashioned single-shot pistol, utilized primarily by juvenile gangs. Frequently these are fashioned from simple pieces of pipe, tubing, and even automobile radio antennas.

A second type of handgun is the *revolver* (Fig. 12–10). The name comes from the cylinder that revolves or rotates within the frame of the gun. The revolving cylinder (which may rotate to the right or the left, depending on the design) has a series of chambers (usually 5 to 9) into which cartridges are loaded. The cocking of the gun causes the cylinder to rotate, bringing one of the chambers in line with the bore of the barrel so that, upon firing, the bullet will leave the cylinder chamber and enter the barrel and exit from the muzzle shortly thereafter. There is, of necessity, a small gap between the cylinder and the barrel from which combustion residues escape. The revolver may be either a single-action or a double-action type. In the single-action revolver, the hammer must be cocked by hand, after which the gun can be fired by trigger pressure, which releases the hammer. In the double-action revolver a single steady pull on the trigger will both cock and release the hammer. The double-action revolver is more difficult to shoot accurately, because greater trigger pressure is needed to cock the weapon while the shooter is at the same time trying to align his sights properly. Some double-action revolvers do not have exposed hammers. Some revolvers are loaded through a loading gate (on the side of a solid frame), some are loaded by unlatching the top of the frame so that the cylinder tips up and exposes the cylinder chambers (top break), and others by swinging the cylinder out to the side on a crane or yoke.

The third basic type of handgun is the *semiautomatic* or *self-loading pistol* (Fig. 12–11). This gun is frequently referred to as an automatic pistol, but the term is not technically correct. The semiautomatic pistol requires a separate pull on the trigger for each shot that is fired; the true automatic is one in which a single pull on the trigger will permit the gun to fire continually as long as the trigger is depressed and the magazine contains ammunition. The semiautomatic pistol must be manually loaded for the first shot. When the trigger is pulled, the firing pin strikes and fires the cartridge, extracts and ejects the fired cartridge case, cocks the hammer or firing pin, and feeds and loads a fresh cartridge

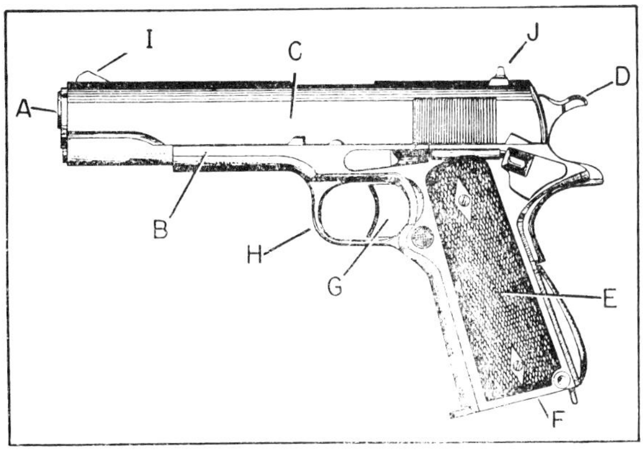

Figure 12–11. A typical semiautomatic pistol. A, Barrel; B, frame; C, slide; D, hammer; E, grips; F, magazine; G, trigger; H, trigger guard; I, front sight; J, rear sight. (Courtesy of the Institute of Applied Science.)

into the chamber. This cycle is repeated each time the trigger is pulled and the gun fired. The extraction, ejection, cocking, feeding, and loading action is all usually the result of the recoil or the blowback operation from the pressure generated in the cartridge on firing. Cartridges are usually fed from a magazine in the grip portion of the frame of the gun.

Rifles

By definition a rifle is, very simply, a firearm intended to be fired from the shoulder. Rifles have bores with rifling grooves running down their length in a spiral fashion to impart spin to the bullet. Short-barrel rifles, usually having a barrel length of less than 22 inches, are generally referred to as carbines.

Like handguns, rifles are made by a great number of different manufacturers, both domestic and foreign. Some of the better-known American manufacturers of rifles are Winchester, Remington, Marlin, Savage, Mossberg, and Ruger.

Rifles can be classified into four common basic types: the slide-action, the bolt-action, the lever-action, and the semiautomatic (Fig. 12–12). The names imply the manner in which the action operates to chamber a cartridge for firing. All four types can be designed to fire either the rimfire or the centerfire cartridge (see later discussion of modern ammunition).

The *slide-action rifle* is frequently referred to as the pump-action, and occasionally as the trombone-action. It is a mechanism in which a manual movement of a slide on the underside of the barrel permits a repeating-type operation. The slide is moved backward and forward to extract and eject a fired case, feed and load a fresh cartridge into the chamber, and cock the gun. The magazine is usually of the tubular type.

The *bolt-action rifle* may be either a single-shot or a repeating rifle. This depends on the presence or absence of a magazine to contain additional cartridges. It is a manually operated rifle in which the bolt and its handle function to open and to close and at the same time lock the breech. The magazine is usually of a box type.

The *lever-action rifle* may be utilized in both single-shot and repeating rifles, but it is more common to the latter. This type utilizes manual operation of a lever usually located beneath the receiver or frame (which also forms the trigger guard). The lever is moved in a swinging and pivoting downward motion and then returned. This acts through a linkage system to open, extract and eject the spent cartridge from, and close and lock the breech block. Unless it is a single-shot version, this action also cocks the hammer and chambers a fresh cartidge. The magazine is usually of the tubular type.

The *semiautomatic rifle* (autoloading, self-loading) very generally operates in a manner similar to the semiautomatic pistol. To function, this type of rifle may employ the recoil or blowback action on firing or it may tap off some

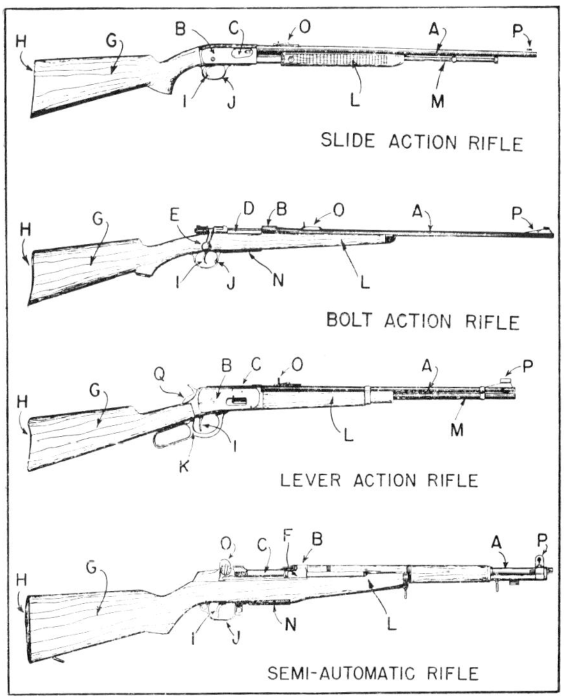

Figure 12–12. Four basic rifle types. A, Barrel; B, receiver; C, breech bolt; D, bolt; E, bolt handle; F, operating handle; G, stock; H, butt plate; I, trigger; J, trigger guard; K, lever; L, forearm; M, tubular magazine; N, box magazine; O, rear sight; P, front sight; Q, hammer. (Courtesy of the Institute of Applied Science.)

of the high-pressure cartridge gases. The magazine may be of either the box or the tubular type.

Shotguns

Shotguns are also shoulder weapons, but normally have a bore with no rifling (smooth bore). Shotguns were originally designed to fire a charge containing one or more round balls or pellets. Special projectiles called rifled slugs have since been designed to be used in shotguns for big game hunting. Shotguns usually have a muzzle constriction at the end of the bore that serves to condense the shot pattern. If the barrel has no constriction at all, it is said to be a cylinder bore. The greatest amount of constriction in a shotgun muzzle is called a full choke. The intermediate type is designated "modified choke." There are variations between these designations also. In general, the greater the amount of constriction, the tighter and smaller the resulting pellet pattern. As with handguns and rifles, there are a great many foreign and domestic manufacturers of shotguns. Some well-known domestic manufacturers are Remington, Winchester, High Standard, Savage (Stevens-Fox), Mossberg, Harrington & Richardson, and Ithaca. There are single-barrel, double-barrel, slide- or pump-action, bolt-action, and semiautomatic or autoloading shotguns; Figure 12–13 shows the more common types. Because the basic actions in shotguns are similar to those previously described for modern weapons, only the *double-barreled shotgun* is described here. As the name implies, the double-barreled shotgun has two barrels, which may be arranged side by side or over and under. The gun is loaded by a break action at the breech in which the barrels, when unlocked by a top lever, pivot upward to permit the cartridges to be inserted. This same action extracts and usually ejects the fired cartridge cases. (The *single-barrel shotgun* usually operates in the same fashion, the barrel chamber being unlatched and pivoting upward.

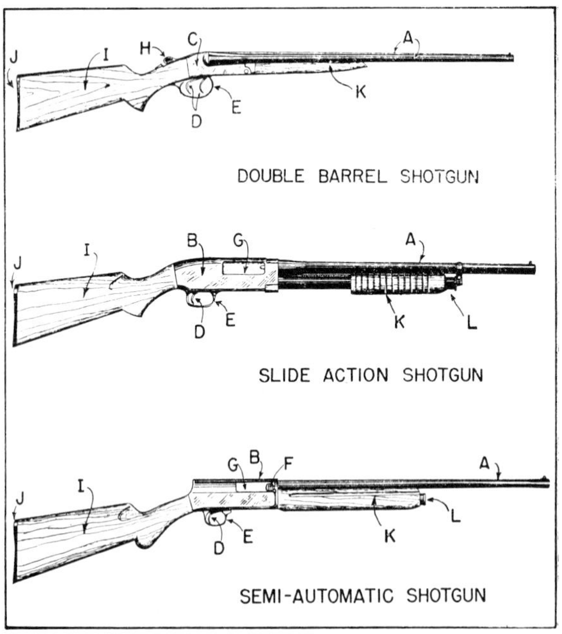

Figure 12–13. Three basic shotgun types. A, Barrel; B, receiver; C, frame; D, trigger; E, trigger guard; F, operating handle; G, breech block; H, top lever; I, stock; J, butt plate; K, forearm; L, magazine. (Courtesy of the Institute of Applied Science.)

Automatic Weapons

The automatic weapon is one that, when the trigger is depressed, will continue to fire as long as the trigger remains depressed and ammunition remains in the magazine. Such weapons are usually for military use, such as machine guns and submachine guns. Fully automatic weapons are sometimes used by the police and quite frequently are found in use among criminals. The famous, or infamous, "Tommy gun" is one of the better-known automatic weapons.

Powder-Actuated Tools (Power Tools)

Modern industry has applied cartridges to the needs of the construction trade in the form of powder-actuated tools, more commonly known as "stud guns." The purpose of these tools is to drive hardened nails, studs, or fasteners into steel and concrete. The total powder-actuated system consists of the tool (the gun), the powder charge, (the cartridge), and the fasteners (the projectile). The cartridges come in various calibers and loadings depending upon the needs of the job at hand. There is also a great variety of fasteners, both threaded and unthreaded. While these tools are made with safeguards, such as muzzle guards and a required minimum pressure against the end of the muzzle or barrel, accidents do occasionally occur, usually when the tool is improperly used or improperly maintained. The number of these accidents is evidenced by the frequency with which wounds received from studs or fasteners are described in the medical literature. Figure 12–14 illustrates the general function, operation, and application of the tool.

MODERN AMMUNITION

Types of Cartridges

During the last 150 years, there have been developed a great many variations in cartridges and their manner of ignition. Insofar as modern ammunition is concerned two methods of cartridge ignition are primarily involved: rimfire ignition and centerfire ignition. The rimfire cartridge gets its name from the location of the priming compound that ignites the cartridge powder around the inside of a hollow cartridge rim. The ignition is accomplished by the firing pin crushing the cartridge rim (Fig. 12–15). The centerfire cartridge, on the other hand, is ignited by means of a primer located in the center of the cartridge head (Fig. 12–16). When we speak of the rimfire cartridge in modern ammunition, we are usually dealing with the .22-caliber rimfire. This cartridge is used in both rifles and handguns. It has been estimated that 6 of every 10 shots fired in the United States is a .22-caliber rimfire; over 3 billion rounds are fired every year. Formerly, there were many calibers of rimfire ammunition. The case formation and the strength are ballistically adapted only to lower pressures and comparatively lower velocity levels, however, and they have been superseded almost entirely (in calibers other than .22) by the modern centerfire cartridge case. Basically, the .22 rimfire cartridge is either the .22 short, the .22 long, or the .22 long rifle. There are also the little-used .22 Winchester automatic and the .22 WRF. While these last two rimfire cartridges mentioned were popular several years ago, they find little usage at present (cf. Figure 12–17 with ballistics tables). There also are special .22-caliber shot and blank cartridges available. The illustrations also show a recent addition to the rimfire field, the 5 mm Remington Magnum rimfire cartridge. Rimfire cartridges are also used in a number of powder-actuated tools.

Essentially, all other modern rifle and handgun ammunition is some form of centerfire ammunition. Centerfire cartridge cases may be either rimmed or rimless. By a rimless case it is meant that the head diameter of the cartridge is approximately the same diameter as the case body. An extractor groove is cut in the head to permit the gun extractor to hook onto the cartridge and pull it from the gun barrel chamber. The rimmed case, on the other hand, has a head or rim of greater diameter than the body of the case. Some less common variations of these two basic types are found in what are called the semirimmed case and the rebated rimless case. The case body in the centerfire cartridge may also be straight, have a straight taper, or be bottlenecked. The names of these case types are very descriptive of their appearance (Fig. 12–18). Some cases, called belted cases, are usually utilized in the so-called magnum rifle cartridges and have a reinforcing band, or belt, around the case wall next to the head. (See Figure 12–19 for typical ballistics tables and illustrations of centerfire rifle and handgun cartridges.)

Bullets and Projectiles

The shapes and sizes of the bullets and projectiles in modern ammunition vary greatly. Round balls or pellets are found in shotgun shells, while cylindrical or semicylindrical projectiles with variably shaped noses and bases are found in rifle and pistol bullets. These variations in shapes and sizes result from the balancing of the intended use of the bullet with the laws of ballistics and physics that govern its flight.

The present-day pistol bullet is generally one of two distinct types, the one the solid lead alloy bullet, and the other a composite of the lead alloy slug with a harder metal attachment. The usual composite pistol bullet is a lead alloy slug with an outer copper alloy jacket. The jacket may cover all of the bullet except the base or, just the reverse, may leave the nose exposed. The nose of a pistol bullet may take several forms, of which the round nose is the most common. The nose may also be essentially flat, as in the "wadcutter" used in target ammunition. The abrupt shoulder tends to cut cleaner holes in a target, thus making for easier scoring. The nose may also be conical or pointed. Some bullets have a hollow point to enhance bullet expansion to make them more effective on game. The bases of the bullets also vary from essentially flat to hollow or convex, with many variations of each. The weights of the bullet vary from 40 grains or less in the .22-caliber to over 240 grains in the .44-caliber (see Figure 12–20 for the common pistol bullets).

Rifle bullets can generally be classified into two categories: expanding or nonexpanding. The expanding bullet is designed to be used against thin-skinned game. The nose formation is made intentionally weak by exposing a soft lead nose or making the point hollow. The objective is to have the nose upset and expand to insure maximum energy transfer to the game animal on impact. Other means of weakening the metal at the nose are to split the jacket at

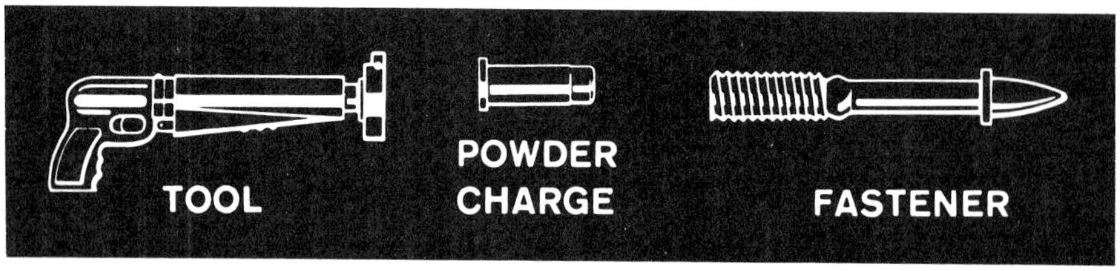

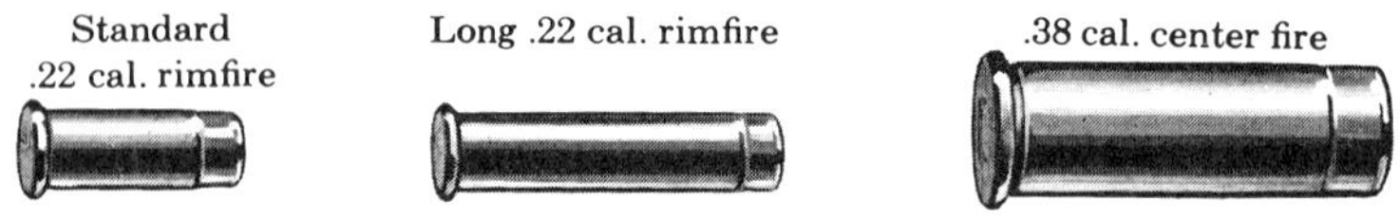

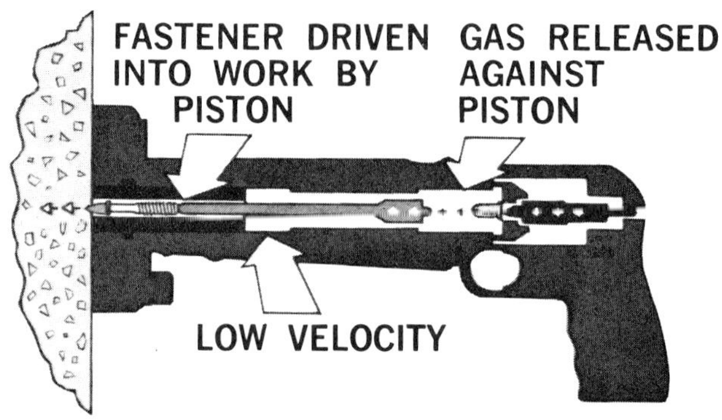

Figure 12–14. *A.* Powder-actuated tools, cartridges, and fasteners employing the low-velocity principle. The energy from a special industrial powder charge actuates a piston inside the tool barrel. The actuated piston fastens drive pins and threaded studs at a low velocity with a hammerlike blow. (Courtesy of Olin Corporation, Winchester Group, Ramset Fastening Systems.)

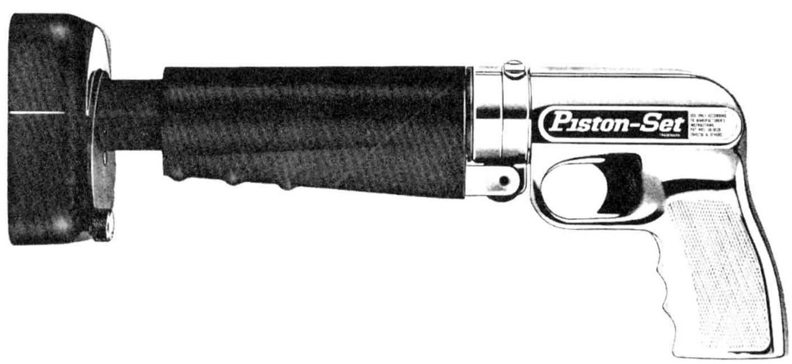

Illustration continued on opposite page

predetermined points, to thin the jacket near the nose, or to insert a hardened metal wedge to rupture the nose on impact. Nonexpanding rifle bullets are commonly military ammunition (as required by the international rules of war) or hunting bullets intended for use against large, dangerous, thick-skinned African and Asiatic game animals. Their construction ensures the deep penetration needed to get through the tough, thick hides and heavy layers of bone and muscle. Such bullets are generally round-nosed with one-piece jackets over a lead core. They are sometimes referred to as "solids."

As with the pistol bullets, the shapes of the rifle bullet bases vary. The flat base is, however, the most common. Boat-tail bases are not uncommon in rifle bullets, the base tapering to the flat with a profile much like the rear portion of a boat. The purpose is to reduce air drag on the base, giving the bullet a longer range. Rifle bullet weights usually run from about 25 grains (.17-caliber) to approximately 500 grains (45-caliber) (Fig. 12–21).

Shotgun projectiles, except for rifled slug loads and other special-purpose projectiles, are round pellets. The shot pellet sizes vary from the small No. 9 shot (.08-inch) to the 00 buckshot (.33-inch). The larger the number, the smaller the shot size. The selection of the shot size to be used, of course, depends on the nature of the game being hunted. The No. 9 shot would typically be used for birds such as quail or pigeons, while the 00 buckshot would be reserved for larger game animals. The 00 buckshot is also utilized in police ammunition.

Text continued on page 550

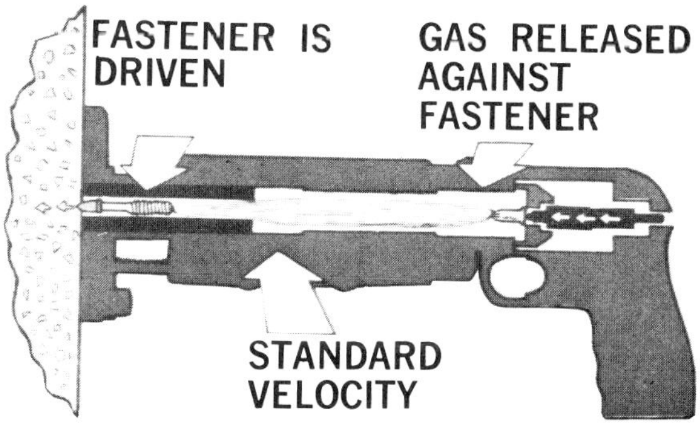

Figure 12–14 *continued. B.* Powder-actuated tools and fasteners employing the standard-velocity principle. The most powerful method in fastening systems. Drive pins and threaded studs are driven directly into concrete by a force provided by a special industrial power load. A powerful column of expanding gas propels the fasteners into concrete or steel to fasten wood and metal to tougher thicker materials. (Courtesy of Olin Corporation, Winchester Group, Ramset Fastening Systems.)

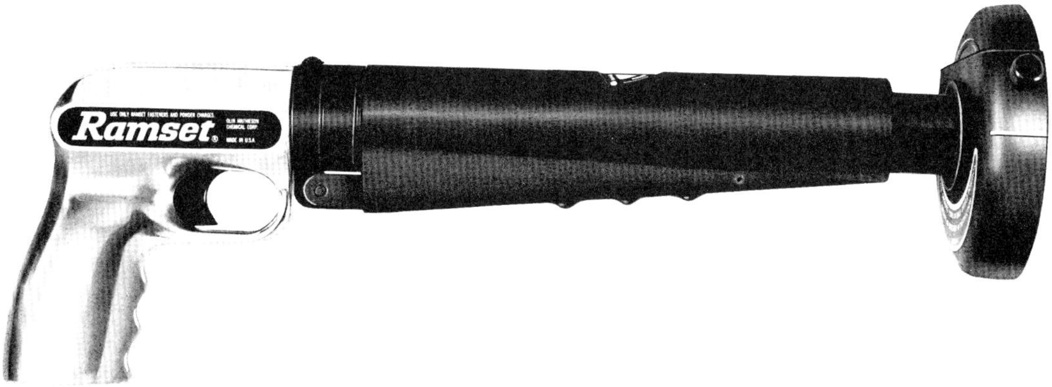

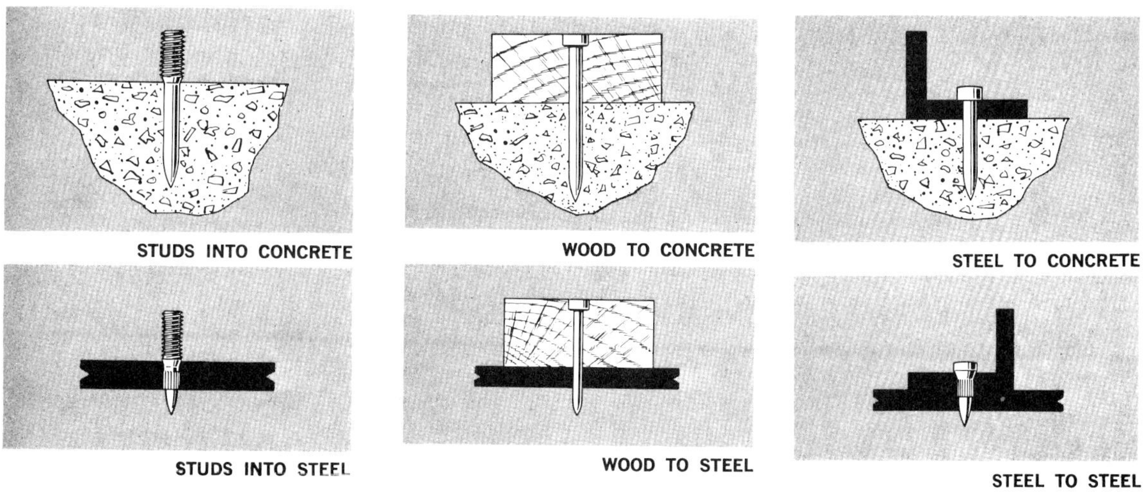

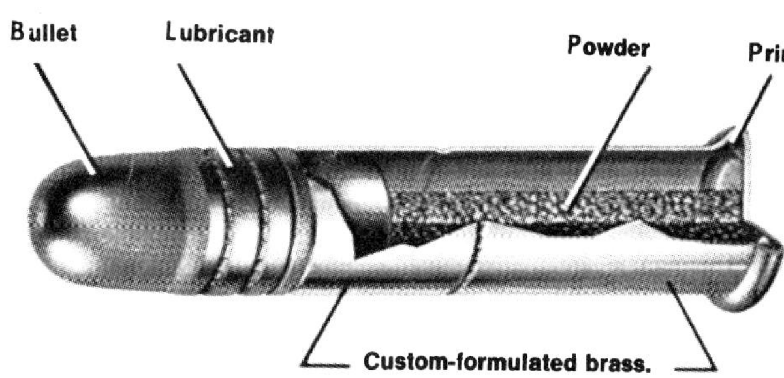

Figure 12–15. Rimfire cartridge construction. (Courtesy of Winchester-Western Division of Olin Corporation.)

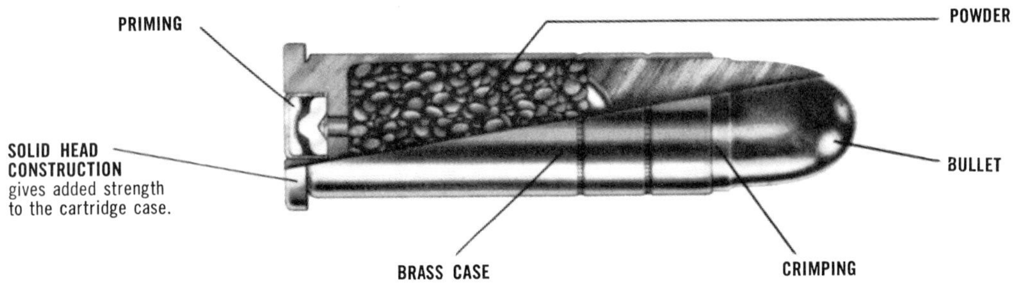

Figure 12–16. Centerfire cartridge construction. (Courtesy of Remington Arms Company, Inc.)

	BULLET Wgt.-Grs.	BULLET Style	VELOCITY — FT. PER SECOND Muzzle	VELOCITY — FT. PER SECOND 100 YDS.	ENERGY — FOOT POUNDS Muzzle	ENERGY — FOOT POUNDS 100 YDS.	MID-RANGE TRAJECTORY 100 YDS. Inches
22 SHORT	29 27	Lead Hollow Point	1125 1155	920 920	81 80	54 51	4.3 4.2
22 LONG	29	Lead	1240	965	99	60	3.8
22 LONG RIFLE	40 36	Lead Hollow Point	1285 1315	1025 1020	147 138	93 83	3.4 3.4
22 W.R.F. (REMINGTON SPECIAL)	45	Lead	1450	1110	210	123	2.7
22 WIN. AUTOMATIC	45	Lead	1055	930	111	86	4.6

	BULLET Wgt. Grs.	BULLET Style	VELOCITY — FT. PER SECOND Muzzle	VELOCITY — FT. PER SECOND 100 YDS.	VELOCITY — FT. PER SECOND 150 YDS.	ENERGY — FOOT POUNDS Muzzle	ENERGY — FOOT POUNDS 100 YDS.	ENERGY — FOOT POUNDS 150 YDS.	TRAJECTORY RIFLE SIGHTED IN AT 100 YDS. 100 YDS. Inches	TRAJECTORY RIFLE SIGHTED IN AT 100 YDS. 150 YDS. Inches
5mm REMINGTON MAGNUM	38	"Power-Lokt" Hollow Point	2100	1605	1400	372	217	165	0	–4.3

Figure 12–17. Rimfire cartridges and ballistic data. (Courtesy of Remington Arms Company, Inc.)

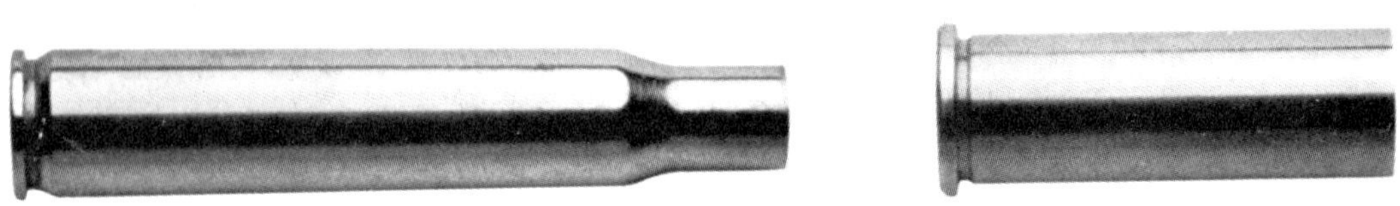

Figure 12–18. Centerfire cartridge case types. *Left,* Rimless bottleneck case; *right,* rimmed straight case. (Courtesy of Remington Arms Company, Inc.)

Cartridge	Bullet Wt. Grs.	Bullet Type	Velocity (fps) Muzzle	Velocity (fps) 100 yds.	Velocity (fps) 200 yds.	Velocity (fps) 300 yds.	Energy (ft. lbs.) Muzzle	Energy (ft. lbs.) 100 yds.	Energy (ft. lbs.) 200 yds.	Energy (ft. lbs.) 300 yds.	Mid-Range Trajectory (inches) 100 yds.	Mid-Range Trajectory (inches) 200 yds.	Mid-Range Trajectory (inches) 300 yds.
218 Bee Super-X and Super-Speed	46	OPE(HP)	2860	2160	1610	1200	835	475	265	145	0.7	3.8	11.5
22 Hornet Super-X and Super-Speed	45	SP	2690	2030	1510	1150	720	410	230	130	0.8	4.3	13.0
22 Hornet Super-X and Super-Speed	46	OPE(HP)	2690	2030	1510	1150	740	420	235	135	0.8	4.3	13.0
22-250 Super-X and Super-Speed	55	PSP	3810	3270	2770	2320	1770	1300	935	655	0.3	1.6	4.4
220 Swift Super-X and Super-Speed	48	PSP	4110	3490	2930	2440	1800	1300	915	635	0.3	1.4	3.8
222 Remington Super-X and Super-Speed	50	PSP	3200	2660	2170	1750	1140	785	520	340	0.5	2.5	7.0
225 Winchester Super-X and Super-Speed	55	PSP	3650	3140	2680	2270	1630	1200	875	630	0.4	1.8	4.8
243 Winchester (6mm) Super-X and Super-Speed	80	PSP	3500	3080	2720	2410	2180	1690	1320	1030	0.4	1.8	4.7
243 Winchester (6mm) Super-X and Super-Speed	100	PP(SP)	3070	2790	2540	2320	2090	1730	1430	1190	0.5	2.2	5.5
25-06 Super-X and Super-Speed	90	PEP	3500	3090	2730	2420	2450	1910	1490	1170	0.4	1.8	4.7
25-06 Super-X and Super-Speed	120	PEP	3120	2850	2600	2360	2590	2160	1800	1480	0.5	2.0	5.5
25-20 Winchester	86	L, Lead	1460	1180	1030	940	405	265	200	170	2.6	12.5	32.0
25-20 Winchester	86	SP	1460	1180	1030	940	405	265	200	170	2.6	12.5	32.0
25-35 Winchester Super-X and Super-Speed	117	SP	2300	1910	1600	1340	1370	945	665	465	1.0	4.6	12.5
250 Savage Super-X and Super-Speed	87	PSP	3030	2660	2330	2060	1770	1370	1050	820	0.6	2.5	6.4
250 Savage Super-X and Super-Speed	100	ST(Exp)	2820	2460	2140	1870	1760	1340	1020	775	0.6	2.9	7.4
*256 Winchester Magnum Super-X	60	OPE	2800	2070	1570	1220	1040	570	330	200	0.8	4.0	12.0
257 Roberts Super-X and Super-Speed	87	PSP	3200	2840	2500	2190	1980	1560	1210	925	0.5	2.2	5.7
257 Roberts Super-X and Super-Speed	100	ST(Exp)	2900	2540	2210	1920	1870	1430	1080	820	0.6	2.7	7.0
*257 Roberts Super-X	117	PP(SP)	2650	2280	1950	1690	1820	1350	985	740	0.7	3.4	8.8
264 Winchester Magnum Super-X and Super-Speed	100	PSP	3700	3260	2880	2550	3040	2360	1840	1440	0.4	1.6	4.2
264 Winchester Magnum Super-X and Super-Speed	140	PP(SP)	3200	2940	2700	2480	3180	2690	2270	1910	0.5	2.0	4.9
270 Winchester Super-X and Super-Speed	100	PSP	3480	3070	2690	2340	2690	2090	1600	1215	0.4	1.8	4.8
270 Winchester Super-X and Super-Speed	130	PP(SP)	3140	2880	2630	2400	2850	2390	2000	1660	0.5	2.1	5.3
270 Winchester Super-X and Super-Speed	130	ST(Exp)	3140	2850	2580	2320	2850	2340	1920	1550	0.5	2.1	5.3
270 Winchester Super-X and Super-Speed	150	PP(SP)	2900	2620	2380	2160	2800	2290	1890	1550	0.6	2.5	6.3
284 Winchester Super-X and Super-Speed	125	PP(SP)	3200	2880	2590	2310	2840	2300	1860	1480	0.5	2.1	5.3
284 Winchester Super-X and Super-Speed	150	PP(SP)	2900	2620	2380	2160	2800	2290	1890	1550	0.6	2.5	6.3
7mm Mauser (7x57) Super-X and Super-Speed	175	SP	2490	2170	1900	1680	2410	1830	1400	1100	0.8	3.7	9.5
*7mm Remington Magnum Super-X	150	PP(SP)	3260	2970	2700	2450	3540	2940	2430	1990	0.4	2.0	4.9
*7mm Remington Magnum Super-X	175	PP(SP)	3070	2720	2400	2120	3660	2870	2240	1750	0.5	2.4	6.1
†30 Carbine	110	HSP	1980	1540	1230	1040	955	575	370	260	1.4	7.5	21.7
30-30 Winchester Super-X and Super-Speed	150	OPE(HP)	2410	2020	1700	1430	1930	1360	960	680	0.9	4.2	11.0
30-30 Winchester Super-X and Super-Speed	150	PP(SP)	2410	2020	1700	1430	1930	1360	960	680	0.9	4.2	11.0
30-30 Winchester Super-X and Super-Speed	150	ST(Exp)	2410	2020	1700	1430	1930	1360	960	680	0.9	4.2	11.0
30-30 Winchester Super-X and Super-Speed	170	PP(SP)	2220	1890	1630	1410	1860	1350	1000	750	1.2	4.6	12.5
30-30 Winchester Super-X and Super-Speed	170	ST(Exp)	2220	1890	1630	1410	1860	1350	1000	750	1.2	4.6	12.5
30 Remington Super-X and Super-Speed	170	ST(Exp)	2120	1820	1560	1350	1700	1250	920	690	1.1	5.3	14.0
30-06 Springfield Super-X and Super-Speed	110	PSP	3370	2830	2350	1920	2770	1960	1350	900	0.5	2.2	6.0
30-06 Springfield Super-X and Super-Speed	125	PSP	3200	2810	2480	2200	2840	2190	1710	1340	0.5	2.2	5.6
30-06 Springfield Super-X and Super-Speed	150	PP(SP)	2970	2620	2300	2010	2930	2280	1760	1340	0.6	2.5	6.5
30-06 Springfield Super-X and Super-Speed	150	ST(Exp)	2970	2670	2400	2130	2930	2370	1920	1510	0.6	2.4	6.1
30-06 Springfield Super-X and Super-Speed	180	PP(SP)	2700	2330	2010	1740	2910	2170	1610	1210	0.7	3.1	8.3
30-06 Springfield Super-X and Super-Speed	180	ST(Exp)	2700	2470	2250	2040	2910	2440	2020	1660	0.7	2.9	7.0
30-06 Springfield Super-Match and Wimbledon Cup	180	FMCBT	2700	2520	2350	2190	2910	2540	2200	1900	0.6	2.8	6.7
*30-06 Springfield Super-X	220	PP(SP)	2410	2120	1870	1670	2830	2190	1710	1360	0.8	3.9	9.8
30-06 Springfield Super-X and Super-Speed	220	ST(Exp)	2410	2180	1980	1790	2830	2320	1910	1560	0.8	3.7	9.2
*30-40 Krag Super-X	180	PP(SP)	2470	2120	1830	1590	2440	1790	1340	1010	0.8	3.8	9.9

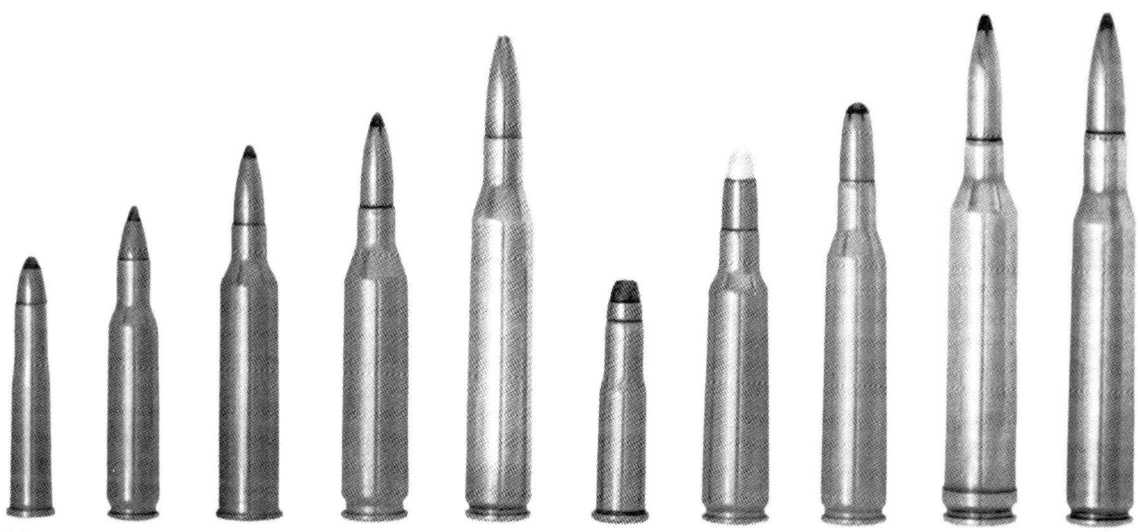

Figure 12–19. *A.* Centerfire rifle cartridges. (Courtesy of Winchester-Western Division of Olin Corporation.)

Illustration continued on following page

Cartridge	Bullet Wt. Grs.	Bullet Type	Velocity (fps) Muzzle	Velocity (fps) 100 yds.	Velocity (fps) 200 yds.	Velocity (fps) 300 yds.	Energy (ft. lbs.) Muzzle	Energy (ft. lbs.) 100 yds.	Energy (ft. lbs.) 200 yds.	Energy (ft. lbs.) 300 yds.	Mid-Range Trajectory (inches) 100 yds.	Mid-Range Trajectory (inches) 200 yds.	Mid-Range Trajectory (inches) 300 yds.
*30-40 Krag Super-X	180	ST(Exp)	2470	2250	2040	1850	2440	2020	1660	1370	0.8	3.5	8.5
*30-40 Krag Super-X	220	ST(Exp)	2200	1990	1800	1630	2360	1930	1580	1300	1.0	4.4	11.0
300 Winchester Magnum Super-X and Super-Speed	150	PP(SP)	3400	3050	2730	2430	3850	3100	2480	1970	0.4	1.9	4.8
300 Winchester Magnum Super-X and Super-Speed	180	PP(SP)	3070	2850	2640	2440	3770	3250	2790	2380	0.5	2.1	5.3
300 Winchester Magnum Super-X and Super-Speed	220	ST(Exp)	2720	2490	2270	2060	3620	3030	2520	2070	0.6	2.9	6.9
300 H&H Magnum Super-X and Super-Speed	150	ST(Exp)	3190	2870	2580	2300	3390	2740	2220	1760	0.5	2.1	5.2
300 H&H Magnum Super-X and Super-Speed	180	ST(Exp)	2920	2670	2440	2220	3400	2850	2380	1970	0.6	2.4	5.8
300 H&H Magnum Super-X and Super-Speed	220	ST(Exp)	2620	2370	2150	1940	3350	2740	2260	1840	0.7	3.1	7.7
300 Savage Super-X and Super-Speed	150	PP(SP)	2670	2350	2060	1800	2370	1840	1410	1080	0.7	3.2	8.0
300 Savage Super-X and Super-Speed	150	ST(Exp)	2670	2390	2130	1890	2370	1900	1510	1190	0.7	3.0	7.6
300 Savage Super-X and Super-Speed	180	PP(SP)	2370	2040	1760	1520	2240	1660	1240	920	0.9	4.1	10.5
300 Savage Super-X and Super-Speed	180	ST(Exp)	2370	2160	1960	1770	2240	1860	1530	1250	0.9	3.7	9.2
303 Savage Super-X and Super-Speed	190	ST(Exp)	1980	1680	1440	1250	1650	1190	875	660	1.3	6.2	15.5
†303 British Super-Speed	180	PP(SP)	2540	2300	2090	1900	2580	2120	1750	1440	0.7	3.3	8.2
308 Winchester Super-X and Super-Speed	110	PSP	3340	2810	2340	1920	2730	1930	1340	900	0.5	2.2	6.0
308 Winchester Super-X and Super-Speed	125	PSP	3100	2740	2430	2160	2670	2080	1640	1300	0.5	2.3	5.9
308 Winchester Super-X and Super-Speed	150	PP(SP)	2860	2520	2210	1930	2730	2120	1630	1240	0.6	2.7	7.0
308 Winchester Super-X and Super-Speed	150	ST(Exp)	2860	2570	2300	2050	2730	2200	1760	1400	0.6	2.6	6.5
308 Winchester Super-X and Super-Speed	180	PP(SP)	2610	2250	1940	1680	2720	2020	1500	1130	0.7	3.4	8.9
308 Winchester Super-X and Super-Speed	180	ST(Exp)	2610	2390	2170	1970	2720	2280	1870	1540	0.8	3.1	7.4
308 Winchester Super-X and Super-Speed	200	ST(Exp)	2450	2210	1980	1770	2670	2170	1750	1400	0.8	3.6	9.0
32 Winchester Special Super-X and Super-Speed	170	PP(SP)	2280	1870	1560	1330	1960	1320	920	665	1.0	4.8	13.0
32 Winchester Special Super-X and Super-Speed	170	ST(Exp)	2280	1870	1560	1330	1960	1320	920	665	1.0	4.8	13.0
32 Remington Super-X and Super-Speed	170	ST(Exp)	2120	1760	1460	1220	1700	1170	805	560	1.1	5.3	14.5
32-20 Winchester (Oilproof)	100	L, Lead	1290	1060	940	840	370	250	195	155	3.3	15.5	38.0
32-20 Winchester (Oilproof)	100	SP	1290	1060	940	840	370	250	195	155	3.3	15.5	38.0
†8mm Mauser (8x57; 7.9) Super Speed	170	PP(SP)	2570	2140	1790	1520	2490	1730	1210	870	0.8	3.9	10.5
338 Winchester Magnum Super-X and Super-Speed	200	PP(SP)	3000	2690	2410	2170	4000	3210	2580	2090	0.5	2.4	6.0
338 Winchester Magnum Super-X and Super-Speed	250	ST(Exp)	2700	2430	2180	1940	4050	3280	2640	2090	0.7	3.0	7.4
338 Winchester Magnum Super-X and Super-Speed	300	PP(SP)	2450	2160	1910	1690	4000	3110	2430	1900	0.8	3.7	9.5
†348 Winchester Super-Speed	200	ST(Exp)	2530	2220	1940	1680	2840	2190	1670	1250	0.7	3.6	9.0
35 Remington Super-X and Super-Speed	200	PP(SP)	2100	1710	1390	1160	1950	1300	860	605	1.2	6.0	16.5
35 Remington Super-X and Super-Speed	200	ST(Exp)	2100	1710	1390	1160	1950	1300	860	605	1.2	6.0	16.5
351 Winchester Self-Loading (Oilproof)	180	SP	1850	1560	1310	1140	1370	975	685	520	1.5	7.8	21.5
358 Winchester (8.8mm) Super-X and Super-Speed	200	ST(Exp)	2530	2210	1910	1640	2840	2160	1610	1190	0.8	3.6	9.4
358 Winchester (8.8mm) Super-X and Super-Speed	250	ST(Exp)	2250	2010	1780	1570	2810	2230	1760	1370	1.0	4.4	11.0
375 H&H Magnum Super-X and Super-Speed	270	PP(SP)	2740	2460	2210	1990	4500	3620	2920	2370	0.7	2.9	7.1
375 H&H Magnum Super-X and Super-Speed	300	ST(Exp)	2550	2280	2040	1830	4330	3460	2770	2230	0.7	3.3	8.3
†375 H&H Magnum Super-Speed	300	FMC	2550	2180	1860	1590	4330	3160	2300	1680	0.7	3.6	9.3
38-40 Winchester (Oilproof)	180	SP	1330	1070	960	850	705	455	370	290	3.2	15.0	36.5
*44 Magnum Super-X	240	HSP	1750	1350	1090	950	1630	970	635	480	1.8	9.4	26.0
44-40 Winchester (Oilproof)	200	SP	1310	1050	940	830	760	490	390	305	3.3	15.0	36.5
†45-70 Government	405	SP	1320	1160	1050	990	1570	1210	990	880	2.9	13.0	32.5
†458 Winchester Magnum Super-Speed	500	FMC	2130	1910	1700	1520	5040	4050	3210	2570	1.1	4.8	12.0
†458 Winchester Magnum Super-Speed	510	SP	2130	1840	1600	1400	5140	3830	2900	2220	1.1	5.1	13.5

*—Western Brand Only; †—Winchester Brand Only; HSP—Hollow Soft Point; PEP—Positive Expanding Point; PSP—Pointed Soft Point; PP(SP)—Power-Point Soft Point; FMC—Full Metal Case; SP—Soft Point; HP—Hollow Point; L—Lubaloy; OPE—Open Point Expanding; ST(Exp)—Silvertip Expanding; FMCBT—Full Metal Case Boat Tail

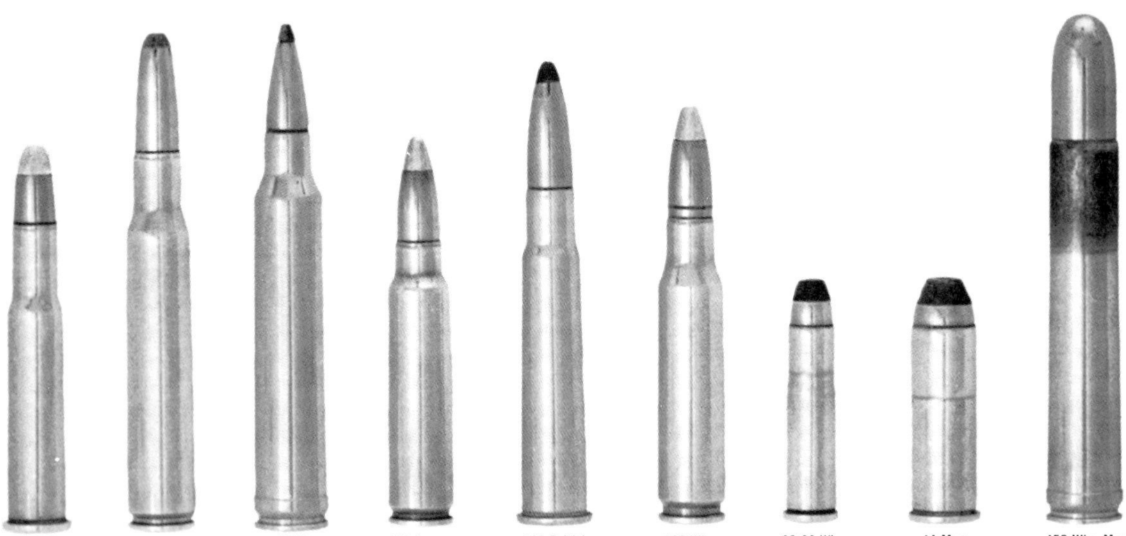

Figure 12–19 *continued.* *B.* Centerfire rifle cartridges. (Courtesy of Winchester-Western Division of Olin Corporation.)

Illustration continued on opposite page

Cartridge	Bullet Wt. Grs.	Bullet Type	Barrel Length	Muzzle Velocity (fps)	Muzzle Energy (ft. lbs.)
25 Automatic (6.35mm) (Oilproof)	50	FMC	2″	810	73
*256 Winchester Magnum Super-X	60	OPE	8½″	2350	735
30 Luger (7.65mm) (Oilproof)	93	FMC	4½″	1220	305
32 Automatic (Oilproof)	71	FMC	4″	905	130
32 Smith & Wesson (Oilproof) (inside lubricated)	85	L, Lead	3″	680	90
32 Smith & Wesson Long (Oilproof) (inside lubricated)	98	L, Lead	4″	705	115
*32 Short Colt (Oilproof) Greased	80	Lubaloy	4″	745	100
*32 Long Colt (Oilproof) (inside lubricated)	82	Lubaloy	4″	755	105
†32 Colt New Police (Oilproof) (inside lubricated)	98	Lead	4″	680	100
32-20 Winchester (Oilproof) (inside lubricated)	100	L, Lead	6″	1030	235
32-20 Winchester (Oilproof)	100	SP	6″	1030	235
357 Magnum Jacketed Hollow Point Super-X (Oilproof)	110	JHP	8⅜″	—	—
*357 Magnum Super-X (Oilproof) (inside lubricated)	158	Lubaloy	8⅜″	1410	695
*357 Magnum Metal Piercing Super-X (Oilproof) (inside lubricated, lead bearing)	158	Met. Pierc.	8⅜″	1410	695
*357 Magnum Jacketed Hollow Point Super-X (Oilproof)	158	JHP	8⅜″	1450	740
*357 Magnum Jacketed Soft Point Super-X (Oilproof)	158	JSP	8⅜″	1450	740
†9mm Luger (Parabellum) (Oilproof)	115	FMC	4″	1140	330
†9mm Luger (Parabellum) (Oilproof)	100	PP	4″	1325	390
38 Smith & Wesson (Oilproof) (inside lubricated)	145	L, Lead	4″	685	150
38 Special (Oilproof) (inside lubricated)	158	L, Lead	6″	855	255
38 Special (Oilproof) (inside lubricated, lead bearing)	158	Met. Pt.	6″	855	255
†38 Special (MS) Police	158	Lead, HP	6″	1060	395
38 Special Super Police (Oilproof) (inside lubricated)	200	L, Lead	6″	730	235
†38 Special Semi Wad Cutter Super-Speed (Oilproof) (inside lubricated)	158	Lead	6″	1060	395
*38 Special Super-X (Oilproof) (inside lubricated)	150	Lubaloy	6″	1060	375
*38 Special Metal Piercing Super-X (Oilproof) (inside lubricated, lead bearing)	150	Met. Pierc.	6″	1060	375
38 Special Super-Match and Match Mid-Range Clean Cutting (Oilproof) (inside lubricated)	148	Lead	6″	770	195
*38 Special Super-Match (Oilproof) (inside lubricated)	158	Lead	6″	855	255
*38 Short Colt (Oilproof) Greased	130	Lubaloy	6″	730	150
*38 Long Colt (Oilproof) (inside lubricated)	150	Lubaloy	6″	730	175
38 Automatic Super-X and Super-Speed (For use only in 38 Colt Super and Colt Commander Automatic Pistols)	130	FMC	5″	1280	475
38 Automatic (Oilproof) (For all 38 Automatic Pistols)	130	FMC	4½″	1040	310
380 Automatic (Oilproof)	95	FMC	3¾″	955	190
38-40 Winchester (Oilproof)	180	SP	5″	975	380
†44 Smith & Wesson Special (Oilproof) (inside lubricated)	246	Lead	6½″	755	310
*44 Magnum Super-X (Gas Check)	240	Lubaloy	6½″	1470	1150
44-40 Winchester (Oilproof)	200	SP	7½″	975	420
45 Colt (Oilproof) (inside lubricated)	255	L, Lead	5½″	880	410
45 Automatic (Oilproof)	230	FMC	5″	850	370
*45 Automatic Super-Match Clean Cutting	185	FMC	5″	775	245

*—Western Brand Only; †—Winchester Brand Only; Met. Pierc.—Metal Piercing; FMC—Full Metal Case; SP—Soft Point; L—Lubaloy; JHP—Jacketed Hollow Point; JSP—Jacketed Soft Point; Met. Pt.—Metal Point; OPE—Open Point Expanding; HP—Hollow Point; PP—Power Point

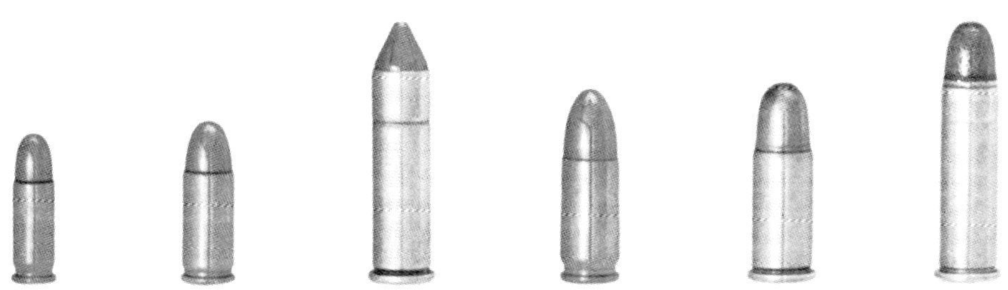

Figure 12–19 *continued.* C. Centerfire handgun cartridges. (Courtesy of Winchester-Western Division of Olin Corporation.)

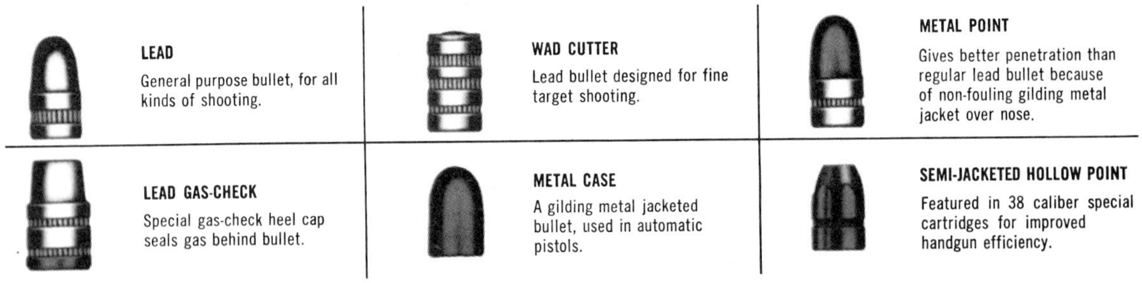

Figure 12–20. Handgun bullet types. (Courtesy of Remington Arms Company, Inc.)

A very small shot (No. 12) is used in special .22-caliber rimfire shot shells. (See Figure 12–22 for shot sizes.) Special rifled slugs are available for deer hunters. The rifled slug projectile appears similar in general shape to a blunt bullet with a deep hollow cavity in the base. The sides commonly have angularly inclined fins, or ribs, that somewhat resemble very coarse rifling marks on a bullet. Their purpose is to add stability to the slug during its flight and thereby make it more accurate. The slugs are usually a little smaller in diameter than the shotgun bore itself. Some slugs, especially foreign-made ones, have wadding fastened to the base on a barrel gas seal. Rifled slugs are commonly available in 12 gauge (7/8 oz), 16 gauge (4/5 oz), 20 gauge (5/8 oz), and 410 bore (1/5 oz). The American manufacturers of the great bulk of ammunition for the American market are the Federal Cartridge Corporation, Remington Arms Company, Inc. (Remington-Peter Brands), and Winchester-Western Division of Olin Corporation.

Primers and Propellants

The purpose of the primer or priming compound used in modern firearms is to ignite the powder or propellant charge in the cartridge case. With the exception of a rather rare electrically primed French shotshell, modern primers are ignited by impact (percussion) of the gun's firing pin. In rimfire cartridges the priming compound is contained within the hollow rim of the cartridge and ignited when it is crushed between the rim walls of the cartridge head by the impact of the firing pin. Centerfire rifle and pistol primers are small metal cups usually held in place in the cartridge head primer pocket by friction. The primer cup contains the priming mixture and an anvil positioned so that the blow of the firing pin on the primer cup will crush the priming compound against the anvil center and ignite it. The ignited priming compound then flashes through the flash hole in the centerfire case head to ignite the powder charge. Figure 12–16 shows the approximate shape and position of the anvil within the primer pocket. The primer utilized in shotgun shells is called a primer battery cup. This consists of a battery cup into which a primer cup fits. The battery cup provides the support for the anvil and provides a flash hole. It is also held in place by friction. The difference in construction is due to the basic makeup of the shotshell and the lack of a primer pocket or flash hole. The rate of primer activation is very fast—approximately 0.00001 second. A number of ingredients make up the various priming mixes in modern ammunition. Lead styphnate is frequently the basic ingredient. Tetracene is used to control sensitivity, and barium nitrate is added as a moderator and oxidizer with minor amounts of other ingredients to act as fuels and create friction.

While black powder was the main propellant used in great-grandfather's day, smokeless powders are the principal present-day firearm propellants. Black powder is, however, still used by certain individuals who find pleasure in shooting the old percussion-type firearms. Smokeless powder used in small arms has been

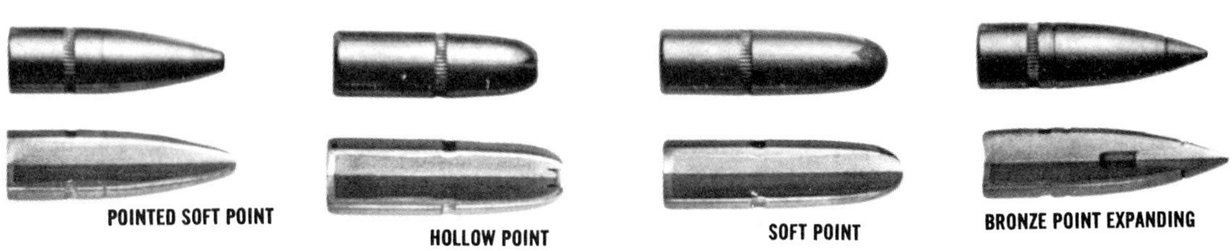

Figure 12–21. Rifle bullet types. (Courtesy of Remington Arms Company, Inc.)

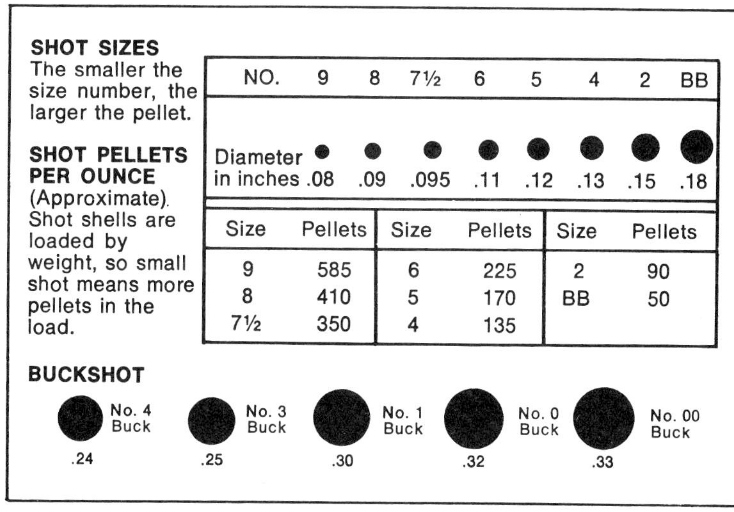

Figure 12–22. Shot size and diameter chart. (Courtesy of Federal Cartridge Corporation.)

estimated to have an energy content of approximately 1,155,000 to 1,246,000 ft-lb per pound of powder, or energy of about 165 to 178 ft-lb per grain weight. The rate of conversion of this huge amount of energy to bullet energy in a gun is only about 30 to 32 per cent. The loss of efficiency and energy is due to many things, of which the following are the principal factors: energy required to force the bullet out of the cartridge case and into the rifling, friction of bullet and barrel during the bullet's travel down the barrel, heating of the barrel and chamber, and the acceleration of the powder gases. Modern powder types are single-base and double-base. In the former, nitrocellulose is the base; in the latter, nitrocellulose and nitroglycerine make up the base. Double-base powders are usually considered to be of higher potential and hotter burning than single-base powders. A cartridge powder charge can be burned in approximately 0.001 sec or less. The shapes and sizes of powder grains vary greatly between types and brands. Some grains are circular disks, others are square or rectangular, some are cylindrical, some spherical, some are perforated, and others are irregularly shaped. The burn rates are controlled in many ways. Perforation and control of grain size and the coating of grains are the typical ways. Powder may be described as degressive, neutral, or progressive burning. In degressive powders the outer surface of the grain burns away, the exposed surface gets smaller, and the speed of burning decreases. This produces peak pressure close to the breech and low muzzle pressure in the gun. Neutral burning is accomplished by putting a hole or perforation in a grain of powder, which permits it to be ignited inside at the same time as outside, the outside burning to a smaller diameter while the inside counterbalances it by burning to a larger diameter. For progressive burning the outside of the grains are coated to retard the rate of burning until the coating is burned through. This gives maximum pressure further along the gun bore and higher muzzle pressure. The smaller the grains, the more surface exposed to ignition and the faster the powder burns. In general, pistol cartridges call for fast-burning powders because of the short barrels. Large-caliber rifles usually call for large grains of coated powders.

The Shotshell and Its Components

The modern shotshell is a self-contained unit consisting of a tube of plastic or paper (most current shotshells have plastic tubes), a metal head (usually brass), a battery cup with primer in the head, a smokeless powder charge, wadding, and a shot charge. A few shotshells are being made that have both tube and head of plastic and are of one-piece construction. Wadding at one time consisted of an over-powder wad, filler wads, and an over-shot or end wad with a rolled crimp to hold it in place. The wads were constructed of paper or fiber. The present trend in the industry is toward plastic wads, and in some cases, a one-piece construction combining all wads into a single plastic wad column including a shot cup or wrapper (Fig. 12–23). The purpose of the shot cup or wrapper is to protect the shot from being deformed by the sides of the barrel during its travel down the barrel. The plastic cup or wrapper cushions the outer shot layers, resulting in more uniform shot pellets, better accuracy, and better patterns. The over-shot or end wad has been replaced for the most part by a folded crimp or the pie crimp utilizing the end of the shotshell tube itself. In the United States

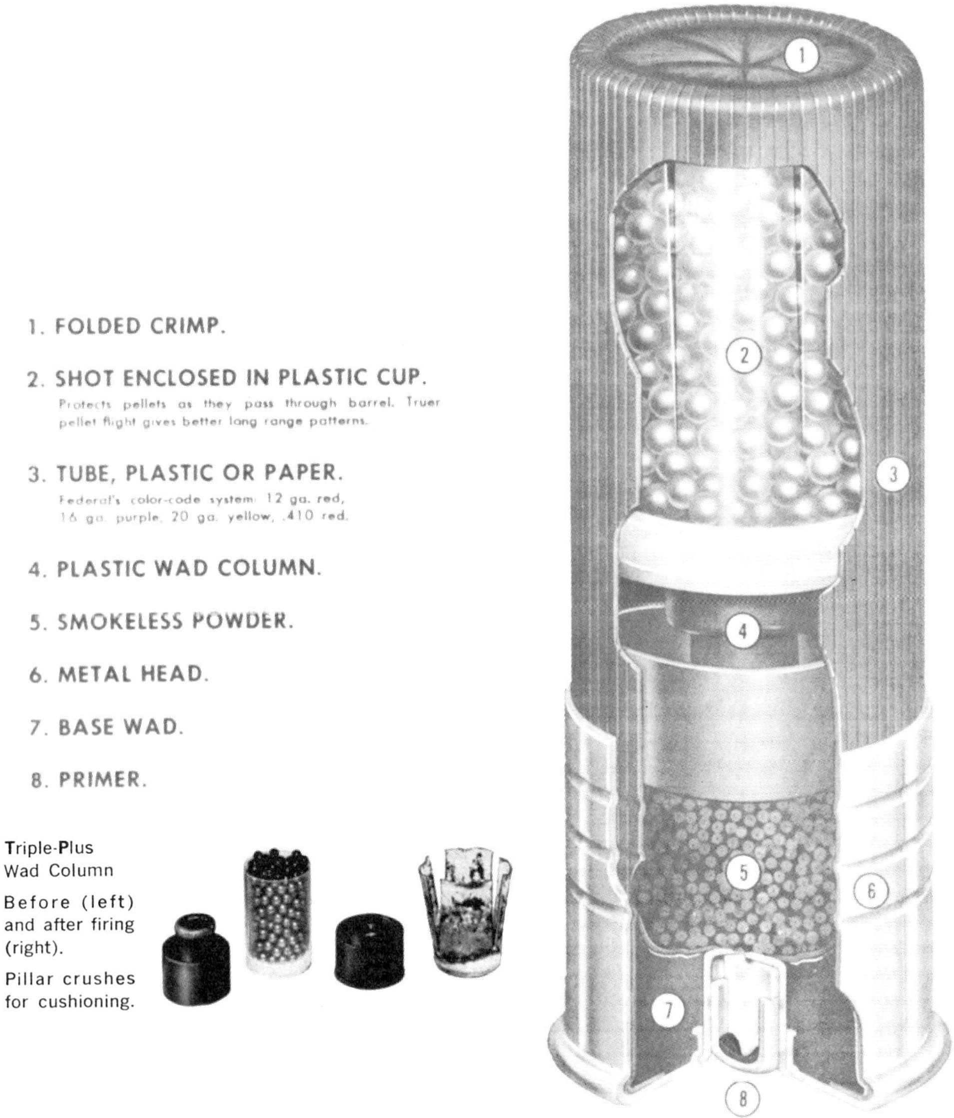

Figure 12–23. Shotshell identification. (Courtesy of Federal Cartridge Corporation.)

shotshells are currently produced in lengths of 2¾ and 3 inches. The 410-bore cases are 2½ and 3 inches in length. While 2¾-inch shotshells can be fired in guns with 3-inch chambers, the 3-inch shotshells should not be fired in guns chambered for the 2¾-inch shell because of the resulting increase in chamber pressure. Some old American shotguns and some European shotguns do have shorter chambers than those just mentioned. The amount of wadding, or the length of the one-piece wad depends on the type of charge powder and shot being loaded into the shell. The one-piece wad and the combination wad come in differing lengths and many variations and styles. Some typical shotshell loads and velocities are given in Table 12–1.

Manufacturers' Markings

The manufacturers, as a general rule, mark the heads of their cartridge cases with certain identifying data. These markings are called headstamps and the data serve two purposes. Commercially made ammunition generally has the caliber of the cartridge, along with the identity or the brand of the maker (Fig. 12–24). Military ammunition usually has the identity of the manufacturer (initials or a code) and the year and sometimes the month of manufacture. The caliber usually does not appear on military ammunition headstamps. In the case of the small .22 rimfire cartridge, only the maker's symbol, brand, or initials appear. There are literally thousands of different headstamps

TABLE 12–1. TYPICAL SHOTSHELL LOADS AND VELOCITIES*

Gauge	Federal Load Number	Shell Length Inches	Powder Drams Equiv.	Ounces of Shot	Shot Sizes
MAGNUM LOADS					
12	F131	3	4	1⅞	BB, 2, 4
12	F129	3	4	1⅝	2, 4, 6
12	F130	2¾	3¾	1½	2, 4, 5, 6
16	F165	2¾	3¼	1¼	2, 4, 6
20	F207	3	3	1¼	2, 4, 6, 7½
20	F205	2¾	2¾	1⅛	4, 6, 7½
HI-POWER LOADS					
12	F127	2¾	3¾	1¼	BB, 2, 4, 5, 6, 7½, 9
16	F164	2¾	3¼	1⅛	4, 5, 6, 7½, 9
20	F203	2¾	2¾	1	4, 5, 6, 7½, 9
28	F283	2¾	2¼	⅞	6, 7½, 8
410	F412	2½	Max.	½	6, 7½, 9
410	F413	3	Max.	11/16	4, 5, 6, 7½, 9

12, 16 and 20 Gauge Hi-Power loads have Triple-Plus wad column. 28 Gauge load has a plastic shot cup and conventional "Altite" filler wads. The F412 and F413 have all-plastic wad column. Magnums have plastic shot cup and conventional "Altite" filler wads.

Gauge	Federal Load Number	Shell Length Inches	Powder Drams Equiv.	Ounces of Shot	Shot Sizes
FIELD LOADS					
12	F124	2¾	3¼	1¼	7½, 8, 9
12	F123	2¾	3¼	1⅛	4, 5, 6, 7½, 8, 9
16	F162	2¾	2¾	1⅛	4, 5, 6, 7½, 8, 9
20	F202	2¾	2½	1	4, 5, 6, 7½, 8, 9
GAME LOADS					
12	F121	2¾	3¼	1	6, 8
16	F160	2¾	2½	1	8
20	F200	2¾	2½	⅞	8
BUCKSHOT					
12	F131	3	Sup. Mag.		00 Buck—15 Pellets
12	F131	3	Sup. Mag.		4 Buck—41 Pellets
12	F130	2¾	Magnum		00 Buck—12 Pellets
12	F127	2¾	Max.		00 Buck— 9 Pellets
12	F127	2¾	Max.		0 Buck—12 Pellets
12	F127	2¾	Max.		1 Buck—16 Pellets
12	F127	2¾	Max.		4 Buck—27 Pellets
16	F164	2¾	Max.		1 Buck—12 Pellets
20	F203	2¾	Max.		3 Buck—20 Pellets

APPROXIMATE **SHOT SHELL VELOCITIES**

Gauge	Length	Powder Chg. Drs. Equiv.	Oz. Shot	Muzzle Velocity
12	2¾″	2¾	1⅛	1145
12	2¾″	3	1	1290
12	2¾″	3	1⅛	1200
12	2¾″	3¼	1⅛	1255
12	2¾″	3¼	1¼	1220
12	2¾″	3¾	1¼	1330
12	2¾″ Mag	4	1½	1315
12	3″ Mag	4¼	1⅝	1315
12	3″ Mag	4½	1⅞	1255
16	2¾″	2½	1	1165
16	2¾″	2¾	1⅛	1185
16	2¾″	3¼	1⅛	1295
16	2¾″ Mag	3½	1¼	1295
20	2¾″	2¼	⅞	1210
20	2¾″	2½	1	1165
20	2¾″	2¾	1	1220
20	2¾″ Mag	3	1⅛	1220
20	3″ Mag	3¼	1¼	1220
28	2¾″	2½	⅞	1260
410	3″	Max	¾	1135
410	2½″	Max	½	1135

*Courtesy of Federal Cartridge Corporation.

world-wide. A ballistics laboratory would normally maintain as extensive a list or index of headstamps as possible for ammunition identification.

Hand Loading

Hand loading or reloading of cartridges is a very popular hobby among shooters and hunters. This is particularly true of target shooters such as trap and skeet shooters and centerfire pistol target shooters. The economic saving to a large-volume shooter is very substantial. Centerfire hunters also have their pet loads. Many companies manufacture reloading equipment; a few of the common brands are RCBS, Lee, Lyman, Pacific, Belding & Mull, and Herters. All the large ammunition manufacturers make reloading components (bullets, shot, cases, primers, and powders) available to hand loaders. There are also companies that specialize in the

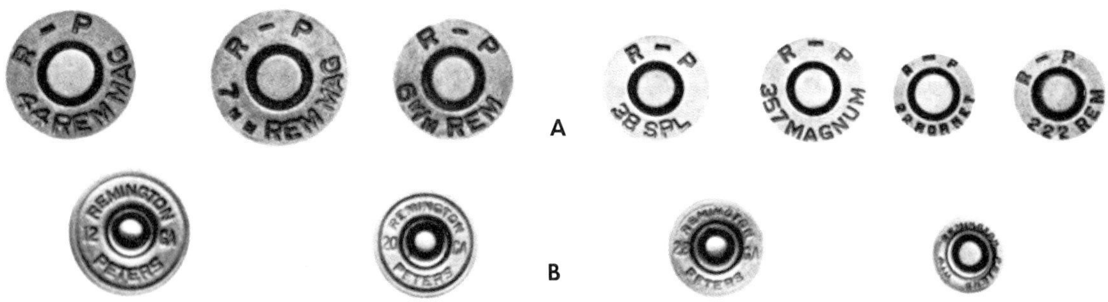

Figure 12–24. Typical commercial headstamps. *A.* Centerfire rifle and pistol cartridge; the "R-P" stands for Remington-Peters. *B.* Shotshells. (Courtesy of Remington Arms Company, Inc.)

production of bullets for reloaders, such as the Sierra Company, the Speer Company, and Hornady. Powder companies such as Hercules and DuPont make their products available to the reloader. While it would be possible to hand load the .22-caliber rimfire cartridge, technical difficulty and economics make it impractical to do so.

One should never overlook the possibility that a hand-loaded cartridge was involved in a shooting incident. In most cases the ballistics laboratory can determine from striations on the case wall, differences in components, primer internal construction, and the like whether a cartridge was reloaded. Hand-loading or reloading errors (e.g., wrong powder, overloads) may be the cause of accidents involving burst cartridge cases or blown-up guns. While the hobby of reloading is generally a safe one if reasonable care is exercised, unfortunately careless errors do occur because of unwise experimentation with components.

MANUFACTURE OF MODERN FIREARMS

It would be impossible to cover the entire manufacturing process of a complete firearm with all its parts in this rather limited discussion; to do so would require a textbook in itself, and would provide a vast bulk of information having little relevance to the pathologist's needs. Our purpose is to cover the manufacture of the barrel, the breech face, and associated parts that are of forensic interest because of their role in producing identifying marks on the bullets and cartridge cases fired in the gun.

A great many different machine-tool operations go into the production of a firearm: turning (lathe), grinding, filing, milling, broaching, drilling, and other processes. The basic forming (both rough and finished) is done by forging, stamping, swaging, and casting. In general, most of the processes leave on the finished parts microsopic imperfections that in turn are passed on to the fired bullets and cartridge cases.

Generally, various steel alloys are the basic material used in a gun, with wood for stocks and grips and plastic reserved for some handgun grips and rifle or shotgun butt plates. At the present time, some aluminum alloys are being used for firearms receivers and frames. Plastics are occasionally used to replace wooden stocks and parts such as trigger guards.

The Gun Barrel

The steel used in gun barrels is generally of good quality. Its exact type varies between manufacturers according to their preferences on suitability. Chrome-molybdenum, low- and medium-carbon steel, sulfurized carbon steel, and manganese steel barrels are common, and a few are made of stainless steel. The steel is subjected to special heat treatment to give it the required hardness for strength and durability.

The first step in making the gun barrel is to drill the bore in a solid barrel blank to the approximate caliber size required. The drilling is done by a special deep-hole drill with a hollow shank through which oil comes in under high pressure and flushes out the steel chips. Modern methods of deep-hole drilling have greatly improved the finish on the inside of the bore following the drilling operation. Reaming has usually been necessary to bring the inside diameter to the proper finish and size, but a few manufacturers, at the present time, do not find any reaming necessary following the drilling process. Some shotgun barrels are now being produced from a new high-quality seamless heat-treated alloy tubing instead of being drilled from solid stock.

The rifling of handguns and rifle barrels at the present time is almost entirely done by a cold forming process. Originally, rifling grooves were cut one at a time with a single blade (hook or scrape cutter). Several passes of the cutter through the barrel were necessary to produce a single groove, a time-consuming process that has been almost entirely eliminated. This was followed by the broach method in which all grooves were cut simultaneously with a single pass of a gang broach through the barrel. The gang broach had several cutting edges spaced close together on a single stem or rod, so that each cutting edge removed a little more metal than the previous one until the final one had cut the grooves to the required dimensions. This method is still being used but has largely been replaced by the cold forming process. One method of cold forming, the button process, uses a tungsten-carbide "button" with a cross-section representing a negative of the desired finished rifle bore. This button is then forced through the bore and swages or cold forms all rifling grooves in a single pass (Fig. 12–25). The other cold forming process is the "hammer" process. In this, the barrel has an oversized bore diameter into which is placed a mandrel containing a negative of the finished rifling cut into it. The outside of the barrel is then swaged down around the mandrel by radial hammer blows. The breech end of the barrel has an unrifled portion called the chamber into which the cartridge case seats. The chamber is cut to fit the dimensions of the particular cartridge case and type to be used in the gun being manufactured, but is slightly larger than the cartridge case to permit ease in loading and to accommodate the various makes and brands of ammunition (Fig. 12–26). The rifling at the edge of the chamber is tapered from normal height to the chamber case mouth dimension. This portion is referred to as the chamber leade or throat. In revolvers, the cartridge chamber is located in the rotating cylinder, which has five to nine chambers, depending on the caliber and the manufacturer. Cocking the revolver rotates the cylinder and aligns one of the chambers with the gun barrel bore.

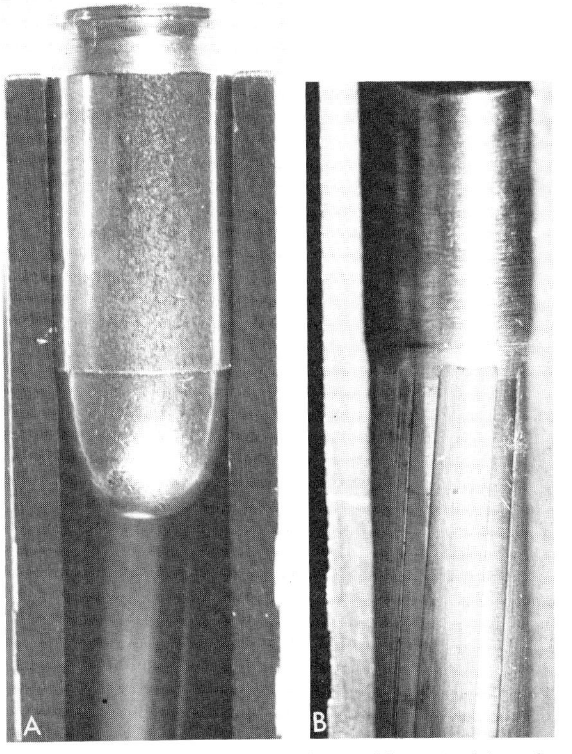

Figure 12–26. Two sectioned .45-caliber pistol barrels. *A.* A .45 ACP cartridge in the chamber. *B.* No cartridge in the chamber; the focus is on the barrel rifling.

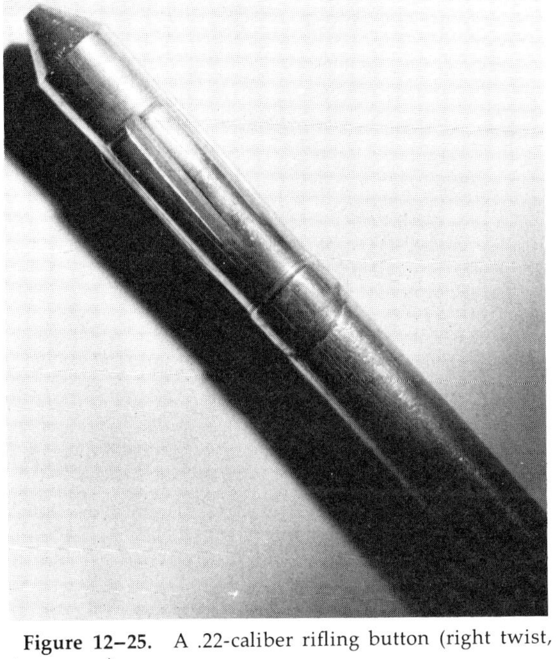

Figure 12–25. A .22-caliber rifling button (right twist, six grooves).

Breech Face or Bolt Face

The breech face or bolt face, along with the barrel interior, has the greatest forensic significance in identifying fired bullets and cartridge cases with a particular gun. The purpose of the breech face or bolt face is to support the head of the cartridge at the time of firing. Breech pressures generally run from approximately 8,000 lb per square inch to over 50,000 lb per square inch, depending on caliber and type of cartridge being fired. The breech face or bolt face also contains the firing pin and usually the extractor or extractors and the means of ejection (ejector) of the fired cartridge cases.

Because of the significant breech pressures developed by the cartridge on firing, the small imperfections and tool marks appearing on the breech face or bolt face are usually imprinted on the softer metals of the head and primer of the cartridge. This imprinting action is similar to the action of a die.

Many of the machine tool operations described in the beginning of this section are utilized in producing the surface finish on the breech face or bolt face (e.g., milling, broaching, filing). Figure 12–27 shows three different breech and bolt faces with assorted firing pins, extractors, and ejector positions. The firing pins are usually produced on automatic screw machines that give them their basic shape and size. This is usually followed by a milling process to bring the firing pin blank to final shape. Some flat firing pins are produced on punch presses, and in some cases, the final finish on the striking surface is done by a grinding operation. The finished firing pin is then heat treated to give it sufficient hardness and durability. All these various operations leave microscopic tool marks and imperfections on the firing pin.

Most centerfire firing pins have a hemispherical point, tip, or striking surface. There are, however, a few centerfire pistols that have rectangular firing pins.

The .22-caliber rimfire firing pin presents the greatest variety of geometric shapes and sizes in the firing pin tip. The six basic types or shapes and the approximate percentage of their frequency of occurence are shown in Figure 12–28. The firing pin imparts (by die action) its general shape, size, and tooling imperfections to the primer surface.

The same general manufacturing processes are used to produce the extractor and the ejec

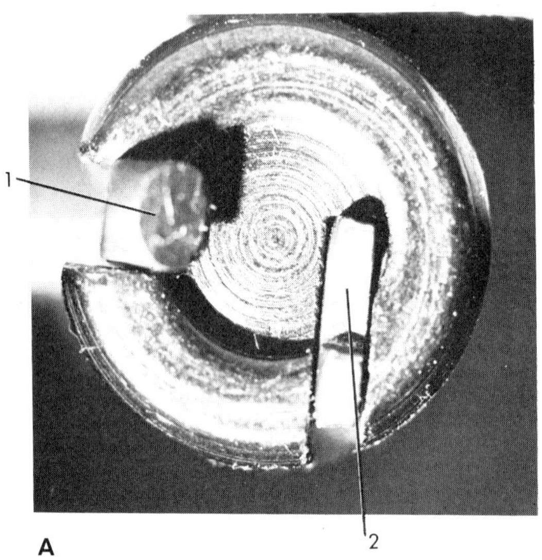

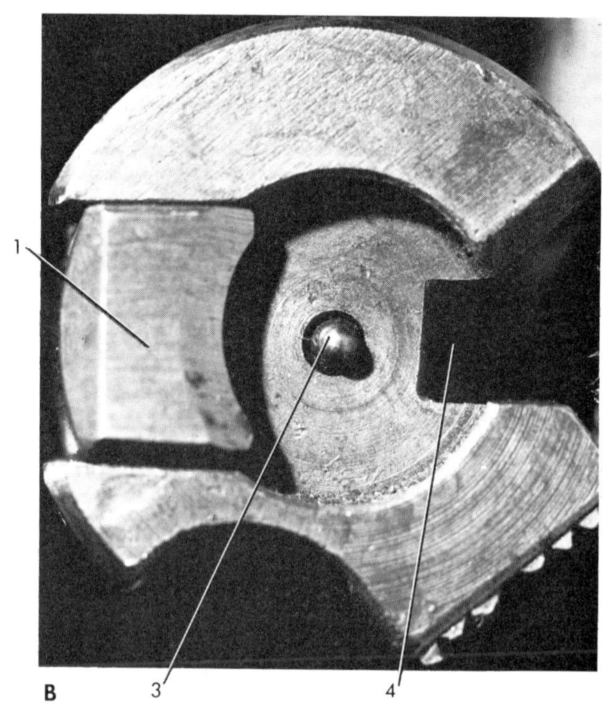

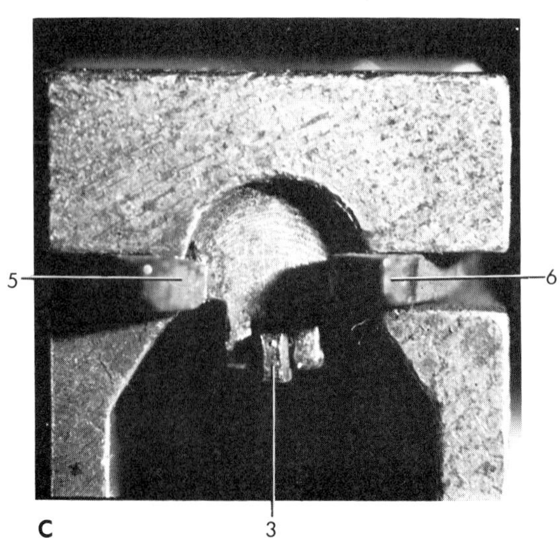

Figure 12–27. Breech faces (bolts). *A.* A Stevens model 15 rifle (.22-caliber). *B.* A German MP 44 automatic rifle (7.92 mm short). *C.* A Marlin .22-caliber model 989M2 carbine. 1, Extractor; 2, combination firing pin and ejector; 3, firing pin; 4, ejector slot; 5, right extractor; 6, left extractor.

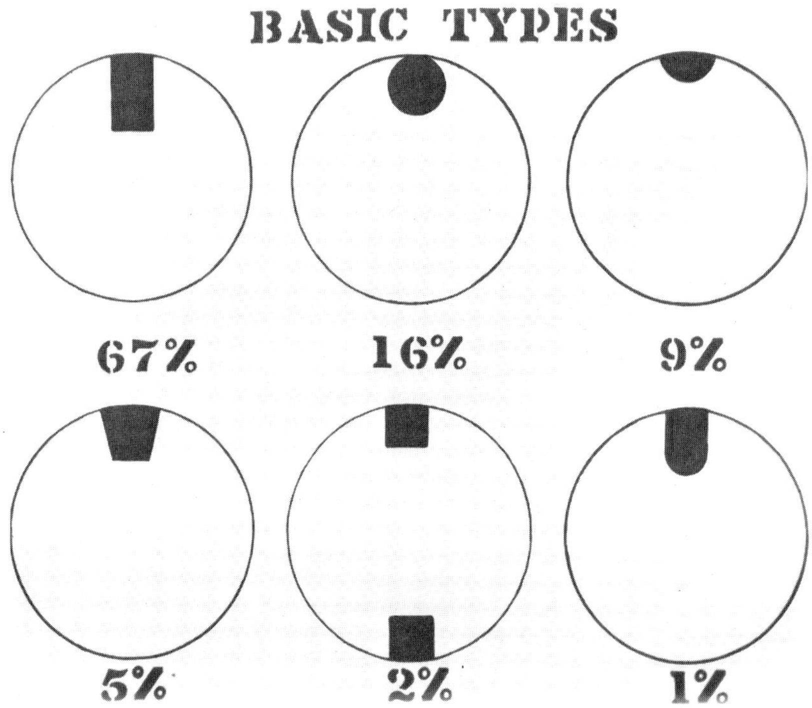

Figure 12–28. Diagram of the six basic types of .22 rimfire firing pin impressions (of which there are variations and subtypes). Rectangular type, approximately 67 per cent frequency of occurrence; circular type, approximately 16 per cent frequency of occurrence; semicircular type, approximately 9 per cent frequency of occurrence; wedge type, approximately 5 per cent frequency of occurrence; double type, approximately 2 per cent frequency of occurrence; and the odd type (combinations of other basic types), which accounts for only about 1 per cent of noted firing pin impressions.

tor. These parts also leave characteristic markings on the softer cartridge case metals during the feeding, firing, extraction, and ejection processes.

BULLET AND CARTRIDGE IDENTIFICATION

Inasmuch as the preceding section on the manufacture of firearms ended with a discussion of the breech and bolt faces and their associated parts, it is appropriate to discuss fired cartridge case identification principles and procedures next and then to move on to fired bullet examination and identification, class and individual characteristics (common to both cartridge and bullet identification), and the types of markings to be found on fired cartridges and fired bullets.

Cartridge Case Examination and Identification

From careful examination of a fired cartridge case, useful facts and items of information frequently can be ascertained. The caliber and type of cartridge, as well as its manufacturer, usually can be determined from the shape and size of the case as well as the manufacturer's stampings on the case head. From the markings left on the cartridge head and primer by the firing pin, extractor, ejector, magazine, and breech face, and their comparison with known standards of reference, it is sometimes possible to determine the make and model of gun in which the case was fired.

In many instances, this identification involves several possibilities. Frequently, the markings are common to a great many guns and no useful determinations are possible. When two fired cartridge cases are available, it is usually possible by examining their markings to determine if they were fired in the same gun. When one or more evidence cartridge cases and an evidence gun are available, it can usually be determined whether those cartridge cases were fired in that gun. This is decided by test firing the evidence gun and comparing the markings on the test-fired cartridge cases with those on the evidence cartridge cases.

Class and Individual Characteristics

The identification of cartridges is based on the examination, observation, and analysis of the class and individual characteristics of marks found on the fired cases. The class characteristics (sometimes referred to as primary or gross characteristics) are those peculiar to all guns of a certain make and model or to all guns in a certain group or class. For example, semiautomatic arms will leave markings characteristic of that class or group of firearms. Revolvers as a group also have their distinguishing characteristics. Individual (sometimes referred to as secondary or accidental) characteristics, on the other hand, are those peculiar to only one gun. Whereas class characteristics are determined before manufacture of the gun and result from manufacturing specifications, design, and dimensions, individual characteristics result accidentally during manufacturing processes, are usually microsopic in nature, and have random distribution. Individual characteristics may also be acquired after manufacture of the gun through wear, abuse, and corrosion. Class characteristics are most useful in identifying the make and model of gun involved; individual markings can serve to identify one specific gun to the exclusion of all others.

There are many examples of class and individual characteristics to be found on fired cartridge cases. The shape and size of a firing pin impression is a class characteristic that is especially apparent in rimfire cartridges. A wide variety of shapes and sizes of firing pin impressions may be found, varying from rectangular, square, and wedge-shaped, to circular and semicircular, depending on the design of the manufacturer (see Fig. 12–28).

In centerfire cartridges, the firing pin impression on the primer is almost always circular, but the diameter varies. A few centerfire guns, however, have rectangular firing pins. The microscopic tool markings found on the end of the firing pin striking surface are an individual characteristic.

Ejector and Extractor Markings

Other class characteristics are the location of the extractor and ejector markings. The extractor usually marks the rim of a cartridge case while withdrawing the cartridge from the chamber, but may also make marks as it snaps over or slips over and engages the cartridge rim or at the time of disengaging the rim. The end of the extractor hook may bear against the case wall next to the head and produce markings there. This may also produce microscopic markings that are usable as individual characteristics, although the general location of the extractor marking is a class characteristic. Some manufacturers locate the extractor in the 3 o'clock position on the rim, others at the 2 o'clock or 5 o'clock position. Some makers design their guns with two extractors, and both leave markings on the cartridge case.

The ejector strikes the rim or head of the cartridge sharply during ejection and usually leaves a mark, the location of which is a class characteristic. Individual characteristics may also result. In certain model guns (notably rimfire), the firing pin does double duty by also acting as the ejector.

The magazine or clip may leave both class and individual characteristics, as may the process of chambering the cartridge. In semiautomatic and repeating firearms the bolt face or breech face strikes the cartridge head while moving it into the chamber, necessarily marking it in the process. Lips of a magazine usually mark the rim edges of cartridges as they are stripped from it and chambered.

Imperfections at the edge or mouth of the chamber will also mark the cartridge case as it is moved into and out of the chamber in loading and extraction. In automatic arms, the loading, extraction, and ejection may be quite violent, resulting in more pronounced markings than those found in other arms.

Many individual characteristics are imparted to a cartridge case by the internal pressure in firing. This acts in all directions, forcing the case hard against the breech face and sides of the barrel chamber. The breech or bolt faces and the chamber act as dies to impress their tool marks and manufacturing imperfections onto the cartridge case head and sides. Outlines of the firing pin hole as well as other breech face openings can frequently be seen impressed on the cartridge case by this pressure.

Types of Markings

Individual characteristics or markings can be divided into two basic types.

The first are *impression-type markings*, also called stampings. These are formed as their name implies by the forcible application of a hard surface against a soft one, leaving an impression of the harder. This may result in an obvious dent on the softer surface, or in many instances, only in very subtle markings. Impression-type markings result from the steel firing pin striking the primer in centerfire cartridges or case rim in rimfire cartridges. Also the internal pressure of firing forces the soft brass head of the cartridge case against the steel breech or bolt face, transferring to the brass some of the milling, turning, and filing marks left when the gun was made. Impression-type markings actually produce a combination of both individual and class characteristics.

The second type of individual markings are the *striations*. These can also be described as abrasions or simply scratches. They are produced by a harder surface scraping, dragging, sliding, or slipping across a softer one, leaving a series of abrasions, scratches and scrapes, or striae, from microscopic irregularities of the harder surface. As the cartridge is chambered, striations are caused by the lips of the magazine as the cartridge slides against them and, again, by the edge of the chamber as the cartridge slides into place. The extractor also produces striations as it slips over the cartridge rim. The ejector may produce a combination of impression and striation markings as the cartridge case is ejected from the gun.

Examination and comparison of all these individual markings and class characteristics is the basis for identification of a cartridge case as having been fired from a certain gun. An evidence cartridge case is closely examined under a microscope for the individual markings. The same is done with cartridge cases that have been test fired in the suspected gun. The actual comparison procedures are similar to those utilized in bullet identification.

The standard method is to use a comparison microscope, essentially two microscopes joined together with a single eyepiece. This permits simultaneous observation of half the view of each microscope, side by side in the eyepiece. A line in the center of the field of view separates the views of the two microscopes. If two cartridge cases can be brought into position under the respective objectives so that their individual markings appear to flow from one to the other at the dividing line, an identification is made (Fig. 12–29).

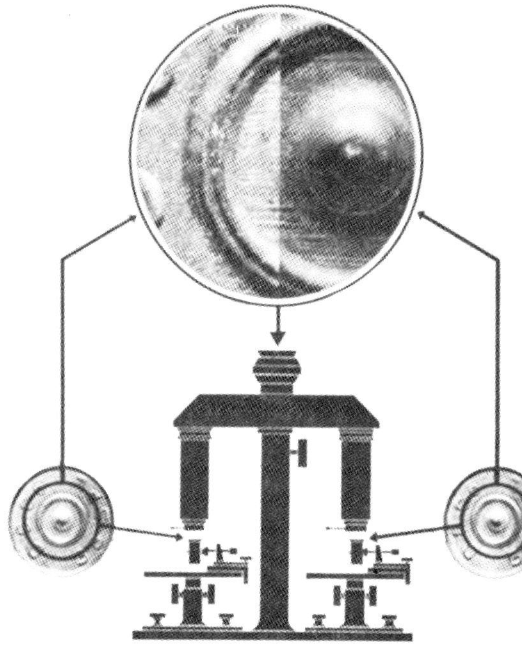

Figure 12–29. Cartridge case identification with a comparison microscope. The view through the comparison eyepiece proves that both cases were fired in the same gun. The left half of the comparison photomicrograph shows a portion of the left-hand cartridge case, while the right half of the comparison view is of the primer area on the right-hand cartridge case. (Courtesy of the Institute of Applied Science.)

An identification may sometimes be accomplished with photomicrographs of the heads of the test and evidence cartridge cases. The photographs are cut and superimposed to demonstrate the flow of the individual markings from one cartridge case to the other.

There are many problems and pitfalls for the firearms examiner in the area of cartridge identification, and considerable experience and skill are needed to understand and overcome them. For example, the tool markings on the breech or bolt face are not always impressed into the cartridge case clearly enough for use. In centerfire cartridges, the breech face markings are most readily apparent on the primer, including the area surrounding the firing pin impression. This is because the primer is of much softer metal than the cartridge head and, therefore, more impressionable.

It is extremely important in test firing (of both centerfire and rimfire cartridges) always to use the same brand and type of ammunition as the evidence cartridge. Brass hardness varies among brands of cartridge cases, which therefore differ in their ability to receive usable individual markings. Different types of loadings may also produce different pressure levels and again affect case markings. The smoother the finish on the bolt and breech face, the less apparent the breech face markings on the fired cases. With any given quality of finish, the markings are most apparent in high-velocity rifle cartridges, since these guns have the highest breech pressures.

Manufacturer's headstamps on both centerfire and rimfire cartridges tend to interfere with production and observation of breech face markings. Many times the markings left on cartridge cases from their manufacturing processes resemble the individual characteristics left on them by the gun in firing; these can confuse the uninitiated. Accidental abrasions can result from the cartridge being roughly handled, dropped, or carried about, and such markings can be confused with those left by the gun. Cartridges may have been worked through a gun action in loading and unloading before they were eventually fired in the gun, acquiring more than the normal number of extractor, ejector, and magazine markings on the case. This can be confusing to the examiner attempting to identify the make and model of a gun by its class characteristics.

Reloaded Cases

In centerfire cartridges, there is always the possibility that the cartridge case has been reloaded once or several times before the last firing. It may have been fired in different makes and models of gun of the same caliber, each of which will have left its own set of class characteristics and some individual characteristics on the cartridge case. Here, close attention to the primer markings (both firing pin and breech face) are most helpful, as a primer is replaced with each loading.

One must always be mindful of the possibility that intentional alterations have been made in the suspected gun to prevent identification. These could take the form of changes in the breech or bolt face surfaces as well as replacement of the original firing pin with a different one.

Other Stumbling Blocks

One cannot always conclude that finding an automatic pistol cartridge case means it was fired in a self-loading pistol. As one example, special half-moon retaining slips to hold three .45 automatic pistol cartridges were made during World War I to facilitate firing the .45 automatic pistol cartridge in the Smith & Wesson and Colt cal. .45 M1917 revolvers. A cheap single-shot pistol firing the same cartridge was specially made for use by underground forces during World War II. It is also possible to peen the rim edges of certain semiautomatic pistol cartridges so they can be fired in revolvers.

Bullet Examination and Identification

The principles of fired bullet identification are similar to cartridge case identification. As in cartridge case identification we are interested in both the class characteristics and the individual characteristics. These are imparted to the bullet by the barrel. The class characteristics in fired bullet identification would be: (1) *caliber* (see earlier definitions); (2) *number of lands and grooves*, usually varying from 2 to 20 (see earlier definition of rifling); (3) *direction of twist of the rifling* (left or right); (4) *rate of twist or rifling* (angle of the lands and grooves; some rifling may have a very fast twist and would make a complete revolution in 10 inches or less, but other rifling would have a slower twist and would make a complete revolution in up to 24 inches or more); and (5) *width of the lands and grooves*. The first step taken by a firearms examiner is to determine whether the class characteristics of the bullet under examination are the same as those of test bullets fired for comparison or of other evidence bullets being compared with it. As previously pointed out, the class characteristics are peculiar to all guns of a certain make and model. Manufacturers, however, frequently make changes in the rifling specifications of the same model gun over a period of years. Therefore, it is possible for an early specimen of a certain make and model to have different class characteristics from a gun of the same model produced at a different time. The change most frequently found is in the width of the rifling lands and grooves. Change in number of lands and grooves is, however, not uncommon. Change in the direction of twist is the least common.

The class characteristics are most useful in eliminating certain guns from further consideration. If the class characteristics of a suspected gun are different from those of the evidence bullet, then the possibility of that gun having fired the evidence bullet is eliminated. If the class characteristics on an evidence bullet are peculiar or unusual, it may be possible to determine the exact make and model of the gun from which the bullet was fired. In most cases, however, it is only possible to say that the bullet came from one of a number of makes and models of guns having approximately the same class characteristics. The crime laboratory normally maintains records of manufacturers' class characteristics and as extensive as possible a

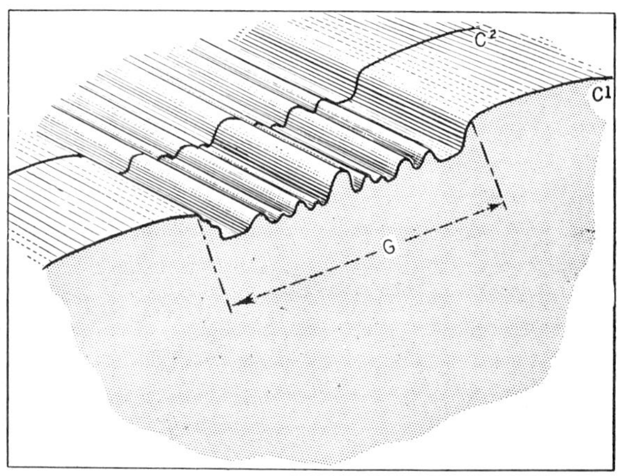

Figure 12–30. Diagrammatic view of the cross section of a portion of a bullet shows a part of the surface view and the "end" view of a portion consisting of a single groove G. The line C¹ represents the cross-sectional view. It consists of the contour line of the striations that form the groove marking (made by the rifling lands). Line C² is a similar line across the groove at a different point. Both C¹ and C² have the same general contour. (Courtesy of the Institute of Applied Science.)

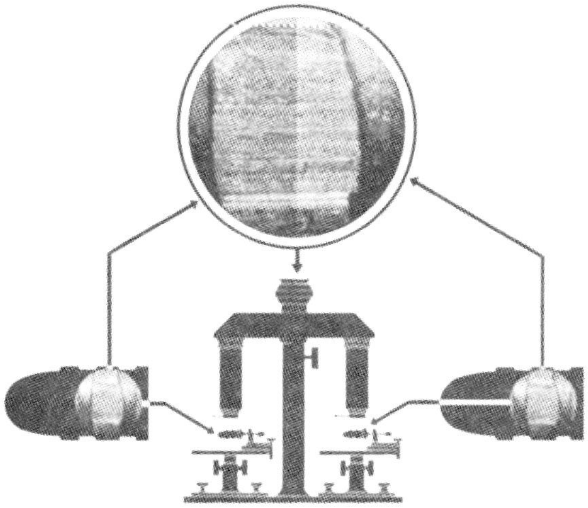

Figure 12–31. Bullet identification with a comparison microscope. The view through the comparison eyepiece shows a portion of each of the two bullets, which in this illustration were fired from the same weapon. The left half of the comparison photomicrograph is of the left half of the left-hand bullet specimen, and the right half of the comparison picture includes the right half of the right-hand bullet. (Courtesy of the Institute of Applied Science.)

collection of specimens of fired bullets (and cartridge cases) from different makes, models, and calibers of guns.

If the examination of the fired bullet reveals that the class characteristics closely match those of the test-fired bullets, or other evidence bullets being compared, the examiner would then compare the individual characteristics (those peculiar to only one gun).

The individual characteristics found on fired bullets consist essentially of striations. These are imparted by the rifling as the bullet passes through the bore of the barrel, the lands cutting into its sides and making grooves in the bullet as they force it to follow the spiral path of the rifling down the gun barrel. The rifling then acts as a die to reproduce all the microscopic tool markings and imperfections of the rifling on the sides of the bullet in the form of striations of varying depth, width, and contour (Fig. 12–30). As with cartridge case identification, the standard method of making the comparison is to use the comparison microscope. If two bullets can be brought into position under their respective microscope objectives so that, when viewed in the eyepiece, their individual markings appear to flow from one side to the other at the dividing line, an identification is made (Fig. 12–31).

Also as with cartridge case identification, there are certain stumbling blocks that may be encountered. In automatic pistols it is usually rather easy to replace the original barrel with a new barrel. In other types of guns the barrel may also be changed, but it is much more difficult and usually requires the services of a gunsmith. The gun barrel on a rifle or revolver may have been shortened, and in the process the resulting individual markings grossly changed. Such cases are rare but within the realm of possibility.

CRIME OR ACCIDENT SCENE FIREARMS EVIDENCE

This section contains some guidelines for gathering, handling, and interpreting firearms evidence found at the scene of a crime or accident. It is more oriented toward the preservation of firearms evidence and its significance than toward crime scene investigative processes in general.

If physical evidence is to be used in court proceedings, the court must be satisfied that the item to be introduced in evidence is the same item found at the scene of the shooting. There must be an unbroken chain of custody of the evidence from the scene to the courtroom. Testimony must be available as to the circumstances under which the evidence was gathered, its condition, and who has had possession or custody of it in the interim. Any alterations must be justified and accounted for.

Recovery, Marking, and Preservation of Evidence

The usual items of firearms evidence to be found at the scene of a shooting may be a bullet or bullets, fired and unfired cartridges and cases, and the firearm or firearms involved. (Powder residues and shot patterns are discussed later.)

Firearms

A firearm found at the scene should normally not be moved until it has been properly photographed in position. A written record should also be made. The crime scene investigator would also want to protect it for possible latent print evidence. Under no circumstances should a gun be cleaned on either the exterior or the interior. Some consideration should also be given to the safety of the persons moving a gun that is loaded and ready to fire because of possible accidental discharge. This might require uncocking visible hammer guns or placing the gun on safety if such a mechanism is available. The gun is normally unloaded after receipt in the laboratory; the recommended method of transporting it to the laboratory is in a plastic bag. A record should be made of the gun's make and model, the type, any serial numbers, and the location of the gun when found. Identifying initials should normally be scribed onto the gun's frame, receiver, or slide and on the gun barrel; they should not be placed on easily removable parts such as grips. Such marks should also be made as small as possible while still retaining their legibility and should be placed on such parts so that they are not readily apparent. In order to diminish the value of the firearm as little as possible, the underside of the frame and the underside of the barrel are places recommended for such markings. The owner may later be entitled to the return of the weapon and would not look kindly on large, carelessly and openly scrawled initials across the gun's surface. The laboratory personnel, when unloading a loaded gun, should record and number the position of the fired and unfired cartridges in a revolver cylinder as well as noting the maker's headstamps on each. A record should also be made of any ammunition found in a gun's chamber or in the clip or magazine.

Fired Bullets

Bullets should be handled with care to avoid damage. Every effort should be made to avoid damage in the removal of bullets from either a body or other lodging place. Particular care should be taken to safeguard the rifling area surfaces (sides of the bullet) against mutilation or damage of any kind. The bullet should be marked for later identification with an initial or other identifying mark scratched or scribed on the metal. There are differing opinions as to the proper place to mark a bullet. Obviously it should not be marked on the sides or the rifling surfaces. Recommendations have been made both for marking the bullet on the nose and for marking it on the base, but the author recommends that the base not be used. It frequently will have the manufacturer's identifying marks or other markings that might identify the type of powder being used, and to mark it may well obliterate them. Instead, the author recommends marking the bullet just above the rifling marks on the ogive but not squarely on the end of the nose. The nose of a bullet frequently picks up trace evidence that may have significance. For instance, lead bullets often pick up the pattern of the weave of fabric through which they have passed (Fig. 12–32). When more than one bullet is recovered, they can be numbered for identification and record

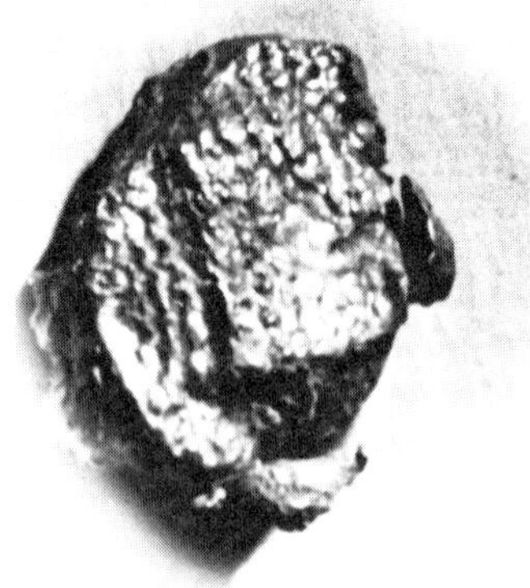

Figure 12–32. The mushroomed nose of a .22-caliber bullet showing the weave pattern of the cotton undershirt through which it had passed.

keeping, the number following the identifying initial, such as A–1, A–2,. . . The properly marked bullets should be placed in separate small plastic bags and rolled up and placed in sealed and marked envelopes or wrapped in cotton and placed in small cardboard pill boxes that are properly marked for identification. Identifying data should include date and place of recovery, name of person recovering evidence, and how bullet was marked for identification. If a bullet has any special identifying peculiarities or characteristics they should be noted.

Bullet Trace Evidence. It is also necessary to handle bullets carefully to avoid the loss of trace evidence that may be important to the investigation. Bullets frequently have areas on which there is dried blood, tissue, and body fluids. If the bullet in question was not recovered in the body, perhaps these dried body fluids and material have some special significance. It may be that additional serologic examinations would be helpful to the investigation.

In addition to body fluids and tissue, a bullet frequently carries traces of material through which it has passed. A bullet mushrooming in or passing through wood frequently has compacted wood fibers in and around portions of the mushroomed nose. This is also true of plaster, drywall, and other construction materials. On occasion, clothing fibers are attached to a bullet. Sometimes ricochet bullets have grains of sand imbedded in the surface that struck the ground. It was mentioned earlier that the nose of a soft lead bullet will on occasion pick up a print of a fabric weave. Frequently similar patterns are picked up when a bullet passes through screen materials in a screen door or window.

Whenever any foreign substances are noted

on a bullet, great care should be exercised not to dislodge this material but rather to preserve it and to get it into the hands of the laboratory examiner for analysis.

Fired Cartridge Cases

Fired cartridge cases should receive the same general care and precaution in handling as fired bullets. The identifying initials or marks should be made near or preferably inside the mouth of the case. Never mark the head of the fired case. Packaging and record keeping are similar to those for a bullet. Manufacturers' headstamps and other markings should be recorded. If a revolver is involved, the fired cartridge case will probably still be in the gun. It would be unusual for all cartridges in the revolver cylinder to have been fired, the fired cartridge cases removed, and the gun reloaded. In the case of repeating weapons, semiautomatic and automatic fire arms, however, the fired cases may be located at some distance from the point of firing. This is particularly true in connection with the semiautomatic and automatic weapons. The fired cartridge cases may be ejected with considerable violence and land from a few to several feet from the position of the gun at the time of firing. They may also roll for some distance. The most common direction of ejection is to the right side at right angles to the gun. The design of the extractor and ejector locations determines the approximate direction of ejection. The great variety of designs results in many different ejection angle and direction possibilities. Some firearms eject the fired cases almost straight to the front, and others at an angle to the rear. Because of the possible angles and distances of ejection, careful examination and inspection of the scene are necessary to locate all fired cartridge cases; their location should be carefully recorded.

Shot Wads and Pellets

It is not necessary to mark recovered shot pellets or wads individually. They should be placed in a small plastic or paper envelope and sealed. Glass vials with cotton packing may also be used for pellets, and pill boxes can be utilized for wadding. Identifying data should be recorded on the envelope, vial, or box, and should include location, date, and other pertinent information.

Loaded Cartridges

Loaded cartridges should be marked for identification on the side of the case. The handling, preservation, and packaging are similar to the methods utilized for bullets and cartridges. Again, careful records should be kept of the origin and location of the cartridges, as well as of the manufacturer's markings.

Firearms Combustion Residues and Patterns

This discussion of firearms combustion residues is limited to the mechanics of their formation and the characteristics of their patterns; Dr. Knight's discussion of firearm injuries covers their appearance on and in actual wounds. Firearms combustion residues often have great value in helping to answer the question "What distance was the gun from the victim at the time it was fired?" This question is frequently of critical importance in cases of questionable suicide or murder or self-defense. As indicated in the earlier discussion of ammunition, present-day propellants are almost always one of the several types of smokeless powder. When a firearm is discharged, certain combustion residues are formed and expelled from the muzzle of the gun with, and immediately following, the bullet. These residues can be placed in three categories, by weight.

The lightest residue is a sooty, smoky deposit that travels a very short distance. Next in weight would be consumed powder particles in the form of ash. These residues have irregularly shaped bodies and are of greater weight than the sooty deposits. They travel greater distances. The third type of deposit consists of partially burned and unburned powder particles. These particles have the greatest weight and travel the greatest distance. Minute amounts of primer residues are also mixed with the powder residues, and there may be other particles expelled with the combustion residues. Little bits of metal may become dislodged from the bullet, as may bullet lubricating grease or waxes.

Several factors affect the amount of combustion residues that are produced as well as the amount of residues that reach the target. The type and brand of ammunition being used account for differences in residues. It is always important in making comparative tests to use *exactly* the same type and brand of ammunition. Different manufacturers use different types of powder and load the cartridges with varying volume of powder depending on the ballistic requirements of their particular cartridge. It is not enough that the brand be the same, but the type must also be the same. (See Figure 12–33 for a dramatic demonstration of this point.)

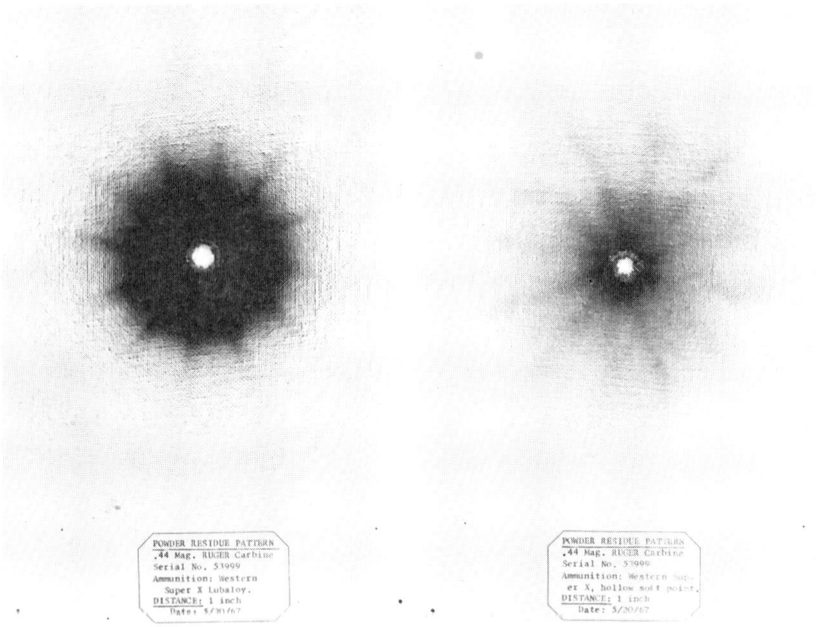

Figure 12–33. Photo comparison of two powder patterns fired from a .44 Ruger magnum carbine at a distance of 1 inch. Both were Western Super-X brand ammunition. One, however, was a loading with a lubaloy lead bullet, *left,* and the other, *right,* was with a hollow soft-point bullet. The slightly different loadings of the same brand produced greatly different patterns. The radiating pattern from the 12 rifling grooves in the gun barrel can be clearly seen.

Other factors are the length of the gun barrel (shorter barrels usually produce greater deposits over larger areas), humidity and temperature (humidity and temperature affect the rate of burn and the amount of resulting residue), distance from the gun muzzle to the target (discussed later), winds and wind velocity (blowing and scattering residues in the direction of the wind), and angle of the gun barrel to the horizontal or vertical. At a given distance more particles will reach a target when a shot is fired vertically downward than when fired horizontally. The particles have weight and tend to fall in an arc. Depending on the distance, some will fall short; if the distance is great enough, all will fall short of the target.

The combustion residues are deposited on the target in a definite pattern depending on the distance of the gun muzzle from the target. Size and density of pattern are the important factors in distance determination. As the distance between the gun muzzle and the target increases, the pattern size also increases and the density decreases until a point is reached where deposits no longer reach the target. Contact shots usually result in gaping entrance holes in clothing (destructive force of high-pressure gases), with the residues passing through and into the wound. Close shots usually result in the residues being confined to a small area. Sooty deposits are found only in cases in which the barrel was a few inches from the target (because of the lightness of the sooty material). As the distance increases the soot is no longer found in the pattern, only the ash and partially burned or unburned particles reaching the target. At the greatest distance only the heavier particles (usually the unburned or partially burned particles) reach the target. As a general rule, very little evidence of residue will be found beyond 20 to 25 inches. This will vary, however, the greater or lesser distance depending on the caliber, type of ammunition, and weapon involved. Figures 12–34 and 12–35 show examples of firearms discharge residues at varying distances with a .22-caliber and a .38-caliber weapon.

In trying to interpret the evidence of firearm discharge residues, it must be kept in mind that additional factors affect the amount of residues remaining on the victim, clothing, or target. Rough handling may have caused the loss of residues due to their becoming dislodged and falling away from the surface. Many of the residues are not found on clean white surfaces; most often the clothing is dark in color and tends to disguise their presence. The laboratory is normally equipped to detect the presence of firearm discharge residues. This is done by microscopic examination with a stereomicroscope, or by chemical processing (Walker test and "H" acid tests) of the clothing in a fashion that will transfer the residue pattern to photographic paper as a color pattern.

The detection of firearm residues on the person is also obviously of significant importance in the investigation of firearms incidents. The value is obvious in questions of murder or suicide. There are at present a few methods in use to test for the presence of firearm dis-

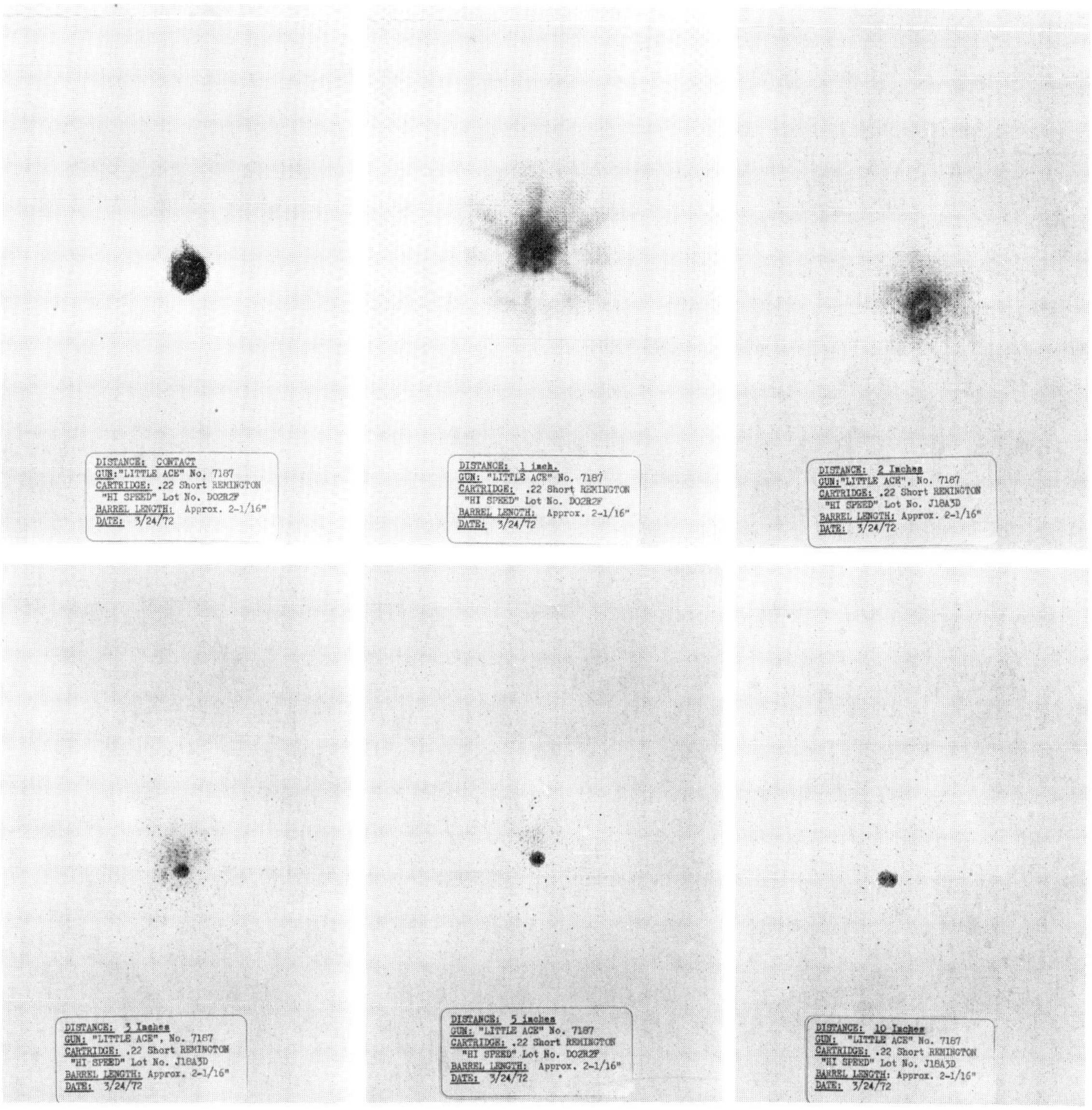

Figure 12–34. Firearms discharge residues from a .22 Derringer (.22 short) at distances of contact, 1, 2, 3, 5, and 10 inches.

charge residues on the person (hands) to determine if the person has fired or handled a firearm. When a gun is fired, residues are, in addition to being propelled from the barrel, also released from the ejection port in automatic and semiautomatic weapons and between the cylinder and barrel in revolvers. The handling of the weapon can also tranfer the residues to the hands.

Traditional Paraffin Test

The name of the paraffin test (also called the Gonzalez test, the dermal nitrate test, or the diphenylamine test) is somewhat of a misnomer because the paraffin is simply used to remove residues from the skin for later testing. (A paraffin cast is made of the hand. The cast is treated with a solution of diphenylamine, and the resulting color reaction is noted.) The purpose of the test is to detect the presence of nitrates and nitrites on the hands of the person. Firearms combustion residues contain nitrates and nitrites, but the test is specific for detecting not firearms discharge residues but only the nitrates and nitrites found in them. Unfortunately the detection of such residues, a positive reaction, does not mean that the person actually fired or handled a gun. There are a number of substances that a person may handle in the course of his daily living that will give

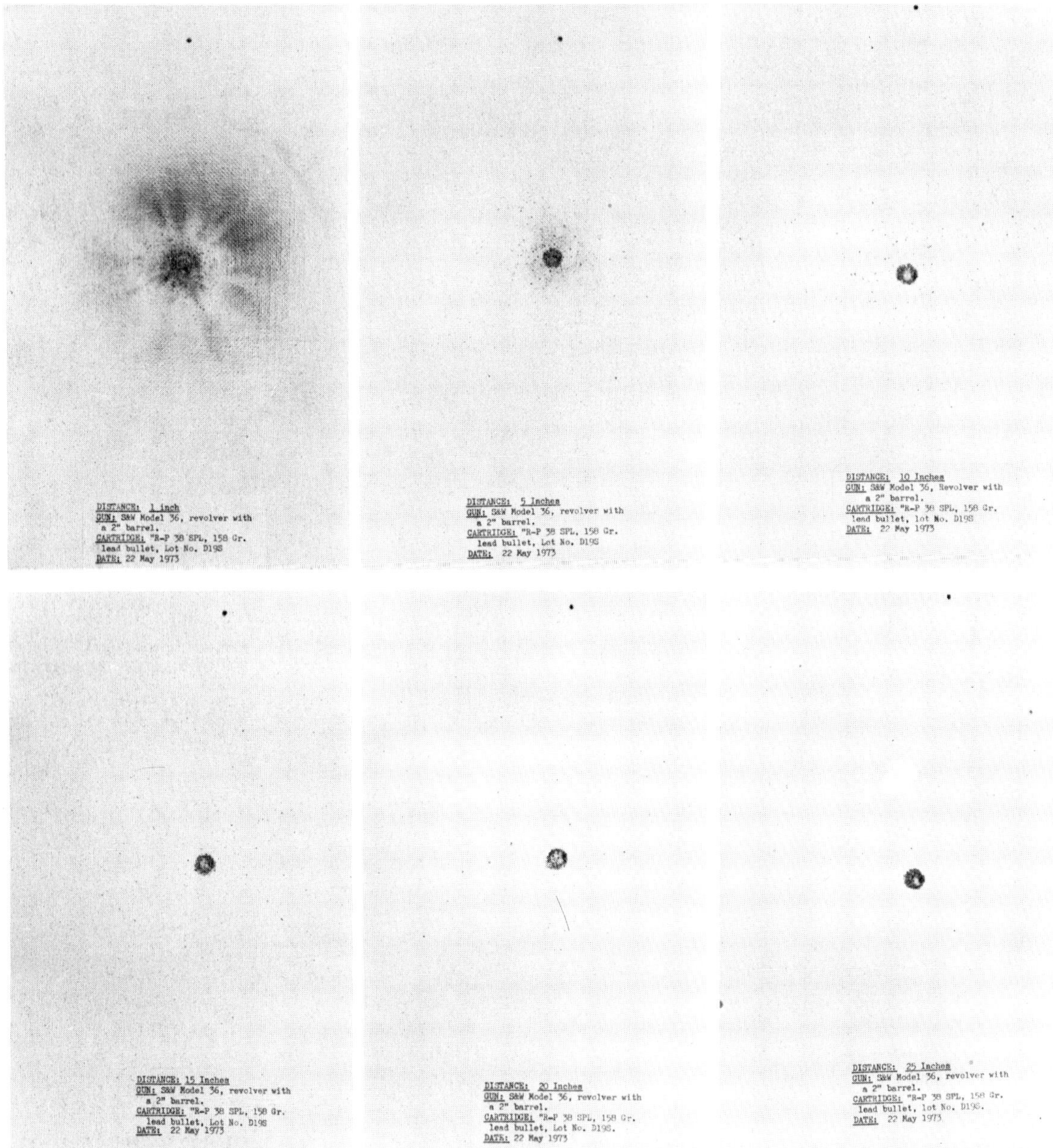

Figure 12–35. Firearm discharge residues from a .38 special revolver (2-inch barrel) at distances of 1, 5, 10, 15, 20, and 25 inches.

the same positive reaction to the test, common examples of such substances being tobacco, fertilizers, pharmaceuticals, leguminous plants, and many others. Twenty-one countries participated in the first Interpol Seminar on Scientific Aspects of Police Work in 1964. The following statement concerning the paraffin test resulted:

> The seminar did not consider the traditional paraffin test to be of any value, neither as evidence to put before the courts, nor even as a sure indication for the police officer. The participants were of the opinion that this test should no longer be used.

Harrison and Gilroy Test

This is also a chemical reaction test. It differs widely, however, from the foregoing test both in the manner of collecting the residues for testing and in the elements or compounds tested for. Again, this test is not specific for firearms discharge residues but only for certain elements or compounds to be found in such residues. In the paraffin test, melted paraffin is utilized as the means of collecting the residues. Harrison recommends the use of a cotton swab moistened with .1 molar hydrochloric acid. The paraffin test is used to detect the presence of nitrates and nitrites. Harrison and Gilroy's test (Harrison's test) specifically detects the presence of antimony, barium, and lead. (These are commonly found in firearms discharge residues.) Whereas one reagent is used in the paraffin test, three reagents are used in the Harrison test. The Harrison test is considered far superior to the paraffin test because the likelihood of an individual who has not fired or handled a gun having traces of barium and antimony on his hands is rather remote or rare compared to the likelihood of his having nitrates or nitrites on his hands. The Harrison test does not appear to enjoy any substantial utilization by criminalistics laboratories in spite of its superiority as a test and Harrison and Gilroy's literature on the subject published in 1959.[5a] The fact that one of the reagents (triphenylmethylorsonium iodide) is not available commercially but must be synthesized may be one reason. Because of the large amount of residues emitted between a revolver cylinder and barrel, tests involving such weapons are frequently more successful than others, but success has been achieved with most types of firearms.

Neutron Activation Analysis

This method involves the collection of the residues, their activation in a nuclear reactor, and their identification by gamma-ray spectrometry. The method of collection is either by the paraffin cast method or by the use of cotton swabs. The detection of antimony, barium, and copper is the intended end result. It is a highly sensitive test, the most sensitive of any considered. Again, it is not specific for firearms discharge residues but rather for certain elements or compounds to be found in such residues. Because of its uniqueness and the required instrumentation as well as the expense, this test is not widely available to law enforcement people. Considerable publicity has been given to it, however, and experimentation has been and is being done by Gulf General Atomic, the Internal Revenue Service, the Post Office Department laboratories, and others. This has resulted recently in utilization of this method by more and more law enforcement agencies, so it can no longer be called an unusual procedure.

Atomic Absorption Spectroscopy

The most recent methods of analysis in use in the larger, better-equipped laboratories are atomic absorption spectroscopy (AAS) and flameless atomic absorption spectroscopy (FAAS). These procedures are suitable for the measurement of barium, copper, and antimony in gunshot residues. Atomic absorption spectroscopy lacks the sensitivity of neutron activation analysis, but flameless atomic absorption spectroscopy is said to afford sensitivity comparable to that of neutron activation analysis. Advantages of these methods over neutron activation analysis are far lower cost of operation, availability, and rapidity of output.

Shot Patterns

Shot patterns were described earlier in this chapter in the sections on modern firearms and modern ammunition. Their value as evidence is much like that of firearm discharge residues. They provide significant information on the distance involved between the shotgun muzzle and the victim or target (shotgun wounds are discussed in Chapter 11).

As a very general statement, it can be said that a shot charge, after leaving the gun barrel, tends to remain together as a cylindrical cluster for a short distance (approximately 3 ft), after which the pattern starts to open up or spread. As the distance increases, the pattern gets progressively larger and less dense. The amount of spread is roughly proportional to the range involved. For a rule of thumb that is good only as a general guide, the shot pattern diameter for a full-choke shotgun is approximately 1 inch for each 3 ft of distance between the muzzle and the target. For example, a distance of 30 ft would give roughly a 10-inch diameter of spread. Again it must be cautioned that this is only a general rule and the best evidence is to

TABLE 12–2. APPROXIMATE PATTERN DIAMETERS OF SHOTGUNS AT VARIOUS RANGES AND CHOKES

Approximate Circle Diameter in Inches to Include 95% of Pellets—No. 6 Chilled Shot				
Range (yd.)	Full Choke	Modified	Improved Cylinder	Cylinder Bore
10	9	12	16	18
15	13	18	24	28
20	19	24	32	38
25	24	31	41	48
30	31	38	50	58
35	38	46	60	68
40	46	55	70	80
45	54	64		
50	64	74		
55	74	85		
60	85	96		

*Courtesy of Winchester-Western Division of Olin Corportion.

test fire the gun involved over various distances, using the same brand and loading of shotshell. Table 12–2 gives approximate circle diameter of shotshell patterns at varying distances and chokes.

There are a number of variables that affect the size of the shot pattern. The most obvious of course are the distance and the degree of shotgun choke. Other variables consist of differences in shotshells (e.g., gunpowders, types of wadding, shot loadings, pressures). Differences in the shotgun barrel length and barrel conditions in addition to the choke may also result in variations. Shotshell wadding will follow the shot charge for a distance. At close ranges of a few feet, the wadding will probably enter the same hole as the main shot charge. As the distance increases the wadding tends to be diverted to the side and soon falls to the ground. This is due to the relatively light weight of the wadding and the proportionately heavy resistance of the air to the large surfaces presented by the wadding. The modern one-piece plastic wadding tends to have greater range due to its greater weight. A typical shot pattern at varying distances is shown in Figure 12–36.

As a rule, the large United States manufacturers of shotshells utilize plastic wads (Fig. 12–37). Remington-Peters utilizes a one-piece wad

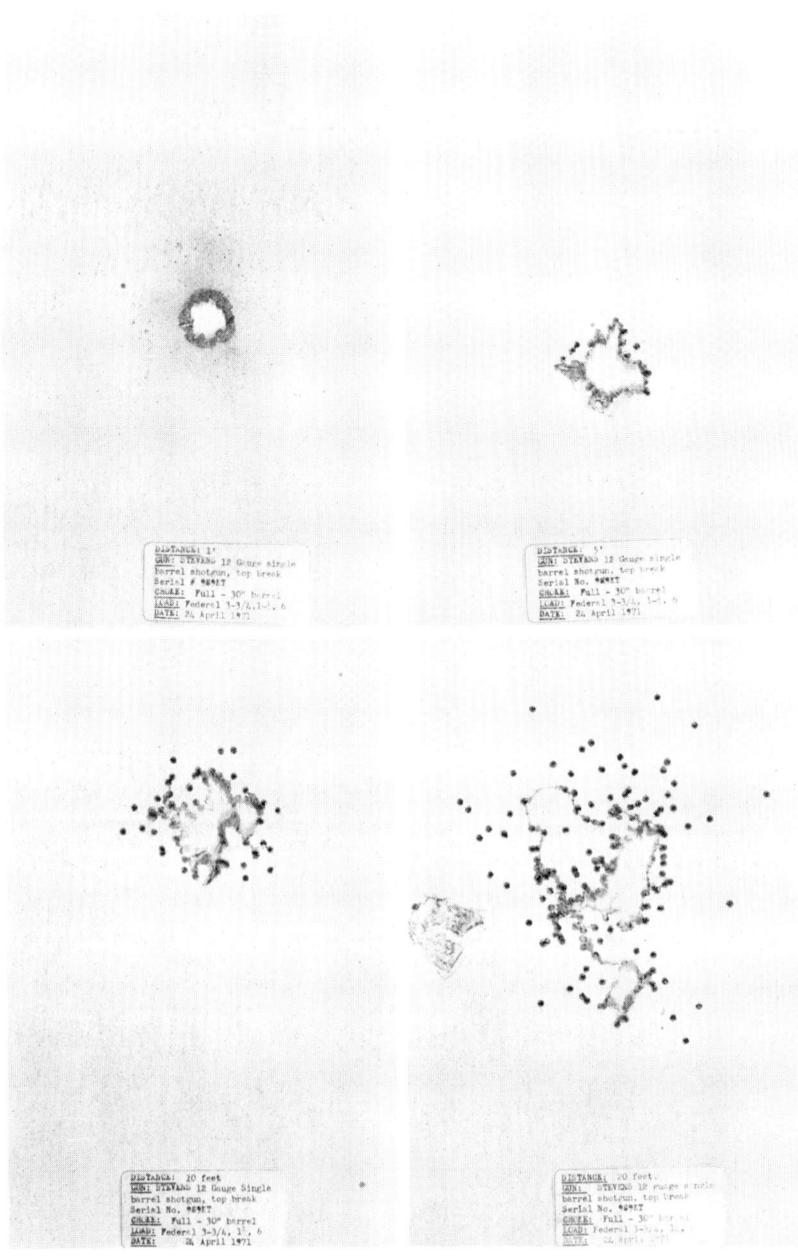

Figure 12–36. Shotshell pellet patterns (12-gauge full-choke gun) at distances of 1, 5, 10, and 20 ft. Note impact mark from plastic shot wad on 20-ft pattern.

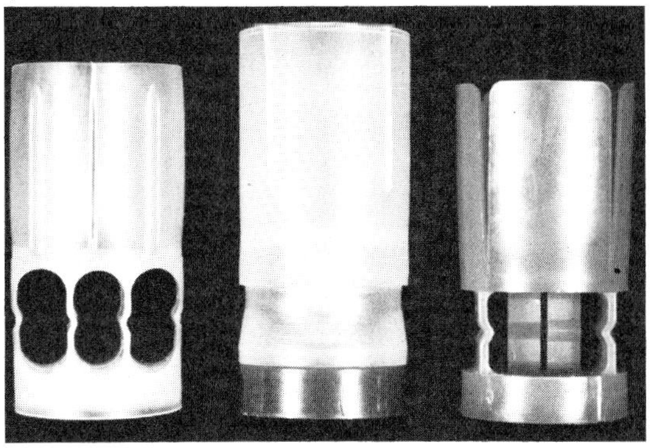

Figure 12–37. Three styles of plastic one-piece shotshell wads. *Left to right,* Remington Power Pistol, Federal Champion, and Winchester-Western Double A wads.

column that they call Power Pistons. Federal Cartridge Corporation uses their all-plastic Triple-Plus and Champion wad columns. Winchester-Western uses a one-piece plastic wad column in their target loads called Double A wads. They utilize fiber wads in their hunting loads, but use a wraparound plastic shot wrapper to protect the shot charge during its passage down the gun barrel. The collection and preservation of wad evidence is very important. The identification of the brand and type of shotshell being used is frequently possible because of the distinctive differences between the modern plastic wads. The firearms or ballistics laboratory normally maintains a reference collection of different types and styles of domestic and foreign shotshell wads for identification purposes. Fiber and paper wads (once the predominant style) are not as distinctive and easily identifiable.

SELECTED READINGS

1. Bearse, R.: *Centerfire American Rifle Cartridges 1892–1963*, South Brunswick, N. J., A. S. Barnes and Co., Inc., 1966.
2. Burrard, G.: *The Identification of Firearms and Forensic Ballistics, 3rd Edition.* New York, A. S. Barnes and Co., 1962.
3. Butler, D. E.: *The American Shotgun*, New York, The Winchester Press, 1973.
4. Davis, J. E.: *An Introduction to Tool Marks, Firearms and the Striagraph.* Springfield, Ill., Charles C Thomas, 1958.
5. Gunther, J. D., and Gunther, C. O. : *The Identification of Firearms.* New York, John Wiley & Sons, Inc., 1935.

5a. Harrison, H., and Gilroy, R.: Firearms discharge residues. J. Forensic Sci., *4*:184, 1959.

6. Hastings, M.: *The Other Mr. Churchill—A Lifetime of Shooting and Murder.* New York, Dodd, Mead & Co., 1963.
7. Hatcher, J. S., Jury, F. J., and Weller, J.: *Firearms Investigation, Identification and Evidence.* Harrisburg, Pa., Thomas C. Samworth, 1957.
8. Houts, M.: *From Evidence to Proof.* Springfield, Ill., Charles C Thomas, 1956.
9. Jones, L. V.: *Scientific Investigation and Physical Evidence.* Springfield, Ill., Charles C Thomas, 1959.
10. Josserand, M. H., and Stevenson, J.: *Pistols, Revolvers and Ammunition.* New York, Crown Publishers, Inc, 1972.
11. Kirk, P. L.: *Crime Investigation.* New York, Interscience Publishers, Inc., 1953.
12. Krcma, V.: *The Identification and Registration of Firearms.* Springfield, Ill., Charles C Thomas, 1971.
13. Mathews, J. H.: *Firearms Identification.* Springfield, Ill., Charles C Thomas, Vols. I and II, 1962, Vol. III, 1973.

13a. Midkiff, C. R.: Detection of gunshot residues: modern solutions for an old problem. Police Sci. Administration *3*:1:77, 1975.

14. Moenssens, A. A., Moses, R. E., and Inbau, F. E.: *Scientific Evidence in Criminal Cases.* Mineola, New York, The Foundation Press, Inc., 1973.
15. Munhall, B. D., and White H. P.: *Cartridge Identification.* Vol. 1, *Centerfire Metric Pistol and Revolver Cartridges;* Vol. 2, *Centerfire American and British Pistol and Revolver Cartridges.* Washington, D.C., The Combat Forces Press, 1950.
16. Munhall, B. D., and White, H. P.: *Cartridge Headstamp Guide.* Bel Air, Md., H. P. White Laboratory, 1963.
17. National Rifle Association Staff: *NRA Firearms & Ammunition Fact Book.* Washington, D.C., The National Rifle Association, 1970.
18. Nonte, G. C.: *Firearms Encyclopedia.* New York, Harper & Row, 1973.
19. O'Hara, C. E., and Osterburg, J. W.: *An Introduction to Criminalistics.* New York, The MacMillan Co., 1949.
20. Osterburg, J. W.: *The Crime Laboratory.* Bloomington, Ind., Indiana University Press, 1967.
21. Richardson, J. R.: *Modern Scientific Evidence.* Cincinnati, The W. H. Anderson Co., 1961.
22. Smith, J. E., and Smith, W. H. B.: *Small Arms of the World.* 7th Edition. Harrisburg, Pa., The Stackpole Co., 1962.
23. Smith, J. E., and Smith, W. H. B.: *The Book of Rifles.* 3rd Edition. Harrisburg, Pa., The Stackpole Co., 1963.
24. Smith, J. E., and Smith, W. H. B.: *Book of Pistols and Revolvers.* 7th Edition. Harrisburg, Pa., The Stackpole Co., 1968.
25. Smith, S.: *Mostly Murder.* New York, David McKay Co., Inc., 1959.
26. Snyder, L.: *Homicide Investigation.* Springfield, Ill., Charles C Thomas, 1959.
27. Soderman, H., and O'Connell, J. J.: *Modern Criminal Investigation.* 4th Edition. New York, Funk & Wagnalls Co., 1952.
28. Steindler, R. A.: *The Firearms Dictionary.* Harrisburg, Pa., The Stackpole Co., 1970.
29. Svensson, A., and Wendel, P.: *Techniques of Crime Scene Investigation.* 2nd Edition. New York, American Elsevier Publishing Co., Inc., 1965.
30. Thorwald, J.: *The Century of the Detective.* New York, Harcourt, Brace & World, Inc., 1964.

SECTION 2. INJURY BY FIREARMS, BOMBS, AND EXPLOSIVES

chapter 13

INVESTIGATION OF BOMBS AND EXPLOSIVES

by Derek McVitty and Robert Alan Hall

Explosives constitute a major category of physical agents capable of causing death or a wide variety of injuries to mind, body, and property. The effects of the trauma are generally similar and pose similar problems to pathologists wherever they occur; blast injuries to individuals in one country do not differ significantly from those in another. The causative agents, however, may differ markedly, and bomb investigation in any country is necessarily limited by the opportunities afforded to investigators within that country by the criminal activities of its people. The construction of a bomb is a function of the knowledge and skills of the criminal individual or group operating within the constraints of the supply of materials and the level of law enforcement, and is conditioned by the social and physical environment within which the product is used. It is not surprising, therefore, that the knowledge and skills of investigators differ from one country to another nor that the material in this chapter is necessarily incomplete, since the authors do not pretend to have worldwide experience of this problem.

Our experience of terrorist activity, extending back over nearly 20 years but mostly gained quite recently, leads us to presume, however, that the content of this chapter will interest and assist those who may at some time be involved in the investigation of bombing incidents or the pathologic examination of those who are killed or injured in them. The treatment of the subject is partial rather than general, emphasizing matters within our personal experience. This is not a serious limitation, since bombs are bombs wherever they are made, and although there is much scope for variation and improvisation in their construction and manner of use, the end products exhibit a degree of similarity that may, in part, result from parallel development in technology in this field but more probably results from the direct and indirect free exchange of information among subversive elements around the world. There is little know-how in the field that is not now the common property of those everywhere who wish to use it against society, and this increases the urgency and importance of becoming more fully aware of the real or potential threat and better prepared to meet it. This can best be facilitated by improved communication between those who have to deal with the problem of this particularly damaging expression of deviant behavior wherever it arises.

The methods of investigation are essentially the same everywhere except when constrained by lack of knowledge and experience on the part of the investigators, or by limitations of financial and human resources, or by both. A complete treatment of the subject is beyond the firsthand experience of any single authority and could not be contained in a single chapter. Within these constraints, we aim to convey the dynamic quality of the problems and practice of this aspect of forensic science in a real life setting in which time and change are major dimensions.

In recent years Northern Ireland has suffered a campaign of terrorism so intense and prolonged as to be almost unique in modern times. Even within its political, social, and economic context, which in turn is capable of varied interpretation and explanation, the complexity of the problem there defies the understanding of most observers and, indeed, of many of those who suffer its effects. Apart from the rights or wrongs of the situation, the present campaign of violence is the most serious since, in 1921, Ireland was partitioned and Northern Ireland established as an integral part of the United Kingdom with control of many of its governmental functions devolved on a Northern Ireland Parliament subordinate to the Westminster Parliament in London. We confine ourselves to the effects of this situation that have been manifested in the bombing campaign of the recent past, while noting that bombing is only one expression of the terrorist activity.

After three years of growing tension punctuated by political demonstrations and isolated sectarian murders, violence erupted on a massive scale in Northern Ireland in August 1969. From that time until March 1976, over 1,500 persons were killed and over 10,000 injured of a population of only 1.5 million. More than 350 people were killed by explosions, of which there were over 5,000. The magnitude of the problem is not conveyed by absolute numbers, however. The sheer size of many of the bombs, the number of incidents to the square mile, and the number of victims relative to those at risk distinguish the Northern Ireland problem from that of, say, the United States, where a similar absolute number of bombing incidents occurs but results in a smaller absolute number of deaths and injuries spread over a country some 650 times as great in area and a population about 130 times as large as that of Northern Ireland. Immense difficulties face the investigators, who are often unable to benefit from the sources of information usually available in criminal investigations. Whole districts have been, at times, "no-go" areas for the police and the army; witnesses have been afraid to come forward; and terrorists have been sheltered and assisted by sympathizers in their own communities. Nor are the terrorists identifiable by any obvious racial or ethnic characteristics; in appearance and speech they are indistinguishable from their victims. With direct evidence often lacking, increased reliance has had to be placed on indirect or circumstantial evidence, and this leads to a further distinction of some importance. Whereas in the United States, for example, responsibility for the investigation of bombing incidents is spread among many law enforcement agencies, in Northern Ireland there is only one polic force, the Royal Ulster Constabulary, and one forensic science laboratory, in which the experience of bomb investigation is concentrated.

CLASSIFICATION OF BOMBS

Depending on their active ingredients, bombs are often described as either incendiary or explosive, but this simple classification ignores the fact that they may have both explosive and incendiary properties, e.g., an explosive charge may be used to ignite an incendiary substance. Explosive substances themselves are classified as high explosives or low explosives according to their composition, but some incendiary materials can be used to produce explosive effects.

A second method of bomb classification is by their manner of use: those that are projected and those that are placed or laid. Thus an incendiary device may be thrown like the small petrol bomb or may be laid and so constructed as to ignite after a time delay. Similarly, explosive bombs are divided into types that are commonly lobbed at the target and types that are placed where they can exert the maximum effect. Here again there is some overlap, for many devices can be employed in either way.

In a third way of categorizing bombs, according to the intentions of those who employ them, they can be described as antipersonnel or antiproperty devices, though here also there is no hard and fast line since many are used for a dual purpose or have a dual result.

Many divisions and subdivisions of these sys tems can be elaborated: projected bombs can be activated by a fuse or by impact; laid charges can be arranged to operate on a short fuse or after a longer preset time delay. Most practical preset delay devices that require some degree of timing precision incorporate a clockwork mechanism, but time delay can be achieved with less noise, though with greater uncertainty, by chemical or other means. Similarly, laid bombs may lie quiescent until they are operated remotely on command from the bombers, or left as booby traps to be set off by the intended victim. Command-controlled bombs require either extension wiring to a remote switch or wireless control from a position of concealment. Booby-trap bombs can be mechanically or electrically operated, and there are many variations of each type.

Extensive systems of classification of bombs can be devised to embrace their major and minor characteristics. Such systems are useful in organizing knowledge and enhancing understanding of the relationships between the various types within the system, and are particularly helpful in training bomb investigators. It is difficult, however, if not impossible, to devise a universally acceptable system for any area of inquiry, and this is certainly true of bomb technology. There is no particular merit in quoting any particular system nor in adding to the list by constructing a new one. Such systems are artificial, necessarily arbitrary and short-lived, and require constant modification in the light of new technology and experience.

DATA COLLECTION AND USE

More concerned with practice than with theory, however, those who are concerned with bomb investigation find that as the number of incidents increases, it is very helpful to have a satisfactory method of organizing the accumulating mass of data. A practical, low-cost method of data control can perhaps be best achieved by using a multiple-entry punched-card system in which all the known possible features can be listed. Such a system not only facilitates rapid information retrieval but is sufficiently flexible to permit the information to be retrieved under whatever headings are from time to time considered necessary. More ambitious and less cost-conscious authorities might consider a computerized system of data control justified.

A practical difficulty with such a system is that, since information gathering is itself time consuming and expensive and it is not easy to identify the stage at which bombings are frequent enough to warrant this expenditure of scarce resources, by the time a decision is taken to implement an effective system, much of the early information may be unavailable. A practical point in its favor is that several different authorities may, for various good reasons, wish to keep a record of events, and some coordination of these activities can ensure not only that there is no duplication of effort but also that the several systems are interlocking and compatible. Coordination permits overall control and rationalization of procedures, sometimes leads to large economies, and encourages cooperation and the exchange of information between the different parts of the law enforcement structure, whether it be at the county, state, or national level. Full investigation, good record keeping, and information exchange can help to identify trends in bomb technology and criminal activity, alerting those whose function it is to initiate or implement control procedures. Geographic areas of great activity that demand closer police supervision can be recognized; similarities of constructional detail or manner of use may indicate a common source of components or the existence of a central assembly or manufacturing point; laboratory analysis may demonstrate a growing dependency on certain explosive substances, highlighting the need for legislation to control their availability; and the coexistence of two or more quite different technical approaches in the same area can suggest or confirm the existence of different, perhaps opposing, subversive groups and may even permit an incident to be attributed to one or another of them. Finally, proper investigation of incidents and effective record keeping may lead to the linkage of events and perhaps to the identification of a suspect, at which time the accumulated circumstantial evidence may be used in criminal proceedings.

INCENDIARY BOMBS

Background Events in Northern Ireland

Every year, the "Apprentice Boys," a Protestant organisation, commemorate the shutting in 1688 of the city gates of the old walled city of Londonderry in the face of the advancing Catholic army of King James I, the French-supported pretender to the British throne. In August 1969 this traditional annual parade through Londonderry, the second largest city in Northern Ireland, led to disaster. The Catholics claim that they were insulted by the Apprentice Boys, or by some of them, who were alleged to have thrown down pennies from the walls of the old city in a gesture of contempt toward the people in the Catholic Bogside district. The Protestants claim that they were insulted and jeered at by the minority elements. There is probably some truth on both sides. The march was broken up by stoning, and the day ended in tragedy when a major confrontation developed between the police and the inhabitants of the Bogside. This was no skirmish; it developed into a battle that

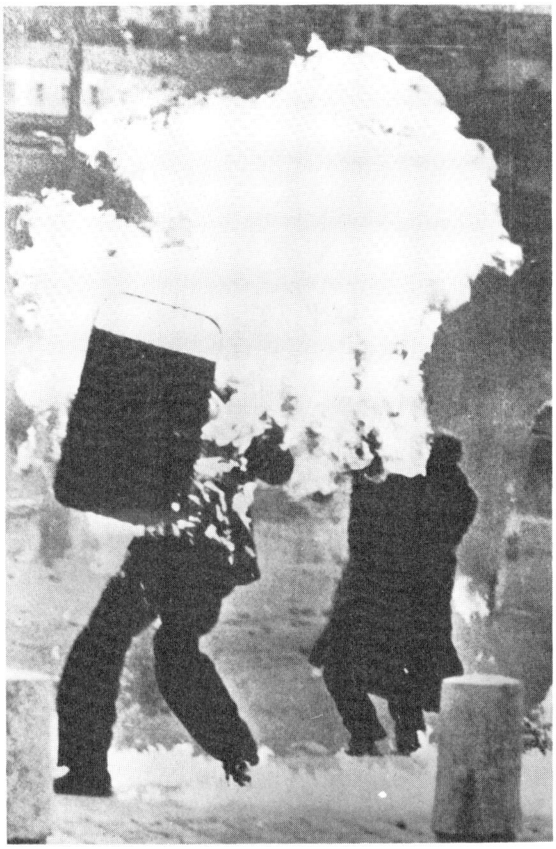

Figure 13–1. Human torch. A policeman carrying a riot shield is the victim of a petrol-bomb attack. Londonderry, 1969.

lasted three days. The police, armed with batons and riot shields, made several sorties into the area but were met by determined resistance from the inhabitants, who were clearly operating from prepared positions and armed with a seemingly endless supply of petrol bombs, some of which they aimed very effectively from the commanding heights of the tops of blocks of flats (Fig. 13–1). Police reinforcements were brought in from all over the country, but the police organization was not prepared for battle on the scale that developed, and the men, untrained in riot control, suffered heavy casualties as a result of the bombardment with petrol bombs and stones. It was later estimated that one tenth of the entire force of approximately 3,000 was injured in the first days of the campaign of violence that started at that time.

The petrol bombs, simpler to prepare and use than the old-fashioned Molotov cocktails, consisted of nothing more complicated than a milk bottle full of petrol with a cloth wick protruding from the neck. One had only to touch a light to the wick and hurl the bottle at the foe. They were extremely effective.

At the height of the battle of Bogside, a call went out for simultaneous risings elsewhere to relieve pressure on the Bogside, and major rioting, burning, and shooting flared up between the Protestant and Catholic communities in Belfast,. the capital city. The police were exhausted, and at the request of the Northern Ireland government, the government in London ordered the army into Northern Ireland to quell the disturbances. Peace of a kind was restored, but the army, at this time less skilled in dealing with civil conflict, attempted to keep the combatants apart—even erecting, along a "peace line," a semipermanent high barrier in the small streets of West Belfast and so separating the Protestant and Catholic areas by a structure reminiscent of the Berlin Wall. This action provided opportunity and perhaps even encouragement for the demarcation, designation, and development of the Catholic "no-go" areas of Belfast and Londonderry. "Free Belfast" and "Free Derry" were created under the uncomprehending eyes of the British Army and in the face of rising anger among the Protestants.

The Protestants themselves were not slow to use fire as a weapon in 1969. The retail liquor trade in Northern Ireland was almost a Catholic monopoly, even in Protestant areas, and public houses were an easily identifiable target for Protestant mobs. Many were petrol bombed, and Protestant licensees hurriedly began to display the Union Jack as a protective symbol. Nor were the Protestants less guilty than the Catholics in burning the homes of those of the opposite religion who found themselves living on the wrong side of the line in this new expression of sectarian bitterness.

The rioting of 1969 was largely spontaneous, or at best, loosely organized. The underground Irish Republican Army (IRA) was at low ebb and in no condition to assume a dominant role in the fighting. During the months that followed the arrival of the British Army, the uneasy peace continued, broken only by occasional isolated acts of violence, while in the Catholic areas the IRA built up its strength. Internal dissension split the IRA into two factions, the Officials and the Provisionals. The Officials, perhaps more closely representing the traditional IRA, played little part in the subsequent events. Indeed, their reluctance to commit themselves to a direct confrontation with the British Army at this stage may have led to the emergence of the Provisionals. Organizing along military lines, the latter set up brigades, battalions, and company staff. Volunteers joined in large numbers, and the

"Provos" quickly became a force to be reckoned with.

Construction and Delivery of the Bomb

The year 1970 was to become the year of the incendiary bomb. The typical device consisted of a small, crudely made cardboard box bound with electrical insulating tape (Fig. 13–2). From a small hole in one side projected a short length of wooden dowel rod through the end of which was a finger ring of wire to facilitate easy removal. Inside the box, the other end of the dowel held open the jaws of a spring clothespeg furnished with drawing pins to act as electrical contacts. From these terminals, wires led to two small 1.5-v penlight (torch) batteries, connected in series, and to a simple heating element embedded in a small polythene-wrapped packet of sodium chlorate and sugar. The heating element was typically a strand or two of wire wool joining the ends of the circuit wires, which were strapped to the sides of a short length of lollipop stick. The bomb was armed by withdrawing the dowel rod through the hole in the box, but an ingenious arrangement prevented the jaws of the clothespeg from closing at once. The other ends of the peg had been squeezed together and wrapped with solder wire. When the bomb was armed, the spring of the clothespeg tried to close the jaws, but the solder wire provided an effective delay. Gradually the strength of the spring overcame the resistance of the ductile solder, which stretched, allowing the jaws to close and complete the circuit. The full voltage was dropped across the high-resistance element, which quickly got red hot, igniting the incendiary mixture. Varying the tightness of the solder wire binding made different time delays possible, and on many of the recovered devices an optimistically estimated delay was found written on the sides of the clothespegs. An ounce or two of the incendiary mixture (sodium chlorate and sugar) was usually employed, sometimes with the addition of a small amount of crumbled, solid paraffin firelighter to prolong the resulting blaze. (Used alone, the chlorate and sugar produces an intense but short-lived ball of fire.)

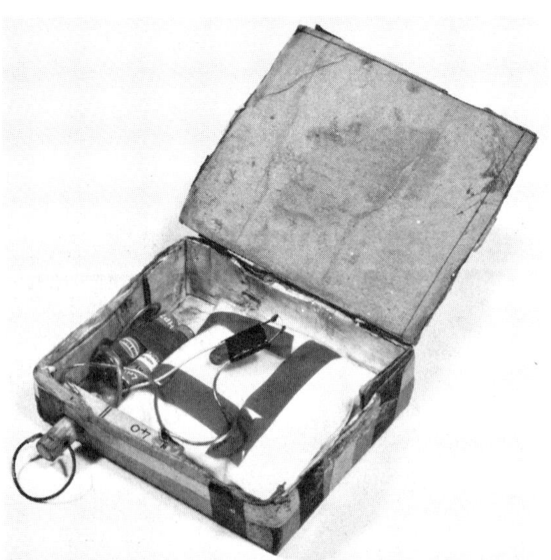

Figure 13–2. Improvised incendiary device, partly dismantled. Note batteries, clothespeg switch held open by dowel rod with finger ring, and heating element displayed on packet of incendiary mixture.

Throughout 1970, some hundreds of these delayed-action devices were placed in department stores, shops, and offices, often just before closing time, causing many fires. At this time security measures were nonexistent and the small incendiary bombs, sometimes housed in empty cigarette packets, could be delivered to their targets with impunity; a woman with a shopping basket could carry and plant a dozen bombs within an hour. Slipped inside furniture on display, placed between piles of bedding, or thrown into boxes of waste paper, they would lie until the fire started or until they were discovered accidentally. When the full seriousness of the fire bombs was realized a poster campaign was introduced to educate the public, and regular searches of shops and offices by employees began to lessen the incidence of fires. Customer searches at store entrances were instituted and have since become part of the way of life.

The story of the bombing campaign by the IRA and the efforts of the Royal Ulster Constabulary army to combat it is essentially one of action and counteraction. As each new ploy of the bombers was recognized and countermeasures were introduced, the IRA in turn developed new techniques requiring further countermeasures by the security forces. A substantial proportion of the clothespeg bombs failed to ignite because of faulty construction or because they were found and disarmed before the time delay expired. The reply of the IRA was to post incendiary bombs through the letter boxes of business premises after they had closed for the day. These letter bombs were a variation of an old IRA technique used in the 1930s. In a stout Manila envelope were two polythene packets, one containing an incendiary chlorate and sugar mixture and a wax capsule of acid in a deflated and tied-off rubber balloon or contraceptive sheath, and the other containing a sponge soaked in petrol to provide a reservoir of fuel. Just before the envelope was "posted," the wax capsule was crushed, releasing the acid, which gradually penetrated the rubber balloon to react with the incendiary mixture, instantly producing fire. Usually a shortage of inflammable material behind the door of the premises prevented development of a major fire, and even the added petrol failed to prolong the initial fire long enough to cause any real damage. Many letter boxes were sealed up at this time to foil the IRA mailmen. Between 1970 and 1973 incendiary bombing lessened considerably, but in 1974, 1975, and 1976 hybrid explosive/incendiary bombs were in regular use.

Investigation of Fire Bombings

Inquiries into the causes of fires are notoriously difficult. Complete burn out and collapse of a building may destroy the evidence entirely or render its discovery almost impossible. Even when a fire is brought under control quickly, the cause may remain uncertain despite the most painstaking investigation. This is particularly true of a deliberate fire when the firesetter has used readily combustible materials such as waste paper and empty cartons—to be found in almost any commercial building. Even in the midst of a wave of fire bombing, however, the investigator cannot assume that any particular fire was deliberately caused; although arson may be suspected or indicated, there is still the problem of whether the fire was the result of ordinary criminal activity or was started for political reasons. Only the most careful examination of the scene can sometimes resolve the issue.

In petrol bombings fragments of the bottle may be found, perhaps in association with the charred remains of a twisted cloth wick. Occasionally, when the fire has been discovered early or perhaps has failed to spread, a quickly mounted investigation may allow the recovery of material close to the burned area that may still bear traces of the inflammable liquid. Preserved in sealed containers, such material can later be examined by gas chromatographic techniques. When there is no obvious cause of fire, a slow and usually prolonged search of the debris must be made. After the complete burnout of a fashionable Belfast furniture store, preliminary investigation revealed the approximate center of origin of the fire at street level. The upper floors had collapsed, but all the burned material in the area was collected and inspected piece by piece. Finally the debris was sieved and a clothespeg spring was found. On other occasions clothespeg springs, burned wiring, and charred remains of small batteries have even more clearly indicated the causes of major fires. To show that an incendiary device is the cause of a fire is a positive contribution, but the forensic scientist can assist the courts even more directly, as the following example demonstrates.

At the height of the fire-bomb campaign in 1970, the police received information that a man had been seen acting in a suspicious manner in the vicinity of a derelict house. A search of the house resulted in the discovery of the two small incendiary bombs shown in Figure 13–3, unarmed but ready for use, and these were brought to the laboratory for examination. They were alike in construction but differed in detail from others that had been seen before. Their outer covering was of thin cardboard formed into a packet some 6 inches by 4 inches by 1 inch and bound with both red and black electrical insulating tape. Inside, the heating element of wire wool strands was tied between two panel pins knocked into a short length of dowel (Fig. 13–4). The thin black polyvinyl chloride–covered wire to the panel pins was secured to the dowel by candle wax. The flying leads from the clothespeg completed the circuit, which was powered by a small 9-v battery. The heating element was wrapped in a small packet of chlorate and sugar primer, and there were two larger packets—one containing chlorate and sugar; the other, crumbled white solid paraffin firelighter. The arming pins, not shown in Figure 13–3, were also short lengths of dowel. They were drilled to take a finger ring, but no ring was present.

Among the tasks of the forensic scientist is participation in the police education program. This program helps ensure that the police are fully aware of the laboratory's needs and potential, and frequently pays handsome dividends.

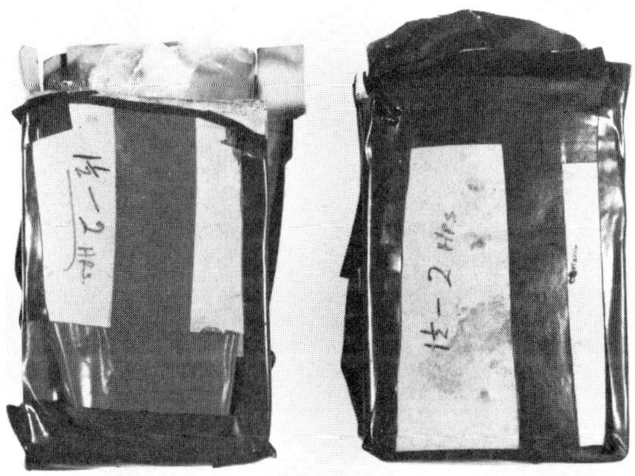

Figure 13–3. Two improvised incendiary devices found by police in Belfast.

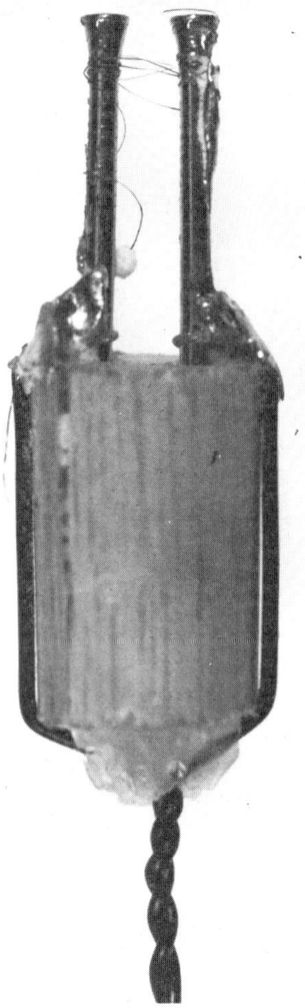

Figure 13–4. Heating element used in incendiary devices shown in Figure 13–3.

A few weeks after the discovery of the two incendiary bombs, the police raided a house in West Belfast. Among the items they seized was a school exercise book containing handwritten instructions on bomb making and sabotage, but they also took possession of other items that many policemen might have overlooked. The items brought to the laboratory included a large partially used sheet of thin cardboard, a haversack of tools, a solder wire dispenser, a reel of electrical wire with black polyvinyl chloride covering, a box of panel pins, a reel of red electrical insulating tape, a box of screws, several boxes of small batteries, and a reel of nylon fishing line. Although they had not known of their existence, these police officers had found the source of the two incendiary bombs and the evidence to prove it.

The bomb coverings were the same material as the sheet of thin cardboard. When one of them was flattened out it exactly fitted a cut edge of the large sheet, and moreover, when the two pieces were examined under ultraviolet light, a fluorescent stain was seen to lie half on one and half on the other side of the matching edge. The red insulating tape was 1 inch wide and similar in all respects to that used to wrap the bombs, but a search for matching ends was unsuccessful.

Fifty-five small batteries were found in the house, an unusually large number if they were being used for an innocent purpose. Ten of them were small 9-v batteries of the type used in the two bombs, and the other forty-five were 1.5-v batteries, the type more commonly used in incendiary bombs. Significantly, many of these 1.5-v batteries were wired in series pairs and strapped together with insulating tape, exactly as in the great majority of IRA incendiary bombs.

The solder dispenser was equally interesting. It contained, not a coil of wire, but many pieces bent into a rectangular shape with the ends twisted together. Identical in every way to the solder-wire ties used to pinch together the ends of the clothespegs in IRA incendiary bombs, they were, perhaps, evidence of practice in bomb construction or experimentation with time delays.

The black polyvinyl chloride–covered electrical wire was identical to that used as circuit wiring to the heating element in the two bombs shown in Figure 13–4.

The box of panel pins provided further evidence. Not only were the pins in the box similar in size and shape to those used in the two bombs, but a comparison of the irregular pattern on the heads of both sets of pins showed them to be identical (Fig. 13–5). Because the value of this evidence was uncertain, test purchases of panel pins were made throughout the city, with particular coverage of hardware shops near the suspect's home. In every box purchased, the pins had similar head patterns, but in no case did those in one box resemble those in any other, and no pins were found with a head pattern like that on the pins from the bombs and the suspect's home. Clearly the unique head pattern was an accidental imperfection caused by the particular machine on which the pins were made. This evidence was another valuable link.

The haversack contained an assortment of hand tools of no particular interest. They would have been useful in bomb construction, but were just as suitable for many legitimate uses. But the haversack did not contain only the tools; the dust and debris from it were examined microscopically and found to contain fragments of candle wax, wire wool, solid paraffin firelighter, and crystals of sodium chlorate and sugar—all components of the two bombs. Crystals of sodium chlorate and sugar and fragments of wire wool were also found in the box of screws and on a sticky label on the reel of fishing line. The debris from the haversack also contained two interesting pieces of thin-gauge galvanized wire (Fig. 13–6).

At about the same time as the raid on the suspect's home, a search of an empty house proved rewarding; a Thompson submachine gun, a favorite weapon of the IRA, other weapons, and a large assortment of ammunition were found under the floorboards. With them was a polythene bag containing a quantity of clothespegs made up with terminals and flying leads, several heating elements,

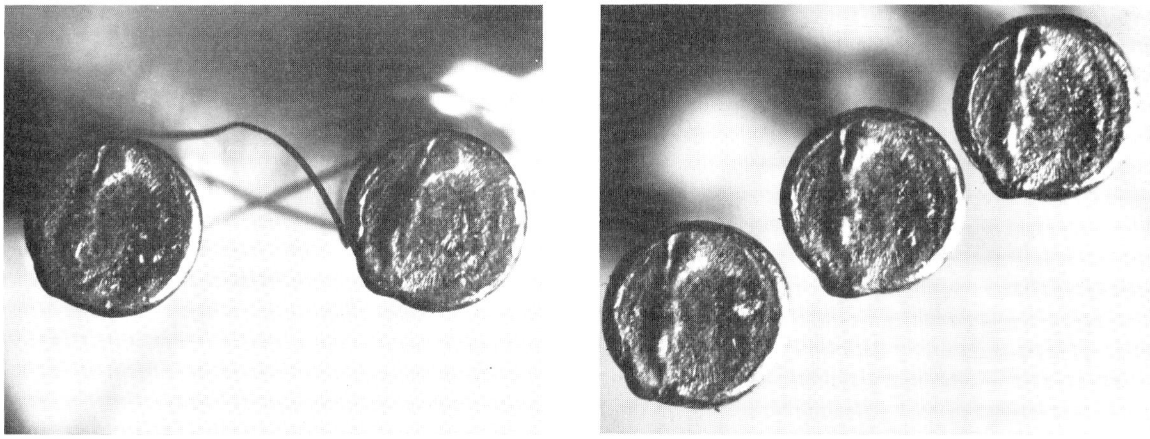

Figure 13–5. Head end comparison of the two panel pins shown in Figure 13–4 with three pins from the box of panel pins found in the suspect's home.

and a number of arming pins made of the usual short lengths of wood dowel and complete with finger rings. All were ready for incendiary bomb construction. The finger rings were of the same thin galvanized wire as the two pieces of wire from the haversack, and interestingly, those in this second find were fastened in two different ways. In some the two ends were overlapped and soldered together after the wire had been passed through the hole in the dowel. Once soldered, such a ring could be removed only by desoldering the joint or, more easily, by cutting the wire. In the other rings the two ends of the wire had been clenched back, close to the dowel, but not soldered. The two pieces of wire found in the haversack had clearly been made up as finger rings—one of each type. Their condition indicated that they had been removed from their dowel rods after fabrication, for the soldered ring had been cut at a point away from the soldered joint, and the unsoldered ring had simply been pulled out, its shape distorted but still showing turned-over ends. When these two pieces of wire were reformed into a circle they made rings of the same size as all the others.

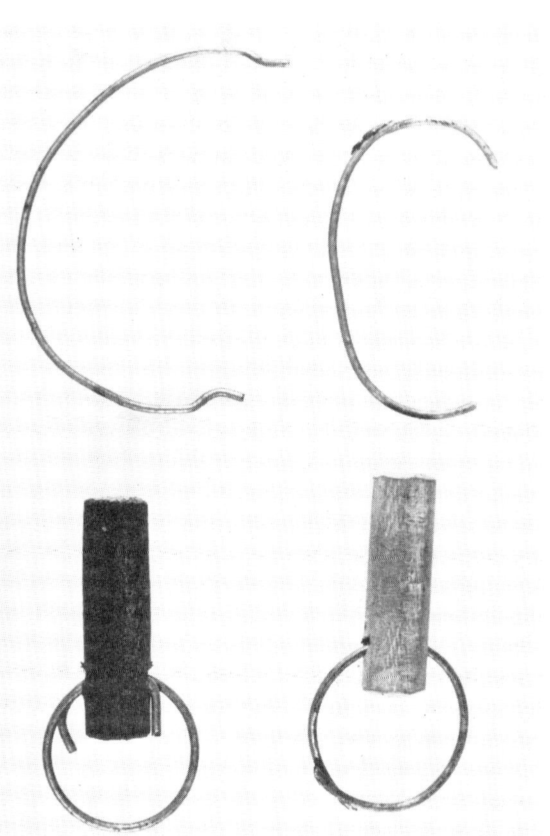

Figure 13–6. Two pieces of thin galvanized wire were found in a suspect's haversack, and two arming pins equipped with finger rings were recovered from another source. One of each pair is soldered, but the others have clenched ends.

An obvious question is, "Why should the two rings have been removed from their dowel rods?" The answer lies in the manner of construction of the bombs, and its discovery further strengthened the evidence. During assembly of the bombs, the jaws of the clothespegs have to kept open by the arming pin to prevent the chlorate and sugar mixture from igniting. Once the assembled components are enclosed in the outer cover, however, the arming pin must protrude through the small hole in the packet made for this purpose (see Fig. 13–2). Clearly the person who had made up these two bombs had found, when wrapping the completed assembly, that the rings on the arming pins were too big to pass through the hole from the inside of the packets and, since they were not really essential, had removed them. This would explain the absence of finger rings on the two bombs and also the two dismantled rings in the haversack. Presumably, with the more common box container, the correct assembly procedure would be to insert the dowel rod through the hole from the outside and into the jaws of the clothespeg at an early stage of construction when the size of the finger ring presented no problem.

A comparison of the dowel rods from the bombs

with those in the second find revealed evidence of a common origin. This evidence (matching machine marks along the surface and even matching cell patterns on the transverse surfaces) was ruled inadmissible, and a charge of possession of the weapons, ammunition, and other items was withdrawn. The trial jury found the defendant guilty of possession of explosive substances, however, and he was sentenced to eight years' imprisonment.

CLASSIFICATION OF EXPLOSIONS

Although in retrospect the criminal events of 1970 appear to have been dominated by the widespread use of incendiary devices, explosions also were common. Even during the political unrest of the late 1960s Protestant groups were responsible for several bombing attacks on major public utility installations such as water pipelines and electricity pylons in country districts close to Belfast. The IRA, however, has a longer tradition of using explosives and, at the beginning of the present campaign, included in its ranks many older men who had been active in earlier years. It was not long before the sound of explosions became commonplace in urban areas.

An explosion can be simply defined as the sudden release of previously confined energy, and the easily recognizable characteristics of this process are the production of heat, large quantities of gas, and plenty of noise. There are three basic types of explosion: atomic, mechanical, and chemical.

Atomic Explosions

Atomic nuclei can be regarded as stores of highly condensed energy, and the uncontrolled release of this energy constitutes an atomic explosion, the devastating effects of which need no elaboration. At the present time this subject is outside our terms of reference.

Mechanical Explosions

A mechanical explosion occurs when greater pressure is suddenly created than can be readily dissipated by the immediate environment. A common example, frequently encountered in building fires, is the rapid conversion to steam of the moisture in concrete floors or asbestos roofs. The steam, produced too rapidly to escape from its surroundings, causes a build-up of pressure that is released by an explosion, with mechanical rupture of the material. Pressure systems are subject to mechanical explosions, and the simplest example is the bursting of a toy balloon. More serious consequences result from the bursting of metal containers such as the liquefied petroleum gas cylinders now widely used domestically and in industry. Accidental explosions are not uncommon, even though these containers are designed with reasonable safety margins. The cause is usually to be found in the application of excess heat, in which case the term "cook-off" is appropriate.

The ingenuity of terrorists is often demonstrated in their ability to work with readily available materials, as our experience shows, and an explosion in Belfast at the home of a well-known politician illustrates this point.

The house was in the hands of builders who were carrying out renovations. A loud explosion was heard one night, and considerable damage was found to have been done. Among the debris was a ruptured gas cylinder. Inquiries revealed that the cylinder belonged to the builders, who kept it connected to a portable gas ring used for making tea. When examined, it was seen to have been burned on its base, and closer inspection of the distorted base showed that it bore three regularly spaced indentations. These were found to fit the kettle supports on the top of the gas ring, and the cause of the explosion then became clear. The person responsible had lighted the gas fire and stood the cylinder on top of it so that it would self-destruct. The force of the mechanical explosion had driven the base of the cylinder downward against the gas ring, providing an unusual example of the industrial technique of explosive forming of metals.

Chemical Explosions

Chemical explosions occur when a chemical reaction produces heat and gas faster than the surroundings can dissipate it. At the start of the reaction the initial heat or gas pressure increases the rate of reaction, which progresses at a faster and faster rate until an explosion results. There are two distinct types of chemical explosion, dispersed and condensed.

Dispersed Explosions

Dispersed explosions are those in which the reactants are unconfined. When a jet of flammable gas burns, a chemical reaction takes place between the gas and the oxygen in the atmosphere. Heat is produced, but there is little change in volume, since both the reactants and the products are gaseous. The heat is easily dissipated in the surroundings because only limited quantities of the reactants are together at any given time. If, however, the gas and air are mixed in the correct proportions and then ignited, the immediate total reaction results in the sudden production of heat, and therefore of pressure, sometimes greater than even the open environment can easily accommodate. The result is a relatively mild blast of hot gases capable of causing serious burns. When such a reaction takes place in a confined space, the heat and resultant pressure cannot be dissipated quickly, the rate of reaction increases, and an explosion ensues. The most common example of a dispersed gas explosion is in the internal combustion engine, where the pressure produced by the explosion of a petrol and air mixture drives a piston and hence propels a motor vehicle.

The burning of gas and air mixtures occurs only within well-defined limits of concentration. These are known as the "explosive limits," outside which no reaction will take place. Some examples are given in Table 13–1.

In recent years the greater use of gases such as propane and butane has increased the incidence of dispersed gas explosions. The petroleum gases are heavier than the older gases produced from coal and tend to settle in hollows, basements, and badly ventilated areas. A typical accidental explosion occurred in a trailer park.

As darkness fell, the gas supply from a cylinder was turned on and two gas mantles about head high on the walls of the trailer were lighted. Some time later the occupants, a man and a woman, prepared for bed. The woman was in her nightdress and the man was just removing his shirt when an explosion blew the woman's nightdress off and hurled her through the door of the trailer. She died immediately. The man was thrown to the floor but suffered only superficial burns and shock. The trailer was damaged only slightly, perhaps because the door acted as a pressure valve. An examination of the vehicle provided a simple explanation for the accident. The gas pipe from the cylinder ran horizontally at floor level beside a fitted bunk before rising to the wall lights. A T-joint connection on the horizontal section of the pipe was provided for a gas heater. The tap on the T-joint was turned off, but when the supply from the cylinder was turned on, gas escaped from the ends of the T-joint, which was too large for the gas pipe itself. When the gas mantles were lighted, gas escaped from the faulty compression joint and built up at floor level. By the time the occupants were ready to retire they must have been wading in the heavy gas, and when the man removed his shirt, gas was swirled upward, forming an explosive mixture that was ignited by the flame of the gas mantle.

TABLE 13–1. EXPLOSIVE LIMITS FOR SOME COMMON GASES*

GAS OR VAPOR	PERCENTAGES OF GAS IN THE ATMOSPHERE CREATING AN EXPLOSIVE MIXTURE
Ammonia	16.0–27.0
Acetylene	2.5–80.0
Benzene	1.4–7.1
Carbon monoxide	12.5–74.2
Hydrogen	4.0–74.0
Methane	5.0–15.0
Petrol	1.4–6.0
Propane	2.1–9.3

*From *Handbook of Chemistry and Physics*. 42nd Edition. Cleveland, The Chemical Rubber Publishing Co., 1960. Reprinted by permission.

A similar method of causing explosions has been used by terrorists during the present campaign. For example, an explosion in a church was contrived by terrorists who carried a gas cylinder into the church, opened the valve, and set a small incendiary device with a time delay. This later initiated a much larger dispersed-gas explosion that completely destroyed the building.

It is worth noting in passing that a less obvious but equally important source of accidental dispersed explosions is suspended dust. The finely divided dust takes the place of gas, igniting and propagating in the same way. Among the most common inflammable and finely divided dusts are coal, sugar, flour, aluminum, and fiber. Many very serious explosions have occurred from these materials, and all that is required is a stimulus to raise the dust from the beams and ledges on which it has settled, and a source of ignition. An old flour mill in Belfast was badly shaken by such an explosion some years ago (Fig. 13–7).

Condensed Explosions

Condensed explosions, the second category of chemical explosions, occur when large quantities of heat and gas are produced as a result of a very rapid chemical reaction in a solid or liquid material. Another specific feature is that such an explosion has a point of origin, so the most severe damage is caused closest to the source and the effects diminish as the distance from the center of the explosion increases. The third characteristic of condensed explosions is that no atmospheric oxygen is required; if oxygen is required in the reaction it is incorporated into the explosive.

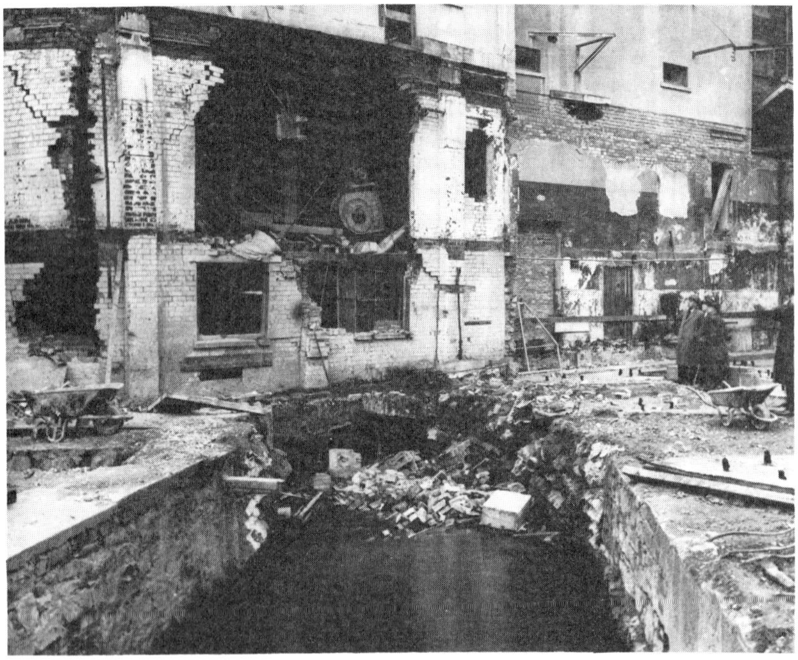

Figure 13–7. A Belfast flour mill was badly damaged by a dust explosion.

CLASSIFICATION OF EXPLOSIVES

There are two main categories of explosives, low explosives and high explosives.[3]

Low Explosives

Low explosives, or deflagrating explosives, are those that rely on burning and confinement to produce an explosion. When unconfined they burn rapidly, but as in unconfined dispersed explosions, the heat and pressure are produced slowly enough for the energy to be dissipated safely in the surroundings. When the reaction is confined, the build-up of heat and pressure causes the reaction rate to increase rapidly to an explosion. Up to an optimum, the greater the confinement the better will be the explosion. Gunpowder is the best-known low explosive, consisting of an intimate mixture of potassium nitrate, charcoal, and sulfur. The oxygen supply is in the potassium nitrate, and the other ingredients supply the fuel. After its discovery in the thirteenth century, gunpowder came to be used, as its name suggests, as a propellant in firearms, and it was not until the seventeenth century that its value as a means of rock breaking and earth moving was recognized. Low explosives produce a slow heaving action very suitable for some forms of blasting when large pieces of rock are required rather than small fragments.

High Explosives

High explosives detonate. Detonation is a phenomenon characterized by very high pressures and very fast reaction rates. A shock wave passes through the explosive, causing molecular disruption and producing heat, gaseous products, and enough energy to propagate the shock wave. It is this shock wave, spreading out from the explosion, that causes the disruptive effects of high explosives.

The difference between low explosives and high explosives can be understood by imagining a very long tube of explosive in which the explosion starts at one end. With a deflagrating explosive, the explosion travels along the tube at speeds up to 300 m per second (600 mph), whereas with a high explosive the speed may be 7,000 m per second (14,000 mph) or more.[1] The pressure of a low explosion can reach 50,000 psi, but in high explosions the pressure developed may range from 50,000 to 4,000,000 psi. High explosives are subdivided into two subcategories, primary and secondary high explosives.

Primary High Explosives. Primary high explosives are extremely sensitive materials that detonate if ignited. They are too sensitive to use in bulk but are ideal for the construction of detonators. Mercury fulminate and lead azide are the best examples.

Secondary High Eplosives. Secondary high explosives are much less sensitive. When ignited they do not explode and often do not burn well. To produce an explosion they must be subjected to a shock wave from another detonating explosive, usually supplied by a detonator, or blasting cap.

Most commercial secondary high explosives are based on nitroglycerin, a yellow viscous liquid explosive that is too unstable to be used alone. When mixed with nitrocellulose (gun cotton), they form a stable gel, and this mixture, called blasting gelatin, is the basis of all nitroglycerin explosives. Ammonium nitrate, a very insensitive secondary explosive, is used as an additive in most formulations, and by varying the proportions, a whole range of explosives with widely differing velocities of detonation can be prepared. Commercial explosives also contain a range of other additives: wood meal, starch, aluminum, other nitro bodies, and waterproofing agents. Recent developments in explosive technology have centered round nonnitroglycerin explosives, and ammonium nitrate slurries are being investigated by many explosives manufacturers.

TERRORIST USE OF COMMERCIAL EXPLOSIVES

Large quantities of explosives are used legally in mining, tunneling, and quarrying, and smaller amounts are employed in explosive welding and forming, demolition, and seismic investigations. The use of explosives for minor agricultural tasks is not without significance. A few years ago many farmers in Northern Ireland had a few pounds of gelignite for removing rocks or tree stumps from their land. In Northern Ireland, 3,000,000 lb of explosives were used commercially in 1968, so it was not surprising that some of this found its way into the wrong hands. Even had security measures been 99 per cent effective, some 30,000 lb could have gone astray, and in a community in which opposing groups were bent on violence, explosives were available to those who sought them. So, too, were the necessary accessories, fuses and detonators.

By 1970, the army came to realize that the real threat of violence was offered by the IRA, which had taken over de facto leadership of the Catholic community in the poorer districts of Belfast and Londonderry and in many rural areas. When the Protestant community saw that the army understood the situation, their own aggressive activity virtually ceased.

The Nail Bomb

Confrontations between the army and the Catholic mobs were now daily occurrences, and with the army cast by the politicians in the role of peace keepers, the advantage lay with the mob. Shouting abuse and wielding hurley sticks and throwing stones, they harassed army patrols whose only defense lay in their plastic visors and riot shields. The nail bomb was used freely. IRA bombs come in many sizes and in

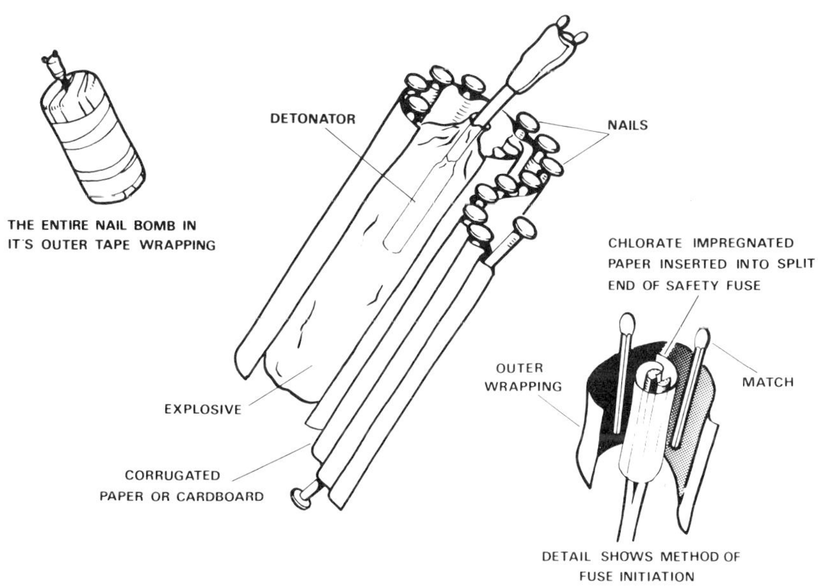

Figure 13–8. Construction of an IRA nail bomb.

many guises to suit the particular purpose, and the nail bomb is a small, convenient antipersonnel device (Fig. 13–8). It consists of a 2-oz stick of gelignite wrapped around with corrugated cardboard. Three-inch nails are pushed into the corrugations, and the cardboard is bound with strong adhesive tape. A plain detonator is inserted into the charge from one end, and to this is attached about 3 inches of safety fuse. Several nail bombs can be carried in the pockets of one person, and when the enemy is within range it is easy to light a fuse and lob the bomb over the heads of the crowd so that it lands among the soldiers. After much restraint and many warnings, the army announced that anyone seen throwing bombs would be shot. In Catholic districts street lighting had been put out of action early in the campaign to enable the gunmen and the bombers to move from cover and to get away again without being sighted. During the hours of darkness, then, a match struck to light the fuse on a nail bomb was more easily seen by the security forces, and for those few seconds the bombers were easy targets for army rifles. After the IRA had suffered a few casualties in this way they reacted by fitting igniters to the safety fuses on their nail bombs. These were simply a ring of red-headed matches taped around the fuse end so that the bomber had only to scrape the igniter against a wall and throw the bomb. Ignition of the fuse took place in flight. Many minor casualties were caused by nail bombs, but the soldiers quickly learned to avoid them.

The Nail Mine

The nail mine, shown in Figure 13–9, was a logical development of the nail bomb. A small wooden box was constructed with two compartments of unequal size. In the larger compartment a stick or two of gelignite was surrounded by nails. An electric detonator was pushed into the explosive, and the detonator wires led into the second compartment, which contained a 4.5-v battery and an instantaneous clothespeg switch. A dowel-rod arming pin, complete with finger ring, was inserted through a small hole in the box to keep the jaws of the clothespeg open, and one end of a long length of nylon fishing line was tied to the ring. This device could be left in a shop doorway or any other concealed position to await the arrival of an army foot patrol, when the bomber would tug on the line and pull out the arming pin, detonating the charge. Alternatively, the line could be used as a trip wire with the same effect.

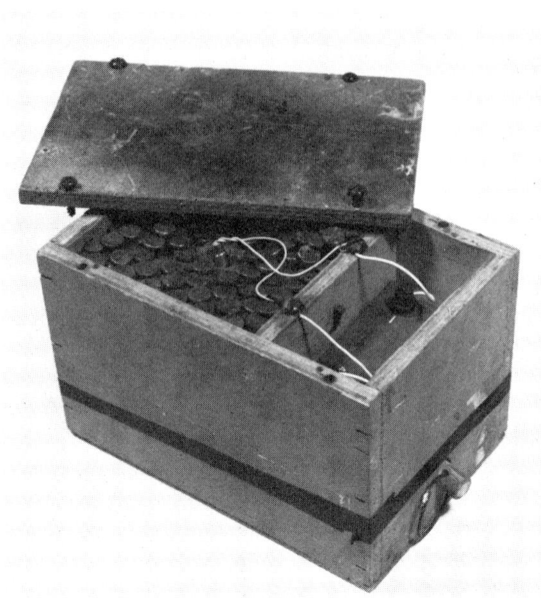

Figure 13–9. IRA nail mine.

The Claymore Mine

Still bigger was the IRA version of the claymore mine, also a two-compartment box with one half packed with explosive and the other half packed with short lengths of steel rod to act as shrapnel (Fig. 13–10). Usually these were operated only by a length of safety fuse leading to a detonator, but sometimes an additional time delay device was incorporated. One example, which failed to explode, had an acid and balloon delaying device inside a twisted sheet of newspaper that was impregnated with sodium chlorate, and this was wrapped around the safety fuse. The acid had failed to penetrate the balloon, and in later examples of this

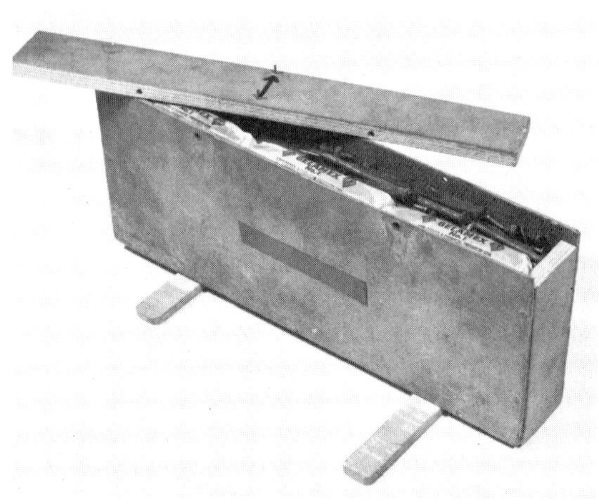

Figure 13–10. IRA claymore mine.

time delay technique, thin contraceptive sheaths were usually substituted for balloons.

The value of preserving material from the scene of a bombing was demonstrated very clearly in the case of this same unexploded claymore mine:

Some time after a claymore mine was found, a patrol from the Special Patrol Group of the Royal Ulster Constabulary observed an automobile traveling along a border road. When they pursued it, the driver abandoned his vehicle and made off across the fields toward the border. The police searched the automobile and in the trunk found a box containing 60 lb of gelignite manufactured in the Republic of Ireland. Within a few hours of a vehicle license check, they searched a house where they found 29 wooden boxes identical to the claymore mine box. In the laboratory a careful comparison produced conclusive evidence of a common origin. Marks left by the planing machine on the surface of some of the pieces used to make the bases and lids of these boxes exactly matched planing marks on similar pieces from the bomb box; the wood had been planed on the same machine (Fig. 13–11). After further scrutiny the lid from the bomb was fitted to the base of one of the boxes by matching the longitudinal and end grains of the wood. They were thus proved to be adjacent pieces cut from the same length of wood.

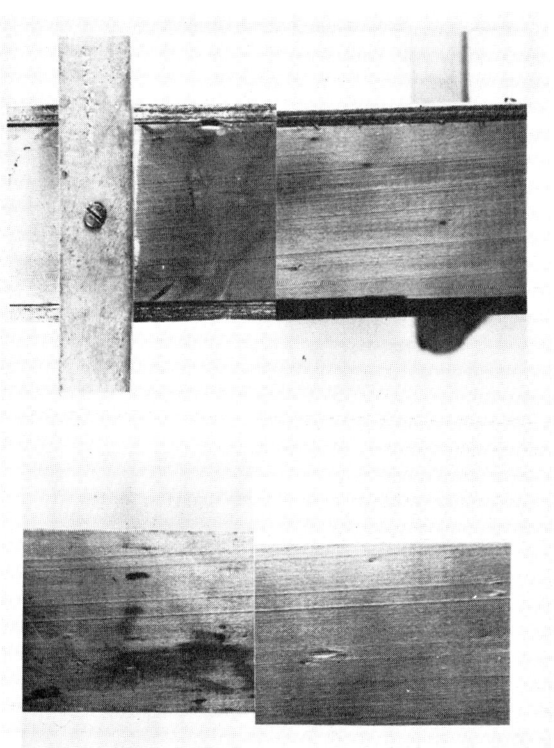

Figure 13–11. Planing machine marks on wood from an unexploded claymore mine (left) matching similar marks on wood from boxes of similar construction found in a suspect's house.

Attacks on Civilian Targets

The investigation of bombing incidents must, of course, involve a search of the scene for fragments of the device so that evidence can be gathered and the nature of the device can be determined. This requires the attendance of police officers and perhaps of forensic scientists. The possibility of fire means that the fire brigade also should be in attendance. Because gas, water, and electricity installations may have been damaged, repair crews are called. Army bomb disposal men and armed troops have their duties to perform, and curious onlookers gather to inspect the damage and watch the show. The opportunity to create panic in situations like these has not been overlooked by the IRA, and on some occasions a second, bigger bomb has been timed to explode a suitable time after the explosion of the first one, the so-called "invitation bomb." In one such case, it was discovered during the investigation that many people at the scene of an explosion had escaped death or injury by a lucky chance; the explosion had severed the fuse leading to another concealed bomb perhaps intended for the investigators.

The first use of high explosives to attack the civilian population in the center of Belfast directly occurred in 1970. There was an explosion in a busy city bank in which several customers were injured, one of them seriously. An examination of the scene proved that the bomb had been placed in a garbage bin in an alcove near the bank entrance. Before this incident explosions had always occurred away from the downtown area, which had suffered only incendiary attacks. Indeed, bombs containing high explosives had for the most part been laid in country districts, especially along the border with Eire, where British customs posts and Royal Ulster Constabulary stations in border towns and villages were the favored targets. From this time onward the central business districts of Belfast and Londonderry were to receive the increasing attention of the IRA in a bid to bring the commercial life of these cities to a halt.

At first the bombers usually came by night, placing bombs in the doorways of bars, shops, and office buildings. Small charges of a few pounds of explosive were used, and the bombs were simple in construction, initiated directly by detonator and safety fuse. Confirmation of the type of bomb construction could often be gained by a careful search, which might reveal fragments of burned-out safety fuse, fragments of detonator, or even small lumps of unconsumed explosive plastered onto walls that had been in the line of the blast. The bombers exhibited little skill in placing the bombs, and although a lot of damage was done, the explosions were often less destructive than they might have been.

Very few arrests were made at this time, and as its confidence grew, the IRA became bolder. By the summer of 1971 members began to deliver their bombs during business hours. Two or three armed men, driving a stolen car, would arrive at a chosen target, perhaps a shop or warehouse, and carry a bomb into the building, holding the staff and customers at gunpoint. After lighting a fuse, they would announce that the occupants had three minutes to get out and would then make their escape in the stolen car, which they later often abandoned. Most people facing a bomb with a lighted fuse will get out of the building at top speed, but sometimes an owner or an employee more brave or stubborn than the rest would pick up the bomb and carry it out into the street. Occasionally the IRA retaliated. A second bomb, perhaps with a shorter fuse, was sooner or later carried into the same premises, and at times, bombs were stuck down with contact adhesive to make their removal more difficult. One man who had successfully removed a bomb from his premises was killed some months later while trying to carry another out. Selected targets have often been bombed repeatedly, even after rebuilding has been completed.

Deliberate disregard for human life was very evident in the way that bombs were laid. Attacks on police stations, army posts, and commercial property were carried out regardless of the danger to the occupants. It is true that IRA explosions have often been preceded by a telephoned warning, but such messages are notorious for their inaccuracy. In August 1971, for example, a bomb was planted in a locker on the second floor of the headquarters building of the Electricity Board for Northern Ireland, and a telephone call warned that the bomb would go off in 15 minutes. Immediate evacuation was ordered, but a few minutes later, just as the landing was crowded with typists and clerks hurrying to get out, the bomb exploded. One person was killed; many were injured, some of them seriously. In other incidents bombs have exploded in public bars, killing or maiming anyone within range. One of the worst of these direct attacks on civilians was the explosion at the Abercorn Restaurant in Belfast.

A fashionable restaurant patronized by shoppers and business people, the Abercorn was crowded one day in the spring of 1972 when a bomb exploded among the diners. Two young girls were killed and many persons were very grievously injured. One girl lost both legs and one arm. Her sister lost both legs, as did a male victim. One woman lost an arm and a leg, another a leg, and three people were blinded. A telephoned warning received just minutes before the explosion occurred had identified only the street where the bomb had been laid. At the scene, enough fragments of the device were recovered to show that it was a time bomb in which a foreign-made alarm clock had provided the time delay. The remains of an identical clock were recovered from the scene of the explosion at the Electricity Board headquarters building. The IRA had accepted responsibility for this bomb, but denied causing the explosion at the Abercorn Restaurant. The evidence suggests that both explosions were caused by the same group.

Time Bombs

Time bombs are a favorite weapon of the IRA, and the use of a particular make of cheap watch or alarm clock often helps to identify a series of bombs as the work of the same technician. Further indications are given by the way the necessary modifications are carried out, by the materials used for the circuitry, and by the construction of the container.

Quantity production of bombs is common. The first example of one series was found in the summer of 1971.

A new government building was almost ready for occupancy when it was badly damaged by an explosion, and a forensic scientist was called to the scene. The contractors on the site were anxious to begin clearing operations, and a bulldozer driver was already maneuvering his machine into position to clear the debris. After a quick inspection of the damage, the scientist formed a definite opinion about the probable location of the center of the explosion, but this area was covered by a fallen wall. He explained the situation to the bulldozer driver and obtained his willing cooperation. With delicate movements of his machine, the driver carefully scooped away the overlying debris to reveal the bomb timing mechanism, still in fairly good condition. It was housed in a small, crudely made hardboard box and proved to be of a novel type. Any time delay up to two hours could be chosen by setting a modified pocket timer of the sort used by motorists as a key-ring parking time reminder (Fig. 13–12).

The warning clapper mechanism had been removed and replaced by a pair of contacts that closed when the set time had expired, and these completed a circuit to the detonator. Protection for the bomber was provided by a primary circuit containing a special type of electrical fuse that operated like a nonreturn changeover switch. When the parking timer had been set and the ticking could be heard,

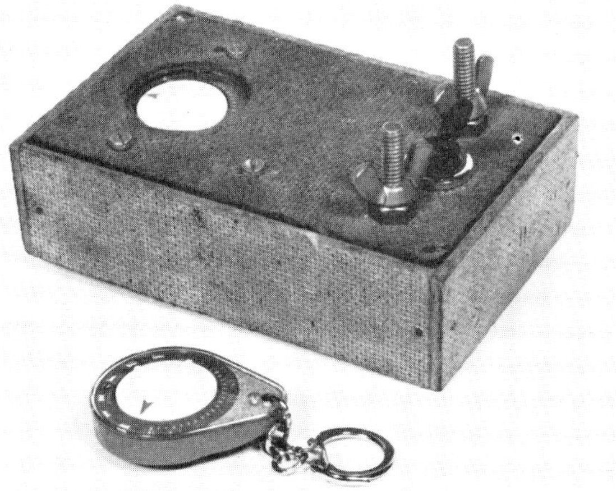

Figure 13–12. IRA bomb timing mechanism incorporating a modified parking timer. An unmodified timer is shown separately.

the bomber switched on a simple toggle switch in the primary circuit, and all the battery voltage was dropped across the special fuse switch, which immediately blew, completing the detonator circuit up to the points on the timer. Switching off the toggle switch on the outside of the box would then have no effect on the operation of the timer.

Some 10 or 12 of these timing devices were recovered from unexploded bombs, and these unsuccessful incidents could most often be attributed to the failure of the timer to close the points. The bombs were very dangerous in this condition, since any movement could restart a faulty timer, perhaps with only a few seconds to go before the contacts came together. How many bombs of this series were exploded successfully cannot be known, since not every scene could be properly investigated, but the wholesale nature of their manufacture was revealed after search of a house that appeared to be the center of operations: 265 key rings and chains, 209 redundant clapper mechanisms, 32 partly modified parking timers, and 6 unmodified parking timers were found. Many other bomb components were collected and so was all the debris from a workbench. It contained many small strips of metal about 2 inches long, similar to the metal strips used as contacts in the bomb timing mechanisms. A microscopic comparison of the cut edges of these strips and the metal strips in the bombs proved that they had all been cut with the same tool (Fig. 13–13). In this way, bombs recovered intact from three areas in which different IRA units were operating were shown to have a common origin.

The job of the Ammunition Technical Officers of the Royal Army Ordnance Corps is to render bombs harmless. Pitting their skill against the terrorists day by day, examining and disabling bombs, and achieving many successes (more than 1,600 bombs have been neutralized), they inevitably became prime targets of the IRA, and the weapon chosen was, appropriately enough, the bomb itself. Many of the subsequent developments in bomb technology appeared to be designed to kill army personnel, and an early victim was claimed.

In the autumn of 1971 a young army captain, newly arrived from England, was sent out to deal with a suspicious looking object reported lying outside an Orange Hall in a rural location close to Belfast. (Orange Halls are meeting places for members of the Orange Order, a Protestant organization committed to the defense of the faith and the retention of Northern Ireland's position within the United Kingdom.) The object proved to be a homemade wooden box, measuring about 6 inches square by 12 inches high, with a thin metal rod projecting through a small hole in the lid. The captain began his examination, but as he was working at it the box exploded and he was killed instantly. He was one of many bomb disposal experts who have been killed in Northern Ireland.

In the days that followed, several similar boxes were laid by terrorists, but their secret was soon uncovered. Each box incorporated a microswitch under the lid and another in the base, and the switches were wired in parallel to the detonator circuit, which was powered by a

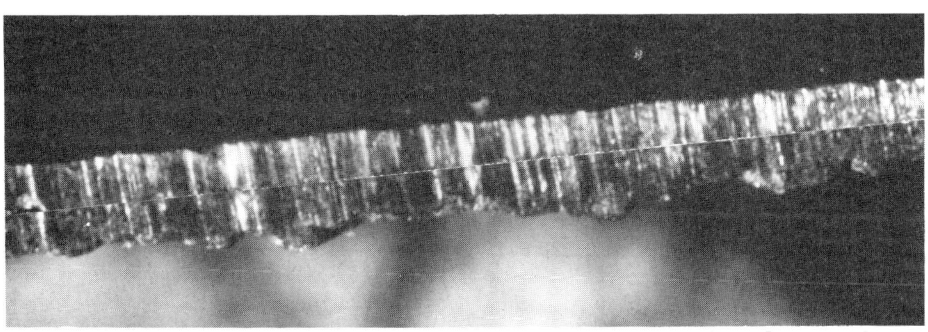

Figure 13–13. Comparison of striations on the cut edge of a contact strip from a bomb timing mechanism with similar marks on a metal strip found in a house search.

small battery. Once armed, the bomb would explode if the lid was prized up or if the box was tilted, thus relieving the pressure on either microswitch. The person laying the bomb was protected by a now familiar arrangement of the circuitry, a third switch that enabled the bomber to place the box in safety. It consisted of the special type of electrical fuse in a primary circuit that has already been described. The metal rod was the means of completing the primary circuit once the bomb was in position. Inserted through the small hole in the lid, it was passed through two loops of copper strip screwed to the inside of the box. These were terminals in the primary circuit, and once they were bridged by the rod, the fuse blew, breaking the primary circuit but arming the secondary or detonator circuit. It now only required the operation of one of the microswitches to set off the explosive charge. The circuitry of this bomb was successfully elucidated by constructing a working model in which a small flashlight bulb was substituted for the detonator (Fig. 13–14). Such laboratory reconstructions of terrorist devices are greatly assisted by careful searching at the scene of explosions and the recovery of all fragments that might have been part of a bomb.

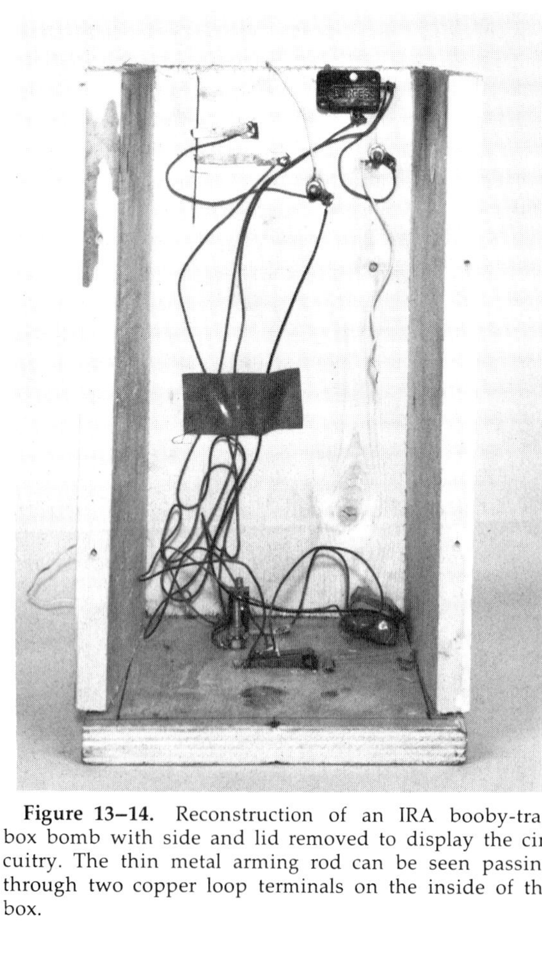

Figure 13–14. Reconstruction of an IRA booby-trap box bomb with side and lid removed to display the circuitry. The thin metal arming rod can be seen passing through two copper loop terminals on the inside of the box.

The electrically detonated bombs in which microswitches were used to confer antihandling properties made it unsafe for any untrained person to interfere with a bomb once it had been placed and armed. Only bomb disposal experts could hope to disable such bombs, and they soon developed the necessary techniques. The weakness of this particular type of booby-trap bomb was that it remained safe unless it was moved or interfered with, giving the bomb disposal team time to deal with it effectively. The army successes prompted the IRA to develop a more complex bomb.

The new bomb incorporated the same antihandling switches as the earlier one, but a change in circuit design and additional components were included. Now, when the bomb was armed, the coil of a relay drew current from a battery. The points on the relay were connected independently to the detonator wires and held open as long as the relay coil was energized. The small battery gradually was exhausted, the points closed, and the detonator fired. This arrangement meant that the bomb would explode after a time interval that depended on the resistance of the relay coil and the type of battery employed. The time available for disabling the bomb was now finite but unknown.

The design of these "collapsing" circuits, as they are called, is subject to many variations, and in late 1971 the battle of wits between the army and the explosives experts of the IRA continued. One very complex device contained in a travel bag was left in a ladies' hairdressing salon, presumably by a customer. Fine circuit wiring was taped over the inside surface of the bag and threaded through the zipper fastener. Breaking this wire by cutting open the bag or by working the zipper would cause the bomb to explode, and collapsing circuitry ensured that the bomb would eventually detonate if left alone. Finally, if the bag was lifted, an antihandling microswitch in the base closed a time-delay circuit calculated to fire the detonator after an interval of several minutes. This last provision may have been added to convince anyone pulling the bomb out with a rope and hook that it was safe to approach. Fortunately this overelaborate device did not explode because of a fault in the wiring, and its recovery was swiftly followed by laboratory examination. The investigation exposed the level of technology that the terrorists had reached and the type of components they were using. Such discoveries provide new intelligence about improvised explosive devices and a further supply of physical material for possible comparison with bomb-making materials found in house searches.

X-ray examination of bombs is sometimes used to help determine their internal structure so that the correct disabling technique can be applied.

A large bomb in a wooden box, deposited by armed men in the foyer of a large new hotel in the center of Belfast, was carefully x-rayed before being dealt with by a bomb-disposal officer. Television cameras captured the drama for home viewing as it unfolded behind the all-glass frontage of the brightly illuminated hotel. The very next day, in a daring repeat of tactics, another box bomb was placed in the same hotel. This time the x-ray examination showed a very different picture. Many more wires and components could be seen, and the device looked much more complex than its forerunner. After long deliberation, however, it was judged to be of fundamentally similar construction and was successfully disarmed. When opened, it was found that an unnecessary amount of wiring and components had been packed into the bomb. Not part of the bomb mechanism, they had apparently been added in an attempt to confuse the x-ray picture and render interpretation impossible.

Letter Bombs

Although in Northern Ireland the mail service was used to deliver an explosive device to an intended victim as early as 1969, it was not until 1973 that the terrorists realized the potential of this method. The Arab-Israeli conflict, in which many letter bombs were used in 1972 and 1973, may have revived interest in it, or it may have just been part of the increasing attempts to kill selected individuals. Whatever the reason, on April 17, 1973, several members of the Royal Ulster Constabulary stationed in Londonderry received envelopes through the mail that, when opened, were found to contain a small package of commercial explosive, a plain detonator, and a needle fixed in a harness. The device was so constructed that withdrawing the contents of the envelope would drive the needle against the initiating compound in the detonator. Not surprisingly, none of the five letter bombs received during April functioned as intended, but like so many other terrorist ideas, the design was soon improved and effective bombs were produced. The new design made its appearance in the same district less than a month later.

Two prominent legal personalities received registered letters. One, a magistrate, became suspicious when he opened the envelope. Instead of removing the contents he went into his garden and, holding the envelope by the sealed end, flung out the contents. There was a loud bang, and the contents disintegrated just after they left the envelope. Fortunately the magistrate received only slight injuries. The second recipient, also suspicious of his letter, informed the police. When examined, the envelope was found to contain a thin booklet, the center of which had been cut out and refilled with commercial explosive, electric detonator, and a slim battery. Removal of the booklet triggered the device, bringing together two foil contact strips fastened to adjacent pages but insulated from each other by a card glued to the bottom of the envelope and completing the circuit to the detonator.

This was a much much more effective letter bomb, and the design remained unchanged in the later attacks directed against Establishment individuals such as members of the part-time Ulster Defence Regiment, the British Army, the Royal Ulster Constabulary, the Police Authority, and prison warders.

Of the 21 letter bombs in this series, only 4 exploded, 1 causing slight injuries to the magistrate already mentioned, 1 blowing off part of one hand of the mother of a prison warder as she opened it, 1 causing slight facial and hand injuries to a member of the Police Authority, and 1 injuring a Post Office sorting clerk.

By late summer the letter bomb campaign had moved to England and abroad. Over a period of four months, devices were posted to Establishment individuals in the London area and in British embassies in Europe and the United States. These devices were identical in design and construction to those used in Northern Ireland and their similarity once again demonstrates the need for close collaboration between investigating agencies. Few of these devices exploded, and those that did caused relatively minor injuries, with one or two exceptions.

The IRA achieved considerable success with these insidious antipersonnel bombs, disturbing normal commercial and business life, and spreading alarm among secretaries, postal staff, and those persons having official connections with Northern Ireland affairs. The letter bomb is an efficient device in that it uses a very small quantity of explosive and is delivered to the target by an innocent and unwitting accomplice, leaving the sender more or less free from risk. Investigational procedures include the search for fingerprints on the envelope and contents, a comparison of the contents and of the handwriting on envelopes sent to different addresses, and basic detective work to discover the source of the various materials.

Control of Commercial Explosives

Not unnaturally, the extensive use of commercial explosives by terrorists provided a sharp stimulus for the tighter control of explosives bought for legitimate purposes. Stricter security of explosives storage and closer supervision of shot firing in quarrying operations helped to prevent losses. Control of detonators by the police until the time of their use became routine. The border between Northern Ireland and the Republic of Ireland, however, is easy to cross, and there is a long tradition of smuggling of goods and cattle from one country to the other. Prices, subsidies, and taxes fluctuate independently in each country, and there is always a profit to be made by the illegal movement of some commodity across the border. When the control of explosives was improved in the North, increased smuggling of commercial explosives from the South helped to maintain IRA supplies. Tighter security measures in the Republic of Ireland reduced the flow, however, so the IRA came to rely more and more on improvised explosives.

TERRORIST USE OF IMPROVISED EXPLOSIVES

Improvised explosives were already in common use of course, particularly for incendiary devices and for small devices such as pipe bombs and homemade hand grenades. The pipe bomb typically is made from a length of iron piping sealed at both ends. A small hole is drilled in one end for filling, usually with sodium chlorate and sugar, and to allow a length of safety fuse to be inserted. When ignited by the safety fuse, this mixture burns fiercely and quickly, consuming its own oxygen supply, to produce gas pressures that explosively rupture the metal pipe. These bombs can be thrown or laid and are capable of doing considerable damage to persons and property.

A wooden box containing at least five pipe bombs was left in an alley against the wall of a public bar. Each bomb was made from 2½-inch diameter heavy iron pipe some 18 inches long with ¼-inch thick steel plates welded to each end, and probably contained about 3 lb of the explosive mixture, which was identified by laboratory analysis of the residues. In the explosion a hole measuring 3 ft by 4 ft was blown in the 18-inch thick wall and the inside of the bar was wrecked. The jagged iron casing of one bomb, weighing several pounds, traveled a horizontal distance of 114 yd. In its flight the missile must have reached a considerable height, for it cleared a three-story building on the other side of the alley and only 10 ft away from the wall of the bar.

The power of this lethal mixture of sodium chlorate and sugar was demonstrated again in a fatal explosion in Belfast.

Despite an allegation that a bomb had been thrown through a rear ground-floor window of a house, investigation revealed that the explosion center was in the bedroom above. The back of the house was virtually demolished, and two men were killed. In the search, enough evidence was found to indicate that this was an accidental explosion in a pipe-bomb home industry. Nine prepared pipes were recovered, together with fragments of many more. Analysis of the explosive residues proved that this was a sodium chlorate and sugar explosion.

The dead men were Protestants, and this incident confirmed that some Protestants were still making pipe bombs as late as 1971, although Protestant violence was hardly noticeable by this time. The pipe bomb had been used mostly by militant Protestants as an antipersonnel weapon. The IRA had made more use of improvised hand grenades. These were similar in their action to the pipe bomb, but in appearance they sometimes resembled the military hand grenade, being deeply cut to assist fragmentation (Fig. 13–15).

When the supply of commercial explosives was no longer sufficient, the IRA began to employ improvised explosives more often for bigger bombs. The year 1972 was notable for this development, which opened the door to death and destruction on a still larger scale. Sodium chlorate and sugar mixture is a low explosive, and then only when it is confined, but other mixtures of easily available chemicals form high explosives that detonate with velocities comparable to those of commercial high explosives.

One such mixture is sodium chlorate and nitrobenzene. Nitrobenzene is a yellowish liquid used in the preparation of aniline dyes, in the manufacture of shoe polish, and in the tanning industry. Although there is a small tanning industry in Northern Ireland, dyestuffs and boot polish are not manufactured, and the annual demand for nitrobenzene for industrial use would not exceed a gallon or two. The situation in the Republic of Ireland is not much different, yet an English manufacturer unwittingly supplied 5 tons of nitrobenzene to an address in the Republic and became suspicious only when a second order for a similar amount was received. When one realizes that 5 tons of

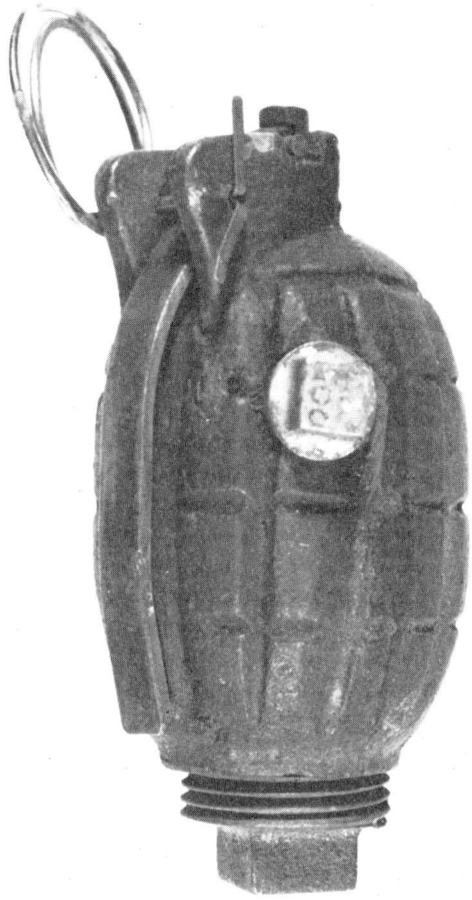

Figure 13–15. Improvised IRA hand grenade.

nitrobenzene can be combined with sodium chlorate, a very common agricultural chemical, to make 55 tons of high explosive, it is clear that IRA problems with the supply of explosives were being overcome. It was not long before this mixture was in widespread use. It was christened "co-op sugar" because it was first detected following an explosion in a store owned by the Belfast Co-operative Society.

The important characteristic of a condensed explosion is its independence of an external oxygen supply, and many common oxidizing chemicals can be used as the basis of explosives, ammonium nitrate being particularly suitable. Staggering amounts are used in agricultural fertilizers, and it needs only the addition of a suitable fuel to form a highly explosive mixture. Ordinary diesel oil will suffice. The IRA's discovery of the effectiveness of mixtures of these universally available materials ended the scarcity of explosives and the need for economy in their use as a weapon of violence.

The Car Bomb

In retrospect, it is tempting to regard the success of the authorities in controlling the availability of commercial explosives as the precipitating factor in the search for substitutes and the success of the terrorists in finding substitutes in great quantities as the stimulus for the development of the car bomb early in 1972. As long as commercial explosives could be obtained they were used in the limited quantities available, and the size of bombs was constrained. Agricultural chemicals are supplied by the sackful, however, and the terrorists soon realized that there was no need to use less than this amount for each bomb. Motor cars were already being stolen or hijacked for transporting the smaller bombs of 20 to 40 lb, which were then carried into buildings or placed against targets by volunteers. Much bigger bombs could be accommodated in the trunks of motor cars, but they would obviously be difficult to manhandle from the car to the target. The solution was to abandon the car, with the bomb inside it, at the target. The automobiles were expendable anyway, and with this new technique, large bombs containing over 100 lb of explosive could be delivered without risk to the bomber, who had only to park the vehicle, arm the bomb, and walk away. Electrical initiation would follow in due course.

In the months that followed the introduction of the car bomb the destruction of life and property increased and became even more indiscriminate. Particularly horrific was the car bomb explosion on March 10, 1972, in Donegall Street, a narrow and busy shopping and business street in the center of Belfast. This was one of the first car bombs, and it shocked a community already hardened by years of violence.

> A telephoned warning was received that there would soon be an explosion in a little street off Donegall Street and a hasty evacuation of shoppers and office workers was begun. Many of these people hurried into Donegall Street, where, in fact, the car bomb had been parked. Another warning, received too late, referred to Donegall Street itself, but a few minutes later the bomb exploded, killing 7 people and wounding 154 others. Among the dead were two policemen who had been checking the car when it exploded and two city sanitation men who had been collecting garbage. The fronts of buildings were destroyed, and many victims who escaped the blast were injured by flying glass and other missiles.

Investigation of this incident (and others like it) was made difficult by the clear need to sub-

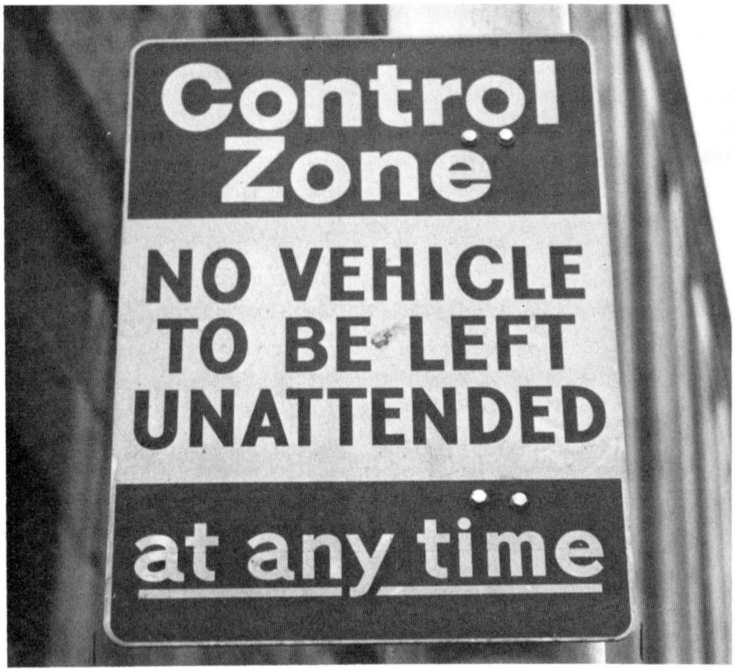
Control Zone
NO VEHICLE TO BE LEFT UNATTENDED
at any time

Figure 13–16. Street poster to remind motorists that cars must not be parked and left unattended in the street. An anti–car bomb precaution.

ordinate the preservation of the scene to the care of the injured and the prevention of further damage by fire or gas explosions. There were strong pressures to clear the scene, to allow buildings to be made safe and secure, and to let commercial life begin again.

Countermeasures to lessen the death and destruction caused by the car bombs were soon introduced. A complete ban on the parking of unattended vehicles was imposed in the center of Belfast (Fig. 13–16). Already many protected segments of the city were closed to traffic by railings across the entrances to side streets. Gateways were left for pedestrians, and these checkpoints were initially manned by troops who searched those going through to make sure they were not carrying small bombs or weapons. Later a special force of uniformed civilian searchers was established for this work. The danger and the inconvenience to shoppers in Belfast was reflected in the decline of trade. Many people transferred their custom to the smaller towns nearby, but the huge mobile bombs followed, and soon the ban on parking was extended to the outlying towns as well. Complete protection was impossible short of banning traffic altogether, and the explosions continued. Car bombs left in the controlled zones were now obvious immediately, an unattended car in an otherwise empty street being too conspicuous to be overlooked, but in the smaller towns and villages where restrictions were not in force, car bombs were unexpected and more likely to take life.

Car bombs also added a new dimension to the work of the bomb disposal teams. In one sense the car bomb is like any other enclosed bomb; the car itself is the container. It can incorporate a time delay in the detonator circuit or be booby-trapped in many ways. In 1970 two young policemen had been killed when they were about to bring in a stolen car found abandoned near a border village. The investigation of that incident revealed that the bomb was wired to the door-operated light switch. With speed and care, an expert can usually hope to beat the time limit and avoid a booby trap, but the car bomb, being out on the street, gives the bombers the opportunity to choose the moment of detonation. Using inexpensive radiotransmitters (the sort used to control model aircraft, readily available in hobbies shops) to close a switch in the detonator circuit, they can watch and wait until the bomb-disposal officers are in the most vulnerable position before transmitting the lethal signal.

Special techniques have been developed for the remote inspection and treatment of car bombs and, indeed, for dealing with bombs in buildings. Remotely controlled trollies carry television cameras for close inspection. Car doors, windows, and trunks can be opened remotely by mechanical or explosive forces; and bombs can be neutralized by burning or by controlled explosions initiated from a safe distance.

Control of Chemicals

The wholesale use of agricultural chemicals for bomb making posed a new problem for the authorities. Agriculture is a major industry in Northern Ireland, and an immense tonnage of chemicals is used each year in ground clearing, crop growing, and harvesting. Nevertheless, action was necessary, and in June 1972 the government made it illegal to sell or possess, without a license, sodium chlorate or any fertilizer containing more than 79 per cent ammonium nitrate. These decisions were taken following the advice of forensic scientists involved in the investigation of bombs and explosives. Laboratory analysis and field trials had shown that the lower the percentage concentration of ammonium nitrate, the less suitable would fertilizers be for bomb making. The percentage allowed was a compromise achieved in collaboration with the agricultural interests and represented a useful improvement in security. A great deal of fertilizer with a high concentration of nitrogen was still available in farm barns, however, and the illegal border traffic still could not be entirely prevented. Routine analysis of samples of fertilizers now became part of a laboratory program that constantly monitored the chemical composition of improvised explosive devices in a bid to identify trends in terrorist technology.

Direct Rule

Because of the Northern Ireland government's inability to find a political solution to the violence and the Westminster government's constitutional difficulty in working through the local administration in many matters of policy, the Northern Ireland Parliament was suspended and direct rule from London was imposed for a period of one year. A Secretary of State for Northern Ireland was appointed, and assisted by a small team of ministers and senior civil servants, he took office on March 24, 1972, just four days after the Donegall Street explosion. The political story concerns us, however, only insofar as it impinges on the level of terrorist activity. The new administration was determined to use the law to its full extent in prosecution of suspected terrorists, and the security forces worked hard to uncover hidden stores of arms and explosives, but the emphasis was placed on achieving a political solution. Following secret talks between the British government and the leaders of the Provisional Irish Republican Army, the IRA announced that a truce would go into effect on June 26, 1972. The conditions were not made public, but the news that the British government had actually negotiated with the IRA infuriated many Protestants to the point of violence, and matters were not helped by the punitive intensification of IRA terrorist bombing in the last few days before the truce.

For over two and a half years the Protestant community had patiently watched the efforts of the security forces to contain and subdue the urban guerrillas. As many as 20,000 troops were stationed in Northern Ireland, in constant danger from the invisible enemy. "Free Belfast" and "Free Derry" still existed as barricaded areas from which the terrorists operated almost with impunity, and the Catholic community either supported them or was powerless to intervene. Protestant anger was for the most part expressed in verbal terms, but a militant fringe was losing patience. Direct rule and the secret negotiations with the terrorists were seen by Protestant hard liners as final indignities that demanded a physical response. Already suspicious of London's political intentions, they were now openly alienated from Westminster's policies and confirmed in their opposition by the intransigence of the IRA, which broke the truce after only two weeks, when the renewed violence became even more intense than before.

In July 1972, a record-breaking month, there were 184 explosions. The worst day in Belfast was Friday, July 21, when in just over one hour on a lovely summer afternoon, 19 bombs exploded, killing 9 people and injuring more than 100 others. The life of the city was brought to a halt, its people shocked by the senseless horror. On the morning of July 31, 1972, three car bombs exploded in 11 minutes on the main street of the tiny village of Claudy in County Londonderry. Of the population of Claudy, 410 at the last census, 7 died and 30 were injured. Main Street was devastated.

By coincidence, on the same day as the Claudy disaster, many hundreds of troops were deployed in "Operation Motorman." This was the code name for the action to regain the no-go areas of Belfast and Londonderry that had been in the grip of the IRA for nearly three years. Little opposition was offered, many of the IRA leaders slipped quietly away across the border, and from this time on the government scored increasing successes. The urban areas were still dangerous, they still harbored many terrorists, but the advantage lay more and more with the security forces. The number of arrests for shooting and bombing, previously very few, began to grow. Confidential telephone lines were advertised and increasingly used to give information about hidden arms and explosives. The success of this campaign for Catholic cooperation depended on the army's maintaining a low profile in the former no-go areas, but the lack of obvious military activity angered Protestant militants. They wanted to see the immediate military defeat of the IRA, whose bombing campaign had now reached a crescendo.

Working-class Protestants began to organize. The Ulster Defence Association was allegedly committed to the protection of Protestant families and their homes. The Ulster Volunteer Force, more openly concerned with attack than with defense, began to carry the war to the enemy. Unhappily for many innocent people, the real enemy could not be distinguished, and there began a period of assassinations justified on the sole grounds that the victims were of the opposite faith. Warned that the murders would continue unless their activity ceased, the IRA simply retaliated in kind, and the militant Protestants finally adopted the bombing tactics of the IRA.

CONTROL OF CHEMICALS

Protestant Improvised Bombs

Apart from a few isolated instances there had been little to suggest "loyalist" (Protestant) involvement in bombing incidents before June 1972, when the first of what was clearly a new and not very effective series of bombs went off like damp squibs. Two metal beer kegs were used as containers, and these were found only partly exploded on the back seat of a car. The kegs were filled with a mixture of ammonium nitrate and fuel oil (ANFO), and a small booster charge of commercial explosive was included to promote the detonation of this relatively insensitive but potentially destructive improvised explosive. Although the booster charge exploded, it merely burst open the kegs, scattering the ammonium nitrate and fuel oil. Later the same day, in a repeat performance, the contents of two more beer kegs, about 90 lb of explosive mixture, were harmlessly scattered.

These two attacks in a staunchly republican area were made without warning, and this was to become a feature of Protestant bombings. Allegedly a counterterrorist campaign against the supporters of the IRA, the whole Catholic population as seen by the militant Protestants, it developed into a widespread series of somewhat amateurish attacks on Catholic bars, churches, and schools. The Protestant bombings were, however, much less frequent than those of the better organized and more experienced terrorists of the IRA.

It was obvious that the loyalist groups had, like the IRA, stockpiled ammonium nitrate fertilizer prior to the time that the controls became effective. For several months, device after device was constructed with one, two, or even three beer kegs of ammonium nitrate and fuel oil, the ammonium nitrate being the pure variety supplied as prills in the now illegal fertilizer. Fortunately the bombers had little knowledge of explosives. In the first 18 incidents only two bombs detonated properly. In the remainder, either the ammonium nitrate and fuel oil was scattered or the vehicle was set on fire. Of 44 Protestant bombings in 1972 only 17—employing small bombs—were successful. Toward the end of the year, however, several beer-keg devices exploded, causing considerable damage and the loss of several lives.

A new series of smaller bombs made its appearance in the latter part of 1972. These were based on the 7-lb carbon dioxide cylinder that is normally used to pressurize and carbonate many draught beers. These cylinders will accept about 10 lb of explosives, are ideal for low explosives (which depend on confinement), and produce large pieces of shrapnel. Sodium chlorate and sugar mixtures were used at first, but as the June controls began to take effect the sodium chlorate supply decreased and finally stopped.

Control of the composition of fertilizers or the availability of other chemicals was a predictable response by the authorities to the criminal misuse of these substances, but it was not the end of the story. Just as the shortage of commercial high explosives was successfully overcome, so now the new controls would not be allowed to restrict the bombing campaign.

In March 1973, a strong smell of chlorine at the scene of several explosions that were apparently the work of the Protestant terrorists indicated very clearly that a new explosive was in use. No identification was made until a month later, when a military patrol chased and stopped a car after a bomb had been thrown into a Catholic club. A second unexploded bomb found in the car was found to contain a mixture smelling strongly of chlorine. On analysis, the explosive was identified as a mixture of sodium dichloroisocyanurate and sugar.

Sodium dichloroisocyanurate is a commercially available chemical supplied for purifying the water in swimming pools, for disinfecting milking parlors, in household abrasive cleaners, and for similar purposes. Although we are aware that most of the improvised explosives used in Northern Ireland are also used by other subversive groups around the world, we believe that this compound has not been mentioned previously in the literature on the subject and probably has not been used elsewhere as an explosive substance. Its use should serve to remind investigators that the list of substitute explosives available to the bomber may be long. It certainly includes materials that would be unlikely to arouse suspicion even in security checks, especially if they were labeled with chemically uninformative trade names.

Protestant extremists, although more given to shooting than to bombing, were enterprising in the quest for new substitute explosives. Sodium chlorite (a bleaching agent used in Northern Ireland's famous linen industry) mixed with sugar and detonated in the confinement of a carbon dioxide cylinder was another successful mixture, as was sodium nitrate (used in the cured meat industry) and icing sugar.

In mid-1973, after many trials, the Protestant terrorists finally perfected a beer-keg explosive consisting of a mixture of crushed ammonium nitrate prills, sodium or potassium nitrate (another fertilizer available in bulk as Chile saltpeter), and icing sugar. Use of this mixture is now established, and although it produces only a low-order explosion, it has proved very effective for demolition.

Continuous monitoring of the composition of terrorist explosives exposed the technologic changes in their formulation and indicated what new controls were necessary. Sodium chlorite, for instance, was usually sold to industrial users as a solid, in which form it was suitable for incorporation into an explosive mixture. Arrangements were made for an international chemical firm to supply the sodium chlorite in solution. Sodium nitrate, normally added to sodium chlorite to prevent the corrosion of stainless steel tanks, could no longer be added to the sodium chlorite solution without the premature evolution of chlorine dioxide. To overcome this problem the sodium nitrate had to be supplied separately. As a solid, however, sodium nitrate was already a security risk. Once again the chemical manufacturers cooperated by producing sodium nitrate paste.

Further Controls

The persistent use of sodium chlorite in explosive mixtures led to the introduction in December 1973 of controls similar to those imposed 18 months earlier for sodium chlorate, ammonium nitrate, and nitrobenzene. Orders controlling the supply or possession of sodium and potassium nitrates were issued in April 1974. This move led to the substitution of sodium nitrite in terrorist explosives, and this in turn was controlled by a new order in 1976 (Fig. 13–17). It is obviously impossible to proscribe completely chemicals that are essential to industrial production, but the firms involved were encouraged to use safe formulations (such as sodium chlorite in solution) and if this was not possible, licenses to use the controlled material were granted only to those who complied with stringent security precautions. In spite of these precautions, chemicals were stolen at gunpoint by terrorists who wished to avoid having to formulate new mixtures. Three tons of pure ammonium nitrate, enough for 60 car

STATUTORY RULES OF NORTHERN IRELAND

1976 No. 51

EXPLOSIVES

Control of Sodium Nitrite
Explosives Regulations (Northern Ireland) 1976

Made . . . . . . *13th February* 1976
Coming into operation . . . *22nd March* 1976
To be laid before Parliament

WHEREAS it appears to the Secretary of State(**a**) that the substance specified in these regulations is likely to be used whether by itself or in combination with other things for unlawful purposes as an explosive:

NOW, THEREFORE, in pursuance of section 3 of the Explosives Act (Northern Ireland) 1970(**b**), and article 3 of the Explosives (Northern Ireland) Order 1972(**c**) the Secretary of State hereby makes the following regulations:

Citation and commencement

1. These regulations may be cited as the Explosives Regulations (Northern Ireland) 1976, and shall come into operation on 22nd March 1976.

Control of Sodium Nitrite

2. Subject to regulation 3, a person shall not manufacture, sell, acquire, transfer, store, transport, handle, use, or dispose of sodium nitrite or any mixture or solution which contains sodium nitrite in combination with any other substance or substances except under and in accordance with a licence from the Secretary of State.

Exemption

3. These regulations shall not have effect in relation to any manufactured goods containing not more than 5 per cent by weight of sodium nitrite.

Merlyn Rees
Northern Ireland Office — One of Her Majesty's Principal
13th February 1976 — Secretaries of State

Figure 13–17. Substitution of sodium nitrite for other chemicals in terrorist explosives led to its control in 1976.

bombs, was stolen in a single raid, but was later recovered.

The IRA has shown little inclination to change its explosive mixtures and has used its energies to beat the controls rather than to search for effective substitutes. Ammonium nitrate has been recovered in very large quantities from legal fertilizers whose other principal constituent is calcium carbonate. The fertilizer is mixed with water, the ammonium nitrate is dissolved, and the chalk is allowed to settle before the supernatant solution is removed and evaporated to recrystallize almost pure ammonium nitrate. Nitrobenzene and sodium chlorate, the ingredients of co-op sugar, also are still available to the IRA, which can bring supplies along "Ho Chi Minh" trails from the south.

In a modern economy, many chemicals with intended and unintended explosive potential are in daily use for peaceful purposes. An effective program for investigating bombs and explosions must reveal which of them are being used so that countermeasures can be introduced. Since one of the aims of terrorism is to disrupt industry and trade, controls must be carefully designed to defeat the terrorists without damaging the economy. Our experience in Northern Ireland has shown that administrative and legislative measures, properly thought out, can effectively and selectively restrict, but not completely eliminate, the supply of explosive substances for terrorist use.

BOOBY TRAPS

The searching of homes and empty or derelict houses has been a routine security procedure, and army search teams have been specially trained for this work. Explosives, weapons, and ammunition are frequently stored in unoccupied property so that in the event of their discovery no one can be charged with possession. Huge quantities have been found, but at a cost; the IRA, knowing that its caches were vulnerable, has often sought to protect them with booby traps. Anonymous tip-offs about the location of dumps of explosives and weapons have been used to lure troops to booby-trapped buildings. Trip wires, pressure switches, and tilt switches are commonly used to trigger bombs. Searchers must tread carefully and be wary of opening doors, cupboards, and drawers. During the hours of darkness, it might seem sensible to use a flashlight to avoid trouble and assist in the search. Knowing this, the terrorists have employed light-sensitive devices as switches for electrically detonated bombs, in one case leaving a light-sensitive cell poking out of a partly opened drawer.

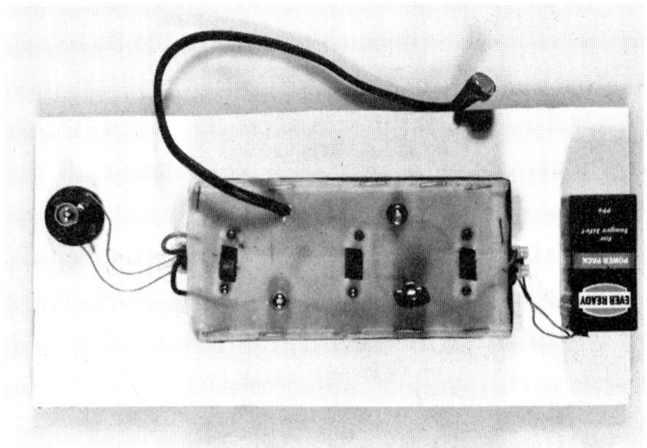

Figure 13–18. Light-sensitive cell and control box for an IRA bomb.

A soldier saw the device in the light of his torch and fortunately became suspicious before the full beam illuminated the cell and triggered the bomb. Recovered for examination, the electrical mechanism displayed circuitry designed to protect the bomb planter who had to arm the bomb. Three switches were provided on the small box containing the electronic device (Fig. 13–18). Closing the first switch simply connected the battery supply to a primary circuit containing a photocell, a variable resistor, and a thyristor. Firing the thyristor powered a secondary circuit containing a small bulb, but only if the second switch was closed. By adjusting the variable resistor, one could fire the thyristor, and thus light the bulb, only when light fell on the photocell. Opening the second switch and closing the third switch substituted the detonator for the bulb, the two being wired in parallel. With all the adjustments made, the bomb could be planted in a dark place, switched on, and left to be activated by daylight or a searcher's torch.

In another similar device added protection was afforded by the inclusion of a modified parking timer to switch on the power after a suitable getaway time had elapsed, and so a link was established between the manufacture of the light-sensitive devices and of the time bombs that incorporated the parking timers.

Variations in circuit design were seen in other examples of the light-sensitive switch. Sometimes the circuits included unnecessary components, and these provided a clue to one source of wiring circuits used by the IRA. It became clear that they had been copied from popular journals on electronics, which provide an endless supply of circuit ideas for the amateur to build. For somewhat different applications, the terrorists sometimes seemed to have selected them with little understanding of the purpose of some of the components; appropriate modifications were not made. Many simple electronic circuits have switching functions, and it requires little knowledge or imagination to employ them in improvised explosive devices.

Booby traps designed to be initiated by the victim have been placed indiscriminately, many in places where they could be triggered by children at play. Booby-trapped flashlights and fountain pens have been left where they can be found and picked up by any curious individual. Perhaps intended for army patrols, they are just as likely to be found by anyone else. Switching on the light or removing the cap from the pen detonates a charge powerful enough to remove a hand or to kill the victim.

ROCKETS AND MORTAR BOMBS

One result of the losses suffered by the IRA in its direct confrontations with the army was the development of missiles that could be delivered from a greater distance than the hand-thrown nail bombs.

The first attempt made use of the bow and arrow. A small tin can filled with explosives and complete with the usual fuse and detonator was fastened to an arrow and fired from a bow in Red Indian style. The arrow grenade was quickly superseded by the spigot grenade, a similar small bomb on a length of 3/4-inch diameter stick fired from a shotgun. These spigot grenades were directionally unpredictable and might have done more damage to noncombatants outside the target area but that few of them exploded. Their use continued sporadically for several months until September and October of 1972.

In May 1972 the IRA produced its first mortar bomb. It was about 16 inches long, with a body section of copper piping with metal fins as stabilizers. The filling was commercial explosive, and impact initiation was dependent on the nose-end firing pin striking the target. Since the nose end was flat, this seldom happened. The bomb was projected from a homemade mortar by a .303 rifle round incorporated in the tail section. Four bombs were fired in the first attack with this new weapon, but a short time later six such bombs and a mortar were found in an empty house. After this no more bombs of this particular type were used.

Two months later the IRA successfully fired several 3.5-inch rockets of military origin. Only one of these exploded on impact—against a protective wire mesh screen around a police station in West Belfast. The bazooka-type launcher was found in a house search during September. In November a military patrol found the tail section of a 3.5-inch rocket in an alley. While this was being handled it exploded, killing a senior noncommissioned officer. Subsequent examination established that the propellant had been replaced by a high explosive, a good enough indication that the find was a booby trap.

In November 1972 the IRA first used the Russian RPG7 rocket launcher to fire the PG7 high-explosive antitank (HEAT) rocket shown in Figure 13–19 against police stations and army posts. On impact, the detonation of a shaped charge in the nose of the rocket propels a jet of molten metal that is capable of penetrating 12 inches of armor. On the first day that the weapon was used, a rocket exploded against the steel shutters covering a window of a border police station, and the molten slug passed through it easily, killing a policeman in the room behind.

These Russian rockets, which the IRA is thought to have acquired in considerable numbers from a North African state, have been used regularly since that date. About 150 had been fired by the end of 1973, but in IRA hands, with no great accuracy. Perhaps half these rockets have struck some part of the chosen targets, usually the protective wire mesh antibomb screen that has become a feature of police station architecture in Northern Ireland. There has been only one additional death, that of a soldier, but 37 people have been injured. The callous disregard for civilian casualties was evident, as the attacks continued after direct

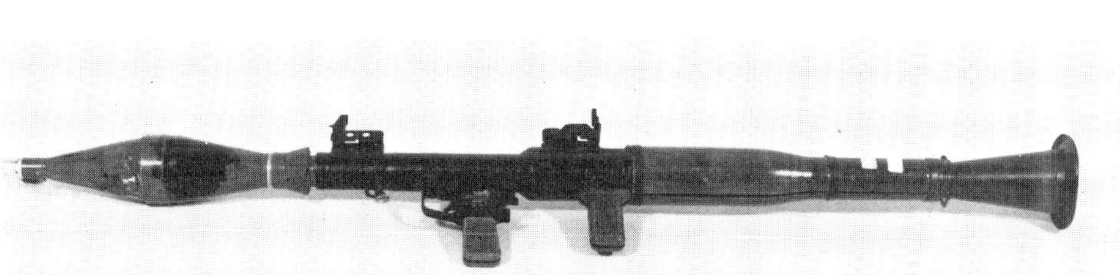

Figure 13–19. Russian-made RPG7 rocket launcher with PG7 high-explosive antitank rocket loaded ready for firing. This was an IRA weapon widely used in the terrorist campaign.

hits on a school, a nurses' home, and other civilian buildings.

Many rockets and launchers have been recovered by security forces. Examined and test fired for evidence to use in court, this has been shown to be an accurate, highly sophisticated weapon with a range of about 1,000 yd. Proof of its use by terrorists is based on recognition of the characteristic damage it does and the recovery of fragments identifiable by shape, size, color, and surface texture. Tail-end parts of the rocket are particularly likely to survive the explosion, which causes discrete rather than general destruction.

The Mark II

Continuing development of the homemade product led to the appearance of an improvised Mark II version of the IRA mortar bomb in December 1972, when in concerted attacks on targets in four towns, 26 mortar bombs were fired. One, which missed the target, seriously injured a mental patient. An army officer who picked up an unexploded bomb was killed instantly when it exploded in his hands. Nine mortar bombs and two launchers were recovered by security forces after being abandoned by one group of terrorists.

The Mark II mortar bomb, about 16 inches long and more robust than its predecessor, was made from steel pipe with a finned tail assembly containing the propellant, a shotgun cartridge. On impact, a .22-caliber cartridge in the pointed nose cone fired a 2-inch length of safety fuse inserted in a plain detonator buried in the charge, a pound or two of commercial explosive. Laboratory study of its design, chemical identification of the explosive, and field trials of its effectiveness followed quickly. The bomb had no power to penetrate solid obstructions such as brick walls, but when lobbed high into the air it could fall through a roof and explode within a building. The fragmentation pieces were larger and lighter than the ideal, but the design of the weapon was reasonably successful. Whole bombs and component parts have been found in the possession of terrorists, and tail assemblies have been recovered in debris searches following explosions.

After 18 months of IRA attempts to produce a reliable mortar, it was not surprising that the Protestant militants should copy their tactics. The first Protestant-designed mortar bomb was found in a burned-out car in February 1973 in Shankill Road, the Protestant heartland of Belfast. Measuring about 12 inches long, it was made from cast-iron pipe connectors, to which were added a pointed nose at one end and tail fins at the other. On impact the striker in the nose was to fire a small-bore cartridge, which in turn was supposed to ignite a length of detonating fuse leading into a main charge of improvised explosive. This was not a practical design, since the fuse cannot be detonated in this way. Later specimens of these mortar bombs showed that the construction had been simplified by using a .22-caliber cartridge fitted into the end of a plain detonator as the striker.

At the end of March 1973 police raided an Ulster Defence Association training ground outside Belfast where training with mortars was in progress. They found five mortars, one of them burst apart, eight complete mortar bombs, many fragments of bombs, and a variety of adapted cartridges. Seven men were arrested and three of them were subsequently convicted of possession of explosive substances. Trials with the captured mortars showed their range to vary up to 300 yd according to the loading of the propellant cartridge, but the more propellant used, the greater the risk of a burst barrel. The accuracy was moderately good.

During the next two months there were sporadic and ineffective mortar attacks against a Catholic enclave in Protestant East Belfast, but they ceased when five mortars and one mortar bomb were found in the headquarters of the Ulster Defence Association a short distance away. Nine days later several Association mortar bombs were fired into the Catholic Ardoyne district of Belfast. This was the last known use of mortars by the militant Protestants.

The Mark III

The very next day the IRA introduced a much improved mortar bomb, which became known as the Mark III. More than 30 of these were fired in the next 10 days, and then the army recovered one mortar and 10 bombs in a house search. The bombs were about 22 inches long, weighed about 7 lb, and were made of heavy steel pipe. The tail section, made from 1-inch-diameter perforated steel pipe, was packed with a cloth that had been soaked in sodium chlorate and allowed to dry. In the base was a .22-caliber cartridge. Dropping the bomb into the mortar barrel fired the .22 cartridge and thus ignited the sodium chlorate, which burned fiercely, serving as a propellant. From the tail section, a 10-inch length of safety fuse passed through a plug and terminated in a plain detonator buried in the main charge. This was contained within the body section of $2\frac{1}{4}$-inch-diameter steel pipe and consisted of a mixture of ammonium nitrate and aluminum flake. No stabilizing fins were necessary, since the propellant ignited the fuse to the detonator in flight. The mortar itself was stable and adjustable for range. It could be dismantled for easy transport and concealment. In trials, the weapon was found to be reasonably accurate up to about 300 yd.

Before the end of 1973, more than 100 of these Mark III mortar bombs had been fired, mostly at police stations and army camps across Northern Ireland. In keeping with IRA policy of doing everything possible to disrupt commercial life and spread terror, Belfast Airport also was chosen as a target. The most dramatic incident, however, was the attack on the Pomeroy Police Station on August 17, 1973.

After 10 mortar bombs had been fired at the station, the IRA broke off the engagement and made off. In a follow-up search, a lorry was found abandoned at the roadside; on it were a burst mortar, 16 mortar bombs, and the dead bodies of two IRA men. Possibly one of the bombs had jammed in the barrel after firing, the inevitable ignition and detonation sequence being completed seconds later, but the deaths may well have been caused by a flash-through from the propellant chamber to the explosive chamber, by-passing the fuse and so eliminating the time delay.

These two deaths on the platform of the "mobile launching pad" were the only ones caused by this version of the IRA mortar during the six months in which it was used, although two other IRA men had a narrow escape when they got a hangfire in a mortar barrel during an attack on an army camp. They quickly got out of range of the expected explosion, which in fact did not materialize. Obviously deciding that discretion was the better part of valor, they did not return to collect the mortar and the rest of their bombs.

The popularity of the Mark III mortar with the IRA volunteers at this time was thought to have decreased, and there were reports that guerillas who refused to use the weapon because of the danger to themselves had been deliberately crippled—a traditional punishment, effected by shooting through the kneecaps, used as a form of disciplinary action against IRA men who refuse to carry out their orders or who act unwisely on their own initiative or for their own profit. The discovery of seven Mark III mortars and 70 mortar bombs in searches, almost as many as were fired successfully during this six-month period, gives some indication of the rate at which intelligence was being gathered by the security forces.

The Mark IV

After a few months for redevelopment, a Mark IV mortar bomb appeared early in 1974. Some 22 of the new bombs were fired in a border attack on British troops from Lifford in County Donegal, which is part of the Irish Republic. Although none of them was recovered in an unexploded condition, enough fragments were found to allow a laboratory reconstruction and elucidation of the new mechanism by experienced scientists.

In the new bomb a triangular protective cover surrounded the previously exposed propellant firing cap (Fig. 13–20). This may have been designed to prevent accidental explosions resulting from dropping or careless handling. More significant was the new fusing mechanism. A solid metal plug with a firing pin on the rear end fitted loosely into a tube projecting from the front end of the mortar bomb and was held in place by a transverse shear pin passing through the tube and the plug. The firing of the propellant charge drove the bomb out of the mortar with such acceleration that the inertia of the metal plug caused the shear pin to break. This allowed the firing pin to strike a cap and ignite a length of safety fuse leading into the open end of a plain detonator buried in the main charge.

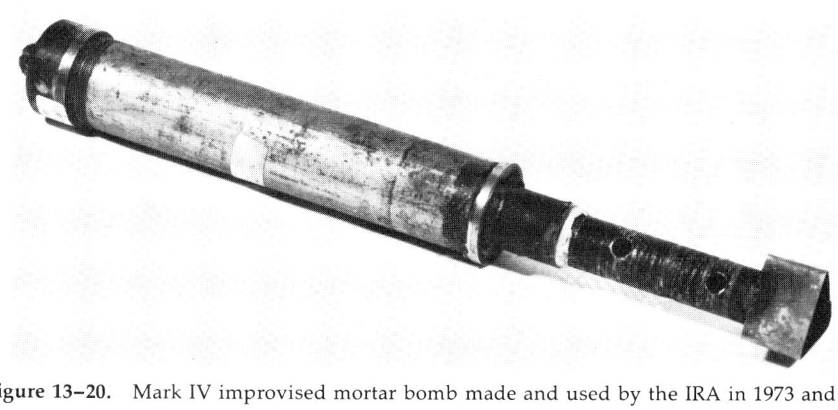

Figure 13–20. Mark IV improvised mortar bomb made and used by the IRA in 1973 and 1974.

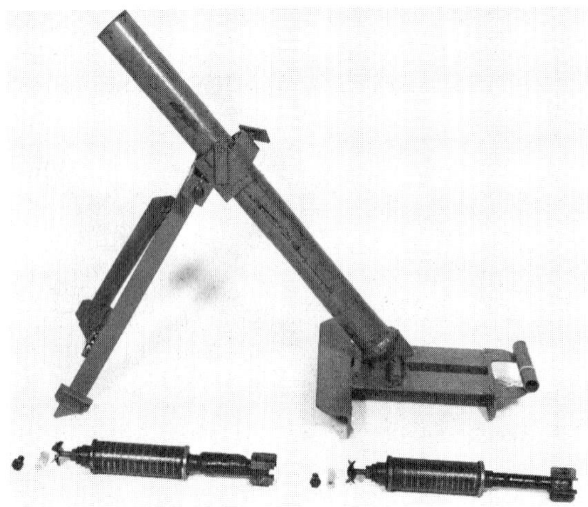

Figure 13–21. Mark VI mortar bomb, with a range of about 1,200 m, was fin stabilized and armed during flight by a propeller in the nose that screwed a firing pin into position to strike on impact.

The Mark VI

Further development work produced an unsuccessful Mark V and then a more sophisticated and successful Mark VI version (Fig. 13–21). This mortar bomb, with a range of about 1,200 m, was fin stabilized and armed only during flight by the action of a small propeller in the nose. This screwed a firing pin into the firing position, ready to strike on impact. In an attack on Belfast Airport in March 1976 a lorry loaded with 14 mortar bombs in disposable mortars embedded in sand was parked outside the airport perimeter. The propellant in the bombs was electrically ignited by a wiring device with a time delay that allowed the driver of the lorry to make good his escape. Little damage was done, and nobody was injured.

Although the Protestants did not fire any more mortar bombs after their abortive attempts in the spring of 1973, information was received in the autumn of that year that a new Protestant mortar was being manufactured in large quantities. A search was organized in a country district south of Belfast, and in a workshop ostensibly devoted to the production of radio equipment, the security forces uncovered enough mortars to equip a small army.

Of a completely new design, this mortar bomb was simply a screw-topped tin, to the base of which were fastened wooden stabilizing fins (Fig. 13–22). No detonating mechanism was found, and no explosives. The bomb was fired when a spring-loaded firing pin struck the base of a 12-bore cartridge in a metal breech section of the mortar, but the barrel was just a length of plastic rainwater pipe. During the firing trials that followed the seizure, several barrels disintegrated, spraying jagged plastic shrapnel around. After the action was cocked, the firing pin was released by pulling sideways on a trigger. A small hole in the trigger allowed one to attach a thin line and stand well away from the weapon, pulling the trigger from a distance. This was a safety feature much appreciated by those engaged in the test firing.

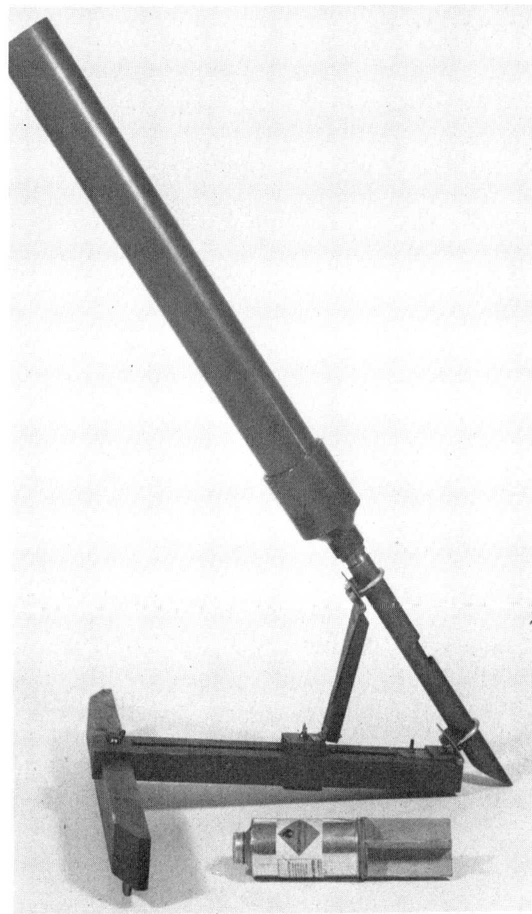

Figure 13–22. Mortar manufactured in large quantities by Protestant militants but never used. The barrel is a length of plastic rainwater pipe. The mortar bomb is a screw-top tin with wooden fins.

It was apparent that much care had been taken with the design and construction of this weapon. About 250 of them had been manufactured, and it was later discovered that they had been distributed to three other areas. There has been no evidence of their use, however, and it is assumed that the weapons have been stockpiled against the possibility of civil war. It is surprising that those responsible seem to have overlooked the danger to the users from the plastic barrel; possibly they had not tested any of the weapons. Not every trial ended in disaster, however, and enough results were obtained to suggest that the mortars may have a maximum range of over 300 ft.

IRA DEATHS

The victims of the IRA bombing campaign have not all been innocent civilians or members of the security forces. More than 25 per cent of all deaths from explosions have been of the bombers themselves. Lacking adequate training, they have been careless in handling explosive substances or, harassed by the security forces, have made mistakes. The arrest or detention of hundreds of IRA members has pressed younger and less experienced volunteers into use in the manufacture, transport, and laying of bombs whose nature and potential they do not fully understand. Even the absence of effective coordination between different units has led to unexpected consequences.

Two groups separately planned to attack the same target, a British Customs Post on the main road to the south. This Customs Post has been destroyed and replaced so many times that it is without doubt the most symbolic target in all of Northern Ireland, and it was perhaps inevitable that a mistake would occur eventually. The first group was inside the building preparing its destruction when the second group arrived and set it on fire. One of the first group was burned to death.

On another occasion, two arsonists entered an Orange Hall and sprinkled it liberally with petrol. One climbed out through a window, and the second passed him the empty petrol tin. Before climbing out himself, he stopped to light a match and was killed in the explosion that followed.

Investigations of these and similar incidents have posed no special problems. Careful examination of the scene and laboratory analysis of samples collected have usually produced a convincing explanation of the events. Signs of forced entry, the deliberate accumulation of combustible material, the presence of several centers of fire, or the typical signs of a dispersed-gas explosion are easy to read. Traces of a vehicle that has been removed from the scene and empty containers or other material abandoned in flight suggest the escape of accomplices. Identification of flammable solvents or other incendiary agents reveals the means employed.

Sometimes the cause of the terrorists' misfortune is obvious:

Four men on a bombing mission arrived by car at a suburban bar. The first one to enter was recognized immediately by an off-duty policeman, and the bombers retired in haste to their car and sped off. A few hundred yards from the bar the car disintegrated in a violent explosion, and the mutilated bodies of the four bombers were distributed over a considerable area. Probably the bomb had been armed on arrival at the target, and either the set time expired during the flight or one of the men was attempting to defuse it under difficult and dangerous circumstances.

Many members of the IRA have died in similar circumstances. Improvised explosive devices, imperfectly constructed and containing large quantities of chemically unstable substances, have been handled too casually or transported in unsuitable vehicles. Jolting when the vehicle is driven over potholes in the road may be enough to initiate an explosion.

In Northern Ireland there are ramps across roads wherever there is a police station, an army post, or another likely terrorist target. These ramps must be negotiated at almost zero speed to avoid damage to the vehicle. Two young IRA volunteers died instantly when a bomb exploded in a van that was being driven too fast over a ramp. The evidence suggested that the bomb was between them on the front seat. A few minutes before the explosion they had tried unsuccessfully to carry the bomb past a security guard and into a store close to an army post. The young couple were given the usual quasi-military IRA funeral, and the coroner returned an open verdict.

Occasionally it is alleged that the dead were innocent victims of raiders from another district. Rapid, impartial investigation is necessary to forestall an immediate hostile reaction by local sympathizers. (In these tense situations the danger to the investigators themselves is usually another good reason for speed.)

An explosion in a small street in an area of Belfast dominated by the IRA killed six people in a small house. Inhabitants of the street alleged that a bomb had been thrown from a passing white car. This version of the incident, with its implication of anti-Catholic action, received immediate publicity, and the examination of the scene had to be conducted among hostile neighbors, some of whom assisted in the search for bodies. The investigators, for their own safety, were allowed only a limited stay by the army escort but were able to establish that the seat of the explosion had been in a ground-level room at the rear of the house. The house had collapsed and those on either side had fallen in on the scene so that the search had to be conducted with the aid of a bulldozer. Explosive residues were found and later identified. The possibility of an outside attack was discounted, a premise that was confirmed by death notices that appeared in a morning newspaper claiming the dead as members of the IRA. It is believed that the explosion occurred after IRA explosive officers arrived at the house to disarm a bomb that two unsuccessful bomb planters had brought back from target premises.

In another strongly Catholic part of Belfast eight people were killed in a large explosion that demolished several small houses. The bang was heard at 2:00 A.M. It was established that a large bomb had exploded at the rear of a parked car. The mutilation of the bodies suggested that they had all been close to the center of the explosion, some of them very close, and it was surmised that the bomb had been dropped as it was being manhandled into the trunk of the car. The examination of the scene was conducted under very difficult circumstances. Army protection was provided, but nail bombers harassed the investigators, who were unable to extend their stay in the area. Nevertheless, a search for bodies was completed and an indication of the size of the bomb was obtained when the trunk of a body was found about 120 yd from the seat of the explosion. Death notices of six of the eight dead persons acknowledged their membership in the IRA.

INVESTIGATION OF EXPLOSIONS

Examination of the Scene

The basic rules for investigation of any scene of criminal activity apply equally to the examination of the scene of an explosion: always verify that a crime has been committed, look for signs of how it was committed, and search for evidence that might lead to the arrest and conviction of the guilty.

In every case priority must be given to the care of the injured and to any action designed to prevent further casualties. After an explosion the scene must be declared safe by the explosive and ordnance disposal (EOD) team, who may have to deal with more unexploded bombs. There may be fires to fight or buildings to be made safe. Subject to these essential services, the scene must be protected against the intrusion of any unauthorized persons. Strict crowd control is necessary to prevent looting or the destruction of evidence.

General Techniques

Before there is any further disturbance, the scene must be carefully photographed from several angles, since the subsequent search and clearance may reveal evidence that can be interpreted only by reference to the condition of the scene immediately after the explosion. Record photographs should then be taken of any items of interest as they are discovered and before they are moved. The disposition of objects thought to be significant should be shown on a sketch or plan of the scene, and new information can be added as the search develops. Care in taking measurements is important.

Whenever it is relevant, the investigator should look for the usual indications of criminal activity. Signs of forced entry, tool marks, hairs and fibers, footprints, vehicle tracks, bloodstains, or fingerprints may be found, perhaps in an area that has escaped destruction.

Investigators should question anyone who might possess useful information. Local residents, workers from nearby shops and offices, doormen, and the inhabitants of the bombed building should all be asked if they saw anything unusual prior to the explosion and if they can describe what they saw, heard, or felt during the explosion. Information should be gathered about the plan of the building, the means of access, and the existence of possible hazards from gas or chemicals. When mines have exploded in rural areas the questioning should bring to light unusual activities even days before the incident. Multiple ambush mines take time to lay and to connect. The terrorists must be prepared to wait for many hours until a suitable target vehicle approaches. Country people notice strangers in the district and are curious about their reasons for being there. Time spent in talking to people with local knowledge is often well spent.

Dispersed Versus Concentrated Explosions

In practice, one of the first tasks of the expert is to determine whether the explosion was dispersed or concentrated; the evidence will be provided by the nature of the damage. In a dispersed explosion, the resulting pressure may be distributed over a wide area and is applied more evenly to all parts of the damaged structures than is the case in concentrated explosions. The damage is more haphazard or diffuse. The same is true of the injuries suffered by victims, who may be burned on all exposed skin surfaces. By contrast, a concentrated explosion, whether mechanical or chemical, will by definition have a point source from which heat and pressure radiate, the greatest damage being found closest to the center of the explosion. At the very center a cavity may be found where the bomb was resting.

The nature of the premises or the type of business being carried on may indicate that the requirements for an accidental dispersed explosion were already present. Flour mills and factories engaged in sack making or using wood-cutting machinery typically have fine organic dust widely distributed on exposed ledges. When the dust is raised and suspended in air, a spark or flame may cause it to explode.

Fractured gas pipes or petrol spillages can lead to dispersed-gas explosions. A gas explosion, even when it does not lead to a general fire, often ignites the leaking gas so that a flaming jet identifies the source of the leak. In the absence of such obvious signs, the characteristic smell of town gas, of liquid petroleum gases, or of the stenching agent added to them, should warn the investigator that gas is still leaking. Portable gas detectors can be used to identify the presence of an explosive mixture. A sample of the atmosphere can be collected by emptying a bottle full of water and then sealing the bottle to await laboratory examination by gas chromatography or another method. When the explosion results from petrol spillage or from the vapors of volatile solvents, a search for containers is essential and the source of ignition should be found. It should be self-evident that naked flames or electrical equipment liable to arcing must never be used when gas or vapor leaks are suspected.

The possibility of an accidental or contrived secondary dispersed explosion following a primary concentrated explosion should not be overlooked. The IRA has, several times, hijacked fuel tankers and abandoned them on busy streets with high-explosive bombs on board. Most have been disarmed. One exception was a bomb attached to a tanker containing nearly 6,000 gallons of low-distillate fuel destined for the Londonderry gasworks. It exploded, bursting the tanker and causing serious secondary damage.

Concentrated explosions of the mechanical type that burst metal containers are identified by the discovery of the damaged containers, which may show clear signs of the application of external heat and sometimes outward splaying, or "banana peeling," of the metal edges around the point of rupture. The distinction between an accidental and a deliberate mechanical explosion must be made after considering all the circumstances. This frequently requires an investigation into the cause of a preceding fire. The explosion of liquefied petroleum gas cylinders, tins of paint, or drums of petrol is often the inevitable consequence of an accidental fire in domestic premises, shops, and warehouses and is a hazard well known to professional fire fighters, but deliberately started fires can produce such mechanical explosions as bonus. Proof of the deliberate use of fire to initiate an intended mechanical explosion can be difficult and may depend upon the ability to establish that the criminal has gathered the necessary materials together in one place. Containers may be found that are foreign to the scene or there may be evidence of the deliberate accumulation of combustible material around or beneath containers in a store. The example cited in the discussion of mechanical explosions (the liquefied petroleum gas cylinder placed on a lighted gas ring fueled by the cylinder gas) illustrates both the basic requirements of a mechanical explosion and the convincing nature of the evidence of criminal intent that can sometimes be found.

Concentrated explosions of a chemical nature, for which we have used the term "condensed explosions," require both an explosive substance and a means of initiation. Low explosives also need to be confined. When either low or high explosives are used for criminal purposes there may be wrappings or a harmless-looking container for disguise. There may also be a time-delay mechanism. High-explosive devices frequently incorporate provision for booby trapping or command control. The possibility of finding parts of some or all these accessories, which may themselves be legally defined as explosive substances when they are used with intent to cause an explosion, should provide adequate incentive for the investigator. The chances of finding them, however, depend to some extent on the size of the explosion. The bigger the explosion, the more completely fragmented and widely dispersed the bomb components will be, and the smaller the hope of finding them, especially when the scene is covered with the rubble of destroyed buildings. If the investigators are further hampered by the danger of attack by bomb or bullet a successful outcome is even less assured.

Search of the Debris

Before any attempt is made to search the debris, valuable information can be gained from an overall assessment of the scene that takes into account the extent and directional effects of the blast damage. The radial nature of blast damage emanating from the explosion center may be distorted by rigid obstacles that set up reverberations and redirect the blast force over other structures or around corners. The partial vacuum created by the violent outward pressure is quickly filled by an inrush of air that may cause further damage, sucking objects toward the center. An experienced investigator may attempt to estimate the size of the explosive charge, but a wide margin for error must be allowed. It may be possible to determine which type of explosive was employed, since the slower, heaving action of low explosives differs from the shattering action of high explosives.

After the preliminary survey has been completed and the necessary photographs taken, the physical search can begin. Its nature is determined by the extent of the damage, the available resources, and the importance attached to the discovery of the explosive. The extent of the area to be searched depends on the size of the explosion, and investigators must be prepared to range widely from the damaged area in the search for flying debris. Ideally the preliminary survey will have delineated the possible area within which evidence might be scattered, and this area, perhaps a circle with a radius of 150 yd, should be searched systematically for bomb fragments and other material. Most of this will be found in a smaller central area. In buildings, parts of bombs can be found embedded in woodwork, furniture, partitions, or ceilings. Some will be in the bodies of the victims and will be recovered during treatment or autopsy.

Whenever circumstances have permitted, our practice has been to divide the rubble-strewn area into numbered segments of convenient size and to collect separately all the debris in each segment, putting it into numbered containers for examination elsewhere. This procedure calls for organization of both men and equipment, and requires shovels, brushes, machinery, and the preparation of maps or sketches on which is imposed the grid pattern of the segments. After the debris has been cleared the nature and position of any craters are more easily seen.

At a suitable place, the contents of the containers are examined by a team instructed in the method to be employed and the possible nature of the fragments sought. Larger pieces, perhaps brick or stone, are put to one side, and the smaller debris is passed through sieves of several sizes. The material retained in each sieve is spread out on a search table, and all items that might be significant are picked out for closer scrutiny. Fragments of burned safety fuse, torn and twisted pieces of clock mechanism, parts of batteries, short bits of wire, clothespeg springs, parts of switches, fragments of electrical insulating tape, and pieces of container are examples of the types of fragments that can be recovered and studied for some indication of the nature of the device. These fragments are compared with the components of other devices that have been recovered, more or less intact, and with material found on suspects, in their vehicles, or in house searches.

Although this somewhat elaborate procedure has often been successful we have often had to content ourselves with a less comprehensive search. When time for the examination of the scene is limited, when bombings are numerous, or when manpower is scarce, the costs of this technique may outweigh the benefits. The search is not always productive and, even when it is, the success is likely to be confined to identification of the mechanism and perhaps, by inference, of the group responsible. Seldom, at least in urban guerilla warfare, is evidence found that points to the guilt of particular individuals, unless there is other supporting testimony. This other evidence may be direct or circumstantial. Eyewitness descriptions of the bombers have sometimes led to the detection of suspects who have then been further implicated by scientific evidence, and sometimes fingerprints have been found on the remains of bomb wrappings, particularly on adhesive tape.

The examination of an explosion scene does not always end when the outdoor investigational work appears to have been completed and site clearance has begun. It is advisable to have the rubble taken to a secure area and isolated in case the need arises to examine it further in the light of subsequent developments.

When two armed men carried a bomb into a public bar in a provincial town some 20 miles from Belfast it might have been another successful IRA incident had not the bomb exploded prematurely, killing one of the terrorists and wounding the other. The survivor was believed to have been standing on a flight of stairs leading down from the entrance hallway to the bar, covering his companion who was placing the bomb, when the blast of the explosion blew him through the doorway into the street, a distance of 14 or 15 ft. His overcoat was blown off and landed some yards away from where he fell. A gun was found in the pocket of the coat. The man received hospital treatment for his injuries and was later charged with causing the explosion, but he immediately raised the defense that he was simply an innocent passerby who had been injured by the blast. He claimed that he had not been inside the bar and that the incriminating coat was not his. In the light of this statement, the scene was re-examined.

When found, the man was wearing a sweater. The man, his sweater, and the disputed coat all showed signs of flash burns, indicating that they had been near the center of the explosion. Just how near could not be estimated sufficiently accurately to resolve the doubt created by his statement. The wreckage of the door and its frame were recovered and repositioned at the exit from the bar. The inner surfaces of the door, the frame, and the walls of the narrow passageway inside the door were free from scorching by the fireball. In view of his burns, the man's claim appeared to be unlikely, but it was decided to set up experiments to determine the severity of flash damage at varying distances from the center of a similarly large explosion. Clothing was fixed at measured intervals from the charge, and after the test explosion, this was compared with the sweater and the coat in question. Clothing that was placed as far from the test bomb as the man claimed to have been from the bomb in the bar was undamaged. Only the clothing placed much nearer to the center of the test explosion showed flash burns comparable to those on the coat. The man's ownership of the coat was then proved by the discovery of a two-way transfer of fibers between the sweater and the coat.

He was subsequently tried, convicted, and sentenced to 14 years' imprisonment.

Biologic Evidence

The forensic biologist may be needed to answer some of the difficult questions that can arise after an explosion. The number of dead may be in doubt. Not infrequently it is necessary to decide whether injured people could have been responsible for explosions. Evidence from hairs and fibers and from increasingly accurate discrimination between the blood types of different people has often provided decisive answers to such questions.

The bodies of persons close to the center of an explosion may be so disintegrated that the investigators cannot tell how many people have died.

At one scene fragments of scalp were shown, by comparison of the hair, to be from two people; most of two scalps were reassembled by fitting the pieces together. Clothing fragments collected at the scene were examined and sorted. It was determined that they were parts of not more than two sets of clothing. A reasonable assumption in this case was that only two people had died.

Police called to the scene of an explosion in an outbuilding of a farm found only small pieces of flesh, some bearing hair, all of which were collected in a small polythene bag. The number of victims was uncertain. Macerations of the several pieces of tissue were subjected to blood group analysis and found to be identical in each of five blood group systems. The particular combination of groups found in the tissue fragments occurs in approximately 1 in every 1,000 of the Northern Ireland population, so the odds were in favor of a single victim. Hairs found on one piece of tissue matched hairs on a jacket found inside the farmhouse and helped to identify the dead man.

Two people were killed when a bomb exploded in a car in Newcastle, County Down. The dead were found lying beside the car. A third person, found injured nearby, denied having been in the car but was suspected of having been the driver; there was ample scientific evidence to support this view. The injured man was wearing only one shoe, and the missing shoe was found in the car, in front of the driver's seat. Red fibers on the front of his jacket and trousers were microscopically and chemically similar to the red fibers of the carpet from the car. Clumps of white cotton fiber on his jacket and trousers were similar to the filling of the damaged car seats. Samples of blood from the two dead people and from the injured man, when compared with each other and with bloodstains found inside and outside the car, could be differentiated by at least two of the five blood group systems examined (Table 13–2). Blood similar to that of each of the victims was found inside or close to the remains of the car; bloodstains beside the driver's seat matched the blood of the suspect. The deceased man was believed to have been sitting in the rear seat, cradling the bomb with his left arm, which was found severed on the opposite side of the car. The deceased woman appeared to have been the front seat passenger.

IDENTIFICATION OF EXPLOSIVES

Not the least important aspect of the investigation of the bombs and explosives is the detection and identification of the explosives. There are no serious difficulties when bulk quantities of explosives are discovered in a house, when bombers are intercepted on their way to a target, or when a bomb has been successfully disarmed. Adequate samples can be taken for laboratory analysis. Even after an explosion, unconsumed explosives may be found. Imperfect mixing of the ingredients of improvised explosives, loose packing of commercial ones, or another fortuitous circumstance can result in incomplete detonation that scatters some of the explosive. In many cases the samples available for analysis are small, perhaps contaminated, and possibly unrepresentative. Very small amounts of explosive may be

TABLE 13–2. ANALYSIS OF BLOOD SAMPLES BY GENETIC MARKERS

		Blood Elements					
Sample No.	Source of Blood	ABO	Phosphoglucomutase	Adenylate Kinase	Adenosine Deaminase	Erythrocyte Acid Phosphatase (EAP)	Haptoglobin
1.	Male deceased	0	1.1	1.1	1.1	B	2.2
2.	Roadway on rear far side of car	0	1.1	1.1	1.1	B	2.2
3.	Female deceased	0	1.1	1.1	1.1	A	1.1
4.	Roadway beside front near side of car	0	1.1	1.1	1.1	A	1.1
5.	Injured suspect	0	2.1	1.1	1.1	BA	2.1
6.	Inside car beside driver's seat	0	2.1	1.1	1.1	BA	2.1

recovered from the dust and debris of a suspect's clothing, his vehicle, his workbench, or his tool bag. A preliminary visual examination is usually enough to allow the explosive to be classed as either improvised or manufactured.

Positive identification of explosives may be obtained even when discrete fragments cannot be seen. Invisible traces, in some cases very small ones, on containers, on clothing, and on the skin of suspects, as well as postexplosion residues from surfaces (in our experience, only nonabsorbent surfaces) exposed to the explosion can be detected.

The correct treatment of the contaminated material is vital for successful identification. Clothing items should be packed separately in sealed airtight containers, carefully labeled, and sent to the examining laboratory within 24 hours. The same treatment should be given to selected surfaces from the scene when this is possible. Samples from large or immovable objects must be taken in situ by wiping with small cotton wool swabs on sticks. Commercial swabs for medical use should be avoided unless it is known that they have not been pretreated with substances likely to interfere with the subsequent tests. Dry swabs or swabs soaked in distilled water are used first to collect inorganic residues; and then the area is swabbed again with new swabs soaked in ether or acetone to remove organic compounds. The swabs are then put into sealed containers.

The hands of suspects are treated similarly. After a careful visual inspection, particulate matter, perhaps from between the fingers or under the nails, is removed and put into clean vials that are then sealed and labeled. Then the hands are swabbed as already described. Usually some time elapses between detention of the suspect and the hand-swabbing operation. During this time the suspect must not be allowed to wash, wipe, or rub his hands. It is not good practice to cover the suspect's hands with polythene bags, since this will cause them to warm up and sweat, increasing the rate of loss of volatile substances from the skin surface.

Inorganic Compounds

The methods used to identify the inorganic chemical compounds in improvised explosives are quite straightforward. For each inorganic anion, preexplosion and postexplosion tests are given. Also included are some of the more common cations. Tests for sugar, so commonly used to fuel the oxidative improvised explosions, are discussed in the following section on organic compounds.

A small quantity of the explosive is dissolved in water. The dry or aqueous swabs or selected areas of clothing suspected of bearing invisible traces are extracted with water. The solution, or aqueous extract, is tested as follows.

Chlorate. *Preexplosion tests* include:

1. The addition of concentrated sulfuric acid to the extract produces a yellow-orange color, owing to the liberation of chlorine dioxide. Care should be taken, however, since in the presence of an organic fuel, a violent reaction may occur.
2. To 1 drop of the extract add 1 drop of a 1:1 mixture of saturated manganous sulfate solution and syrupy phosphoric acid, and allow to stand for five minutes. The development of a violet color indicates the presence of chlorate. Chlorite, bromate, and iodate interfere with the test.
3. To 1 drop of the extract add 1 drop of 5 per cent aniline sulfate solution followed by 1 drop of concentrated sulfuric acid. A violet color indicates the presence of chlorate. Chlorite, persulfate, bromate, iodate, and nitrite interfere with the test.

The *postexplosion residues* of a chlorate explosive consist of chlorides.

1. The addition of 1 drop of 5 per cent silver nitrate solution and 1 drop of dilute nitric acid produces a curdy white precipitate soluble in ammonia.

Chlorite. *Preexplosion tests* for chlorite, whose presence will have been indicated by the clorate tests and only requires confirmation are:

1. One drop of extract is mixed with 1 drop of acidified potassium permanganate. Chlorites decolorize the permanganate.
2. Add 1 drop of the extract to a mixture of 1 drop of 0.6 per cent solution of nickel sulfate and 1 drop of 0.1N sodium hydroxide. Heat at 40 to 50° C for two minutes; the presence of black flecks or a black coloration in the green mass confirms chlorite. Persulfate interferes with the test.

The *postexplosion residues* of a chlorite explosive mainly consist of chlorides, and therefore differentiation from chlorate explosives relies on the presence of unchanged chlorite or chlorate.

Perchlorate. The *preexplosion test* for perchlorate is:

1. To 1 drop of extract add 1 drop each of a saturated solution of zinc sulfate, a 20 per cent solution of potassium nitrite, and a 0.03 per cent solution of methylene blue. The development of a purple color indicates the presence of perchlorate. Persulfate interferes with the test.

Again, the *postexplosion residues* consist mainly of chloride, and differentiation from chlorate and chlorite depends on the presence of unchanged perchlorate.

Bromate. This will have been indicated by the chlorate tests and requires only confirmation. The *preexplosion test* is:

1. To 1 drop of extract add 1 drop of a saturated solution of phosphomolybdic acid and approximately 10 mg of sulfosalicylic acid. After warming for five minutes in a boiling water bath the development of a blue or green color confirms the presence of bromate.

The main *postexplosion residue* will be bromide, the presence of which can be identified by the silver nitrate test for chloride. Bromides produce a creamy precipitate less readily soluble in ammonia.

Nitrate. *Preexplosion tests* are:

1. Test for the presence of nitrite by adding to 1 drop of extract 1 drop each of a 1 per cent sulfanilic acid in 30 per cent acetic acid solution and a 0.03 per cent solution of *N*-1-naphthylethylenediamene dihydrochloride in 30 per cent acetic acid. The presence of nitrite is indicated by a red coloration.
2. In the absence of the red color in the first test, add 2 mg Devarda's alloy. The gradual development of a red color indicates the presence of nitrate.

The presence of nitrates, nitrites, and ammonium salts have been detected *after the explosion* of improvised explosives based on nitrates even when the nitrate used was the sodium or potassium salt.

Peroxide. For *preexplosion identification* of peroxide:

1. A drop of the neutral or slightly acid extract is dropped onto lead sulfide–impregnated filter paper. The appearance of white flecks or a white circle indicates the presence of peroxide.

There are no significant detectable *postexplosion anions,* but most of the peroxide used in Northern Ireland is in the form of the magnesium salt, and the presence of magnesium may indicate the use of magnesium peroxide.

Perborate. *Preexplosion tests* for perborate are:

1. Hydrolyze the extract by heating with 1 drop of 5 per cent sodium hydroxide solution and test for peroxide as already described.
2. To 1 drop of the hydrolysate add 1 drop of concentrated sulfuric acid and 5 drops of methyl alcohol. Ignition of the solution produces a green flame in the presence of borate.

A *postexplosion indication* of the use of perborate-based explosives is the presence of borate in the explosion area.

Persulfate. *Preexplosion tests* include:

1. The nickel hydroxide test as applied to chlorites to give an indication.
2. To 1 drop of the extract add 1 drop of 5 per cent barium chloride and 1 drop of dilute hydrochloric acid. The formation of a white precipitate on heating indicates the presence of persulfate.

A *postexplosion test* for the use of persulfate-based explosives is the presence of sulfate in the explosion area.

Permanganate. *Preexplosion tests* are:

1. The color of the extract is highly indicative of the presence of permanganate.
2. The addition of 1 drop of hydrogen peroxide to 1 drop of the extract results in decolorization of permanganate.

A *postexplosion indication* of the use of permanganate is the presence of manganous salts in the explosion area.

1. To 1 drop of the extract add 1 drop of concentrated sulfuric acid, 1 drop of 4 per cent silver nitrate solution, and 2 mg ammonium persulfate. Heat gently. The formation of a red-violet color indicates the presence of manganese.

Dichromate. *Preexplosion tests* are:

1. The strong color of an extract.
2. To 1 drop of the extract add 1 drop of a saturated solution of chromotropic acid in water and 1 drop of dilute nitric acid. A red coloration indicates the presence of a chromate.

The *postexplosion presence* of chromium salts in the area indicates the use of dichromate.

1. To 1 drop of the extract add 1 drop of sodium hydroxide solution and 2 drops of hydrogen peroxide solution. Warm, acidify with nitric acid, and apply the chromate test.

Sodium. The presence of sodium is indicated by:

1. The flame test, in which an intense and persistent yellow flame is produced.
2. To 1 drop of neutral test solution add 8 drops of zinc uranyl acetate reagent. The formation of a yellow crystalline precipitate indicates the presence of sodium. This standard reagent may be purchased already prepared or prepared as directed in any standard analytical reference book. The results should be interpreted with caution, since sodium is a common ion.

Potassium. Tests for the presence of potassium include:

1. The flame test, in which the production of

a lilac flame indicates the presence of this element.

2. To 1 drop of neutral test solution add a crystal of sodium cobaltinitrite. A precipitate or turbidity indicates the presence of potassium. Lithium, thallium, and ammonium ions interfere with the test.

Calcium. Tests for the presence of calcium include:

1. The flame test, in which the production of a brick red flame indicates the presence of the element.
2. To 1 drop of neutral test solution add 2 drops of saturated potassium ferrocyanide solution. A precipitate or turbidity indicates the presence of calcium. Magnesium interferes with the test.

Ammonium. Tests for ammonium include:

1. The evolution of ammonia gas when several drops of the test solution is warmed with 1 drop of sodium hydroxide solution indicates the presence of ammonium ions.
2. To 1 drop of test solution add 1 drop of Nessler's reagent. The formation of a brown precipitate indicates the presence of ammonia. Many metals interfere with this test.

Organic Compounds

Sugar. *Pre-* and *postexplosion tests* are:

1. Molisch's test. To 1 drop of extract add 1 drop of 15 per cent 1-naphthol in ethanol and layer 1 drop of concentrated sulfuric acid under the mixture. A purple ring indicates the presence of carbohydrate. This test is unreliable in the presence of oxidizing agents.
2. A drop of the extract is spotted onto an Eastman Chromagram sheet 6065 (cellulose) and developed in ethanol, ethyl acetate, and water, 12:3:6. After drying, the developed plate is sprayed with a solution containing 5 ml *p*-anisaldehyde, 5 ml concentrated sulfuric acid, and 90 ml 95:5 ethanol and water. It is then heated for 10 minutes at 100°C. A blue-purple spot at R_f approximately 0.7 indicates the presence of sucrose.

Sodium Dichloroisocyanurate. *Preexplosion tests* for this compound are:

1. The solid and aqueous solutions smell of chlorine.
2. To the dry residue produced by the evaporation of 1 drop of test solution add 3 drops of 5 per cent isopropylamine in methanol and 1 drop of 1 per cent cobalt acetate in methanol. A violet coloration indicates the presence of the compound. Other isocyanurates and cyclic urea condensates such as the barbiturates interfere with the test.
3. Larger amounts can be confirmed by infrared spectrophotometry.

Postexplosion tests include:

1. The most significant feature, the presence of a strong smell of chlorine in the explosion area.
2. The presence of chloride, which may be a further indication.

Commercial Explosives

For the identification of visible amounts of manufactured gelignite explosives we use the method of Amas and Yallop, which avoids the need for successive solvent extractions followed by qualitative and quantitative examination of the fractions.[4] It is based instead on simple spot tests for the separate organic and inorganic ingredients, can be amended to accommodate the range of formulations likely to be encountered, and when necessary can be supplemented by a limited quantitative analysis. It quickly leads to the identification of most commercial and many military explosives.

To detect invisible amounts of organic explosives or their residues, selected areas of clothing or the ether swabs are extracted with more ether, and the concentrated extract is examined by gas chromatography. The presence of the various nitro compounds and nitrate esters produces peaks in certain positions in the output signal, but the peaks are not unique to these compounds. Therefore the suspected nitroglycerin peak or the ethylene glycol dinitrate peak is confirmed by a test that is specific for nitrate esters. The method of choice is governed by the amount of the substance available.

Nitroglycerin and Ethylene Glycol Dinitrate

1. Millimicrogram amounts of nitroglycerin are confirmed by a gas-liquid chromatography method. One drop of nitrogen-free sulfuric acid, 2 drops of sodium dried ether, and 10 μl of the ether extract are mixed. After 5 minutes, 5 μl of toluene is added and the mixture is shaken gently for 15 minutes. Dilute sodium carbonate is added carefully until the sulfuric acid is neutralized, when 1 ml of ether is added. After extraction, the ether layer is separated, dried with sodium sulfate, and evaporated to reduced bulk, and a sample is introduced into the gas chromatograph. The presence of a nitrotoluene peak con-

firms the original presence of a nitrate ester. The limit of detection is 5 mμg.

2. An alternative confirmation procedure is to dilute the concentrated ether extract with dry ether to 1 ml and to add 2 to 3 mg lithium aluminum hydride followed by 1 drop of acetyl chloride. After filtration and concentration a sample is introduced into the gas chromatograph; the presence of peaks corresponding to glycerol triacetate and ethylene glycol diacetate confirms the original presence of nitroglycerin. The limit of detection is 100 mμg.
3. If microgram amounts are available, a thin-layer chromatography procedure based on the method of Lloyd may be used. A sample is spotted onto an Eastman 6060 silica gel sheet and developed in toluene. After development and drying the sheet is sprayed with 1.0N sodium hydroxide solution, heated at 100°C for 10 minutes, and then sprayed with Griess's reagent (0.25 per cent sulfanilic acid and 0.1 per cent 1-naphthylamine in 1:1 aqueous acetic acid). The appearance of a red spot indicates the presence of a nitrate ester, and the specific identification is determined by the R_f. The limit of detection of nitroglycerin is 200 mμg for this simpler but coarser technique, which is unsuitable for the detection of ethylene glycol dinitrate.[5]
4. Urbanski and Kraziejko reported a more sensitive detection system in which the developed thin-layer chromatography plate is treated with a 0. 5 per cent solution of tetramethyl-*p*-phenylenediamine in hexane followed by irradiation with ultraviolet light. Nitrate esters appear as violet-blue spots, and again the R_f determines which one is present. The limit of detection is reported as 20 mμg.[6] In practice, however, with swabs from dirty hands and other surfaces, we have found 100 mμg to be a more reasonable lower limit. This reaction has the advantage of detecting the di- and polynitro aromatics in the same examination.

Nitrobenzene. Nitrobenzene is detectable by the initial gas-liquid chromatography examination. It is a most important constituent of improvised explosives in Northern Ireland. When mixed with sodium chlorate it forms "co-op sugar." Once again the confirmation procedure depends on the amount of material available.

1. Levels from 1 to 1,000 mμg can be confirmed by a reaction reported by Masson and Hanby. Three drops of iodyl sulfate in concentrated sulfuric acid suspension are mixed with an aliquot of the ether extract and allowed to react for two minutes. The reaction is terminated by the addition of 0.5 ml water, and the liberated iodine is removed with a few drops of sodium thiosulfate solution. The resultant clear liquid is extracted with 1 ml ether, and the ether layer is separated, washed in turn with a saturated sodium carbonate solution, sodium thiosulfate solution and water, dried, concentrated, and introduced into the gas chromatograph. The presence of a peak of *m*-iodonitrobenzene confirms the presence of nitrobenzene in the original extract. The iodyl sulfate is prepared by powdering and mixing 1 g iodine and 2 g iodine pentoxide and shaking with 20 ml concentrated sulfuric acid. A gradual separation of the pale yellow iodyl sulfate occurs, and this can be retained in the refrigerator as a stock suspension. For use, 2 or 3 drops of the suspension is removed, washed with nitrogen-free sulfuric acid, and centrifuged; the sulfuric acid is decanted; and the iodyl sulfate is suspended in 2 or 3 drops of nitrogen-free sulfuric acid. This suspension is now ready for the addition of the ether extract.[7]
2. For levels above 1 μg, thin-layer chromatography in which Eastman 6060 silica gel sheets are used and developed with hexane is suitable. Visualization of the spots under ultraviolet radiation is followed by spraying with a solution of stannous chloride in hydrochloric acid, then with the mixture of nitrogen oxides produced by the action of concentrated nitric acid on copper, and finally with a 1 per cent of 2-naphthol in 2.5N sodium hydroxide. The production of a red-orange spot with the correct R_f confirms the presence of nitrobenzene in the ether extract.

Gas-Liquid Chromatography Equipment

In all these tests, the gas chromatograph we have used is the Perkin-Elmer F11, with electron-capture detector and a 2-m-1/8-inch inside diameter glass column packed with 7 per cent E 301 on Chromosorb W. The column temperature is 140°C, the injection temperature is 180°C, the detector temperature is 170°C, and the carrier gas is nitrogen at a pressure of 25 psi.

Explosive Vapor Analysis

Some explosives have characteristic odors. Dogs are used to search for hidden explosives, and with patience they can be taught to discriminate between somewhat similar types. Some investigators set store by their own sense of smell, but few would claim the sensitivity and selectivity of the dog's olfactory organ; finding nothing but the smell of an explosive, they might hesitate to be "dogmatic" about its composition. The possibility of positively identifying an explosive from its smell alone, however, has at last become a reality. Our first use of the method relied on an instrument known as the "sniffer."

The instrument was produced and marketed as a leak detector, suitable for the detection of sulfur hexafluoride and other refrigerant gases, but it was found to react also to nitroglycerin, ethylene glycol dinitrate, and some of the lower nitroaromatics. Several of these instruments were introduced into Northern Ireland in mid-1971 to be used by specially trained troops in screening large numbers of rioters after nail bombs had been thrown and in examining cars in random road checks. With them, an experienced operator could, to a reasonable degree, discriminate between nitrate esters and nitro compounds on the one hand and tobacco smoke, dry cleaning fluids, and air fresheners on the other. The "sniffer" was little more than a self-contained electron-capture detector monitoring those components of the atmosphere that could pass through a silicone rubber membrane. Such a membrane will not delay the passage of most molecules absorbed by it, but the nitro compounds and nitrate esters and some other compounds of no consequence are delayed sufficiently to make the signal slower to build and of longer duration.

The equipment was used for screening purposes only, and positive reactions were taken as indicators for close search of vehicles and for hand swabbing or clothing examinations of individuals. In practice the "sniffer" was not wholly reliable, but although many false positive results were obtained, it was a valuable asset at a time of serious rioting when means were needed to control the easy transport of illegal explosives by road.

The partial success of the first instrument in an unplanned application encouraged its development for the specific task of detecting the volatile organic constituents of explosives, and a new model is now in use in the Northern Ireland Forensic Science Laboratory. This new instrument, shown in Figure 13–23, is much more sophisticated than its predecessor. It has two modes of operation. In the search mode, it samples the atmosphere in a bag of clothing, in a box of debris, in the trunk of a car, or in a room in a building, giving a visible and audible warning whenever it detects certain groups of compounds. The instrument can then be switched to the analysis mode, in which the questioned atmosphere is analyzed by the built-in gas chromatograph and the results are displayed on a chart recording. The equipment is battery- or main-operated and, being mounted on luggage casters, is entirely self-contained and very mobile when working from the battery. It is therefore eminently suitable for use at scenes of explosions or riots, and a valuable addition to the equipment of an explosive and ordnance disposal team.

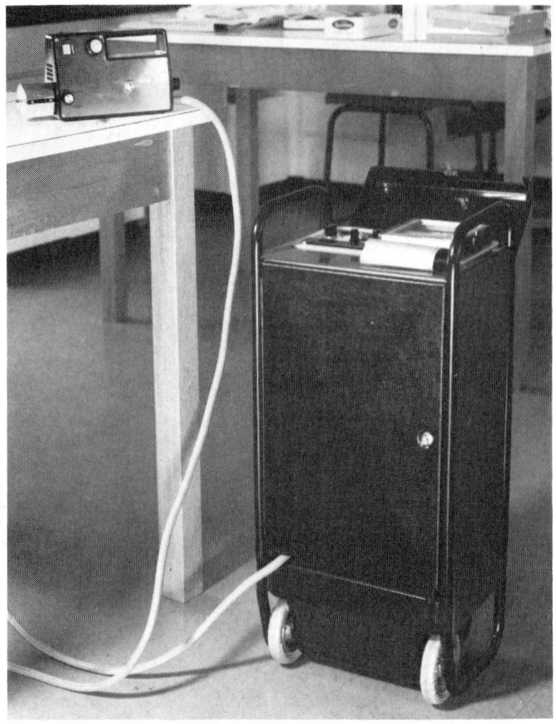

Figure 13–23. Portable main- or battery-operated equipment for the specific detection of the vapors of organic explosives.

Equipment based on similar operating principles might in the future be built into aircraft, enabling the crew to sample the atmosphere in the cabin and luggage compartments before takeoff.

BORDER PROBLEMS

In Northern Ireland, the population living close to the border of the Republic of Ireland is predominantly Catholic and, once merely sympathetic to, is now dominated by, the IRA. The border areas are subject to frequent incursions by guerillas operating from bases in the south, using minor unapproved roads or crossing the fields.* Country roads must be patrolled regularly by the security forces if even nominal control is to be maintained in territory that has always been republican in sentiment. Whereas in the cities, towns, and villages the terrorist campaign is largely designed to lay waste commercial property, to intimidate the civil population, and generally to disrupt the urban scene, in the rural areas the frank aim is to attack and kill as many as possible of the army, the police, for the Ulster Defence Regiment, a part-time force of volunteers recruited to guard vital installations and to carry out vehicle searches at impromptu checkpoints.

Operating in more or less friendly territory, the IRA can prepare unhindered for the passing patrols on border duty. Cleverly concealed booby traps and elaborate ambushes are the principal methods of attack. Huge land mines in culverts under narrow roads have contained hundreds of pounds of high explosives.

A mine for which the IRA openly claimed credit was detonated remotely by the terrorists as a patrol in a Saracen armored vehicle passed over the spot where it was concealed. The 13-ton vehicle was flung 20 yd, three young Scottish soldiers were killed, and four more were injured. The crater in the ground measured 30 ft across and was nearly 20 ft deep. Shortly after the explosion a woman in a small car drove straight into the crater and was lucky to escape with minor injuries.

Normally, investigation of these incidents would involve searching the surrounding area for fragments of the device and for the command wires leading back to the cover used by the terrorists, but sometimes the explosion is only the first phase of an ambush. It may be used to attract new targets for gunmen hiding, possibly on the other side of the border, where they are immune from pursuit. Consequently, the first task of the relief column, apart from attending to the injured, has been to deploy into a protective screen, ready to return the enemy's fire. Seeing this, the IRA began to lay booby-trap mines in areas of good cover near the first bomb, in the expectation that the troops would walk into these traps and be blown to pieces. Acres of ground have sometimes been covered with a network of booby traps, mines, and command wiring. Pressure mats and trip wires linked to milk churns packed with explosives, hidden under walls and in ditches, or buried in the ground make searching hazardous.

In reaction to these tactics, the army visits immediately only those explosion sites where men must be removed from danger or given urgent medical attention. In other cases no action is taken during the hours of darkness. In daylight the whole area is searched from the air by observers in low-flying helicoptors, and only then do the troops move in on the ground if this is thought to be necessary. The battle of wits has produced many variations of this deadly game.

A hijacked lorry left athwart the main railway line at first looked like a simple attempt to block the line but in reality was carrying a load of explosives to be detonated by a wireless signal from a hidden terrorist when the army arrived.

The dead body of a man missing for days and believed to have been assassinated was discovered bound and hooded in a field. The corpse had been boobytrapped to explode when the body was moved.

The army is seldom caught in traps like these now. Aerial reconnaissance of the scene and stakeouts on the ground reduce the possibility of being caught in an ambush, while specialized search teams and trained dogs are better able to avoid the danger of the booby trap. Explosive and ordnance disposal teams always blow up or dismantle any device they discover, but an explosion in a dangerous or hostile border area is not necessarily followed by immediate examination of the whole area for fragments if it is considered unsafe for investigators. The land mine concealed in a culvert or a hedgerow anywhere along hundreds of miles of country roads is almost impossible to anticipate, but one way of avoiding this hazard is to reduce the number of road patrols and substitute helicopter patrols, which are more effective in covering any type of ground.

Some idea of the importance of the border problem is conveyed by an estimate that in 1973 almost 500 attacks were launched from Eire. In that year 21 members of the security forces were killed within 12 miles of the border.

*Major roads crossing the border are approved for crossing and are customs controlled. Minor roads are unapproved and signposted to that effect. For the last six years the army has been putting up obstacles or blowing up minor roads, and the local population has been removing the obstacles or filling the craters up again. (Apart from hindering terrorists, the army action interferes with the "respectable" operation of ordinary commodity smuggling.)

LATER DEVELOPMENTS IN NORTHERN IRELAND

The intensification of the border campaign in 1973 reflected the growing pressure on the IRA in the urban areas, particularly in Belfast and Londonderry, and caused an increasing number of terrorists to seek sanctuary in the south. At the end of 1973 and in early 1974 however, the urban bombing compaign suddenly rose again to a high level.

The car bomb has been by far the most significant weapon of urban destruction, and toward the end of 1973 the terrorists found a new way of putting it to use.

In Omagh, the principal town of County Tyrone, an IRA gang held up a Post Office mail van, loaded up a 400-lb bomb, and instructed the driver to drive the van to the police station and park it outside. He was told the bomb would be detonated by wireless signal if he failed to obey. The driver complied, but when he stopped outside the police station, he was challenged by the guard. He shouted that there was a bomb in the van and the station was quickly cleared of men. The massive bomb went off shortly afterward, demolishing the station. Not surprisingly, such bombs delivered to the target on behalf of the IRA by innocent people acting under duress were soon to become widely known as "proxy" bombs.

A similar sequence of events resulted in the destruction of the police station at Lurgan, in County Armagh. In Belfast, at the height of the Christmas shopping, in separate incidents, the IRA hijacked a double-decker Corporation bus and a taxicab, loaded them with explosives, and made the drivers abandon them in central shopping streets, where they caused widespread damage.

In 1974, using a further development of the same tactics, the IRA managed to get car bombs into protected segments.

In Dungannon, a major town in County Tyrone, a Post Office mail van and its driver, allowed into the segment on official business, were captured by gunmen within the segment and then taken back to a vehicle barrier in a quiet street. Some 600 lb of explosives were manhandled over the barrier and loaded into the van. The Post Office employee was then forced to drive to the market square and abandon the van close to the police station, where it exploded doing vast damage to the property.

Pillar boxes (mailboxes) on city streets are provided with posting slits large enough to admit small packages, and in 1974, the IRA revived an old habit of attacking the mail. In the 1930s incendiary bombs were slipped into the pillar boxes, but in this latest move explosive bombs were preferred. A 5-lb time bomb in one pillar box exploded without warning, fragmenting the cast-iron box and injuring 12 people, including some passengers on a passing bus. After a spate of such explosions the Post Office authorities responded by closing all the mailboxes, but then relented to the extent of leaving slits large enough to allow the posting of thin envelopes.

The IRA made several attempts at aerial bombing. In one, using a civil helicopter hijacked in the Republic of Ireland, they flew over Strabane, a border town in Northern Ireland, and dropped two bombs, milk churns packed with high explosives. Fortunately, neither of them exploded.

Very considerable damage was caused to the center of Belfast in a new wave of incendiary attacks on shops in early 1974—with time bombs combining both explosive and incendiary elements.

Some of the combination time bombs were smuggled into Woolworth's largest store. A warning was given that they would explode at intervals. A serious fire followed the first explosion, and firemen were unable to enter the building for fear of further explosions, which did follow in due course. The store was largely destroyed in spite of the efforts of some 70 firemen using 10 pieces of fire-fighting equipment during the five-hour blaze.

A blockbuster car bomb, estimated at 500 lb, exploded outside the Grand Central Hotel on Belfast's Royal Avenue in early March 1974. The particular significance of this incident was that the hotel was the headquarters building of the army in Belfast. Damage to the hotel and surrounding property was estimated at over £1,000,000.

It is easy to underestimate the difficulty of preventing the urban terrorist from planting bombs, even in those areas to which only pedestrians are allowed access. Patient queues of men and women move slowly through the checkpoints, while troops search endlessly for suspicious material. The job of frisking men and women, young and old, prodding parcels, and dipping deeply into shopping bags and ladies' handbags requires substantial manpower, but not even all these precautions can prevent destruction within the heavily protected shopping areas. Customers entering shops along the main thoroughfares forming the perimeters of these areas face less wholehearted searching by civilian security guards, sometimes elderly, untrained, and diffident, and often cursory in the performance of their boring and unrewarding task. Total security is not compatible with the continuance of trade, and the terrorist with ingenuity can penetrate the defensive screen. The female terrorist poses a special problem. Bombs have been taken into stores concealed in prams, and on at least one occasion it was suspected that a "pregnant" woman entered a store, "delivered" a bomb, and left again much thinner.

INTERNATIONAL ASPECTS OF TERRORIST BOMBING

In the years of violence since 1969, almost every possible type of terrorist bomb has been used in Northern Ireland, most of them in considerable quantity. A prodigious amount of commercial explosives and of a wide variety of improvised ones have been used. Great damage has been done, costing many millions of pounds. Neither a political nor a military solution has yet been found, although the terrorists stand condemned by the church, the state, and most of the people in Ireland, north and south. They have long since lost the propaganda battle, and although the bombing and the shooting continue unabated, it is inconceivable that they will ever achieve their extremist aims through force alone. The IRA is not yet beaten; it still retains the power to inflict more suffering and destruction. Already over 1,500 people have died. A proportionate loss of life for the United Kingdom as a whole would be 60,000 and for the United States, 195,000—comparisons that indicate all too clearly the magnitude of the problem in human terms.

The need for investigational know-how and resources is not peculiar to any one country. The IRA has known links with similar organizations around the world, and law enforcement agencies in many countries face the task of combating terrorist bombing campaigns. Techniques of violence used in Northern Ireland are used elsewhere; improvised explosive devices made by the IRA in Belfast are similar to those made, for example, by the Bader Meinhof in West Germany, by the Cubans in Florida, and by the FLQ (Quebec Liberation Front). At the investigational level this is an international problem demanding international awareness and cooperation if it is to be contained. Distance may divide us; heredity, culture, and environment may make us different; but the traumatic effects of a bomb are the same for all of us.

REFERENCES

1. Cook, M. A.: *The Science of High Explosives*. New York, Reinhold Book Corp., 1958.
2. Handbook of Chemistry and Physics. 42nd Ed. Cleveland, The Chemical Rubber Publishing Co., 1960.
3. Fordham, S.: *High Explosives and Propellants*. Oxford, Pergamon Press Ltd., 1961.
4. Amas, S. A. H., and Yallop, J.: The identification of industrial blasting explosives of the gelignite type. J. Forensic Sci. Soc., *6*:185, 1966.
5. Lloyd, J. B. F.: Detection of microgram amounts of nitroglycerine and related compounds. J. Forensic Sci. Soc., 7:198, 1967.
6. Urbanski, T., and Kraziejko, T.: A method for the detection of nitrate esters. J. Chromatogr., *84*:218, 1973.
7. Masson I., and Hanby, E.: The iodous cation as an agent for aromatic substitution. J. Chem. Soc., p. 1699, 1938.

SECTION 2. INJURY BY FIREARMS, BOMBS, AND EXPLOSIVES

chapter 14

EXPLOSION INJURIES

by T. K. Marshall

Explosions are uncommon, and few doctors have much experience of them. Most of our knowledge has been gained in wartime and concerns the explosion of shells, ammunition dumps, torpedoes, and atomic bombs, but there have been some notable explosions affecting civilians not engaged in wartime activity. Among these are colliery disasters such as the one at Hulton in 1911, when 343 persons lost their lives, and disasters such as that in Texas City in 1947, when a ship loaded with ammonium nitrate fertilizer exploded at the docks, killing 561 people and injuring 3,000.[1, 2] Within recent years, terrorist activity in many parts of the world, but particularly in Northern Ireland, has added a new dimension to "civilian" explosions; the parcel bomb, letter bomb, and car bomb have become a daily potential hazard in many communities.

When an explosion occurs, the explosive material is suddenly converted into a large volume of gas with the release of a tremendous amount of energy. Pressures of up to 1,000 tons per square inch (up to 150,000 atm) can be generated, and the temperature of the explosive gases can rise to 3,000°C. A person in the vicinity can experience a number of effects: (1) If he is very near the seat of the explosion, he can be blown to pieces and scattered by the force of the explosion gases. (2) If he is near enough for the skin to be in contact with the explosion flame, he can sustain the usual kind of flame burn. This type of burn is also caused by contact with clothing or other material ignited by the explosion. At greater distances, exposure to the momentary heat radiation causes "flash" burns, which can be equally serious. (3) The person can be injured by the wave of pressure, called the shock wave, which spreads concentrically from the blast center. When the explosion is in air this pressure wave is referred to as air blast and it is followed by a postblast wind that also does damage. When the explosion is in water, the pressure changes are called underwater blast, and when it forces a solid material such as the deck of a ship against the body, the effect is called solid blast. (4) The person can be struck by flying missiles propelled by the explosion. (5) He can be injured or crushed by debris, usually of buildings demolished by the explosion. (6) He can be overcome by fumes formed as a result of the explosion.

The degree to which each of these effects is present in any particular explosion varies, and this accounts for what is sometimes a remarkable difference in the effects experienced by victims of the same explosion.

DISRUPTIVE EFFECTS OF BLAST

When a person is in the immediate vicinity of an explosion his body may be disrupted. He may be literally blown to pieces, and small parts of the body may be scattered over a wide area. This occurs in wartime when a high-explosive shell lands nearby or an explosive store is detonated. In today's terrorist situations it occurs when someone is carrying a large bomb that explodes or when a victim is blown up by a land mine. Little of the body may be recovered.

particularly if a building is demolished simultaneously and there is a large amount of rubble. When the area is scoured by untrained persons, the parts that are collected are usually the fairly obvious portions of the body such as a segment of spine or a foot, and pieces of scalp and skin. The internal organs are less frequently found.

When the explosion is small or when the victim is a little distance away from a large one, injury may be limited to the blowing off of the head or a limb or the mangling of a localized area. The mangled area is heavily soiled; when it is on a limb, immediate amputation is the only treatment.

When people are blown up in a civilian situation, as by a terrorist bomb, it is usually necessary to ascertain the number of victims. Most of the dead will be sufficiently intact to be counted, but some near the explosion center may have been disintegrated. A search of the area, for 100 yd or more from the seat of the explosion, must be made for human tissue, and whatever is recovered must be washed and carefully examined.

First, nonhuman tissue must be identified and discarded. It is surprising how often animal tissue is present. Some might be expected when a bomb explodes in a farmyard (in one such instance, the pile of soft tissue contained a small ball of muscle that turned out to be a gizzard stuffed full of seeds). Yet even in an urban situation, animal tissue is frequently recovered in the search—usually small bones. These are not difficult to identify as animal by those with experience; some may have obviously been cut with a butcher's saw.

Whenever differentiation between animal and human tissue is important, yet impossible by naked-eye examination, it can be achieved by an antigen-antibody reaction.

The next step is to segregate those parts that will help to establish the number of victims. Pieces of scalp, skin, jaw, joints, spine, pelvis, hands, and feet are put into separate piles (Fig. 14–1). The hair on the pieces of scalp is compared for length, color, and texture. The pieces of skin are separated according to color. The joints are identified and separated into right and left; the hands and feet compared for size, general configuration, and skin color and texture. A simple examination of this kind will at least indicate the *minimum* number of bodies—there is always the chance that there were more.

Careful examination of the residual tissue scraps might seem unrewarding, yet it is surprising how frequently the tissue yields important clues.

On one occasion a terrorist bomb exploded as it was being loaded into a car, demolishing a nearby house and scattering human remains for a distance of 100 yd. Four identifiable bodies were recovered in addition to a mound of flesh that, piled high, was more than one mortuary trolley would hold. When this was sorted, there was a female face that appeared to pose no serious problem in identification. Before it was correctly identified, however, a young man wrongly identified the victim as his sister. There were also numerous recognizable pieces of human body, including scalp of two different kinds, a mangled trunk, 6 shoulder joints, 2 elbow joints, 6 hands, 3 hip joints, 5

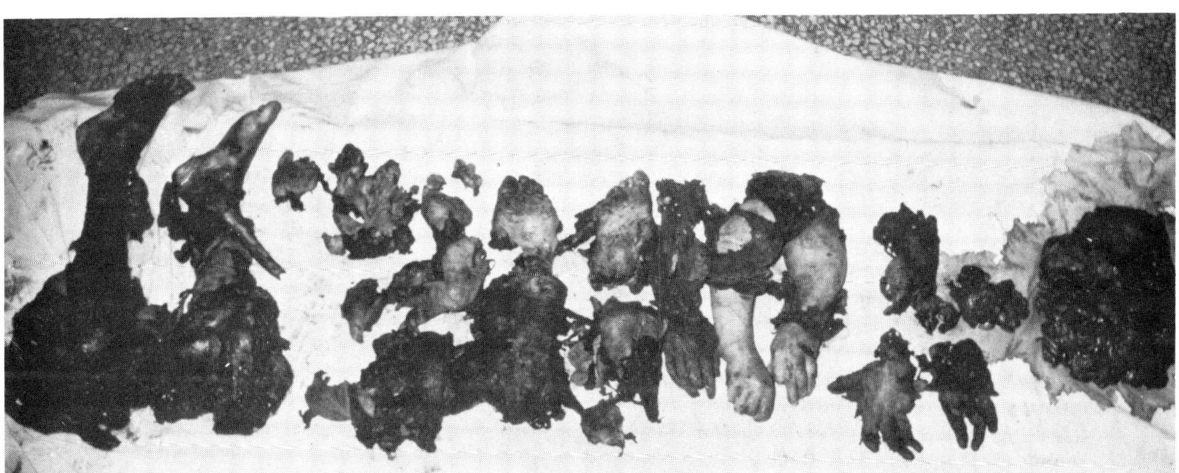

Figure 14–1. Some of the recognizable parts recovered after an explosion that disintegrated four adults and killed four others. They represent about a quarter of the remains brought to the mortuary. They have been washed and sorted prior to a detailed examination.

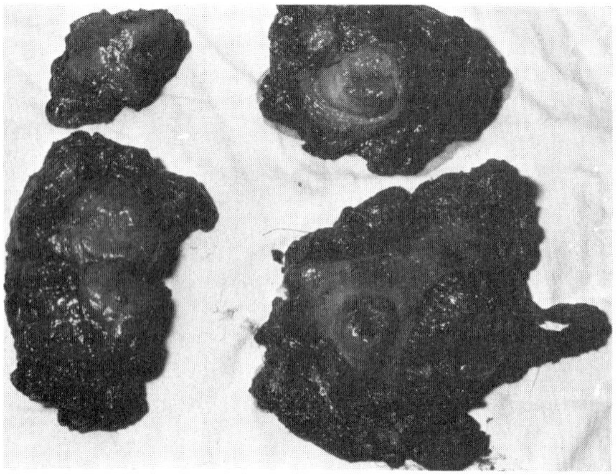

Figure 14–2. Parts recovered after an explosion that disintegrated four adults and killed four others. A detailed examination of the mound of apparently unidentifiable soft tissue revealed these two prostate glands *(left)* and two uterine cervixes *(right)*. This evidence gave at least the sex of the disintegrated victims.

knee joints, 2 legs, and 27 recognizable pieces of viscera. Finally, a mound of scraps, some 47 lb in weight in all, was examined. In spite of the unpromising nature of the material, careful inspection revealed two uterine cervixes and two prostate glands (Fig. 14–2). Although these disintegrated remains, other than the face, could not be identified, nor could the pieces be apportioned to individual bodies, at least there could be no doubt that two men and two women were involved. Subsequently, death notices in the newspaper revealed the identity of the four disintegrated victims and inferred that no one else had died.

On another occasion terrorists entered a customs shed with a bomb that went off prematurely. Eight mangled bodies were recovered; they were of four customs officers, two lorry drivers, and two terrorists. Many pieces of human tissue were collected, and the recognizable portions were being apportioned to the eight victims when, among the scraps, there was a penis. This was only just recognizable because it was stripped of skin and heavily soiled by dirt, but close examination revealed the corona, glans, and meatus. It was not from one of the eight victims; it became the only clue to there being a ninth victim. He must have been carrying the bomb and been completely disintegrated.

The discovery of genitalia obviously establishes the sex of the victim. On other occasions the sex might be inferred from the hair. This can prove misleading, of course, as can a portion of breast. After an explosion that killed two people, some more tissue was recovered from the rubble and it became evident that there had been a third victim. A piece of skin with a very prominent nipple suggested that a woman had been killed, but when all the evidence came to hand there was no doubt that the victim was a man. In problem cases one might have to resort to determining the sex by microscopic examination of the tissue, mucosa, or skin.

Next comes the identification of the bodies. Apart from the difficulties introduced by injuries, dismemberment, or mangling, the principles are no different from those of the identification of any human corpse (Fig. 14–3). Visual inspection is the first step once the body has been cleaned. As in all instances of identification, the evidence of lay people must be accepted with caution because such complicating factors as deformity of the skull or facial injuries may mislead them. Clothing is very helpful, of course, but when the person was close to the explosion, most of this may have been burned or blown off and what remains on the

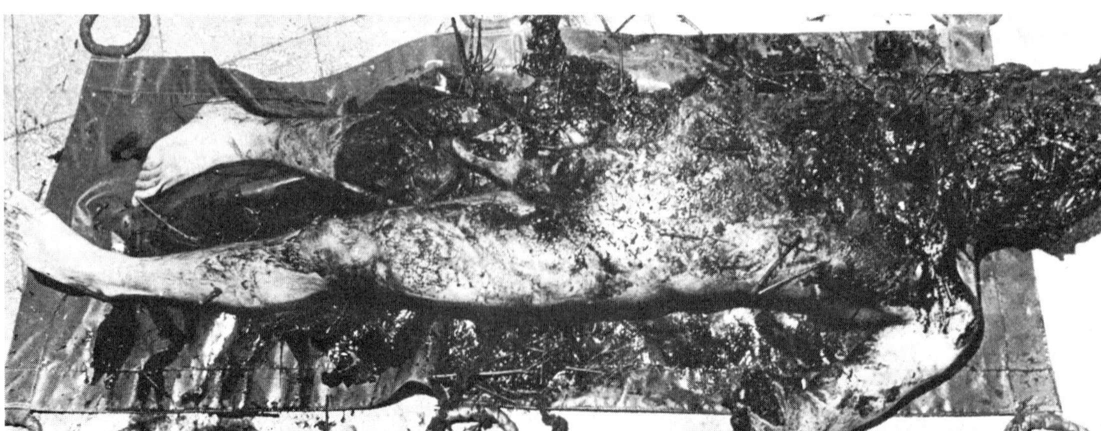

Figure 14–3. A victim of a terrorist bomb explosion. Owing to the injuries, visual identification is very difficult.

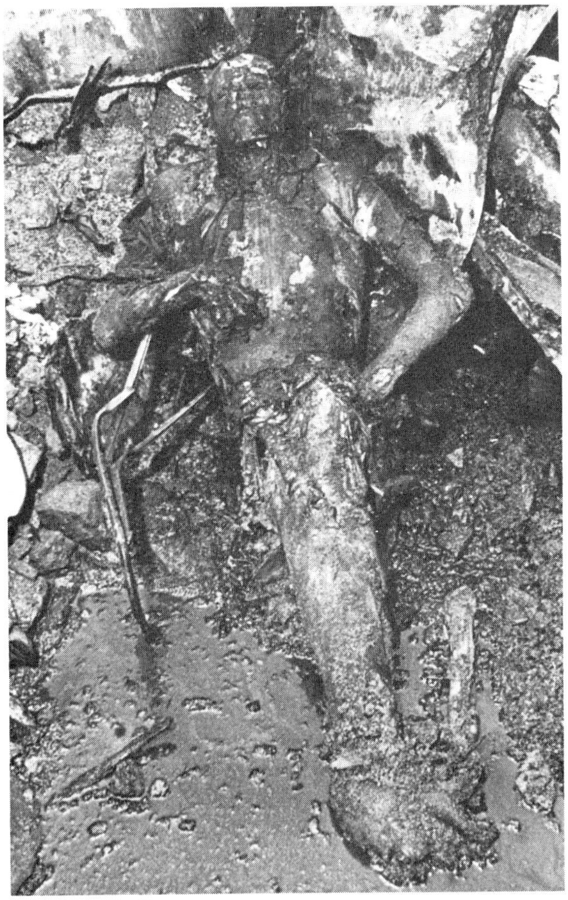

Figure 14–4. The victim of a terrorist bomb. Identification is difficult because of soiling of the body.

body may be so stained with blood and oil, soaked with water, or soiled by cement dust and dirt as to be unrecognizable before thorough cleaning (Fig. 14–4).

Fingerprinting must never be omitted, since it can prove identity in many cases. If the victim is a terrorist, his fingerprints may be available in police records. If an explosion victim has not previously been fingerprinted, the fingerprints taken after death may still confirm identity once this has been suggested and his prints have been found on articles he has handled at home or at work. The dentition and artificial teeth too can establish certain identity provided a good dental record is available. It is important to have the mouth examined by a dental surgeon so that as much detail as possible can be recorded. Scars, tattoos, and deformities also help, and a complete x-ray of the body may reveal old fractures, bony changes, and stones that an alleged victim was known to have.

Finally there is the question of the cause of death. The immediate inference is that it was the explosion, and this is usually correct. It is nevertheless possible for someone to be shot dead, perhaps while trying to prevent the planting of a bomb, and for his body to be mangled when the bomb exploded (Fig. 14–5). It is also possible for a dead body to be blown up deliberately. This might be to obliterate the corpse and prevent identification (with a modicum of luck on the side of the investigators this is unlikely to succeed). More likely, however, the dead body will have been charged with explosive as a booby trap for security forces. To be aware of these possibilities is not to accept the cause of death at its face value and so be misled.

FLAME AND RADIANT HEAT

When a bomb explodes, the temperature of the explosive gases can rise to 3,000°C. Contact with the momentary flame causes burns, and people outside this range can be burned by the

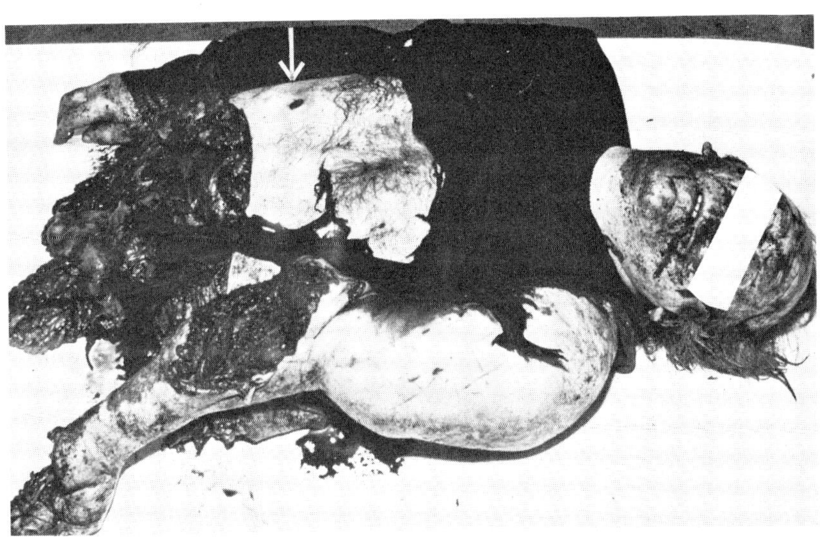

Figure 14–5. The upper half of an adult body recovered from a building blown up by a terrorist bomb. The arrow points to a fatal bullet wound inflicted before the explosion.

radiated heat. The burning effect of radiated heat depends not only on the total thermal energy received but also on the rate at which the energy is supplied. The rate of heat transfer depends in turn on the duration of the explosion. For a given heat output, the more rapid the explosion the more it will cause burns. The thermal radiation received increases directly with the weight of the explosive and inversely with the square of the distance from it; because of this inverse square rule, a person has to be within feet of an ordinary bomb to sustain radiant heat burns. These burns are usually referred to as "flash burns" to distinguish them from the "flame burns" due to the flame at the explosion center, to burning clothing, and to environmental fire.

A radiant heat dose of 1.5 cal per square centimeter on bare skin will just cause pain. A dose of 2 cal per square centimeter will cause reddening like sunburn, often referred to as a first-degree burn. Twice this dose, 4 cal per square centimeter, will cause a second-degree burn characterized by blistering, and a dose of 6 cal per square centimeter will cause a burn of third degree in which the full thickness of the skin is involved and skin grafting is required in treatment.

Heat radiation of this intensity can be stopped by solid objects and by clothing. A person crouching behind a wall is thus protected, and others tend to sustain burns only on the unclothed parts of the body—usually the head and hands. White outer clothing gives better protection than darker clothing, which absorbs more of the heat, and two or more layers of loosely draped clothing is best.

In an incident in which terrorists were mak ing bombs in a small room of a house, something went wrong and there was an explosion that scorched parts of the room and blew out the windows. A young woman, 19 years old, staggered outside. She had sustained third-degree burns on 80 per cent of the body surface and, after a stormy course during which the burns became infected, she died 10 days later. At autopsy the distribution of the burns showed clearly the protective effect of her bra, pants, and footwear (Fig. 14–6).

Flash burns usually affect an area, perhaps the face or one side of a limb, more or less uniformly, sparing those areas shielded in any way from the direct heat. When death occurs fairly quickly, these areas dry, becoming reddish brown and parchmentlike. Flame burns from burning clothing and objects tend to be less uniform in degree. The clothing is often set alight by fire in the vicinity, but it can also be ignited by the heat radiated by a large explosion if it is of an easily combustible material. Dark-colored clothing is more likely to ignite than light-colored clothing. Burns from clothing, unlike most flash burns, occur on both clothed and unclothed areas. When the environment is set on fire the whole of the body may be burned.

AIR BLAST

Exposure to blast must have occurred ever since man first made gunpowder, but a full appreciation of its effects is of relatively recent date. Even as late as the 1914–1918 War, air blast was poorly understood; it was recognized that it could perforate the eardrums, but in general it was not until the Spanish Civil War when bombs had become larger that it was realized that air blast could kill without producing external injuries by splinters or secondary missiles. How air blast could do this was discovered by clinical observation and experiment during the Second World War.

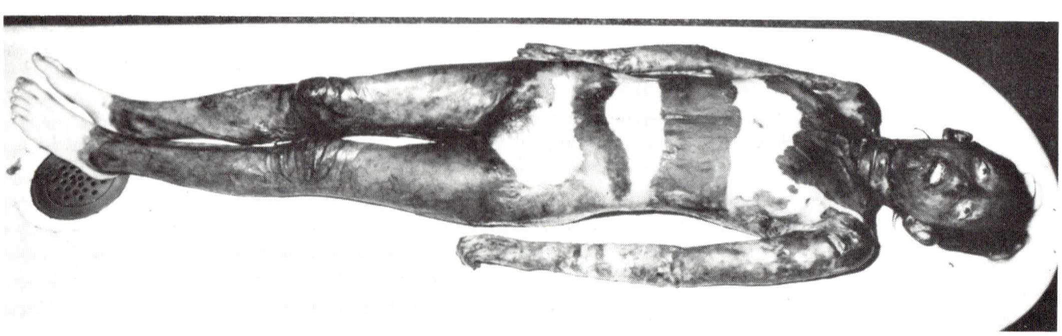

Figure 14–6. Flash burns on a victim of an explosion. She survived a few days, and the burned areas became parchmented. The protective effect of some of her clothing is clearly shown.

Physical Principles of Air Blast

The shock wave, which spreads concentrically from the blast center, is a sound wave of a very high pressure that moves past a person, temporarily engulfing him, as a bather is washed over by a sea wave breaking in the surf. Beyond the violent changes in the vicinity of the explosion, the velocity of this shock wave soon decreases to about the speed of sound in air (1120 fps), but near the explosion it is many times faster, since the velocity increases with increased air pressure. The shock wave has never the smooth form of a sound wave; the wave front is steep, rising suddenly to peak pressure in less than a millionth of a second and then falling away steadily, finally becoming negative, a suction, for a period of time (Fig. 14–7). The total duration of the shock wave is brief. For instance, at 30 ft from a 70-lb charge the pressure component lasts about 5 msec and the suction component 30 msec. As the distance from the explosion is increased, the pressure component lasts longer because the front of the wave where the pressure is highest always travels faster than the tail of the wave where the pressure is lowest. The duration of the suction component remains more or less constant, however, at up to five times the duration of the pressure component.

The blast wave can knock a person down, move objects, and demolish buildings. These effects are usually due to the impact of the steep pressure wave front, which, at pressures of 2 psi and above, is felt as a sudden blow. Williams states that a pressure of 6 psi at right angles to the muzzle of a ship's gun lifted an officer off his feet.[3]

The movement of air particles within the blast wave, owing to its varying pressures, also produces a blast wind that pushes in one direction in the pressure phase and pulls in the other direction in the suction phase. With ordinary explosions the particle movement is so momentary as not to be felt as a wind. It is different with atomic explosions, however, in which the two phases of the blast wind may operate over a period of seconds; these winds can be of exceptional force and do serious damage. In very big explosions we must also take account of winds that follow on the heels of the blast wave. These are generated by the outward push of the tremendous volume of explosive gases liberated at the explosion center. In atomic explosions a wind is also generated by the subsequent rush of air back to the explosion site as the hot cloud ascends.

These various winds that accompany a shock wave decay more rapidly than the pressure front as the distance from the explosion increases, but they can displace objects at considerable distances. In the Texas City disaster people up to 3,000 ft from the explosion were displaced from a few feet to several hundred; for instance, one man standing 500 ft from the ship was blown horizontally for 10 ft.[2] The direction of translation was haphazard and unpredictable, however. Some were blown away from the explosion, some toward it, others vertically, and some first in one direction and then in another. Many persons, even those inside buildings, had most or all of their clothing blown off.

Obviously the force of the shock wave or the postblast wind can knock buildings down, but with buildings, another force called ground shock can be involved. This arises when an explosion occurs in the ground, as when a bomb dropped from an aircraft penetrates the earth. This generates a complex train of shock waves similar to those of an earthquake, and buildings can be tumbled in a capricious way depending on their natural frequencies.

Displacement and crushing of the body by disintegrating buildings cause injuries that are discussed subsequently. The injuries caused by air blast that have occasioned most interest are those specific to the momentary pressure to which the body, even when it is restrained from movement, is subjected by the shock wave. These effects are the ones that can cause death without any external signs. They depend on three main features of the shock wave: pressure, impulse, and duration.

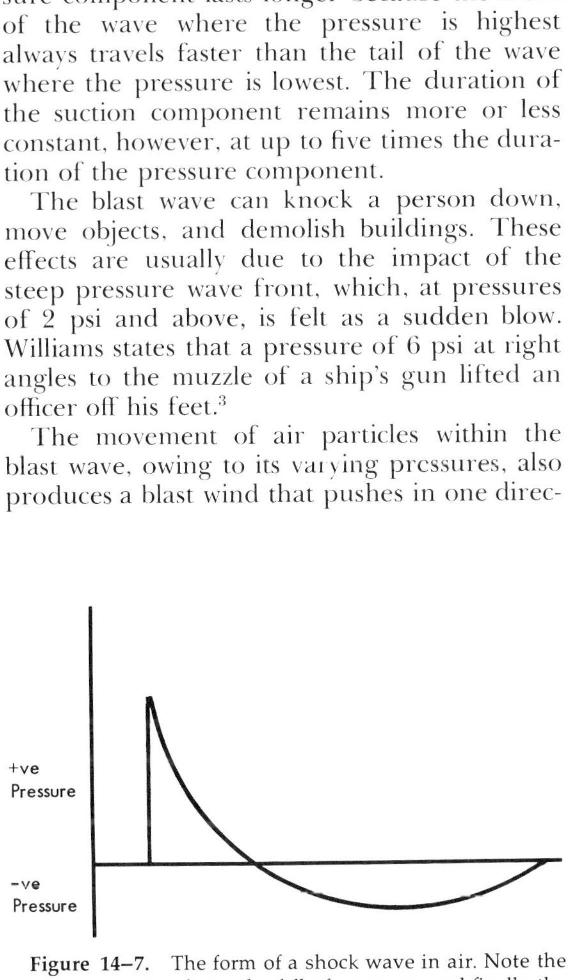

Figure 14–7. The form of a shock wave in air. Note the steep-rising wave front, the fall of pressure, and finally the phase of negative pressure or suction.

Peak Pressure

The hydrostatic, or air, pressure is highest in the region of the explosion and it falls rapidly,

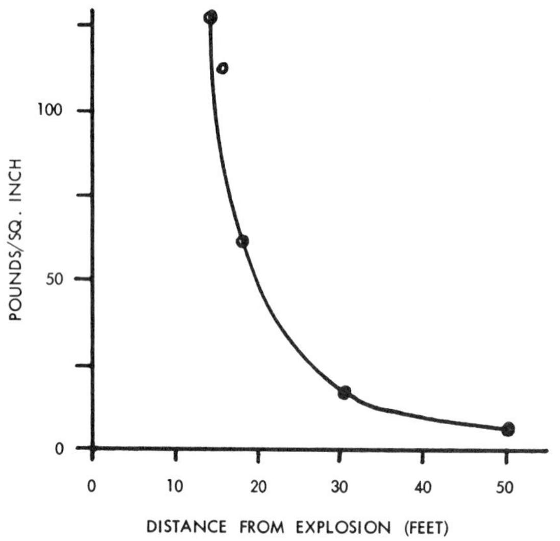

Figure 14–8. This curve relates the peak pressures from the explosion of a 70-lb charge measured at distances of 14 to 50 ft from the explosion. Note how the peak pressure is rapidly reduced as the distance from the explosion increases.

almost exponentially, as the distance from the blast center increases (Fig. 14–8). Thus, in the case of a 70-lb charge the excess air pressure in pounds per square inch (psi) over the normal atmospheric pressure of 15 psi was 110 at 14 ft, 60 at 18 ft, 15 at 30 ft, and 6 at 50 ft, although when a shock wave strikes a flat surface at right angles and is reflected, the pressure experienced by the surface can be twice as great.[4] Whereas pressure of 1 psi is able to break windows and of 3 psi to break walls, the air pressure must reach the vicinity of 100 psi (or 6 atm) to endanger the life of human beings.[5] Because the suction component is always weaker (and in no case can it be greater than 15 psi in air, since this would produce a perfect vacuum), it is unlikely that the suction wave would have any serious effect on a human being. Window panes that are pulled out by the suction have usually been first fragmented by the pressure pulse.

Impulse

This is the time integral of the pressure and it is represented by the area under the pressure curve (the shaded areas in Figure 14–9). It depends on the peak overpressure and the duration and rate of decay of the shock wave. Two explosions can produce shock waves of the same peak pressure, but one in which pressure falls quickly over a short period of time (Fig. 14–9*A*) will have a smaller impulse than one in which pressure is better sustained for a longer time (Fig. 14–9*B*). The crack from a rifle and the boom from a 12-inch gun are good respective examples. A greater impulse is to be expected when an explosion occurs inside a building. An atomic explosion is the extreme example of the high-impulse explosion, and the persistence of its pressure over a comparatively long period of time makes its damaging effects far more dependent on its impulse than on its pressure peak.

Duration

This quality of the shock wave has received the least attention, but a study was carried out in 1954 by Celander and his co-workers. They showed that this factor was not as important as the peak pressure but found, nevertheless, that the longer the duration of the shock wave, the greater was the injury inflicted.[6] It is likely that in the human, the lethal effect of an overpressure of 100 psi acting for 5 msec is equal to that of an overpressure of 60 psi acting for 20 msec. The influence of the duration is greatest in those cases in which an only moderate peak pressure would cause only moderate injury.

In practice, the damaging effect of an explosion depends principally on both pressure and impulse. A high peak pressure is of little importance if it is not sustained long enough to disturb a structure beyond the point of its elastic recovery. On the other hand, a large impulse means little unless the peak pressure rises above what the structure is able to withstand. Since both impulse and peak pressure decay rapidly as the distance from the seat of the explosion increases, only those persons close to the explosion are likely to be seriously affected by blast.

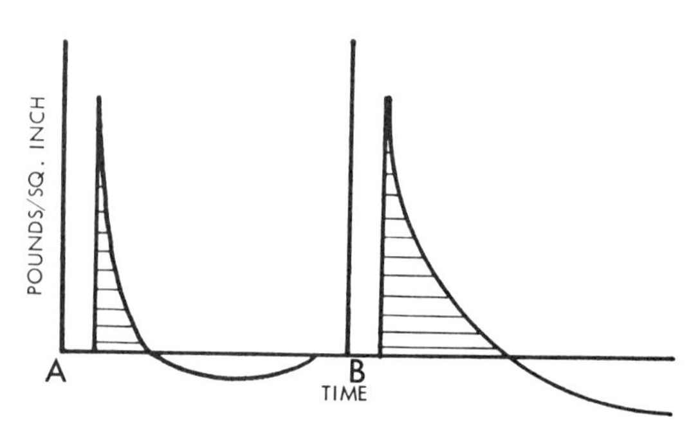

Figure 14–9. The meaning of impulse. Curve *A* shows a quick fall of shock wave pressure. Curve *B* shows the same peak pressure but a slower decay; the impulse of this explosion, represented by the shaded area, is greater than that of explosion *A*.

Biophysics of Air Blast Injury

Most of our knowledge of the action of air blast on the living body stems from animal experiments, notably those carried out by Zuckerman during the Second World War and the more recent experiments by Clemedson and his colleagues at the Research Institute of National Defence in Sweden.

When a shock wave strikes the body surface, part of it is reflected, part is deflected, and the rest is absorbed. The absorbed fraction of the shock wave is then propagated throughout the body in a complex way that depends to a large extent on the structural differences of the tissues. Broadly speaking, however, the shock wave passes through relatively homogeneous tissues such as the heart, the thigh, and the solid organs without much modification apart from a decrease in the steepness of the wave front, and it does not damage them. Air-containing organs are very vulnerable, however. For instance, in its passage through the unhomogeneous lungs there is considerable damping of the wave, this damping being achieved by movements of the lung tissue.[7] The acceleration of parts of different density and the compression and reexpansion of alveoli as the pressure wave passes through them are thought to be among the causes of the lung damage that is universally recognized as a constant and significant feature of air blast injury and that can occur at peak pressures of 15 psi. Another cause is the shredding or bursting effect that occurs when a pressure wave breaks out of the liquid medium of the lung tissue into the gaseous medium of the alveolus. Whatever the relative importance of these, and perhaps other, mechanisms, there is no doubt that the structural damage due to a shock wave is confined mainly to air- or gas-containing organs and, in particular, the ears, the lungs, and segments of the large bowel. It must be stressed that the effects of pure air blast diminish rapidly as the distance from the explosion is increased and that little physical damage is to be expected at distances greater than 30 to 50 ft. Barcroft exposed goats to 500-lb bomb detonations in the open and found that only animals within 15 ft of the explosion suffered ill effects.[8] In Zuckerman's experiments with animals placed between 13 and 70 ft from a 70-lb charge of high explosive, no animals were killed at distances over 18 ft and none was affected at a distance greater than 50 ft. Humans might be even less susceptible. Tolerance is greater to a shock wave that rises slowly to a peak pressure; it is minimal to the fast-rising long-duration wave form.

Tissue Damage Due to Air Blast

Ear

Since a blast wave is a sound wave of high intensity, it is obvious that the ear, built specially for the reception of sound, is likely to be damaged by exposure to blast overpressures. Whether the ear is damaged depends on many factors. Blast is always capricious in its effects, and injury to the ear is no exception; it is well recognized that the ear damage sustained by different persons exposed to the same explosion varies considerably. Much depends on the intensity of the blast, the proximity to the source, the orientation of the axis of the external auditory canal to the wave front, the duration of exposure, the awareness of the explosion, protection afforded by any object between the explosion and the ear, and preexisting aural disease.

A pressure pulse approaching the human ear is concentrated as it passes down the external auditory canal so that the pressure on the tympanic membrane is about 20 per cent higher than that just outside the ear.[10] Wax that occludes the canal yet remains separated from the eardrum by an air space will attenuate the blast wave and reduce damage. On the other hand, if the plug is near to or touching the eardrum, it can be forced through the drum by the blast wave and may disrupt the ear ossicles. This is more likely to happen when the shock wave lasts for a relatively long time. The reactions of the middle ear ossicles to the shock pulse of a blank cartridge were investigated and described by Perlman.[11]

Clinical examination of those who have been exposed to blast reveals effects on the ears that can be graded thus: (1) Hyperemia of the intact tympanic membrane, (2) punctate bruising of the intact tympanic membrane, (3) rupture of the tympanic membrane, and (4) damage to the cochlea.

Experiments and clinical data concerning rupture of the tympanic membrane appear to indicate that a fast-rising pressure pulse such as occurs in explosions ruptures some eardrums at an overpressure of 5 psi. When the pressure rises to 15 psi, about 50 per cent of eardrums are ruptured.[12] The tear involves the pars tensa, and any quadrant can be torn. The tear is usually associated with bleeding into the middle ear. One or both ears may be affected. The drums of children resist perforation better than those of adults.[13]

Damage to the cochlea is said to occur more frequently when the tympanic membrane remains intact, but experience with explosions in Belfast throws some doubt on this.[13] There is a sudden severe deafness followed by a period of recovery during which acuity for all frequencies is depressed. Any residual deafness tends to be greater in the high frequencies. Slight hemorrhage into the scala tympani near the round window, hemorrhage into the basal coil of the cochlea, and hemorrhage in the fundus of the internal meatus have been described.[14]

The prominent symptom of ear damage is, of course, deafness. At the time of the explosion this is frequently complete and associated with tinnitus. Some recovery usually occurs within the next few hours, however, and any residual deafness takes one of three forms. The first is a sensorineural deafness. When the pressure wave is of relatively short duration, as it is from the muzzle of a rifle or antiaircraft gun of less than 3-inch caliber, the acoustic loss is called "report deafness" and it is characterized by a depression in hearing around 4,000 cycles (the so-called C^5 dip) with retention of good hearing for frequencies below and above this level. This deafness is similar to the occupational noise-induced deafness as experienced by, say, boilermakers. When the pressure wave lasts longer, as it does with large guns and bombs, the pressure peak may be the same, but the greater impulse and the greater content of low-frequency tones cause a loss of auditory acuity for all high tones, that is, approximately 4,000 Hz and above. These forms of deafness are not dependent on damage to the middle ear structures. The second form of deafness, conductive, involves all frequencies and is associated with rupture of the eardrum and sometimes with dislocation of the middle ear structures. When the drum alone is affected, there is good recovery of hearing after healing. When the ossicles are damaged, the hearing loss can only be reversed by surgery. The third form of deafness is a mixture of these sensorineural and conductive types.

Lung

Hooker first drew attention to the important role of lung damage in the blast syndrome, and it was Zuckerman who first showed by animal experiments that the lung lesions of air blast were due to the direct impact on the body wall of the pressure component of the shock wave.[9, 15] Previously some had argued that the lung damage was due either to a wave of pressure traveling down the trachea or to the suction component of the wave acting likewise through the trachea, but these mechanisms have now been discredited.

The lung lesion takes the form of alveolar hemorrhage, its severity varying directly with the size of the explosive charge and becoming greater the nearer the victim is to the explosion (Fig. 14–10). When it is severe, the respiratory

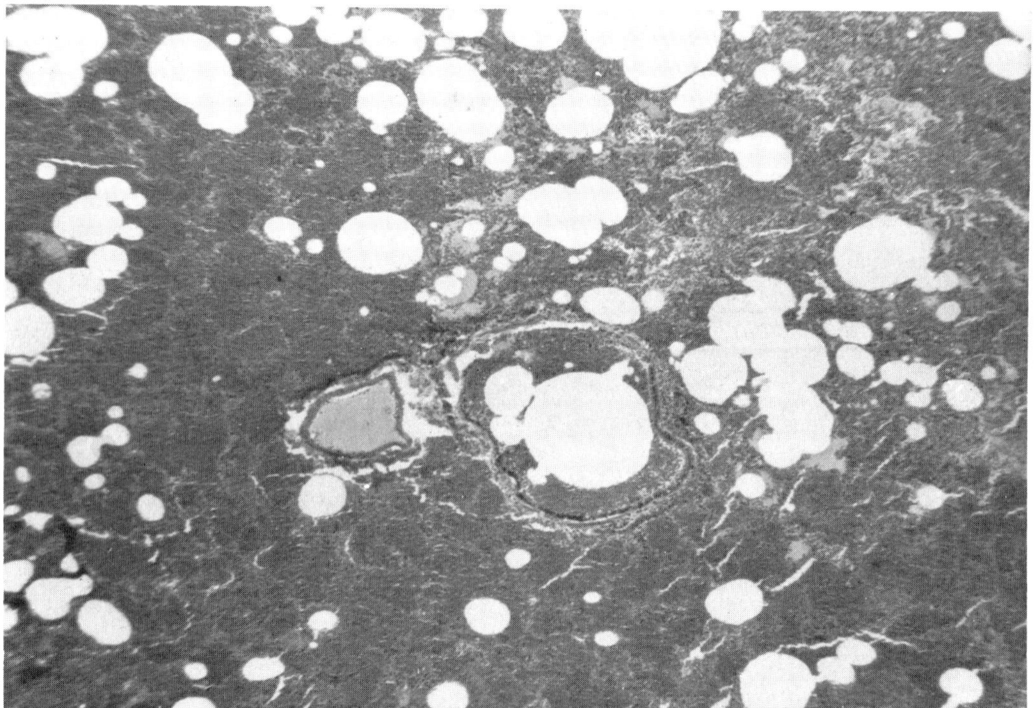

Figure 14–10. Photomicrograph of lung damaged by blast. The alveoli are filled by hemorrhage, and the alveolar septa are ill-defined. The hemorrhage has gained the bronchiole.

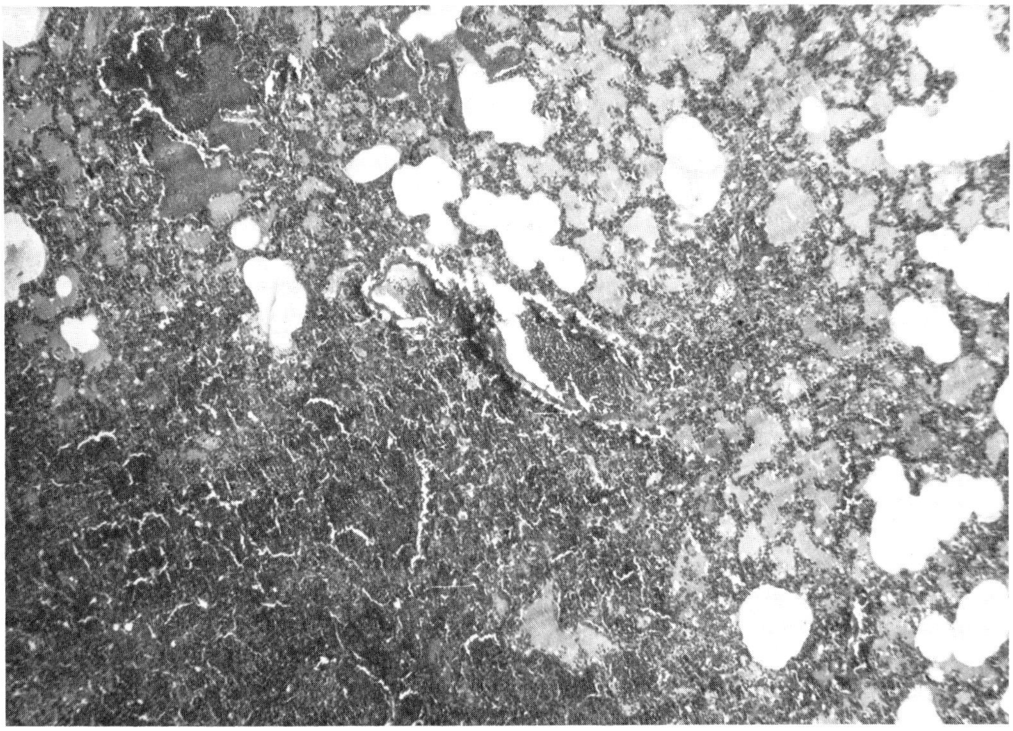

Figure 14–11. Photomicrograph of lung damaged by blast. This was the periphery of an area of confluent hemorrhage. Intraalveolar hemorrhage, blood in the bronchioles, edema, and dilated alveolar ducts are clearly shown.

passages may be filled with blood and froth, causing suffocation. The hemorrhages are due to tearing of the alveolar septa and they arise in each lung immediately after the explosion, but if the person survives they can probably extend during the next few hours. At autopsy some of the hemorrhages may be visible on the surface of each lung as subpleural patches of purple-red color and varying size. Usually they are scattered at random, but occasionally they cross the lung surface in the line of the ribs and at other times are grouped near the anterior and costophrenic margins. Section of the lungs reveals more discrete hemorrhages here and there in the tissue, often with a tendency to be more central than peripheral. The rest of the tissue is patchily edematous.

Microscopically, fresh hemorrhage may occupy clearly defined alveoli, but sometimes there is a large confluent hemorrhage and the alveolar septa are not discernible. Hemorrhage extends into the bronchioles in places. There is a variable amount of edema fluid in the alveoli and emphysematous dilation of some of the alveolar ducts (Fig. 14–11). Hemorrhage may also be seen in the interstitial tissue. In the bronchioles sheets of epithelium may be loosened or shed into the lumen, and pink-staining fluid and red cells may be found between the epithelium and the lamina propria, which is sometimes infiltrated by neutrophils. This differentiates epithelial detachment from the postmortem artifact with which all pathologists are familiar. In those who survive for some hours, a neutrophilic inflammatory reaction is often superimposed in the areas of alveolar hemorrhage and may progress to bronchopneumonia.

Not all pulmonary hemorrhage after explosions is due to air blast. Sometimes the lungs are bruised by direct blows on the chest by bomb fragments and debris. Frequently, a lobe or lung may be fairly uniformly mottled with hemorrhagic areas about 1 cm in diameter from aspiration of blood down the trachea. Other hemorrhagic areas, usually larger, in which the tissues appear rather blurred to the naked eye and poorly defined under the microscope, frequently arise from aspiration of stomach contents. This can occur after death. In fact, when one considers that blast injury is only likely at distances from a moderate explosion at which chest injury from flying missiles is very likely, it must be uncommon for pulmonary hemorrhage to be caused by blast alone.

Gastrointestinal Tract

Compared with the lung damage, gastrointestinal tract injury is very inconstant. When it occurs it usually takes the form of hemorrhages beneath the peritoneum of the gut and into the mesentery and omentum. These hemorrhages can vary in size from small punctate spots to quite extensive areas, although the majority are perhaps 1 cm across. On the intestine they often extend circumferentially as annular bands. They tend to occur mainly on the cecum and colon, the small intestine and stomach being less frequently affected. Unlike the pulmonary hemorrhages, there is no close correlation between the abdominal hemorrhages and the peak pressure or impulse of the blast wave although the injury in both regions is regarded as due to the impact of the wave on the body wall. Occasionally the gut ruptures, and this is most likely in an air-filled segment; in rabbits, for instance, the large and air-filled cecum is vulnerable.

Other Organs

Other injuries from air blast are uncommon, although a review of the many reports reveals occasional damage to most organs. Hemorrhage on the surface of an organ such as the liver, spleen, or kidney or within its substance is found once in a while; more rarely a laceration is found. No specific changes have been detected in the brain, but Zuckerman has described extradural hemorrhages around the nerve roots of the thoracic spine, sometimes continuous with hemorrhage along the intercostal nerves, hemorrhage in the posterior columns of the spinal cord, and edema around the central canal.[4]

Clinical Effects of Air Blast

It is understandable that attention has been directed principally to tissue damage as a result of blast, but our present-day knowledge of this does not explain all the clinical signs and symptoms. Experiments with animals have shown that, when the explosion occurs, various reflex mechanisms slow the heart and it may soon stop beating altogether and remain so permanently. The breathing often ceases at the moment of the explosion, but after a period of apnea lasting up to two minutes, the respirations recommence in a slow, irregular, jerky fashion and then, because of vagal reflexes initiated in the damaged lungs, become regular and rapid for up to 24 hours. The animals are never concussed, but they are frequently sluggish as if dazed and have a low blood pressure. Human victims of explosions are frequently profoundly shocked, pale, cyanotic, and restless. The blood pressure is low, the pulse fast and thready, and there is dyspnea, perhaps with pain in the chest, widespread rales, and hemoptysis. As in animals, a dazed lethargy or apathy sometimes overtakes them. These are the effects of organic blast (or shell) concussion, which should not be confused with the psychogenic war neurosis called blast (or shell) shock that is characterized by anxiety symptoms, confusion, muscular and mental weakness, stammering and jerking, hysterical blindness, dumbness, and paralysis.

Death within an hour of the explosion may be due to many different factors. When pulmonary hemorrhages are extensive or give rise to a copious bloody froth in the air passages, the victim may suffocate. Pulmonary edema has also been incriminated, but it is more likely that this arises as a result of a fatal circulatory failure. Such profound circulatory changes may result from obstruction of the respiratory passages or the pulmonary circulation or from lethal reflexes initiated in the vagus nerves or the pressoreceptors of the pulmonary artery. Another factor that operates in some deaths is systemic air embolism, a result of air gaining the pulmonary veins after blast damage to the lungs. Air has been found in lethal quantities in the arteries of animals that have been killed by explosions; it has been found especially in the coronary arteries, the left chambers of the heart, and the basal arteries of the brain.[16] Air embolism might account for those deaths that occur soon after the explosion in which the more obvious pathologic changes are not sufficient to account for the fatal outcome. In other cases blast "shock" must be implicated, but as yet we know little about it.

IMMERSION BLAST

This refers to the blast effects of an explosion in water as is often experienced in wartime by those who abandon a sinking ship. The ship might be a member of a convoy and the explosion due to torpedoes or bombs directed at other vessels or to depth charges dropped by escort ships. Alternatively, if the sinking ship is a warship, the explosion might be of one of its own depth charges already primed to explode at a certain depth. Injury can be expected within 150 ft of a 300-lb charge of TNT exploding at a depth of 50 ft.

The physical changes brought about by the explosion are essentially similar to those accompanying an explosion in air, but there are a few notable differences. The explosion converts the charge into gas of a very high temperature and pressure, which expands, pushing the surrounding water radially. As it does so, a shock wave, the initial pulse, extends outward from the expanding gas bubble. The gas bubble itself expands to a point at which the pressure within it becomes less than the hydrostatic pressure of the water. Then the enveloping water reverses the process and recompresses the gas. When the gas bubble reaches a minimum size, a second shock wave called the first bubble pulse is emitted.

The form of the initial pressure pulse or shock wave is similar to that in air; it rises to its maximum pressure almost instantaneously and then decays over a period of a few milliseconds. Near the seat of the explosion, where the water pressure is high, the shock wave travels radially at high speed, but beyond this immediate area its velocity falls to near the velocity of sound in water, about 5,000 fps. As the shock wave travels outward, its width, perhaps 15 ft, widens as it does in air because the high-pressure face travels faster than the low-pressure tail. Also the peak pressure decreases as the shock wave gets farther away from the seat of the explosion; its decay is not linear like small-amplitude sound waves, but more exponential in form.

If the water is relatively shallow, the shock wave is reflected by the sea bed and a person floating at the surface experiences both the direct and reflected pulses separated by a short interval of time (Fig. 14–12). When a shock wave reaches the water surface it can produce very interesting changes.[17] A relatively small shock wave is reflected as a tension wave, which has the effect of cutting short the pressure pulse experienced just below the water surface and converting it into a pulse of tension (Fig. 14–13). With higher pulse pressures the water surface breaks and the top layer is thrown into the air as a "dome" of spray. This happens because water can only withstand a sustained tension of about 100 psi, and when the direct pressure pulse and the reflected pulse added together exceed this value, the pressure breaks out into the air and is dissipated. This would happen, for instance, if a 300-lb charge of TNT exploded at a depth of 100 ft, when the peak pressure experienced at the surface could be of the order of 1,000 psi. The sudden dissipation of pressure as the spray dome is formed produces pressure changes just under the water surface similar to those shown in Figure 14–14. The spray dome is due entirely to the shock wave; it is not caused by the expanding gas bubble. This bursts through the surface much later, throwing the water upward as a "plume," but this contributes little to the damage that has already been done by the shock wave.

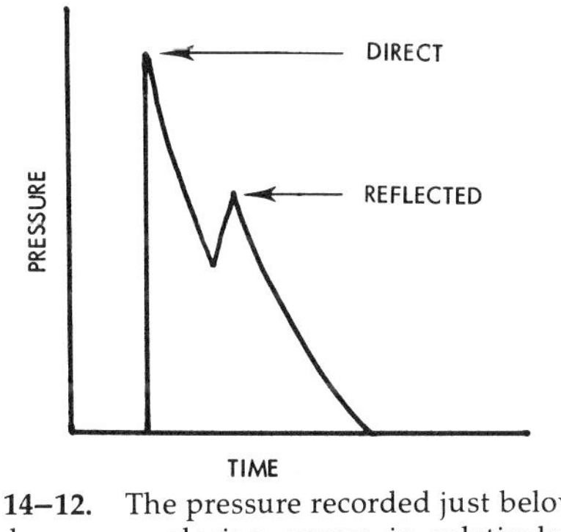

Figure 14–12. The pressure recorded just below the sea surface when an explosion occurs in relatively shallow water. The shock wave produces a steep rise in pressure, and its decay is interrupted by a second pressure pulse reflected from the sea bed.

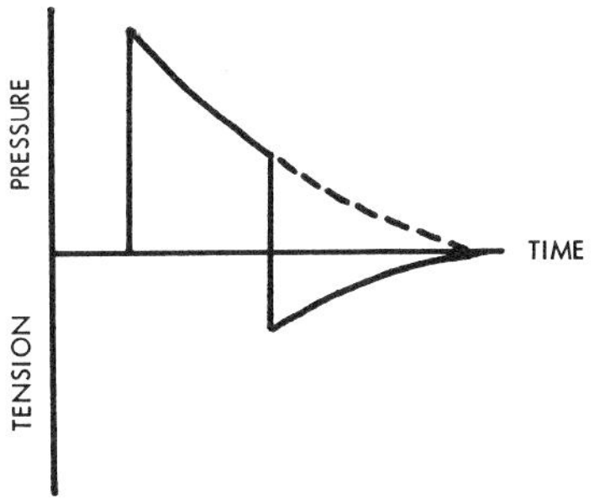

Figure 14–13. The pressure recorded just below the sea surface when a small explosion occurs in deep water. The relatively small shock wave, reflected at the sea surface as a tension wave, neutralizes the decaying pressure pulse and converts its last part into a pulse of tension.

The pressure of underwater explosion experienced by those floating in the water might well be 1,000 psi. When the pressure wave reaches the body, which is largely water, it will pass through the solid tissues unimpeded and do little damage. In an air-containing viscus, however, its transition from the wall to the cavity causes disruption at the interface, and the injuries are therefore found to be predominantly in the gastrointestinal tract and less constantly in the lungs. This predilection of sites is the reverse of that found in air blast, and there is also evidence to suggest that most of the lung injury, when it occurs, is due to pressure transmitted from the abdomen through the diaphragm.

When survivors recount the effects of the blast wave in water they describe a sudden tight constriction of the trunk or a kick in the ab-

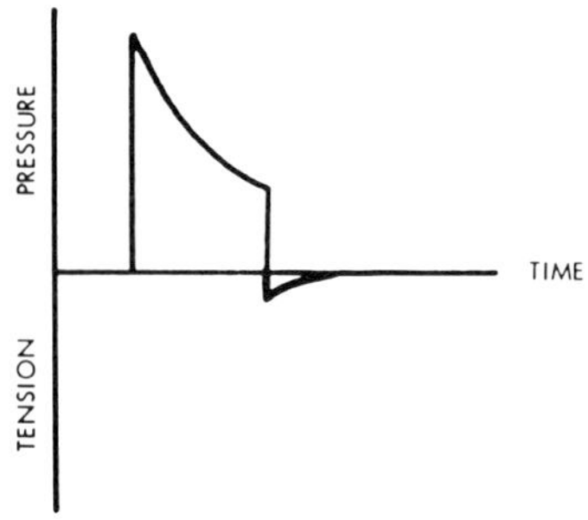

Figure 14–14. The pressure recorded just below the sea surface when a large explosion occurs in deep water. The shock wave breaks through the water surface, producing a dome of spray, and the pressure pulse is suddenly dissipated.

domen or back, followed at once by abdominal pain that in its milder forms lasts only a few minutes and causes only momentary cessation of swimming. In more serious cases, however, the victim's legs are paralyzed and he floats listlessly in the water. Yet even these people often recover movement to a large extent within half an hour. When rescued, most of the victims are shocked. The abdominal pain frequently returns, and testicular pain is an occasional complaint. Some then develop nausea, vomiting (sometimes with blood), and diarrhea (sometimes with blood). Symptoms referable to the respiratory tract are relatively mild, although some blood-stained sputum may be coughed up.

Examination reveals no external marks on the trunk. There is a variable amount of abdominal tenderness and rigidity, and the problem is to identify those with perforations. These patients, who require operation, are the ones who remain shocked and have persistent abdominal tenderness and rigidity and an increased pulse rate.

At operation or necropsy there are two principal findings: hemorrhages and perforations.

Hemorrhages occur beneath the peritoneum of the abdominal wall, in the intestinal mesentery, beneath the serous coat of the gastrointestinal tract, and beneath the mucosa of the intestines. They are multiple and can be widespread, the majority being up to 3 cm in diameter. The wall of the intestine is also frequently edematous. The submucosal hemorrhages account for the blood found in the lumen of the gut and for the hematemesis and melena that sometimes occur. It has been argued that subsequent bacterial invasion of a hemorrhagic area of gut wall might account for the cases of peritonitis and subphrenic and pelvic abscess that occur occasionally after an operation has revealed no perforation, but it is more likely that in these cases a minute perforation has been overlooked.

Perforations have been found in the small and large intestine. They are usually circular, 1/2 to 1 inch in diameter, with a prolapsed mucous membrane. There can be as many as 20 at times. They can occur anywhere, but the antimesenteric border of the ileum and the outer side of the cecum are said to be sites of predilection. Gas-filled segments of the bowel are particularly vulnerable, especially to pressures over 250 psi.

Other findings are less common. Injury to solid organs such as the liver can be said to be rare unless the victim is within a few yards of the explosion, when he is usually killed outright. Lung injury is more common, and in experiments with animals pulmonary hemorrhage with blood-stained fluid in the air passages and alveolar and interstitial emphysema have been reported.[18] There can be varying degrees of air embolism, which may be a significant factor in those who die soon after the explosion.[19] Pulmonary hemorrhage can occur even when the thorax is not immersed or is protected by an air-inflated life jacket. It is in the basal parts of the lungs, and it seems to be due to force transmitted through the diaphragm when the blast wave forces the abdominal organs violently against it rather than to the force of the blast wave acting directly on the chest wall.

SOLID BLAST

This refers to the wave of energy that spreads through a rigid structure when an explosion is detonated near it. People in contact with the structure can be injured. Wood conducts the shock wave poorly, but the steel construction of tanks and warships conducts it extremely well and, while protecting personnel from bullets and shell fragments, causes solid blast injury.

An explosion beneath a tank or ship causes an initial movement of small displacement but very swift acceleration. A person standing on the deck of a ship, for instance, could experience a blow as if the soles of his feet had been struck by a steam hammer. Bones break and the skin and subcutaneous tissues burst, producing compound fractures. These are solid blast injuries. Following on this shock wave, there may be flexion and oscillation of the entire ship's structure. These movements are of considerable magnitude and can throw a person a great distance. He can then sustain serious injuries, but these are secondary and should not be confused with thc injuries specific to solid blast.

Solid blast injuries are very different in character from those caused by air blast or immersion blast.[20] They are predominantly skeletal and their situation depends on the position of the subject at the time. The person who is standing sustains injuries to the lower limbs mainly, while the one seated in a chair avoids serious injury to the legs but sustains fracture of the vertebral column. Lying on the deck would probably be the most dangerous position. Those lying in their bunks seem to suffer least injury.

Most commonly the calcaneus, the astragalus, and the lower ends of the tibia and fibula are fractured. In half the cases the fractures are multiple, comminuted, and compound. The skin of the ankles and feet is bruised, and lacerations, sometimes with fractured bone projecting through them, are found chiefly around the ankle and on the weight-bearing surface of the heel. The shafts of the tibia and fibula may break, but more frequently the fractures are found in the tibial condyles and they involve the knee joint. The knee is often dislocated, with or without a fracture, and often when this happens the popliteal vessels are torn or thrombosed so that amputation becomes necessary. Fractures of the femur and pelvis are less common, but the spine is vulnerable and fractures here, usually between the ninth dorsal and fourth lumbar vertebrae, are sometimes associated with partial or complete paraplegia. When other fractures occur they are usually found to be secondary to the body being thrown against other structures. An interesting delayed injury is aseptic necrosis of the articular surfaces of the joints of the lower limbs, which arises as a result of damage to the cartilage—laceration and partial detachment from the subjacent bone—by the solid blast impact. Partial or complete ankylosis of the joint may be the result.

Many of these victims lose consciousness at the time of the explosion. This is often the result of a secondary head injury, but in some cases it appears to be caused by a primary blast injury and it must then be attributed to cerebral concussion as a result of a blow transmitted up the spine. Other persons are just dazed. Most of those injured are profoundly shocked.

FLYING MISSILES

Blast is the primary effect of an explosion, but it becomes important only when explosive devices reach a considerable size. Even then, the victim of pure blast has to be relatively near the center of the explosion.

It has always been much more common for explosions to injure and kill in a secondary way by means of the solid material they propel in all directions. This material is frequently the fragmented container of the explosive; it may be the metallic casing of a shell or, in a terrorist situation, a car filled with explosive. On the other hand, the explosion may be meant to propel missiles as in the hand grenade, the casing of which is specially designed to fragment into lethal shrapnel, and the nail bomb in which many large nails are bound round a stick of gelignite. Other kinds of solid material propelled by the explosion consist of the remains of the explosive mixture itself and debris from the surroundings—e.g., earth, brick, plaster, wood—varying from reasonably large fragments to dust. In general, the larger the fragment the deeper it will penetrate the body and the more lethal it is likely to be.

Explosion missiles follow the general rules of ballistics, their impact energy being a function of their mass and the square of their velocity. Because they are accelerated more slowly than

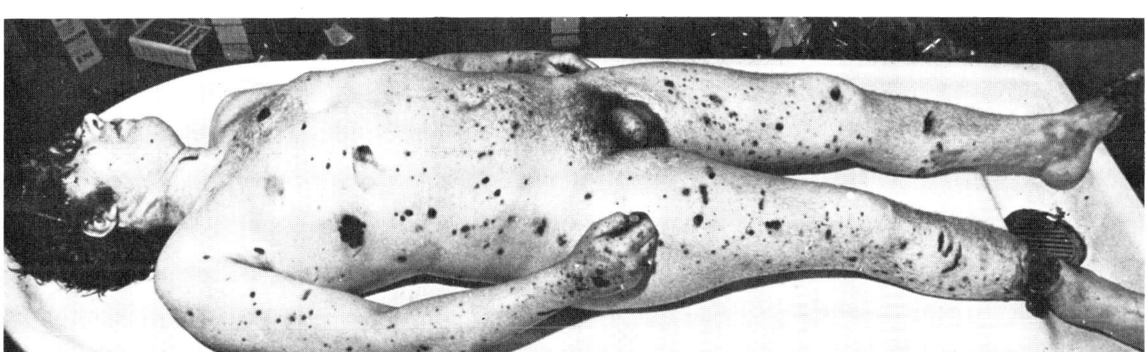

Figure 14–15. The victim of a terrorist bomb explosion. Note the peppering of the body with small bruises, abrasions, and puncture lacerations, a characteristic triad.

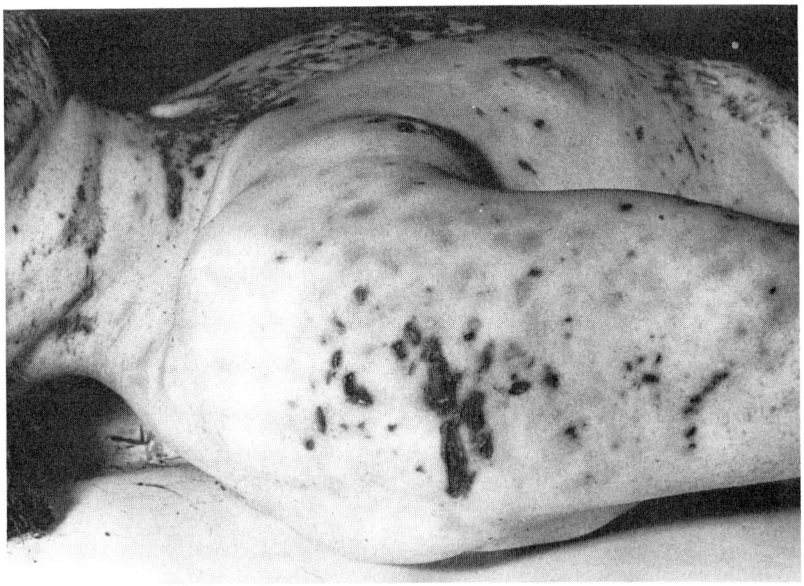

Figure 14–16. The victim of a terrorist bomb explosion. The injuries are mainly small bruises and abrasions.

the associated gases, they lag behind the blast in the early stages of the explosion. Because of their momentum, however, they tend to be more damaging at a distance.

The common basic injury due to fragments propelled by an explosion is a triad of small lesions—bruises, abrasions, and puncture lacerations—which are intimately mixed on the skin and can, when close together, give it a purplish color (Fig. 14–15). The bruises and abrasions are quite small, generally 1 to 10 mm in diameter, and the puncture lacerations, usually surrounded by an irregular zone of bruising and abrasion, are up to 3 cm in diameter. The conjunction of these injuries produces an appearance that is diagnostic (Figs. 14–16, 14–17, and 14–18). Some of the puncture lacerations contain obvious fragments of metal, clothing fibers, or debris, but in most the fragment that caused the injury can only be detected by x-ray. Then it is surprising how minute the fragment is—often too small to be recovered by dissection even though the puncture laceration and surrounding bruised abrasion are perhaps 1 cm across. The reason, of course, is that the size of the wound is a function of the energy surrendered to the tissue by the penetrating fragment, and since its energy varies with the square of its velocity, minute fragments traveling at very high speeds cause relatively large wounds.

Superimposed on this triad of small lesions there may be larger lacerations due to the penetration of fragments of greater size (Fig.

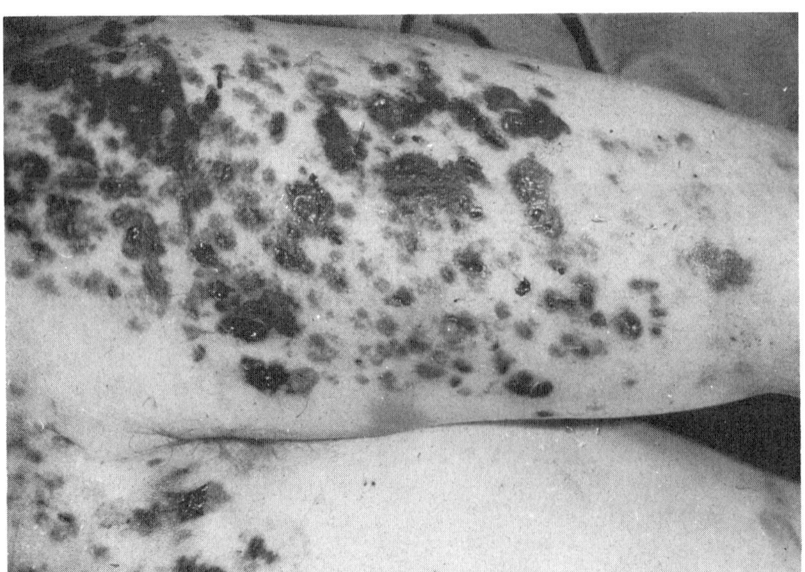

Figure 14–17. The victim of a terrorist bomb explosion. The injuries consist of small bruises, abrasions, and puncture lacerations, the characteristic triad.

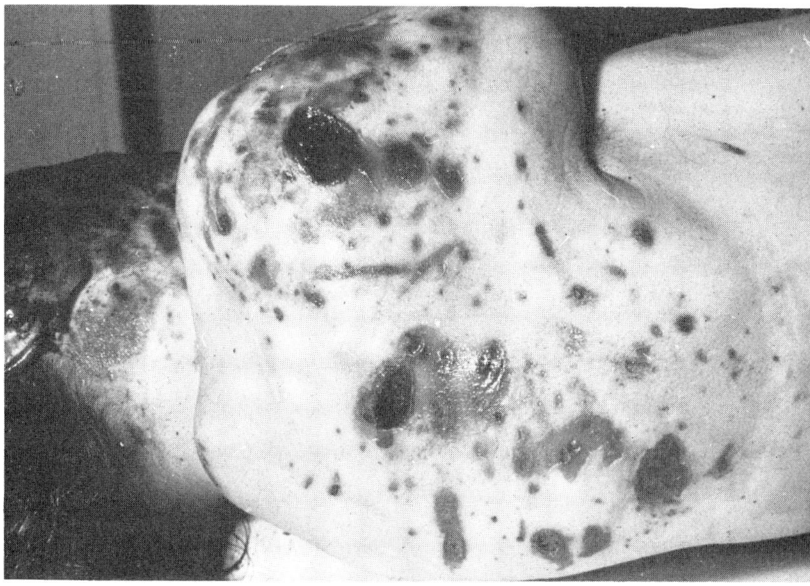

Figure 14–18. The victim of a terrorist bomb explosion. There are small bruises and abrasions, but the puncture lacerations are more notable.

14–19). Some large fragments can travel a long way and can penetrate a victim some considerable distance from the explosion. They are to be reckoned with because they can perforate the neck, damaging the carotid arteries or the airway; they can perforate the chest and abdomen, where their dirty state will compound any physical injury to the viscera; or they can penetrate a limb and sever a major blood vessel. When the person dies it is usually obvious that the injuries were the cause, but there are some deaths in which the injuries are not so serious and one must surmise that an element of explosion shock played an important contributory role.

Of less importance from a clinical viewpoint is the dust that is propelled by the explosion. When there is a lot of it, it can be driven into the skin to cause a fairly uniform tattooing. The skin is darkened, and this provides a background for the triad of small bruises, abrasions, and puncture lacerations. Whereas these lesions can occur beneath clothing, the fragments that cause them having sufficient momentum to perforate clothing, the dust tattooing is only seen on exposed skin (Fig. 14–20). It stops abruptly at the shirt collar, the rolled-up shirt sleeves, or the jacket sleeves at the wrists.

The force of an explosion is difficult to comprehend by those who have no firsthand experience of explosive substances. For instance, people find it hard to appreciate the serious injury that can result from a letter bomb. It is just as hard to imagine the penetrating force of a small explosion fragment. A small piece of metal can penetrate bone quite cleanly, as it did when a piece of light alloy 4 cm long with a triangular cross section (the sides being about 7 mm long) was blown off a motor car and was found deep within the brain of a 16-year-old boy. It had struck the skull end-on and had traversed 3 mm of skull bone, leaving only a

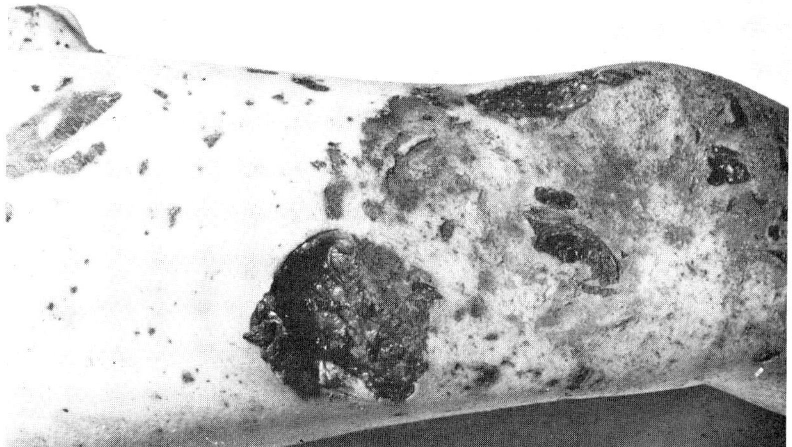

Figure 14–19. The victim of a terrorist bomb explosion. The limb bears a large ragged puncture laceration, and the perforating fragment severed an artery. Note the particles of dirt driven into the skin.

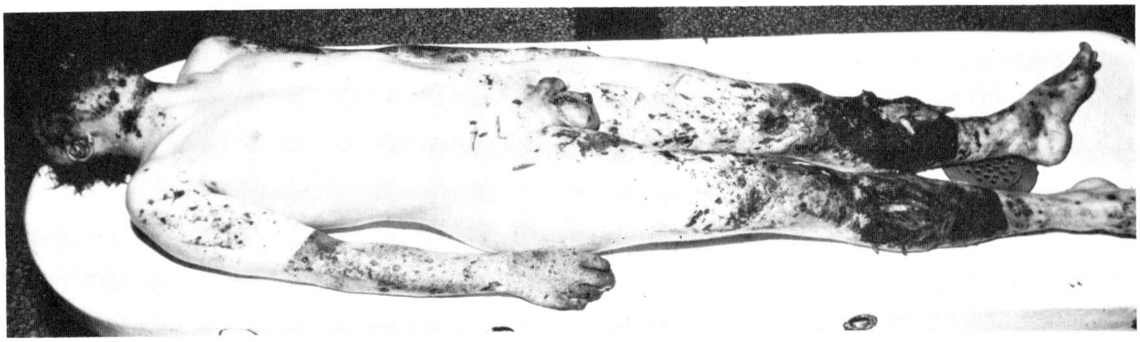

Figure 14–20. The victim of a terrorist bomb explosion. Note the dust tattooing of the right elbow, forearm, and hand, its upper limit at the level of the rolled-up shirt sleeve.

small hole (Fig. 14–21). In another death, a nail from a nail bomb had obviously penetrated the skull without difficulty (Fig. 14–22). Even fragments of minute size can penetrate the soft tissues of the body quite deeply, their momentum being obtained not from their mass but from their velocity. These minute fragments are not often of significance because the victim has usually been injured simultaneously by fragments of larger size. Occasionally, however, the internal injury due to a minute fragment is the important one. Then the surgeon can be in difficulty; the fragment and its track are too small to trace and yet it may have perforated an important structure. In one victim, a minute fragment penetrated the left flank and traveled to the right through the abdomen to perforate the bile duct. The injury was not detected by the surgeon, and the patient died later from biliary peritonitis.

The distribution and pattern of the bruises, abrasions, and puncture lacerations may help to determine the relationship of the victim to the explosion. At times of civil disturbance this is often important. When a bomb goes off prematurely, perhaps while being manufactured or loaded into a vehicle, it may be alleged by relatives of the victim that he was an innocent passer-by. When a bomb goes off while being transported, it may be said that the victim, known by the police to have been a passenger in the car, was an innocent pedestrian. When a bomb goes off prematurely in a bar, some of the injured or dead may be those who were carrying or handing over the bomb, while others are innocent victims; the distinction is important. When army personnel are killed by an explosive laid as a terrorist trap, it is often important to know how the soldiers were positioned at the time.

These questions may be answered by comparing the injuries of the victims, particularly their severity, distribution, and pattern. Those carrying a bomb are disintegrated or have the arms and midtrunk blown away. A terrorist

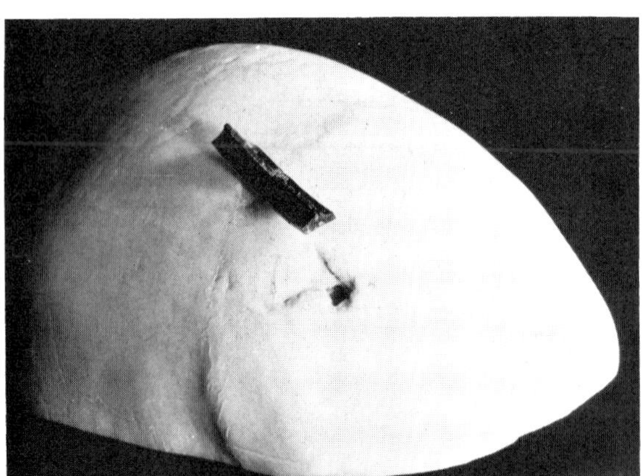

Figure 14–21. A small piece of alloy from a motor car and the hole it made as it entered the skull of a 16-year-old boy when a terrorist car bomb exploded near him. The metal fragment was found deep within the brain.

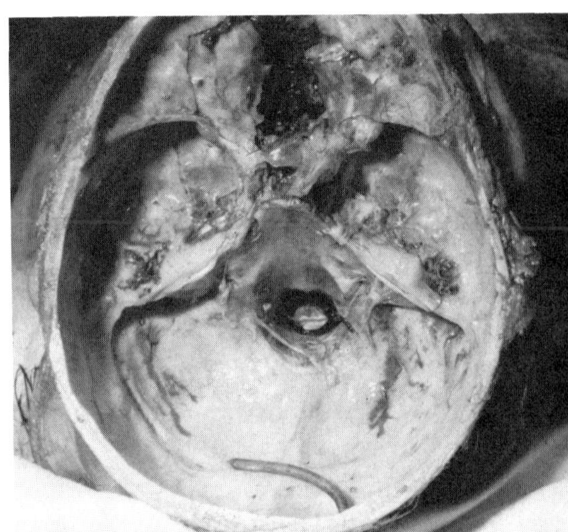

Figure 14–22. A nail from a terrorist nail bomb driven into the skull of an adult when the bomb exploded near him.

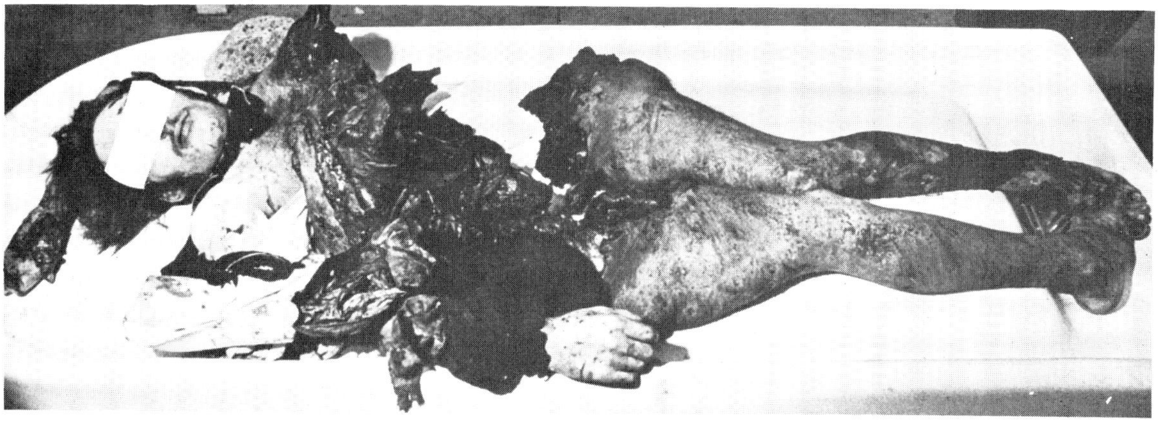

Figure 14–23. Midtrunk injuries sustained when a parcel bomb exploded in the victim's lap.

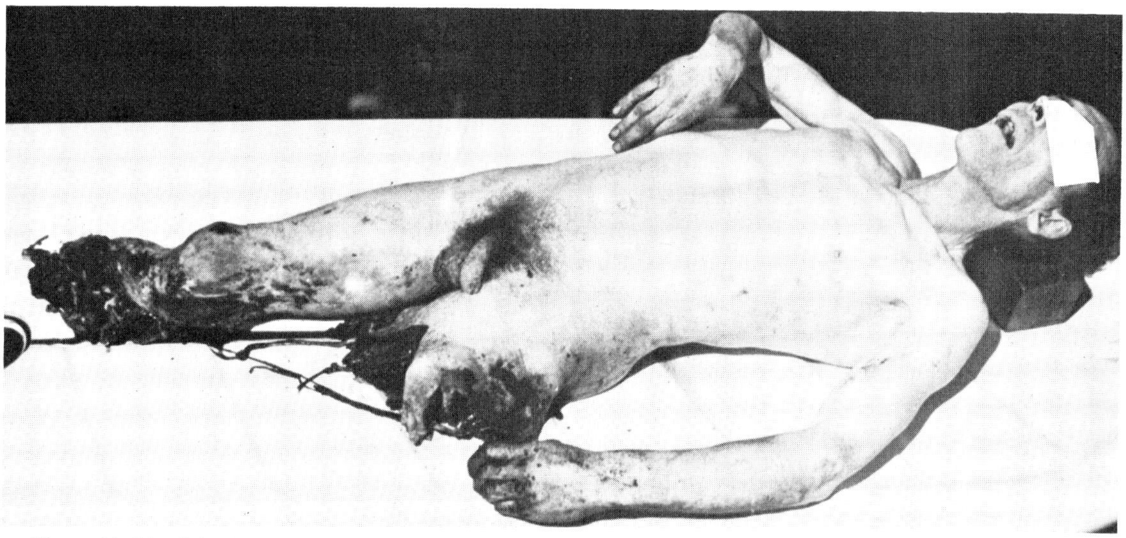

Figure 14–24. Injuries practically confined to the lower limbs due to an explosion near the victim at ground level.

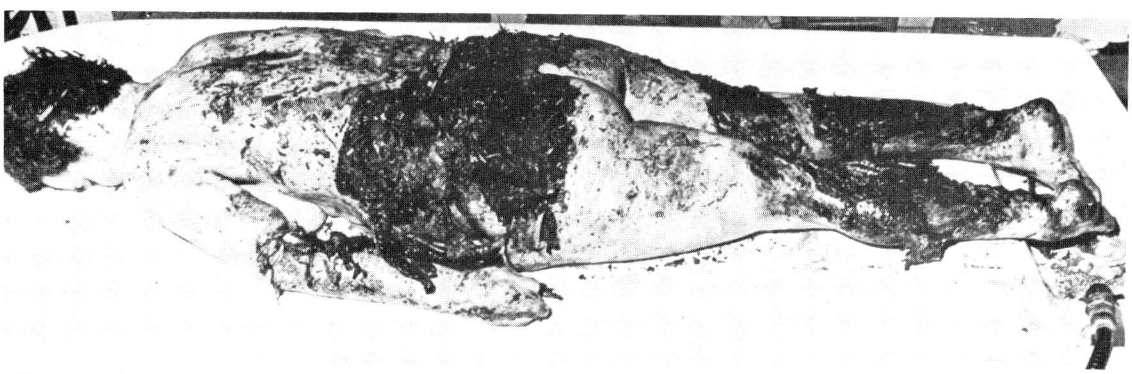

Figure 14–25. Injuries principally on the back after a bomb exploded behind the victim as she was seated in a bar.

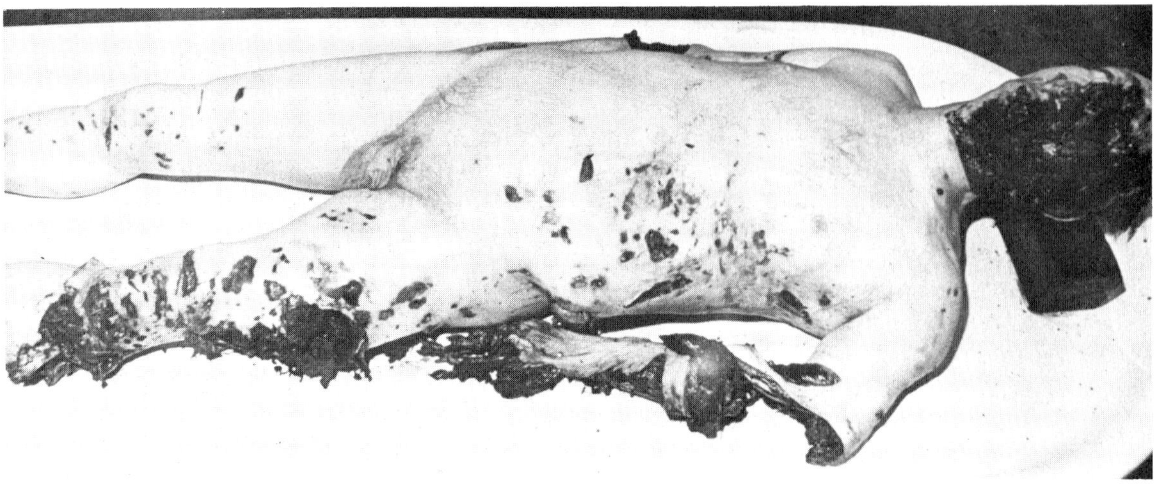

Figure 14–26. Explosion injuries so distributed that there can be no doubt that the victim had his left side facing the blast.

carrying a bomb on his lap in a car has injuries centered on the pelvis (Fig. 14–23). An explosion at ground level injures the legs of those nearby more than other parts of the body (Fig. 14–24). An explosion behind a person injures the back more than the front, and one at the side injures that side more than the other (Figs. 14–25 and 14–26). Sometimes the abrasions and lacerations are linear in type, radiating from the source of the explosion (Fig. 14–27). An intelligent assessment of this kind is often invaluable in the investigation. A word of warning is needed, however; unless the significance of the features is really obvious, this kind of evidence should be used with care in court because unusual things can happen in explosions and a pattern of injuries sometimes proves misleading.

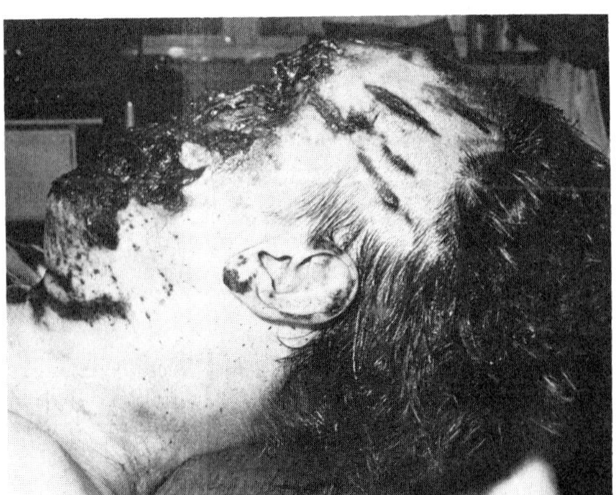

Figure 14–27. This victim of a terrorist parcel-bomb explosion was examining the parcel when it blew up. Note the linear injuries radiating from a point in front of his face.

Eye Injuries

When fragments and debris impelled by an explosion strike the head they frequently injure the eyes. Isolated injuries of the eye are less common; there are usually associated injuries elsewhere, and when these other injuries on the body are not rapidly fatal they are often of a severity to take precedence over the eye injuries in treatment.

The bulb is frequently ruptured, the penetration of particles of metal, glass, wood, and other debris causing ragged wounds of the cornea and sclera. These pose a problem in treatment; many of the foreign bodies are nonmagnetic, and intraocular hemorrhage and cataract usually make their removal under direct vision impossible.

FALLING MASONRY

A person removed from a building demolished by an explosion is likely to have sustained multiple injuries caused by the collapsing masonry; on many occasions these injuries are the only effects of the explosion on the body. The body and its clothing are soiled by dust from brick, cement, or plaster, and the extent and nature of the injuries are only revealed when the clothing has been removed and the body thoroughly washed (Fig. 14–28). Then the injuries are often found to be sufficient to account for death. There are occasions, however, when there are no injuries to vital structures and death is due to crush asphyxia. Usually signs of crush asphyxia are quite clear—purple discoloration of the upper parts of the body with petechial hemorrhages

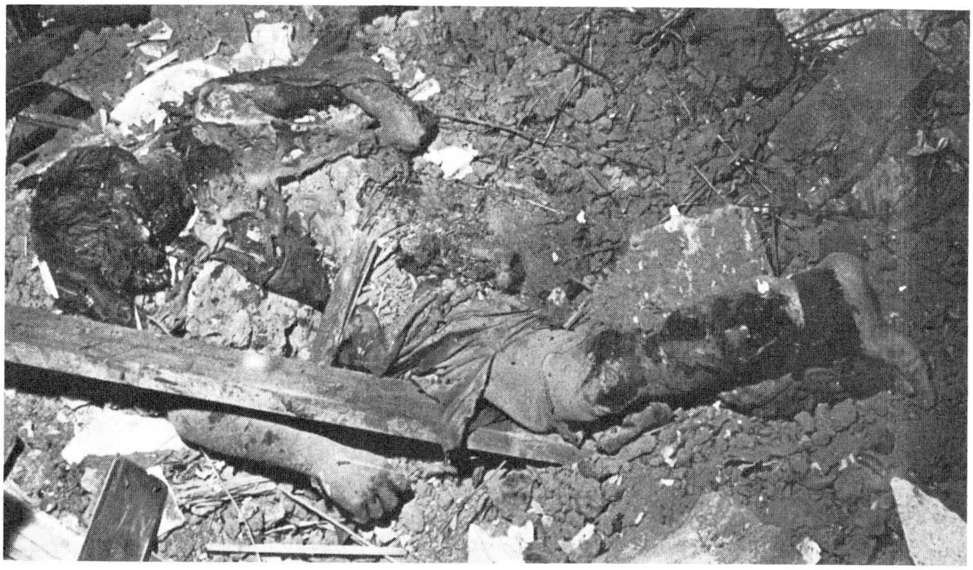

Figure 14–28. The victim of a terrorist bomb. Note the soiling of the body. In these circumstances, death is likely to have been caused by falling masonry.

in the skin and the conjunctivae, edema of the conjunctivae, and perhaps some congestive hemorrhage from the nose or ears. There are other times, however, when these classic features of crush asphyxia are absent but death from crushing can still be inferred either from the account of how the person was lying in the rubble or from injuries on the skin of the trunk that indicate the pressure of, say, a beam. When there are neither multiple injuries nor evidence of crush asphyxia, consideration must be given to the blast effects of the explosion and shock.

POISONING BY FUMES

Toxic fumes are evolved in any explosion, but it is only in an enclosed space that they become harmful. Thus there is danger in wartime when an aerial bomb penetrates an underground shelter or when someone is trapped by debris in a pocket of fumes. Terrorist bombs are not large enough or used in situations in which the explosion fumes are likely to do serious harm, but there is always the danger that damage is done to a domestic gas supply and that people immobilized by the explosion are poisoned before being extricated. The greatest danger from fumes after explosions, however, is in mining accidents when the afterdamp, as the gaseous products of the explosion are called, often proves lethal to those lying injured and also to the rescuers. Thus, in the Darran colliery explosion in 1909 in which 22 miners and 5 rescuers died, all but one of the victims was thought to have been killed by inhaling afterdamp.[21] It is generally agreed that over 80 per cent of deaths in mining disasters occur from the inhalation of fumes.

Afterdamp consists of a mixture of gases—carbon monoxide and dioxide and hydrogen sulfide—with a deficiency of oxygen. The principal constituent is carbon monoxide, and thus the fumes are not dissimilar to those produced by an explosive. Exposure to a carbon monoxide concentration of 1 to 10 per cent causes death within a few minutes; hence the danger of the fumes can be readily appreciated. When the bodies of these victims are recovered, the faces retain a normal skin color, and when the postmortem lividity develops, it is a uniform pink color, even in the most intensely stained colors. Examination of a drop of blood with a reversion spectroscope will confirm the diagnosis in a few minutes.

EXPLOSIONS OF SPECIAL TYPE

The damaging effects of explosions in general have been analyzed, but as was mentioned at the outset, not all these effects operate at any one time; much depends on the distance from the explosion center, the medium in which the explosion occurs, and whether debris is flung about or buildings toppled. Quite apart from these factors, some explosions have specific peculiarities and they deserve brief mention.

Coal Mine Explosions

There is always danger of an explosion in a coal mine. Gas can seep into the workings and is easily ignited. For this reason miners are not allowed to take matches down the pit and they use safety lamps in which the flame is specially screened so as not to be a danger. Nevertheless, explosions occasionally occur, perhaps because a lamp is defective or because a spark is generated from some electrical gear. The flame or spark ignites the gas locally in the atmosphere, and the flame then spreads along the workings with extreme rapidity by igniting the very fine coal dust in the atmosphere and on the walls and timbers. An area perhaps a mile square can be affected practically simultaneously by the momentary fire.

Some miners die at once from the blast without any external signs. Some die from injuries sustained when they are hurled by the blast or buried under roof falls. Some die from the effects of the momentary fire, having sustained burns; since the flame travels nearer the roof than the floor, the upper half of the bodies is burned more than the lower half. Most, however, die from the inhalation of the postexplosion fumes called afterdamp, the principal poisonous constituent being carbon monoxide. Many victims have first been immobilized by blast, injuries, or burns.

In a mine explosion with many dead there are difficulties in examining the bodies; it may not be safe to enter some of the workings, which may have to be sealed off, or there may be a delay of days or weeks in recovering the bodies, during which time decomposition takes place. This interferes with the pathologist's assessment, but fortunately, even after some weeks, it is still possible to diagnose carbon monoxide poisoning with sufficient accuracy.

Domestic Gas Explosions

The commonest form of domestic explosion is that due to leaks in the gas supply. The prerequisites for such an accident are an explosive proportion of gas and air together with a source of ignition. Manufactured gas, or town gas, varies somewhat in its composition, but an explosion is possible whenever its proportion in the atmosphere lies between 4 per cent and 40 per cent, with optimal chance at about 25 per cent. Natural gas, which is practically all methane, explodes at concentrations in air between 5 and 15 per cent. Ignition is often caused by matches or candles, fires, pilot lights, and sparking electric switches; natural gas requires a slightly hotter spark than town gas.

The gas and air mixture may fill only one room or it may overflow into others. In either event, the mixture varies from place to place, and an explosion occurs when the mixture at the ignition source reaches optimal proportions. Its explosion is accompanied by a momentary flame that can set furnishings alight and melt lampshades (Fig. 14–29). The air pressure could theoretically rise to 100 psi, but it is very much lower in practice, perhaps less than 10 psi, owing to venting through broken windows and doors. The peak pressure depends to a large extent on the burning velocity of the gas, and since natural gas has a burning

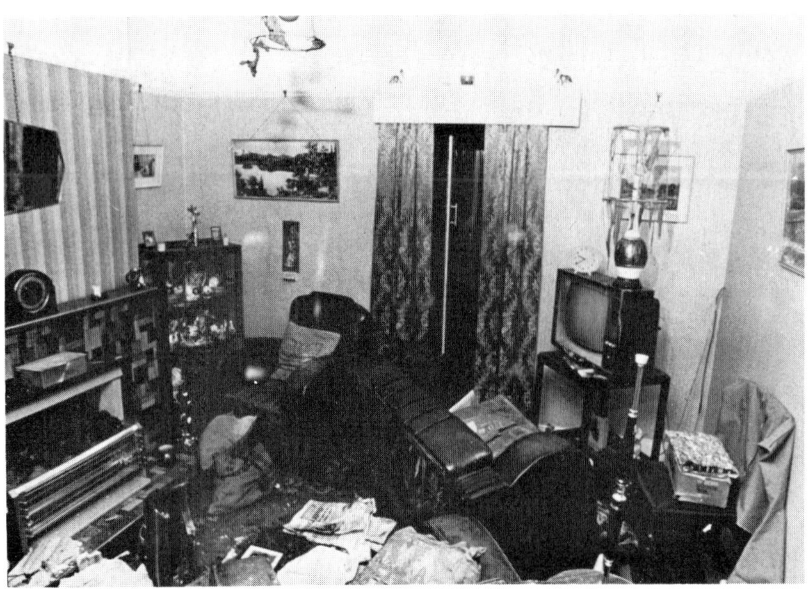

Figure 14–29. A room of a dwelling house after a domestic gas explosion. Note the overturned settee and the melted lampshades. A man and woman were found dead in the room, but neither bore any significant burns. A high level of carboxyhemoglobin in each person indicated that they had succumbed to the inhalation of gas before the explosion.

velocity only one third that of town gas, it produces much lower pressures.

Experience has shown that people involved in these explosions are rarely killed by the explosion itself. They can be thrown off their feet and injured. The momentary flame, of longer duration than that produced by a solid explosive, can singe hair and produce localized superficial scorching, but it has not the temperature to do more in the short time. Most danger arises when the building collapses and the victim is buried in the rubble. There are occasions when, a person having been found dead in a room after an explosion but having sustained little injury, spectroscopic examination of the blood reveals a fatal level of carboxyhemoglobin. A careful assessment of events then usually indicates that death occurred from carbon monoxide poisoning due to the accidental inhalation of town gas before the explosion occurred.

Nuclear Explosions

The effects of a nuclear bomb explosion have been described in detail by Glasstone.[22] Only a few important features are mentioned here. The fission of about 100 lb of uranium liberates energy equal to that of a million tons (one megaton) of TNT. Within a few millionths of a second of such a bomb's exploding in the air, the gases, as hot as the sun and at a pressure of millions of pounds per square inch, expand as a luminous ball of fire that to an observer 60 mi away would appear about 30 times as bright as the sun at noon. The flash can cause blindness for an hour or two, and a person looking at the fireball can sustain a retinal burn that leaves a small permanent blind spot. The fireball contains the radioactive fission products and the bomb materials in the form of vapor, and if it touches the earth's surface, it has been estimated, more than 20,000 tons of vaporized soil or 100,000 tons of water could be added to it. As the fireball grows rapidly in size, a shock wave extends radially in front of it and is about 3 mi ahead by the time the fireball reaches its maximum diameter of some 7,200 ft after 10 sec. The fireball is then rising at about 300 mph. After about a minute, at a height of 4½ mi, the fireball has cooled sufficiently to become invisible. During this time it has emitted what is known as the "initial nuclear radiation" consisting of neutrons, gamma rays, and alpha and beta particles, but only the neutrons and gamma rays extend a significant distance. As the fireball fades, it is replaced by condensing vapors that form a "mushroom" cloud of solid particles and water droplets. This hot cloud continues to ascend and draws air inward and upward rather like the draught up a chimney, producing strong "afterwinds" of 200 mph or more, which raise dirt and debris from the earth's surface to form the stalk of the mushroom cloud. This cloud persists for about one hour before it is dispersed by winds. The condensation products and debris in the cloud are contaminated with radioactive fission products and when a megaton explosion occurs nearer than 3,000 ft from the earth's surface, giving a large particle content to the mushroom cloud, there is a substantial fallout that, depending on the winds and rain, can contaminate the earth's surface over an area of many thousands of square miles. This starts after several hours and can last many hours.

The nuclear bomb differs from the conventional high-explosive bomb in three ways. First, it is many thousands of times as powerful, and the effects of blast are very prominent. Second, a large proportion of its energy is emitted as thermal radiation, causing skin burns and starting fires at considerable distances. Third, the explosion emits a highly penetrating and harmful radiation, and the substances remaining after the explosion continue to emit radiation over a long period of time.

Most of the material damage caused by a nuclear bomb bursting in the air is due to blast; among survivors, 70 per cent will have injuries of one kind or another. After a 1-megaton air explosion, the pressure front will reach a point 1 mi away in about 4 sec, and the pressure phase here, peaking at about 20 psi, will last about 2 sec. Reflection of the pressure wave by the earth's surface can set up complicated pressure fronts, including the laterally moving Mach front, with pressures much greater than the original incident pressure. The blast wave is of sufficiently long duration to be accompanied by transient blast winds of up to 350 mph, and the pressure and winds cause considerable and widespread damage to buildings, a "mass distortion," and a tremendous amount of debris is flung about. Then come the winds due to the radial displacement of air as the explosion gases expand and finally a wind in the opposite direction as air is sucked back by the rising fireball and mushroom cloud.

Among the survivors of such an explosion, blast injury is essentially the same as that caused by high-explosive bombs, but the greater impulse of the nuclear bomb blast means that more damage will result from lower peak overpressures. The high wind pressure will displace the body more easily, but by far the greater danger is from the collapsing buildings and flying missiles. Owing to the coincident radiation and the disorganization of medical facilities, wounds heal slowly and become infected.

One third of the energy of a nuclear explosion is emitted from the fireball in the form of thermal radiation consisting of ultraviolet, visible, and infrared rays. During its transit through the atmosphere at the speed of light most of the ultraviolet radiation is absorbed or scattered; the other radiations, also attenuated to some extent in this way, lose energy in proportion to the square of the distance from the explosion. Nevertheless, the thermal radiation remains of high intensity, and a 1-megaton explosion could cause fires up to 10 mi away. Thermal radiation of this order easily causes flash burns, mainly on people exposed in the open; about 75 per cent of survivors will have burns, and third-degree flash burns can be expected 8 mi away from a 1-megaton air explosion. Thus flash burns are more common than with conventional high explosives, but more thermal energy is required to produce them since the rate of energy release in a nuclear explosion is relatively slow. Clothing tends to protect the skin; but dark clothing absorbs radiation, heats up, and can char so that in certain circumstances skin can be burned by clothing instead of being protected. Objects that throw shadows across the body also protect the shaded area from thermal radiation and, because the intensity is only momentarily high, a clean shadow-shaped area of normal skin can be encountered in the flash burn area. Some remarkable examples of this were seen after the nuclear explosions in Hiroshima and Nagasaki. Interest in this type of burn should not overshadow the fact that after a nuclear explosion a large area around ground zero will be set alight and most burns sustained by people here will be ordinary flame burns. These victims do not survive, however.

The initial nuclear radiations penetrate a few miles from the explosion center, and fairly thick layers of high-density material are needed to absorb them. At 1 mi from an air burst of 1 megaton, about 1 ft of steel, 4 ft of concrete, or 5 ft of earth would be required to provide a safe shield against the gamma radiation, and of those shielded by less than half of this, 50 per cent would die. Neutron shielding is a more difficult problem, but 4 ft of concrete would provide satisfactory attenuation. The harmful effects of these radiations arise from their ionization of the body cells, which are thus damaged or destroyed; injury depends on both the amount of radiation absorbed and the rate of its absorption. Whether or not it is reparable depends on the particular tissue. The proportion of the body surface irradiated is also important, for 700 R over the whole body will cause death, while if concentrated on one part, it will cause only local damage. The effects of excessive radiation doses are discussed in detail in Chapter 18. Appreciable residual nuclear radiation from fallout is to be expected only with a low air burst or a surface burst, and the radiation from it arises mainly from the bomb residues. Even when spread over hundreds of square miles, these can emit gamma radiation of very high intensity during the first day or two, when most of the harmful dose is received. Some of the radiation is in the form of beta particles, which will cause "beta burns" if material contaminated with these emitters soil the skin. More injury is caused by radioactive contamination of food, water, and air whereby fission products gain the interior of the body. The harmful effects of these radiations, too, are discussed in Chapter 18.

REFERENCES

1. Hatton, W. A.: The Hulton colliery explosion. Br. Med. J., *1*:1164, 1911.
2. Blocker, V., and Blocker, T. G.: The Texas City Disaster. Am. J. Surg., *78*:756, 1949.
3. Williams, E. R. P.: Blast effects in warfare. Br. J. Surg., *30*:38, 1942–3.
4. Zuckerman, S.: Discussion on the problem of blast injuries. Proc. R. Soc. Med., *34*:171, 1941.
5. Bernal, J. D.: The physics of air raids. Nature (Lond.), *147*:594, 1941.
6. Celander, H., Clemedson, C.-J., Ericsson, U. A., and Hultman, H. I.: A study on the relation between the duration of a shock wave and the severity of the blast injury produced by it. Acta Physiol. Scand., *33*:14, 1955.
7. Clemedson, C.-J., and Pettersson, H.: Propagation of a high explosive air shock wave through different parts of an animal body. Am. J. Physiol., *184*:119, 1956.
8. Barcroft, J.: Cited in Blast injuries. Br. Med. J., *1*:89, 1941.
9. Zuckerman, S.: Experimental study of blast injuries to the lungs. Lancet, *2*:219, 1940.
10. Golden, P. M., and Clare, R.: The Hazards to the Human Ear from Shock Waves produced by High Energy Electrical Discharge. Atomic Weapons Research Establishment Report No. El/65, Aldermaston, 1965.
11. Perlman, H. B.: Reaction of the human conduction mechanism to blast. Laryngoscope, 55:427, 1945.
12. Hirsch, F. G.: Effects of overpressure on the ear—a review. Ann. N.Y. Acad. Sci., *152*:147, 1968.
13. Kerr, A. G., and Byrne, J. E. T.: Concussive effects of bomb blast on the ear. J. Laryngol. Otol., *89*:131, 1975.
14. Fraser, J. S., and Fraser, J.: The morbid anatomy of war injuries of the ear. Proc. R. Soc. Med., *10*:56, 1916–7.

15. Hooker, D. R.: Physiological effects of air concussion. Am. J. Physiol., *67*:219, 1924.
16. Clemedson, C.-J., and Hultman, H. I.: Air embolism and the cause of death in blast injury. Milit. Surg., *114*:424, 1954.
17. Wakeley, C. P. G.: Effect of underwater explosions on the human body. Lancet, *1*:715, 1945.
18. Cameron, G. R., Short, R. H. D., and Wakeley, C. P. G.: Pathological changes produced in animals by depth charges. Br. J. Surg., *30*:49, 1942–3.
19. Gouze, F. J., and Hayter, R.: Air embolism in immersion blast. U.S. Nav. Med. Bull., *43*:871, 1944.
20. Barr, J. S., Draeger, R. H., and Sager, W. W.: Solid blast personnel injury: a clinical study. Milit. Surg., *98*:1, 1946.
21. Llewellyn, T. L.: The Darran explosion from the medical standpoint. Br. Med. J., *1*:1399, 1910.
22. Glasstone, S.: The Effects of Nuclear Weapons. Washington, United States Atomic Energy Commission, 1957.

SECTION 3. BAROTRAUMA (DYSBARISM)

chapter 15

INJURIES FROM INCREASED ATMOSPHERIC PRESSURE

by William G. Eckert

The physical effects related to increased pressure are referred to as barotrauma.[1] This occurs most frequently under water, and in order to study this problem one must appreciate that the pressure of an underwater environment is always greater than that of the atmosphere and that the actual pressure levels may fluctuate but they are always higher than the atmospheric pressure. Problems of this type arise when the pressure of the air or gas in a cavity of the body becomes different from that of the surrounding tissues. This failure to maintain equality of pressure between the body and the surroundings may be due to the weakness of the individual himself or to the inadequacy of protection available to him, to his equipment, or to the handling of the equipment by other people. In its simplest basic circumstances, the problem is exemplified in the free dive in which the individual inhales a lungful of air and plunges into the aquatic environment. The limitations of a free diver are dependent on the length of time that the individual can hold his breath. Occupational use of this technique requires a rapid descent to the bottom, as for pearl diving or salvage or treasure recovery. The diver who enters the water with fully expanded lungs, in the absence of any pulmonary disease, has a total lung volume of approximately 6 liters. As he descends into the water the pressure on his chest increases with the increasing depth. The volume of air in the lungs is decreased as the pressure increases. At about 100 ft the total respiratory volume may be reduced to that of the residual volume. As the descent continues, the air in the lungs remains at a constant volume and pressure while the pressure of the pulmonary circulation and tissue wall continues to increase, thus creating a pressure difference. This state will result in pulmonary edema by fluid transfer from the alveolar capillaries into the alveolar spaces, to be followed by vessel rupture and hemorrhage. The chest wall may also be crushed. When divers are equipped with suits, a situation may arise in which air pressure in the lungs is greater than the depth pressure as a result of inflation of the suit; a diver's suit may be "blown up," and rapid-decompression sickness or even rupture of the lungs may result. In the latter, gross distention of the lung follows the relative increase of intrapulmonary pressure that occurs when the lungs are full of air and the air is not released as the surrounding pressures decrease. As the ascent continues, the pressure of the air becomes increasingly higher than that of the tissues. The point is reached at which pulmonary tissue ruptures, and the air may escape into the interstitial tissue or the pleural cavity, or be drawn into the circulation. This situation occurs during training when an inexperienced diver descends without releasing the air in his lungs or when, in an actual escape from a sunken ship or submarine, the individual does not release air while he rises. It may be seen when a scuba diver releases his equipment and returns to the surface without releasing air. Breath-holding as environmental pressure decreases predisposes to burst lungs. The hazard increases when nearing the surface, as the relative pressure volume changes are greatest at this point. Lambert pointed out that in 35,000 ascents only 12 cases of pulmonary barotrauma were seen.[2] Lung damage is caused by overdistention and stretching rather than by direct effects of increased pressure.

SYNDROMES OF BAROTRAUMA

Pulmonary Barotrauma. The three syndromes in which pulmonary barotrauma is manifest are pneumothorax, interstitial emphysema, and air embolism. They may be present individually or as mixed syndromes. Air embolism represents the most important and the one in which immediate attention is most needed. The clinical effect of air embolism depends directly upon the actual site of the bubble collection. If it is in the brain, convulsions, visual changes, spastic or flaccid paralysis, or less dramatically, tingling in the limbs and vertigo may occur. Pneumothorax and interstitial emphysema cause chest pain and abdominal pain. Nose bleeds, hemoptysis, and coughing may be present, as may cyanosis. Immediate recompression is mandatory to shrink the embolism bubble mass.

Barotalgia. The second location in which injury from barotrauma is seen is the middle ear, where the air pressure differs from that in the external ear and the nasopharynx. If the air pressure in the middle ear cannot be kept in equilibrium with that in the nasopharynx, for instance, because of inflammation of the eustachian tube, the eardrum may bulge inward, with resulting stretching, pain, hemorrhage, and ultimate perforation. This is a problem in sudden descents from high places such as mountains, or in landing in an aircraft, and it becomes a much more acute problem in diving because there are greater pressure gradients. The acute pain, however, may prevent the diver from going deep enough to produce a perforation in his ear. Difficulty may also arise in situations in which air may be trapped in the external canal when an individual is wearing a tight fitting cap. The water pressure, upon rising, compresses the hood against the ear until the air volume can shrink no further. If the eustachian tube opens, this pressure is passed to the middle ear. The drum will bulge outward because of the pressure differential, and edema may develop, as may large bloody blisters on the meatus.

Barosinusitis and Barodontalgia. There are many occasions when divers experience vertigo or dizziness under water. Those suffering from sinusitis or polyps of the nasopharynx may experience a very painful condition owing to the variation in pressure between the surrounding tissue and the sinuses.

Small pockets of gas resulting from fermentation in the roots of teeth may shrink during compression, and the space may become occupied by blood or fluid. This will cause increased pressure and pain when the diver returns to the surface.

Intestinal Complications. As the result of increase in the volume of the gaseous content of the intestinal tract, which ordinarily is decreased by the pressure of a dive, continued fermentation may produce additional gas, which will cause abdominal distention, discomfort, and embarrassing flatulence upon return to the surface. Miles relates that meals taken under pressure in the chamber have produced so much distention on decompression as to cause syncope.[1] This could also result from the swallowing of large volumes of air by inexperienced or anxious divers before and during the dive.

In aviation there are parallel pressure problems, the difference being that the directions are reversed. There is a decrease in pressure first, then an increase on return to ground level, causing respiratory and aural problems. In addition, the aviator who leaves the ground with large quantities of gas in his gastrointestinal tract will have considerable discomfort from abdominal distention when the environmental pressure is reduced. Decompression sickness is a hazard in both fields—diving and aviation.

NITROGEN NARCOSIS AND OXYGEN POISONING

Although nitrogen has been considered an inert gas, Carpenter has noted, in a paper on inert gas narcosis read at a symposium on underwater physiology held in Washington in 1955, that "despite their chemically unreactive nature, the noble gases at certain pressures display all the typical properties of anesthetic agents."[3] Nitrogen, which makes up approximately 79 per cent of the air we breathe, has been demonstrated by Cousteau in 1954 to produce an effect that he referred to as "rapture of the deep."[4] The so-called narcosis is preceded by euphoria. If alcohol has been taken prior to pressurization, the effect of nitrogen is greatly enhanced, the two being almost additive. Usually, upon release of the pressure, excess nitrogen leaves the tissues and recovery is complete. In severe cases, however, there may be some temporary amnesia. Helium has been used in place of nitrogen in the breathing mixture, which allows for a much deeper diving potential.

The problem of hyperoxia (oxygen poisoning) is a factor and has been discussed in detail by Donald.[5] The effects may result from prolonged exposure to low oxygen concentration or brief exposure to very high tensions (1,500 mm of mercury). Acute oxygen poisoning is a much more common danger in diving, and convulsions have been reported when divers have breathed pure oxygen at a pressure of 4 atm (partial pressure of 3,040 mm of mercury).[6] Degree of exertion and depth must be considered. At depths greater than 25 ft, pure oxygen is not currently used. The mechanism of oxygen poisoning includes an excessively high partial pressure of oxygen, which produces sufficient concentration in tissues to produce acute effects, especially in the central nervous system, where, however, there is no permanent damage. There may be an irritant effect on the lung tissue from smaller excess pressure for a considerable time. This is chronic oxygen poisoning.

SCUBA DIVING FATALITIES

The term "scuba" refers to self-contained underwater breathing apparatus. The diver is supplied by one or more tanks strapped to his back, which enable him to remain submerged for indefinite periods of time. "Skin diving," in contrast, refers to swimming with a breathing tube that has a mouthpiece at one end. The other end of the tube remains above the surface of the water unless the diver submerges, when the spherical float attached to it keeps the water from entering it. The diver holds his breath for the length of time he remains under water. This is also called "snorkeling."

In Los Angeles County a very active program is maintained by the County Department of Parks and Recreation in an effort to provide instruction and support to the many thousands of divers who take advantage of the waters in this county and along the ocean front. A committee also reviews the deaths of and accidents to divers and recommends improvements in the safety measures required of diving enthusiasts. In the six-year period from 1965 through 1970, 63 deaths associated with underwater activity occurred, 90 per cent of which (or 57) involved scuba diving and 6 per cent (4) free diving; there were 2 involving unknown cause or unknown activity, and one in a submarine. The Los Angeles County Coroner's Office is responsible for investigation of deaths in this category, and they recognize four basic groups of factors contributing to the fatalities. These include panic in minor emergencies such as the loss of a mouthpiece or face mask, or entrapment in kelp or a gill net, and poor judgment in estimating the distance from safety.[7]

Improper use or maintenance of equipment is a serious factor. This includes insufficient servicing and the use of defective components. Occasionally regulators are defective, and water may be inhaled instead of air. The third group of fatalities are caused by acute alcoholism; judgment is impaired and inhibitions are lost as a result of the intoxicant.

The fourth group includes fatalities caused by organic disease. Cardiovascular disease, specifically severe coronary sclerosis, may be evident and suggestive in the absence of any definitive contributing cause of drowning. It is well known that hypoxia is associated with increased susceptibility to the effects of alcohol, impairment of coordination of muscular activity, and decreased perception of depth and color. Newman has demonstrated that a concentration of alcohol in the blood that is incapable of producing measurable signs of intoxication when an individual is at sea level produces deterioration of performance at an altitude of 18,000 ft. Unconsciousness may be the result of either an increase in carbon dioxide tension or a decrease in oxygen tension, and loss of consciousness may be associated with hyperventilation.

Water Accident Investigation Team

The medicolegal investigation technique for water accidents developed by Noguchi is known as "WAIT" (Water Accident Investigation Team). It consists of a forensic pathologist and his medical and paramedical support team, including a diving expert who may be a medical officer who has sufficient experience in hyperbaric medicine. The work of this team is coordinated, by means of a liaison officer, with that of the investigative team of an agency such as a department of beaches, parks and recreation, the Coast Guard, law enforcement agencies, and rescue and fire departments.[9]

It is advisable that every scuba fatality be very thoroughly investigated and documented. It is also advisable that a hearing be held to determine what happened, the circumstances surrounding the death, and what recommendations should be made to prevent such incidents as well as to improve training, licensing, and maintenance of diving gear. A coordinated effort should be made, with the active sports diving equipment manufacturers as well as representatives of commercial interest (diving shop, charter boat) invited to help formulate the recommendation. In Los Angeles County the Underwater Safety Committee was first established in 1961 following a large number of fatalities in 1960. Every year a review is made.

The medicolegal autopsy in fatal water accidents including scuba deaths should include the following steps:

1. *Do not* remove the masks or any gear from the deceased divers, as equipment should be examined for flaws. Absence of a weighted belt is significant.
2. Photograph the tank and send it to a proper testing facility.
3. Leave the wetsuit undisturbed until the autopsy begins.
4. Document the time of notification, arrival time, diving time, and conversations with witnesses such as the skipper and other divers and diving instructors.
5. Photograph the body in the position in which it was found underwater (face down, face up) as soon as possible. Note rigor mortis. There should be minimum disturbance of the position of remains, diving gear, wetsuit, and safety equipment.
6. Transfer the body to the examining room without delay to prevent artifacts' being increased by putrefaction.

Photograph each step of the undressing.

External examination should follow in the usual fashion from top of head to tip of toe without missing any of the surface of the skin. Evidence of squeezing or pressure on the skin should be looked for as well as evidence of air embolism. The eyelid, conjunctiva, sclera, neck, and thoracic wall should be examined for subcutaneous emphysema.

X-rays of the chest in the standing position will indicate a fluid level in the chest cavity or the presence of a pneumothorax or pneumomediastinum. Radiographs of the knees may show nitrogen bubbles in the joint, indicating a long diving period.

In a case of air embolism, air samples should be removed with a syringe lubricated by oil for gas chromatographic or electron mass spectrometer analysis of the gas components. Theoretically if a person dies of a massive air embolism from rupture of the lung the proportion of oxygen to nitrogen would be 20 per cent to 80 per cent. A larger portion of nitrogen, such as 95 per cent, indicates with a degree of certainty that the person suffered from nitrogen narcosis.

It is preferable that when the deceased is found at or below the level of 16 ft, the autopsy be performed in a decompression chamber maintained at the same depth as that at which the body was recovered in order to determine the degree of tissue damage. If this facility is not readily available for the study, however, then the examiner should determine the total air in the blood vessels and should then recalculate, according to Boyle's law, the amount that it would be at the depth where the body was found.

When the skin incision is made, it is important not to overlook the small air bubbles that come out from subcutaneous tissue. This is another sign that there is an abundance of air in the general circulation. Blood is generally fluid, it is not coagulated. The heart need not be opened under water as previously recommended in most textbooks. It is more important to measure the total amount of air in the chambers of the heart and to find out the air composition.

The contents of the stomach are important and must be examined in order to determine the presence of food, drugs, or alcohol.

SUMMARY

Problems related to pressure may be found whether the individual is involved in free diving, snorkeling, scuba diving, or diving into depths using full diving suit and hard hat.

The major forms of barotrauma include effects on specific body organs. In the lungs, for instance, there may be a resulting pneumothorax, interstitial emphysema, air embolism, or any combination of these. The middle ear may be affected, with subsequent rupture of the eardrum, vertigo, or dizziness. The teeth may be the site of gas collection and might explode under certain conditions. Nitrogen narcosis may be found in which increased nitrogen accumulation may have caused disorientation and the fatal consequences. This may be enhanced by accompanying alcohol consumption. Oxygen poisoning from prolonged exposure to higher levels of oxygen may result in acute neurologic problems from central effects.

Scuba diving fatalities should be investigated in an organized way with the investigation beginning, preferably, on the ocean floor with initial examination of the victim. One agency equipped to do so is the WAIT—Water Accident Investigation Team.

REFERENCES

1. Miles, S.: *Underwater Medicine*. 3rd Edition. Philadelphia, J. B. Lippincott Co., 1969.
2. Lambert, R.: Submarine escape. Proc. R. Soc. Med., *51*:824, 1958.
3. Carpenter, F.: Inert gas narcosis. Symposium on Underwater Physiology, Washington, D.C., 1965.
4. Cousteau, J. I., and Dumas, F.: *The Silent World*. London, Hamish Hamilton Ltd., 1954; New York, Harper & Row, Inc., 1953.
5. Donald, K. W.: Oxygen poisoning in man. Br. Med. J., *1*:172, 1947.
6. Thomson, W. A. R.: The physiology of deep sea diving. Br. Med. J., *2*:208, 1935.
7. Noguchi, T. T., and Moore, S.: Scuba Diving Fatalities. Med. Arts Sci., 81–87, 3rd Quarter 1962.
8. Newman, H. W.: Effect of altitude on alcohol tolerance. Q. J. Stud. Alcohol, *10*:398, 1949.
9. Los Angeles County Underwater Safety Committee Report. Sept. 1974.

SECTION 3. BAROTRAUMA (DYSBARISM)

chapter 16

INJURIES RELATED TO LOW ATMOSPHERIC PRESSURE

by William G. Eckert

Serious injuries and fatalities have resulted from exposure to decreased pressure. This may occur during flights at high altitudes or during simulated high-altitude conditions in a decompression chamber.[1]

An understanding of the nature of the environment is important to any attempt to study this problem. Those responsible for investigating injuries or deaths of persons exposed to high altitude should have information concerning the particulars of the flight or the conditions in the decompression chamber. The temperature, pressure, and humidity are important in this situation.

The barometric or atmospheric pressure at sea level is above 760 mm of mercury. This pressure is referred to as standard or 1 atm if the temperature is 0° C. Pressure may also be expressed as pounds per square inch (psi) or grams per square centimeter. Thus 1 atm equals 760 mm of mercury, 34 ft of fresh water, 33 ft of salt water, 14.7 psi, or 1,033.3 g per square centimeter.[2] Atmospheric pressure plus gauge pressure equals absolute pressure. At various altitudes pressure is decreased as follows: up to 5,000 ft, the pressure is 1 atm; at 10,000 ft it is 0.83; at 20,000 ft it is 0.69 atm; at 30,000 ft it is 0.30 atm of absolute pressure.

MECHANISMS OF HYPOBARIC INJURY

High-altitude decompression sickness has symptoms similar to those of caisson disease. There are, however, differences between the two in the circumstances of development and in the progression of the process. Armstrong, in his experiments in the decompression chamber, observed a syndrome, which he labeled as "aeroembolism," that was due to nitrogen bubble emboli formed in the blood vessels when the blood, because of the nitrogen physically dissolved in it, became supersaturated with respect to ambient nitrogen pressure.[3]

Dysbarism consists of those disturbances in the body, exclusive of hypoxia and air sickness, that result from the existence of a pressure differential between the total ambient barometric pressure and the total pressures of dissolved and free gases within the body tissues, fluids, and cavities. In altitude dysbarism the total change in pressure is less than 760 mm of mercury.

Adler classifies dysbarism symptoms into those due to hypobarism and those due to hyperbarism. Hyperbaric effects result from an excess of ambient gas pressure over that within the body fluids, tissues, and cavities. These are exemplified by barotalgia and barosinusitis (aerosinusitis) and are discussed in Chapter 15. Hypobaric effects result from an excess of gas pressure within body fluids, tissues, and cavities over ambient gas pressure. These effects are subdivided into the evolved gas types and the trapped gas types.[4] Both hyperbaric and hypobaric effects could be suffered during a single flight, the latter being noted on the ascent and the former being noted on the descent.

The evolved gas types of dysbarism are the bends, characterized by joint pains caused by evolved gas bubbles within the joints; the chokes, with cough, chest pain, and dyspnea due to pulmonary intravascular evolved gas as well as mediastinal emphysema from evolved gas bubbles; central nervous system symptoms caused by evolved gas pressure on or in the brain as well as embolic phenomena; and skin disturbances (the itches) due to evolved gas bubbles under the skin and to neurocirculatory phenomena due to bubble pressure on nerves and blood vessels.

The trapped gas types include abdominal distention and barodontalgia.

The problems of hypobarism are related to its causation by evolved gases or by trapped gases.

Evolved Gases. Gases are evolved and form bubbles when, with a rapid decrease in ambient pressure, tissues saturated with a dissolved gas may become supersaturated Nitrogen is implicated in most cases, but oxygen and carbon dioxide bubbles may also form and cause dysbarism. Nitrogen may total 1,000 to 1,500 ml in solution in the body, representing saturation of the tissues at sea level. Most is in the tissues, with little in the blood. In the body, nitrogen is transported in simple solution according to Henry's law. It enters into and is removed from the body by the establishment of one equilibrium between nitrogen pressure in the alveolar air and the venous blood, and another between the tissues and the arterial blood.

During an ascent, ambient nitrogen pressure is reduced and nitrogen transport is directed toward its removal from the lungs. Nitrogen in tissue, then being higher in pressure than that in the arterial blood, is transported to the blood, then to the alveolar air, and is expired. As only a small amount of nitrogen can be transported by a given amount of blood, the rapid reduction in ambient pressure results in supersaturation of the tissues with resultant bubble formation. The nitrogen bubbles can form in any tissue, including blood, and their effect depends on the location of accumulation.

Trapped Gases. Gases may be trapped in hollow viscera, teeth, or body cavities, with resultant pain and the possibility of rupture. Thus there may be gases trapped in the sinuses, middle ear, teeth, joints, beneath the skin, or in the intestinal tract.

CLINICAL MANIFESTATIONS OF HYPOBARISM

Individual susceptibility to hypobarism varies widely. This may be considered in selection of candidates for aviation training by utilizing a standard stimulus to rule out symptomatic candidates. There are also predisposing factors that must be considered in the production of injury. These include age, obesity, exercise, rate of ascent, attained altitude, increased tissue pressure of nitrogen prior to ascent, decreased nitrogen pressure prior to ascent, recent scuba diving, previous injury, repeated exposure, temperature, and total dissolved gas tension.[5] The age of the person exposed to high altitude is shown as a factor by Fryer and Roxburgh. In the obese occupant of a plane, both the probability and the frequency of dysbarism are greater. Fatty tissue contains less blood than muscular tissue, and nitrogen is five times as soluble in fat as in muscle. Thus the combination of larger stores and poor transport of nitrogen makes the plane occupant who is more liberally endowed with fatty tissue also more capable of suffering from dysbarism than his leaner companion. Exercise at altitude increases the incidence of dysbarism, possibly because of the concomitant increase in tissue metabolic carbon dioxide. Exercise causes symptoms to occur at a lower altitude and after a shorter time than they do at rest.[6] Dysbarism does not usually occur during flights at altitudes under 20,000 ft, but cases have been experienced at lower altitudes when individuals had been scuba diving within 12 hours of the flight. The United States Navy has adopted the "rule of 12" to cover this circumstance: no flight above 12,000 for 12 hours following a scuba dive of 12 ft or more. The physiologic reason for this rule is that enough time must be allowed at sea level, breathing air, to complete respiratory washout of the excess nitrogen stored in the tissues during the dive. "Excess" is defined as the amount present over and above that required to produce nitrogen saturation at 1 atm. The other factors affecting altitude dysbarism are (1) previous injury (bubbles tend to form at sites of recent injuries in some cases); (2) repeated exposure (some individuals who have once had an attack of dysbarism may be more susceptible to another such attack); (3) total dissolved gas tension (implicated as the cause of dysbarism, rather than simply nitrogen tension, which accounts for the increased incidence following exercise but leaves other questions unanswered); and (4) lower ambient temperatures (dysbarism occurs with greater frequency, possibly because of decreased nitrogen transport associated with peripheral vasoconstriction due to cold).[5]

The clinical features of hypobarism include joint symptoms and pain in muscles and long bones. This condition is referred to as "the bends." The onset follows the ascent with a variable lag period. The areas involved are first the knee, then the shoulder, elbow, wrist, hand, and fingers. The bends are not serious per se and may be relieved on descent. "The chokes" are characterized by substernal distress, nonproductive cough, and respiratory distress accompanied by a sense of apprehension and suffocation. More serious than the bends, the chokes result from bubble formation and accumulation in the pulmonary capillaries or from the effects of extravascular mediastinal bubbles exerting pressure on mediastinal contents and adjacent pulmonary tissue. It may be a solitary manifestation of hypobarism or it may accompany the bends. When the chokes occur in an individual they are found later in the flight than bends and become progressively more disabling. The cough and the substernal distress are markedly aggravated when an attempt is made to take a deep breath, resulting in decreased pulmonary ventilation and thus hypoxia. This may be followed by syncope and collapse. The onset of chokes demands prompt attention and return to normal pressure by way of descent to lower altitude or termination of the flight of the aircraft or removal from the low-pressure chamber. The symptoms of central nervous system involvement are usually referable to the senses, especially vision, and to disturbance in orientation. They are related to the bubble size and the location of lodging in the arterioles and capillaries of the brain. These symptoms are an indication for mandatory hospitalization—as on occasion sudden and severe neurocirculatory collapse may occur without warning. Hypobaric collapse is preceded by bends and chokes and may occur later in the flight. It frequently follows central nervous system manifestations. Skin manifestations are due to pressure on dermal nerve endings. Subdermal emphysema may occur and is revealed by crepitation on palpation. The latter two phenomena may be the first manifestations of gas hypobarism.

The trapped-gas type of hypobarism may result in the doubling of the hollow viscus volume at 18,000 ft and its quadrupling at 33,000 ft. Stomach expansion, if not relieved, may cause diaphragmatic herniation.

RAPID AND EXPLOSIVE DECOMPRESSION

Rapid decompression and explosive decompression result from mechanical failure of the aircraft's pressurization system or from external or internal perforation of the plane's hull. Loss of pressure in less than a second is referred to as explosive decompression; if longer, it is referred to as rapid decompression. The classic examples of air crashes involving explosive decompression were the 1954 Comet disasters in the sea off Italy; a defective part in a portion of the fuselage had provided a point of weakness. Armstrong reported the findings in the victims.[7] Mason and Tarlton reported a similar case of explosive decompression that was initiated by an explosive device.[8] Mason and Reals, in their excellent monograph, have suggested the following criteria to aid the pathologist who may have to distinguish between injuries resulting from impact and those arising from a catastrophe at altitude: (1) a grading of injury pattern is probable, as the effects of turbulence are unlikely to be identical in all parts of the aircraft; (2) some passengers may well have died from hypoxia, in which case anomalous heavy congested lungs may be found in bodies subjected to severe secondary impact trauma; (3) ruptured eardrums may be present in the absence of basal skull fractures; and (4) microscopic examination of the lungs will almost certainly reveal the presence of bone marrow emboli resulting from nonfatal injuries sustained before ground impact.[1]

DEATHS DUE TO DECOMPRESSION TO SUBATMOSPHERIC PRESSURE

The number of deaths due to decompression to subatmospheric pressure has been low. Fryer reports 17 cases, of which 10 occurred in the decompression chamber and 7 occurred in actual flight.[9] This does not include the deaths of three Russian cosmonauts during the reentry of Soyuz II.

In Fryer's cases the maximum chamber altitude was 35,600 ft, and in jet aircraft it was 30,400 ft. Time of exposure was approximately one hour. The common finding in those who died was overweight. Clinically, hyperpyrexia was common, as were leukocytosis and hemoconcentration. Hyperglycemia, hyperkalemia, mild uremia, albuminuria, and increased protein in the spinal fluid have been reported.

The postmortem features, as stated by Mason and Reals, have been those of shock, pleural effusion, pulmonary congestion, and pulmonary edema. Patent foramen ovale is seen frequently. Histologically, pulmonary and systemic congestion has been confirmed almost always and a severely fatty liver has been reported with frequency. Accelerated autolysis or tubular necrosis in the kidney was found as well as ischemic foci in the brain. Presence of antecedent disease is more frequent than would be expected. Fat embolism is seen frequently without trauma. Systemic fat embolism is found only in the clinical syndrome of fat embolism and is rarely reported unaccompanied by trauma except in postdescent shock.[1]

The determination and establishment of the cause of death in postdescent shock has never been clearly established. Philp and co-workers in Canada suggest that gaseous embolism and traumatic shock are operating jointly in the genesis of fatal postdescent shock. They have shown that the presence of gas in the circulation leads to the formation of microthrombi and blood sludging at the blood-gas interface. They further believe that this complex stimulates the coalescence of plasma lipids with the formation of lipoid emboli.[10]

SUMMARY

It is essential that those investigating injuries related to exposure to low atmosphere pressure should have the benefit of detailed information on the circumstances of the flight or decompression chamber run. In addition the profile of experience and behavior of the victim should be understood.

Clinical manifestations of this problem are related to the formation of bubbles and their accumulation in loose soft tissue, cavities, or hollow viscera. Thus involvement of the joints results in the bends with excruciating pain as a prominent symptom; involvement of the mediastinum may produce the picture of chokes with difficulty in breathing and severe coughing; and a spectrum of neurologic symptoms may be related to vascular location of the bubble formation and involvement of the skin, which produces subcutaneous emphysema. Trapped gases produce abdominal distention and barodontalgia.

Predisposing factors that may affect the injury potential include age, obesity, exercise, ascent rate, attained altitude, nitrogen pressure before descent or ascent, recent scuba diving, previous injury, temperature, and total dissolved gas tension.

Rapid and explosive decompression have produced tragic consequences, as evidenced by the Comet crashes of 1954. The pathologist may lend valuable assistance to the investigation of the cause of the crash if he can distinguish between injuries resulting from impact and those arising from a catastrophe at high altitude.

Postmortem examination by a properly trained pathologist can be of extreme importance in establishing the cause of the air crash as well as the means required for prevention when hazards have been shown to exist.

REFERENCES

1. Mason, J. D., and Reals, W. T.: *Aerospace Pathology*. Chicago, College of American Pathologists, 1973.
2. Miles, S.: *Underwater Medicine*. 3rd Ed. Philadelphia, J. B. Lippincott Co., 1969.
3. Armstrong, J.: The ideal relationship between inspired oxygen concentration and cabin altitude. Aerosp. Med., *4*:991, 1963.
4. Adler, H. F.: Dysbarism Review 1–64. Brooks Air Force Base, Texas, USAF School of Aerospace Medicine, 1964.
5. U.S. Naval Bureau of Medicine: *U.S. Naval Flight Surgeon's Manual*. Washington, D.C., U.S. Government Printing Office, 1968.
6. Fryer, D. I., and Roxburgh, H. L.: Decompression sickness. In *Textbook of Aviation Physiology*. Edited by J. A. Gillies. New York, Pergamon Press, 1965, pp. 122–151.
7. Armstrong, J. A., Fryer, D. I., Stewart, W. K., and Whittingham, H. E.: Interpretation of injuries in the Comet aircraft disasters. Lancet, *1*:1135, 1955.
8. Mason, J. K., and Tarlton, S. W.: Medical investigation of the loss of the Comet 4B aircraft, 1967. Lancet, *1*:431, 1969.
9. Fryer, D. I.: Pathologic findings in fatal subatmospheric decompression sickness. Med. Sci. Law, *2*:110, 1962.
10. Philp, R. B., Inwood, M. J., and Warren, B. A.: Interactions between gas bubbles and components of the blood: implications in decompression sickness. Aerosp. Med., *43*:946, 1972.

SECTION 4. INJURY BY ELECTRICAL FORCE

chapter 17

by Endre Somogyi and C. G. Tedeschi

PHYSICAL PRINCIPLES IN ELECTROTRAUMA

Of all categories of injuries produced by physical agents, probably none is ruled by the laws of physics more strictly than that induced by electrical force. Whether or not an injury will occur and, if it does, its extent and degree of severity depend on well-defined factors: (1) the nature of the current (DC, pulsating, AC); (2) the voltage to which the victim of the accident was exposed; (3) the frequency, if AC; (4) the amount of current (amperage); (5) the length of time the victim was in the circuit; (6) the condition of the earth (moisture), if the shock was from conductor to earth; (7) the presence of uninsulated points in the electrical system or (8) intervening material between the source of voltage and the victim; (9) the transformer connections; and (10) the direction of the force (as established by the points of entrance and exit of the current); and (11) the resistance offered by the body at the time of the accident. Finally, the route followed by the current within the body is of paramount importance in determining the final outcome of the accident.

The physician trained in the forensic sciences rarely masters the principles of physics well enough to answer many questions that arise in an investigation of electrical injury. Not infrequently the answers are provided by the evidence presented by the electrical expert. Furthermore, in many cases of accidental electrocution, data that are essential for an exact reconstruction of the events are unknown or cannot be established. This is well exemplified by the fatal shock concurrent to lightning in which the amount of electrical force, amperage, resistance, and duration of flame cannot be measured and therefore remain unknown factors.

As a general rule, the extent of the injury is proportional to the amount of current measured as amperes. The latter can be calculated by dividing the potential (measured as volts) by the resistance (measured as ohms).[1] Thus, as the current flows through the body and becomes part of the circuit, its amount can be determined by the formula:

$$C \text{ (current)} = \frac{V \text{ (voltage)}}{R \text{ (resistance)}}$$

Direct and Alternating Current

Direct current is broadly applied in industry in which electrolytic activity is required, for instance, in the purification of metals (e.g., production of aluminum from bauxite), in plating (e.g., silver and chrome plating), and in galvanoplasty. High-voltage direct current also is extensively used in railway operations. Accidents with direct current are relatively infrequent, but when they do occur, are usually severe. This is explained by the electrolytic action.

It is well substantiated that the human organism is four to six times as sensitive to alternating as to direct current; the greater incidence of fatal outcomes is due to the tetanoid effects elicited by alternating current that prevent the victim of the accident from taking his hands off the charged wires. An alternating current of 70 to 80 ma may be lethal, whereas a direct current with an intensity of 250 ma may be tolerated without damage.

The greater risk attends alternations between 39 and 150 cycles per second, and the danger decreases with the increasing number of cycles; a 60-cycle alternating current may cause death if the heart or brain stem lies in its path.

Voltage

The borderline between low-voltage (low-tension) current and high-voltage (high-tension) current is conventionally placed at the 1,000-v level. Whereas the distinction between the two types of current is important from the standpoint of physical properties, it has no bearing on biologic implications. Contact with a low-tension current of 100 v or less may prove fatal, while the shock from a discharge of 10,000 v may be survived. Approximately 60 per cent of all fatalities by electricity are caused by currents of 115 v. Children's electric toys are considered to be safe within a voltage of 24; the safety limit is set higher—42 v—for domestic appliances.

Death in low-voltage accidents is primarily due to ventricular fibrillation, whereas in high-voltage accidents the major threat is provided by the ensuing electrothermal injury, the severity of which bears a direct relation to the duration of the contact.

The heating effect of a current is ordinarily calculated by the formula:

$$H = C2R/4.187$$

in which H stands for gram calories per second, C for current in amperes, and R for resistance in ohms.[1]

Arc Current

Body injury may occur without direct contact with the conductor of the electric current. As a body approaches a high-voltage line, an electric arc may pass through it; in relation to the voltage, injury may occur at the following distances:

1,000 v	Few mm
5,000 v	1 cm
20,000 v	6 cm
40,000 v	13 cm
100,000 v	35 cm

The temperature generated by arc current may be as high as 4,000°C. Thus, according to Joule's law, electrical force is changed into thermic energy, and the effects essentially duplicate those of a flame from other sources.

Accidents due to arcing occur most frequently on exposure to high-voltage current, but they may take place as well in the presence of low-voltage current whenever the body resistance is low.

Resistance

In accordance with Ohm's law, amperage is inversely proportional to resistance. The resistance of the human body to the passage of electric current varies from tissue to tissue; variations are primarily determined by the water content of the tissues. On the whole the conductivity of tissues is significantly less than that of metals.

The most resistant tissular layer of the body is the skin, followed in order of decreased resistance by bone, fat, nerve, muscle, blood, and body fluids.

Within the tegumental layer there are variations in the degree of resistance that depend on the thickness of the skin and the relative number of hair follicles and sweat and sebaceous glands. Thick callous skin is more resistant than thin delicate skin. The resistance of damp sweating skin is significantly less than that of dry skin. This explains why accidents occur more frequently during the summer months. Hyperhydrosis may be a decisive factor. Daily oscillations have also been registered, with peak resistance in the morning and evening hours.[2] Resistance is decreased by febrile states and by drugs that induce sweat formation. As a general rule, in a healthy individual, resistance is highest in the skin of the back and lower in the forearm, palms of the hands, arm, and scalp, in the order given.[3] Because there are so many variables, there is no reliable method by which body resistance can be determined in the case of a fatal accident.[4] It is worthwhile to point out that resistance is also considerably altered by the postmortem cooling of the body.

In analyzing injuries by electrical force, consideration must also be given to the so-called *transitional resistance,* by which is meant the resistance provided by any material situated between the conductor and the human body or between the human body and the earth. The footwear of the individual exposed to electric current may be of decisive importance in determining the outcome of the accident. The protective rubber gloves and shoes usually worn by electrical technicians provide adequate insulation. The resistance of dry leather soles also provides good insulation, but it is reduced by the presence of nails or iron heels.

Amperage

The outcome of bodily contact with an electric current depends primarily on the amperage affecting the body. Thus, according to the law of Ohm, amperage is determined by the relationship between voltage and resistance. Since body resistance can only be estimated, the retrospective determination of amperage rests primarily on the response to the electrical contact by the victim of the accident.

From a considerable number of observations, Löbl has tabulated the data in Table 17–1. He also states that 30 ma is the upper limit of tolerance for man; 40 ma causes loss of consciousness, and death occurs at 100 ma.[5] Using as criteria amperage, duration of the contact, and path of the current, Koeppen has classified electrical accidents into the following four groups:

Group I. Amperage below 25 ma (in the case of direct current, between 25 and 80 ma); high transitional resistance. No harmful effects can be expected.

Group II. Amperage between 25 and 80 ma (in the case of direct current, between 80 and 300 ma); transitional resistance lower than in Group I. Loss of consciousness, arrhythmias, respiratory spasm.

Group III. Amperage between 80 and 100 ma (in the case of direct current, between 300 ma and 3 amp); transitional resistance lower than in Group II. If the exposure time is between 0.1 and 0.3, the biologic effects are very similar to those in Group II. On longer exposure (above 0.3) irreversible ventricular fibrillation sets in.

Group IV. Amperage exceeding 3 amp. Cardiac arrest.[6]

TABLE 17–1. EFFECT OF AMPERAGE ON BODILY INJURY FROM ELECTRIC CURRENT

AMPERAGE (ma)	EFFECTS
1.0	Sensation, threshhold of current
1.5	Distinct formication; perception of current
2.0	Numbness of hand
3.5	Slight stiffness of hand
4.0	Paresthesia of forearm
5.0	Tremor of hand and spasm of forearm
7.0	Slight spasm extending to upper arm
10.0	May voluntarily let go of electric line
15.0	Contraction of flexor muscles prevents release of electric line
20.0	Painful muscular contraction

*From Lobl, O.: Messungen uber die todliche Stromstark. ETZ-A. *80*:97, 1959. Reprinted by permission.

Path and Density of Current

As a general rule, the sites of entrance and egress of the current determine its path. As shown in Figure 17–1, in the *hand-to-hand* path, both hands come into contact with the conductor under voltage, or one hand touches the conductor and the other simultaneously touches an adequately grounded object, for instance, a water tap. The *hand-to-foot* path is taken when the victim of the accident touches the conductor under voltage with one hand, while his foot is grounded. The *head-to-hand* path is pursued when one hand comes into contact with the conductor under voltage and the head is grounded. The *head-to-foot* path occurs when the head touches the conductor under voltage and the foot is grounded.

The concept is well accepted that the current passes through the body in the shortest path between the points of contact rather than along the areas of weakest resistance.[7] Irrespective of tissular dispersion, the greatest density of current will develop on the shortest path.

Duration of the Contact

The longer the time of contact, the greater the amount of current that will pass through the body and consequently the greater the amount of body damage. To determine the duration of contact in retrospect is a difficult task. In general, the victim of the accident is inclined to overestimate the time, and his statements must be accepted with a great deal of reservation. If he states that he did not become unconscious and was able to interrupt the circuit voluntarily, then one may conclude that the duration of the contact was very short. Conversely, if he reports that he was stuck to the electric line, could not let go of it or free himself in any other way, then it may be assumed

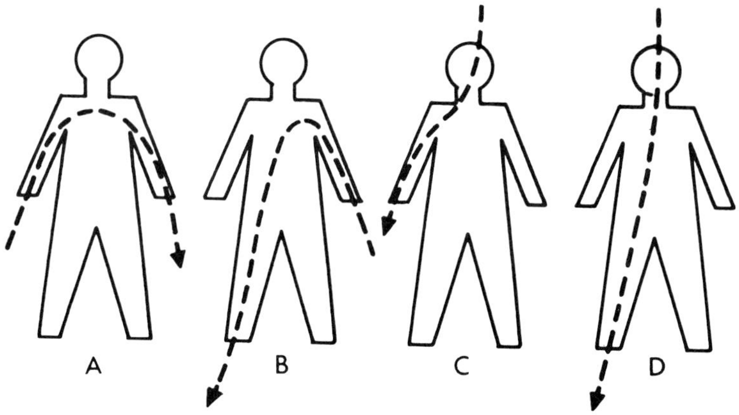

Figure 17–1. Paths of current. *A.* Hand to hand. The victim of the accident contacts the two poles with both hands or touches the conductor under voltage with one hand, and with the other hand simultaneously touches the adequately grounded object, e.g., water supply system. *B.* Hand to foot. The victim of the accident touches the conductor under voltage with one hand while his foot is grounded to earth. *C.* Head to hand. The victim of the accident touches the conductor under voltage with his hand, while his head is near the conductor under voltage. *D.* Head to foot. The head touches the conductor under voltage while the foot is grounded.

that the time of contact exceeded the critical time of two to three seconds.

Finally, if the victim of the accident lost consciousness, the presumed time of contact cannot be established, even with approximation. As loss of consciousness supervenes, as a rule the victim falls to the ground, thus interrupting the circuit. Often the state of unconsciousness, by shortening the time of contact, becomes a lifesaving event.

The deposition of witnesses who intervened, interrupting the circuit or otherwise rendering assistance, is likewise unreliable. Usually, they are inclined to overestimate the time of contact.

As suggested by Incze, perhaps the best method of obtaining a fairly reliable estimate of the period of contact is to ask the witness, if one was present, to reenact the accident while others check the time.[8]

STATISTICAL ANALYSIS OF ACCIDENTS DUE TO ELECTRICITY

Knowledge of the incidence of electrical injuries and underlying causes is of primary importance, the ultimate goal being their prevention. Statistics are not entirely suitable for comparison, however, because the methods of assembling information frequently differ from study to study. In general, the injuries from electrical force that reach the statistics are those that are fatal or that cause disability of some duration. Accounts of industrial accidents are usually accompanied by an investigation report, and this provides useful information. On the other hand, accidents occurring within the home are poorly documented or not reported at all. National statistics show that the absolute number of accidents due to electricity has not increased at the same rate as has the utilization of electric energy, both industrial and civilian. Nevertheless, in spite of intensified preventative measures, the number of disabling or lethal electrical accidents is still very high.

Biegelmeier has tabulated the average number of fatal accidents by electric current in eight different countries (Table 17–2).[9]

DEATH DUE TO ELECTRICITY

In most fatal electrical accidents, death is caused by the electric energy itself. Not uncommonly the electrotrauma becomes associated with mechanical injury; this is the case when the victim of the accident falls from a height, and in this instance, it may be difficult to ascertain the immediate cause of death.

If death is due solely and directly to electrical force, the label generally applied is *electric death* or *death due to electricity.* Death often occurs at once, and no revealing lesions are found at autopsy. The characteristic *current marks* may not be present, and the cause of death must be determined from the findings reported by the electrical expert investigating the case. Occasionally even the technical investigation fails to give an unequivocal verdict. Walther and Sam report the case of a 26-year-old construction

TABLE 17–2. AVERAGE NUMBER OF LETHAL ELECTRIC ACCIDENTS PER YEAR, 1954–1959*

Country	Nonfatal Accidents	Population (Millions)	Lethal Accidents per Million
United Kingdom	150	50	3
Belgium	30	8.5	3.5
Netherlands	35	10	3.5
Sweden	28	7	4
Switzerland	28	5	5.7
German Fed. Rep.	300	50	6
United States	980	154	6.4
Austria	80	7	11.4

*From Biegelmeier, G.: Der vollkommene Fehlerschutz bei Niederspannungsanlagen. Elektromedizin, 4:35, 1959. Reprinted by permission.

worker operating a concrete mixing drum who suddenly uttered a cry and collapsed, dead. Except for acute congestion of the internal organs, no diagnostic lesion and no current marks could be demonstrated at autopsy. Two electrical engineers consulted in the case dismissed the possibility of electric death and assumed that the victim was affected by a heart condition and that death had been precipitated by fatigue and oppressive heat. In the absence of morphologic evidence that could support this contention, the forensic pathologist in the case rendered the opinion that electric death was probable and that the intensity of the current must have been between 16 and 95 ma.[10]

Jellinek has pointed out that death due to electricity does not necessarily take place immediately. In addition to the *exitus momentaneous* (immediate death), he enumerates three other forms of death: *exitus dilatatus* (delayed death), *exitus retardatus* (late death), and *exitus interruptus*. In the latter the victim is made unconscious by the electrical trauma, then regains consciousness, speaks, and walks, only to collapse dead shortly thereafter.[11]

Tappero describes such a situation in a successful suicidal attempt by contact with 9000 v, in which the person, before expiring, was able to walk a distance of 80 m. Cases like this are, however, exceptional, and as a rule the victim of the exposure becomes unconscious and remains unconscious until death occurs during transportation to the hospital, or on arrival. More realistic is the categorization of death proposed by Boemke and Piroth: instant death, death after a short time, delayed death, and death resulting from late complications.[13] The victim can also be found dead, and in this case the reconstruction of events may represent an insurmountable obstacle.

Not infrequently the electrical accident is followed by *apparent death*. The vital functions of the organism are reduced to a minimum, and signs of life cannot be detected by the usual clinical methods of examination. An electrocardiogram may prove valuable in these cases and may demonstrate persistence of cardiac function. In the experience of one of us (Somogyi), in quite a few cases of apparent death, the electrocardiogram may register heart activity one and one half hours after the apparent cessation of somatic functions. As long as respiration does not cease at the cellular level, it is possible to restore to life the victim of an electrocution in whom there have been no apparent signs of life. There is an approximate interval of five minutes between clinical and biologic death; after this time cells—primarily neurons, which are extremely sensitive to anoxia—undergo irreversible damage.

It has been stated that individuals with a preexisting heart condition or with reduced resistance from different causes are more prone to precipitated electric death. Nonetheless, the majority of electric deaths occur in healthy and able-bodied persons while they are at work. Our knowledge of the mechanisms operating in electric death rests on three main sources: results of animal experiments, observations in cases of judicial electrocution, and accidental electrotrauma.

Experimental Investigations

Most of the observations on the experimental animal have been made on the exposed heart. The sheep is probably best suited for the test because its response to electrical stimulation is very similar to that in man.

Experiments indicate that immediate death following electrocution can result either from ventricular fibrillation or from brain-stem injury and paralysis of the respiratory center. It has, however, been shown that ventricular fibrillation is reversible and that it can stop spontaneously.[14]

Ferris and co-workers established the time required for currents of different intensities to induce ventricular fibrillation. Their results are shown in Table 17–3. According to these investigators, ventricular fibrillation develops upon brief electrical stimulation only when the heart is in a refractory state.[15] Wiggers, Wegria, and Pinera called this condition the vulnerable stage of the heart, but there is no consensus on this point.[16, 17]

By the same token, experiments on anesthetized rabbits subjected to impulses of current of varying intensity and duration (220 to 600 ma; 5 to 30 sec; 220 v) indicate that in brain-stem injury respiratory arrest occurs at expiration.[18]

TABLE 17–3. TIME AND CURRENT INTENSITY REQUIRED TO PRODUCE VENTRICULAR FIBRILLATION*

Current Intensity (ma)	Duration (sec)
70– 300	5
200– 700	1
300–1300	0.3
500–2500	0.1
1800–8000	0.01

*From Ferris, L. P., King, B. G., Spencer, P. W., and Williams, H. B.: Effect of Elektroshock and Heart. A.I.E.E. Trans., 55:498, 1936. Reprinted by permission.

Some evidence has been presented that poor meteorologic conditions such as fog, rain, or snow increase the death rate associated with exposure to electric current.[19, 20] This can be interpreted as due to fatigue or better conductivity or both.

Judicial Electrocution

Judicial electrocution was first applied in the State of New York in 1890. At the time this procedure was introduced, knowledge of the effects of electric current on the human body was quite limited. A generally accepted but erroneous assumption was that the lethal effect was directly proportional to the intensity of the voltage.

In the first electrocution performed the metal electrodes were placed on the head and on the sacral region of the condemned. In order to decrease the cutaneous resistance, a sponge soaked with physiologic salt solution was rubbed at the points of application of the electrodes. An alternating current of 1,600 v, 150 Hz was used. The man was declared dead after 17 sec; however, after half a minute respiratory movements were noted, the man groaned, foam appeared at his mouth, and respirations became increasingly deeper. Current was switched on again until the "body of the victim steamed" and finally death occurred.[21] At the second execution, respiration returned for 27 sec after the administration of 1,485 v. In another case, signs of life were noted after 52 sec following the administration of 1,240 v.

After these early experiences, the procedure was modified several times. Alvensleben was present at several electrocutions and has given an accurate account of his observations. The upper and lower extremities of the condemned are fixed to the chair, and the resistance of the scalp is reduced by moistening. One of the electrodes (shaped like a helmet) is applied to the head, and the other is fastened on the right leg. An impulse of 2,000 v is transmitted through the body for three to five seconds. Considering the reduced resistance, this represents an amperage of 2.5. The condemned loses consciousness immediately. After a short interval tension is reduced to 250 to 500 v, and a new impulse is applied, which results in death.

Beneath the electrodes the skin temperature rises as high as 60°C, and third-degree burns may develop. Under the electrode placed on the leg, postmortem rigidity occurs at once within the right crural musculature, to spread gradually to the other parts of the body. Sperm ejaculation is not infrequent.

Werner mentioned that, in autopsies performed after the execution, the brain steamed and its temperature was as high as 63°C. He also described the brain as hyperemic, with the whole cortex covered by blood suffusions.[23] The same description has been given by other authors. Rupture of neuroaxons and blood vessels is the major finding at the microscopic examination of the brain.[21]

Accidental Electrocution

In accidents by exposure to low-voltage current, death as a rule is caused by ventricular fibrillation. Conversely, following exposure to high-voltage current, ventricular fibrillation is uncommon, and the most frequent cause of death is respiratory paralysis followed by contraction of respiratory muscles and acute asphyxia.

In 77 of 103 accidental electrocutions analyzed by Baur and Bissig, cardiac death took place within a few seconds.[25] Neuhold described a case in which the injured survived the accident but died shortly after in uremic coma; at autopsy necrosis of myofibers was demonstrated.[26] Taylor and Stoelting reported the case of a 15-year-old boy who died of rupture of the heart and cardiac tamponade during anesthesia for wound revision, five weeks after accidental electrocution.[27]

Several observations substantiate that ventricular fibrillation takes place predominantly on exposure to between 80 ma and 3 amp for at least one second and that the most vulnerable stage of heart contraction is at the end of systole. Ventricular fibrillation is most frequently elicited by alternating current of industrial frequencies (50 to 60 Hz).

The assumption that ventricular fibrillation induced by electric current is reversible in animals but not in man is not correct. This erroneous view is disproved by a series of observations in cases of accidental electrical trauma, which show that spontaneous reversion of ventricular fibrillation may occur in man also.

Death may also be induced by the hyperthermic effect of the trauma on the vital centers of the brain. As Prinz says, a combination of mechanisms is probably operating in most cases, and it is likely that the complex biologic reactions cannot be explained simply on the basis of physical events.[28]

PHYSIOPATHOLOGY OF ELECTROTRAUMA BY ORGAN SYSTEMS

Skin (Current Marks)

In any attempt to reconstruct the chain of events, careful analysis of the cutaneous lesions may provide the most valuable lead in the investigation of the case. The skin is a relatively thin layer of tissue but highly resistant to the passage of electric current; resistance is not homogeneous, and at certain points insulation is poor. At these points, ion mobilization of cellular fluids takes place, resulting in damage to the cell membranes. The diminished tissue resistance allows the current to "penetrate" the skin.

The higher the voltage, the greater is the chance of skin penetration. The same is true of the length of electric contact, until a point is reached at which cutaneous resistance is reduced to zero. Lesions induced by electrical force are generally known as *current marks*. Not uncommonly they are not detectable. According to Koeppen and co-workers, current marks are not likely to occur if the contact of the current is over a large surface of the body and if the time of impact is only a few seconds and the amperage is 1.5 amp at the most. On practical grounds, reduced cutaneous resistance and low density of current are the two factors that facilitate the traceless passing of the current through the skin. A classic example is provided by the electric death in the bathtub. It follows that a severe or lethal accident is not necessarily associated with current marks; it is therefore inappropriate to draw conclusions on the severity of an accident solely on the basis of the presence or absence of current marks.

Current marks vary from superficial circumscribed lesions to severe burns with full-thickness tissue necrosis. The factors responsible for the injury are generally listed as electrospecific, electrothermic, thermic, and due to secondary trauma.

So far it has not been possible to differentiate the alterations caused by the electrospecific force from those induced by other factors.

According to Joule's law, *hyperthermia* plays a primary role in the causation of the current marks, and not infrequently it is difficult to differentiate a current mark from a burn produced from other causes.[29-31] The only difference is in the origin of the force that is responsible for the injury; in a "burn" (as generally understood) it is of an extrinsic nature, whereas in an electrothermic burn it is produced within the tissue itself.

As a general rule, electric burns are less uniform than common burns, and between the damaged areas one may still note intact areas. The injury is often more severe when there has been simultaneous burning of clothing adhering to the skin (Figs. 17–2 to 17–4).

Current marks give useful information on the path pursued by the current. The lesion may be limited to the epidermis and be characterized by a grayish-white parchmentlike alteration, or it may extend into the corium or even deeper into the subjacent tissues, giving rise to a crater-shaped ulcer with curling borders (Fig. 17–5). Not infrequently the lesion is surrounded by a bright red area of hyperemia including vesicles as seen in a second-degree burn from other causes.

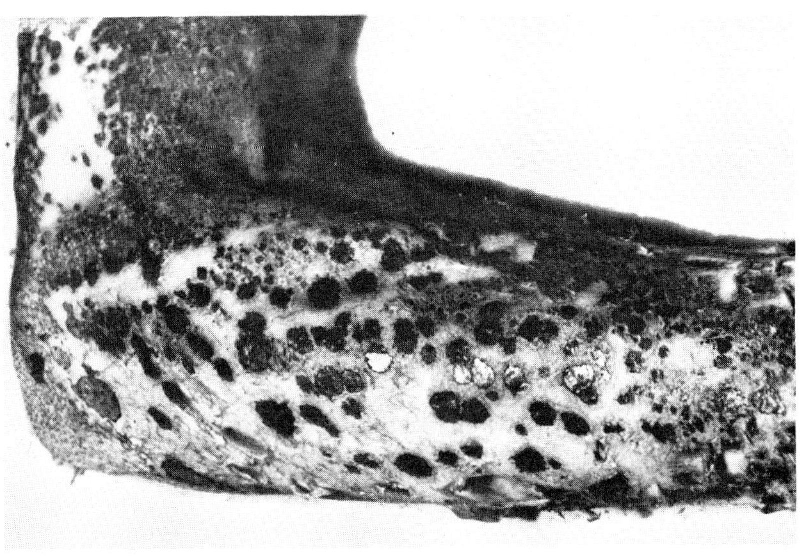

Figure 17–2. Multiple burns on the arm, including vesicular lesions caused by high-potential current.

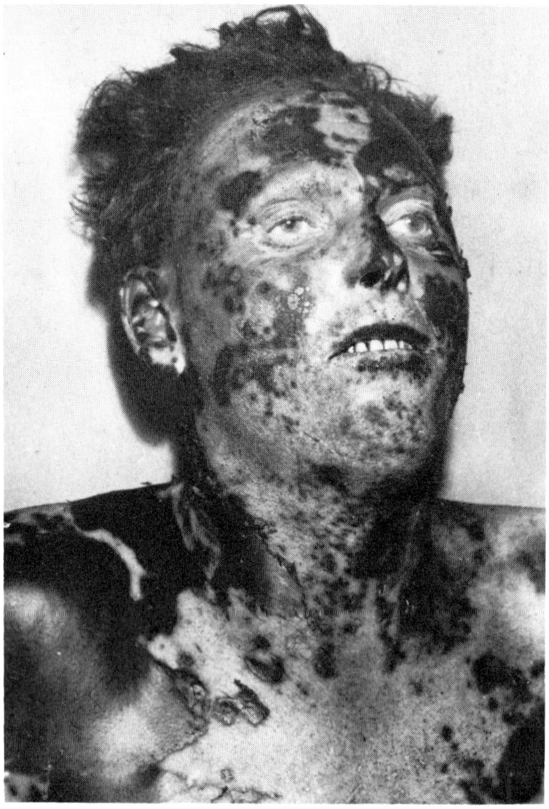

Figure 17–3. Severe burns on the head and upper chest caused by high-voltage current.

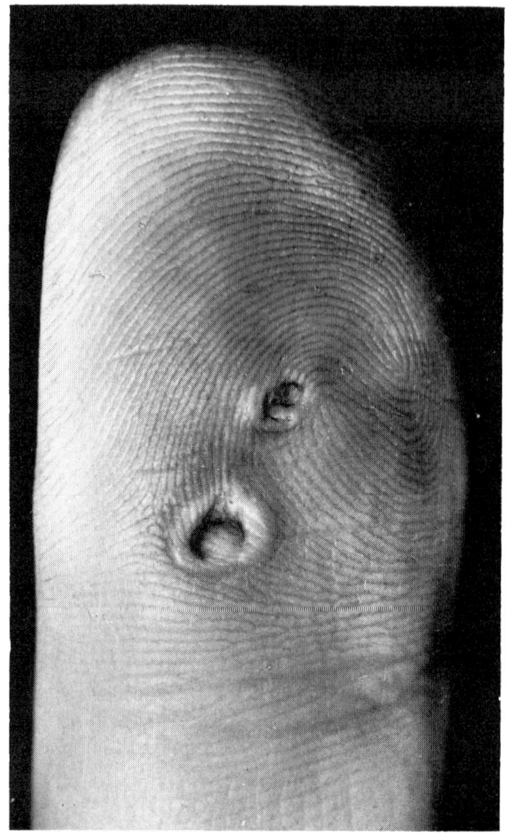

Figure 17–5. Characteristic current mark with round, curved-up borders (finger).

The current mark may be the size of a pinhead or a lentil, but rarely larger. Generally speaking, it is of the same size as the conductor with which the victim comes in contact. The shape of the wound varies and in general mirrors the shape of the object that caused the injury (Figs. 17–6 and 17–7). In some instances, the skin appears linearly divided, mimicking an incisional wound. The smell of recent current marks resembles that of burnt cork.

Current marks are characteristically found at

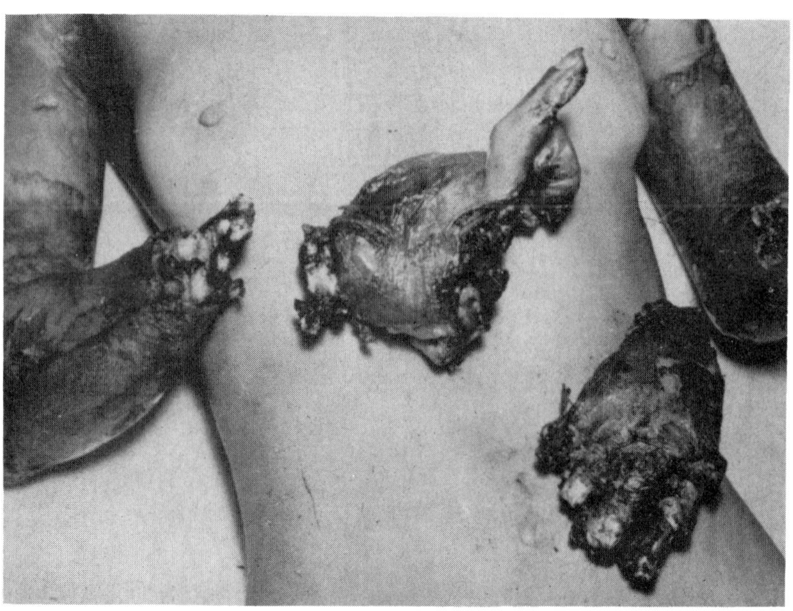

Figure 17–4. Charring and amputation of both hands following contact with current of 10,000 v.

the site of entrance and exit of the electric current (Fig. 17–8). Most fatalities occur when the current passes from hand to hand and from head to foot, namely, when the path of the electric force crosses the heart or the brain stem. Other routes such as hand to foot, foot to foot, and back to front are less inclined to interfere with vital functions.

The current mark may occur under the intact clothing or hair and therefore may remain unnoticed. In a case described by Mueller, current marks were not discernible in a body lying in the rain, but became visible the next day after the body was moved and the skin dried out.[32]

Microscopically the current mark is characterized by separation of cells in the form of sharp slits, attributed by Kaplan to electrodynamic force.[33] This particular pattern has become known as "electric channels." Equally characteristic is the fasciculated arrangement of the cells and the elongation of both cells and nuclei. Using histochemical techniques and electron microscopy methods, Somogyi has contributed detailed observations on the nature of the changes that characterize the current mark, including the progresssive disappearance of dermasome layers, obliteration of cellular and nuclear membranes, destruction of mitochondria, and detachment of basal membranes (Fig. 17–9).[34–38]

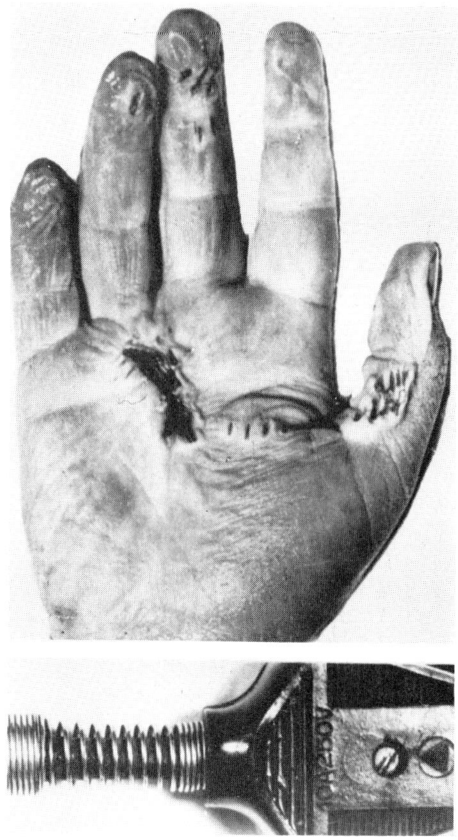

Figure 17–7. Electric shock from defectively insulated wire on electric iron caused the impression of the wire spiral under voltage on the palm and finger tips.

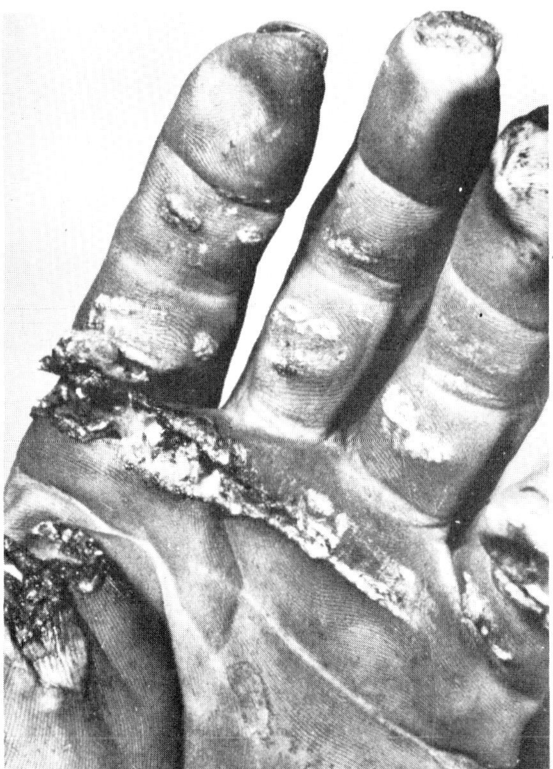

Figure 17–6. Linear and rounded penetrating current marks of the hand and ventral side of fingers.

From the forensic standpoint, it is important to realize that current marks may also be induced postmortem. In their general appearance they correspond to those on a living person. Although the current mark is proof that current passed through the body, only the detection of vital reactions will decide whether the exposure to the current occurred before or after death.

Whenever occult current marks are suspected in a corpse, Prokop recommends the dissection of the carpal flexor muscles. By this method the palm of the hand can be more easily surveyed, and even small current marks can be detected in the folds of the palms or between the fingers.[39]

The current mark is fairly resistant to postmortem decomposition and may be demonstrable for a considerable time on a buried corpse. In questionable cases, it is worthwhile to carry out an exhumation.[40]

Schrader has shown that under the influence of alternating current of 50-Hz frequency, ion migration and electrolysis take place.[41] As this occurs, the tissular acid ions of negative charge combine with the metals of the electrode to form salts that diffuse into the tissue. This process depends both on the density of the current and on the type of metal. From the standpoint of identification, therefore, the most important change at the point of entry of the current is the penetration of metal into the skin that may take place both with direct and with alternating current (skin metallization).

The color of the imprint left by the metal depends on the composition of the electrode: that of iron is brownish black, that of copper is reddish brown, and that of aluminum is silvery. The metallized skin desquamates within a few weeks. In rare cases the metallic coating may also be observed on the nails; usually in this location it disappears progressively as the nails grow. Metallization provides decisive evidence that the burn was produced by electrothermic force. By spectroscopic or histochemical analysis the nature of the metal may be determined. This can easily be accomplished by scraping the metallized epithelium or by obtaining a skin fragment and submitting the sample to spectrographic or histochemical analysis.[42] In every case a similar control specimen from the adjacent normal skin must be obtained and tested.

The polarographic method is suitable for detecting metallic particles even in marks undergoing postmortem decomposition. By spectral analysis in various skin layers, it has been shown that copper, iron, and chromium penetrate 5 mm; and zinc, magnesium, manganese, molybdenum, and aluminum, 3 mm.[43] So far a suitable explanation has not been found for this difference in penetrating power.

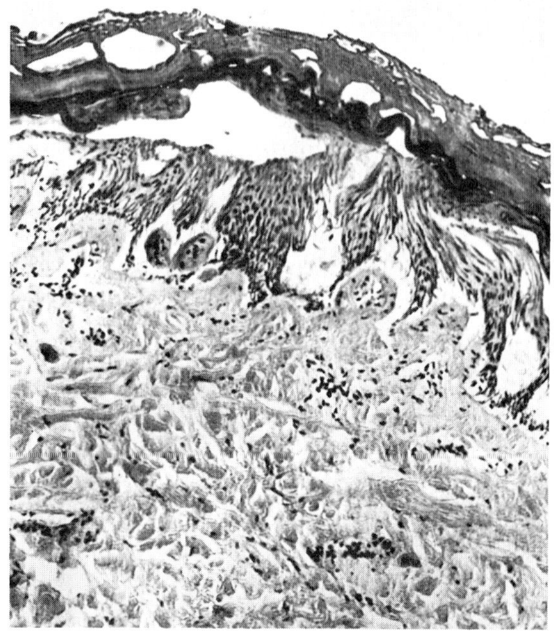

Figure 17–9. Microscopic view of current marks showing lifting of corium, elongation of malpighian cells, and homogenization of subcutaneous tissue.

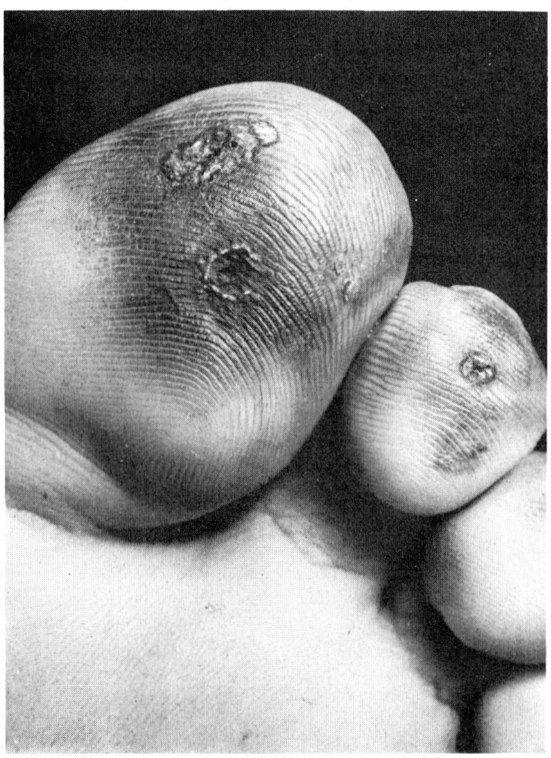

Figure 17–8. Exit current marks (toes).

Other methods are available for the demonstration of the different metals, including the *acroreaction test* devised by Adjutantis and Skalos, which is capable of demonstrating metal particles on skin surfaces by simple color reactions.[44]

Whenever the voltage is high enough to overcome the breakdown potential of the air, an arc may be caused by touching or getting near an electric line under tension. Carriero reported the case of a 28-year-old electrical technician who suffered burns over two thirds of the body surface without contacting the source of the electrical force. The current was transmitted by the ionized air within the transformer.[45]

A typical feature of arcing is that its effects last only for a few seconds. The temperature it can develop may, however, attain 3,000° or 4,000°C, and even this short exposure may produce profound burns. Death may occur, although the current does not pass through the body. In conjunction with the arc effect, a considerable number of metal and gas particles are deposited on the skin, and the vaporized metal metallizes the skin, producing typical marks. Since the *light intensity* of the electric arc is very great, the exposed person shuts his eyes reflexively, and the heat as well as the metallic impurities leads to the formation of a "crowsfeet-like" pattern around the eyes.

The arc of a current of high potential may affect not only the soft tissues but also the bones. If the person exposed to an electric arc simultaneously touches an electric line, the heat produced will be of such a degree as to induce immediate carbonization of the tissue, an occurrence that in some way is beneficial, interrupting the circuit (self-disconnection).

In 15 per cent of electrical accidents there is associated mechanical trauma.[46] The victim of an electric shock often becomes unconscious and falls to the ground, not uncommonly from a height, injuring himself. Thus for a proper reconstruction of the events related to the accident, it is important to differentiate the injuries related to the electric shock from the injuries that have resulted from the fall to the ground.

In electrical trauma involving the face, not only the skin but also the mucous membranes of the oral cavity may become affected. Lesions of the mucous membranes are prominent in small children, who are likely to put every object into their mouths. It is not infrequent that a child puts both poles of an electric plug in the mouth, thus producing a short circuit.

Kaplan studied electrical accidents of the face and oral cavity, which according to his observations represent the second most frequent localization after the upper extremities.[47] A case reported by Schleyer illustrates this situation: A child, three and a half years old, bent down for a drink from a water tap situated in a courtyard. As soon as the tap was opened, the child's jaws became locked on it, and only by forcibly opening his jaws did the child's mother succeed in pulling him away from the tap. The child was blue, his face was swollen, and blood flowed from his mouth. After a few convulsions he expired. Investigation of the accident showed that the water tap was in a circuit of 240 v and that, by opening the water tap, the child had placed himself in the circuit.[48]

Similarly worth reporting is the situation described by DeFazio and Loving in which two small children (aged 14 and 24 months) and an older child (a 10-year-old girl) placed the loose plug of an electric household appliance charged with an alternating current of 125 to 225 v in their mouths. All three children suffered injuries of the oral mucosa, and the tips of the tongues became necrotized. Typical current marks were noted in the resected tissue.[49]

Muscles and Tendons

Among the tissues of the body, striated muscle possesses the greatest electric conducting power. The effect of electric current on muscles is twofold: having components related to the direct stimulation of the motor neuromuscular plaques and components related to the local elevation in temperature. The response to the former is muscular contraction; the latter produces electrothermic injury.

Muscular contraction affects both the agonistic and antagonistic muscles. During voluntary contraction, the effective relation between the function of agonistic and antagonistic muscles is regulated by the central nervous system. Under stimulation by electric current, the central regulation ceases and muscular action is rendered autochthonous. If the power of agonistic and antagonistic muscles were identical, muscle tone, but no contraction, would develop. The power of one of the muscle groups prevails over the other, however. For instance, if the muscles of the hand are relaxed in mid-position and an electric stimulus of identical intensity acts simultaneously upon the tensor and flexor muscles, flexor muscles will prevail and digital flexion will take place.

Experience indicates that electric stimuli rarely affect the muscles in the state of relaxation or mid-position. Therefore the induced contraction is influenced by the momentary state of muscular activity. A person contacting the line under voltage with his hands will keep a tight hold on the line because of the powerful contraction of the flexor muscles. If he does not become unconscious, he may with some effort (depending upon the degree of current) take his hands off the line, but if the intensity of the current is very high (about 15 ma or more), he will not be able to release the line even by exerting maximal effort. To use a generally employed expression, the current "takes hold" of the victim of the accident. According to Maclachlan, in the case of a high-voltage circuit, muscular spasm occurs as soon as the hand reaches the electromagnetic field surrounding the conductor.[50]

Jellinek has pointed out that the effects of the current are greatly influenced by the degree of preparedness of the person involved in the accident; they are more severe if the electric shock is unexpected or unforeseen, and conversely, they will be less severe if some degree of preparedness exists and escape movements are rapidly effected.[51] The functional state of the muscle at the time of impact, the posture of the body, and the speed of escaping movements may influence the outcome of the accident.

The violent and uncoordinated muscular contraction induced by the current may cause alterations in the affected muscles.

A sensation of pain in the muscles, usually described as muscular strain, is a common complaint among surviving victims of an accident. In general, this painful sensation disappears spontaneously within 24 to 48 hours.

Tearing of muscle is a comparatively rare sequel. It may, however, be assumed that it occurs more frequently than is actually diagnosed.

In 62 cases of electric shock with lethal outcome, Incze and Arvay noted muscular rupture in only two. The history of one of these cases is worth reporting:

> A 33-year-old stoker was standing on a coal wagon pushing coal to a locomotive with a long iron shovel. Inadvertently the handle touched the overhead wire carrying 11,000 v, and a voltaic arc burst out. The stoker fell down in the coal wagon, became unconscious, and died three quarters of an hour after the accident. At autopsy, deep current marks (scorched and charred areas) were noted in the palms of both hands. On the soles of the feet current marks of egress were present. Burns were also visible from the region of the right nipple down to the left side of the pubes. On the flexor side of the upper third of the right arm, there were bulging masses covered by intact skin. On dissection these masses were identified as the biceps, severed from the tendinous insertion. A few fresh blood suffusions were also noticeable.[52]

Guglielmetti and co-workers tested the effect of curare in experimental animals exposed to currents of various intensities. The group of animals receiving curare in a dose sufficient to prevent muscular contraction showed a lower level of serum phosphocreatine than the noncurarized electrocuted animals.[53]

The electrothermic action of the current is another cause of muscular damage. This takes place primarily in high-voltage electrical accidents. The muscles undergo various degrees of burns, and as the fluid content of the muscle vaporizes, within milliseconds the muscular tissue becomes "stewed" in the vapor. On cross-section the tissue is grayish white, resembling skinned fish melted into a homogeneous mass. If the temperature exceeds the flashpoint of the muscular tissue, the muscle will ignite and burn until the stage of charring is reached. Severe injuries of this kind are generally observed after protracted contact with the current and as a rule have a lethal outcome.

In contrast to muscle burns from other causes, in electrothermic injury the formation of intense heat takes place within the muscular tissue and affects simultaneously, within a fraction of a second, both superficial and deep layers of tissue.

Microscopically, electrothermic muscular injury is characterized by the spiral or corkscrew-like appearance of muscle fibers, their transformation into bands of hyaline material, loss of striations, granular disintegration, and the patterns of coagulation necrosis.[54]

Large quantities of myoglobin are released from the injured muscles. Myoglobinemia may develop within a few seconds and reach the maximum within one hour. The quantity of myoglobin excreted with the urine may reach several grams and lead to obstruction of renal tubules as seen in the crush syndrome of acute tubular necrosis.[55]

Rupture of tendons is uncommon. The tensile strength of tendons exceeds that of muscles, and the break in tissue continuity takes place at the junction between tendon and muscle.

Bones and Joints

The violent muscular contractions may lead to fracture of bones; this occurrence not infrequently is overlooked because other injuries require more prompt attention.

In one case of personal observation (Somogyi), fracture of the femur was detected five days after the accident, and two fractured ribs were detected three weeks later. In one of the cases reported by Burgel, a fracture was not detected until nine months after the accident.[56]

In general, the portions of bone most likely to break off are the processes or tubercles where large muscles are inserted.

At the level of the shoulder girdle and the upper extremities, the bones most likely to undergo fracture, in order of frequency, are the head of the humerus, the neck of the humerus, and the ulna. Luxation of the shoulder joint is also far from uncommon.[57] According to Jenny, fracture of the coracoid process almost invariably occurs.[58] Thomas indicates that fracture of the humerus is typical in the elderly and luxation of the shoulder girdle is typical in the young.

In the lower extremities, fracture of the femoral neck leads the list. In the vertebral column, fracture of spinal processes is more frequent than compression fracture of the bodies of the vertebrae. According to Bassett the hydroxyapatite crystals present in bone have a piezoelectric property. As a result, during the stress of the trauma, an electric charge is generated within the bone, leading to its deformation.[60]

In high-voltage accidents, bones do not escape electrothermic effects resulting in osteonecrosis and actual "melting" of bone tissue. The characteristic products of "melting" are the so-called "osseous pearls" of phosphoric acid calcium. They are the size of a pea, grayish white, and hollow, and usually are found on the surface of the injured bone. Their formation has been attributed by Pietrusky to fluid vaporization within the spongiosa. When the victim of the accident survives, extrusion of bony sequestra may occur and persist several months after healing of the soft tissues.

On bones adjacent to electrothermic burns involving soft tissues, fissures may be noted. They can be as thin as hair and therefore can be missed at roentgenologic examination. Because of their irregular course they have been compared to the zigzag fissures seen on trees struck by lightning and accordingly labeled *osseous schisis.*

Electrical injury of the skull is rather uncommon; when it does occur, it is in general caused by arcing. This serious injury is most likely to take place when transformer and switch operators and persons working on utility poles inadvertently touch the cable with the vertex of the head. In two cases described by Fritz, following contact with a current of 15,000 v, the skull split open and the orbital contents were extruded through the eye sockets; this explosive effect was attributed to the boiling of the brain and the formation of steam within the skull.[63] Under similar conditions, decapitation has been recorded.[64]

Tissue ischemia from diminished or obstructed blood supply may be responsible for late bone injuries.

Vascular lesions may occur percutaneously as well as subcutaneously, namely, under the intact skin, and the damage can range from massive coagulation necrosis of the entire vessel wall to lesions of microscopic dimensions predominantly affecting the media.[65] Intimal changes as a rule are less prominent, inasmuch as this layer is somewhat protected by the cooling effect of the circulating blood.[66] Hemorrhage and thrombosis are within the natural course of events; delayed hemorrhages, one to six weeks after the accident, have been reported.[67, 68] Expectedly, thrombosis is frequently associated with thromboembolism and related complications.

Tissue edema (edema electricum) is another phenomenon connected with immediate and late vascular injury.

Heart and Circulatory System

Acute Reaction. On brief exposure to low-voltage current, cardiac action may momentarily cease but start again promptly, though with irregularities, and chest pains and dyspnea are among the complaints. A few hours after the accident the heart function returns to normal and the electrocardiogram fails to reveal abnormalities.

The situation is entirely different when there is exposure to a current of greater intensity and following a contact of longer duration. The victim lies unconscious, the skin is cool, the face is pale, occasionally cyanotic, the eyes are fixed, pupillary reaction is absent. If the pulse is not palpable and heart sounds are not perceptible, either ventricular fibrillation or cardiac arrest has taken place. Blood pressure is not measurable, and within a few minutes, after a short period of rattled breathing, respiration stops; however, without the assistance of the electrocardiogram there is no certain way to establish whether death has occurred.

The accident caused by high-potential current and arcing has a different effect on the heart. Ventricular fibrillation does not occur; conversely the electrical insult primarily affects the respiratory center, and in fortunate cases reactivation can be established by prompt resuscitative procedures.

Late Manifestations and Morphologic Changes. The occurrence of pains in the precordial region, exactly mimicking those occurring in angina pectoris (the so-called *angina pectoris electrica*), is frequently listed among the sequelae of electrical injury.[69] Palpitation, sweating, restlessness, and labored breathing are associated manifestations. A preexisting heart condition may accentuate these disorders, but they have, however, been described as well in young and middle-aged people (between 15 and 45 years old). From a medicolegal standpoint, the angina that follows electrical trauma can be considered related to the injury only when the medical history indicates that prior to the accident the individual was free of manifestations of arteriosclerotic heart disease. As a rule the anginal attacks fade away within weeks or months and the electrocardiogram returns to normal. The same is true of auricular fibrillation, sinus tachycardia (less frequently sinus bradycardia), and other manifestations of cardiac arrhythmia. This does not rule out, in individual cases, persistence of electrocardiographic changes and other manifestations of cardiac disorders whenever the heart has suffered ischemic necrosis at the time of the primary electrical injury. By the same token it may be difficult to deny that the electrical injury may deteriorate a preexisting cardiac condition or cause coronary thrombosis, followed by myocardial infarction.[70]

In terms of compensation a prerequisite to fair assessment rests on expert opinion of the nature and severity of the accident, on the age of the victim, and on his physical state prior to the accident. Thus the decision can be based on the comparative evaluation of productivity and working capacity before and after the accident.[71]

The morphologic counterpart of these functional changes lacks specificity. Furthermore, most of the available information is on the hearts of people who succumbed immediately or shortly after the accident, a condition that prevents the development of visible changes. Findings at postmortem examination include dilatation of the auricles and petechial as well as larger hemorrhages on the endocardium, pericardium and myocardium, particularly at the base of the aortic cusps. Fragmentation and twisting of myofibers, interstitial edema, and foci of colliquative necrosis have also been recorded.[72] By electron microscopy, more subtle changes—from detachment of the external mitochondrial membrane to rupture or total disarrangement of myofibers—have been described in rabbits exposed to low-voltage current (Fig. 17–10). Histochemical changes have also been recorded and interpreted as direct manifestations of the passage of the electric current.[73, 74]

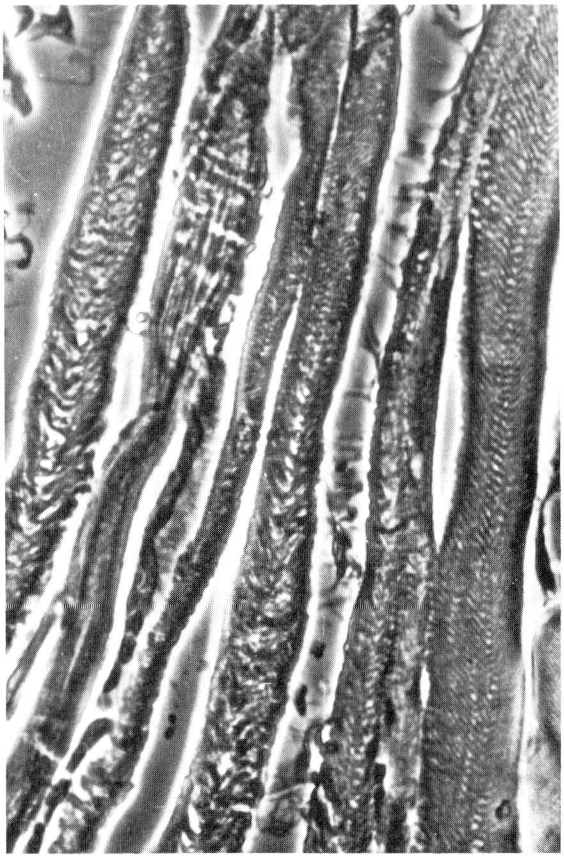

Figure 17–10. Phase-contrast photomicrograph of myocardium showing incipient irregular contraction, homogenization, and incipient disintegration of myofibrils. ×410.

Nervous System

Acute Response. Loss of consciousness frequently occurs. According to Kawamura, this takes place in three fourths of accidents caused by high-voltage current and in one third of accidents caused by low-voltage current.[75] On exposure to a voltage of less than 1,000 v, the duration of unconsciousness rarely exceeds a few seconds, whereas above 1,000 v, unconsciousness is inclined to persist and frequently to progress to coma and death. Other common manifestations, such as persistent headache, somnolence, disorders in cardiac rhythm and respiration, nausea, vomiting, and convulsions, have been linked to cerebral edema and increased intracranial pressure. Patients who did not become unconscious at the time of the accident have described their sensations as painful muscular spasms, darkening of the visual field, loss of hearing, and distorted feelings, such as swelling of the head and shrinking of the body to unrealistic dimensions.[76] Critchley reports that some of his patients recalled feeling pulsating sensations, enabling them to "count the number of alternating current cycles." He also mentions the frequently distorted appreciation of time—for instance, an electric contact of 5 seconds being estimated by the patient as having lasted 10 minutes.[77] Paresthesias are common, particularly a feeling of numbness in the extremities.

In a series of 212 survivors analyzed by one of us (Somogyi), 96 became unconscious at the time of the accident; they just collapsed without emitting a sound. Rarely did the victim either cry for help or utter inarticulate sounds. No correlation was found in this series between loss of consciousness and voltage; conversely, unconsciousness consistently occurred when the head was in the path of the current and did not occur when the current went from hand to hand or hand to leg.

Late Effects. Total or partial loss of memory is a quite frequent sequela, particularly when the victim of the electrical trauma was rendered unconscious at the time of the accident. The amnesia can last days or weeks, or sometimes longer. The patient is unable to give any information on the accident. Often the amnesia is retrograde and involves events prior to the accident. Psychic reactions also occur frequently, such as a feeling of phobia against electric current or equipment, from mild aversion to horror and all grades of fear.

Evidence of localized neurologic deficit is rarely found. In electrical trauma, except for the lethal effects of heat, the passage of the current through the body fails to elicit brain changes of a lasting nature. Death may result from circulatory failure when the current flows through the heart, or from paralysis of the respiratory center when the current flows through the brain stem, and in both instances systemic anoxia is responsible for the fatal outome.

A debated question is whether or not electrotrauma can be responsible for the development of a psychosis. As in the case of mechanical trauma, it is prudent to say that electrotrauma per se is an unlikely cause of mental disorder; however, it may precipitate a psychotic condition in an individual with a preexisting neurotic temperament or personality difficulties. To pursue the comparison to mechanical trauma further, the role of compensation should not be ignored; the differentiation between compensation neurosis and anxiety neurosis applies as well to electrotrauma.

If the victim of accidental electrocution dies immediately, the elapsed time between the passage of the current and death is so short that cell life stops abruptly and visible alterations have no time to become manifest. The situation is different when the victim survives for a period of time. This period, the length of which is variable, allows the development of the secondary changes usually ascribed to cerebral anoxia. Hemorrhages of varying sizes and irregular in distribution, foci of ganglion cell degeneration, demyelination and fragmentation of neuroaxons, and areas of perivascular necrosis may be seen and are generally attributed to hypoxic damage rather than to the direct effects of the current.[78]

Experimental observations have shown that alternating current of 110 v passed through the brains of animals for periods of from one to three seconds may produce a transient constriction of small meningeal arteries.[79] It is not unlikely that larger amounts of current or longer exposures to the current may elicit permanent vascular damage in the human also and possibly be responsible for ischemic necrosis of tissue supplied by the affected vessels.

Equally connected to vascular damage are epidural, subdural, subarachnoidal, intracerebral, and intraventricular hemorrhages. In the presence of any one of these manifestations, the possible role played by mechanical trauma should be taken into account. Not infrequently the victim of the accident falls to the ground, often from a height, incurring mechanical injuries.

The most conspicuous change in the brain at postmortem examination is the absence of the customary flattening out of the base of the encephalon on the dissecting table. This is probably due to coagulation and hardening of the tissue brought about by the high temperature induced by the current. Temperatures as high as 145°F have been recorded.[80]

The spinal cord is infrequently affected by electrical trauma. Available information on the structural alterations of the spinal cord in electrical injury has been drawn primarily from observations in experimental animals. It has been shown that when the current flows from forefoot to forefoot, a significant amount of current passes through the cord, concentrating at the level of the fifth and seventh cervical segments, then fading away both cranially and caudally.[81] This observation correlates with the clinical findings in humans showing that hand-to-hand contacts cause fairly consistent lesions between the fifth and seventh cervical segments—mainly softening with myelin degeneration, small hemorrhages, and cavitating lesions—eliciting an unpredictable variety of lasting disorders in function.[82, 83] Infrequently a condition that Panse labeled "spinal atrophy" and attributed to vascular insufficiency affecting the anterior horns of the spinal cord becomes manifest a few weeks to several months after the accident.[84] Mainly characterized by weakness and paresthesias of the extremities, it seldom progresses and tends to remain stationary or to regress.[85] It has been stated that a milder form of this disorder may occasionally be encountered among electrotechnicians exposed to repeated electrotrauma.[86] The possibility of an independent, preexisting, or concurrent neurologic condition should be ruled out before ascribing this disorder to electrotrauma.

Sympathetic and Endocrine Systems

Disorders vaguely attributed to dysfunction of the sympathetic and endocrine systems have been described. Although as a rule they pass within a few weeks, they may also last for months. In this category is a broad spectrum of disturbances for which a rational explanation is difficult to find, such as paroxysmal perspiration, dehydration of skin, pigmentolysis, herpetic eruptions, graying and loss of hair, disorders in the menstrual cycle, temporary glycosuria, polyuria, and rapid loss or gain in weight. Manifestations of thyroid dysfunction or diencephalon-pituitary disorders as seen in diabetes insipidus have also been reported.[87] Nevertheless, aside from the reaction to stress, which does not differ from that elicited by any other type of trauma, no clear-cut evidence is available that electrical trauma may be responsible for endocrine disturbances.

Peripheral Nerves

The old concept that the current flow is carried in the body along the nerve trunks and large blood vessels has been disproved. It is now generally acknowledged that current flow proceeds by the shortest path, from contact with current source to contact with ground, without being deflected by anatomical structures.

Injuries of the peripheral nerves are infrequent. Possibly the most common situation in which nerve injury may be expected to occur is in conjunction with severe burning of adjacent tissues, overextension of the limbs, rupture of muscle, and fracture-dislocation of bones and joints.[88]

Observations on cats indicate that the amount of current per unit of nerve diameter necessary to produce lasting disorders in function and structure is 40 ma per 3 mm of nerve diameter and five seconds' shock. Temporary disturbances occur on exposure to lesser forces, the duration of which mathematically correlates the amperage of the current and the time of its flow. Exposure to a current of magnitude sufficient to temporarily abolish irritability and conductivity elicits a vasomotor response. It has been suggested that interference with blood flow is responsible for the myelin degeneration and the changes in axis cylinders noted in disabled nerves at critical levels in cases of lasting disturbances.[82, 83]

Blood and Hematopoietic Systems

After fatal accidents culminating in instantaneous death, the blood is characteristically dark and liquid. If the victim of the accident survives, blood hemolysis (because of the thermal effect), anemia, and an elevation in the serum bilirubin level are frequently found.

Lungs

Pulmonary edema and petechial hemorrhages are usually seen in cases of electrocution and have been noticed as well in experimental animals submitted to electric shock.[89] In a victim of high-voltage accident, Custer found burns on the apical lobe of one of the lungs and concurrent pneumothorax, most probably resulting from passage of the current through the victim's lung.[90]

The problem of aggravation of preexisting pulmonary conditions may arise in surviving victims of the accident. The claim can be favorably looked upon whenever it can be demonstrated that: (1) the shock was produced by a current of an intensity sufficient to elicit strong muscular spasm and elevation of blood pressure; (2) the current had passed through the victim's lung; (3) the duration of the contact was long enough to cause direct damage to the lung; and (4) the manifestations of aggravation of the preexisting process became apparent within a short time of the accident, not much beyond a three-week period.

Liver

An elevation in serum bilirubin and bilirubinuria are not infrequently detected after accidental electrocution, but jaundice, as a rule, does not become manifest. In fatal cases no characteristic lesions are found in the liver.

Pancreas

A few cases are on record suggesting that severe electrical trauma directly involving the pancreas may provoke diabetes or activate latent diabetes; the general consensus, however, does not support this concept, and when the problem arises in the course of a medicolegal investigation, as a rule it can be proved that the diabetes existed prior to the electrical accident.

Alimentary Tract

Petechial or larger hemorrhages in the gastrointestinal mucosa are found in 1 of 100 fatal electrocutions.[91] A case is on record of perforation of a preexisting chronic peptic ulcer following the accident.[92] These nonspecific lesions can be categorized as manifestations of systemic anoxia and stress.

Kidneys

Renal failure is a common complication of high-voltage and electric-arc accidents associated with extensive body burns.

Oliguria, rapidly progressing to anuria, rise of nonprotein nitrogen values, electrolyte imbalance, and proteinuria are the usual clinical manifestations; the findings at postmortem duplicate those of acute tubular nephrosis. In conjunction with extensive burning of muscle, myoglobin is released through the kidneys, the urine assumes the reddish brown color associated with myoglobinuria, and numerous myoglobin casts are found in the renal tubules at the microscopic examination of the kidneys.[90, 93-95]

Organs of Sense

Ear

Whenever the ear is in the path of the current, a broad spectrum of lesions and related functional deficits is likely to occur. As a rule the type and severity of the lesions are not directly related to the nature of the current nor to the intensity of the voltage.[96] Any portion of the hearing apparatus, including the acoustic nerve, may be affected. Hemorrhages in the tympanic membrane, middle ear, cochlea, cochlear duct, and vestibular apparatus have been described; among the sequelae secondary infection is not uncommon; mastoiditis, sinus thrombosis, meningitis, and brain abscess have all been recorded. The hearing deficit may become manifest immediately after the accident or shortly thereafter; it can be temporary or permanent.

In matters of compensation it must be ascertained that the patient's hearing was normal prior to the accident, that the clinical symptoms developed immediately after the accident—with no complaint-free period—or at the utmost after an interval not exceeding a few weeks.[97]

Eye

Ocular lesions connected with electrical accidents can be ascribed to two categories of phenomena: electrothermal effect and light effect (arc flash).

Electrothermal burns may affect the eyelids, eyebrows, eyelashes, conjunctiva, and cornea. In the cornea the lesions may range from temporary hyperemia to third-degree burns. Guist has stressed the stripelike opacities on the cornea, likely to progress to circumscribed areas of necrosis and ulceration.[98] There is no portion of the eye that can escape injury. Among the most frequent manifestations, photopsy, strabismus, ptosis, paralysis of ocular muscles, disturbances in accommodation, scotomas, and narrowing of the field of vision have been recorded.[99] Kaplan observed a decrease in ocular tension as a regular reaction to electrical trauma.[33] The list of detectable lesions includes intraocular hemorrhage and thrombosis, uveitis, retinal edema and detachment, papillitis, and atrophy of the optic nerve.

Some of the minor disorders, such as conjunctival congestion or winking spasm, may disappear in a few days and the patient's vision be restored completely. Other disorders appear later and slowly progress to a permanent lesion. This is the case for cataract formation, the development of which may become manifest anywhere from a few weeks or months to several years after the accident.[100, 101]

Cataracts caused by electrothermic injury are generally unilateral—in contrast to the cataracts induced by lightning, in which both eyes are usually affected. It has been suggested that it is prerequisite to cataract formation that the current pass through the eye, but this does not invariably seem to be the case; cataract formation has been described also after the passage of the current through the head or through the body of the victim. Equally variable is the potential of voltage, ranging from 220 to 30,000 v. In the majority of cases the development of the cataract takes from two months to two years, but on occasion the process remains stationary and sporadically regresses. Thus it is difficult to set an exact prognosis on the outcome of the lenticular opacity.

The ocular lesions induced by arc light or electric arc are of a different nature. They are caused solely by the exposure to intense light, including infrared, visible, and ultraviolet rays in different proportions. Each of these rays penetrates the eye to a different depth, in conformity with its own wavelength.[102, 103]

If the eye is not protected, approximately 20 per cent of the energy is absorbed by the lens, 40 per cent is absorbed by the vitreous body, and 12 per cent reaches the retina.

Photopsy appears immediately after the exposure, and after a latent period of 3 to 10 hours, the eyelids become edematous, the conjunctiva become swollen and congested, blepharospasm develops, and the patient is hardly capable of opening his eyes. He complains of pains in the forehead and feels as if his eyes were full of sharp, prickling sand. Although the acute stage of the reaction looks very alarming, as a rule the course is benign; the entire process subsides in two to three days, and the working ability of the victim of the accident is restored within a few days. It is doubtful that a single exposure to an electric arc will lead to cataract formation.

In brief, the reaction of the eye to electric arc is similar to its reaction to excessive exposure to the rays of the sun (retinitis solaris or eccliptica). Many such ocular reactions occurred among the observers of the eclipse of the sun in 1912; fortunately, as a result of an extensive educational campaign stressing prophylactic protective measures, fewer occurred during the similar event in 1954.

Photoelectric ocular disorders often occur among *welders*. Welders usually put on their goggles only when they have placed the soldering iron on the right spot. Any delay in applying this protective measure may lead to "arc eye" injury. After a few hours lacrimation begins, and often the patient sees colored circles around objects—the result of diffraction—caused by swelling of the superficial cells of the cornea. Accidental exposure of the unprotected eye to arc light primarily affects the macula; longer, repeated exposures may lead to retinitis.[102]

The question of whether cataracts are likely to occur among welders has been a source of conflicting reports. According to some investigators, ultraviolet rays are not "cataractogenic"; conversely, others have presented evidence that repeated exposure to infrared rays can damage the lens. This primarily occurs in industrial activities related to metallurgy, and among glass and furnace workers.[99, 103]

ELECTROSHOCK THERAPY

Electroshock therapy, introduced by Cerletti and Bini in 1938, is widely used in treatment of mental disorders.[104] As originally devised, the method consists of the application of electric impulses capable of eliciting tonoclonic convulsions and loss of consciousness. During this period the patient is apneic, but normal respiration is reestablished within 45 seconds. About five minutes after the seizure the patient regains consciousness, then usually sleeps for several hours and on awakening has no recollection of the treatment. During the postseizure period, leukocytosis, hyperpotassemia, and an increase of the serum bilirubin level have been recorded.[105] Electrocardiographic changes have also been described but generally disappear within one to two hours and rarely persist longer.[106]

Fatal complications of electroshock therapy are rare and almost invariably their cause is found in unrelated conditions, most likely a cardiac disorder or the unescapable degenerative disorders associated with the process of aging. It is now acknowledged that in the human no structural alterations or ill effects occur in the brain or in other organs as a result of therapeutic electroshock.

Skeletal fractures and dislocations were not uncommon when convulsions were not controlled. According to Müller, fractures occurred in 2.48 per cent of the patients, and vertebral fractures led the list (1.31 per cent), followed by scapular, humeral and femoral neck, and pelvic bone fractures.[107]

In the vertebral column, compression fractures were more common than arch fractures, and the fifth to the eighth dorsal segments were the ones more frequently affected. Dislocations of ankle, shoulder, elbow, and mandible were also reported, and cases are on record of habitual luxation of the jawbone occurring at each convulsive treatment.

Fatal cases of cerebral fat embolism were also described in conjunction with bony fractures.[108]

With the administration of muscle relaxants and anesthetic drugs, the intensity of the seizures has greatly decreased, and the occurrence of fracture-dislocations has declined in a parallel course. From a practical standpoint they are no longer a matter of concern. Among the complications or side effects, mental confusion and memory defects deserve consideration. As a rule these manifestations are transitory and do not necessitate the interruption of the therapy; however, the patient should be warned in advance that side effects of this type can be expected. Electroencephalographic changes have been described during and immediately after the seizure, to disappear within one to two hours.[109]

In contrast to the observations in humans, which clearly indicate that electric shock is not conducive to organic brain damage, a broad spectrum of lesions has been described in experimental animals submitted to electroshock under conditions comparable to those under which shock treatment is carried out in man. Hemorrhages in various parts of the brain, demyelinization of axis cylinders, vacuolization of oligodendroglia, degeneration of nerve cells, neuronophagia, and gliosis have been described.[110, 111] Differences in animal species and methods have, however, resulted in findings so lacking in uniformity that extrapolation of the results to the human is unreliable.

It is the duty of the physician who is planning to carry out the treatment to inform the patient (or the closest relative if the patient is incapable of making decisions) of the risks (remote as they are) associated with the treatment and to obtain written authorization to proceed. On account of the increased risk, shock treatment should be avoided in elderly people and in people with cardiovascular or respiratory disorders or fragility of bones.

ELECTRIC SHOCK AND PREGNANCY

According to the type and intensity of the current and the duration of the contact, electric shock in pregnancy can lead to one or the other of the following effects: (1) death both of the mother and of the product of conception; (2) survival of the mother and death of the fetus; (3) survival of both mother and fetus, namely, the pregnancy proceeds undisturbed; (4) death of the mother and survival of the fetus if it is promptly removed from the mother at term or close to term; or (5) death of the fetus, with or without spontaneous abortion, hours or days or weeks after the accident.

The positive correlation between the electric shock and the ensuing loss of the product of conception is generally acknowledged under the following conditions:

1. There has been normal pregnancy (pregnancies) and delivery (deliveries) in the past gestational history of the mother.
2. The course of the pregnancy was uneventful until the occurrence of the accident.
3. The accident has been proved.
4. No other factor or factors can be advocated to explain the loss of the fetus or the death of the mother.
5. The stage of development of the dead fetus corresponds to the stage of pregnancy, and the degree and extent of its maceration is proportional to the time that has elapsed between the accident and the death of the fetus.

The fetus is less resistant to electric shock than the mother. Both the hyperemic pregnant uterus and the amniotic fluid are exceptionally good conductors. Fetal skin offers 200 times less resistance to the passage of current than does postnatal skin. According to Dordelmann, exposure of the fetus to 100 to 380 v 25 ma current for 0.3 sec may be regarded as lethal.[112] Postmortem observations on the fetus describe dilatation of the heart chambers and hemorrhages in the brain, kidneys, and liver.[113]

Electrical stimulation may elicit uterine contractions and lead to the induction of labor; however, no case is known in which criminal abortion was induced by exposure to electric current. Years ago galvanic current was used on medical indication to provoke uterine contraction. The cathode was inserted into the cervix and the anode was fastened to the waist or to the abdominal wall of the expectant mother. This procedure is no longer applied because of the hazards related to the use of electric current.

A case is on record of fetal death following electroshock treatment applied in the fifth month of pregnancy.[114] Also documented is the occurrence of temporary disturbance in the fetal heart rhythm after electroshock therapy.[115]

The effects of electroshock on the fetus have been profusely tested in the experimental animal, but results cannot be extrapolated to the human.[110] Enough information is available, however, to conclude that an electrical accident to the pregnant mother can endanger the life of the fetus. Should the fetus survive the accident, late ill effects can be expected, although at present actual documentation is lacking.

INJURIES CAUSED BY ELECTROMAGNETIC WAVES

Physical therapists exposed for a long time to poorly protected shortwave apparatus not infrequently complain of vague general malaise and weakness, apathy, anxiety, and frequent headaches. Similar manifestations have been noted in persons attached to radar stations, in individuals operating radiofrequency generators, and in the technical personnel of broadcasting stations. As a rule, these disturbances disappear after a short period of rest.[116-120]

The effects of electromagnetic waves have been studied in frog nerve-muscle preparations, birds, insects, guinea pigs, plants, and viruses.[121, 122]

Experimental evidence from these different sources indicates that electromagnetic waves of frequencies ranging from short waves to microwaves elicit biologic effects that are proportional to field strength and inversely proportional to wavelength.

As to underlying mechanisms, the majority of investigators favor the theory that the biologic effects are related to the conversion of the absorbed energy to heat.

Efficient prevention of the effects of high-frequency electric waves on the organism rests on the determination of permissible maximal field strength. Field strength, in the case of microwaves, is expressed as power output per surface unit, i.e., as power density (W/cm^2). At the radar stations of the United States Army, no ill effects have been recorded even after prolonged exposure to $10^{-2} W/cm^2$. The twentieth part of that power density, -5×10^{-4} W/cm^2, has been accepted by the North Atlantic Union as the safety limit. The maximum permissible density in the Soviet Union is 10^{-5} W/cm^2.

American airframe manufacturers have defined three danger zones. In the "inner" zone, intensity may reach $1.31 \times 10^{-2} W/cm^2$; exposure to this zone should be avoided. In the "middle" zone the power density is $3.9 \times 10^{-3} W/cm^2$; prolonged exposure to this zone is prohibited. In the "outer" zone, power density is less than that in the middle zone and is considered biologically ineffective; persistent exposure is deemed permissible.

For individual protection, clothing incorporating metallic fiber has been introduced, and in radar zones with a power density of $10^{-5} W/cm^2$, special goggles are recommended.[123]

STATIC ELECTRICITY

A piece of resin or ebonite rubbed with a piece of fur will attract small pieces of paper placed near it. This well-known classroom experiment exemplifies *static electricity*. The phenomenon is explained as the effect of positive and negative charges. It is less widely known that a static charge can also be produced by the separation of two surfaces without rubbing. The human body acts as a conductor, and the charge acquired by the skin is continuously conducted to earth or dispersed in the atmosphere. When a charged insulated person becomes suddenly grounded the discharge is accompanied by a spark, as a rule lacking sufficient energy to ignite the clothes or to harm the individual unless explosive material or inflammable gases are present. Why certain persons are more susceptible than others to the accumulation of static electricity is not known. Everyone has experienced the sensation of being electrified by grasping the handle of a door or a water faucet, or by the simple contact of the hand with someone else's hand.

Air is not a perfect insulator; the extent of its conductivity depends on the number of ions, small and large, positive and negative, for 1 ml, and this varies with place and time. A person's degree of insulation from earth depends first on the material of the soles of the shoes and second on the material of the clothes. Leather footwear is a good conductor and should be avoided where explosive materials or inflammable gases are present. Modern insulated floors favor the accumulation of static electricity. Synthetic fibers used for clothing (nylon, dacron, orlon, and the like) are hydrophobic and therefore excellent insulators; because of their surface properties they adhere to the skin, acquire and maintain a strong charge, and easily become a source of static electricity.

In industry, accidents caused by static electricity are far from uncommon. Materials on belt conveyors may be significantly charged in paper, textile, and rubber factories. Wetting the inner surface of the belt with a mixture of equal portions of glycerin and water at weekly intervals offers effective protection; water alone is not suitable because of rapid evaporation.

Industrial dust from insulating materials, resins, sugar, sulfur, coal, chocolate, flour, and sawdust, when dispersed in the atmosphere by a draught or other means, may become charged, and a spark may initiate a fire. The investigation of a fire of unknown origin in the printing or paper industry should include evaluation of the effects of static electricity.

Charging may also occur when undiluted solvents, highly resistant to electricity, are transferred from one container to another. The mixture of the vapors of inflammable solvents and air is highly explosive, and a spark of static electricity may be sufficient to set them aflame. The hazards of static electricity in connection with solvents have been described by Watson, and Howard has written on the astonishing effects of static electricity on oil refineries.[124, 125]

A situation recorded by Schwanecke illustrates the phenomenon.

Toluol was being transferred by an electric pump from a large container to small cans standing on the ground. A rubber tube mounted on a grounded metal pipe was hanging into the can. When the can was two thirds full an explosion took place, the toluol went up in flames, and the lines disintegrated.

Investigation of the case led to the conclusion that the rubber (usually offering practically infinite resistance) had become charged with static electricity.[126]

Static electricity may also be the cause of material damage and bodily injury in ungrounded disconnected aerial lines. Charging may occur for various reasons. A strong wind may whirl sand or snow, which on contact with the loose wire will generate frictional electricity (the charge of the cable may be as high as 10,000 v). The negative charge of thunderclouds may produce a positive charge in the cable following induction, or the wire may become charged by the static electricity of the earth. Whatever the operating mechanism, the sudden equalization of the charge may cause an accident.

Another accidental cause of fire and material damage may occur in dry cleaning. The clothes acquire a negative charge by friction with the revolving drum, while a positive charge accumulates in the stationary part of the apparatus. When the door of the machine is opened, a spark may ignite the inflammable vapors.

Equally well known is the formation of static electricity by rubber tires on the road. In the presence of suitable atmospheric conditions, a charge will flow to the undercarriage and from there extend to the body of the car. As the passenger enters the vehicle and touches a metal part, he will feel an electric shock. Voltage may be high, but intensity of the discharge is too low and duration too short to cause any organic damage to the body.

Charge has to be continually led off from vehicles carrying inflammable material, either by chains skimming the ground or by the so-called conducting rubber tires, as used in flying vehicles.

SUICIDE AND HOMICIDE BY ELECTRICAL FORCE

Suicide by the use of electrical force has increased with the spread of electrification, but still stands last among the methods of self-destruction. The method has been applied by both male and female, but predominantly by the former; as far as we could determine, only five cases are on record of suicidal attempts by women. Overall statistics indicate that in 90 per cent of the reported cases, the attempt was successful.[127-131]

Suicidal methods can be grouped in the following major categories: One method consists of climbing a pylon and grasping the wire carrying high-voltage current. In this case loss of consciousness occurs immediately, severe burns take place, and equally serious mechanical injuries are sustained during the fall to the ground. Exposure to the current is short, but death is usually instantaneous. According to another method, the person attempting the suicide does not climb on the pylon, but fastens one end of a long wire to one of the limbs (usually the wrist), grasps it strongly in one hand and throws the other end of the wire (strengthened by a heavy object) over the transmission line. The person loses consciousness and falls to the ground. Disconnection of the current is inhibited by the sudden contraction of the flexor muscles to which one pole of the wire is attached. Long exposure to the current is a characteristic feature of this method of suicide, and severe burns are usually found, to the extent that the limb to which one pole of the wire is attached may become detached. In the third group, alternating current is most frequently used. The prospective suicidal person establishes contact with both ends of the electric supply, winds the wires around his waist or limbs, and switches on the current. The fourth group includes a variety of heterogeneous methods, such as placing the end of an electric line in the mouth to ensure the passage of the current through the head, or using an electric saw to simulate an industrial accident (Figs. 17–11 and 17–12).[131, 132]

Investigation of the case almost invariably reveals a psychopathic personality, a depressive state, a motivating or unmotivating emotional disturbance.

Sensational reports by the communications media on the methods of suicide may lead to imitation by highly suggestible individuals and to serial suicides by the same method. Weimann describes three suicides that occurred in West Berlin within a short period, all performed by the same method. Each of the victims had constructed a clock with a complicated electrical device that switched the current on at a set time.[133]

Electric current is equally used in *homicide* attempts: placing a live wire across a road where a prospective victim is expected to walk or drive, or placing in circuit an object that he is

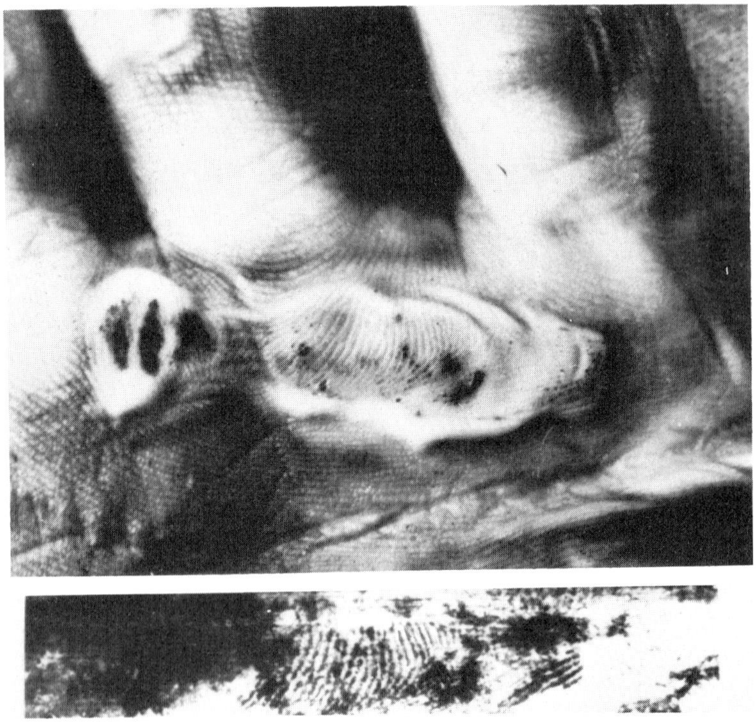

Figure 17–11. Suicide committed by the insertion of tin-lead solder. Notice imprints of the tin-lead solder at the finger root and in the folds of the palm.

expected to touch are well-documented instruments of murder. Bornstein reported a case in which a 22-month-old baby was killed with domestic current by a paranoid schizophrenic who had been living with the child's mother for some months. Cases of women killed by their husbands while taking a bath have not uncommonly been reported in the forensic literature.[134] The investigation of such cases provides a challenge to the investigating team, as the possibility of murder, suicide, and accident may be equally entertained.

LIGHTNING

Lightning, as generally understood, is the discharge of the atmosphere potential between clouds; lightning stroke, in contrast, is the discharge between a cloud and a mass of the earth.[135]

There are many ways by which lightning can induce electric shock: (1) The current of the main discharge may pass directly through the body of the victim (*direct effect*). In this case the intensity of the current may be as high as 30 ka, and the duration of the exposure may be as long as one second. Here death is inevitable. (2) The current of the main discharge may be dispersed in the area where the victim of the accident happened to be. Intensity and duration of the exposure are substantially less, being of the magnitude of 100 a and 0.5 μs. In this situation body damage is induced by the current of counter discharge *(indirect effect)*. Death is probable in this case. (3) The electric shock may be caused by *induced voltage* when the lightning flash strikes a nearby metallic object. In these circumstances, many survive. (4) Lightning shock may also occur inside dwellings at the time of the atmospheric discharge, when the victim of the accident is in physical contact or within arcing distance of an electric iron, electric switch, or loose connection. Any electric apparatus, such as a radio aerial, is a good conductor of lightning; similarly lightning may travel for a long distance on transmission lines. (5) Shock may be sustained when voltage created by dissipated current in the surroundings of the area struck by lightning passes from foot to foot. The relatively innocuous current path is not conducive to serious body damage.

The electric arc of the lightning flash, as well as the radiofrequency electromagnetic waves that are emitted, may spread over several kilometers. This is because the arc is not produced between two metal electrodes, but between two clouds (aerosols) or between a cloud and earth or a cloud and water. Atmospheric gases may become heated to a temperature of 20,000°C, as opposed to the temperature of 3,000°C of technical arc lights.

Rapid heating of gases in the path of light-

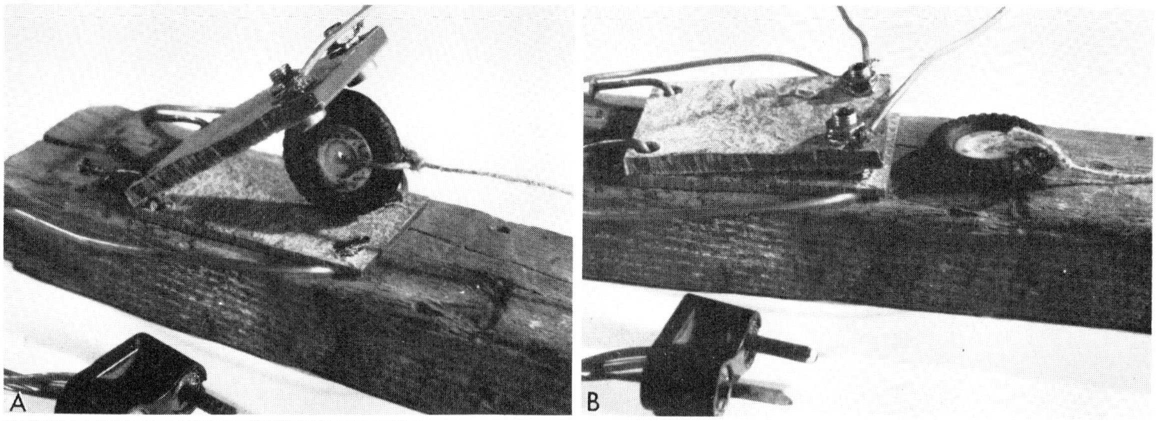

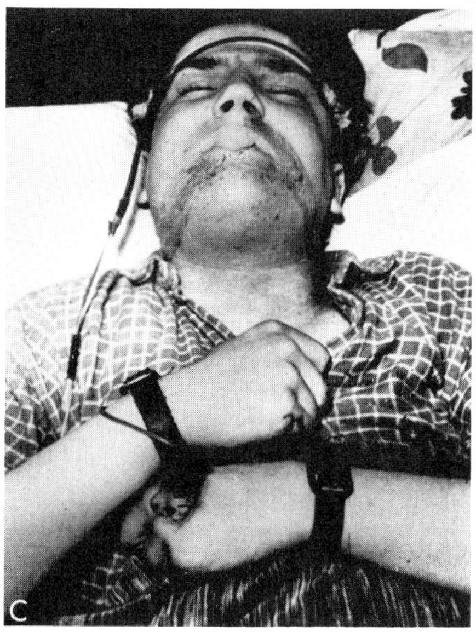

Figure 17–12. *A* and *B*. Instrument used for committing suicide by electric current. The other part of the conductor was attached to the body. The circuit was closed by pulling the rubber out. *C*. Body in the original position. Notice the electrodes fastened to the head and wrists.

ning causes explosive expansion. The resulting compression waves travel in the atmosphere at a higher velocity than acoustic waves. After some kilometers their speed is reduced and they are transformed into acoustic waves. The compressional and decompressional components of the waves vary in proportion to the strength of the explosion and decrease rapidly with the distance traveled. Though the duration of the explosion is no longer than a split second, the blast effect can be devastating. Solid objects can be fragmented and carried far away by the compressional waves.

Rupture of the tympanic membrane and hemotympanum are far from uncommon, and persons standing at a great distance from the explosion can be knocked down by the blast effect or "wind" of lightning. Shallock describes a case in which four individuals were thrown out of their beds while sleeping; he also mentions the fulminating death of a football player who was struck by lightning, while the other players in the same field were thrown to the ground.[136] Similar observations are found in abundance in the literature.

The light produced by the discharge is of great intensity and contains infrared, ultraviolet, and roentgen rays in different proportions. Cataracts may form as a result of a lightning shock and they are regarded as being due to radiation injury.

In about one third of the victims of lightning, death occurs immediately from paralysis of the vital centers. If the victim of the shock survives the immediate effects of the accident, he is likely to develop the so-called *lightning syndrome,* which is characterized by loss of consciousness, occasionally by temporary impairment of peripheral and cerebral nervous function (keraunoparalysis), conduction deafness, and skin burns. Painful sensations and muscular contractions are usually absent, and as a rule the internal organs escape damage.

The incidence of lightning accidents is 30 times as great among farmers as among city dwellers, and the majority of accidents occur in the open fields—53 per cent according to Harms.[137] Mass accidents involving several people simultaneously are on record, such as the one at Ascot in 1955 during the world-famous horse race, in which 4 persons died and 51 required hospitalization.[138]

If the danger of lightning is recognized in time, the best protection is provided by taking refuge in the house. Instruments capable of giving alarm signals are commercially available; they are essentially based on the ability to measure changes in field intensity. As a general rule, if less than 10 seconds elapse between the lightning and the thunderclap, this may be taken as an indication that lightning has struck within the approximate radius of 3 km.

Inside the house one should stay at least 1 m away from electric lines, or appliances, switches or sockets, chimneys, stoves, or fires because of the hazards of secondary discharge. Radio and television sets should be switched off and the aerials should be grounded. It is not advisable to stand near a window. Glass does not offer protection against lightning; conversely, glass splinters from a broken window may penetrate deeply into the eye or the skin. One should also stay at a safe distance from water faucets and avoid taking a bath during an electrical storm.

If one is caught by the storm while in the open and no building is within easy reach, he should seek shelter at the bottom of a cliff, in a deep gully, or in a cave. It is dangerous to stay on the crest of a hill, at the bottom of a haystack, or under a tree. In the open, one is best protected by lying down on the ground, at the farthest possible distance from any metal fence, agricultural machine, or other metal object.[139]

Lightning often strikes over a large surface of water. Sitting in a floating boat during a storm or bathing in a river, lake, or the ocean is a hazard, and shelter should be sought as far away as possible from the shore.

Vehicles with metallic bodies, such as automobiles, railway carriages, street cars, and airplanes, as a rule offer sufficient protection. Several cases are on record of people in a car escaping injury when the car was struck by lightning. The risk of airplanes being struck by lightning is great. According to Few, about 500 airplanes are struck by lightning every year in the United States. This happened to Apollo 12 on landing, but fortunately no one was hurt.

Campers should not place tents on top of hills, under isolated trees, or on the outskirts of a forest. Under the tent, people should sit in the center, without touching the metal rods supporting the tent or any other conducting part.

Medicolegal Evaluation of Lightning Injury

When a person is struck by lightning in the presence of eye witnesses and the weather conditions prevailing at the time of the accident are known, a cause and effect relationship can easily be drawn between the lightning and the injury or death sustained by the victim of the accident. In the absence of witnesses, it is well to keep in mind that lightning can be used to disguise a murder carried out by other methods. Cases are on record in which the perpetrator of the murder set a building afire during an electrical storm for the purpose of destroying the evidence of the crime.

It should also be pointed out that a round well-demarcated hole in window glass at the point of entry of the lightning flash may simulate a bullet hole. The same applies to clothes worn by the victim of the accident, which can be torn or can be found at a distance from the body, thus simulating a physical assault on the deceased.[141] Dependable evidence of a fatal lightning bolt is usually found on the ground, trees, buildings, and objects in the vicinity of the body (Fig. 17–13). Metallic objects may be

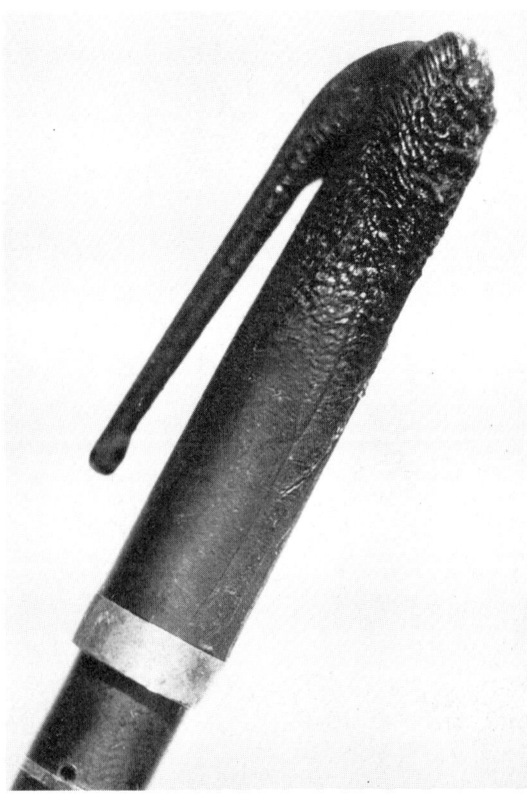

Figure 17–13. Scorched fountain pen in the pocket of a victim of fatal lightning shock.

found fused, walls of rooms split open, and furniture disintegrated.

The presence of marks on the skin and scorched hair on the body gives further support to the conclusion that electric shock was the primary cause of death (Fig. 17–14 to 17–16). There is general agreement that lightning causes death by paralysis of the respiratory center; it is also well substantiated that in the greater number of fatal accidents, lightning passes through the head. Death occurs instantaneously in 44 to 60 per cent of cases, and the body is often found in the position the victim was in when struck by the lightning. In general, those who survive recover completely, and should sequelae develop, they are of a minor nature and do not interfere with the victim's working capacity. Exceptions to this general rule must be made for the temporary or progressive loss of hearing, for the development of cataract, and for the immediate or late effects of mechanical or thermal injuries sustained at the time of the accident.

Though the term "lightning mark" is generally used, it should be made clear that the marks do not differ from those left from a first-degree burn. In the majority of cases the "marks" consist of a red line of varying width—from 2 to 8 cm—extending in craniocaudal direction from the vertex of the head or from the chin to the ankles or heels. "Marks" may likewise appear as disseminated red patches of various shapes, not uncommonly in the form of a swallowtail. They are not detected in every instance; they were missing in 50 victims of lightning in a series of 300 cases analyzed by one of us.[142]

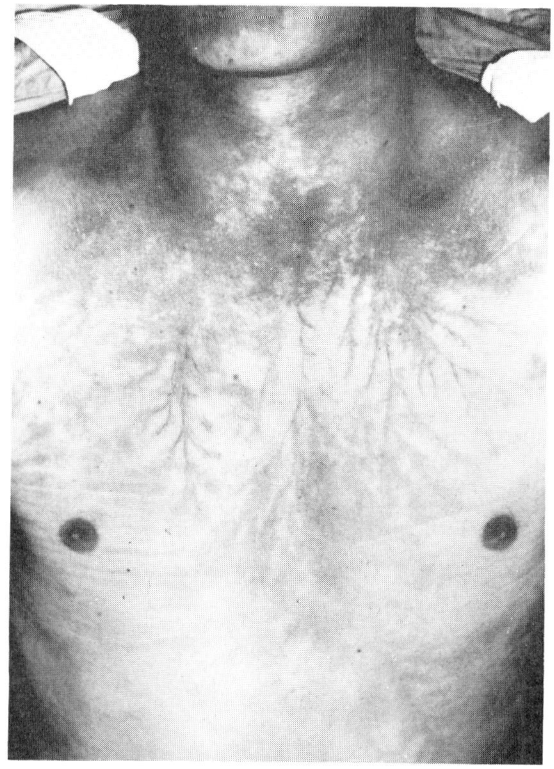

Figure 17–15. Lightning mark resembling a pine bough.

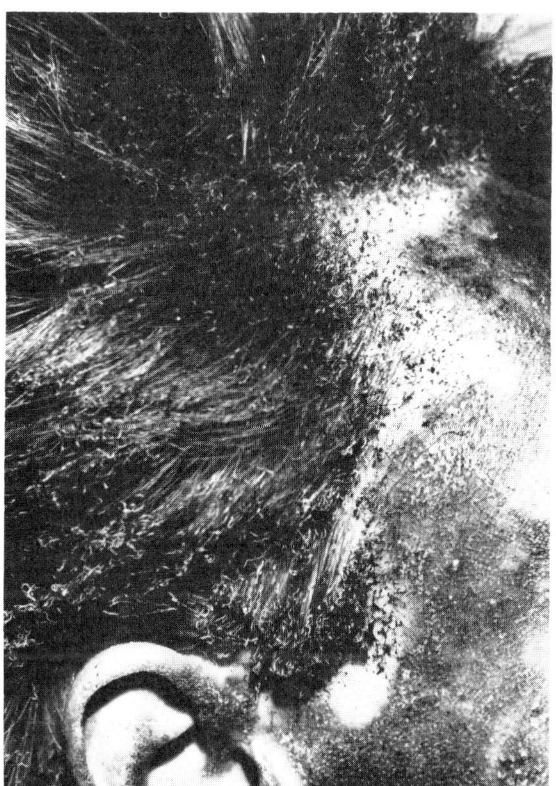

Figure 17–14. Charring of skin and hair by lightning.

Third-degree burns can also be found, as a result of the effects of Joule's heat or arcing; however, in contrast to the burns caused by high-voltage accidents, burns caused by lightning do not extend deep into the subcutaneous tissues, and muscles, tendons, fasciae, ligaments, joints, and bones as a rule escape thermic injury. Whenever bony fractures are encountered (fracture of the skull is not uncommon), it is more likely that they occurred when the victim of the accident was thrown to the ground by the explosion.

A quite common observation is that the clothes worn by the victim of the accident have been scorched although the skin may appear intact. This phenomenon is due to the clothes' having become wet in the thunderstorm and, as such, good conductors.

Usually, no diagnostic findings are disclosed at the examination of the internal organs. Vis-

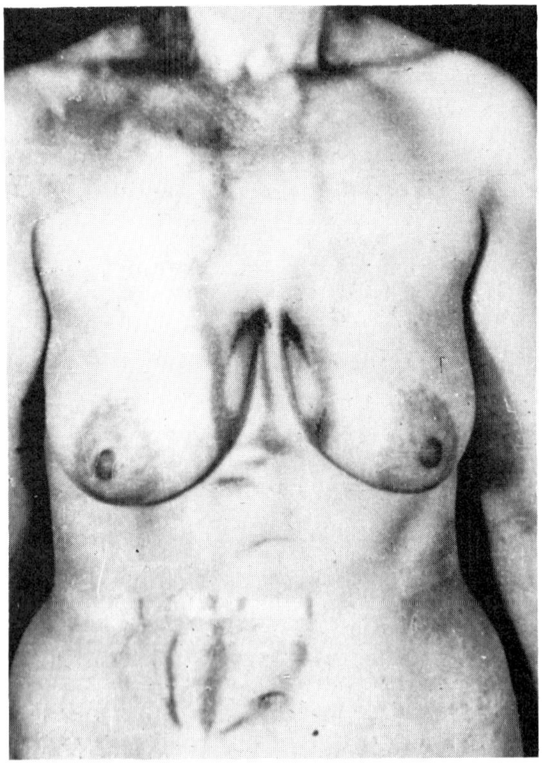

Figure 17–16. Fatal lightning shock. Notice the lightning marks on the anterior surface of the body.

cera are congested, petechial hemorrhages can be noted in the serous membranes, and blood in fluid state is usually present in the heart chambers. Occasional reports, however, indicate that changes of a more complex nature can also be detected. For example, Grand describes the case of a 19-year-old man who developed myocardial infarction 25 hours after being struck by lightning.[143]

Cerebral, epidural, and subarachnoidal hemorrhage, not restricted to old people or people with preexisting atherosclerosis, have also been recorded.[144] In these cases it is not unlikely that the lesions occurred in conjunction with mechanical trauma brought about by the force of the explosion and the fall to the ground.

Owing to the short duration of the exposure, thermal lesions in the brain and spinal cord are only rarely seen in lightning casualties, presumably when the lightning charge passed through the victim's head.[145]

The nature of the disorder underlying the temporary paralysis of motor and sensory peripheral nerves and cerebral nerves as well is not clear. The manifestations of lost neural function as a rule appear immediately, last a few hours or days, and can mimic hemiplegia, paraplegia, or monoplegia. Sensory loss may reach such a degree that the victim sees his burning clothes but does not feel the heat, nor can he move on account of his paralysis. Aphonia, dysphagia, ptosis, hearing defects, pupillary rigidity, and anisocoria are all manifestations of cerebral nerve involvement.[146, 147]

Lightning in Pregnancy

Fifteen cases in which lightning struck pregnant women are on record; fetal loss occurred in seven. Rupture of the pregnant uterus has also been described.[148, 149] Marleschki has presented a detailed study on the effects of lightning on pregnant women.[150]

ELECTRICAL HAZARDS

In Industry

Most of the accidents occurring in industry are due to carelessness. Many occur because a workman touches a live conductor on the assumption that it is not live, or because a machine or part of it becomes live when the circuit is completed and protective grounding is either missing or faulty. It frequently happens that a metal instrument that the workman is using, such as a screwdriver or pliers, completes the circuit. Among machines, drills, electric cranes, and pumps, and even the apparently innocent flashlight, are the most common sources of accidents. About 23 per cent of the accidents occur in industries concerned with production, transformation, and distribution of electric energy, and 77 per cent occur at manufacturing plants in the various branches of industry.

The hazards of low-voltage current are often underestimated. A case is known in which the spark of an electric bell operated at 10 v set fire to a benzine bottle 1 m away, causing serious burns to a person working in the area.

High-voltage accidents occur primarily on the grid system carrying alternating current of 3,000 to 400,000 v. Accidents of this type primarily take place at distributing or transforming stations, where the escape of the victim is very difficult or impossible. Danger is further increased if the workmen's clothes are soaked with oil.

In the majority of cases that come under investigation, the victim is a skilled electrician, and open wires mounted at an accessible height are the cause of the accident. Inadequate insulation of a switch or instrument, faulty grounding, wet soil, or damp clothes or hands may either cause the accident or increase its severity.

In agriculture, inefficiently grounded equipment is often responsible for the accident. Electric fences, commonly used to prevent livestock from going astray, and usually harmless to human beings and animals alike, may also cause accidents, when by coincidence or out of mischief, the fence becomes connected with high-voltage lines.

Operators in the railroad industry belong in a high-risk category. Lambusta and Catalano have investigated 361 electrocutions among personnel in electric railways, 109 of which had a fatal outcome.[151]

In the Home

Domestic accidents are often not recorded and therefore do not appear in the pertinent statistics. The toll of fatalities is, however, high. By far the largest proportion of domestic accidents occur during incompetent manipulation of live conductors at a voltage of 110 v.

As a rule, in domestic premises, the electric wires are nonmetallic (Romex), are inside the wall, and are covered with plaster. Electric appliances are the major source of accidents around the home. A layman attempting to fix a television set takes a risk if he fails to withdraw the plug from the wall socket. The flexible cords of domestic appliances are often wound around the appliance after use, and the plug withdrawn from the wall socket by pulling at the flexible cord, or the appliance is carried about in the room without the plug being withdrawn. All this leads to the flexible wiring being frayed or damaged and to the risk of an accident. The handle of an electric iron is usually well insulated with wood or plastic material; if the handle breaks, however, the contact of the hand with the metal may cause an electric shock. Similar risks are linked to the operation of washing machines, sewing machines, percolators, or vaccum cleaners whenever the apparatus is not properly grounded or the casing is broken. The same is true of carelessly handled electric warming pads, a well-known cause of fires, burns, and even fatal accidents.

In bathrooms, wall sockets are placed close to the handbasin (for use of an electric razor), and the switches placed outside. This precautionary measure has greatly reduced the number of accidents occurring in bathrooms. Still, they do occur, and the following case is an example. A nurse in a hospital washed her hair while she was having a bath and in the course of this procedure connected the electric hairdryer to a lamp socket. She was found dead in the bath, holding the hairdryer close to her body. Under these circumstances current marks are generally absent, and not infrequently loss of consciousness may contribute to secondary drowning. Portable appliances and faulty connections are the most frequent source of accidents in the bathroom.

In the Hospital

Among the accidents likely to occur within the walls of a hospital, those taking place in the operating room deserve primary consideration.[152-154] This has been done in Chapter 35. To round up the subject, the following points deserve further appraisal.

Spark discharges of static electricity or from high-frequency equipment (surgical or otherwise) in the presence of anesthetic gases are the most frequent causes of explosions in the operating room. Use of the cautery is an added risk. The risk depends primarily on the relatively small size of the rooms and on the fact that anesthetic gases are often mixed with oxygen. Some of the gas mixtures used in anesthesiology are flammable and combustible. When these agents are administered in oxygen-rich mixtures, the risk of combustion becomes greater.

Static electricity may come from different sources, such as defective apparatus, the material included in the anesthetizing apparatus, and even from the rubbing of a defective balloon used in anesthesia against the dry trousers of the anesthesiologist.

The moisture content of the atmosphere may also play a role. Where the moisture content in the operating room is very low, accidents are more frequent; conversely if the level of humidity is high the danger of explosion is practically nonexistent. Objects become coated by moisture and thus are in constant equilibrium with the atmosphere; surface resistance is reduced to such an extent that charges are immediately led off, and dielectric constants are equalized.

The question of flooring is extensively dealt with in the technical literature. Nowadays artificial stone floors and conductive tile floors are generally used in operating rooms, and static electricity is led off by iron components built into the floor. Full protection is provided for if the charge is led off as rapidly as it develops.

Protective grounding, by different methods, of the operating table, the anesthetizing apparatus, and the chair of the anesthesiologist guards against the accumulation of static electricity. Portable apparatus should be grounded as well as the patient and the persons working in the operating room. The latter should wear shoes with conducting rubber soles, and their clothes should be made from cotton rather than from artificial materials.

The introduction into the operating room of specific automatic devices signaling the danger of static discharge has decreased the risk of explosion a great deal.

Chernick and Raber have reviewed the subject of electrical hazards in the newborn nursery.[155]

Diagnostic and Therapeutic Cardiologic Procedures

The potential risks linked with cardiologic procedures that are based on the use of electric current have been the subject of a profuse literature.[156-158] The simultaneous use of several types of electric apparatus—for instance, a defibrillator and a recording electrocardiograph—increases the risk. Thus electrocardiographic monitors should be detached while defibrillators are being used. Equipotential grounding should be required and ensured.

Accidents do not occur frequently to patients who are being monitored, but when they do they can initiate fatal ventricular fibrillation.

Ross mentions the case of a patient who was recovering from an infarction and who sustained an electric shock while being submitted to an electrocardiographic determination. As soon as the switch of the machine was turned off the patient regained consciousness; there was no demonstrable cardiac damage.[159]

Ventricular fibrillation has been recorded following the introduction of an intracardiac catheter electrode. Data, either in favor of or against transseptal catheterization, have been presented. The introduction of microcatheterization techniques has considerably reduced the risks connected with this procedure.

Equally well known are the failure, side effects, and complications connected with the application of electric defibrillators, a procedure quite frequently used for regulating the cardiac rhythm. Usually the critical condition of the patient justifies the risks related to the method.

Pacemaker implantation is being applied more and more to the correction of disorders in cardiac rhythm recognized by electronic monitoring. A pacemaker consists of a battery-operated electronic apparatus, no larger than palm-size. The electrodes are brought into contact with the heart by two cables and the apparatus is implanted in the thoracic or abdominal musculature. Technical breakdown of the apparatus (e.g., amputation, corrosion, and dislocation of the electrodes) rarely occurs, and when it does, defects of this type can be corrected. Functional dropout of the pacemaker, preceded by disturbances of synchronization, in general becomes manifest two to three weeks prior to the total dropout.

Damage of the sarcoplasmic reticulum of the myofibers has been observed in the experimental animal following pacemaker stimulation.[160]

INVESTIGATION OF THE ACCIDENT

Investigation of electrical accidents should be carried out in conjunction by the technical and medical experts. It should be aimed at collecting all data that might prove to be of importance in explaining the accident. The purpose of the investigation is not solely to establish the responsibility in a given case; comparative study of a large series of accidents will help to gather scientific knowledge and will contribute as well to the development of improved technical precautionary measures and the elaboration of safety standards. Assessment of the case cannot be made according to a rigid system, and general rules cannot be given; the most important guiding principles are as follows.

The experts identify the victim of the accident and record the evidence given by the witnesses of the scene and time of the accident. Sketches and photographs should not be omitted. Careful examination of the floor (concrete, earth, wood), its state (dry, wet, intact, damaged) and its covering (carpet, plastic) are pertinent parts of the examination. Lighting conditions (natural, artificial, shade) should be mentioned.

The technical expert records the data concerning the electric equipment; he states the voltage, the type of current, and the estimated value of total resistance (in ohms). He also examines the parts of the electric appliance that were liable to have caused the accident; tests the wires, electric lines, insulations; measures the diameter of the electric supply; tests the fuses and switches.

The cause of accidents occurring in the bathtub can often be revealed only after careful examination of the electric appliances. Unusual conditions should also be thought of. It has happened that a circuit was closed by the body of a squirrel. In a case described by Jellinek a child urinated on the overhead feed line of an electric train and was fatally electrocuted.[14] Unusual, "mysterious" accidents often have criminologic aspects.

It must be stated in the report whether rules for testing the apparatus were properly observed, and the time and result of the last test should be registered. It should also be ascertained whether the equipment complies with standard specifications, or in what respect it differs from them.

The experts have to state what work the injured person was performing and after how many working hours the accident occurred. The physiologic conditions of the individual that might have influenced the occurrence of the accident (rested, exhausted, skin dry or sweating) should be recorded. The clothes and shoes of the victim should be examined.

The clothes of the victim of fatal electric shock should be examined with the same meticulous scrutiny as his body. The clothes may get torn and burned during exposure to electric current. At the point of entry of low-voltage current, the material becomes perforated as if pierced with a needle. When examined under a microscope, the ends of the thread are smooth and rounded off, but their structure is not significantly altered. These small perforations must be differentiated from the loss of material caused by mechanical objects or chemicals, or from moth holes. Moth holes are round and reveal parallel passages. When chemicals are involved, the threads become swollen or disintegrated. On exposure to high-voltage current, the clothes get burned and fluids get vaporized. Tears in clothing produced by lightning often cannot be distinguished from those caused by mechanical force.

Meteorologic conditions (e.g., temperature of the surroundings, relative humidity of the atmosphere, wind, fog) should be recorded.

The medical expert makes a record of the injuries and of the treatment adopted, and gives a detailed description of the nature and severity of the lesions.

After assessment of the data, the experts indicate whether an electrical accident can be unequivocally proved; they also determine the probable physical and technical conditions that in their estimation caused the accident.

If possible it should be stated whether contact was powerful (e.g., victim gripped the wire) or only superficial.

The intensity of the current causing the shock can be calculated on the basis of Ohm's law, namely from the voltage and from the estimated value of total resistance. Density and path of the current can be deduced from the size of the contact area.

The duration of exposure can rarely be stated with precision. As a general rule an exposure of long duration, possibly lasting for hours, can be established only approximately. If the injured person was able to let go of a live conductor or lost consciousness and broke the circuit, however, it can be estimated that the duration of the exposure was only one to two seconds.

Accidents may occur for reasons related to the individual, such as inattention, carelessness, irritation, ignorance, haste, alcoholic intoxication, general malaise, or mischief, or because of malfunction of appliances or equipment. Inefficient insulation, lack of protective grounding, faulty grounding, short circuit, inadequate lighting, and faulty or inadequate instruments are examples of the latter.

The possibility of finding evidence of prior planning should always be kept in mind whenever suicide or homicide is suspected.

REFERENCES

1. Moritz, A. R.: Physical Agents in Causation of Injury and Disease. In *Pathology*. Edited by W. A. D. Anderson. St. Louis, C. V. Mosby Co., 1961.
2. Rutenfranz, J.: Der Widerstand der Haut Gegenuber schwachen elektrischen Stromen. Hautarzt, *9*:289, 1958.
3. Pfister, R., and Schultz, P.: Betrachtungen uber Messungen des elektrischen Hautwiderstandes bei gesunder und pathologischer Haut. Med. Welt N.F., *18*:2003, 1967.
4. Gobatto, F., Ruchetto, P., and Zagarese, G.: Variations in the electric resistance of the human body in relation to the site and methods of contact. Lav. Umano, *15*:260, 1963.
5. Löbl, O.: Messungen uber die todliche Stromstarke. ETZ-A, *80*:97, 1959.
6. Koeppen, S.: Der elekstrische Unfall. Elektromedizin, *6*:215, 1961.
7. Weeks, A. W., and Alexander, L.: The distribution of electric current in the animal body: an experimental investigation of 60 cycle alternating current. J. Ind. Hyg. Toxicol., *21*:517, 1939.
8. Incze, G.: Az elektromos aramsujtottak eletmentesi lehetosegeirol. Orv. Hetil., *20*:592, 1952.
9. Biegelmeier, G.: Der vollkommene Fehlerschutz bei Niederspannungsanlagen. Elektromedizin, *4*:35, 1959.
10. Walther, G., and Sam, K.: Zur Problematik der Begutachtung todlicher Elektrounfalle. Lebensversicherung-medizin, *23*:69, 1971.
11. Jellinek, S.: *Elektrische Verletzungen. Klinik und Histopathologie*. Leipzig, J. A. Barth, 1932.
12. Tappero, P.: Another case of suicide by electric current with protracted free interval. Minerva Medicoleg., *89*:25, 1969. (Italian)
13. Boemke, F., and Piroth, M.: Zur Pathologie des elektrischen Stromtodes. Pathologisch-anatomische und

histologische Befunde bei 100 Todesfallen. Frankfurt. Z. Pathol., *70*:1, 1959.

14. Jellinek, S.: *Der elektrische Unfall.* Leipzig, Deuticke, 1925.
15. Ferris, L. P., King, B. G., Spencer, P. W., and Williams, H. B.: Effect of elektroshock and Hearth. A.I.E.E. Trans., *55*:498, 1936.
16. Wiggers, J., Wegria, R., and Pinera, B.: The effects of myocardial ischemia on the fibrillation thresholds and the mechanism of spontaneous ventricular fibrillation following coronary occlusion. Am. J. Physiol., *131*:309, 1940/41.
17. Lown, B., Neuman, J., Amarasingham, R., and Berkovits, B.: Comparison of alternating current with direct current electroshock across the closed chest. Am. J. Cardiol., *10*:223, 1963.
18. Andreuzzi, P.: Pathology from electricity. Ventricular defibrillation. Experimental observations. Folia Med. (Napoli), *42*:806, 1959. (Italian)
19. Frenkel, E. V.: Szovremennüje problemü elektropatologii. I. Konf. elektrotravm. Frunze, Medgiz, 1962.
20. Ljuban, G. L.: *Elektricseszkij sok i mehanizm szmertyi elektrotravme.* Frunze, Medgiz, 1962.
21. Spitzka, E. A., and Radasch, H. E.: The brain lesions produced by electricity observed after legal electrocution. Am. J. Med. Sci., *144*:341, 1912.
22. Alvensleben, K.: Die elektrische Verletzung. In *König and Magnus: Handbuch der gesamten Unfallheilkunde.* Stuttgart, Enke, 1932.
23. Werner, A. H.: Death by electricity. N.Y. Med. J., *118*:498, 1923.
24. Hassin, G. B.: Changes in brain in legal electrocution. Arch. Neurol. Psychiatry, *30*:1046, 1933.
25. Baur, E., and Bissig, H.: Tödliche Elektrounfälle an Hochspannungsanlagen. Elektromedizin, *7*:150, 1962.
26. Neuhold, R.: Zur Morphologie und Histochemie der Herzveränderungen bei Starkstromeinwirkung. Beitr. Pathol. Anat., *116*:594, 1956.
27. Taylor, C., and Stoelting, V. K.: Cardiac rupture following electrocution. J. Indiana State Med. Assoc., *55*:1502, 1962.
28. Prinz, H.: Physikalische Grundlagen der Stromverletzungen. Therapiewoche, *17*:803, 1967.
29. Koeppen, S., Eichler, R., Folz, G., Hoppe, D., Hosang, W., Osypka, P., and Kostka, F.: The electric accident. Anatomical, physiological, clinical, neurological, psychological studies and technical analyses following accidents with AC and DC current. Elektromedizin, *7*:35, 1962.
30. Moncrief, J. A., and Pruitt, B. A., Jr.: Hidden damage from electrical injury. Geriatrics, *26*:84, 1971.
31. Wagner, C. E.: Untersuchungen zur Diagnostik von Stromeintrittsstellen auf der menschlichen Haut. Dissertation, Erlangen, 1961.
32. Mueller, B.: *Gerichtliche Medizin.* Berlin, Springer, 1953.
33. Kaplan, A. D.: Einige neue forensische wichtige Befunde aus der Elektropathologie. Dtsch. Z. Gesamte Gerichtl. Med., *17*:217, 1931.
34. Somogyi, E.: Elektropathologiai vizsgálatok az igazságügyi és szociális orvostan szemlélete alapján. M.T.A. V. Oszt. Közl., *XVI*:2–3:256, 1965.
35. Somogyi, E., Rózsa, G., and Sótonyi, P.: Histochemische und fluoreszenzoptische Untersuchungen der Strommarke. Acta Morphol. Acad. Sci. Hung., *4*:311, 1965.
36. Somogyi, E., Sótonyi, P., and Rózsa, G.: A bör kollagen rostjai elektromos áram hatására történt változásainak polarizációs optikai vizsgálata. Morph. Ig. Orv. Szemle, *3*:186, 1965.
37. Somogyi, E.: Kisérletes áramjegyek szubmikroszkópikus vizsgálata. Morphol. Ig. Orv. Szemle., *4*:256, 1965.
38. Somogyi, E., Rózsa, G., Törö, I., Jr., and Nevelós, A.: Electron microscopic observations on the epidermis of the electrocuted skin of rats. Med. Sci. Law, *7*:155, 1967.
39. Prokop, O.: *Lehrbuch der gerichtlichen Medizin.* Berlin, VEB Verlag, 1960.
40. Dalla Volta, A.: The poorly-defined electric mark and its diagnostic value. Arch. Antropol. Crim. Med. Leg., *51*:604, 1931. (Italian)
41. Schrader, G.: Eperimentelle Untersuchungen zur Histopathologie elektrischer Hautschädigungen durch niedergespannten Gleich—und Wechselstrom. Veröffentlichungen aus der Gewerbe und Konstitutionspathologie. Jena, Fischer, 1932.
42. Gerlach, W.: Die spektrographische Untersuchung von Metallisationen an Geweben und Kleiderstoffen bei elektrischen Unfällen. Dtsch. Z. Gesamte Gerichtl. Med., *22*:433, 1933.
43. Jakob, F. J.: Emissionspektralanalyse als diagnostisches Hilfsmittel bei der Untersuchung von tödlichen Elektrounfällen. Dtsch. Z. Gesamte Gerichtl. Med., *51*:560, 1961.
44. Adjutantis, G., and Skalos, G.: The identification of the electric burn in cases of electrocution by the acroreaction test. J. Forensic Med., *9*:101, 1962.
45. Carriero, F.: Electrocution without contact. G. Med. Leg. Infortun. Tossicol., *12*:1, 1966.
46. Bissig, H.: Über Niederspannungsunfälle. Elektromedizin, *5*:154, 1960.
47. Kaplan, H. D.: Experience de travail dans le domaine de l'électrotraumatologie. Acta Med. U.S.S.R., 620, 1938.
48. Schleyer, F. L.: Eine Stromverletzung der Mundhöhle. Dtsch. Z. Gesamte Gerichtl. Med., *39*:349, 1948.
49. DeFazio, F., and Loving, G.: Electrocution by tongue contact. 151. Med. Leg. 81. 142, 1961.
50. Maclachlan, W.: Electric shock. Interpretation of field notes. J. Ind. Hyg., *12*:291, 1930.
51. Jellinek, S.: Durch Elektrizität verursachte Unfälle. Med. Welt, 661, 1950.
52. Incze, G., and Árvay, A.: Görcs által okozott izomszakadások elektromos áramsujtaskor. Kisérl. Orvostud., *4*:444, 1955.
53. Guglielmetti, P., et al.: Pathology caused by electricity. Boll. Soc. Ital. Biol. Sper., *41*:1491, 1965. (Italian)
54. Somogyi, E., et al.: Polarisationsoptische Untersuchungen der elektrischen Strommarke. Dtsch. Z. Gesamte Gerichtl. Med., *57*:431, 1966.
55. Fischer, H., and Rossier, P. H.: Starkstromunfälle mit schweren Muskelschädigungen und Myoglobinurie. Helv. Med. Acta, *14*:212, 1947.
56. Burgel, E.: Über Knochenverletzungen durch elektrischen Unfall. Fortschr. Röntgenstr., *65*:207, 1942.
57. Harrison, S. H., and Arden, G. P.: Electrical Burns. Br. J. Clin. Pract., *10*:117, 1957.
58. Jenny, F.: Über chirurgische Folgen elektrischer Unfälle. Hefte Unfallheilkd., *44*:49, 1953.
59. Thomas, G.: Stromverletzungen am proximalen Humerusende. Arch. Orthop. Unfallchir., *59*:177, 1966.
60. Bassett, C. A. L.: Electrical effects in bone. Sci. Am., *213*:18, 1965.
61. Reuter, F.: Ein weiterer Fall von tödlicher Starkstromverletzung des Schädels. Dtsch. Z. Gesamte Gerichtl. Med., *1*:362, 1922.
62. Pietrusky, F.: Experimentelle Untersuchungen über

die Wirkung mittel- und hochgespannter elektrischer Strüme auf den lebenden Körper. Dtsch. Z. Gesamte Gerichtl. Med., *6*:535, 1926.

63. Fritz, E.: Eigenartige Befunde bei Einwirkung elektrisches Stromes gegen den Schädel. Dtsch. Z. Gesamte Gerichtl. Med., *34*:177, 1941.
64. Schieche, M.: Dekapitation beim Unfall durch elektrischen Strom. Monatsschr. Unfallheilkd., *66*:239, 1963.
65. Hückel, R.: Zur Frage der Beeinflussung des Blutgefässes durch den elektrischen Strom. Monatsschr. Unfallheilkd., *44*:488, 1937.
66. Robinson, D. W., Nasters, F., and Forrest, W. J.: Electrical burns. A review and analysis of 33 cases. Surgery, *57*:385, 1965.
67. Jellinek, S.: Der elektrische Strom und die Blutgefasse. Wien. Klin. Wochenschr., *65*:137, 1953.
68. Jenny, T.: Betrachtungen zu einer Statistik über elektrische Unfälle. Z. Unfallmed. Berufskr., *42*:22, 1949.
69. Schridde, H.: Elektrische Verletzung und Kreislauf. Dtsch. Z. Gesamte Gerichtl. Med., *24*:101, 1937.
70. Noiret, R., and Boever, J. M.: Infarctus myocardique après électrocution tachycardie électrique externe. Acta Cardiol., *19*:558, 1964.
71. Koeppen, S.: Schäden die durch Elektrizität ausgeslöst werden. Dtsch. Med. J., *16*:256, 1965.
72. Brumstein, M. S.: Zur pathologischen Anatomie des Elektrotraumas. Neuropath., *11*:27, 1940.
73. Bujdosó, G., Fonyó, A., and Somogyi, E.: Structure and biochemical function of mitochondria isolated from heart tissue after electric injury. Zacchia, *44*:232, 1969.
74. Somogyi, E., Sótonyi, P., Bujdosó, G., and Nemes, A.: Elektronenmikroskopische Untersuchung von Herzmuskelveranderungen, die under dem Einfluss von Niederspannungs-Schrittmacher Strom (Pacemaker) zustande gekommen sind. Z. Rechtsmed., *68*:180, 1971.
75. Kawamura, J.: Klinische und experimentelle Elektropathologie. Z. Gesamte Exp. Med., *12*:168, 1921.
76. Maclachlan, W.: Electric Shock. El. Eng., *70*:871, 1951.
77. Critchley, M.: Neurological effect of lightning and electricity. Lancet, *1*:68, 1934.
78. Stevenson, L. D.: Electrical injuries to the nervous system. Arch. Neurol. Psychiatry, *48*:179, 1942. (Discussion of paper by L. Alexander)
79. Echlin, F. A.: Vasospasm and focal cerebral ischemia. Arch. Neurol. Psychiatry, *47*:77, 1942.
80. Tedeschi, C. G. (Ed.): *Neuropathology: Methods and Diagnosis.* Boston, Little, Brown and Co., 1970.
81. Weeks, A. W., and Alexander, L.: The distribution of electric current in the animal body: an experimental investigation of 60 cycle alternating current. J. Ind. Hyg. Toxicol., *21*:517, 1939.
82. Alexander, L.: Clinical and neuropathological aspects of electrical injuries. J. Ind. Hyg. Toxicol., *20*:191, 1938.
83. Alexander, L.: Electrical injuries to central nervous system. Med. Clin. N. Am., *22*:663, 1938.
84. Panse, F.: Die Neurologie des elektrischen Unfalls und des Blitzschlags. In *Klinische Elektropathologie.* Edited by S. Koeppen and F. Panse. Stuttgart, G. Thieme, 1955.
85. Farell, D. F., and Starr, A.: Delayed neurological sequel of electrical injuries. Neurology (Minneap.), *18*:601, 1968.
86. Regli, F., and Haynal, A.: Die Beziehungen zwischen amyotropher Lateralchlerose und Traumata bzw. Elektrotrauma. Z. Unfallmed. Berufskr., *58*:136, 1965.
87. Walther, G.: Zur Frage zentralnervosen Schaden des zentralen Nervenfeibers nach elektrischem Unfall. Klin. Wochenschr., *32*:516, 1954.
88. Barber, J. W.: Delayed bone and joint changes following electrical injury. Radiology, *99*:49, 1971.
89. Neergard, K. V.: Experimentelle Untersuchungen zur Elektronarkose. Arch. Klin. Chir., *122*:100, 1922.
90. Custer, W.: Uber Hochspannungsunfalle. Elektromedizin, *4*:113, 1959.
91. Boemke, Fr., and Piroth, M.: Zur Pathologie des elektrischen Stromtodes. Pathologisch-anatomische und histologische Befunde bei 100 Todesfallen. Frankfurt. Z. Pathol., *70*:1, 1959.
92. Lambusta, A.: Intra-pyloric gastric ulcer perforated by electric current discharge. Minerva Medicoleg., *77*:39, 1957. (Italian)
93. Bywaters, E. G. L.: Ischemic muscle necrosis. J.A.M.A., *124*:1103, 1944.
94. Fischer, H., Huber, P., and Staub, H.: Beitrag zur Nierenpathologie des Starkstromunfalles. Arch. Gewerbepathol. Gewerbehyg., *13*:643, 1955.
95. Sartorius, H.: Nierenveranderungen nach Starkstromverletzungen. Therapiewoche, *17*:839, 1967.
96. Perwitzschky, R.: Uber die Schadigungen des Gehorsund Gleichgewichtsorgenes durch den elektrischen Starkstrom. Arch. Ohren Nasen Kehlkopfheilkd., *134*:345, 1933.
97. Kittel, G. I.: Horstorungen nach Elektrotraumen., Z. Laryngol. Rhinol. Otol., *45*:384, 1966.
98. Guist, G.: Fall von elektrischer Strommarke der Hornhaut. Klin. Monatsbl. Augenheilkd., *71*:775, 1923.
99. Duke-Elder, S.: *Textbook of Ophthalmology.* Kimpton, 1954.
100. Adam, A., and Klein, M.: Electric cataract: notes on cases and review of the literature. Br. J. Ophthalmol., *29*:169, 1945.
101. Long, J. G.: Cataract due to electric shock or arc. J.A.M.A., *221*:721, 1972.
102. Minton, J.: Occupational eye diseases and injuries. Br. Med. J., *1*:392, 1949.
103. Langworthy, O. R., Ortello, R., and Kouwenhoven, W. B.: Injuries produced by contact with electric circuits. Am. J. Hyg., *16*:625, 1932.
104. Cerletti, H., and Bini, L.: L'elettroshock. Atti Accad. Med. (Roma), 64, 1938.
105. Kirilov, Sz. H., and Korocskina, N. M.: Szosztojanyije pecsenyi u pshihicseszkij bolsuh lecsenyijem elektrotokom. Zsurn. Neuropathol. Psychiatr., *3*:31, 1952.
106. Ungvary, L.: *Klinikai kiserleti elektrokardiografia.* Budapest, Medicina, 1961.
107. Müller, E.: Gibt es eine thermoelektrische Encephalopathie? Elektromedizin, *15*:223, 1970.
108. Meyer, A., and Teare, D.: Cerebral fat embolism after electrical convulsion therapy. Br. Med. J., *2*:42, 1945.
109. Meyer, L., and Mickeleitor, W.: Der Weg beim Elektrokrampf des Menschen. Arch. Psychiatry, *183*:12, 1949.
110. Alpers, B. J.: The brain changes associated with electrical shock treatment. A critical review. J. Lancet, *66*:363, 1946.
111. Barrera, S. E., Lewis, N. D. C., Pacella, B. L., and Kalinowsky, L.: Brain changes associated with electrically induced seizures. Studies in Macacus rhesus. Trans. Am. Neurol. Assoc., *68*:31, 1942.
112. Dordelmann, P.: Intrauterin Frucht Tod. Zentralbl. Gynaekol., *79*:1647, 1957.
113. Hrozek, D.: Intrauterines Abstreben der Frucht einer von elektrischen Strom getroffenen Mutter. Zentralbl. Gynaekol., *85*:203, 1963.

114. Nyiro, Gy., Somogyi, E., and Iranyi, K.: A halmozott elektroshock kezeles igazsagugyi orvosi vonatkozasai. Morphol. Ig. Orv. Szemle., *1*:246, 1961.
115. Boyd, D. A., and Brown, D. W.: Electric convulsive therapy in mental disorders associated with childbearing. J. Missouri Med. Assoc., *45*:753, 1948.
116. Lidman, G., and Cohen, C.: Effect of radar emanations on the hemopoietic system. Air Surg. Bull., *2*:448, 1945.
117. Barron, C. J., and Baraff, A. A.: Medical considerations of exposure to microwaves (radar). J.A.M.A., *168*:1194, 1958.
118. Daily, L. E.: A clinical study of the results of exposure of laboratory personnel to radar and high frequency radio. U.S. Nav. Med. Bull., *41*:1052, 1943.
119. Morgan, H.: Microwave radiation hazards. Arch. Ind. Health, *21*:570, 1960.
120. Iranyi, J., Orovecz, B., and Somogyi, E.: Storungen des vegetativen nervensystems bei Arbeitern von Rundfunksendern. Munch. Wochenschr., *102*:140, 1960.
121. Epstein, U. A., and Cooh, H. F.: The effects of microwaves on the Rous No. 1 fowl sarcoma virus. Br J. Cancer, *5*:244, 1951.
122. Fallis, R. H.: Studies on the biological effect of light frequency radio waves. Am. J. Physiol., *147*:281, 1946.
123. Presman, A. S.: Metodij zashchity of deisztvija elektromagnitnuch polei radio csasztot v proizvodsztvennuch uszlovijach. Gig. Sanit., *1*:23, 1958.
124. Watson, C. V.: Static danger of solvents. Saf. Manuf., *119*:43, 1960.
125. Howard, J. C.: The evil genie of petrol. Safety Maintenance, 28, 1953.
126. Schwanecke, R.: Statische Elektrizitat als Ursache einer Verletzung. Zentralbl. Arbeitsmed., *17*:137, 1967.
127. Somogyi, E., Iranyi, K., and Orovecz, B.: Elektromos suicidum sorozat pszirhes infekcio alapjan. Pszichologiai Tanulmanyok., *III*:559, 1960.
128. Somogyi, E., Orovecz, B., and Iranyi, K.: Cas de suicides retires commis par courant electrique dans des villages hongrois. Travaux Prep. IV. Cong. Int. Criminal, La Haye, 1960.
129. Somogyi, E., Orovecz, B., and Iranyi, K.: Angaben zu dem Problem der durch elektrischen Strom begangenen Selbstmorde. Dtsch. Z. Gesamte Gerichtl. Med., *52*:52, 1961.
130. Holder, J. C.: An unusual method of attempted suicide. Med. Leg. J., *28*:41, 1960.
131. Bornstein, F. P.: Homicide by electrocution. J. Forensic Sci., *7*:516, 1962.
132. Manfredi, M.: Suicide by electric saw. Arch. Soc. Lombarda Med. Leg., *3*:391, 1967. (Italian)
133. Weimann, W.: Selbsttotung nach der Uhrzeit. Arch. Kriminol., *127*:127, 1961.
134. Lautenbach, L., and Schwerd, W.: Mord mit elektrischem Strom in der Badewanne. Arch. Kriminol., *126*:33, 1960.
135 Editorial. Lighning shock. Br. Med. J., *2*:1168, 1957.
136. Shallock, G.: Uber eine ungewohnliche Form von Blitzschlagfolgen. Zentralbl. Allg. Pathol., *88*:245, 1952.
137. Harms, W.: Personenblitzschaden 1959 in der Bundesrepublik. Elektromedizin, *6*:44, 1961.
138. Arden, G. P., Harrison, S. H., Lister, Z., and Mandsery, R. H.: Lightning accident at Ascot. Br. Med. J., *16*:14503, 1956.
139. Editorial: Prevention of accidents caused by lightning. Munch. Med. Wochenschr., *112*:1, 1970.
140. Few, A. A.: Lightning and new-generation aircraft. Science, *168*:1101, 1970.
141. Zerndt, B.: Uber den Nachweis von Epidermisresten an Klidern bei Blitzverletzungen. Arch. Kriminol., *129*:27, 1962.
142. Somogyi, E., Horváth, T., Irányi, J., and Irányi, K.: A villam hatastenyezoinek megitelese az orvosszakerto szemszogebol. Morphol. Ig. Orv. Szemle., *7*:99, 1967.
143. Grand, A., Delarbre, A., and Jacques, F.: Coeur et électrocution. Arch. Mal. Coeur, *64*:1516, 1971.
144. Morgan, E. W., Headly, R. N., Alexander, E. A., and Sawyer, C.: Atrial fibrillation and epidural hematoma associated with lightning stroke. N. Engl. J. Med., *259*:956, 1958.
145. Woods, J. D.: Spinal atrophic paralysis following lightning stroke. S. Afr. Med. J., *62*:92, 1952.
146. Shaw, D., and York-Moore, M. E.: Neuropsychiatric sequelae of lightning stroke. Br. Med. J., *2*:1152, 1957.
147. Leyds, D.: Spinal atrophic paralysis (case following lightning shock). Edinb. Med. J., *49*:657, 1942.
148. Samsoenar, J. O.: Rupture of a pregnant uterus by lightning. J. Indones. Med. Assoc., *9*:420, 1959.
149. Rees, W. D.: Pregnant women struck by lightning. Br. Med. J., *5427*:103, 1965.
150. Marleschki, V.: Blitzschlag wahrend der Schwangerschaft. Zentralbl. Gynaekol., *87*:1512, 1965.
151. Lambusta, A., and Catalano, G.: Clinical statistical observations on 361 cases of electrical accidents. Minerva medicoleg., *81*:143, 1961. (Italian)
152. Leonard, P. F., and Could, A. B., Jr.: Dynamics of electrical hazards of particular concern to operating-room personnel. Surg. Clin. N. Am., *45*:817, 1965.
153. Hagelsten, J. O.: Conditions for the formation and elimination of static electricity in a Danish hospital: with particular reference to treatment of the floor with benzalkonium chloride. Br. J. Anaesth., *37*:438, 1965.
154. Lubin, D.: Electrical safety. Hospitals, *43*:57, 1969.
155. Chernich, V., and Raber, M. B.: Electrical hazards in the newborn nursery. J. Pediatr., *77*:143, 1970.
156. Kouwenhoven, W. B.: Effect of capacitor discharges on the heart. Trans. Amer. Inst. El. Eng., *75*:12, 1956.
157. Dalziel, C. F., and Mansfield, H.: Perception of electric current. El. Eng., *69*:794, 1950.
158. Maclachlan, W.: Electric shock. El. Eng., *70*:871, 1951.
159. Ross, D.: Totung Zweier Pferde durch Schrittspannungen. Bull. S.E.V., *41*:705, 1952.
160. Alvensleben, K.: Zusammenhang zwischen kardiovaskularen Reaktionen und Strom-Intensitat. Zentralbl. Chir., *53*:1442, 1928.

SECTION 5. INJURY BY IONIZING RADIATION

chapter 18

EFFECTS OF OCCUPATIONAL AND ENVIRONMENTAL EXPOSURE TO IONIZING RADIATION

by Shields Warren

The injurious effects of ionizing radiation were recognized soon after the discoveries of x-ray and radium. Eight years after his first exposure during a series of experiments with x-rays, Thomas Edison's assistant died of metastases from carcinoma of the skin induced by the radiation exposure. A distressing number of the early workers with roentgen rays and radium died or were severely injured by excessive radiation. The sequence of excessive exposure, radiodermatitis, and cancer became all too familiar not only among radiologists but also among some patients treated too long with too massive doses.

High death rates among researchers working with radium (Madame Curie herself died of radiation-induced aplastic anemia), among medical specialists in its use, and among radium chemists called attention to the danger from another source of radiation—internally absorbed radioactive materials. Full awareness of this danger did not come, however, until Harrison Martland, medical examiner for Essex County, New Jersey, called attention to the lesions that developed in luminous dial painters who tipped their brushes with their lips and ingested small amounts of radium and mesothorium.[1] Martland's studies were followed by the brilliant work of Evans, who laid the foundation for the present ongoing study of internal contamination by radioactive materials at the Argonne National Laboratory of the Energy Research and Development Administration.[2]

As ionizing radiation became a more and more important tool in medicine, as its dangers became better appreciated, and as larger numbers of patients were exposed to it in greater or lesser degree, the need for radiation protection was recognized. An important step was the establishment by radiologists and the radiation industry of a National Committee on Radiation Protection (now the National Council on Radiation Protection and Measurements), which for years set informal but widely accepted standards for the protection of radiation workers and, later, of potentially exposed general populations. Similar organizations have been established in other countries. Their activities are coordinated by an international committee. Radiation standards for the federal government are the responsibility of the Federal Radiation Council. The federal agencies most immediately concerned are the Bureau of Radiological Health in the Department of Health, Education, and Welfare, a related group in the Environmental Protection Agency, and the Nuclear Regulatory Commission. State governments are responsible for standards and regulations regarding potential radiation hazards. These largely follow the recommendations of the national bodies.

With World War II and the international race to develop controlled atomic energy, large numbers of persons were for the first time occupationally exposed to a wide range of radioactive materials. Very fortunately, the potential occupational and public health hazards were appreciated from the start, thanks to earlier experience with therapeutic or occupational exposure, and adequate standards were laid down for the protection of those involved.

The atomic explosions at Hiroshima and Nagasaki revolutionized warfare as they tipped the balance overwhelmingly in favor of the offensive. The efficiency and cheapness of destruction were increased several thousandfold. The death of thousands from radiation, the dramatic surrender of Japan, and the availability of hitherto unknown man-made radioactive sources ranging from atomic reactors to radioactive isotopes led to a great surge of interest in radiation effects and the development of the new fields of radiobiology, nuclear medicine, and health physics. These and other factors that made ionizing radiation of much greater importance in our daily lives, as for example, the growth of nuclear power, altered the attitude of the general public from indifference to almost unduly heightened concern.

Forensic medicine endeavors to detect evidences of radiation injury so that hazards may be prevented or controlled, so that those injured may be helped to whatever extent possible and adequately compensated if compensation is deserved, so that late complications may be avoided through knowledge of the progress of lesions, and so that false compensation claims may be detected and rejected.

SOURCES OF RADIATION

Natural Sources

From his beginnings, man has been exposed to a small amount of background ionizing radiation, of which about half is of cosmic origin (the sun and radiation from outer space) and half is of terrestrial origin (chiefly from elements in the radium-thorium series in granitic rocks and sands and some naturally occurring potassium-40). The average dose of whole-body radiation in the United States is about 100 mrad per year. In a few naturally highly radioactive areas such as Kerala in India and southeastern Brazil, the level is about 10 times as high. In the United States, relatively high levels are found in the Colorado plateau and, owing to increased cosmic radiation at high altitude and to the chemical makeup of rocks and soil there, are over three times as high as at sea level.[3]

Minute traces of carbon-14, too small to be readily detected, are present in food, air, and water. Since the carbon-14 content of living things is in equilibrium with that of their environment, archeologists have been able to make practical use of this fact by determining the carbon-14 content of retrieved organic substances, comparing the level found in them with the current atmospheric level, and so arriving at an estimate of age.[4]

Man-Made Sources

The chief man-made sources of radiation are diagnostic x-ray equipment, clinical nuclear pharmaceutical agents, radiation sources used in industry, and therapeutic radiation apparatus. It is estimated that the genetically significant dose to the United States population from medical and dental sources is about 100 mrem per year.[3] Improvements in technique are leading to reductions in this annual average. In general, man-made devices for the production of ionizing radiation emit radiation only when electric power is applied. Portions of cyclotrons or other complex devices may, however, remain radioactive because of neutron absorption, the length of time depending also on the physical properties (neutron capture cross sections) of the exposed materials. Radioisotopes also may be sources of exposure, depending on their physical characteristics and the degree of control exercised in their use.

Nuclear Sources

Uranium mines and mills provide a potential radiation hazard through associated radon and its daughter products. Uranium is somewhat toxic and as an absorbed chemical poison is injurious to renal tubular cells, but has little radioactivity unless enriched. Carcinoma of the lung has been induced among uranium miners, particularly those who also smoke cigarettes. The transuranic elements, particularly plutonium, are especially hazardous because of their emission of alpha particles.

Nuclear power generating plants and other reactors normally produce three types of radioactive substances as wastes: gases, liquids, and solids.

Gases. Gases such as tritium, krypton-85, xenon-131, xenon-133, and small amounts of the several radioisotopes of iodine, chiefly iodine-131, are emitted in vapor. These are appropriately collected, diluted, and discharged to ensure the safety of both reactor power station personnel and the potentially exposed public.

Liquids. Small amounts of liquid wastes may result from leakage of primary coolant water from a reactor and from other substances exposed to neutron flux radioactivity. Among important radioactive liquid contaminants are tritium, iron-59, strontium-90, iodine-131, and cesium-137. These liquids are for the most part contained, but some are diluted and discharged.

Solids. The chief potential hazards are particles such as inert dust particles that have adsorbed radioisotopes on their surfaces or in very rare instances particles of plutonium that give off alpha radiation. Reactor fuel rods accumulate radioactive fission products as they are used. Used fuel rods are therefore potentially more dangerous than fresh rods. In addition, they contain varying amounts of plutonium, a transuranic element emitting alpha particles, which has been shown to be extremely potent in producing cancer in animals. No such lesions have yet been reported in man. An atomic fuel reprocessing plant may have particularly complex problems in maintaining radiation protection because of the many types of radioactive elements present.

Solid wastes are largely substances that have been exposed to neutron flux, in which radioactivity has been induced within them by neutron capture, as might occur in metal from the reactor core or in substances contaminated by radioactive materials. Radioactive wastes, liquid and solid, are put in containers with adequate shielding and shipped to controlled disposal sites. They are packaged so that, in case of transport accident, the radioactivity would be contained.

Under the established standards the contribution of atomic power plants to the average whole-body radiation dose to the population of the United States is about 1/33,000 of the dose received from the natural background.[5] One argument used by the opponents of nuclear power to delay its utilization is that a major catastrophe due to a runaway reaction might occur, generating great local heat ("meltdown") and liberating large amounts of a variety of radioisotopes.[6] Specifically, a loss of coolant has been hypothesized. The probability of such an event is extremely small and has been compared to that of a meteor striking a populated area of the earth.

Radiopharmaceuticals are now widely utilized in the United States and may contribute about 1 per cent of the average annual whole-body dose of radiation to the population. These substances are usually transported by truck or airplane and are specially packaged to protect those who handle them and the public.

Among the man-made sources that may contribute to accidental occupational exposure are devices for radiologic examination of industrial fabrication such as welds, castings, or pipes. Radioisotopes such as cobalt-60, cesium-137, and others are used as sources.

Fallout from Nuclear Tests

Radioactive materials have been added to the biosphere through surface and atmospheric nuclear tests and, rarely, through accidental venting of underground tests. These fission products are usually in too low a concentration to have detectable pathologic effects. There have been rare events like, for example, the passage of a radioactive cloud over the atoll Rongelap in 1954 following a nuclear test explosion in which both gaseous and particulate materials were present. Radioisotopes of iodine were the most important contributors to the dose in that instance, and because of the avidity of the thyroid gland for iodine, more damage was done to it than to other organs.

If an atomic explosion is sufficiently powerful to project radioactive material into the upper atmosphere and the stratosphere, world-wide distribution of the material may occur. The first studies of the nature and distribution of radioactive fallout were made by the Manhattan Project of the United States following the Trinity Test in 1945. Subsequently, Japanese and American scientists studied fallout after the explosions at Hiroshima and Nagasaki. Since then worldwide studies have been repeatedly carried out in which detailed measurements of radioactivity have been made, and there has also been a very wide range of studies of the distribution of radioactive materials and their entry into the biosphere and particularly into the food chains. The results of these studies have been summarized in reports of the United Nations Scientific Committee on the Effects of Atomic Radiation, the Committee on Biological Effects of Atomic Radiation, the Committee on Biological Effects of Ionizing Radiations, and the Medical Research Council of the United

Kingdom.[7-11] In spite of numerous tests of atomic explosive devices, worldwide distribution of radioactive fallout makes only a slight contribution to the total dose of ambient radiation.

KINDS OF IONIZING RADIATION

Ionizing radiation reacts with matter by the addition or removal of electric charges from atoms or molecules that are ordinarily neutral, thus converting them to electrically charged ions. The six types of ionizing radiation are: *alpha rays*, positively charged particles that are the nuclei of helium atoms and that penetrate poorly but ionize densely, having high linear energy transfer; *beta rays*, electrons that are negatively or positively charged and moderately penetrating; *gamma rays*, a type of electromagnetic radiation of short wavelength, highly penetrating; *x-rays*, a form of electromagnetic radiation similar to gamma rays and also exceedingly penetrating; *neutrons*, uncharged but highly penetrating particles that are basic elements in the nuclei of atoms; and *cosmic rays*, a mixture of highly accelerated heavy particles (stripped elemental nuclei) with different energies, extremely penetrating, and of galactic or solar origin (most are excluded from the earth by the Van Allen radiation belt.)

AVERAGE HUMAN EXPOSURE TO RADIATION

Levels of Radioactive Materials Normally Found in Man

The radium-226 content of the skeleton of an average man is about 30 pc. This represents 80 to 85 per cent of the total radium in the body. The concentration of radium-226 per gram of body ash is constant throughout life. The index of the radium to calcium ratio in body ash is 0.016. The natural skeletal content of thorium-228 is 10 pc. The lead-210 content is about 270 pc. The average total potassium content of the body is 140 g; 0.1 per cent of this is the radioisotope potassium-40. The total dose from this radioactive element is about 11 mrad per year to bone and somewhat more to soft tissues.[12, 13]

As a result of atmospheric nuclear weapons testing, a few atoms of many of the longer-lived radioisotopes are present in the bodies of most members of the world's population, but in insignificant amount so far as effect is concerned. Among those that can be readily detected are strontium-90 and cesium-137. If a body or skeleton does not contain minute traces of either of these isotopes, death probably occurred prior to 1954, when large-scale nuclear weapons testing began. Strontium-90, metabolized like calcium, tends to enter into the crystalline structure of bone and is retained selectively to a considerable degree. The average adult body burden in New York is currently about 1 nc.[14] The levels of cesium-137, on the other hand, tend to be in equilibrium with those in the envrionment.

Population Dose Rates to Critical Tissues

The relative average contributions of the different sources to radiation of the gonads, the bone-forming cells, the bone marrow, and the whole body of man are shown in Table 18–1. These figures refer to contributions to average population doses. Obviously, some individuals (e.g., patients requiring radiation therapy, seriously ill patients requiring multiple diagnostic x-ray studies, and possibly some persons exposed occupationally) may exceed these average levels.[10, 15]

The permissible occupational radiation dose level is arrived at by the formula $N - 18 \times 5$ *rem* = permissible dose, in which N is the number of years of age. Occupational exposure of persons under 18 years of age is not permitted. No unfavorable results have been detected in those who have maintained the accepted occupational safeguards.[16]

TYPES OF RADIATION DAMAGE

Radiation Damage to Cells

Ionization can be produced in almost any element of the cell from the all-pervasive water to complex proteins; hence, every aspect of cellular activity may be damaged. If the dam-

TABLE 18–1. DOSE RATES IN MILLIRADS PER YEAR TO CRITICAL TISSUES

Source of Radiation	Gonads	Bone-forming Cells	Bone Marrow Cells	Whole Body
Natural	94	96	90	102
Medical and dental	11–45	–	32	73
Occupational	–	–	–	0.8
Nuclear power	–	–	–	0.003

age is slight, there may be a latent period before it becomes apparent, and because living tissue is not inert, there is also some degree of repair of radiation damage. This principle is taken advantage of clinically in protracting therapeutic radiation to reduce its injurious effects on normal tissues.

A major early effect is damage to protein and DNA as well as to various enzymes. Since these are controlling mechanisms in the cell, the effect of radiation is usually much greater than would be expected from the mere transfer of caloric energy involved. A particularly important effect is the retardation or inhibition of cell division, often accompanied by structural changes in chromosomes (fragmentation, translocation, or deletion). This chromosomal damage may well be the key factor in injury to the cell.

Large amounts of radiation will produce significant changes. As little as 22 rads of whole-body radiation may produce detectable but probably insignificant chromosomal abnormalities. More extensive changes are induced by doses above 200 rads. Chromosomal changes may be detected in man by a culture study of lymphocytes from the peripheral blood. Fragmentation or deletion of chromosomes is a nonspecific type of injury. The presence of dicentric or ring chromosomes is strongly suggestive of radiation injury. Radiomimetic drugs such as nitrogen mustard may produce chromosomal aberrations similar to those seen following radiation, but do not cause the more localized types of tissue and organ damage produced by radiation.

The structural changes in chromosomes evidence damage to DNA. If these changes occur in cells of germinal epithelium, hereditary effects may be manifest. These are beyond the scope of this chapter. If the damage has been done to somatic cells, a wide variety of changes ranging from prompt cell death to death of cells after several cell divisions have taken place or to varying degrees of impairment of cell function may result.

One of the best indices of exposure to damaging amounts of radiation is the presence of quantitative and qualitative chromosomal abnormalities in circulating lymphocytes in culture. The chromosomes may be studied by appropriate treatment and cultivation of circulating lymphocytes in whole blood. Of the many observed forms of chromosomal damage, such translocations as dicentric chromosomes and ring forms are particularly characteristic of radiation injury. In fact, the absence of such changes in a patient with a history of prior exposure to radiation should raise serious question as to the accuracy of the history. Some of the radiomimetic drugs may induce similar changes. A wide variety of mutagenic substances can cause fragmentation or loss of chromosomes.

The cytoplasm of cells may also be altered by radiation, the changes being chiefly vacuolization in the acute stages of injury and increased evidence of maturation or senescence later. Electron microscopic study of radiation-damaged cells shows, in addition to nuclear damage and vacuolar cytoplasmic changes, dilated cisternae of the endoplasmic reticulum and swelling of mitochondria.[17] These changes, however, are not specific for radiation damage.

Radiation often leads to premature maturation and aging of cells, as evidenced by accumulation of end products such as pigments or keratin granules. The absence or slowing of mitosis may also lead to the formation of giant cells with multiple or large or bizarre nuclei.

Genetic Effects of Radiation

Ionizing radiation is one of the most potent means known for inducing genetic change, as Muller pointed out.[18] It is assumed in planning protective measures against ionizing radiation that there is no dose so small that genetic change may not occur, and that any increase in the exposure of a population will cause a proportional increase in genetic mutations. On this basis a dose of 1 R to 1,000 members of a population would have the same hereditary effect as a dose of 100 R to 10 members. An excellent discussion of genetic changes in man is presented in the reports of the United Nations Scientific Committee on the Effects of Atomic Radiation.[19, 20] Also of value is the comprehensive report of Neel and Schull on the termination of pregnancy among the irradiated survivors of Hiroshima and Nagasaki.[21]

Somatic Effects of Radiation

Somatic effects are determined by the combination of a variety of physical and biologic factors such as the volume of tissue irradiated, the sensitivity of its constituent cells, the dose, the dose rate, and the type of radiation. The broad experience gained in using therapeutic radiation has shown that very large doses aggregating thousands of roentgens can be delivered to a very limited portion of the body without undue general deleterious effect, whereas whole-body radiation is but poorly tolerated. The lethal dose of whole-body radiation for 50 per cent of a given population is about 450 rem (roentgen equivalent, man). Large doses of whole-body radiation may lead to shortening of life in both animals and man. Localized radiation may result in local atrophy or ulceration, and ultimately in neoplasia.

Rapidly growing tissues, such as those of the embryo or the child, are specially susceptible to radiation injury; the effects in infancy and childhood and on the growth of bone, teeth, and soft parts have been discussed by Dawson.[22] The epiphyseal cartilage cells are particularly sensitive to radiation. Damage to the epiphyseal plate interferes with growth of bone and may, under some circumstances, produce osteochondromas. The iatrogenic aspects of radiation carcinogenesis have been presented by Warren.[23]

Irradiation in utero may lead to abortion if the dose is over 200 rem or may cause a wide variety of congenital anomalies. These effects have been discussed in detail by Russell, by Rugh, by Warren, by Kučerová, and by Kato.[24-28]

Radiation damage to various tissues and organs may result in a wide variety of lesions, but all tend to have certain common properties. Since the cells and tissues have varying degrees of sensitivity to radiation, usually greater the more rapidly the tissue proliferates, there tends to be a selective loss of certain structures.[29] Thus, radiation of the skin produces loss of hair follicles while the erector pili muscles remain intact. Because the endothelial cells of capillaries and small vessels are quite sensitive, vascular damage is usually an important component of radiation injury and is shown early by swelling of endothelial cells or even necrosis and thrombosis, and later by the development of large endothelial cells with irregular nuclei and by hyaline or fibrous thickening of vascular walls. Telangiectases may be prominent. Commonly, intercellular substance, chiefly collagen but sometimes elastica as well, is increased. The collagen usually shows some degree of hyalinization. Surviving fibrocytes and at times other cells may have giant and distorted nuclei.

Irradiation of bone may result in two types of change. Osteolytic changes occur if the dose inhibits osteoblastic activity but is not large enough to kill osteoclasts (as sometimes results from a dose of several hundred rads or more). The more common response is increased density or eburnation of bone when the dose has been sufficient (usually several thousand rads) to kill osteoclasts and to damage but not destroy osteoblastic function so that dense bone continues to be laid down without resorption or remodeling. Irradiated bone is always more brittle than normal bone.

CRITERIA FOR IDENTIFYING RADIATION INJURY

There are several types of criteria for identifying injuries caused by radiation. In any case of suspected injury by radiation a detailed history of exposure and an estimate of dose and physical factors are helpful.

Localized Radiation

Acute localized lesions appear at some time within the first two months, first as edema of the skin, usually accompanied or followed by epilation and loss of ability to sweat. When the radiation dose has been heavier (thousands of rads), erythema or even blistering occurs, and may be followed by dry desquamation, moist desquamation, and necrosis and ulceration in that order as the dose increases. These changes are frequently accompanied by itching or pain.

Desquamation and ulceration may appear if mucous membranes are involved. Very rarely the dose may have been large enough to produce necrosis, usually sharply demarcated by the limits of the field of exposure.

Generally, because of the latent period in development of radiation effects, an early radiation lesion only rarely looks as serious as it is. (This is the reverse of injury due to another physical agent, cold, in which the initial frostbite damage tends to appear more extensive than it ultimately proves to be.) After months or even years, delayed lesions may appear. Radiation dermatitis is extremely persistent and usually painful, with patchy keratoses and foci of ulceration. Ultimately, epidermoid carcinoma or basal cell carcinoma may develop in the irradiated epithelium. Very rarely, malignant change will occur in the connective tissue.

Among the milder late changes are hyperpigmentation or depigmentation. Histologic examination reveals hyperkeratinized epithelium and loss of the normal cellular orientation. The sweat glands, sebaceous glands, and hair follicles may show varying degrees of atrophy or may be absent. The fibers of the arrectores pilorum tend to be relatively spared. Collagen is increased in amount and tends to be hyalinized. Focal necrosis accompanied by fibrin deposition may occur. Elastic tissue also is increased. Fibrocytes are decreased in number, and those present may have giant and distorted nuclei. If the lesion is of short duration there are dilatated capillaries with swollen endothelial cells and sometimes even endothelial necrosis with fibrin formation in the lumina. In older lesions telangiectases of varying degrees may be present, and some arterioles show hyaline thickening of their walls.

Irradiated tissue does not repair itself readily after trauma. It is also susceptible to infection, which may be intractable owing to impaired circulation and the reduced viability of the irradiated cells or their dependents.

Generalized Radiation

Such radiation is rarely experienced except in a radiation accident or the blast of an atomic weapon. With doses of 5,000 rads or more, generalized erythema accompanied by disorientation occurs promptly and is followed immediately by coma. Practically no pathologic effects are apparent, as death occurs before recognizable lesions develop. If the patient is kept alive by supportive therapy for a few hours, profound leukopenia will develop. With smaller doses, from 200 to about 5,000 rem, the characteristic evidences of the acute radiation syndrome are found, their severity increasing with the size of the dose.[30]

The course of an uncomplicated case is quite distinctive. With whole-body exposure of 600 rads or more, prompt nausea and vomiting are followed by prostration and rapidly developing and persistent leukopenia. In the next few days the patient will have a rising sustained fever and diarrhea. Death occurs within 14 days. Ulceration of lymphoid tissue, such as tonsils, and a variety of purpuric manifestations may appear as death approaches. If the radiation dose is smaller (about 400 rads), transient nausea and vomiting may develop a few hours after exposure, to reappear some days later. Mild lymphocytopenia may develop with a fluctuating total white blood cell count that becomes low after a few days. Easy fatigability persists. In about three weeks epilation and purpura may appear; there may be bleeding from various body orifices. Oropharyngeal ulcerations are common, as are diarrhea and fever. There is severe leukopenia accompanied by multiple infections, general sepsis, and breakdown of healing wounds.

In milder cases, those receiving from 200 to 300 rads, the early symptoms will be less apparent, often only fatigability and mild nausea, and will be followed by a period of apparent well-being. After about two weeks malaise, sore throat, petechiae, diarrhea, loss of weight, and epilation, largely of the scalp, may appear.[31]

Whether the symptoms related to hematopoietic damage or those related to gastrointestinal injury will predominate appears to depend largely on chance and the intestinal bacterial flora. Components of both are always present.

In an atomic explosion radiation injuries may very well be complicated by burns, by trauma, and by infection because of damage to immune mechanisms.

Most radiation lesions have in common the interplay of three fundamental components—the death or retarded growth of cells or cell groups, changes in intercellular substance and some loss of supporting mesenchymal cells, and damage to blood vessels with all the sequelae of impaired circulation. If the covering epithelium is seriously damaged, ulceration will result and usually be associated with low-grade and localized infection. The change in cellular substance is probably mediated through damage to the supporting cells. It is shown first by localized edema followed by hyalinization of collagen. As time progresses the surviving mesenchymal cells tend to have abnormal shapes and enlarged and often irregular nuclei. Irradiated blood vessels may show distorted endothelial cells. If much endothelial necrosis has occurred, there may be localized thrombosis. In later stages, the vessel wall thickens, largely because of hyalinization of collagen. Some vessels may be completely occluded. Others, predominantly capillaries, become telangiectatic. There may be loss of smooth muscle cells of the media.

The relative contributions of these various types of lesion may vary considerably according to the radiosensitivity of the structures involved. If a given tissue is relatively radiation-resistant, as for example, the striated muscle of the heart, radiation effects will be evidenced largely by diffuse interstitial fibrosis with varying degrees of vascular occlusion. Some atrophy of muscle fibers is usually present and may be accompanied by an increase in the number of nuclei. If the irradiated tissue is relatively sensitive, however, as for example, a lymph node, the bulk of the lymphocytes will be destroyed, although the stroma and some stem cells from which partial regeneration may occur will persist.

Certain specific lesions should lead one to consider the possibility of past radiation injury. Among these are retarded local growth (e.g., a shortened limb due to damage to the epiphyseal plate in a child) or an atrophic defect in musculature or subcutaneous fat, particularly if associated with a soft, pliable, telangiectatic region of skin. Hematopoietic disturbances such as persistent leukopenia or anemia may be the aftermath of hematopoietic damage. Chronic ulceration has already been mentioned. Trauma to a previously irradiated site, whether accidental or operative, heals slowly because of impaired fibroblastic response. Such a wound is prone to sluggish, persistent infection accompanied by gradually progressing ulceration. Localized epilation may be the result of radiation, particularly if the epilated region is also devoid of sweat and sebaceous glands.

There are other less obviously related effects, the most important of which is radiation carcinogenesis.[8] There is overwhelming evidence that a variety of malignant tumors can be induced by radiation. These are not, however, distinctive from spontaneous tumors of the same sites. Therefore, a causal relationship to radiation can usually be determined only by past history or by epidemiologic techniques. The likelihood that a tumor did originate from radiation is strengthened if there is also evidence of radiation changes in otherwise normal body tissues. Cancer of the lung in uranium miners, osteogenic sarcoma and carcinoma of the bony sinuses in radium dial painters, cancer of the skin and leukemia in radiologists, and cancer of the thyroid in those who were irradiated early in life are among the lesions that have long been recognized as radiation effects.

The latent period between exposure to radiation and clinical detection of a radiation-induced tumor is very variable. Among the Hiroshima and Nagasaki survivors, radiation-induced leukemia reached its peak incidence about 10 years after exposure. Cancer of the lung in uranium miners has appeared only rarely within 15 years of occupational exposure, and iatrogenic radiation-induced cancers have been reported 30 years or more after exposure. Although benign tumors have been produced in experimental animals by radiation, their occurrence in man is apparently rare.

There is some evidence of shortening of life owing to radiation, aside from that incidental to induced carcinogenesis. This was noted among some of the early radiologists and followed repeated small accidental overdoses estimated to have amassed a total dose of hundreds or thousands of rads over long periods of time.[32] This shortening may be due to an increase in a variety of immediate causes of death, and the mechanisms are as yet not well understood.

There is no evidence of deleterious effects within present permissible occupational dose levels.

Acknowledgment: This investigation was supported by U.S. Energy Research and Development Administration Contract E(11-1)-3017 with the New England Deaconess Hospital.

REFERENCES

1. Martland, H. S.: The occurrence of malignancy in radioactive persons. Am. J. Cancer, *15*:2345, 1931.
2. Evans, R. D.: The effect of skeletally deposited alpha-ray emitters in man. Br. J. Radiol., *39*:881, 1966.
3. Report of the Advisory Committee on the Biological Effects of Ionizing Radiations: The Effects on Populations of Exposure to Low Levels of Ionizing Radiation. Washington, D.C., Division of Medical Sciences, National Academy of Sciences, National Research Council, 1972, p. 12.
4. Libby, W. F.: Dosages from natural radioactivity and cosmic rays. Science, *122*:57, 1955.
5. Report of the Advisory Committee on the Biological Effects of Ionizing Radiations: The Effects on Populations of Exposure to Low Levels of Ionizing Radiation. Washington, D.C., Division of Medical Sciences, National Academy of Sciences, National Research Council, 1972, p. 19.
6. Ford, D. F., Kendall, H. W., and MacKenzie, J. J.: A critique of the AEC's interim criteria for emergency core-cooling systems. Nucl. News, *15*:28, 1972.
7. Report of the United Nations Scientific Committee on the Effects of Atomic Radiation: General Assembly, Official Records: Thirteenth Session, Supplement No. 17(A/3838). New York, United Nations, 1958.
8. Report of the United Nations Scientific Committee on the Effects of Atomic Radiation to the General Assembly: Ionizing Radiation: Levels and Effects. New York, United Nations, 1972.
9. Committee on the Biological Effects of Atomic Radiation: A Report to the Public on the Biological Effects of Atomic Radiation. Washington, D.C., National Academy of Sciences, National Research Council, 1960.
10. Report of the Advisory Committee on the Biological Effects of Ionizing Radiations: The effects on Populations of Exposure to Low Levels of Ionizing Radiation. Washington, D.C., Division of Medical Sciences, National Academy of Sciences, National Research Council, 1972.
11. Medical Research Council: Statement on the Report of the United Nations Scientific Committee on the Effects of Atomic Radiation. Presented to Parliament by the Lord President of the Council by Command of Her Majesty, August 1958. London, Her Majesty's Stationery Office, 1958.
12. Report of the United Nations Scientific Committee on the Effects of Atomic Radiation: General Assembly, Official Records: Twenty-first Session, Supplement No. 14 (A/6314). New York, United Nations, 1966, p. 25.
13. Eisenbud, M.: *Environmental Radioactivity.* New York, McGraw-Hill Book Co., 1963, p. 160.
14. Personal communication from Drs. J. H. Harley and B. Bennett.
15. Report of the United Nations Scientific Committee on

the Effects of Atomic Radiation to the General Assembly: Ionizing Radiation: Levels and Effects. Vol. I. New York, United Nations, 1972.

16. Warren, S.: The basis for the limit on whole-body exposure—experience of radiologists. Health Phys., *12*:737, 1966.
17. Goldenberg, V. E., Warren, S., Chute, R., and Besen, M.: Radiation pneumonitis in single and parabiotic rats. I. Short term effects of supralethal total body irradiation. Lab. Invest., *18*:215, 1968.
18. Muller, H. J.: Artificial transmutation of the gene. Science, *66*:84, 1927.
19. Report of the United Nations Scientific Committee on the Effects of Atomic Radiation: Chap. VI, Genetic effects of radiation. General Assembly, Official Records; Thirteenth Session, Supplement No. 17 (A/3838). New York, United Nations, 1958, p. 30.
20. Report of the United Nations Scientific Committee on the Effects of Atomic Radiation: Chap. III, The genetic risks of ionizing radiation. General Assembly, Official Records: Twenty-first Session, Supplement No. 14 (A/6314). New York, United Nations, 1966, p. 7.
21. Neel, J. V., and Schull, W. J.: The Effect of Exposure to the Atomic Bombs on Pregnancy Termination in Hiroshima and Nagasaki. Washington, D.C., National Academy of Sciences, National Research Council Publication No. 461, 1956.
22. Dawson, W. B.: Growth impairment in irradiated children. In *Modern Radiotherapy and Oncology—Malignant Diseases in Children.* Edited by T. J. Deeley. London, Butterworth & Co. (Publishers) Ltd., 1974, p. 469.
23. Warren, S.: Iatrogenic effects in radiation carcinogenesis. In *Modern Radiotherapy and Oncology—Malignant Diseases in Children.* Edited by T. J. Deeley. London, Butterworth & Co. (Publishers) Ltd., 1974, p. 484.
24. Russell, L. B.: The effects of radiation on mammalian premature development. *In Radiobiology.* Edited by A. Hollaender. Vol. I. New York, McGraw-Hill Book Co., 1954, p. 861.
25. Rugh, R.: The impact of ionizing radiations on the embryo and fetus. Am. J. Roentgenol. Radium Ther. Nucl. Med., *89*:182, 1963.
26. Warren, S.: Radiation damage in utero. In *Atomic Medicine.* Edited by C. F. Behrens, E. R. King, and J. W. J. Carpender. 5th Ed. Baltimore, The Williams & Wilkins Co., 1969, p. 340.
27. Kučerová, M.: Long-term cytogenetic and clinical control of a child following intrauterine irradiation. Acta Radiol., *9*:353, 1970.
28. Kato, H.: Mortality in children exposed to the A-bombs while in utero. Am. J. Epidemiol., *93*:435, 1971.
29. Bergonie, J., and Tribondeau, L.: Interprétation de quelques résultats de la radiothérapie et essai de fixation d'une technique rationnelle. C. R. Acad. Sci., *143*:983, 1906.
30. Warren, S., and Bowers, J. Z.: The acute radiation syndrome in man. Ann. Intern. Med., *32*:207, 1950,
31. Dunham, C. L., Cronkite, E. P., LeRoy, G. V., and Warren, S.: Atomic bomb injury: radiation. J.A.M.A., *147*:50, 1951.
32. Warren, S.: Longevity and causes of death from irradiation in physicians. J.A.M.A., *162*:464, 1956.

SECTION 5. INJURY BY IONIZING RADIATION

chapter 19

LEGAL PROBLEMS ARISING FROM THE UTILIZATION OF RADIATION

by Paul S. Friedman

GENERAL APPLICATIONS OF RADIATION

Diagnostic Roentgen Radiation

The Radiographic Image

X-rays for diagnostic purposes are produced in an evacuated tube. The filament is heated by a current, so that it emits electrons, which are driven against a tungsten alloy anode target (rhenium and molybdenum may be used) by the application of electric current in the kilovoltage range (Fig. 19–1). A form of electromagnetic energy, x-rays vary in wavelength and ability to penetrate according to the kilovoltage applied. The higher the voltage, the shorter the wavelength and the more penetrating the x-ray. In general, for diagnostic purposes, the wavelength is in the approximate range of 0.1 to 1.0 Å (the Angström unit equals 10^{-8} centimeter).

Diagnostic information is obtained when these x-rays pass through tissue and are absorbed differentially in relation to tissue density (e.g., bone absorbs more of the x-rays than does the air-containing lung). Denser substances such as bones are represented by lighter images on the film, while less dense organs such as the lungs are demonstrated as darker images. Ordinarily, these differential amounts of x-ray reach the film after traversing the film container, a cassette containing intensifying screens that fluoresce (give off light) in proportion to the amount of x-ray that strikes them. This process sensitizes the film, a plastic base coated with silver bromide, so that when it is developed the typical x-ray image appears. Where dense tissue such as bone absorbs much of the incident x-ray the film appears whiter, while

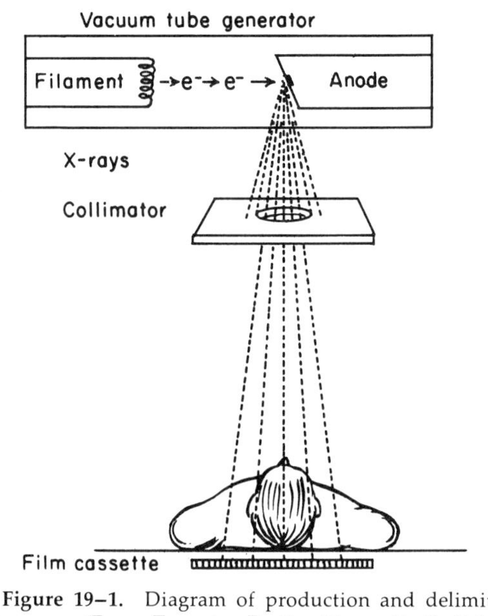

Figure 19–1. Diagram of production and delimitation of x-rays. (From Troupin, R. H.: *Diagnostic Radiology in Clinical Medicine.* Chicago, Year Book Medical Publishers, Inc., 1973. Reprinted by permission.)

where lesser amounts are absorbed, as in the lungs, the film appears darker.

During 1975, a new process, electron radiography, or xonics radiography (XRG), became available for general radiographic use. The standard x-ray unit is used, but the silver halide–coated film is replaced by a sheet of silver-free polyester held in a pressurized metal chamber. The x-rays enter the chamber after passing through the patient and are converted into electrons that accumulate on the film. The image is completely developed within the chamber and without solutions or developing room in less than 90 seconds. On the basis of studies so far, electron radiography gives increased resolution (definition) of images and demonstrates a wider range of tissues on a single exposure. It is cheaper, reduces x-ray exposure from 10 to 30 per cent, and dispenses with solutions and developing units and the developing room.

Similar images are obtained during fluoroscopy, in which the diagnostic x-ray beam that passes through the patient causes an image to appear on a screen. This procedure is valuable for studying physiologic mechanisms involving motion, e.g., swallowing or heart pulsations.

With modern fluoroscopic image amplification, high-intensity images may be obtained with reduced x-ray intensity. These may be viewed directly, through a lens and mirror system, or transferred to film in a cinefluorographic camera. The primary image may be conducted through a television camera to a television receiver, or through a television camera to a television tape recorder.

Research efforts are continually directed toward minimizing exposure during diagnostic studies.

When conventional studies do not give adequate information, contrast studies may be employed. Contrast media include: *iodine compound solutions* to visualize gallbladder, bronchi, uterus and uterine tubes, blood vessels, spinal subarachnoid space and intervertebral disks, and urinary tract; *barium sulfate mixtures* to visualize swallowing and also for the pharynx, esophagus, stomach, small intestine and colon, and on occasion, the bronchi; *air* to visualize intracranial structures, colon, abdominal cavity, retroperitoneal structures, and joints; and several miscellaneous media.

Conventional and Special Diagnostic Procedures

Conventional radiographic studies can be made of every organ and cavity of the body.

The bones and joints are frequently studied for evidence of recent or old trauma. They may show recent or old fractures or dislocations. Fractures may be present that are pathologic, that is, secondary to a preexisting bone lesion such as a metastatic carcinoma (cancer that has spread to bone from another site) or, on occasion, to increased local bone stress. Osteoporosis (loss of bone density), sometimes secondary to injury, may be demonstrated. Infections and tumors, both benign and malignant, may be visualized. Inflammation of the joints (arthritis) may be demonstrated.

Studies of the spine may demonstrate structural abnormalities that relate to pain, either spontaneous or posttraumatic in origin. Metabolic-type osteoporosis may be complicated by demonstrable fractures.

The skull, too, may be studied for evidence of fracture following injury. There may be abnormal intracranial air accumulation (pneumocephalus)—ordinarily the result of a fracture entering a paranasal sinus or the mastoids. Intracranial hemorrhage such as a subdural hematoma may follow injury and may be demonstrated, as may evidence of tumors.

The chest may be studied to visualize rib fractures or their complications, pneumothorax and hemothorax. Mediastinal hemorrhage can be demonstrated, as can infections (such as tuberculosis) and tumors. Abnormalities of the heart may be demonstrated. Pericardial effusion may be visualized. Heart chamber and vascular abnormality can be seen and related to acquired or congenital heart disease.

The abdomen may be studied in detail to demonstrate visceral trauma or rupture following blunt or penetrating injuries. Pelvic fractures may be visualized. Evidence of peritoneal or retroperitoneal bleeding may be present, as well as free intraperitoneal air. Intestinal obstruction or irritation can be visualized. When there is evidence of renal or bladder abnormality, *intravenous urography* may be employed. For further evaluation of the gastrointestinal tract, a contrast water mixture may be administered orally or rectally.

Contrast study of the gastrointestinal tract should include both fluoroscopic and film studies. Irritation, ulceration, or a neoplasm within the intestinal viscera can be demonstrated.

Visualization of the gallbladder and bile ducts may be obtained by *oral cholecystography*—the procedure in which an iodine-containing compound is ingested orally and, by concentrating within them after passage through the liver, opacifies the gallbladder and bile ducts.

The pregnant uterus and the fetus may be examined radiographically. Outline and size of the fetus and the possible mechanism of labor may be determined. *Hysterosalpingography* may be performed by injecting a contrast medium into the uterus; this visualizes the uterus and uterine tubes, and may demonstrate abnormality of the uterus and uterine tubes related to infertility.

The breasts may be examined by techniques using special soft-tissue film designed for this purpose—*mammography*. Hematomas, cystic disease, and benign and malignant tumors may be demonstrated. The breasts may also be studied by thermography, ultrasonography, and xeroradiography. *Thermography* measures infrared emission and results in a recorded image. *Ultrasonography* records the transmission and reflection of sound waves, and gives diagnostic images. *Xeroradiography* is a modified type of x-ray image presentation employing sensitized selenium plates.

The conventional radiographic procedures just described may be supplemented. *Body-section radiography, planography, and tomography* are all terms that refer to a technique in which the x-ray tube and films move in various contrary motions so that small sections of tissue are in focus; on the film image, structures anterior and posterior to the plane of interest are obscured. The kymograph is a device by which the film, during exposure, is moved across a wooden grid containing multiple strips of lead. Motion studies of the heart and aorta, in particular, may be obtained by *kymography*.

With image amplification, bright fluoroscopic images may be obtained and motion studies performed with ease. Alteration in scapulohumeral dynamics in the presence of injury or rotator cuff abnormality may be demonstrated fluoroscopically.

In addition to intravenous urography, there are procedures for studying the kidneys, ureters, and bladder by retrograde injection—*urography* and *cystography*. The urethra also may be studied by anterograde and retrograde methods. Renal cysts may be punctured and injected for diagnosis. For renal visualization, sectional radiography is helpful.

The common bile ducts, in addition to being studied by oral *cholecystography*, may be studied by injecting the contrast agent intravenously, at operation, or into a T tube left in the common bile duct, as well as by percutaneous transhepatic injection.

Opaque material can be injected into the lacrimal duct in *dacryocystography*, into the salivary ducts and glands to perform *sialography*, and into the trachea and bronchi to perform *bronchography*. Contrast visualization of the larynx *(laryngography)* also may be obtained.

At times, injection of gas (carbon dioxide or nitrous oxide) into the abdomen, a diagnostic pneumoperitoneum, may be helpful. *Presacral pneumography*, injection of gas into the retroperitoneal space, primarily to visualize the adrenal glands, can be very useful.

Myelography, in which opaque contrast material is injected to the subarachnoid space, is most helpful in the diagnosis of abnormal intervertebral disks and tumors. This may be supplemented by *diskography*, in which opaque material is injected into the involved intervertebral disk.

Arthrography, in which opaque contrast material as well as gas is injected into a joint, is most contributory in the case of the knee, where it may demonstrate lacerated menisci and torn cruciate ligaments. In the shoulder, a capsular tear may be diagnosed by this method.

Contrast study of the intracranial structures may be performed by injecting air and, occasionally, other dense contrast material. This may be done, as *pneumoencephalography*, by injecting air into the lumbar subarachnoid space, or occasionally, as *ventriculography*, by transcranial injection.

Vascular studies involve the visualization of arteries and veins following injection of an iodine-containing contrast medium. Occasionally, the contrast agent may be injected directly into an artery, vein, or organ such as the spleen, but injection is often performed through an intraarterial catheter introduced percutaneously by the Seldinger technique. This involves transcutaneous cannulation of an artery such as the femoral artery by introducing a needle, passing a guide wire through the needle, withdrawing the needle, and passing a catheter over the guide wire, which is then withdrawn.

The cerebral blood vessels, studied by means of cerebral *angiography*, are visualized frequently. The contrast agent is administered either by direct percutaneous injection of the carotid artery or through a catheter introduced through the femoral artery.

The thoracic aorta may be studied by thoracic *aortography*. At present, a catheter introduced through the femoral artery is most frequently used. Alternatively, however, the brachial artery, the carotid artery, or the axillary artery may be catheterized. Intravenous *angiocardiography* may be employed. On occasion, the contrast agent may be injected directly into the left ventricle of the heart. Similarly, the abdominal aorta may be visualized by lumbar aortography. Injection may be by the translumbar technique or by the femoral artery catheter technique.

In renal *arteriography*, the renal arteries and veins may be studied by injection into an intrafemoral artery catheter. Coronary arteriography visualizes the coronary arteries. This is most commonly done by selective catheterization of the femoral or the brachial artery. The pulmonary arteries may be demonstrated—in pulmonary arteriography—after inserting, usually, a No. 12 Robb-Steinberg needle in an arm vein. The mesenteric, pancreatic, hepatic and splenic arteries may be visualized after administering the contrast medium via a catheter inserted through the femoral artery or, on occasion, through the axillary artery. Peripheral arteries and veins also may be visualized after injection of the opacifying agent.

The lymphatics and lymph nodes may be visualized by *lymphangiography*, which involves injection into a peripheral lymphatic vessel of an oily, iodine-containing contrast material.

Films may be obtained by using rapid-change cassette holders or rapid-motion film changers, which includes cinefluorography, the process in which the cinecamera is used to record the intensified fluoroscopic image.

Nuclear Medicine

This comprises the branch of medicine using radionuclides (radioisotopes) in the evaluation of organ structure and function. A radionuclide is a radioactive form of an element that has an unstable nucleus and emits energy in particles (alpha or beta rays) or high-energy photons (gamma or roentgen rays). Following their introduction into the body, these radionuclides become localized within an organ, which may then be scanned. This produces a two-dimensional image of the organ on which the concentration of the radioactive material within the organ may be evaluated. Two scanning devices are being employed: the *rectilinear scan*, in which the radioactive data is recorded by a detector that inches longitudinally across an organ; and the *scintillation camera*, in which a stationary camera records the radioactivity by producing sequential images.

These procedures are applied to evaluating function and structure of the thyroid, the kidneys, the liver, and the lungs. Scans of the brain, the pancreas, and the bones and joints may also be obtained.

Radionuclide studies are particularly useful in evaluating the size and contour of the organs studied, as well as in demonstrating the presence of neoplasms.

Radiation Therapy

Radiation therapy is performed by using wave energy in the form of particles and short- and long-wavelength roentgen rays, including gamma rays, as a source of energy.

Ray energy extends over a wide spectrum of short and long wavelengths. Those rays originating from radioactive substances are called gamma rays; those originating from electrical machines are x-rays or roentgen rays. The particles originating from radioactive nuclides that produce therapeutic effects are the alpha and beta particles or rays.

Radioactive nuclides are used as unsealed (liquid) sources in treatment. Typically they are iodine-131, phosphorus-32, gold-198, and yttrium-90. Iodine-131, which emits beta and gamma rays, is administered orally to treat hyperthyroidism and thyroid cancer. It is also used to eliminate thyroid function, as for example, in arteriosclerotic heart disease. Phosphorus-32 is given intravenously and orally to treat polycythemia vera and may also be instilled into serous cavities such as the pleural and peritoneal spaces. Gold-198 is instilled into serous cavities to treat cancer, as is also a solution of yttrium-90.

These nuclides may also be used as sealed sources. Radium-226, which emits beta and gamma rays, is used for treatment and is applied in the form of needles and tubes for interstitial-intratissue implantation, intracavitary insertion, and surface application. Radon-222, a derivative of radium, emitting alpha rays, is used in the form of seeds for interstitial and surface treatment. Cobalt-60, emitting gamma rays, is used in place of radium, as needles or tubes. Tantalum-182, emitting gamma rays, is used in the form of flexible wire for implantation to treat cancer of the bladder. Strontium-90, emitting beta rays, has been used for surface therapy, particularly of the eye. Cesium-137, giving off gamma rays, has been used in needles and tubes in place of radium. Iridium-192, emitting gamma rays, is also used in place of radium in tubes and needles. Gold-198, emitting beta and gamma rays, is used as grains for interstitial implantation in cancer. Yttrium-90, giving off beta rays, is used interstitially to eliminate pituitary function. It is inserted as minute pellets or as a rod.

X-Radiation

Radiation that is used for treatment is classified according to the voltage generating the radiation and, correspondingly, its penetration. The higher the voltage applied to the tubes used to generate the roentgen rays, the shorter the wavelength of the emitted radiation and the greater its penetration into tissue before significant absorption occurs. It is convenient to categorize it as: (1) *superficial therapy* (10 to 140 kv); (2) *orthovoltage*, or *kilovoltage, therapy* (about 250 kv); and (3) *megavoltage*, or *supervoltage, therapy* (over 1,000,000 v). The gamma rays originating from cobalt units are in this last wavelength range.

Superficial therapy is usually in the range of 10 to 140 kv. Used to treat skin lesions such as carcinoma, this may be employed as contact therapy in the 45- to 60-kv range. These rays are absorbed superficially and are also used to treat benign lesions such as hemangiomas.

Orthovoltage therapy (approximately 250 kv) has been the basis for most radiation therapy in the past 50 years. It gave adequate penetration of the radiation and accomplished a great deal in tumor therapy.

Orthovoltage units are, however, being replaced by megavoltage and gamma-ray beam (cobalt-60) units. These have greater penetration, increased dosage concentration in the depth of the tissue, sharp margination of the beam, and reduced absorption in and effect upon bone. The linear accelerator is a commonly used megavoltage therapy unit. It gives radiation corresponding to x-rays resulting from a potential of four to eight million volts (4 to 8 Mev). The betatron, less commonly used, can produce x-rays in the range of 15 to 20 mev.

A gamma-ray-beam unit consists of a thick-walled, heavy metal container with an aperture through which the gamma ray beam emerges. There is a radioactive isotope source in the unit. At the present time, cobalt-60 is characteristically used as the source of the gamma rays, which are approximately equivalent to x-rays in the 2,000,000-v range. These units are now being used, in general, as the main radiation source for treatment of malignant lesions.

Contrast Media

Substances Used for Contrast

The opaque media that cause most severe reactions are the iodine-containing substances used intravenously for visualization of the urinary tract and blood vessels. These agents consist of iodine-containing fluids, are injected intravenously, and opacify blood vessels and the urinary tract because of the density resulting from their iodine content.

Contrast media fall into several categories. Two classes are the radiopaques and the radionuclides. Radiopaques absorb radiation, but radionuclides emit radiation. Air and nitrous oxide do neither, but they do change density and so are technically considered contrast media. The major insoluble medium is barium sulfate.

The soluble contrast media, essentially all the rest, are iodine-containing. Their density is related to both the concentration of iodine and the vehicle to which the iodine is attached. Two major materials in this group are the diatrizoates and the iothalamates. They are usually used as sodium salts and methylglucamine salts, the latter possibly being less toxic. Typical examples are meglumine diatrizoate (Renografin) and a meglumine iothalamate (Conray).

In general, the iodinated contrast media are excreted, essentially unchanged, by the liver or the kidneys. The usual sequence for this is rapid dissemination through the body and quick excretion through the kidneys without change in chemical structure. The contrast material has an osmotic diuretic effect that results in loss of fluid through the urinary tract. In addition, because of its hypertonicity, it attracts fluid, either intravascular or intratubular.

Reactions to Contrast Agents

Reactions and complications may follow the use of contrast media, particularly after intravenous or intraarterial injection.

It has been our practice to administer an antihistamine, such as chlorpheniramine (Chlor-Trimeton), 4 mg orally, prior to injecting an iodine-containing medium either intravenously, intraarterially, or at a site where it can be absorbed, such as intrabronchially. If the patient has a history of allergic hypersensitivity, the dose of antihistamine is doubled. In our experience, this preparation has reduced the incidence of reactions.

If a patient has a known iodine hypersensitivity, and if an examination including injection of an iodine-containing material is essential, then administration of prednisone, 40 mg every six hours, for a period of 24 hours prior to and following the examination is indicated.

There is apparently no value in injecting a test dose of the contrast medium. Almost invariably, there is no response to the test dose, even though a severe adverse reaction may follow injection of the major bolus of opaque medium. For this reason and because a very small percentage of patients may have severe reactions after administration of the test dose, there is no medical or legal justification for administering it.

Studies have demonstrated that although an allergic history results in an increased likelihood of a reaction, it does not predispose a patient to a severe reaction. Further, a history of previous reaction to the contrast medium does not necessarily mean that a reaction will recur, nor is there increased severity if it does. Even in the presence of such medical indications, therefore, these patients should not be denied examination by intravenous urography.

It is essential that drugs and equipment be available to treat any severe reactions that may occur. These should include oxygen and a mask, epinephrine (Adrenalin), and chlorpheniramine (Chlor-Trimeton) for intravenous use. The following are the contents of a typical emergency tray that we have available whenever an intravenous injection or other procedure that may cause reactions is performed.

Aromatic spirits of ammonia (1 bottle)
Diphenhydramine hydrochloride (Benadryl) for injection 10 mg per cubic centimeter (1 10-ml vial)
Epinephrine Adrenalin Chloride 1:1000 for injection (130-ml bottle)
Nikethamide (Coramine) (5 1.5-ml ampules)
Methoxamine hydrochloride (Vasoxyl) for injection (12 1-ml ampules)
Norepinephrine (Levophed) (2 ampules)
Aminophylline for injection, 500 mg (3 2-ml ampules)
Metaraminol (Aramine) 1 per cent for injection (2 1-ml vials)
Hydrocortisone (Cortef) 100 mg for intravenous injection (1 20-ml ampule) (Hydrocortone) 100 mg per vial (2 2-ml vials)
Acetylcysteine (Mucomyst) 20 per cent (3 10-ml vials)
Atropine sulfate tablets, 1/100 gr. (1 bottle 100 tablets)
Nitroglycerin tablets, 1/100 gr. (1 bottle 100 tablets)
Glucose, 5 per cent in normal saline (500 ml)
Plastic airways (4)
Venoset (1)
Venopak (1)
Butterfly sets (2)
Syringes, 5-ml (2) 10-ml (2)
Oxygen bottle with face mask (1)
Sterile gauze pads
Tourniquet (1)
Assorted size hypodermic needles

Reactions to contrast media vary in severity. The mild ones include nausea, vomiting, hives, and urticaria, of which nausea and vomiting are the least significant and the most common. They rarely accompany a significant reaction and are related to the hypertonicity of the injected medium.

Hives appear as red papillary lesions, and urticaria as diffuse redness. Marked itching is present. These are significant, as they may precede severe reactions such as cardiac and pulmonary distress. They may be counteracted by an injection of intravenous diphenhydramine (Benadryl); if that does not succeed, then 0.1 to 0.2 ml of diluted epinephrine (Adrenalin), 0.2 ml 1:1000, diluted to 1.0 ml with sterile saline, may be injected intravenously.

Severe reactions are frequently preceded by a feeling of anxiety in the patient. The symptoms fall into several categories. Cardiovascular symptoms are common in the severe response. Syncope associated with transient hypotension occurs; there may be shock, and occasionally cardiac arrest, accompanied by a diffuse eyrthematous rash. Because of these phenomena, pulse and blood pressure should be monitored regularly. An asthmatic syndrome and laryngeal edema may occur. Less commonly, a convulsive seizure of the grand mal type may take place. There may be nasal symptoms, with angioneurotic edema and diffuse swelling of the skin and nasal mucous membrane. Other miscellaneous symptoms may occur—shaking chills with diarrhea and profuse sweating, parotid swelling, and on occasion, restlessness accompanied by severe nausea and vomiting.

Reactions that are associated with nausea and vomiting are almost invariably mild and may be permitted to subside spontaneously. (They are really side effects associated with the hypertonicity of the contrast medium.) They do, however, respond readily to intravenous injection of 10 to 15 mg of diphenhydramine.

Urticaria and hives should be treated by intravenous injection of diphenhydramine in the extremity opposite to the one in which the contrast material was infused. There is, ordinarily, a favorable response within three minutes, during which time the patient's pulse rate and rhythm as well as blood pressure should be monitored. If the hives and urticaria do not regress, 0.2 ml of diluted epinephrine (1:1000 diluted five times with sterile saline; e.g., 0.2 ml 1:1000 diluted to 1.0 ml with sterile saline) should be injected intravenously. The patient should be made comfortable (with pillow removed), and his physician should be notified.

Severe reactions accompanied by respiratory wheezing are initially treated, as just described, with intravenous diphenhydramine followed by epinephrine if indicated. The patient's neck should be hyperextended to maintain an adequate airway. If wheezing persists, 100 of hydrocortisone (Cortef) may be slowly administered intravenously.

If respiratory and cardiac arrest occur, immediate therapy to supply oxygen and restore cardiac function is indicated. Mouth-to-mouth respiration is instituted and external cardiac massage begun. Obstruction of the upper airway should be removed, a plastic airway should be inserted, and oxygen may be used as indicated.

MALPRACTICE

General Features

Malpractice has a well-developed legal background. It falls in the area of the law known as torts (a tort is an injury caused by an act of another). It may be intentional or unintentional, and is an act in violation of a duty that exists between the parties. Intentional torts include assault (threat without contact), battery (contact injury), and interference with peace of mind. The unintentional tort involves negligence and a distinction between danger and risk. Functioning in such a way as to assume unreasonable risk constitutes negligence. The usual criterion of reasonableness is the standard of care in the community. In recent years, this has been modified so that standards are less demarcated geographically.

Malpractice may be defined as practice on the part of the physician that is bad or unskillful, that is not consistent with the generally accepted standards of care, and that results in injury to the patient. In essence, this constitutes professional negligence.

The three basic elements in the occurrence of malpractice are (1) a relationship existed between patient and physician, (2) the physician failed to satisfy a duty that he owed to the patient, and (3) that failure was the proximate cause of injury.

The relationship between the physician and the patient is the result of a voluntary agreement. Unless he is associated with a governmental agency, a physician is not obligated to offer his services to anyone. Such a relationship may arise with minimal verbal contact, without formal agreement, and merely by the giving of advice over the telephone. The doctor may have been engaged for the patient by another person, e.g., a member of that patient's family or a friend.

To quote *Pike* v. *Honsinger:*

> The physician is obligated to possess that reasonable degree of learning and skill that is ordinarily possessed by physicians and surgeons in the locality where he practices and to use reasonable care and diligence in the exercise of his skill and the application of his learning to accomplish the purpose for which he was employed. He is obligated to keep informed and use his best judgment in exercising his skill and applying his knowledge.[1]

It should be noted that the locality rule has now, in essence, been eliminated. In *Carbone* v. *Warburton,* in passing on physician qualifications, the court stated.

> The fact that the doctor is licensed in New York and is not licensed to practice in Patterson (New Jersey) where defendant practices, is not a ground for disqualification.[2]

In *Brune* v. *Beleukoff,* the highest court in Massachusetts abolished the locality rule. It stated that what counts in this modern day, with all the advances in communication and science, is "professional proficiency, not geographic proximity—not place, but proficiency."[3]

Pike v. *Honsinger* further states:

> . . . the rule of reasonable care and diligence does not require the exercise of the highest possible degree of care—it is not enough that there has been a lesser degree of care that some other medical men might have shown, or less than even he might have bestowed but there must be a want of ordinary and reasonable care, leading to a bad result.[1]

It should be emphasized therefore that the duty of the physician is to use ordinary care. Ordinary care may or may not include meeting the accepted standards of practice prevailing in the community at the time in question. It may be that these practices themselves are a breach of ordinary care, in what event compliance with them would constitute negligence, or lack of ordinary care.

There are, consequently, four situations in which malpractice can occur.

1. *Injury resulted from an unintended act.* This constitutes professional negligence. In addition to proving that the demonstrated injury resulted from the physician's actions, there must

be evidence that it was a predictable danger and that there was unreasonable risk involved.

2. *The patient has not extended his informed consent.* For the patient to give informed consent, a careful explanation of the procedure involved, its alternatives, and its risks must be made. In cases of injury, it is often claimed that there was no informed consent. (An intended nonharmful result also may occur in the absence of informed consent.)

3. *The procedure was not authorized.* The result may be as intended but the patient claims the act was unauthorized. This represents battery.

4. *A promised result has not occurred.* When a promised result has been offered to the patient, and he accepted treatment on the basis of this offer, but the result has not occurred, this represents a breach of warranty.

In addition to proving that there has been a departure from proper medical practice, it is essential to demonstrate that the improper practice was the immediate and proximate cause of the injuries sustained. Only then can malpractice be established. It must be established that the malpractice caused or aggravated the patient's condition.

Informed Consent

This doctrine, set forth in *Natansen* v. *Klein*, in 1960, requires that the patient be informed about the nature of his sickness in language as simple as possible.[4] He should also be advised of the nature of the treatment. This doctrine has undergone some evaluation. In the past (circa 1918), it was held that failure to inform was not an act of negligence. Since about 1960 it has been established that there must be disclosure by a physician to ensure intelligent response, or true informed consent.

In the further development of this approach, attention has been directed to the conflict between fully informing and so alarming the patient that the resultant fear and anxiety might unfavorably affect the response to treatment. While failure to obtain informed consent is regarded as a manifestation of negligence, simultaneously there has been cognizance of the "benefit-to-risk" ratio involved. In other words, a balance must be achieved between the desirability of informed consent and the possible emotional consequences that might result from such information. On the one hand, failure to inform represents an act of negligence. To establish such negligence requires expert medical testimony that there was gross risk that should have been disclosed and patient testimony that with full disclosure he would not have consented. On the other hand, this must be balanced against the possibility that a detailed explanation of the risks involved might have caused fear and anxiety in the patient that would have interfered with a favorable response to both diagnosis and treatment. There is some evidence to support the concept that what is visualized mutually is more likely to occur; one might hazard the opinion that a detailed description of the dangerous sequelae that follow a given procedure may contribute to their occurrence.

In spite of these concerns, the practice of informed consent not only constitutes a legal defense against malpractice but establishes a favorable rapport and relationship between physician and patient that is in itself a safeguard against a malpractice suit. In essence, it represents an approach that is good medical practice and is an expression of that personal concern by the physician for the patient that is the core of good medical care.

Res Ipsa Loquitur

In medical malpractice suits, the doctrine of res ipsa loquitur, "it speaks for itself," has assumed greater significance, partly because of the difficulty plaintiffs have faced in obtaining expert medical opinions. This doctrine provides that upon submission of proof of injury to a patient after medical treatment, the burden of presenting further proof that the injury did not result from medical malpractice shifts to the defendant doctor. Two other factors contributed to the development of the doctrine. One was related to the patient who, because of lack of medical knowledge or because he was anesthetized, was not aware of what had happened to him; the other factor was related to the known results of many frequently performed procedures in which both nonmedical and medical observers would be aware that, without negligence, the result would have been a good one.

In essence, this doctrine shifts the burden of proof to the defendant, basically presuming his negligence. It is then incumbent upon the defendant to prove that there has been no negligence.

Case experience suggests, however, that application of the res ipsa loquitur doctrine represents an uncertain basis for a decision favorable to the plaintiff. Juries do not readily accept the concept that the physician defendant is guilty until proved innocent.

Malpractice in Radiologic Practice

Radiologic Diagnosis

Radiologic reports vary in their finality. In certain cases, it may be unequivocally stated that a fracture is present or that abnormal air is present in the pleural space (pneumothorax) or that an ulcer is present in the stomach. On other occasions, although an abnormality or a lesion is present and demonstrable, there may be varying degrees of certitude about its cause. This occurs when a given abnormality has characteristics that may occur in two or more disease states. There may be both differences and similarities that make absolute differentiation difficult. Such difficulties arise in distinguishing certain benign peptic ulcers of the stomach from carcinomatous ulcers, or in distinguishing a benign inflammatory narrowing stricture of the distal esophagus from carcinoma of the esophagus. In such cases, the report may indicate.

> . . . ulcer of lesser curvature of stomach, probably due to benign peptic ulcer. It is not possible to exclude a relation to carcinomatous ulcer. Reexamination after two weeks of medical therapy is recommended.

In other cases, it may not be possible to be sure a lesion is present. The report then may read:

> . . . questionable deossification about the frontal sinuses, such as may accompany frontal osteomyelitis.

When the report is negative and no lesion is demonstrated, on occasion it may be necessary to accept this diagnosis with reservations; the disease process may be present but may not have progressed far enough to be demonstrable by radiographic study. This may occur early in the development of pneumonia, of cancer of the head of the pancreas, and of numerous other lesions. Occasionally there may also be technical factors that obscure a lesion so that it is not demonstrated. Generally, however, exhaustive and detailed examinations should make these instances rare.

Malpractice cases have resulted from improper use of x-rays during diagnostic procedures. Radiation dermatitis (x-ray burn) has resulted from improper fluoroscopic procedures. In *Lamme* v. *Ortiga*, the plaintiff alleged injury to his leg from negligent use of the fluoroscope during location of a bullet.[5]

In *Bowman*, v. *McPhecters*, radiation dermatitis resulted from the process of locating a steel sliver in the patient's arm.[6]

Malpractice cases have also resulted from failure to use radiologic study for initial diagnosis, as in the case of *Friedman* v. *Diesel*, which concerned a fracture of the hip, and in *Gresham* v. *Ford*, in which there was a fragment of hypodermic needle in the plaintiff's arm and the plaintiff had asked the defendant to take localizing x-ray films before proceeding to remove the fragment surgically.[7, 8]

Cases have resulted from inadequate radiographic follow-up of orthopedic problems.

Diagnostic studies must be performed precisely, with proper indications and standard safeguards. Failure to do so consitutes negligence.

Radiologic Consultation

Radiologists are medical consultants and as such have the same responsibility to their patients as do other consultants. Although in most cases they see patients who are referred by other physicians, this is not invariably true; patients may seek a radiologist's help directly. As consultants, radiologists may use radiographic films or fluoroscopic studies to reach a diagnostic conclusion. They may use radioisotopes (radionuclides) for diagnosis or treatment, and may use x-ray units as well as radiation-emitting sources such as cobalt-60 for treatment.

In transmitting the results of consultation, the radiologist frequently communicates his conclusions by telephone and, subsequently, by a written report. Ordinarily, the reports are not given to the patient; this may, however, be done on occasion; it is not unethical or negligent.

The films obtained during a radiologic consultation are the property of the radiologist or the hospital; in practice, however, there is a flexible approach toward availability of films.

Radiation Therapy

Radiation therapy is a frequently used modality in the care of patients. At the present time, it is used primarily to treat cancer and less frequently to treat benign (noncancerous) disease. Its use for the treatment of benign disease has declined because, in many cases, the risk exceeds the possible benefits. For instance, some data have accumulated suggesting that there is an increased incidence of thyroid carcinoma in patients who have received x-ray treatment for enlargement of the thymus.

Irradiation therapy is, however, one of the main modalities of the treatment of malignant disease. It should be administered by a physician-radiologist (not a technician) who has had special training in this area. Proper calibration of the radiation source is essential.

In external irradiation, the dosage emitted from the source must be carefully measured and recorded, as must the size of portals (openings for passage of the beam) and the dosage received at the body surface as well as at depth at the level of the tumor and adjacent to it. Isodose (equal dose) curves are obtained to demonstrate distribution of the dose within the tissues. Body measurements and x-ray film localization are essential. The tissue dose is measured in rads. These data must be recorded. To avoid exceeding tissue tolerance and causing damage where it is not intended, careful calculation and observation during the course of treatment are essential.

With the use of supervoltage external irradiation, the skin effect is diminished because, as the scattering of radiation occurs primarily in the forward direction, most of the dose is received beneath the skin surface. This also permits the accumulation of a larger dose of radiation in and adjacent to the tumor, particularly when one of the various types of rotation is used.

Malpractice has occurred when excessive tissue damage resulted from radiation therapy and there was evidence that usual care had not been exercised in administering it. An example of such negligence would be a case in which a patient received intrauterine and intravaginal radium therapy for carcinoma of the cervix, and vesicovaginal and rectovaginal fistulas resulted from improper positioning of the radium applicator without careful radiologic evaluation of its location.

Complications of Diagnostic Radiology and Their Prevention

Fluoroscopy. In the past, damaging overexposure of the skin has resulted from prolonged fluoroscopic visualization, most frequently in the reduction of fractured bones.

As awareness of this danger has grown, increased filtration in the fluoroscopic tube to reduce the skin dose, image amplification to permit lower x-ray output levels, and sharp collimation to decrease the size of the x-ray beam have reduced the possibility of this occurrence. The use of integrating timers during fluoroscopy has also been helpful.

I recall an experience some years back in which a surgeon who was reducing a fracture under fluoroscopic guidance was not satisfied with the brightness of the image and removed the external filter from the fluoroscopic x-ray tube to improve vision. The patient received a markedly increased skin dose, and a severe radiation reaction, a radiation dermatitis, occurred. This was, of course, negligence. It represented a significant deviation from the accepted standard, it resulted in injury to the patient, and the physician's action was the proximate cause of the injury.

Radiography. In general, the more complex the radiographic procedure, the greater the incidence of complications will be. For instance, a simple radiographic examination of the wrist is less likely to have complications than will performance of an aortogram or cerebral angiogram.

Although oral cholecystography is one of the safest procedures, under certain circumstances it may cause renal damage with acute tubular necrosis. This possibility is increased when large doses of contrast material are administered, particularly in the presence of dehydration, hepatic insufficiency, associated or preexisting hypotension, or accompanying performance of intravenous urography and cholangiography.

Intravenous cholangiography has a greater incidence of complications than intravenous urography. The use of an infusion for injection, by reducing concentration and physiologic effect, may reduce the incidence of complications.

Barium sulfate is essentially nontoxic as it is used in the study of the gastrointestinal tract, but various complications may be associated with its use. On occasion, by error, plaster of Paris has been administered. This usually sets in the stomach, fragments, and is then evacuated. Ohter toxic substances such as x-ray film developer have been administered by mistake, causing serious toxic effects and even death.

Gastrointestinal perforation may occur after oral administration of the barium sulfate and water mixture, but almost exclusively when there is preexisting abnormality or disease in the esophagus or stomach. Large amounts of barium sulfate administered orally, particularly in the presence of dehydration, may become compacted in the colon. Aspiration of barium sulfate will, of course, result in pneumonia. When there is danger of aspiration, water-soluble agents should be used. On occasion, because of their hyperosmolarity, these may cause pneumonia and pulmonary edema.

Barium enema studies may lead to perforation owing to technical errors such as forcible insertion of a firm enema tip or rupture of an overdistended balloon catheter. When segments of the colon are decreased in size or have an altered blood supply, perforation is more likely to occur. The presence of a colostomy predisposes to perforation when a barium enema is performed through it. Tannic acid has been used in barium enemas to improve emptying of the colon; in view of its hepatic toxicity it does not seem desirable to use it.

Arteriography may result in various complications related to the manner in which it is performed. Arterial puncture, direct or for catheterization, may result in local hemorrhage. It may be caused by inadequate compression following catheter removal or by traumatic puncture and catheter manipulation. Hypertension, systemic anticoagulant therapy, and obesity may predispose to such hemorrhage. A hematoma resulting from the hemorrhage may lead to a false aneurysm. When needle injury to both artery and vein occurs, an arteriovenous fistula may follow. Arterial spasm and thrombi may also occur. The latter may become embolic, as may cholesterol plaques that are dislodged by catheterization. The occurrence of arteriospasm and thromboembolism is related to the skill of the arteriographer, the length of the procedure, the size and length and material of the catheter, the degree of muscular spasm, and the character of the muscular compression following catheter removal.

Catheters and metal guides may break while being used. Passage of the guide against resistance is a predisposing factor toward a break and may also rupture a vessel or dislodge atheromatous plaques. Sharp bending during cleaning or use may also cause breakage.

The arterial wall may be penetrated, or dissection of the wall may result from whipping of the catheter tip. Jet dissection is due to splitting of the wall.

Malpractice Suits

Pretrial Aspects of Malpractice

There are common denominators in pretrial preparation both for the defense and in support of the plaintiff.

The most important aspect of a prospective malpractice suit following damage purported to have resulted from a physician's action concerns the patient-physician relationship. First, there is increasing evidence that if the physician has been a solicitous, concerned individual who has given his best scientific and spiritual resources to the patient, there is less likelihood of a suit. The next concerns the behavior of the physician when an accident or untoward result takes place. In the usual case, the physician admits to nothing and breaks off contact with the patient and his family. I have, however, been aware of instances in which the physician involved has assumed full financial and medical supervisory responsibility for the patient with complications that have ensued from his treatment. This, coupled with a warm interest in the patient and family, resolved the issue without a suit.

Radiologists, in particular, must make a special effort to create that type of personally directed atmosphere for their patients. The patient who is receiving treatment should have the benefit of frequent contact with the radiologist, who in turn should exhibit concern for and interest in the patient. Detailed explanations of procedures, effects, and goals of the treatment should be provided. Technicians entrusted with the care of such a patient must be skilled, and in addition, must be trained to be equally solicitous. They must especially be cautioned to be discreet in statements, in the hearing of patients, that could cause concern or could be misinterpreted. Equipment breakdowns in particular should be handled without the patient's being aware of it; such awareness may arouse concern about the efficacy of the procedure and the skill of the staff.

Similarly, when roentgen diagnostic procedures or nuclear medical diagnostic procedures are employed, the presence and care of a radiologist are vital. In many official procedures, the radiologist's presence is required throughout. When that is the case he should create the warm, friendly atmosphere that is so helpful to patients and that prevents suits. It is important to create a personalized environment. The radiologist should introduce himself by name and should also present by name any technicians or other assistants. The patient should be carefully advised about what will occur during the procedure and what its purpose is; with an informed, instructed patient, results will be better and complications fewer. Both radiologist and technicians should carefully monitor statements made during a procedure before they utter them to avoid causing the patient undue concern, anxiety, or apprehension. In particular, no statement should be made that might cause the patient to conclude that an error has been made in the procedure or that he has been injured by it.

A basic component in the physician-patient relationship is the application of the informed consent procedure. Before every procedure performed, the patient should be advised in some detail of what will occur and what information is to be obtained from it. As the procedure takes place, the patient should be told what is expected of him. If a patient indicates before or during a procedure that he does not want it to take place, his wish should be respected—the procedure should not be begun or should be terminated.

There are procedures that have the potential of causing reactions—mild or severe—or damage—mild or severe. Bronchography, myelography, excretory urography, cerebral arteriography, aortography, and arthrography are in this category. In these instances, the patient should be given a verbal description detailing the nature of the procedure, the information to be obtained, and the possible side effects or reactions that may occur. In detailing possible damaging effects, the radiologist must use his judgment concerning the benefit-to-risk ratio. The patient should then sign a form consenting to the procedure. Forms like the accompanying one designed by the American Medical Association are available. These may be modified, but should have certain features. They should describe procedures precisely, yet be flexible enough to permit the physician to alter the approach as indicated and should state the right of the radiologist to have assistance as indicated. A statement that there has been adequate explanation should be included. In the case of therapeutic procedures, it should be stated that no cure has been guaranteed.

Consent to Diagnostic Procedure

PATIENT ____________________ AGE____

DATE ______ TIME ____ A.M. / P.M. PLACE ______

I hereby request and authorize Dr. __________ and whomever he may designate to assist him to perform upon ____________________

(*Name of patient or "myself"*)

the following diagnostic procedure: __________

I have been fully informed of the risks and possible consequences involved and that unforeseen results may occur.

Signature of patient ____________________

When patient is a minor or incompetent to give consent:

Signature of person authorized to consent for patient __________

Relationship to patient ____________________

The foregoing consent was read, discussed, and signed in my presence, and in my opinion the person so signing did so freely with full knowledge and understanding.

Witness: ____________________________

Such forms should be filed with the patient's records. In the performance of any procedure, careful records should be maintained and preserved. They should include a description of the procedure and of the findings. If anything unusual happens, after proper corrective measures have been instituted a detailed record of the occurrence should be made and preserved.

The Medical Expert

The medical expert testifying on behalf of either the defendant or the plaintiff has a special and significant responsibility. Not only must he present the medical data accurately, but he must, in addition, phrase it in such a way as to be most effective. Furthermore, the medical witness should create an atmosphere of integrity and congeniality; his every action, small or large, can contribute to or detract from that impression.

The most basic part of a medical expert's testimony is the preparation that takes place before the deposition or trial. The physician involved should first inform himself fully about all facts relating to the case. This requires that he read and study all related documents. In reviewing medical records, all notes are pertinent. This includes such data as nurse's notes and anything that is entered on the records. During this preparatory procedure, careful notes should be made of significant matters. As this process takes place, a philosophic approach to the case starts to emerge. This will include a set of medical conclusions that support or deny the plaintiff's claim. Concurrently or subsequently, basic anatomical, patholgic, physiologic, and clinical data relating to the problem should be carefully studied and summarized. For instance, in preparing to present medical data supporting a claim of malpractice following radiation therapy for carcinoma of the cervix, the physician should review the entire subject: first the physics of radiation, with attention to such matters as rads (units of absorbed dose), characteristics of orthovoltage versus supervoltage, the measurement of radium dosage and distribution, and related matters; and then biologic features such as tissue tolerance to radiation. The pathologic and clinical features of carcinoma of the cervix should be reevaluated, and a careful analysis of staging should be made. Diagnostic techniques should be summarized. Techniques of radiation therapy should be restudied and compared, both for external irradiation and for intracavitary and intravaginal radium radiation. Both current and former techniques should be reevaluated. A precise reconstruction of the clinical dosage planning should be made and should include the isodose plots. Varying therapeutic approaches, both surgical and radiologic, should be evaluated, and complications of treatment should be analyzed. In the pursuance of such preparation both basic textbooks and current journals should be read. Many data, of course, can be gleaned from personal experience.

In a personal injury case the preparation involved may not be as extensive. It is essential, however, that the subject be carefully reviewed before any testimony is given.

Frequently, a report from the medical expert is submitted before testimony is given. This should be carefully worded in precise medical terminology. No statement should be made that cannot be precisely supported and documented. It is only natural, of course, that such a report be prepared so that it supports the established basic philosophy of the discipline.

Testimony, in a sense, begins as soon as one appears before a jury or judge. Immediately upon entry into the courtroom, the expert witness should regard his every act and gesture as contributing to the image he wishes to create—integrity, dignity, politeness, and congeniality. When called to testify, as one proceeds to the witness box, it is appropriate to say, "Good morning, your honor." After the witness is sworn in, he should respond and say "Thank you" distinctly. His "thank you" for any courtesy that is extended to him should be audible, and it is appropriate to use the word "sir" in responding to questions. It is very important to address the members of the jury directly when speaking and responding to questions. When demonstrating x-ray films make sure the judge and jury can see them; it is appropriate to ask the presiding judge politely whether he or she can see the films adequately. When presenting testimony, speak slowly in a clear, distinct voice. Whenever a medical term is used, paraphrase it carefully in nonmedical terms for clarity. The basic anatomy should be reviewed whenever necessary to clarify subsequent comment and statements.

The expert should analyze the opposing lawyer's questions carefully to evaluate their precise meaning and to avoid acceding to a question that, in its body, attributes to the witness statements that he did not make. When the meaning of a question is not clear, the witness should say so and ask that it be restated or clarified. On occasion, a similar request may be made when one wishes further time to respond to a question. Have in mind the main conclusions that you wish to reach the judge and jury effectively. Such data should be introduced into the body of your statements and repeated at least once in the form of a conclusion. When the medical data are presented they should always be explained and translated into nonmedical terms. Choose words carefully so that they present the information precisely and cannot be misinterpreted or misunderstood. Always present only information that is demonstrably true.

Certain procedures greatly assist a medical expert witness to establish his special capacities. First, when qualifying his medical expert, the lawyer should permit full exploration of the physician's professional qualifications because, on many occasions, the opposing lawyer will offer to waive their presentation. This should not be done. The best way to present qualifications is to combine the use of specific questions with the opportunity for the physician to respond to the broad question, "Doctor, what has been your medical education and training?" This combination of specific and broad questions helps to create an image of skill and good training rather than one of boastfulness and egotism.

Second, in initiating direct questioning, when the medical expert is skilled and well informed it is frequently wise to begin with a broad question such as, "Doctor, what were the main findings demonstrated by your examination of James Brown?" This may then be supplemented by specific direct questions. This tends to create a more professional atmosphere and also to make presentation of the findings appear less forced.

It is advisable that the lawyer, in both direct and redirect questioning, be restrained, terminate his questioning when the main issues have been clarified, and emphasize those findings that have been agreed upon as essential at the pretrial conferences. It is always important to emphasize those findings that have unequivocal support.

One can best contribute as a medical expert witness by having a sense of inner ease and composure fortified by proper preparation and reports that are factually accurate and contain material that can be readily supported. In addition, psychologic preparation before presenting such testimony is most helpful. By developing such a sense of inner composure and confidence, a witness can stay at ease even if the opposing lawyer attempts intimidating tactics such as yelling, sarcasm, or similar devices. If one learns to be psychologically prepared for such approaches, they will have no effect. Inner emotional stability, fortified by comprehensive knowledge and experience and a basically truthful presentation, is the hallmark of an outstanding expert witness.

Within this same framework, a medical expert witness must be prepared to be an adversary. Without discarding his professional dignity or departing from the essentials of the medical testimony, he must strongly attempt to clarify, support, and defend his basic medical theses in the case—and further, so proceed as to contradict the contrary medical claims. This last may frequently be done indirectly.

Personal Injury

Radiologic study constitutes a most significant component in the evaluation of personal injury resulting from physical trauma, industrial trauma, and industrial environmental exposure. In many cases, the radiologic evidence is essential in establishing the causative relationship between the physical agent and the injury experienced, and just as basic in establishing the presence, quality, and degree of abnormality that has occurred. The musculoskeletal system is the most common area that is so injured.

In such a case, radiologic study uses the radiographic procedure in multiple planes and includes comparison of the normal with the abnormal when symmetrical structures such as wrists and elbows are involved. These films may be supplemented by fluoroscopic studies, particularly for functional evaluation.

The presence or absence of fractures is most important to establish. These appear as linear defects in bone. Usually readily demonstrable when multiple-plane exposures are made, on occasion they can be difficult to visualize. Careful clinical evaluation of the patient by the radiologist, in conjunction with the radiographic procedure, gives the best results and greatly improves diagnostic information.

There are certain fractures that are sometimes difficult to demonstrate. The scaphoid (carpal navicular) bone must be studied carefully to demonstrate or exclude fracture; this requires films of the wrist in ulnar deviation, both on an angle board and, also in ulnar deviation, with cephalad angulation of the projecting ray. These views are made in addition to the standard anteroposterior, lateral, and oblique projections. Comparison with the opposite wrist is obtained. A delayed study may sometimes be helpful, as may densitometric demonstration of reduced density at the site of fracture. Dislocation of the lunate frequently occurs in conjunction with scaphoid fracture and should be carefully evaluated.

Rib fractures may be difficult to demonstrate because of rib curvature. Multiple-plane studies must be made, including tangential views through the site of possible fracture. Once callus develops, delayed studies may demonstrate undisplaced fractures.

Not only must the fracture and its characteristics—linear, avulsion, comminuted (multiple fragments), or compound (bone extending through the skin)—be demonstrated, but the precise location of the fracture and its position must be carefully obtained. The fracture defect must be measured both in extent and in relation to the ends of a long bone or other landmarks, and its precise course must be described.

The position of the major fracture fragments must be carefully measured with ruler and protractor, and the precise angle between them should be obtained. The amount of overriding of the major fractured fragments and the resultant shortening should be measured. The fractured member should be compared with the normal one. This is important because a fracture of the distal radius with resultant dorsal inclination of the distal articulating surface of the radius (instead of the normal volar inclination) will, if not corrected, reduce mobility at the wrist and predispose the patient to subsequent posttraumatic arthritis. Similarly, fractures of the neck of the femur exhibit varying degrees of obliquity. The resulting angle between the fracture and the horizontal plane affects the shearing stress, and in turn is related to the possibility of nonunion, to the prognosis, and to the type of treatment.

The age of fractures can be estimated radiologically. Old fractures can usually be distinguished from more recent ones. A recent fracture exhibits fracture surfaces that are not sharply defined and are relatively radiolucent, owing to osteoporosis, and is usually accompanied by soft-tissue swelling, edema, and other alterations. The older fracture has well-defined, dense osseous margins at the fracture surfaces, and the acute type of soft-tissue abnormality just described is absent.

Information can be obtained about delayed union and nonunion. These are manifested radiologically by persistence of the fracture defect, increasing smoothness and sclerosis of the fracture margins, absence of internal bony callus, and usually incompleteness and discontinuity of external bony callus.

Infection resulting in osteitis or osteomyelitis can be demonstrated. This is manifested by periostitis, apparent as linear periosteal new bone. This is accompanied by adjacent local deossification demonstrated as irregular focal radiolucency. As the disease process progresses, both features become more prominent. Eventually, with subacute and chronic changes, irregular sclerosis and deossification occur, and areas of sequestration can be seen.

Osteoporosis (loss of bone trabeculation with reduced density of bone) follows a reduced fracture, but may also occur as a direct result of injury without fracture. In each case, there is a neurotrophic abnormality. This type of osteoporosis occurs, principally, adjacent to joints. There is an intermediate type, neurotrophic in origin, exhibiting similar roentgen changes but associated with brawny edema and pain the so-called Sudeck's atrophy. Another more diffuse type occurs as a posttraumatic osteoporosis.

Soft-tissue injury is a common occurrence and may be evaluated radiologically. The soft tissues, comprising skin, subcutaneous tissues, connective tissues, and muscles, may be directly demonstrated, may be indirectly demonstrated, or may be evaluated through the effects they produce. Such muscles as the psoas or the gastrocnemius and its tendon may be visualized directly. The pylorus, however, must be visualized indirectly as an indentation of the variance contour of the distal end of the stomach. Spasm or hypertrophy make it more prominent and delay gastric emptying. The musculature of the cervical area may be evaluated by the effects that are produced. Following injury, cervical muscle spasm results in reduced cervical lordosis in the neutral position and reduction in cervical spine flexion and extension when these positions are voluntarily assumed. There may be associated cervical scoliosis. This can be demonstrated by multiple radiographic film studies, or by cineradiography.

REFERENCES

1. Pike v. Honsinger, 155 N.Y. 201, 49 N.E. 7601 (1898).
2. Carbone v. Warburton, 11 N.J. 418, 94 A. 2d 680 (1950).
3. Brune v. Beleukoff, 354 Mass. 102, 235 N.E. 2d 793 (1968).
4. Natansen v. Klein, 187 Kansas 186, 354 P. 2d 670 (1960).
5. Lamme v. Ortiga, 129 Colo. 149, 267 P. 2d 1115 (1954).
6. Bowman v. McPhecters, 77 Cal. App. 2d 795, 176 P. 2d 745 (1947).
7. Friedman v. Diesel, 139 Cal. App. 2d 333, 293 P. 2d 488 (1956).
8. Gresham v. Ford, 192 Tenn. 301, 241 S.W. 2d 408 (1951).

SELECTED READINGS

9. Abbuhl, R. W., Bradford, R. T., Rhem, et al.: The doctor in court. J. Leg. Med., 2:17, 1974.
10. Berman, E. Z., Biskind, E. L., et al.: *Examination of Medical Experts* New York, Matthew Bender & Co., 1968.
11. Charfoos, L. S.: *The Medical Malpractice Case.* Englewood Cliffs, N.J., Prentice-Hall Inc., 1974.
12. Fletcher, Gilbert H., M. D. *Textbook of Radiotherapy.* 2nd Ed. Philadelphia, Lea & Febiger, 1973.
13. Hassard, H. (Ed.): *Medical Malpractice.* Oradell, N.J., Medical Economics Book Division, 1966.
14. Horsley, J. E., and Carlova, J.: *Testifying in Court.* Oradell, N. J., Medical Economics Co., 1974.
15. Hutton, G. L.: *Legal Considerations on Ionizing Radiation.* Springfield, Ill., Charles C Thomas, 1966.
16. Kramer, C: *Medical Malpractice.* Rev. Ed. New York, Practicing Law Institute, 1972.
17. Kramer, C.: *Evidence in Negligence Cases.* New York, Practicing Law Institute, 1973.
18. Lanzl, L. H., Pingel, J. H., and Rust, J. H.:. *Radiation Accidents and Emergencies in Medicine Research and Industry.* Springfield, Ill., Charles C Thomas, 1965.
19. Louisell, D. W., Williams, H., and Kalisch, J. R.: *Medical Malpractice.* Rev. Ed. New York, Mathew Bender & Co., 1974.
20. McCabe, J. M.: What to do if you are sued for malpractice. J. Leg. Med., 2:21, 1974.
21. Meany, T. F., Lalli, A. F., and Alfidi, R. J.: *Complications and Legal Implications of Radiologic Special Procedures.* St. Louis, C. V. Mosby Co., 1973.
22. Troupin, R. H.: *Diagnostic Radiology in Clinical Medicine.* Chicago, Year Book Medical Publishers Inc., 1973.
23. Thomson, T. T.: *Primer of Clinical Radiology.* Boston, Little, Brown and Co., 1973.
24. Weigen, J. J., and Thomas, S. F.: *Complications of Diagnostic Radiology.* Springfield, Ill., Charles C Thomas, 1973.

SECTION 6. THERMAL INJURY

chapter 20

SYSTEMIC AND LOCALIZED HYPERTHERMIC INJURY

by C. G. Tedeschi

SYSTEMIC EFFECTS OF HYPERTHERMIA

HEAT REGULATION IN MAN

Thermal homeostasis is maintained by a delicate balance between heat load and heat dissipation. In both, environmental and internal (bodily) factors are involved.

Internal heat identifies itself with the amount of temperature generated by the oxidation of metabolic products. The quantity of heat produced by the individual under conditions of rest and normal thermal balance constitutes the so-called *basal metabolism.*

Environmental heat comes from the sun, and its effects are influenced by the moisture content of the air; by its wavelength, spectral distribution, absorption by ozone and dust, reflection, and absorption by skin and clothing; and by other factors that can be quantitated approximately.

Both environmental and internal heat are measured in calories. A calorie represents the quantity of heat needed to raise a kilogram of water from 0° to 1°C.

Heat load results from the combination of environmental and internal heat. Whenever the heat load exceeds heat dispersion, body heat rises and heat dispersion occurs. This takes place primarily through evaporation of sweat. Each liter of sweat accounts for 580 kilogram calories of heat. At the upper limits of temperature tolerance, sweat can amount to 3.5 liters per hour. Vaporization from the respiratory passages, insensible perspiration, and the trifling loss through excretion are relatively minor channels of heat dispersion.

Insensible perspiration is the term given to the loss of moisture from the nonsweating body. There is considerable variation in the percentage of heat lost by this mechanism; in a cool or neutral environment it can produce a loss of approximately 24 per cent of metabolic heat. The skin vapor pressure, the vapor pressure of the air, and the air motion determine to a large extent the rate of escape of moisture from the skin. If the pressure gradients are reversed, the skin can take up, as well as lose, water. The other half of the insensible perspiration comes from the respiratory tract. Panting, under resting conditions, is not as prominent in man as it is in many animals. On exposure to extreme heat, however, or during heavy exercise, ventilation rate increases in direct proportion to body temperature elevation, and quite independently from alveolar P_{CO_2}. A 1°C rise in body temperature leads to an increase in ventilation rate of about 11 liters per minute.[1] Ingestion of hot or cold substances has little effect on body temperature.

Internal heat is brought to the surface of the body by molecular conduction, according to the specific conductivity of the tissues. The quantity carried by circulating blood depends primarily on the blood temperature and the volume of flow to the skin.

Transportation of heat from the interior of the body to the body surface is one of the homeostatic functions of the blood stream. Evidence has been presented that direct venous convection of heat from the working muscle to the skin is the principal agent of heat transfer.[1] The presence of vasodilator nerves, primarily in muscle tissue, is important in thermic regulation inasmuch as it increases peripheral conductivity up to sixfold during rest and up to twentyfold during exercise.[1] The control of vasomotor regulation is both hormonal and neural. The hormonal control involves the pituitary-adrenal axis. Thus thyroxine influences body temperature by its direct action on body metabolism; corticoids maintain a normal level of carbohydrate metabolism, one of the major sources of caloric production; epinephrine assists in keeping a constant body temperature, on one side by mobilizing hepatic glycogen and on the other by constricting the lumina of the peripheral blood channels and therefore reducing heat dispersion. Thermodispersion is further regulated by vasopressin (Pitressin), a product of the posterior lobe of the pituitary gland, also a vasoconstricting agent.

At neural level the responses are local, segmental, and suprasegmental as well. The parts of the central nervous system most involved in temperature control are the hypothalamus, the spinal cord, and the intervening connecting pathways that are related to the vasomotor system. Experimental evidence points to the preoptic region (between the anterior commissure and the optic chiasma) as the site of suprasegmental regulation; evidence has also been presented that on structural loss of regular thermoregulatory centers, other areas in the brain stem and spinal cord are able to take over, at least to some extent, temperature regulatory functions.[1] Temperature regulation at the neural level implies the existence of temperature-sensitive cells, a kind of biologic thermostat whose response to variations in temperature takes the form of nerve discharges.

The following equation expresses clearly the laws governing heat regulation in man: $M-W-E\pm R\pm V\pm D\pm X=O$, in which M=metabolism, W=work of a physical nature, E=heat loss through evaporation, R=radiation heat (gain or loss), V=convection (gain or loss), D=conduction (gain or loss), and X=ingesta or excreta or unevaporated sweat (gain or loss). Any departure from this equilibrium indicates a state of either heat dispersion or heat retention.

Two temperature scales are customarily used to measure bodily heat levels: the centigrade and the Fahrenheit. In the centigrade scale the interval between the freezing point and the boiling point of water is divided into 100 degrees, with 0° representing the freezing point and 100° the boiling point. In the Fahrenheit scale, the boiling point of water is 212 degrees above zero of the scale; the freezing point is at 32 degrees above the zero point, and the zero point approximates the temperature produced by mixing equal quantities by weight of snow and common salt at standard atmospheric pressure.

The temperature of the normal human body is 37°C (98.6°F). This value is, however, only approximate. There are physiologic variations from individual to individual, and individual variations as well according to age, the state of rest or physical exertion, the time of day, and other factors. The maximal deviation between normal individuals, in excess or in deficit, is 0.4°C. In the newborn, temperature averages 1°C higher, and a similar trend is present in old age. An elevation of 2°C may occur during heavy physical stress, and in children during severe emotional strain. Daily cyclic variations also take place: in the night (around 1 to 2 A.M.), under complete resting conditions, there is a decrease in body temperature of about half a degree, followed by a slight elevation early in the morning and again in the latter part of the afternoon. There are no differences between male and female, except for a slight increase in temperature during ovulation.

Temperature varies in the different parts of the body. The deepest parts are warmer than the superficial ones, and among the latter those lying on a muscular layer are warmer than those that lack muscle. Thus, for example, the teguments over the ears, nose, and testes are cooler than the teguments over the limbs. Rectal temperature mirrors the "internal" body temperature. It is more elevated (about 0.2° to 0.6°C) than oral or axillary temperature; its uniformity and reproducibility have made its recording desirable in controlled temperature studies.

SYSTEMIC HYPERTHERMIA

Normal thermal homeostasis depends on the preservation of the physiologic mechanisms responsible for the loss of heat, namely, sweating, adequate circulation, and acclimatization. We are not concerned in this context with other factors such as congenital absence of sweat glands, as in ectodermal dysplasia, or impairment of circulation, as in congestive heart failure.[2,3]

The human body is far more susceptible to an elevation than to a diminution of temperature. When the environmental temperature increases to the point that cooling by radiation and convection is not sufficient to eliminate the metabolic heat, sweat is evoked. Under resting conditions, sweating is initiated when the environmental temperature reaches 30°C (±1°C). Sweat is more than 99 per cent water. Since as much as 5 to 10 liters of sweat can be lost in a 24-hour period, however, under persistently unfavorable environmental conditions, the overall loss of urea, salts, and other plasma elements can be considerable. It has been estimated that the quantity of urea eliminated with sweat in a 20-minute period parallels that excreted by one kidney in the same period of time. In the unacclimatized individual participating in physical activities in extreme heat, salt losses up to 20 g per day have been registered.[1]

Bradykinin, a substance that is produced by the sweat glands and has prominent vasodilator activity, may play an important role in increasing the blood supply to the gland and therefore its secretion.[1]

Sweat loss is compensated for by decreased rate of urine formation and increased water intake. With very high sweating rates (1,000 to 1,500 g per hour), however, after four to six hours a condition of fatigue supervenes in the overworked sweat glands, sweat ceases, and body temperature rises.

For each degree of rise in body temperature there is an increase of 5 to 14 per cent in metabolic rate. Oxygen utilization increases proportionately, and in contrast, the oxygen-combining capacity of hemoglobin decreases; the greater stability of oxyhemoglobin in association with alkalosis further impairs the release of oxygen to the tissues. Higher rate of blood flow also reduces the oxygen available for tissue transfer. In severe hyperpyrexia the arterial oxygen saturation decreases by approximately 25 per cent, and venous oxygen saturation increases in proportion.[4-6]

Systemic hyperthermia can be caused by four basic conditions: (1) an intolerable elevation of environmental temperature (exogenous or nonfebrile hyperthermia); (2) a rise in body temperature in conjunction with an endogenous disorder, an infection for example, (endogenous or febrile hyperthermia); (3) an accidental, unpredictable febrile state coincidental to administration of drugs (drug fever) or purposely induced for therapeutic reasons (pyretotherapy); and (4) overwhelming heat exposure incidental to a fire (conflagration hyperthermia).

Exogenous or Nonfebrile Hyperthermia

The human body reacts to an environmental elevation of temperature by reducing thermogenesis and by increasing heat dispersion. The decrease in thermogenesis is attained by reducing the metabolic rate to the minimum required to sustain vital functions; thermodispersion is achieved by peripheral vasodilation and profuse sweating, evaporation converting the sweat to water vapor. High relative humidity and lack of air movement hamper the sweating mechanism. When sweating ceases, the manifestations of the hyperthermic syndrome become manifest.

Diseased states due to the effects of excessive heat are customarily divided, in progressive order of severity, into heat cramps, heat exhaustion, thermogenic anhydrosis, and heatstroke. Ultimately all result from the loss of equilibrium between heat load (metabolic and climatic) and the capacity of the organism to eliminate heat. The clinical manifestations of the relatively less severe forms—heat cramps, for instance—are prominent enough to warn the individual of the impending threat and to make him cease any physical activity, thus preventing the occurrence of the more serious heat disorders that, if not promptly recognized and treated, may pursue a fatal course.

Heat Cramps (Miners' Cramps, Stokers' Cramps)

As the term indicates, the major manifestation of this condition is painful spasm of voluntary muscles, especially those of the extremities and the abdominal wall, during or after physical activity in a hot environment. The predisposing role of excessive alcohol intake and ill health is acknowledged; conversely, there is some doubt that salt depletion is the only cause of this condition. Nevertheless, the administration of physiologic saline solution intravenously gives dramatic relief, and prophylactic use of salt tablets and water is common in industry and among sportsmen as a measure to prevent salt depletion and the occurrence of the cramps.[7]

Heat Exhaustion

The manifestations of heat exhaustion are not dissimilar to those elicited by protracted physical exercise in a comfortable climatic environment, brief exhausting exercise, or any physical activity under conditions of severe caloric excess. Prodromic symptoms include thirst, nausea, vomiting, headaches, mental fogginess, dizziness, irritability, and a subjective feeling of exhaustion and incapacity to work. Fainting and manifestations of peripheral vascular collapse not uncommonly follow, in the absence of physical findings of special note. Temperature may or may not be slightly elevated, and in contrast to heatstroke, the skin is not dry and there is sweating.[8]

Thermogenic Anhydrosis

Knowledge of this syndrome (also known as desert syndrome, anhydrotic heat exhaustion, tropical anhydrotic asthenia) rests on a detailed study by Wolkin, Goodman, and Kelley of eight soldiers who, toward the end of a summer spent in the American desert, developed manifestations that in a broad sense duplicated those of heat exhaustion.[9] There were, however, some distinctive features. After profuse generalized sweating for several days, perspiration ceased suddenly in all parts of the body below the neck region; nevertheless, it persisted in the face and neck. Another unusual characteristic was that the unbalanced distribution of sweat was preceded by or coincided with an eruption of prickly heat rash—a kind of miliaria profunda.

The soldiers affected by this condition complained of weakness, headache, dizziness, and shakiness. Bodily temperature elevation was minimal or absent, and with rest and return to a cool environment all symptoms disappeared.

Additional cases fitting this description have been reported by other investigators.[10-12] The condition is not uncommon among Bengali children, and it has been shown to occur in an approximate incidence of 4 per cent among tanker personnel returning from the Persian Gulf.[13, 14]

This syndrome has still not been suitably explained. Among the possibilities, primary consideration has been given to either hyperkeratotic plugging of sweat glands or functional failure of the sweat apparatus, or to a combination of both.

Heatstroke

Complete absence of sweating and an increase in body temperature above an arbitrary level of 106°F (41°C), in the presence of environmental heat stress and the absence of any other cause of pyrexia, constitute heat hyperpyrexia. By common consent, when concurrent with varying manifestations of cerebral deficit, this condition merits the label of heatstroke.

Several investigators have pointed out that fixing the critical body temperature at the arbitrary level of 106°F (41°C) is unsatisfactory. Cases have been recorded in which the typical manifestations of heatstroke occurred at lower body temperature levels.[3, 7, 15, 16]

Hot and dry skin, increased depth of respiration simulating Kussmaul breathing, rapid pulse with a rate of 160 to 180 beats per minute, and severe asthenia are the major characteristic features of this condition. Manifestations of cerebral deficit, such as convulsions (either generalized or jacksonian in type), delirium, or stupor (in time progressing to coma), are poor prognostic signs. There were 12 deaths among the patients who were comatose on admission in Austin and Berry's series.[3] Among the disorders of the central nervous system, disturbances in muscle tone, pyramidal signs, opisthotonos, tetany, and decerebrate rigidity have been recorded. Poor prognosis is also attached to hypotension, hyperpotassemia, and an increase in blood urea nitrogen.[17]

In almost all fatal and severe cases, 1- to 3-plus proteinuria and abundant urinary casts are found; liver damage is evidenced by elevated levels of serum bilirubin and serum iron.

Equally poor prognostic signs are elevated levels of serum enzymes, including glutamic oxaloacetic transaminase (SGOT), which may reflect muscle or liver damage, lactic dehydrogenase (LDH), and hydroxybutyric dehydrogenase (HBD).[16] Eventually, shock ensues and the concurrent peripheral vasoconstriction further impairs heat loss.

The first 24 hours following the early manifestations of distress are the most critical, and death generally occurs within a week.

Predisposing Conditions. The importance of predisposing conditions and individual susceptibility is brought out by the fact that usually only one of a group of people exposed to the same unfavorable environmental conditions falls victim to heatstroke. The factors involved are largely dependent on mechanisms that compromise physiologic heat dispersion.

Alcoholism and preexisting or concurrent disease, primarily cardiovascular and cerebral arteriosclerosis, predispose to the occurrence of this condition and increase the risk of a fatal outcome.

Individuals over the age of 60 constitute the largest group of heatstroke victims. In Austin and Berry's series 70 per cent of the patients were in this age group, and fatalities were equally more frequent.[3] An unusual increase in deaths among the elderly, especially those taking diuretic hypotensive agents, is also shown in the study Schuman and associates made of the Michigan heat wave of 1962 and 1963.[18] The heat chamber studies of Gold similarly show that healthy subjects over the age of 40 are less able to make compensatory circulatory adjustment than younger subjects.[8] The increased susceptibility of older people is explained by the fact that during a given exposure they absorb more heat from the environment; they are also unable to utilize ice water administered for the purpose of heat dissipation as younger individuals do.

By the same token, infection and gastrointestinal upsets carry an extra risk. Fever almost regularly occurs in conjunction with infection. The concurrent anorexia reduces salt and water intake, and vomiting or diarrhea increases loss of water and salt.

Obesity also is considered a factor able to enhance the development of heatstroke. Capillary-poor adipose tissue creates an increased demand on the heart; furthermore, the thick panniculus provides extra insulation for the body. Since metabolic heat is produced in proportion to the bulk of tissue and is lost in proportion to surface area, the large volume-to-area ratio creates an added risk in the obese.[19]

Prodromic Symptoms. The manifestations of heatstroke may come on suddenly or be preceded by prodromic symptoms—nausea, vomiting, vertigo, muscle cramps, dyspnea, and a feeling of hotness. These vague symptoms, in unduly sustained hot weather, should warn the physician of the impending threat of a preventable medical catastrophe.

Gold's description of subjective impressions in 250 healthy adult human volunteers placed in a heat chamber provides a useful guide to the stage-by-stage progress of events that precede the critical phase of outright heat hyperpyrexia: Ability to concentrate begins to wane, and there is a vague feeling of impending physiologic deterioration. Awareness of body heat and profuse perspiration is replaced by the realization that sweating has diminished and then suddenly ceased. The face feels dry and hot, and concurrently the patient mentions feeling a film of dried salt on the cheeks and forehead and at the corners of the mouth. Soon after come realization that the slightest movement of the body produces an increase in heart rate and the premonition of a fainting spell. Paresthesias, particularly in the hands, wrists, feet, ankles, and forelegs, develop at this point, and the face, until now pinkish-red in color, abruptly turns ashen gray—an indication of impending cardiocirculatory collapse. At this stage, Gold says, the volunteer must be removed from the heat chamber because, "were he not, he would become stuporous, faint, and eventually lapse into the coma of heatstroke."[8]

Geographical Considerations. Two of the most thorough reports on the clinical and climatic aspects of heatstroke come from two different continents several thousand miles apart. One, by Austin and Berry, analyzes 100 cases of heatstroke drawn from over 1,000 heat victims admitted to St. Louis City Hospital (St. Louis, Missouri) in the summers of 1952, 1953, and 1954.[3] The other, by Leithead and others, concerns 128 cases of heatstroke arising in the summer months in ships' personnel sailing in the Red Sea, the Gulf of Aden, and the Persian Gulf.[7]

By mere coincidence, the two studies were carried out in about the same years and in the same months of the year. Whereas the cases included in Austin and Berry's report mirrored an unusual climatic condition in St. Louis in three of the six hottest summers in the past century and a quarter, those described by Leithead and associates resulted just from the effects of the usual climatic condition.

Weather Bureau data in the two series correspond very closely and reflect the atmospheric conditions most likely to elicit one or another of the hyperthermic syndromes: shade temperatures of 95° to 120°F (35° to 49°C) in the Persian Gulf, and an average sustained temperature of over 90°F in St. Louis.

Although there is no restricted geographical distribution, heat illness has always been prevalent in Arabia and the Middle East. Heat and fever probably killed more Crusaders than the scimitars of the unfaithful. Poor acclimatization and unsuitable clothing were equally responsible for the heavy death toll (no fewer than 425 in a single month according to Wilcox) suffered by the British Expeditionary Force in Mesopotamia during the first World War and by army personnel in Iraq during the second World War.[12, 20]

It must be realized that although heat casualties arise most frequently in coincidence with adverse climatic conditions, they may occur as well whenever environmental heat stress exceeds the level compatible with balanced thermoregulation. Far from the tropics, cases of heatstroke have been described among those engaged in a variety of occupations, for instance, boiler room and coal mine workers. Cases are also on record of heat hyperpyrexia in the operating room or in a Turkish bath.[22, 23] Therapeutic lamps and any other heat-producing apparatus are equally important hazards.

Physiopathology of Hyperpyrexia. The mortality rate in heatstroke is high. Figures range

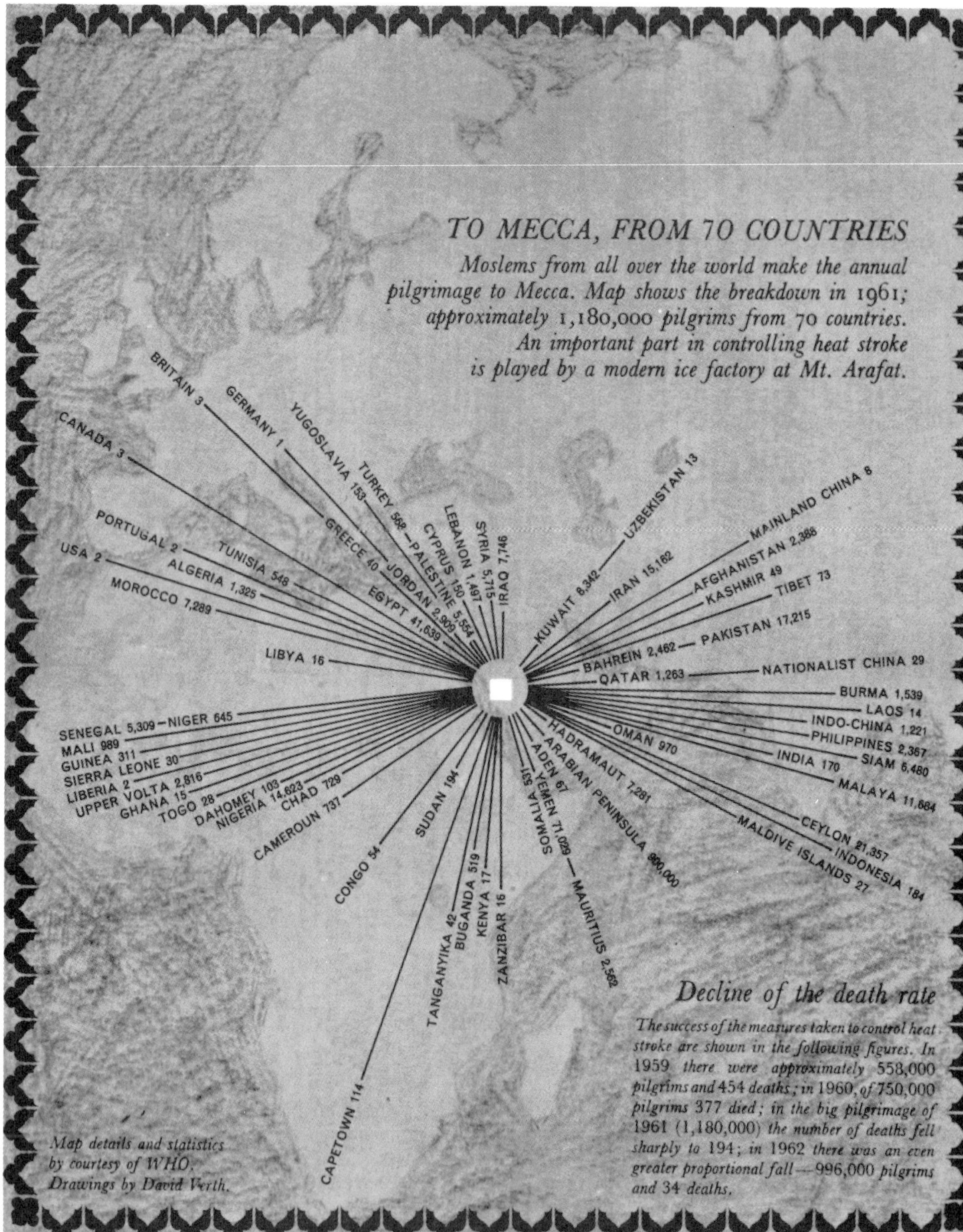

Figure 20–1. Map and statistical details indicating decline of death rate by heatstroke following progressive introduction of preventative and therapeutic measures. (Courtesy of World Health Organization.)

from 70 per cent in older series to 17 per cent in more recent ones.[3] The deceased mortality rate is unquestionably due to better understanding of the problems involved and more effective methods of treatment (Fig. 20–1). For instance, a clinic and a heatstroke treatment room are available to the crews of the tanker fleet berthed at the pier of Mina al Ahmadi (State of Kuwait) where heat casualties occur frequently (approximate incidence index of 1 of 850 seamen).[7]

A general rise in the temperature of the

circulating blood to a level higher than 42.4°C leads to generalized vasodilation, in turn causing an effective reduction in blood volume; to cardiac dilatation; and to stimulation of the respiratory centers and, ultimately, suspension of respiratory activity. Which one of these altered physiologic responses is responsible for somatic deterioration and death is not entirely clear; however, it is generally agreed that the syndrome is the manifestation of a generalized process of cellular damage.

The cardiovascular system apparently takes the brunt of hyperpyrexia. According to Daily and Harrison, the mechanism of circulatory collapse is peripheral; however, the weight of present evidence favors the view that the primary event is high-output cardiac failure.[23] Accordingly, it is postulated that the primary functional pathologic factor in heatstroke is the greatly diminished peripheral resistance that leads to increased and rapid venous return and increased cardiac output as well. As the left side of the heart cannot keep pace with the right, the increase in venous return results in an elevation of venous pressure that triggers high-output cardiac failure and circulatory collapse.[8]

During the stage of hyperpyrexia short of collapse, a massive cutaneous circulation arises that is the functional equivalent of an arteriovenous shunt. The resulting tissue anoxia may explain the paresthesias commonly felt by the victims of heat hyperpyrexia. By the same token it has been suggested that the same increase in venous pressure is ultimately responsible for the cessation of sweating seen at the peak of the heatstroke syndrome.

> As the venous pressure increases, the sweat rate begins to drop off; as the venous pressure decreases, the mechanism of sweating is restored.[8]

Supporting this concept is the observation that the rate of water loss in patients with severe congestive heart failure in a hot and humid environment is only 27 to 47 per cent of that of normal subjects under similar climatic conditions.[24]

Ultimately, oxygen deprivation rather than the direct effect of the increased heat load is the factor that is responsible for the manifestations attending the heatstroke syndrome.

The autopsy findings in heatstroke lack specificity and basically do not differ from those found in death from cardiac failure. An additional feature is the presence of visceral hemorrhages, which some investigators have attributed to thrombocytopenia and the decrease in plasma fibrinogen and prothrombin levels that occur in conjunction with the hyperthermic state.[25, 26]

Hepatic damage has been implicated as a cause of the prothrombin abnormality and of the frequent visceral hemorrhages; however, the extravasations of blood can equally be explained by the increased capillary fragility coincidental to anoxia and circulatory collapse.

In patients who survive more than 24 hours, other commonly encountered changes include degeneration of megakaryocytes, lobular pneumonia, acute tubular necrosis of the kidneys, adrenal hemorrhage, frank adrenal cortical necrosis, and centrilobular necrosis of the liver.[27]

Subendocardial hemorrhage and degenerative changes in myofibers are far from uncommon, and massive extravasation of blood into the myocardium has been recorded.[27] A case has been reported of transmural infarction in which no abnormalities could be found in the coronary arteries.[28] These cardiac changes well explain the frequent detection of electrocardiographic abnormalities, primarily T-wave and conduction defects.

Brain and leptomeninges are congested and edematous, the convolutions flattened, and scattered petechiae are found, most frequently in the walls of the third ventricle and in the floor of the fourth ventricle.

In the classic study by Malamud, Haymaker, and Custer, degenerative changes in cortical neurons were seen as early as 11 hours after the hyperthermic injury; at 24 hours the number of neurons was reduced, and there was already evidence of both glial and microglial mobilization (Figs. 20–2, 20–3, and 20–4).

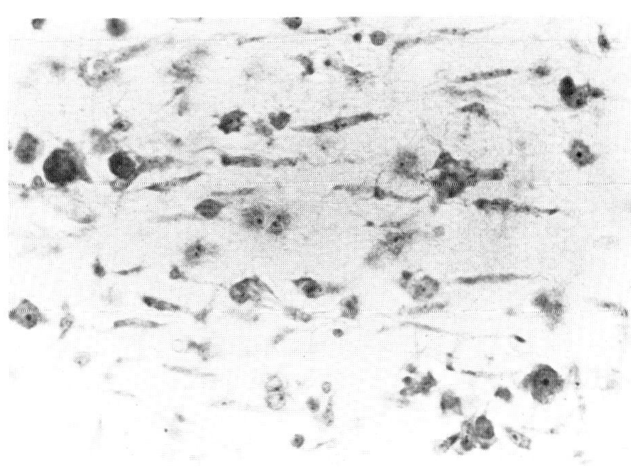

Figure 20–2. Heatstroke. Dropping out and degeneration of neurons with concurrent microglial reaction. Duration of illness, 276 hours. (From C. G. Tedeschi (Ed.): *Neuropathology, Methods and Diagnosis.* Boston, Little, Brown and Co., 1970. Reprinted by permission.)

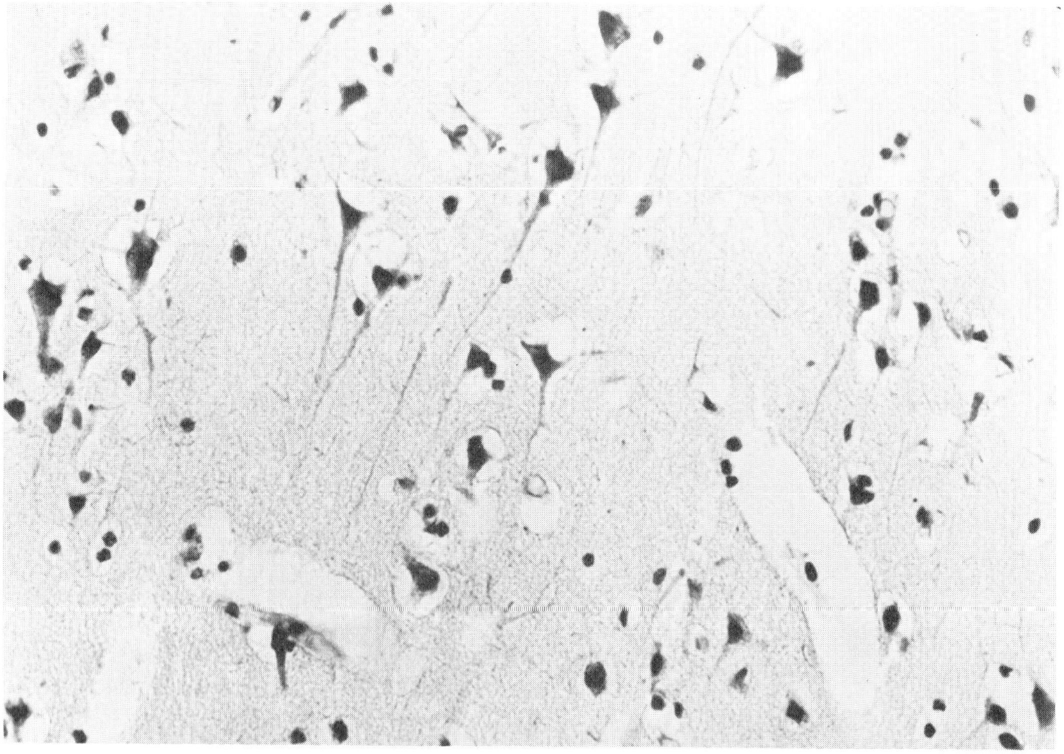

Figure 20–3. Heatstroke. Shrinking and hyperchromasia of cortical nerve cells. Duration of illness, 72 hours. (From C. G. Tedeschi (Ed.): *Neuropathology, Methods and Diagnosis.* Boston, Little, Brown and Co., 1970. Reprinted by permission.)

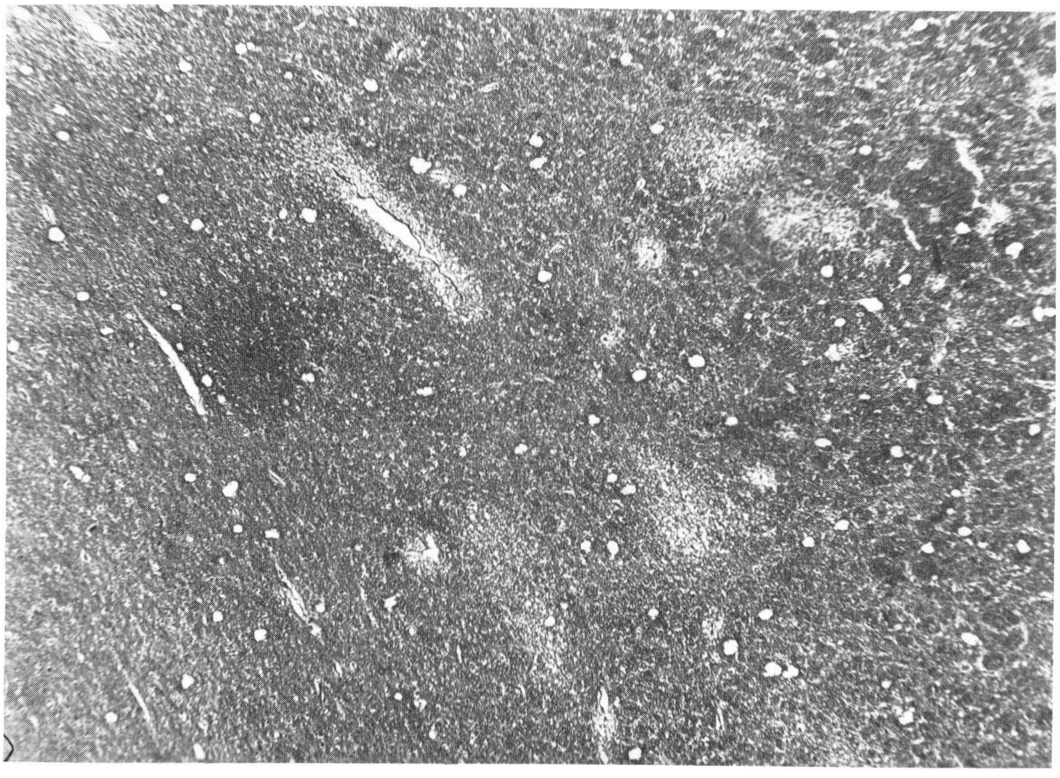

Figure 20–4. Heatstroke. Perivascular foci of rarefaction scattered throughout cerebral white matter. Duration of illness, 12 hours. (From C. G. Tedeschi (Ed.): *Neuropathology, Methods and Diagnosis.* Boston, Little, Brown and Co., 1970. Reprinted by permission.)

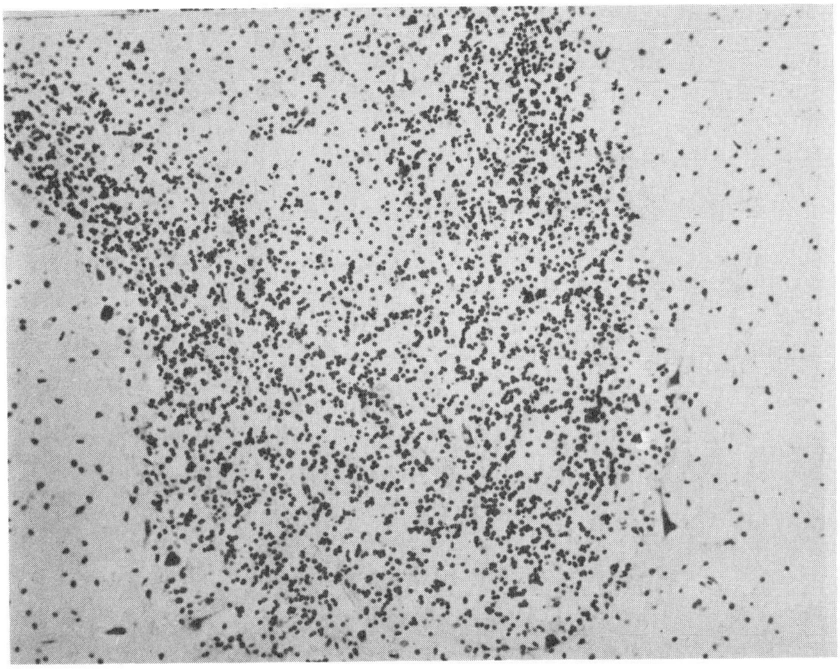

Figure 20–5. Heatstroke. Cerebellum. Notice almost total absence of Purkinje cells. Duration of illness, 49 hours.

Degeneration of myelin was minimal or absent. The globus pallidus was the least affected, and in contrast, the cerebellum was the site of the most striking changes, particularly affecting the Purkinje cell layer (Fig. 20–5).

The heat-dissipation center (preoptic and supraoptic regions), and the heat-conservation and heat-production centers (caudolateral portion of the hypothalamus) have been subjected to extensive investigation, but there is no general consensus about the incidence of demonstrable alterations.[29–31]

The "Sauna Bath." The hot-air bath is a unique tradition of the Finns. Popular opinion holds that bathing in a sauna has a variety of beneficial effects for the healthy and the sick as well. The procedure consists of exposing the body to a hot and relatively dry atmosphere.[32]

Bathing takes place in a special cabin with thick walls of wooden boards or logs and containing a stone stove heated to several hundred degrees centigrade. Wooden benches are fastened to one of the walls at various heights from the floor. As the bather ascends from each bench to the next, the ambient air temperature increases—from 60°C to 120°C. On the average the bath is taken once a week and lasts 10 to 30 minutes each time.

The beneficial or deleterious effects of sauna bathing are difficult to assess because parallel studies in a control population are not available. In general, however, the bathers report a feeling of relaxation, calmness, and lassitude.

This unique national custom has provided the equally unique opportunity to study the physiologic response to ambient heat.

Under identical conditions, marked individual differences have been noticed in the amount of sweat lost. During a sauna bathing session, sweat losses up to 3,000 g have been registered. It is well known that boxers, wrestlers, and weight lifters, whose weight determines their competitive class in contests, use the sauna bath to induce quick weight loss before a competition. Even as the amount of sweat loss varies from individual to individual under the same sauna conditions, there are also differences in the electrolyte content of the sweat; these differences probably reflect variations in the adrenocortical regulatory response. As a general rule, the chloride content increases in proportion to the rate of sweating and the skin temperature, and it decreases as water intake increases. The sodium and chloride contents are less than those in blood plasma; conversely, potassium levels in sweat and plasma are within the same range, and lactic acid in sweat exceeds that in plasma. Small amounts of histamine and other imidazole compounds have been found in sweat.

As water and salt are lost from the body through sweating, a reduction in the output of urine takes place. Infrequently, the presence in the urine of albumin, hemoglobin, porphyrins, casts, and other abnormal elements has been registered on exceptionally intense exposure to heat and has been interpreted as due to altered glomerular and tubular mechanisms.

The respiratory rate increases to 20 to 30 cycles per minute, a phenomenon that implies increased total oxygen consumption (about 20 per cent), and carbon dioxide production. Heart rate also increases, values ranging from 100 to 160 beats per minute. Physical fitness, extent of exposure to hot environment, constitutional characteristics, age, and sex probably have a bearing on the degree of cardiac rhythm acceleration. The decline of pulse rate following repeated sauna bathing may be interpreted as an indication of acclimatization. The heart rate begins to decline immediately when the bather leaves the sauna chamber. Cardiac output increases moderately, and in patients with hypertension, a substantial decrease in arterial pressure may occur and even persist for a while after the exposure. Increased heart rate, rising blood temperature, and concomitant humoral and nervous influences may explain the occasional occurrence of electrocardiographic changes of doubtful significance. A flattened T wave was found by Lundgren in approximately one third of his subjects, but the change disappeared rapidly after the subject left the bath.[33]

Since sauna bathing is particularly popular with sportsmen, the study of its effects on striated muscles has been given much consideration. Results of ergographic observations indicate that the bathing session does not influence the mechanical efficiency of muscle.

Hemoconcentration occurs as a direct consequence of prolonged sweating, and a mild increase in circulating neutrophils and a decrease in lymphocytes and eosinophils have been recorded by some investigators. The statistical significance of these blood changes, however, remains questionable. Equally vague and controversial are the data on plasma electrolytes, except for the increase of chloride content.

The overall findings indicate that alterations in endocrine function take place, but so far they have not been measured directly. It is worth mentioning that old reports in the Finnish literature relate sauna bathing to increased milk secretion. This observed effect can be attributed to an increased oxytocin secretion by the posterior hypophysis, which stimulates lactation. It is interesting, also, that in earlier times the sauna room was used by Finnish country women as the place for delivery of their children.[32]

Observation of the effects of sauna bathing has added considerable knowledge to the understanding of the process of acclimatization.

Acclimatization. This term is used synonymously with physiologic acclimatization to heat. Experience earned the hard way from two world wars has taught us a good deal on the prevention of heatstroke.

It is well known that individuals not acclimatized to the tropics are inclined to develop manifestations of heatstroke upon minimal exertion, whereas acclimatized individuals can withstand a far greater amount of work without ill effects.

Acclimatization is accompanied by a series of physiologic adaptations, the most important of which include: (1) retention of fluid and a concomitant increase in blood volume, which restores cardiovascular stability; (2) a more rapid onset of sweating in response to an elevation in body temperature; (3) an actual increase in the rate of sweating; and (4) a decrease in the elimination of sodium chloride, through both sweat and urine. Another important feature is the reduction in metabolic heat production; this can be achieved by reducing dietary carbohydrates and fats that increase the endogenous heat load.[34]

The process of acclimatization is rapid and may be completed within a week; however, physical fitness increases with long-term acclimatization, which requires months or even years of residence in a hot climate.

There is no agreement about the mechanisms operating in the acclimatization process, but the fluid retention, which precedes the increase in blood volume, indicates that the adrenal gland must play a primary role.[7] Urinary excretion of aldosterone increases during acclimatization.

Looking into the methods of preventing the deleterious effects of environmental heat hyperpyrexia, one is reminded of Bertrand Russell's statement that whereas the man of older civilizations tried to adapt himself to the environment, modern man directs his efforts to adapting the environment to suit himself.[35] Appropriate in this respect is Leithead's comparison of the nomadic Bedouin wearing long robes to protect himself from the fierce heat of the sun and resting in meditative immobility in the shade of his tent at the hottest part of the day, and the lightly clothed Western man taking periodic rest in his bungalow supplied with fans, air conditioning, refrigerators, and ice-cold water fountains.

Endogenous or Febrile Hyperthermia (Fever)

This type of elevation in body temperature is the result of a dissociation between thermogenesis and thermodispersion due to intrinsic rather than environmental causes, and is therefore a subject not strictly pertinent to this chapter. It is sufficient to say that many different endogenous agents can be responsible for an elevation in body temperature.

Hyperpyrexia can be elicited by: (1) the parenteral injection of foreign proteins—a phenomenon that is utilized in pyretotherapy; (2) pyrogenic substances elaborated by bacteria; (3) products of tissular degeneration; (4) an elevation in intracranial pressure; and (5) certain endocrine disorders. For instance, postthyroidectomy heatstroke is a well-documented syndrome of systemic hyperthermia induced by an endocrine-related metabolic disturbance.

The elevation in temperature may take place in gradual fashion or rapidly, reaching the peak in one to two hours, as in tertian malaria. Quite often, the hyperpyrexia is preceded by chills and is associated with a subjective sensation of cold. This sensation, which results from peripheral vasoconstriction, provokes a reduction in thermodispersion; the concurrent contraction of voluntary muscles contributes to the increase in thermogenesis.

Recognition of the pattern—continued, quotidian, remittent, intermittent, relapsing, recurrent, ambulatory, or the like—of the hyperpyrexia constitutes an important clue to the disease that is responsible for the fever. The same consideration applies to the characteristics of the defervescence period, which can occur gradually or by crisis.

According to one favorably received view, endogenous hyperpyrexia results from two major factors: an elevation in basal metabolism and an alteration of the thermoregulatory mechanism provoked by pyrogenic substances. (An elevation in body temperature of 1°C leads to an approximate increase of 13 per cent of the basal metabolic rate; as the temperature of the body increases, there is a parallel increase in basal metabolism to levels from 30 to 40 per cent above normal at a temperature of 39°C to 40°C).

The exact nature of the endogenous pyrogen has not been ascertained as yet; however, present evidence points to the bacterial endotoxins, blood leukocytes, and products of cell degeneration, either singly or in combination, as the agents able to alter the thermoregulatory mechanism.

A new avenue to the understanding of pyrogen-produced fever has been opened by the demonstration that pyrogens have the ability to increase synthesis and release of prostaglandins and that antipyretic and antiinflammatory drugs bring fever down by inhibiting prostaglandin activity. Prostaglandins are natural constituents of brain tissue and have been identified in tissue extracts of the hypothalamus as well as in cerebrospinal fluid. This important discovery is a step toward the understanding of the relations between pyrogens and the thermoregulatory centers.[36]

Drug Fever

Febrile reactions following administration of drugs are part and parcel of the unpredictable side effects inherent in drug administration. In some cases the pyrogen is released from the cells injured by the toxic effects of the drug, while in some others a hypersensitivity mechanism is operating; in still others the culprit can be an accidental contaminant. None of these speculative mechanisms can be generalized, and individual modi operandi can be conceived in particular situations. Drug fever as the only manifestation of adverse drug reaction is uncommon; it has been estimated that it accounts for only 3 to 4 per cent of all reactions.[37] More often, fever is associated with a broad spectrum of other systemic disorders, including skin manifestations, which not infrequently are the first indication that an adverse drug reaction exists.

Pyrogens associated with drug fever may act in one of two ways: either by increasing the rate of heat production or by decreasing the rate of heat loss. Dinitrophenol, which stimulates tissue metabolism, exemplifies the former; epinephrine, which induces peripheral vasoconstriction, illustrates the latter.

Drug fever may be caused by a number of agents: barbiturates, antihistamines, penicillin, sulfonamides, salicylates, diphenylhydantoin (Dilantin), and cocaine, to mention just a few.[37, 38] In some instances the febrile reaction to the drug is not consistent; in others it has the characteristics of a "fixed" response. This often occurs with methyldopa, a drug widely used in the treatment of hypertension. Several cases are on record of recurrence of fever after reinstitution of methyldopa treatment.[39]

Hyperthermia contributes significantly to the lethal effects of *1,1,1-trichloro-2,2-bis(p-chlorophenyl)ethane (DDT)* poisoning.[40] Equally well known are the toxic reactions, including fever, that follow the use of the various *sulfonamides*. Fever may occur alone, with a skin eruption, or with other manifestations of drug intoxication or hypersensitivity. It is commonest after sulfathiazole and least common following sulfadiazine administration.[41]

Since many of the drugs able to induce fever

are administered as part of the treatment of infections, recognition of the cause of the fever is important. This point is illustrated by the following personally observed case.

A 28-year-old Caucasian man sought medical advice for a painful swelling in the right knee following a fall five days previously while playing football. The knee was markedly reddened and tender on palpation, and the skin was abraded over the patellar region. Oral temperature was 99.4°F. Systemic examination failed to reveal any other abnormal condition. On the assumption that an infection was developing in the injured knee, sulfathiozole therapy was instituted. The fever went higher, to 101° to 102°F, and was accompanied by a chill and a skin eruption. Since there was no improvement, the sulfa treatment was intensified. Puncture of the knee joint failed to yield any exudate, and no bacterial growth was obtained by culture. Oliguria and neutropenia soon developed, progressing to anuria and agranulocytosis, and death occurred six days following the beginning of the sulfa treatment. Unfortunately, permission for postmortem examination was not granted.

An important practical aspect of this case is that the tragic course of events could have been prevented by the prompt recognition that the fever was a manifestation of drug sensitivity rather than due to infection.

Fever may equally result from a *sterile abscess* following intravenous or intramuscular administration of a drug or from the release of microbial antigens in the circulation, as in the Herxheimer reaction. Most cases of drug fever are due to hypersensitivity response, however. This situation is best exemplified by serum sickness in which the immunologic mechanism responsible for the fever is the release of pyrogens from activated leukocytes in the blood or from cells of the reticuloendothelial system. Endogenous pyrogens are proteins associated with small amounts of carbohydrate and lipid (molecular weight of 10,000 to 20,000), which can be activated by soluble or insoluble antibody-antigen complexes.[42]

The mechanism by which endogenous pyrogens increase body temperature is stimulation of the thermoregulatory center of the hypothalamus, which initiates heat production by shivering and heat conservation by vasoconstriction.

Though iodide itself is not immunogenic, *iodide fever* has been recorded. In this case, the immunogen is most likely a conjugate of iodide with large molecules of plasma proteins that act as carriers.[43, 44]

Systemic reactions are not uncommon following *blood transfusions*, and a rise in body temperature is the commonest manifestation, particularly in children. In a recent analysis of 246 blood transfusions in children, Sidhu and coworkers cite an overall incidence of 6.5 per cent of pyrogenic reactions. In this series febrile reactions occurred in 16.2 per cent of patients who were pyrexic before the initiation of transfusion, as against 1.2 per cent of those who were afebrile. Malignant disease, burns, anemia, and multiplicity of transfusions increase the probability of a pyrogenic reaction that has been variously attributed to the formation of leukocyte and platelet antibodies, to local infection and thrombosis (thrombophlebitis) at the site of an indwelling plastic catheter, or to the introduction of foreign particles in the blood stream.

Equally difficult to classify, according to underlying mechanisms, is the fever described in conjunction with *splenectomy*, an annoying side effect that may persist for one or two months.[46]

A severe and sustained rise in body temperature, associated with hyperkalemia, metabolic acidosis, and generalized muscle rigidity, characterizes the abnormal response in man and the pig to halogenated anaesthetic agents, either alone or in combination with suxamethonium chloride. This condition is generally known as *malignant hyperthermia*. Although the pig has proved to be a valuable experimental animal for the study of malignant hyperthermia, caution has been suggested in transposing results from one breed or strain of pig to another (Poland-China pigs, Pietrain pigs, Landrace cross pigs) and even more so to the human.[47]

Hyperthermia in an anesthetized patient is infrequent but potentially life-threatening. Its incidence has been shown to be 1:10,000 with a range of 1:5,000 to 1:70,000. Patient ages have ranged from six months to 58 years.[48, 49] To date over 120 cases have been recorded.[50] It seems likely that the increased incidence of malignant hyperthermia in the last decade has paralleled the development and use of more potent anesthetics.

The rise in temperature—insidious, progressive, and accompanied by profuse sweating—occurs 30 to 90 minutes after the induction of the anesthesia. Then sweat ceases, body temperature becomes further elevated, the skin becomes mottled, and tachycardia or bradycardia progressing to cardiac arrest usually follows. The first indication of an untoward reaction is often tightness of the jaw muscles that proceeds to affect all skeletal musculature. Not infrequently this manifestation goes unrecognized because of surgical draping. Disseminated intravascular coagulation may occur concurrently with the hyperthermic state.[51] This condition has been seen to develop following the administration of a variety of anesthetizing agents ranging from halothane to nitrous oxide and oxygen. All the halogenated hydrocarbon inhalants have been incriminated.

The cause of the hyperpyrexia is unknown. In the past it was attributed to the debilitated state of the patient, heavy draping, elevated room temperature, or prolonged surgery. Actually the hyperpyrexial reaction may occur during anesthesia for a minor surgical procedure in an otherwise healthy individual. A disturbance of oxidative phosphorylation has been postulated, but this has been found to be unacceptable, as at least 75 per cent of the heat produced comes from anaerobic sources.[50, 51] Mitochondrial degeneration has been noted, but this is probably a secondary effect. The bulk of present evidence points to the occurrence of malignant hyperpyrexia as a manifestation of an inherited muscular abnormality with autosomal dominance. Individuals affected by this abnormality can be identified by the demonstration of a very high serum creatine phosphokinase (CPK) level. The prevalence of this disorder is well substantiated by the increasing number of reports in the literature of high creatine serum phosphokinase levels in siblings of victims of malignant hyperpyrexia.[50, 53, 54]

The practical conclusions that can be drawn from this relatively new information are: (1) that all relatives of patients who have had malignant hyperpyrexia should be screened by serum creatine phosphokinase determinations so that affected individuals can be warned not to have general anesthetics, and (2) that all individuals undergoing general anesthesia should receive serum creatine phosphokinase determinations.

Induction of controlled hyperthermia in the treatment of disease *(pyretotherapy)* was abandoned a long time ago and has been replaced by the much more efficient antiphlogistic drugs (sulfonamides) and antibiotic agents. Parenteral injections of foreign proteins, malaria parasite inoculations, and bacterial toxin injections were the pyrogens most frequently used when pyretotherapy was in vogue. The debilitating effects of the treatment in an already ill patient and the difficulties in raising the temperature to the desired level hampered clinical application of the method.

Pyretotherapy as a palliative still finds advocates, however. The observation that tumor cells are more easily destroyed by heat than are normal cells has led to the introduction of controlled hyperthermia in the treatment of cancer. Malignant cells are destroyed by temperatures in excess of 40°C, whereas normal cells survive. The earliest clinical evidence of this came from the apparently complete regression of tumors following concomitant attacks of erysipelas. Thereafter methods were devised (arteriovenous shunt, heat exchanger, hot bath, paraffin wax bath) to raise the body temperature as a palliative in terminal stages of malignant disease. Expectedly, results have been conflicting, but claims are not lacking of great reduction or complete loss of pain, of a feeling of well-being, and even of radiologic regression of tumors.[55] Equally conflicting are the results of pyretotherapy applied to another condition—rheumatoid arthritis—in which other treatments often fail and risks are not lacking.[56]

Conflagration Hyperthermia

The forensic, chemical, and thermal attributes of conflagration are so important and complex as to deserve separate consideration. This is being given in the second part of this chapter. The discussion of some of the pertinent problems is, however, likewise appropriate in the context of a survey of systemic hyperthermic trauma.

The extent to which the energy of environmental heat affects the human rests primarily on: (1) the rate at which heat is conveyed to the external surfaces of the body, (2) the rate at which the temperature of the skin rises, (3) the extent of the insulation provided by clothing, and (4) the thickness of the envelope of air that surrounds the body.

Each of these factors is variable; furthermore, heat is only one of the many problems that arise in conjunction with conflagration. In the Cleveland Clinic disaster in 1929, for example, the heat was not excessive, and most of the casualties were attributed to the breathing of chemical irritants given off by burning nitrocellulose x-ray films.[57] In an equally tragic national disaster, the Cocoanut Grove fire in 1942, thermal as well as chemical trauma was considered to have caused most of the deaths. Many aspects of that holocaust are still shrouded in mystery.[58]

The nature of the chemical irritants in smoke is essentially determined by the nature of the materials being burned; carbon monoxide saturation is frequently a contributing agent. Other factors involved include the amount of oxygen available at different times during the fire and the overall temperature that is attained. Aldehydes and acid anhydrides are among the more dangerous products of combustion.[59]

Since no two fires are likely to be alike, the question often arises about the proportion to which chemical or thermal injury has been responsible for the fatal outcome of the exposure. The alterations in the respiratory passages mirror primarily the effects of the chemical injury, whereas thermal injury is measured in terms of the extent of body burns and related systemic effects.

In reference to the effects of inhaled heat on the air passages and lungs, the conclusion drawn by Moritz and co-workers from experiments in the laboratory is that any temperature of the air high enough to produce almost instantaneous burning of the skin and upper respiratory mucosa is also able to produce pulmonary injury. The same study indicates that a temperature able to injure the lungs is more than sufficient to induce a rapidly fatal obstructive edema of the glottis, and that the most vulnerable portion of the lung is the central parenchyma, where bronchioles and alveoli have the most direct connection with the primary bronchi. Equally important is the demonstration provided by the same investigators that moist air is more likely to produce thermal injury than dry air; inhaled steam has 4,000 times the heat-carrying capacity of dry air.[59]

Observations in humans support the conclusions drawn from the experimental laboratory.[60–64] Of the 2,297 patients with thermal injury treated at the Brooke Army Medical Center, 2.9 per cent had inhalation injury.[65] In most of the cases the history was of inhalation of large amounts of superheated smoke in a closed area, resulting in oropharyngeal and facial burns. The concurrent symptoms were cough, hoarseness, bronchospasm, and bronchorrhea with carbon particles in the secretions.

With house fires in the lead, other causes of thermal inhalation injury include mattress fires (jail fires), fumes of sulfur dioxide or refrigerants or phosgene, scald burns from ruptured steam pipes, hyperbaric chamber explosions, and an endless list of other accidental occurrences.

Motorized vehicles hitting land mines and helicopter crashes account for the larger number of thermal inhalation injuries among military personnel. In the case of the land mine, its explosion ignites the gas tank, thus exposing the persons trapped inside the vehicle to thermal cutaneous injuries and to inhalation of acrid irritant fumes leading to respiratory damage. This situation is duplicated in a helicopter crash, in which the men trapped inside the aircraft inhale large amounts of smoke and carbonaceous products.

The strongest pathologic evidence for inhalation of toxic fumes lies in the characteristic eschars within the nares, the black membranous exudation in the larynx and trachea, and the diffuse membranous bronchitis, which is similar to that described as one of the characteristic effects of several of the war gases (phosgene, mustard gas, chloropicrin) and nitrogen dioxide as well. A combination of anoxemia and inhalation injury may explain the frequently associated massive pulmonary edema.[58]

Although inhalation injury plays a major role in the effects of conflagration, evidence has been presented that tracheobronchitis and pneumonia may be complications of tracheostomy, a procedure common in the immediate postburn period. It is equally difficult to differentiate respiratory distress directly related to factors inherent in conflagration from that due to the cardiovascular or metabolic disorders that are sequelae of severe burns.[64] Independently of the effects of asphyxia, carbon monoxide poisoning, the inhalation of flame or fumes, or other factors, cutaneous burns can lead equally rapidly to death. In pigs, a relatively brief (75 sec.) exposure of the skin to a sufficiently high temperature can cause almost immediate death.[66] In this case, the operating mechanism is overheating of the blood as it circulates through the extensive superficial network of subcutaneous vessels. No data are available to show to what extent sweating may be capable of protecting human skin against thermal injury. In relatively low-intensity hot air exposure (below 120°C), man can lose sweat at the rate of approximately 1 liter per hour. This corresponds roughly to a heat loss of 0.5 to 1.0 cal per square centimeter of cutaneous surface per minute. Heat loss of porcine skin through loss of moisture is considerably less, about 0.1 cal per square centimeter per minute. Provided that sweating is already established, therefore, it seems likely that the time threshold for cutaneous burning is higher for man. Equally unpredictable is the degree of protection afforded by clothing. This depends primarily on the degree of thermal resistance of the fabrics involved. With these reservations, there is no reason to believe that man and pig differ greatly in respect to the effects of excessive circumambient and circumradiant heat.

Information gained from the experimental animal indicates that

> . . . source temperatures of approximately 90°C can be tolerated for 45 minutes without

burning, whereas at 100°C burning occurs in 12 minutes and at 180°C, 30 seconds is the longest exposure that can be tolerated without irreversible cutaneous injury.[66]

Experience gained from human disasters is supported by animal experiments simulating conflagration. Observations indicate a correlation between the extent of cutaneous burning and the severity of the systemic disturbances that result from exposure to excessive heat. As in heatstroke, rapidly fatal systemic hyperthermia may result from relatively long exposure to temperatures insufficient to cause cutaneous burning. Conversely, extensive cutaneous burns may occur in conjunction with higher-intensity exposure too short to cause a significant rise in body temperature. Increase in body temperature is ultimately the key to the development of the systemic disorders and the rapidly fatal circulatory failure.

Apart from the cutaneous burns, the visceral alterations at autopsy duplicate the nonpathognomonic changes associated with systemic hyperthermia, namely, stasis of blood in the peripheral vascular bed, dilatation of the right atrium, subendocardial ecchymoses, persistent fluidity of the blood, fragmentation of erythrocytes, and degenerative changes in the cells of the renal tubules, adrenal cortex, and liver.

A finding in conflagration injury that is worth mentioning is the epidural hematoma caused by the sudden expansion and rupture of the intracranial blood vessels. The absence of reactive changes differentiates this hematoma from the epidural hematoma attending head trauma and foul play. The same consideration applies to the far from uncommon splitting of the abdominal wall, usually along the midline, followed by eventration of the bowels, an event that probably results from expansion of the gases within the intestines (see Fig. 20–8*B*).

LOCALIZED EFFECTS OF HYPERTHERMIA (BURNS)

Among all the discoveries made by men, only a few, such as cultivation of the soil, speech, and writing, have borne such eventful developments as has finding out how to make a fire. Manufacturing, transportation, practically all phases of modern industrial life, sprang from the discovery of fire and its tremendous force.

It can be assumed that the earliest fire man encountered was generated by natural events—falling meteors, lightning, material ejected from volcanoes. Probably it took many thousands of years for man to learn to cherish fire of his own making, and almost every country has a different legend about how the discovery of fire was effected.

According to a North American legend, it was the buffalo that gave fire to man. As herds of buffaloes raced across the plains at night, the darkness was lighted up and brush set afire by the sparks from their hoofs' hitting the rocks. A friendly panther, its claws striking a stone, takes the place of the buffalo in the Dakota Indian legend. Not an animal, but a god (Tohil) shaking his sandals, was the donor of fire to man, according to a South American legend. It is not accidental that the symbol of this god, like that of the Mexican god Quetzalcoatl, is a flint.

The conclusion that can be reached from an attempt to interpret these legends is that man, with his perspicacity and curiosity, grasped the fact that sparks capable of igniting grass or leaves may be caused by percussion, friction, or attrition of rapidly moving solid objects. One may assume that in parts of the earth where rocks and dry grass were abundant, the first fire sprang up when, perhaps unintentionally, flint and iron pyrites were made to strike together; whereas in other parts, where vegetation was dense and flinty rocks not present, it is not unlikely that dead branches of trees, in a hot summer, rubbed each other in the wind and took fire.

Whereas it took man a long long time to understand, appreciate, and reproduce these natural occurrences, it took him no time at all to realize that fire can hurt and hurt badly. And so the search for remedies got under way.

Interest in injuries caused by fire certainly dates back to the early days of mankind. The course of history has been elegantly pursued by Shedd, by Cockshott, and by Artz and Moncrief in their monograph *The Treatment of Burns*.[67–69] The trail starts with Hippocrates about 430 B.C. He offers the alternative of several preparations to be applied to the burned area, such as dressings of melted old swine's seam mixed with resin and bitumen or warm vinegar or oak bark solution.

Greco-Roman thoughts on burns are mirrored by the writings of Paulus of Aegena (seventh century A.D.), who advocates various emollient preparations. The Arabic view is related to us by Rhazes and Avicenna, who recommend the local use of refrigerants.

William Clowes's Treatise, *A Profitable and Neccessarie Booke of Observations, for all those that are burned with the flame of Gun Powder* (1596), presents Paré's ideas on the use of ointments, mostly drawn from Greco-Roman, Arabic, and Egyptian sources.

Fabricius Hildamus's *De Combustionibus* (1607) brought forth the first attempt at classification of burns by degree into the classic three categories. This attempt was pursued further by Dupuytren (1832), who recognized six degrees of burns according to the depth of injury. At approximately the same time the first "burn hospital" was erected in Edinburgh under the direction of Dr. Syme, the proposer of the use of dry cotton-wool dressings applied with firm pressure.

Relevant to present-day concepts is Curling's recognition, in 1842, that gastroduodenal ulcerations, now bearing his name, frequently occur as complications of severe burns.

Advancements in the understanding of the pathophysiology of burn injury mark the end of the nineteenth century. The need for intravenous fluid replacement therapy was pointed out by Tappeiner, who stressed the concentration of the blood that occurs in coincidence with extensive burns (1881). The use of intravenous fluids was further advocated by Parascandolo in 1901, but not until 1921 was the rationale of compensating for fluid and protein losses demonstrated by Underhill's enlightening studies.

In the year 1925, tannic acid spray was introduced by Davidson on the assumption that it decreased the fluid loss, relieved pain, and produced a better eschar. Soon this treatment fell into disuse when McClure, in 1944, showed that tannic acid is toxic to the liver.

Emphasis on the systemic effects of burns, removal of the eschar and closure of the burn wound, the "surface area–weight formula" for computing fluid replacement, the understanding that septicemia is the major threat to the life of the burn patient, and ultimately, the introduction of skin grafting belong to the advancements made in our times.

Also of our times is the realization that the treatment of burn injury requires a multidisciplinary approach, best attained by burn teams. The outstanding contributions on treatment and fundamental research brought forth by the United States Army Surgical Research Unit at the Brooke Army Medical Center and by the Shriners Burn Institutes at the University of Texas, the University of Cincinnati, Harvard University, and a few others substantiate the point that the approach is rewarding and worth pursuing.

INCIDENCE OF BURNS

It is apparent that data on the incidence of burns do not take into account minor injuries. Indeed, every one of the burns recorded in vital statistics represents a catastrophic injury:

> . . . catastrophic in the overwhelming insult to the patient, catastrophic in its psychological aspects and catastrophic in cost and suffering to the family involved.[69]

A National Health Survey for the years 1957 to 1961 indicated an annual average number of burn injuries of 1,973,000, of which 268,000 were classified as bed-disabling and 937,000 as activity restricting. A study by the United States Department of Health, Education, and Welfare (Public Health Service, Division of Vital Statistics) for the year 1962 listed 7,534 deaths caused by fires and explosions of combustible material and 849 accidental deaths caused by electric current. According to these figures, 4.1 per cent of the deaths were caused by fire. The young and old are the two age groups most frequently involved in fatal fire accidents. Among the overall deaths by fire in the same series, 29

TABLE 20–1. THE NUMBER OF DEATHS BY FIRE AND THE RATE BY GEOGRAPHICAL AREA FOR THE YEAR 1960*

Area	Number of Deaths	Rate (per 100,000 population)
New England	394	3.7
Middle Atlantic	1,144	3.3
East North Central	1,174	3.2
West North Central	543	3.5
South Atlantic	1,509	5.8
East South Central	901	7.5
West South Central	1,105	6.5
Mountain	225	3.3
Pacific	650	3.1

*From C. P. Artz and J. A. Moncrief: *The Treatment of Burns.* Philadelphia, W. B. Saunders Co., 1969. Reprinted by permission.

per cent were children under 15 years of age and 18 per cent were persons over 65.

These figures compare closely with another analysis by the United States Department of Health, Education, and Welfare (Accidental Deaths and Injury Statistics) for the year 1960, citing 7,645 deaths due to accidents caused by fires and explosions, a rate of 4.3 deaths per 100,000 population. For reasons difficult to explain, the death rates differed considerably in the different geographical areas of the United States, as is shown in Table 20-1.

CAUSES OF BURNS

A classification of burns according to causes leads us to consider two alternate approaches: on one side, the nature of the burning agent, whether physical (thermic, electrical, thermonuclear) or chemical (acid, alkali, magnesium); on the other, the location where the injury occurred, whether in the home, while at work, or in combat. (Burns coincident to conflagration make a distinct category, as discussed earlier in this chapter.) The second approach is chosen here, and since about 80 per cent of burn accidents occur in the home, they are given consideration first.

In the Home

Stoves and gas heaters, open fires and inflammable material, and scalding liquids are the most frequent causes of domestic burns. Data from a few recorded series are worth reporting. Among the 166 thermal injuries (over 15 per cent of body surface) cited by Moyer (Dallas, Texas), about a third resulted from the direct contact of clothing with an open flame.[70] Equally impressive in this respect are Bull's figures of 615 patients admitted to the Birmingham Accident Hospital in England in a 10-year period with burns that were caused by ignited clothing.[71]

There were 231 burned patients hospitalized at Oklahoma State University Hospital between 1945 and 1959; stoves were responsible for the injury in 69 cases, ignition of inflammable material in 43, open fires in 49, scalding liquids in 33, and miscellaneous factors in 29.[72] Remarkably, in this series also, in 153 (66 per cent) of the cases, the burns were caused by burning clothing. In Skoog's series (Sweden) of 789 patients, the cause of the burn injury was scalding in 299 cases, fire in 265 cases, hot objects in 135 cases, chemical agents in 31 cases, and electricity in 53 cases.[73] In Sweden, electricity is the predominant source of power.

An analysis of these series by age groups indicates scalding to be the leading cause of burns under 3 years of age, ignited clothing from 3 to 14 years, industrial accidents from 15 to 60 years, house fires and accidents connected with momentary blackouts over the age of 60 years. Among children, clothing burns are more common in girls and scalds (hot liquids and grease) in boys.

If the search for the causes of burns is to serve the primary purpose for which the investigation is devised, namely, prevention of their recurrence, statistics must point to the major causes of fire in the home. There are two: inadequate heating appliances and flammable fabrics used for clothing. Thus prevention of burns calls for improvement in the manufacture of household heating units, safer noninflammable clothing, and above all, the awareness that children, like primitive man, are fascinated by the flames and sparks of a fire, but are not conscious of its power and of the extraordinary suffering induced by a burn.

A new law (Chapter 650 of the Acts of 1973) requiring physicians to report burns due to fabric ignition has been introduced in the Commonwealth of Massachusetts, effective November 18, 1973. The law reads as follows:

> Any physician, intern or medical assistant, registered as provided in section nine A of chapter one hundred and twelve, public health nurse or any other person who professionally examines or treats a person with a burn injury affecting five per cent or more of the surface area of his body, and who knows, or has reason to know, that such injury arose from or was caused by fabric ignition, shall report such injury to the department of public health in accordance with the rules and regulations of the department. Such reports shall be made on forms prescribed by the commissioner, and shall be submitted not later than three days after said physician, intern, medical assistant, nurse or other person first examines the injured person.
>
> The department shall maintain comprehensive records of all reports submitted pursuant to this section. Such reports and records shall be open to public inspection and constitute public records. The department shall annually compile such records and reports and publish a statistical abstract thereof which shall also be a public record and open to inspection by the public.

In Industry

Fires and explosions are among the industrial and agricultural hazards, particularly in the chemical industry, in mining, in railroading, and wherever high-pressure equipment is involved (see Volume II, Hazards, Part I). Not infrequently occupational burns result from a combination of thermal and chemical trauma, and as in the case of phosphorus burns, the thermal component is the major factor. The distribution and effects of acid and alkali burns depend primarily on the nature of the exposure, its duration, and the concentration of the injuring agent. Acid burns are caused by spill or splatter resulting in spotty burns or burns in the shape of rivulets coursing down the body. This type of burn can occur in the home or laboratory or be produced purposely in a criminal assault. Sulfuric, nitric, trichloroacetic, and hydrofluoric acids and phenol are the most frequent agents of acid burns.

Whenever alkalis are involved, the circumstances of burning are essentially the same as those of acid burns. Potassium and sodium hydroxide, lime, ammonia, phosphorus, mustard gas, and tear gas belong to the category of the burn-producing alkali. Phosphorus burns characteristically emit smoke when exposed to the air and glow in the dark with a bluish-green tinge.

In Warfare

Excluding thermonuclear injuries, burns are quite uncommon in modern warfare as compared to other types of trauma. For the major part, burns seen in military life result from plane crashes, from buildings catching fire, from gasoline explosions, and from the handling of field stoves.

Mustard gas, a vesicant gas that causes rapidly enlarging blisters when it comes in contact with the skin, fortunately has not been used in recent wars. Phosphorus burns still occur, but less commonly than in the past. Burns from flame throwers usually produce instantaneous death.

In contrast to the most common burns, which are due to direct contact with the source of heat (flame, heated object), the predominant thermal injury from thermonuclear blasts is the flash burn caused by heat radiated in the form of electromagnetic waves. The combination of thermal and radiation injury expectedly leads to a greater incidence of death by sepsis.

In the new "culture" of our times, tear agents are being used by law enforcement authorities to disperse or subdue "demonstrating" crowds. Attention has been called by the medical profession to the effects of one of the newest agents, "chemical mace," presumably a nonlethal weapon. The active ingredient of the agent is chloroacetophenone, and since it is disseminated as an aerosol, its action is almost instantaneous and detoxification is equally rapid under open-air conditions. The major effects are on the lacrimatory apparatus and respiratory system. Skin erythema and vesiculation have been recorded when it was applied to previously abraded skin.[74]

Special Types of Electrical Burns

Deep burning is among the effects of electrical injury (see also Chapter 17, Injury by Electrical Force). The characteristics of burns associated with electricity may differ according to the type of accident. Three main types are generally acknowledged: burns by contact, electrothermal burns, and flame burns.

Burns by contact occur at the sites of entrance and exit of the current (Fig. 20–6). Damage at the site of entry is generally more severe than at the exit site. It is debated whether the injury is due to heat generated by the passage of the current or, rather, to some specific effect of the current itself.

Electrothermal burns (flash or arc burns) result from electrical generation of heat outside the skin. They are mainly associated with high-tension current, and since an electric arc has a temperature of approximately 2,500°C, the ensuing lesion as a rule is deep and severe. Under ordinary atmospheric conditions arcing on a

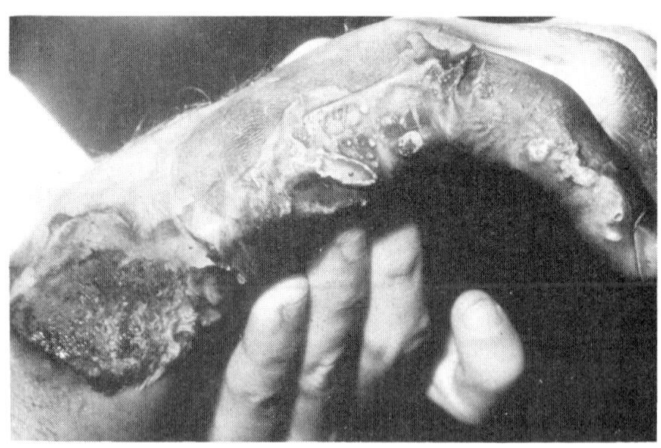

Figure 20–6. A 28-year-old man accidentally electrocuted while at work on a construction site. The tip of his metal shovel cut wires, and the electric current entered his body through both hands, passed through it, and caused instant heart failure. Exit marks at the site of grounding were noted in both feet. Secondary "flash burns" were present on the right side of chest and abdomen where his clothes caught fire. Gross and microscopic examination of viscera revealed acute congestive changes. Notice the extensive third-degree burns on the side of the hand.

high-tension line can span approximately 1 inch for each 20,000 v.

Flame burns are related to the ignition of clothing by electrical sparks and arcing.

With the increased use of electrical equipment and electronic monitoring aids, electrical hazards in hospitals have become a matter of increasing concern. When two or more instruments are used at the same time, interactions may occur, further increasing the risk. Whenever an injury caused by electrical equipment takes place in the hospital, the ultimate responsibility rests on the instrument manufacturer, the hospital administrator, the architect and builder, and the user, be it physician, nurse, or technician.[75]

Burns caused by electrocautery used in conjunction with electronic monitoring equipment have been recorded.[76] The cause of these misadventures is frequently found in faulty equipment and inadequate safety precautions.

Thermal Contact Burns from Streets and Highways

Walking in bare feet is fashionable these days among young people. They should be alerted to the fact that thermal burns have been recorded following contact with hot pavements.[77] Temperature and duration of the contact are the fundamental underlying factors. Burns, as a rule, are caused by short exposure to high temperatures. In contrast, contact burns on streets and highways occur at relatively low temperatures but with relatively long exposure.

Readings taken with a bimetallic surface temperature gauge from pavement in Phoenix, Arizona, were as high as 167° and 172°F on different occasions. Even higher temperatures (178° to 180°F) have been obtained in similar measurements in Yuma, Arizona. Temperatures within these ranges, caused by direct solar radiation, can be expected in summer months on the pavements in many parts of the world. It is well to remember that the exposure of the skin to 158°F for 1 sec results in tissue damage.[78]

ESTIMATION OF EXTENT OF BURNS

The extent of the burn is usually indicated as the percentage of the total body surface area (BSA) involved by the thermic injury. According to a commonly applied method, *head* and *neck* and the *upper extremities* each constitute 9 per cent of the total body surface area; *anterior trunk, posterior trunk,* and *lower extremities* each constitute 18 per cent; and the *perineum* makes up the remaining 1 per cent. Specially designed charts are available for recording the extent of the burn, and they are usually incorporated in the patient's clinical record.

The extent of the area of body surface involved is the most important single factor influencing prognosis and corrective treatment.

PATHOPHYSIOLOGY OF BURNS

Evaluation of the morphologic alterations attending localized hyperthermic injury entails the realization that the effects of the injury extend far beyond the burn area. Indeed, the pathophysiology of thermal injury involves a complex metabolic response that ultimately is responsible for the outcome of the injury.

The Local Lesion

The various physical factors that affect the transfer of heat to and through the skin have been successfully explored both in man and in the experimental animal.[78] The time and temperature thresholds for varying degrees of cutaneous burns are shown in Table 20–2.

A cutaneous burn can be characterized both quantitatively and qualitatively: quantitatively according to the depth to which tissue has been destroyed, and qualitatively according to the nature of the changes that have occurred in the burned tissue. On these criteria rests Dupuytren's classification of burns into six distinct categories: skin erythema characterizes category one; erythema, detachment of the epidermis from the dermis, and vesication are distinctive of category two; destruction of the upper part of the dermis distinguishes category three; involvement of all the dermis, down to the subcutaneous tissue, delineates category four; total necrosis of soft tissues, including muscle, to variable depths constitutes category five; and carbonization in depth delineates category six.[79] Dupuytren's six categories have been narrowed down to three in our times (Fig. 20–7).

First-degree burns are chiefly characterized by a vascular reaction, with dilatation of arterioles and capillaries, resulting in reddening of the skin. This type of lesion is transitory, and if not so extensive as to threaten the life of the patient, as a rule regresses within a few days, with complete return to normal conditions.

Detachment of the epidermis from the dermis, the presence of dead or dying epider-

TABLE 20–2. TIME AND SURFACE TEMPERATURE THRESHOLDS FOR THERMAL INJURY OF HUMAN SKIN‡

		Duration of Exposure			Subthreshold Exposures	Threshold and Supra-threshold Exposures
Subject	Temperature at Surface (°C)	Hours	Minutes	Seconds	First-Degree Reactions—Hyperemia Without Loss of Epidermis	Second- and Third-Degree Reactions—Complete Epidermal Necrosis
1	44	5			x	
2*		5			x	
3		6				x
4*		6				x
5*	45	2			x	
6*		3				x
7		3				x
8*†	47		18			x
9*			20		x	
10*			20		x	
11*			20		x	
12†			25			x
13*			40			x
14			40			x
15†			45			x
16	48		15		x	
17			15			x
18			18			x
19*	49		8		x	
20			8		x	
21			9	30		x
22*			10			x
23			11			x
24			15			x
25	51		2		x	
26			4			x
27			6			x
28	53			30	x	
29			1	30		x
30	55			20	x	
31				30		x
32*	60			3	x	
33*				5		x

*Oil used instead of water as source of heat.
†Subject was atypical in that his threshold for thermal injury was significantly lower than that of other experimental subjects.
‡Slightly modified from A. R. Moritz and F. C. Henriques, Jr.: Studies of thermal injury: the relative importance of time and surface temperature in the causation of cutaneous burns. Am. J. Pathol., *23*:695, 1947.

mic tissue, edema, outpouring of fluid from the dermal capillaries, and vesication are the major components of the second-degree burn. Vesication and edema obviously indicate that the heat has caused an alteration in the walls of arterioles and capillaries, promoting increased permeability. Occasionally, after a thermal exposure sufficient to produce a second-degree burn, vesication does not occur or is delayed. Absence or delayed appearance of vesication may indicate either inadequate dermal hyperthermia or the opposite, namely, overwhelming hyperthermia resulting in almost immediate occlusion (thrombosis, coagulation) of superficial capillaries. Delayed vesication occurs most frequently after hyperthermia of long duration at relatively low temperatures or after brief exposure at high temperatures.

In the third-degree burn the involved tissues undergo massive necrosis. Since the tissues are superficial, exposed to the air they become desiccated, forming eschars from the dehydrated residue of the necrotic tissue. Carbonization occurs when the organic matter un-

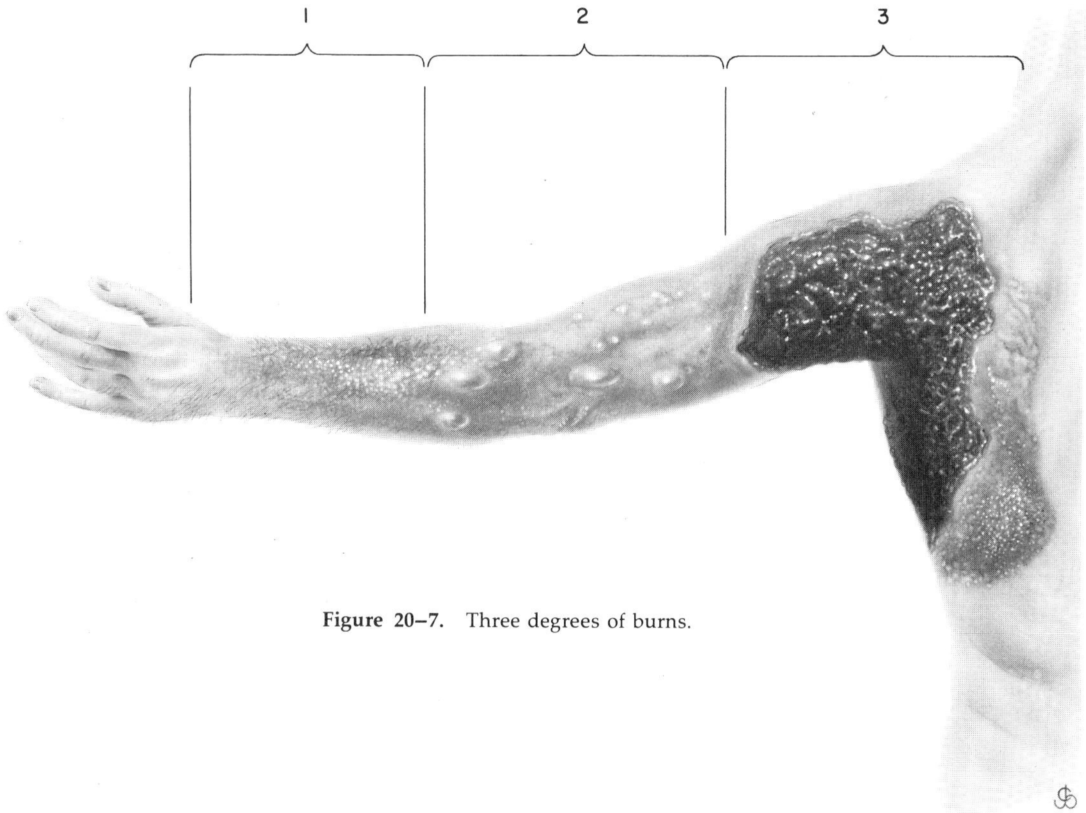

Figure 20–7. Three degrees of burns.

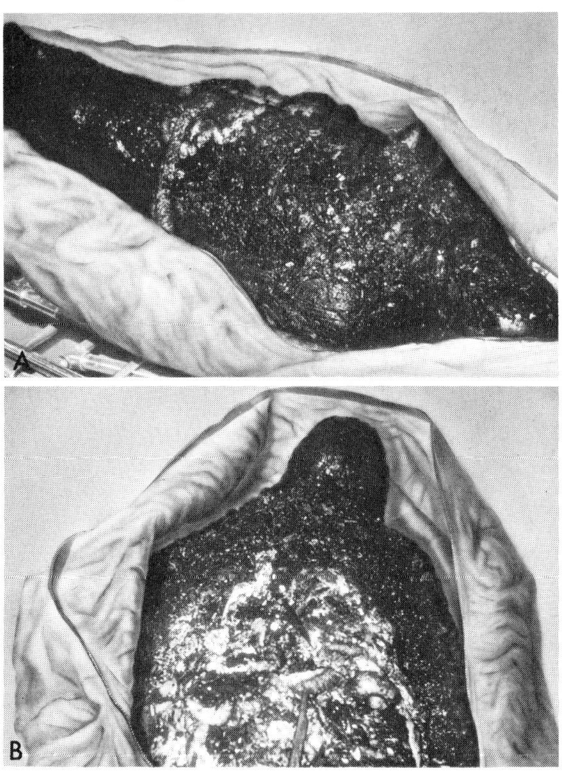

Figure 20–8. *A.* Massive carbonization of entire body. *B.* Notice the bursting of abdominal wall and protrusion of intestines. This 61-year-old man was identified by odontologic studies.

dergoes a chemical transformation, a phenomenon that in general takes place on exposure to temperatures about 300°C (Fig. 20–8).

Irreversible damage to all dermal elements consitutes a *full-thickness burn.* Characteristically the nuclei of the epithelial cells display karyolysis and karyorrhexis, clear indications of irreparable cell injury. Conversely, potential regenerative capacity is retained in a *partial-thickness burn* in which some dermal epithelial elements have survived.

Decreased rate of blood flow at the site of the burn is followed by stagnation and intraluminal agglutination of red blood cells in arterioles, venules, and capillaries. These observations are the basis for Sevitt's concept that the necrosis associated with severe thermal injury is caused by two major events, the direct effect of the heat on the exposed tissue and the concurrent stasis of blood flow leading to stagnant anoxia and complete slough of overlying skin.[80] Intra- and intercellular edema of epidermic cells and subcutaneous tissue, nuclear vacuolization of epidermic cells, separation of dermis from epidermis, and disorganization of the cellular architecture of the dermal appendages are the major microscopic components of the burn lesion. The dermal collagen fibers are spread apart by intervening edema fluid, or fused and homogenized, with increased refractivity and loss of eosinophilia.

Basically, the same type of alteration is shown in the chemical burn. In this category of burn, however, the lesion is characteristically extremely painful, and the pain persists for a long time, owing to the continuing chemical reaction. This is particularly the case with magnesium burns, in which the lesion gradually enlarges and penetrates deeper and deeper until all magnesium is removed.

Data have been presented for and against the existence of a hypothetical "burn toxin," and the deleterious effects on the organism as a whole of proteolytic enzymes and other products of cell breakdown released from the burned area into the blood stream.[81-83] Though conclusive evidence has not yet been presented, one must concede that the pathophysiologic factors responsible for the metabolic and circulatory imbalance of the severely burned patient often are not satisfactorily explained by anatomical alterations.

Systemic Effects of Burns

The pathogenetic mechanisms underlying the immediate and delayed lethal effects of localized hyperthermic injury are not yet entirely understood. The old concept that any burn involving a third of the body surface represents a threat to the life of the patient is no longer tenable in the light of the observation that death can occur rapidly in concurrence with relatively moderate superficial lesions.[84] Acute myocardial insufficiency and, not infrequently, cardiac arrest play a major role in the immediate death of the burned patient. The cardiac effects are probably related to the hyperkalemia that is associated with the massive liberation of potassium by the hemolyzed erythrocytes.

The other major threat comes from secondary shock. The correlation between hemoconcentration, hypovolemia, and the extent of burned body surface is well established. The equation between these three values is currently used as a guide in transfusion therapy. Associated with diminution in total blood volume, the concentration of red blood cells (inspissatio sanguinis) not infrequently reaches values of 10 million erythrocytes per cubic millimeter (hypovolemic polycythemia). The hypovolemia in turn contributes to the development of renal ischemia (tubular nephrosis) manifested by oliguria, anuria, proteinuria, and uremia.

Intercurrent infection and sepsis (discussed in a following section), anemia, and hypoproteinemia further contribute to the occurrence of systemic disorders that endanger the life of the patient. Anemia can be directly related to the diminished production of erythrocytes in the bone marrow and to the alterations taking place in the erythrocytes circulating in the surface areas at the time of the hyperthermic injury; hypoproteinemia can be attributed to the loss of plasma through the burned area and through the urine as well. The loss in albumin comes first (one to two hours) and is greater than the globulin loss.

Metabolic Response

Fluid administered to prevent shock, and extracellular fluid retention are responsible for the early gain in weight that almost regularly takes place in the first few days after burn injury. Thereafter, with the establishment of diuresis, the body weight starts to diminish. Not until the phase of wound closure does the weight curve take an upward trend.

Protein loss and reduced nitrogen intake cause the negative nitrogen balance associated with the early postburn period. Fifteen to twenty per cent of the nitrogen loss takes place through the wound exudate and the rest through the urine in the form of urea. Inadequate protein intake combined with muscle catabolism and anabolism further explains the loss of muscle far more severe than that expected from mere inactivity.

The extent of fat loss depends primarily on the type of nutritional regimen prescribed for the patient. Fat loss, as a rule, parallels the protein loss, but it can persist after return to a positive nitrogen balance. Losses as large as 600 g per day have been recorded.

Diminution in sodium concentration in the blood serum, and hyperkalemia are the major components of electrolyte imbalance. Body metabolism behaves as it would in potassium saturation; the quantity excreted with the urine is equivalent to the total intake plus the amount liberated by protein metabolism.

Epinephrine is the principal hormone secreted by the adrenal medulla, and norepinephrine is the neurohormone of the sympathetic nerve. The stress elicited by thermal burn is attended by prominent activation of the sympathoadrenal medullary system and release of large quantities of both epinephrine and norepinephrine. The degree of elevation of both hormone levels roughly parallels the severity of the burn.

Burn pseudodiabetes is an uncommon manifestation of stress associated with extensive burns. Hyperglycemia, glycosuria without acetonuria, severe diuresis, and high urine specific gravity are the major manifestations that identify this condition. The diuresis is responsible for the marked dehydration and the elevation of the hematocrit and the serum nonprotein nitrogen, sodium, and chloride levels. Unless promptly recognized and corrected, pseudodiabetes can contribute to the death of the patient.

Hypercalcinuria and hyperphosphaturia are commonly detected and can best be explained by prolonged immobilization and high phosphorus and calcium content in the diet. The metabolic rate in general is elevated and pursues a curve that parallels the excretion of epinephrine and norepinephrine.

Burn Wound Sepsis

The burn wound constitutes an excellent medium for bacterial growth. Bacterial colonization may take place on the surface of the wound (supraeschar colonization), within the pits of destroyed hair follicles (intrafollicular colonization), or within the heat-coagulated dermis and subjacent hypodermal fat (intraeschar colonization). The terms "invasion," "burn wound sepsis," and "burn wound infection" are used when bacterial growth extends into the subjacent viable tissue.[69]

For the first one or two days after the injury, the surface of the burn is generally sterile. Then with the passage of time, bacterial colonization begins, proceeding from the surface to the depth of the eschar. The source of the bacterial contamination is often difficult to establish. It may be traced to self-contamination, namely, to the patient's skin flora prior to the burn, or to supervening bacterial invasion.

As for the nature of the bacteriologic flora, *Pseudomonas aeruginosa* is being recognized with increasing frequency as the most important colonizer, particularly of burns sustained in accidents at sea. Both sea water and fresh water contain massive numbers of Pseudomonas (about 100,000 per milliliter of sea water). *Proteus, Escherichia coli, Aerobacter,* staphylococci, and streptococci occupy less important positions in the list of the deadly invaders. Among the fungi, *Candida* is frequently found, and systemic infections by *Candida* and *Mucor* are recorded.

Diffusion of bacterial toxins from the eschar into the subjacent viable tissue and capillary bed may conceivably occur and be responsible for some of the systemic manifestations of the thermal burn illness.

Pus in the burn wound is a clear indication of burn infection. The same is true for the neutrophilic response, the microscopic counterpart of the purulent discharge. Nevertheless it is well to keep in mind that both pus formation and neutrophilic infiltration can be absent in the presence of massive bacterial invasion. The rapid development of a dark tortuous rim or of papular or pustular hemorrhagic lesions between the burn wound and surrounding normal skin (satellite ecthyma gangrenosa) is a pathognomonic manifestation of *Pseudomonas* burn wound sepsis.[69]

Wound sepsis can also be responsible for delay or even absence of granulation tissue response. It can cause poor graft take or slough as well.

The term "septicemia," as commonly used, connotes a systemic dissemination of bacteria; this in contrast to the concept of sepsis that is generally applied to infection at a primary site. Observations by Teplitz support the generalization that septicemia and metastatic visceral lesions caused by staphylococci and gram-negative bacilli play an important role in the death of the burn victim.[85] Conversely, the paucity of blood-borne bacteria in *Pseudomonas* infection seems to indicate that death concurrent to *Pseudomonas* sepsis is more often related to the liberation of bacterial toxins from the site of primary infection than to bacterial dissemination.

Other common sources of generalized infection include sepsis at surgical cutdown sites, bacterial invasion following escharotomy, and infected erosions induced by tracheostomy tube.

EVALUATION OF BURN DEATH

Except for changes at the site of the hyperthermic injury, there is no pathognomic lesion associated with burn death. In order to improve the usefulness of the autopsy, Teplitz has suggested a number of helpful procedures that usually are not applied in the routine postmorten examination.[85]

The Autopsy

Since at the present state of knowledge, sepsis is conceived to be the most important factor in burn death, assessment of the burn wound becomes one of the most essential aspects of the autopsy. Accordingly, the family of the deceased should be informed of the desirability of making multiple incisions throughout the full extent of the burn wounds. A written consent to this procedure should be included in the autopsy permission. Prosectors should be aware that incisions into the skin of a cadaver are an implied autopsy restriction unless otherwise specifically indicated. Considering that elucidation of burn death lies primarily in the evaluation of the presence or absence of infection, a prerequisite to adequate appraisal is a thorough bacteriologic study.

This can be attained by making long, closely spaced parallel incisions over the entire wound, down to the depth of the underlying subcutaneous tissue. Once the subcutaneous bed of the wound is exposed, it also is incised in a similar manner. The blocks of tissue for microscopic study are selected from the areas that are grossly indicative of or arouse suspicion of bacterial colonization. Each block of tissue must be placed in a separate container and labeled with the site from which it was taken. Tissue for bacterial cultures must be obtained from the surface burn as well as from the subjacent subcutaneous tissue.

In order to eliminate accidental contaminants the following procedure is recommended by Teplitz. A cube-shaped block of subcutaneous tissue beneath the eschar is excised with scalpel and forceps. Then the tissue cube is rapidly immersed in 95 or 100 per cent alcohol and ignited for approximately five seconds. This procedure is aimed at destroying the bacteria at the surface of the block of tissue. Subsequently the tissue is placed in a sterile Petri dish and transected with an equally sterile scalpel blade. Culture material is then taken from the cut surfaces, and in order to establish a precise correlation between histologic and bacteriologic findings, sections for microscopic study are taken from the contiguous segments of subcutaneous tissue.[85]

For the demonstration of bacteria in the tissue sections, the best results are obtained by using a modified single-step phosphate-buffered Giemsa stain that does not require differentiation by acetic acid.

Since postmortem cultures from heart blood and viscera often yield a mixed bacterial flora, results are frequently not meaningful. When septicemia is suspected, however, the routine postmortem procedure of taking culture samples from heart blood, basal lung, liver, and spleen is worth pursuing. Because the threat of bacterial contamination increases in direct proportion to the death-to-autopsy interval, the autopsy should be performed as soon as possible.

Respiratory tract alterations are frequently implicated in burn death, particularly in the presence of severe burns in the respiratory area of the face. This requires careful evaluation of respiratory passages and lungs.

Finally, since the pathophysiologic disorders responsible for the circulatory and metabolic imbalance attending the burn death are not, in most of the cases, fully and satisfactorily explained at the postmortem table, objections have been properly raised to the use of the phrase "anatomical causes of death." In the light of the fact that the "pathologist cannot state conclusively what a patient dies *from* but can only indicate what he dies *with*," the customary autopsy protocol should purposely be limited to the classic anatomical enumeration of findings.[85]

Findings at Postmortem Examination

Respiratory System

Obstructive edema of the laryngopharynx, tracheobronchitis, patchy areas of pneumonia, pulmonary congestion and edema, and carbon pigment in alveolar phagocytes are listed among the respiratory lesions that occur in conjunction with thermal injury.

Such injuries can be anticipated in patients who are burned in fires in enclosed spaces, or exposed to inhalation of steam or smoke containing toxic products of combustion. In contrast, except possibly in patients with severe facial burns, damage in the upper respiratory passages is rarely found in the victim of superficial burns. Several carefully analyzed autopsy series indicate a shift from invasive burn wound infection to pulmonary lesions among the fatal complications of superficial thermal injury.

The lungs are heavy, airless, and consolidated and, on microscopic examination, show diffuse interstitial edema with hyaline membrane formation. Cellular debris from necrotic alveolar epithelium and evidence of alveolar epithelial regeneration (granular pneumocytes) are found concurrently. These changes lack specificity and can be found as well in patients who die with posttraumatic respiratory insufficiency (shock lung or adult respiratory distress syndrome). By the same token, these lesions are not limited to the lungs of patients with superficial burns or other types of trauma but can be seen with equal frequency in a broad category of unrelated conditions such as oxygen intoxication, rheumatic pneumonitis, influenzal and mycoplasma pneumonia, uremic pneumonitis, radiation pneumonitis, and the respiratory distress syndrome of the newborn.

The decline in burn wound infection can be attributed to more effective topical chemotherapy. The apparent increase in pulmonary complications makes it imperative to differentiate respiratory distress directly due to thermal injury from that caused by extrinsic factors. For example, pulmonary edema and congestion can reflect an alteration in cardiovascular hemodynamics rather than an inhalation injury. They can equally represent the response to acid-base imbalance. Atelectasis, as a rule, is not associated with bronchial or bronchiolar mucinous plugs, but rather, bears the gross characteristics of the so-called congestive atelectasis.[85] These characteristics may also be linked to mechanical restriction of chest expansion caused by a constrictive full-thickness burn of the thoracic cage. By the same token, bronchopneumonia can be a complication of tracheostomy or be linked to metastatic pulmonary sepsis.[86-89]

In elderly patients, unrecognized as well as overt preexistent cardiorespiratory disorders must be taken into account, and indeed pulmonary complications are listed more frequently in the elderly. Thromboemboli of microscopic dimensions are not uncommonly found in the pulmonary circulation, but as a rule the phenomenon is limited and does not play a major role in the death of the burned patient. The same consideration applies to megakaryocytosis of the septal capillaries of the lungs, probably a nonspecific feature of severe infection.

Heart

In conjunction with septicemia, metastatic septic foci in the myocardium, the endocardium, or both have been recorded. Interstitial edema and myocardial fiber fragmentation have also been reported.[85] The extent of these changes is, however, no greater than frequently found in the hearts of patients dying from a broad spectrum of other conditions.

Liver

Fatty metamorphosis, necrosis, congestion, and enlargement of the liver have been described in victims of superficial burns, but probably they are due to a nonspecific response to injury, to an independent concurrent condition, or to a preexisting disease state rather than to the thermic insult.

Fatty metamorphosis can be linked to suboptimal nutrition. Necrosis is a relatively uncommon finding and when present is of the centrilobular hemorrhagic type, as seen in conjunction with prolonged shock, hypoxemia, and the congestion of circulatory failure. Hepatomegaly, in the absence of significant gross or histologic alterations, has been mentioned in concurrence with marked hypoalbuminemia and attributed to decreased plasma osmolarity and resultant parenchymal edema.[85]

Spleen and Lymph Nodes

Weiskotten's early study of the adrenals in fatal superficial burns describes the collateral finding of edema and necrosis of lymphoid germinal centers and their replacement by macrophages in both spleen and lymph nodes.[90] This observation has been confirmed by Sevitt.[91]

Another investigator has pointed out the not uncommon finding of subintimal deposits of mucopolysaccharide and protein complexes similar, but not identical, to amyloid in splenic arterioles, possibly resulting from the combination of altered permeability of vascular endothelium and circulating infused serum protein and colloid material. Plasma cell immune response from slight to marked is quite consistently found and has been proved, by immunofluorescent studies, to be indicative of active antibody formation.[85] Sevitt has interpreted splenic eosinopenia as an indication of adrenal hyperactivity.

Kidney

Thermal injury per se has no direct effect upon the kidney. It is well documented, however, that acute tubular necrosis leading to acute renal insufficiency is a common sequela of the prolonged shock associated with burn injury. The basic pathologic change is essentially the same as that characteristically found in hemorrhagic or traumatic shock (discussed in Chapter 4). In one of the most thoroughly studied burn series, a consistent morphologic feature was the presence of heme casts in the medullary tubules.[85] According to other investigators, this occurrence is the most important pathogenetic factor in acute tubular necrosis; the intrarenal obstruction leads to microcirculatory insufficiency and ultimately to renal ischemia.[92, 93] Significant as well is the observation that nephromegaly is quite common in patients with fatal burn injury and associated hypoalbuminemia.[85]

The genitourinary tract is one of the potential sources of infection in burn patients. The threat of superimposed infection is particularly great in patients with indwelling catheters. The bacterial population is basically the same as that colonizing the burn wounds: *Pseudomonas*, *Aerobacter*, *Staphylococcus*, and *Proteus*. Hematogenous bacterial dissemination as well as ascending infection can cause pyelonephritis.[94]

Gastrointestinal Tract

A remarkable feature of burn injury is the occurrence of acute ulcers in the mucosa of the upper alimentary tract (Curling's ulcers). Although Curling's original study (1842) dealt with the description of acute ulcerations in the duodenum, ulcerations of the same type are found predominantly in the stomach and not infrequently in the lower esophagus as well.[95] Not uncommon is the occurrence of multiple ulcerations, simultaneously involving esophagus, stomach, and duodenum. The morphologic similarity of the Curling's ulcer to the so-called Cushing's neurogenic ulcer and the stress- and steroid-induced ulcers suggests that the pathogenesis of the lesion is probably the same for all. As indicated in Chapter 4, no single theory has so far been presented that is capable of satisfactorily explaining the complex mechanisms underlying this disorder.

Of clinical significance is the fact that the lesion may represent a serious threat to the life of the patient; profuse bleeding frequently occurs, and perforation of the gastrointestinal wall at the site of the mucosal ulceration is far from uncommon.

Endocrine Glands

Thyroid. Increased weight and histologic evidence of increased activity of the thyroid have been noted after burns. Cope and his associates have assessed metabolic rate and thyroid function in burned patients. A contrast was noted between the markedly elevated metabolic rate (up 30 to 60 per cent) and the protein-bound iodine content of the serum and the rate of uptake of iodine-131 that were within normal limits. Thus their conclusion that although the elevated metabolic rate may be responsible for some of the wasting that occurs in severely burned patients, the increased metabolic rate is not due to thyroid gland dysfunction.[96]

Thymus. A case is on record of a three-week-old infant with a roentgenologically demonstrated enlarged thymus gland that spontaneously shrank to normal dimensions following a burn involving 20 per cent of the body surface.[97]

Involution of the thymus occurs with any major stress. It is most likely that the diminution in size of the gland in this case was mediated by adrenal hyperactivity, a phenomenon that almost regularly takes place in response to nonspecific stress.

Adrenals. Elevation of urine and blood steroid levels following thermal injury is well documented. Increased functional activity is usually paralleled by an increase in size of the adrenal gland. Lipid depletion is commonly found, and cortical or medullary sinusoidal congestion is among the common pathologic findings. This in conjunction with autolysis may simulate hemorrhage. Hemorrhage, not infrequently massive and bilateral, may actually occur in fatal burn injury, and fibrin thrombi are frequently found in the sinusoids. Most likely a correlation can be drawn between this lesion and fulminant sepsis by gram-negative bacilli.

Central Nervous System

Since the majority of burned patients are subjected to thermal injury for a brief period of time, most burns probably do not raise the body temperature more than a degree at most. This explains why the brain, as a general rule, escapes thermal injury. Edema, congestion, increased intracranial pressure, and herniation of cerebellar tonsils through the foramen magnum have been recorded, but it would seem likely that these changes are secondary to water and electrolyte imbalance rather than to thermal injury.[98, 99] Metastatic cerebral microabscesses and hematogenous meningitis have been reported in conjunction with burn sepsis. The neurons, in general, show no abnormalities with the possible exception of the cerebellar Purkinje cells, which occasionally can show degenerative changes.

Musculoskeletal System

Late Effects. Except in conflagration, muscles, tendons, and bones are rarely initially affected by thermal insult. Subsequent alterations are far from uncommon, however. Pathologic fractures head the list, and probably their occurrence can be traced to bone atrophy from long confinement and protein deficit. Confinement and faulty early positioning may be equally responsible for joint dislocation, most frequently of the hip, or for joint fixation (ankylosis). The latter may result from an intraarticular process, such as destruction of the articular surfaces in conjunction with previous joint infection, or from an extraarticular process, such as periarticular calcification or ossification.

No clear explanation is available for the formation of these periarticular deposits of calcium or bone (heterotopic ossification). Their continued growth as long as the wound persists, however, and their progressive reabsorption once the skin lesion has healed underscore the importance of local and humoral factors. It is of interest that heterotopic ossifications with the same behavioral characteristics occur in patients with transient paralytic disorders.

In young patients with joint anklyosis, epiphyses may close prematurely, resulting in arrested growth and disparity in length of limbs. Amazingly, the opposite condition, namely, accelerated growth, has been recorded.[100]

As the skin of burned areas undergoes excessive scarring and contracture, the spinal column can develop transient distortion (scoliosis) that usually disappears as the skin regains elasticity.

REFERENCES

SYSTEMIC EFFECTS OF HYPERTHERMIA

1. Hardy, J. D.: Physiology of temperature regulation. Physiol. Rev., *41*:521, 1961.
2. Jager, H. de: Congenital anhidrotic ectodermal dysplasia: case report. J. Pathol. Bacteriol., *90*:321, 1965.
3. Austin, G. M., and Berry, J. W.: Observations on one hundred cases of heatstroke. J.A.M.A., *161*:1525, 1956.
4. Bazett, H. C.: Circulation in pyrexia. J.A.M.A., *97*:1217, 1931.
5. Kissin, M., and Bierman, W.: Influence of hyperpyrexia on velocity of blood flow. Proc. Soc. Exp. Biol. Med., *30*:527, 1932–1933.
6. Cullen, S. C., Weir, E. F., and Cook, E.: The rationale of oxygen therapy during fever therapy. Arch. Phys. Ther., *23*:529, 1942.
7. Leithead, C. S., Guthrie, J., De La Place, S., and Maegraith, B.: Incidence, aetiology and prevention of heat illness on ships in the Persian Gulf. Lancet, *2*:109, 1958.
8. Gold, J.: Development of heat pyrexia. J.A.M.A., *173*:1175, 1960.
9. Wolkin, J., Goodman, J. I., and Kelley, W. E.: Failure of the sweat mechanism in the desert (thermogenic anhydrosis). J.A.M.A., *124*:478, 1944.
10. Horne, G. O., Mole, R. H.: Anhidrotic heat exhaustion. Trans. R. Soc. Trop. Med. Hyg., *44*:193, 1950.
11. O'Brien, J. P.: Tropical anhidrotic asthenia; its definition and relationship to other heat disorders. Arch. Intern. Med., *81*:799, 1948.
12. Ladell, W. S. S.: Disorders due to heat. Trans. R. Soc. Trop. Med. Hyg., *51*:189, 1957.
13. Jelliffe, D. B.: Miliaria in Bengali children in Calcutta City. Trans. R. Soc. Trop. Med. Hyg., *52*:71, 1958.
14. Smith, F. E.: Analysis of the sickness returns from H.M. ships for the period October 1948 to September 1952. Medical Research Council Report R.N.P., *57*:883, 1957.
15. Romeo, J. A.: Heatstroke. Milit. Med., *131*:669, 1966.
16. Shibolet, S., Coll, R., Gilat, T., and Sohar, E.: Heatstroke: its clinical picture and mechanism in 36 cases. Q. J. Med., *36*:525, 1967.
17. McLean, R., Moritz, A. R., and Roos, A.: Studies of thermal injury. VI. Hyperpotassemia caused by cutaneous exposure to excessive heat. J. Clin. Invest., *26*:497, 1947.
18. Schuman, S. H., Anderson, C. P., and Oliver, J, T.: Epidemiology of successive heat waves in Michigan in 1962 and 1963. J.A.M.A., *189*:733, 1964.
19. Cook, E. L.: Epidemiological approach to heat trauma. Milit. Med., *116*:317, 1955.
20. Wilcox, W. H.: The nature, prevention, and treatment of heat pyrexia; the clinical aspects. Br. Med. J., *1*:392, 1920.
21. Harris, T. A. B., and Hutton, A. M.: Heatstroke during and after anesthesia. Lancet, *2*:1024, 1956.
22. Stoddart, J. C.: Heat hyperpyrexia following a Turkish bath. Br. Med. J., *1*:443, 1958.
23. Daily, W. M., and Harrison, T. R.: Study of mechanism and treatment of experimental heat pyrexia. Am. J. Med. Sci., *215*:42, 1948.
24. Burch, G. E.: Influence of environmental temperature and relative humidity on rate of water loss through skin in congestive heart failure in subtropical climate. Am. J. Med. Sci., *211*:181, 1946.
25. Wilson, S. J., and Doan, C. A.: The pathogenesis of hemorrhage in artificially induced fever. Ann. Intern. Med., *13*:303, 1940.
26. Wright, D. O., Reppert, L. B., and Cuttino, J. T.: Purpuric manifestations of heatstroke. Studies of prothrombin and platelets in twelve cases. Arch. Intern. Med., *77*:27, 1946.
27. Malamud, N., Haymaker, W., and Custer, R. P.: Heat stroke—a clinico-pathologic study of 125 fatal cases. Milit. Surg., *99*:397, 1946.
28. Knochel, J. P., Beisel, W. R., Herndon, E. G., Gerald, E. S., and Barry, K. G.: The renal, cardiovascular, hematologic and serum electrolyte abnormalities of heatstroke. Am. J. Med., *30*:299, 1961.
29. Zimmerman, H. M.: Temperature disturbances and the hypothalamus. Assoc. Res. Nerv. Ment. Dis. Proc., *20*:824, 1940.
30. Morgan, L. O.: Cell changes in some of the hypothalamic nuclei in experimental fever. J. Neurophysiol., *1*:281, 1938.
31. Morgan, L. O., and Vonderahe, A. R.: The hypothalamic nuclei in heatstroke. Arch. Neurol. Psychiatry, *42*:83, 1939.
32. Hasan, J., Karvonen, J. J., and Phrones, P.: Physiological effects of extreme heat as studied in the Finnish "sauna bath." Am. J. Phys. Med., *46*:1126, 1967.
33. Lundgren, R.: The influence of the Finnish bath on the heart, an electrocardiographic study. Acta Med. Scand., *89*:236, 1938.
34. Bass, D. E., Kleeman, C. R., Quinn, M., Henschel, A., and Hegnauer, A. H.: Mechanisms of acclimatization to heat in man. Medicine (Baltimore), *34*:323, 1955.
35. Russell, B.: Quoted by Leithead et al., Ref. No. 7.
36. Feldberg, W., and Gupta, K. P.: Pyrogen fever and prostaglandin-like activity in cerebrospinal fluid. J. Physiol., *228*:41, 1973.
37. Seidl, L. G., Thornton, G. F., Smith, J. W., et al.: Studies on the epidemiology of adverse drug reaction. Bull. Hopkins Hosp., *119*:299, 1966.
38. Cluff, L. E., and Johnson, J. E., III: Drug fever. Prog. Allergy, *8*:149, 1964.
39. Klein, H. O., and Kaminsky, N.: Methyldopa fever. Recurrence of symptoms with resumption of therapy. N.Y. State J. Med., *73*:448, 1973.

40. Woolley, D. E.: Studies on 1,1,1-trichloro-2,2-bis(p-chloro-phenyl)ethane (DDT)-induced hyperthermia: effects of cold exposure and aminopyrine injections. J. Pharmacol. Exp. Ther., *184*:261, 1973.
41. Keefer, C. S.: Toxic reactions following sulfonamide treatment. N. Engl. J. Med., *226*:266, 1942.
42. Root, R. K., and Wolff, S. W.: Pathogenetic mechanism in experimental immune fever. J. Exp. Med., *128*:309, 1968.
43. Horn, B., and Kabins, S. A.: Iodide fever. Am. J. Med. Sci., *264*:467, 1972.
44. Bystryn, J. C.: Drug fever. Am. J. Med. Sci., *264*:473, 1972.
45. Sidhu, A. K., Bhakoo, O. N., Jolly, J. G., and Walia, N. S.: Blood transfusion reaction in children. Indian Pediatr., *9*:271, 1972.
46. Ottolenghi, A., Chiamenti, C., and Bettili, G.: Complicanze della splenectomia. Chir. Patol. Sper., *19*:443, 1971.
47. Hall, L. W., Trim, C. M., and Woolf, N.: Further studies of porcine malignant hyperthermia. Br. Med. J., *2*:145, 1972.
48. Ryan, J. F., and Popper, E. M.: Malignant fever during and following anesthesia. Anesthesiology, *32*:196, 1970.
49. Britt, B. A., and Kalow, W.: Hyperrigidity and hyperthermia associated with anesthesia. Ann. N.Y. Acad. Sci., *151*:947, 1968.
50. Isaacs, H., and Barlow, M. B.: Malignant hyperpyrexia during anesthesia: possible association with subclinical myopathy. Br. Med. J., *1*:275, 1970.
51. Pollock, R. A., and Watson, R. L.: Malignant hyperthermia associated with hypocalcemia. Anesthesiology, *34*:188, 1971.
52. Wilson, R. D., Nichols, R. J., Jr., Dent, T. E., et al.: Disturbances of the oxidative phosphorylation mechanism as a possible etiological factor in sudden unexplained hyperthermia occurring during anesthesia. Anesthesiology, *27*:231, 1966.
53. Denborough, M. A., Forster, J. F. A., Hudson, M. C., and Carter, N. G.: Biochemical changes in malignant hyperpyrexia. Lancet, *1*:1137, 1970.
54. Denborough, M. A., Ebeling, P., King, J. O., and Zapf, P.: Myopathy and malignant hyperpyrexia. Lancet, *1*:1138, 1970.
55. Henderson, M. A., and Pettigrew, R. T.: Induction of controlled hyperthermia in treatment of cancer. Lancet, *1*:1275, 1971.
56. Serre, H., Simon, L., and Bajon, C.: La place de le pyrétothérapie dans le traitement de la polyarthrite rhumatismale. J. Méd. Lyon, *53*:362, 1972.
57. The Disaster at the Cleveland Hospital Clinic, Cleveland, Ohio, on May 15, 1929. Proceedings of a Board of the Chemical Warfare Service. Washington, D.C., U.S. Government Printing Office, 1929.
58. Mallory, T. B., and Brickley, W. J.: Management of the Cocoanut Grove burns at the Massachusetts General Hospital: with special reference to the pulmonary lesions. Ann. Surg., *117*:856, 1943.
59. Moritz, A. R., Henriques, F. C., Jr., and McLean, R.: The effects of inhaled heat on the air passages and lungs. An experimental investigation. Am. J. Pathol., *21*:311, 1945.
60. Phillips, A. W., and Cope, O.: Burn therapy. II. The revelation of respiratory tract damage as a principal killer of the burned patient. Ann. Surg., *155*:1, 1962.
61. Pruitt, B. A., Jr., Flemma, R. J., DiVincenti, F. C., Foley, F. D., and Mason, A. D., Jr.: Pulmonary complications in burn patients. A comparative study of 697 patients. J. Thorac. Cardiovasc. Surg., *59*:7, 1970.
62. Sochor, F. M., and Mallory, G. K.: Lung lesions in patients dying of burns. Arch. Pathol., *75*:303, 1963.
63. Taylor, F. W., and Gumbert, J. L.: Cause of death from burns. Ann. Surg., *161*:497, 1965.
64. Foley, F. D., Moncrief, J. A., and Mason, A. D., Jr.: Pathology of the lung in fatally burned patients. Ann. Surg., *167*:251, 1968.
65. DiVincenti, F. C., Pruitt, B. A., Jr., and Reckler, J. M.: Inhalation injuries. J. Trauma, *11*:109, 1971.
66. Moritz, A. R., Henriques, F. C., Jr., Dutra, F. R., and Weisiger, J. R.: Studies of thermal injury. IV. An exploration of the casualty-producing attributes of conflagrations; local and systemic effects of general cutaneous exposure ot excessive circumambient (air) and circumradiant heat of varying duration and intensity. Arch. Pathol., *43*:466, 1947.

LOCALIZED EFFECTS OF HYPERTHERMIA (BURNS)

67. Shedd, D. P.: Historical landmarks in the treatment of burns. Surgery, *43*:1024, 1958.
68. Cockshott, W. P.: The history of the treatment of burns. Surg. Gynecol. Obstet., *102*:116, 1956.
69. Artz, C. P., and Moncrief, J. A.: *The Treatment of Burns.* Philadelphia, W. B. Saunders Co., 1969.
70. Moyer, C. A.: The sociologic aspects of trauma. Am. J. Surg., *87*:421, 1954.
71. Bull, J. P.: Causes, prognosis and prevention of burns. Med. Press, *239*:205, 1958.
72. Foerster, D. W., and Richardson, W. R.: Causes of burns in Oklahoma. J. Okla. State Med. Assoc., *52*:713, 1959.
73. Skoog, T.: *The Surgical Treatment of Burns.* Stockholm, Almqvist and Wiksells, 1963.
74. Forberg, P. K., and Byers, W. L.: Chemical mace: a non-lethal weapon. J. Trauma, *9*:339, 1969.
75. Von der Mosel, H. A.: Electrical safety and our hospitals. J. Assoc. Adv. Med. Instrum., *4*:2, 1970.
76. Mee, A. S. W., Mazzia, V. D. B., and Spenser, F. C.: Accidental burns associated with electrocautery. J.A.M.A., *217*:916, 1971.
77. Berens, J. J.: Thermal contact burns from streets and highways. J.A.M.A., *214*:2025, 1970.
78. Moritz, A. R., and Henriques, F. C., Jr.: Studies of thermal injury: the relative importance of time and surface temperature in the causation of cutaneous burns. Am. J. Pathol., *23*:695, 1947.
79. Dupuytren, G.: *Leçons Orales de Clinique Chirurgicale.* Paris, Germer-Ballière, 1832.
80. Sevitt, S.: Local blood flow changes in experimental burns. J. Pathol., Bacteriol., *61*:427, 1949.
81. Zamecnik, P. C., Stephenson, M. L., Cope, O.: Peptidase activity of lymph and serum after burns. J. Biol. Chem., *158*:135, 1945.
82. Beloff, A., and Peters, R. A.: An investigation for the presence of a skin protease inhibitory factor in burn skin. J. Physiol., *105*:54, 1946.
83. Davis, J. H., and Abbott, W. E.: The pathology of thermal burns. Changing concepts. A review of the literature since 1945. Surgery, *40*:788, 1956.
84. Bergman, H. C., Kruger, H. E., and Prinzmetal, M.: The mechanism of delayed death following thermal trauma. J. Lab. Clin. Med., *33*:506, 1948.
85. Teplitz, C.: Pathology of burns. In *The Treatment of Burns.* Edited by C. P. Artz and J. A. Moncrief. Philadelphia, W. B. Saunders Co., 1969.
86. Foley, F. D., Moncrief, J. A., and Mason, A. D., Jr.: Pathology of the lung in fatally burned patients. Ann. Surg., *167*:251, 1968.
87. Finland, M.: Respiratory injuries in man resulting from severe burns. In *National Research Council, Symposium on Burns,* 1950, pp. 91–95.

88. Teplitz, C., Epstein, B. S., Rose, L. R., and Moncrief, J. A.: Necrotizing tracheitis induced by tracheostomy tube. Arch. Pathol., *77*:14, 1964.
89. Sochor, F. M., and Mallory, G. K.: Lung lesions in patients dying of burns. Arch. Pathol., *75*:303, 1963.
90. Weiskotten, H. G.: Fatal superficial burns and the suprarenals. J.A.M.A., *69*:776, 1917.
91. Sevitt, S.: *Burns. Pathology and Therapeutic Applications.* London, Butterworth and Co., Ltd., 1957.
92. Goodpastor, W. E., Levenson, S. M., Tagnon, H. J., Lund, C. C., and Taylor, R. H. L.: A clinical and pathologic study of the kidney in patients with thermal burns. Surg. Gynecol. Obstet., *82*:652, 1946.
93. Haynes, B. W., Jr., DeBakey, M. E., and Denman, F. R.: Renal function studies of severely burned patients. Ann. Surg., *134*:617, 1951.
94. Tepliz, C.: Observations on the normal genitourinary tract in bacteriuria and bacteremia. A quantitative bacteriologic and anatomic autopsy study on young fatally burned cases. U.S. Army Surgical Research Unit Res. Rep., *228*:43, 1963.
95. Curling, T. B.: An acute ulceration of the duodenum in cases of burns. Med. Chir. Trans. London, *25*:260, 1842.
96. Cope, O., Mardi, G. T.. Quijano, M., Rovit, R. L., Stanburn, J. B., and Wight, A.: Metabolic rate and thyroid function following acute thermal trauma in man. Ann. Surg., *137*:165, 1953.
97. Davis, J. H., Reiss, E., Artz, C. P., and Amspacher, W. H.: Involution of the thymus after a burn. U.S. Armed Forces Med. J., *5*:545, 1954.
98. Gibson, T.: Studies of Burns and Scalds. VI. Post-mortem Findings in Thirty Fatal Cases of Burning. Med. Res. Coun. Special Report Series (Lond.), *249*:192, 1945.
99. Walker, J., Jr., and Shenkin, H.: Studies on the toxemia syndrome after burns. II. Central nervous system changes as a cause of death. Ann. Surg., *121*:301, 1954.
100. Evans, E. B.: Musculoskeletal changes secondary to burns. In *The Treatment of Burns.* Edited by C. P. Artz and J. A. Moncrief. Philadelphia, W. B. Saunders Co.. 1969.

SECTION 6. THERMAL INJURY

chapter 21

ARSON INVESTIGATION

by Nils-Åke Ek, Andreas Maehly, and Erik Rudh

BACKGROUND INFORMATION

The use and control of fire constitutes one of the earliest and most essential achievements of man. Uncontrolled fires, on the other hand, have always been a serious threat to all living beings. Strangely enough, the English language lacks two simple, separate nouns for discriminating between the wanted (controlled, useful) and the unwanted (destructive) fire. In other languages such distinctions exist (Table 21–1).

This chapter can give only a brief survey of some aspects of our knowledge of fire and of the fundamental physical and chemical phenomena leading to and sustaining fires, the causes of unwanted fires, the course these take, and their technical investigation. Certain legal aspects are touched upon, and for those readers who wish to penetrate more deeply into the subject, a short list of specialized literature in this field is given at the end.

The term "fire" can be defined in a number of ways. In the widest sense fires are exothermic chemical reactions, generally accompanied by flames, the glowing interphase between gases reacting with each other. Thus, for example, hydrogen can "burn" in an atmosphere of chlorine, and metallic magnesium can be "ignited" in nitrogen. Here only oxidation reactions and only those oxidations that lead to visible "destructive" processes are considered as fires. This excludes oxidations of metal surfaces, biologic oxidations, and the like.

In the normal atmosphere (containing 20.95 per cent oxygen, 78.09 per cent nitrogen, 0.03 per cent carbon dioxide, and 0.93 per cent noble gases, predominantly argon) a large range of substances are subject to destructive oxidation when brought to the necessary ignition temperature. In Table 21–2, the ignition temperature and heat of combustion for a number of elements are given. The list is by no means complete, since other elements can react violently with oxygen in the air (e.g., cesium at

TABLE 21–1. THE TERM "FIRE" IN SEVERAL INTERNATIONAL LANGUAGES

LANGUAGE	TERM FOR CONTROLLED FIRE	TERM FOR UNCONTROLLED FIRE
English	fire	fire
French	feu	incendie
Spanish	fuego	incendio
Italian	fuoco	incendio
Russian	ОГОНЬ	ПОЖАР
German	Feuer	Brand
Dutch	vuur	brand
Swedish	eld	brand, eldsvåda

TABLE 21–2. IGNITION TEMPERATURE AND HEAT OF COMBUSTION FOR A NUMBER OF ELEMENTS

REACTION	IGNITION TEMPERATURE (°C)	HEAT SET FREE (kcal) Per Mole of Oxide	Per kilogram of Oxide	Per Equivalent of Oxygen
$2\ Mg + O_2 = 2\ MgO$	480°	144	3,580	144
$4\ Al + 3O_2 = 2\ Al_2O_3$	515°	380	3,730	127
$2\ H_2 + O_2 = 2\ H_2O_{liq}$	590°	68	3,800	68
$4\ Fe + 3O_2 = 2\ Fe_2O_3$	–	198	1,240	66
$C + O_2 = CO_2$	700°	94	2,140	47
$S + O_2 = SO_2$	250°	71	1,110	35
$2\ C + O_2 = 2\ CO$	700°	26	940	26
$2\ CO + O_2 = 2\ CO_2$	640°	42	950	21
$2\ P + 5O_2 = 2\ P_2O5$	60°	–	–	–

room temperature; finely divided zinc, iron, and related metals at elevated temperatures; silicon, and the like), but these reactions are not usually met with in the more common fires, especially in their initial stages. (Corresponding data for organic compounds and for various materials like paper, wood, and plastics are listed later in Table 21–8.)

The great majority of combustible compounds and complex organic materials are essentially made up of carbon, hydrogen, and nitrogen, and the interest of the fire investigator is focused on these substances.

The Metastable Biosphere of the Earth

The biosphere of the earth consists almost entirely of combustible organic compounds. A priori, one could therefore expect it to have burned up in the atmosphere as soon as it was formed. This is obviously not the case, and the biosphere-atmosphere system is said to be in a metastable condition in which combustible matter can exist surrounded by 21 per cent oxygen. The reasons for this phenomenon may be numerous, but two of them play a decisive role. One is the retardation of the oxidation reactions due to the temperature dependence of their rates (temperature coefficients); the other is their inhibition by the existence of an energy threshold (energy wall) that has to be overcome by an activation reaction.

Observations have shown that the rate of chemical reactions increases by a factor of 1.7 to 3 as the temperature is raised by 10°C, all other conditions remaining constant. The effect of this increase can be shown by considering the burning rate of a match. Dry firewood is ignited in air when it is heated to about 280°C. If a match needs 10 seconds to burn up at that temperature (actually the temperature increases to several hundred degrees during burning), one can estimate the time that would be needed for oxidizing the match at room temperature. As the temperature is lowered by 260°C, the reaction rate decreases by a factor of about 2^{26} or 10^8, and at room temperature the process theoretically would require some 30 years. Knowledge of the temperature coefficients of oxidation reactions is of great importance in understanding the course and the spreading of a fire, as well as in combating a fire by decreasing its temperature (cooling by water).

The decisive reason for this metastability is the existence of an energy wall, symbolized in Figure 21–1. The energy necessary for lifting

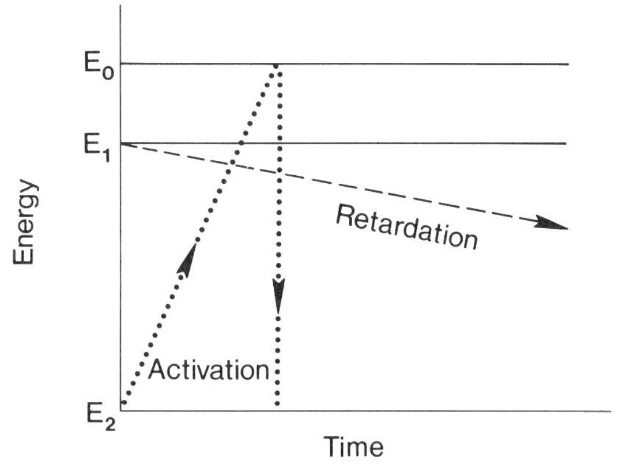

Figure 21–1. The two main reasons for the metastable condition of the biosphere. E_1 is the potential energy of a system before its oxidation, E_2 is the potential energy of the oxidized system, and E_0 is the potential energy of the activated system.

the system across this wall ($E_a = E_o - E_1$) is designated as activation energy. The addition of E_a to the system produces "active" molecules, or rather, increases the ratio of "active" to "inactive" molecules. This activation can be brought about by a variety of energy forms, and one speaks of thermal, mechanical, photochemical, or electrical activation.

A well-known example of photochemical activation is the reaction

$$H_2 + Cl_2 \rightleftharpoons 2\ HCl \qquad \text{(Eq. 1)}$$

A mixture of equal parts of the two gases is metastable in the dark; ultraviolet light activates the reaction, which then takes place explosively. Electric discharges activate the reaction

$$3O_2 \rightleftharpoons 2O_3 \qquad \text{(Eq. 2)}$$

which can play a role in the rare cases in which ozone is involved in starting a fire.

Thermal activation is by far the most common and is probably also the real cause of activation by mechanical means (friction, collisions). The necessary heat can be transported to the critical site by radiation, conduction, or convection. The activation or—pragmatically speaking—ignition process is of paramount interest in the search for causes of conflagrations.

Since carbon is a constituent of all organic compounds, the activation of its combustion is of special interest. A number of mechanisms have been suggested, and the authors do not claim to be familiar with all of them. One possible process provides an example of how activation could proceed. According to this scheme, the essential steps are the following (free radicals are designated by *):

$$\begin{array}{lll} H_2O & \rightleftharpoons H^* + OH^* & \text{(Ia)} \\ H^* + O_2 & \rightleftharpoons OH^* + O^* & \text{(Ib)} \\ C_{solid} + OH^* & \rightleftharpoons CO + H^X & \text{(IIa)} \\ C_{solid} + O^* & \rightleftharpoons CO & \text{(IIb)} \\ & & \\ 2\ C_{solid} + O_2 & \rightleftharpoons 2\ CO & \text{(II)} \\ 2\ CO + O_2 & \rightleftharpoons 2\ CO & \text{(III)} \\ \text{and, over } 1{,}500^\circ\text{:} & & \\ C_{solid} + CO_2 & \rightleftharpoons 2\ CO & \text{(IV)} \end{array}$$

MOTIVATION AND ORGANIZATION FOR INVESTIGATING FIRES

Reasons for Investigation

Before entering into a more detailed discussion of the ignition phase of fires it is valuable to consider the reasons for investigating their causes. Like other accidents, conflagrations and also explosions often lead to considerable damage to property and can cause injury or death to humans and other living organisms. Their investigation aims to clarify the following issues:

1. Has a crime been committed, i.e., is the fire due to arson? If so, in what manner and by whom?
2. Is there any evidence that negligence caused the fire? If so, in what manner, by whom, and to what extent?
3. Can we learn from the fire in question how to prevent or limit future conflagrations?

Deliberate *arson* can be committed for a number of reasons, such as obtaining fraudulent insurance, covering up another crime (murder, manslaughter, robbery, theft), psychologic reasons (revenge, jealousy, hatred, envy, misplaced ambition as a fireman), political reasons (as a weapon directed against an individual, organization, government, creed, or race; this includes terrorist actions and sabotage), pathologic reasons ("pyromania" [a collective term for a variety of psychopathic conditions], hysteria, paranoia, sexual abnormalities, and the like), and committing suicide, even though this is relatively rare.

Negligence leads to many disastrous fires in homes, on farms, and in industrial buildings, as well as in forests and prairielike regions. There are, obviously, various degrees of negligence, ranging from deliberate disregard of fire regulations (e.g., lack or state of disrepair of fire fighting equipment, storage of excessive amounts of inflammable materials, improper "homemade" electrical wiring, short-circuiting of fuses, faulty and leaking gas connections) to plain carelessness and lack of common sense (allowing children to play with matches, smoking in bed, failing to control the temperature of stacked hay or to install lightning rods on exposed buildings, using open fires in garages). Damage to one's own property is a personal matter or the concern of insurance companies. Injury to other persons (or animals) and damage to the property of others, however, can have serious legal consequences, and thus "mere" negligence can amount to a crime.

One of the most rewarding consequences of a properly carried out fire investigation is the discovery of *potential fire hazards*, conditions that may exist in other buildings or installations and whose detection may lead to preventive measures. This pertains especially to faulty construction or installation of electrical and heating equipment as well as to other structural details in private homes, public buildings, farms, and industries. Shortcomings and dangers may include the lack of safe escape routes, fire extinguishers, fire blankets, sprinklers, and alarm systems. The investigation and correction of such hazards, though not the direct responsibility of the fire investigator, is still part of the preventive activities of legal medicine and criminalistics.

Statistical Data

It is of interest to note the incidence of arson and negligence in actual cases of fire. Statistics seem not to be easy to come by and give an incomplete picture at that, mainly because many cases of arson are not recognized as such. Nevertheless, the accompanying fire statistics from Sweden are shown for the record and may contribute to a discussion of statistical evaluations in this field (Tables 21–3 and 21–4).

As these data show, the investigation of fires covers much more ground than merely the discovery and proof of arson. Indeed, the tracing of negligence and the discovery of potentially dangerous construction are very important as preventive measures. They must be brought to the attention of equipment manufacturers, of construction firms, and of organizations that are responsible for fire laws and regulations. It must furthermore be understood that the three main causes for fires (i.e., arson, negligence, and hazards for which preventive measures are needed) can rarely be excluded a priori in a given fire. This means that the majority of fires require investigation even if there is no prior

TABLE 21–3. CAUSES OF FIRE IN SWEDEN DURING THE PERIOD 1960 TO 1966*

Causes	Number of Fires	Per Cent of Total
Chimney fires	1,109	9.8
Other fires in fireplaces or stoves	24,160	21.5
Electrical causes	17,636	15.7
Lightning	16,234	14.4
Children playing with fire	3,529	3.1
Smoking	4,808	4.3
Spontaneous combustion	1,123	1.0
Welding	2,815	2.5
Blasting	7,591	6.7
Arson and safe-blasting	1,412	1.3
Other known causes	16,982	15.1
Unknown causes	5,182	4.6
Totals	102,581	100.0

*Courtesy of Central Office for Swedish Fire Statistics.

evidence that one of these causes is involved. It must be kept in mind that major fires lead to considerable losses, not only to the owner of the property and the insurance company involved but also often to adjoining property and the community at large, because of fire fighting and police efforts, care of homeless citizens, and medical care of the injured. In some cases, loss of life is involved, which aggravates the situation. These considerations strengthen the cause for having fire investigation organizations of high quality, efficiency, and sufficient size.

Organization of the Investigation

The organization of fire investigation varies from country to country and from region to region. It depends further on the population density (large city, small town, rural region, large forest district) and the character of the region (industry, farming). By tradition the police, the fire departments, and—in regard to electrical installations—underwriter associations have carried the responsibility for the investigation of fires. In some countries, the district attorney's office is in charge of this task.

Of the three main instruments for clarifying crimes or accidents, i.e., confession of the perpetrator, statements of witnesses, and physical evidence, the last mentioned has been growing in importance. The courts nowadays expect physical evidence to be presented in a competent and objective manner whenever such evidence is available. Contrary to popular belief,

TABLE 21–4. STATISTICAL BREAKDOWN OF FIRES IN SWEDEN DURING FOUR YEARS (1967–1970) IN WHICH INSURANCE WAS PAID

Causes			Number of Fires	Per Cent
I. Arson and other crimes			3,734	4.1
A. Arson		3,231		
B. Other crimes (safe-breaking, etc.)		503		
II. Lightning			11,882	13.1
III. Predominantly electrical causes (except for II)			15,428	17.0
A. Household appliances		6,971		
B. Heating devices, stoves, furnaces		6,250		
C. Industrial installations		1,204		
D. Lighting fixtures		1,003		
IV. Predominantly chemical causes (except for I)			45,818	50.5
A. Spontaneous combustion		1,196		
B. Open fire and the like		31,396		
1. Ovens, stoves, etc.	16,133			
2. Candles	3,229			
3. Cigarettes (except for IV D)	2,564			
4. Welding	2,554			
5. Chimney fires	2,446			
6. Blasting	1,739			
7. Industrial installations	1,088			
8. Matches (except for IV D)	631			
9. Hot cinders	511			
10. Pyrotechnical material	374			
11. Other causes	127			
C. Molten metals, glass, etc.		341		
D. Childrens' play, smoking in bed, trespassers' and animals' activities		12,885		
V. Unknown causes			13,866	15.3
Totals			90,728	100.0

*Courtesy of Central Office for Swedish Fire Statistics.

fires very often lend themselves to such means of proof. One has to know where, when, and how to look for this proof, however, and therefore the demands on the competence of the investigator are increasing.

The investigator in the field is usually a member of a team of policemen who specialize in the search of crime scenes and participate in the investigation of a large number of fires; he will usually not be exclusively a fire specialist. This need not be a drawback, since the scene of a fire has also to be searched for evidence of such things as forced entry, theft, and at times robbery and murder. Team members are usually police officers who have shown special ability and interest for this job and have been trained in special courses, either at a police academy or at various schools of engineering. In some countries (e.g., England), civilian crime scene teams have been formed; they are, however, part of the police organization. In this work, experience is of particular importance and cannot be replaced by theoretical course work.

In a forensic science laboratory, investigators working exclusively or predominantly with fire problems should have a good basic education, a logical way of reasoning, a clear and correct manner of expressing themselves, and a well-developed sense of responsibility. Integrity of character, objective reasoning, healthy judgment, and especially a clear insight into the limitations of his own knowledge and experience are necessary prerequisites for the specialist in this field. He should have formal education at either a university, a school of technology, or an engineering school, and must then acquire practical experience in scene-of-crime and laboratory investigation pertaining to fire cases, both by attending courses and by working under the supervision of an experienced investigator. Thus prepared, he will be accepted as an expert in court.

The investigation of fires can be divided schematically into three separate but interrelated tasks: *Phase 1* includes the collection of facts and witness testimonies concerning the time period prior to and during the fire; *phase 2*, the technical examination at the site after the fire has been extinguished; and *phase 3*, the laboratory work on physical evidence sent or brought from the site of the fire. Within this sequence there is a progression from general to specialized tasks. Phase 1 is usually carried out by the local police with or without the assistance of their criminal investigation division. Phase 2 requires cooperation with a team of officers trained and experienced in crime scene investigation. In large police organizations, there may be technical personnel available who have specialized in work on fires and who can, on request, be delegated to other districts. On the recommendation of this technical team, the district attorney or his equivalent has to decide if still other specialists are required, either calling them to the scene of the fire or sending them pertinent objects as physical evidence. This leads to phase 3: investigation at the specialized laboratory. This laboratory could be attached to a major fire department, to a forensic science institute, or to another organization connected with fire research and investigation.

As in other fields of forensic science, the question arises whether such laboratory work should be carried out at a number of local smaller centers or at one or a few large institutions. Both systems have their advantages and drawbacks, and various countries have chosen different solutions. In Sweden, which has 8 million inhabitants and is administratively divided into 24 provinces, a stepwise procedure is used. Minor or relatively clear-cut fire matters

TABLE 21–5. ORGANIZATION AND TASKS OF FIRE INVESTIGATIONS IN SWEDEN*

Organization	Phases of Investigation (cf. text)	Summary of Work Involved
119 local police departments	Phase 1 (all fires)	Investigation of small or clear-cut fires
29 technical squads (as a rule one per province) trained for work at crime or fire scene	End of phase 1, all of phase 2	Complicated fire investigations at site
National Laboratory of Forensic Science (center has fire specialists)	Sometimes phase 2, most of phase 3	Laboratory work; sometimes visits to fire site
Specialists (called in by any of the aforementioned organizations)	Phase 3, rarely phase 2	Investigation of special problems, usually by theoretical work

*In major fires, and always when a crime is suspected, the district attorney's office is notified and is usually in charge of operations.

are handled by the local police, but in cases of greater complexity, the services of technical police groups (each province has at least one such group) or the National Laboratory of Forensic Science are used (Table 21–5).

A thorough or complicated search for the cause of a fire may not end at this level, but may require help from specialists in particular fields (e.g., city gas handling, electrical engineering, gasoline usage, manufacture of apparatus, plastics, building materials, matches, cigarettes). During the progress of such a fire investigation, each expert involved must exercise great care not to overstep the area of his special knowledge. As soon as the limit of his competence is reached, he must refer the issue to an individual with better knowledge of and more experience in the special problem involved. There are instances in which not even the combined efforts of all these agents and agencies unequivocally establish the true cause of a particular fire. In such a case, neither expediency, prestige, vanity, nor misdirected zeal must be allowed to distort the findings; it must be stated that the result of the search has been inconclusive. Not infrequently, further facts or evidence emerge later and can then clarify the case unless the issue has been muddled.

The investigation should, on the other hand, always be carried to the end, irrespective of admissions of guilt from a suspect—these admissions can always be withdrawn in court.

TECHNICAL CAUSES FOR THE OUTBREAK OF FIRES

For a fire to start, three conditions must be met: combustible material and oxygen must be present, and the system must be activated. Since in an actual fire the first two conditions have obviously been met, the search for the cause of the conflagration must necessarily con-

TABLE 21–6. COMMON TECHNICAL CAUSES FOR FIRES

Predominantly Thermal Processes

- Sunlight if focused by mirrors, lenses, or the like
- Nonoxidative exothermic chemical reactions: CaO and water, halogens and various materials, certain polymerizations, exothermic decompositions, chemical reactions in which cooling fails
- Heat from electrical equipment like radiators, irons, heating pads, coffee cookers, immersion heaters, stoves, grills, infrared heaters, induction furnaces, unprotected handlamps, soldering irons
- Hot stove pipes and industrial pipes
- Friction heat from brakes, automobile parts in collisions, malfunctioning machinery, overheated bearings and transmissions
- Contributing or releasing factors: covering of heat sources, closing or clogging of vents, failure of cooling systems, drying of water or oil baths

Predominantly Chemical Processes

- Open fires, including fireplaces, ovens, stoves, matches, candles, fireworks
- Smoking, e.g., in bed, in garages or dangerous industrial locations, carelessness with cigarette butts (forests, wastepaper baskets, trash cans, laboratory sinks)
- Spontaneous combustion by reaction with air, e.g., unsaturated oils (linseed oil), paint sprays, roasted organic materials (wood, coffee), coal in large piles, phosphorus, silicon, alkali metals, pyrophoric metals, pyrite (FeS_2), etc.
- Spontaneous combustion involving oxidizing compounds (peroxides, nitric acid, chromates, chlorates, perchlorates, permanganates, nitrates, etc. when mixed with organic substances such as sugar, starch, paper, wood, plastics), reactions of alkali metals with water
- Spontaneous combustion by microbiologic action, especially in haystacks, fertilizers, and the like
- Contributing chemical hazards (leaking pipes or containers with inflammable liquids or gases, explosive mixtures of air and gases or mists or dusts, faulty construction of industrial apparatus, improper use of fire extinguishers)

Predominantly Electrical Processes

- Lightning
- Sparks from static electricity (charging by walking with rubber shoes on plastic floors, driving on rubber tires [cars], in dry cleaning, in industrial processes [paper and textile machines, printing presses, belt transmissions, spraying of finely divided material, piping of liquids, movement of powders])
- Defects in electrical apparatus (faulty construction, faulty assembly, sparks from brushes and circuit beakers, insulation failures in motors or transformers, wobbly contacts, short-circuited resistors or condensers, portions of wiring of insufficient diameter leading to local heating)
- Breaking of hot light bulbs and gas discharge tubes
- Improper modification of electrical installations (short-circuiting of fuses, nailing of wires, too thin wire material, bad and loose connections, old and cracked wiring, improper material in wet surroundings)
- Electrolytic production of gases (such as hydrogen) without precautions

Other or Combined Causes

- Radiation effects
- Natural phenomena (volcanic action, earthquakes, rock slides, avalanches, meteors, storms, even floods and freezing can directly or indirectly cause fires)
- Animals, (rats or mice gnawing at lead insulations and matches, pets upsetting lamps)
- Numerous combinations of dangerous conditions (explosive air mixtures and an electric spark, a gasoline leak and a discarded match)
- Improper construction of buildings and industrial installations (an important contributing factor)

centrate on the third condition, even though other factors such as the speed and direction of the blaze, its temperature, and the behavior of various materials are often of great importance. We have seen that the activation energy necessary to overcome the energy barrier can be of thermal, electrical, or other nature. The overcoming of this barrier constitutes the ignition phase. In actual practice, the investigator is not unduly concerned about the theoretical background of the ignition process but follows a more pragmatic course. Thus, if a building was set on fire by a stroke of lightning, the question of whether the electrical discharge or the heat developed furnished the activation energy is of secondary importance. In Table 21–6 more or less common technical causes for ignition are classified as thermal, chemical, electrical, and others. Clear discrimination between these groups is not possible; there are many instances in which they overlap.

Chemical Causes

Inflammable Liquids and Gases

Inflammable liquids and gases often play a major role in the start and the propagation of fires. They can be ignited on purpose (arson), by negligence, or by accident. Such liquids or gases can also contribute to the spreading or the intensification of fires that started in other ways.

The arsonist, in his wish to start or to intensify a fire, often uses inflammable liquids that are normal for the location where the fire was started—but sometimes he picks whatever is available for his purpose. Experience has shown that the inflammable liquids most frequently found in arson cases are the common ones, typically gasoline, white spirit, kerosene, heating oil, and diesel fuel oil, as well as denatured alcohol, acetone, and various kinds of thinner. Less frequently one finds benzene, toluene, ether, turpentine, carbon disulfide, and alcohols other than ethanol. The rare occurrence of some of these less common liquids in arson cases may be a statistical artifact due to the difficulties in isolating and identifying some of them.

Contrary to widespread belief, even highly volatile liquids can often be located, isolated, and identified after a major fire. There can be a number of reasons for this. The fire may have gone out locally, owing to lack of oxygen, to fallen debris, or to the efforts of the fire department. The liquid can have run through cracks under the floor or can have been soaked up in the soil next to a building. In addition, the insulating properties of porous materials (wood, cork, rock wool) can have retarded evaporation.

The possible role of inflammable gases in starting or spreading a fire is more difficult to evaluate. It is necessary to test thoroughly all gas containers, piping, valves, stopcocks, and the like and to study the dynamics of the fire and its effects on various materials.

Degree of Inflammability. The definitions of inflammability vary somewhat from country to country. The various systems, however, commonly classify inflammable liquids according to their flash points. For a liquid, this is the lowest temperature at which it gives off vapor sufficient to form an ignitable mixture with the air near the surface of the liquid or within the vessel used.

Determination of the flash point should be carried out in standardized apparatus (e.g., Abel-Pensky, Pensky-Martens). The method used must be stated when values for the flash point are published.

The flash point is a good measure for determining the ease of igniting a liquid by an open flame, but it does not indicate the liquid's inflammability upon contact with hot surfaces. This latter property is determined by the liquid's ignition temperature.

Ignition Temperature. The ignition temperature of a substance, whether solid or liquid or gaseous, is the minimum temperature to which the substance must be heated in order to initiate or cause self-sustained combustion independently of the heating or heating element.

It must be noted, however, that the ignition temperature is not an absolute figure, but depends to a high degree on factors such as the composition of the vapor (or gas) and air mixture, the duration of heating, the temperature of the heating source, the size of the space or container in which the reaction takes place, and the presence of catalysts. For example, the ignition temperature for pentane in air has been found to be 548°C for mixtures containing 1.5 per cent, 502°C for 3.75 per cent, and 476°C for 7.65 per cent of pentane, all other conditions being equal. In another series of experiments carbon disulfide caught fire at 120°C in a 200-ml flask, at 110°C in a 1000-ml flask, and at 96°C in a 10-liter container, all other conditions being equal.[1]

For each inflammable gas or vapor there exists an inflammable range, or explosive range, expressed for vapor or gas in per cent by volume, and for dusts in grams per cubic centimeter. Table 21–7 gives the flash point, ig-

TABLE 21–7. FLASH POINT, IGNITION TEMPERATURE, AND EXPLOSIVE RANGE

Liquid	Flash Point (°C)*	Ignition Temperature (°C)	Explosive Range (vol %)
Gasoline	−25	315	1–7
Benzene	− 8	562	1–8
Ethyl ether	−30	180	1–51
Ethanol (95%)	+14	423	3–20
Cabon disulfide	−25	100	1–50

*Measured in standard Abel-Pensky apparatus.

nition temperature, and explosive range for some common liquids. One has to be aware that the flash point is not the only factor determining the degree of inflammability of a given liquid; the ignition temperature and inflammable range, the density of the vapor, the vapor pressure, the miscibility with water, and other factors are also of importance. The surface area of the liquid also plays an important role. If a substance is distributed on a wick, for instance, or present in small droplets (paint sprays, contents of spray bottles of all kinds), the danger (or ease) of its ignition is increased considerably. Table 21–8 lists the approximate ignition temperatures for a range of solid materials.

Spontaneous Combustion and Dangerous Chemicals

In addition to the inflammable liquids and gases already discussed, many other materials and chemicals are able to start or to intensify a fire or are otherwise of importance in fire investigations. They can be dangerous because: (1) they are easily ignitable; (2) they spontaneously react with water or oxygen in exothermic processes; (3) they are oxidizing agents and can therefore intensify fires; (4) they are unstable, leading to spontaneous and exothermic decomposition or polymerization under certain conditions; and (5) they are explosive when exposed to heat, pressure, or impact. Naturally, there are materials that have several of these properties. Also, one must keep in mind that certain compounds, harmless by themselves, can become dangerous when mixed with each other. The following discussion is limited to materials and compounds that are subject to spontaneous reaction with atmospheric oxygen (spontaneous combustion) and to a few examples of dangerous chemical mixtures.

Unsaturated Oils. A number of oils containing double bonds are capable of reacting with atmospheric oxygen, producing considerable

TABLE 21–8. APPROXIMATE IGNITION TEMPERATURE FOR A RANGE OF SOLID MATERIALS*

Material	Approximate Ignition Temperature °C	°F
Yellow phosphorus	60	140
Nitrocellulose	135	275
Paper (newspaper)	185–230	365–445
Wood	220–340	420–645
Hay	230	445
Cotton (loose)	230–275	445–525
Paper (wrapping)	230–280	445–535
Straw	240	465
Sulfur	250	480
Coal (low-grade)	250–280	480–535
Cellulose	270	520
Linoleum	300 -400	570–750
Black powder	310	590
Paraffin	310–325	590–620
Coal (high-grade)	330–440	625–825
Rubber	360	680
Stationery	360	680
Coke	400	750
Sugar	410	770
Wheat flour	410–500	770–930
Linseed oil	440	825
Tin	450	840
Cotton fabric	450	840
Nylon	480	890
Tobacco	485	900
Asphalt	485	900
Lucite	485	900
Tar	505–600	940–1110
Wool	570	1060
Silk	585	1080
Heating oil	600	1110
Teflon	600	1110
Zinc	670	1240

*Data from list in M. Frei-Sulzer and A. Suter: *Leitfaden zur Bearbeitung von Brandursachen und Explosionen*. Hamburg, Kriminalistik Verlag, 1971.

heat. The double bonds occur, for example, in linoleic, linolenic, and oleic acids, the esters of which are components of oils from linseed, chinese wood, poppy seed, sunflower seed, walnut, hemp seed, perilla, seal, whale, and herring.

If unsaturated oils of this kind are dispersed on fibrous materials with large surfaces (such as cotton waste, cellulose wadding, sawdust, or rags) in such a way that there is free access to air but heat conductivity is poor, the heat produced can accumulate and can ignite the material. The kinetics of this process depend on the kind and amount of the oil and the porous carrier, the presence of drying agents (siccatives), solvents (turpentine, white spirit), and other compounds (e.g., paint pigment) as well as on the temperature and the air turbulence.

One of the most common spontaneously oxidizable oils, boiled linseed oil, can normally start a fire two to eight hours after exposure to air. The process starts slowly, but accelerates rapidly as the temperature increases. During the final stages of the reaction, eye irritants such as acrolein are produced in appreciable amounts and cannot fail to be noticed by any person in the vicinity. Experiments have shown that balls of cotton waste weighing as little as a couple of grams, and containing 30 per cent of boiled linseed oil by weight can ignite spontaneously when enclosed in a small space (pocket of clothing or the like).

Phosphorus. This element occurs in several allotropic modifications. Among these, white (yellow) phosphorus is the most poisonous and, considered as a fire hazard, the most reactive and dangerous modification. Its ignition temperature is as low as 60°C, but if finely dispersed (e.g., on filter paper, rags, or the like) it catches fire at room temperature. Because of its ready oxidation and spontaneous ignition in air it must be stored under water.

White phosphorus is used in industry, in chemical laboratories, and in conjunction with other chemicals as a rodenticide. Red phosphorus is less dangerous, but in combination with oxidizing agents such as chlorates, it acquires explosive properties. Such mixtures explode upon the slightest jolt (children's percussion caps).

Alkali Metals. The alkali metals lithium, sodium, potassium, rubidium, and cesium react with water with increasing violence, producing hydrogen gas. This gas is usually ignited in the case of sodium and always in that of potassium, rubidium or cesium. In spite of their rare occurrence (mostly in chemical laboratories), fires and explosions due to alkali metals are not uncommon, often as a result of youngsters' pranks.

Quicklime. Quicklime (calcium oxide, CaO) reacts with water, producing considerable heat ($CaO + H_2O = Ca\ (OH)_2 + 15.5$ kcal). If ignitable material is present, a fire can start in this way. Cases are known in which calcium oxide was used as an admixture to floor fillings; when they were exposed to water, spontaneous combustion occurred.

Carbides. Calcium carbide (Ca_2C) formerly found extensive use in carbide lamps since, in contact with water, it produces acetylene. The heat of reaction ($CaC_2 + 2\ H_2O = H_2C_2 + Ca(OH)_2 + 30.4$ kcal) is sufficient to ignite acetylene and air mixture if the ratio of water to carbide is not so high that cooling takes place. The carbides of lithium, sodium, potassium, and barium have similar properties.

Peroxides. Hydrogen peroxide has been used to drive directional jets in space missions since it spontaneously decomposes in contact with metals or metal salts when its concentration exceeds 90 per cent. Even at 50 per cent concentration, this action can take place, whereas the 30 per cent hydrogen peroxide used in industry and laboratories is not dangerous in itself.

Organic peroxides, such as benzoyl peroxide (used as polymerization reaction initiator and catalyst) and ether peroxides (formed in most ethers when they are allowed to stand) are subject to explosive decomposition. In the laboratory, the danger in evaporating old samples of pure ethyl ether is well known. Technical ether contains stabilizers, preventing or slowing down the formation of peroxides.

Nitrates. Since inorganic nitrates are strong oxidizing agents and are widely used in industry, and especially in agriculture, they frequently come to the attention of the fire investigator. They are not especially apt to undergo spontaneous combustion, but like other oxidizing chemicals, they intensify fires and under fire conditions they release the very poisonous nitrous oxides.

Saltpeter or nitre (potassium nitrate, KNO_3) and caliche or Chile saltpeter (sodium nitrate, $NaNO_3$), used as fertilizers, are often transported in jute sacks. If such sacks get wet and then dry again, they become great potential fire hazards in ships or warehouses.

Concentrated nitric acid can spontaneously ignite organic material (excelsior, sawdust) and reacts vigorously with turpentine.

Chlorates. Chlorates are another group of widely used oxidizing agents (in chlorate explosives, in the match industry, and in easily accessible weed killers). Mixtures of chlorates and organic material (fabrics, wood, flour) are easily ignited by friction. Mixtures popular with youngsters are chlorate and sugar and chlorate and sulfur. These start burning vigorously or explode by reaction with, for example, a few drops of concentrated sulfuric acid; many serious accidents have occurred with them.

Dangerous Mixtures

Many chemicals that are relatively inert and not especially prone to start fires by themselves can become great fire hazards when combined or mixed with each other. The following are some examples (some of them not generally known) of such dangerous mixtures.

Chlorine and Acetylene. The halogens fluorine, chlorine, and bromine are very reactive agents. The most common one of these, chlorine (Cl_2), reacts violently with finely dispersed metals, with ammonia, with hydrogen, and with hydrocarbons such as ethene (C_2H_4) and acetylene (C_2H_2). When chlorine comes in contact with acetylene (most likely to happen in industrial installations), ignition is instantaneous.

Glycerol, Glycol, or Formaldehyde and Permanganates. When glycerol or glycol comes in contact with solid permanganate, an exothermic reaction occurs that can ignite the mixture and start a fire. A similar reaction occurs upon mixing potassium permanganate and aqueous formaldehyde solutions (formalin). This reaction has been used by farmers for killing rodents in stables and under floors. In Sweden, a farmer placed 300 g of potassium dichromate and 0.5 liter of formalin in a rat-hole in his stable. A fire started and destroyed the building.

Potassium Bromate and Thioglycolic Acid. Potassium bromate ($KBrO_3$) is an oxidizing agent similar to potassium chlorate. Thus, a mixture of potassium bromate and sugar burns fiercely when ignited or upon contact with concentrated sulfuric acid.

Less known is the spontaneous ignition of potassium bromate and thioglycolic acid. This seems to be a rare and unlikely combination; it is, however, the base of certain types of home permanent processes. The hair is first treated with a solution of thioglycolic acid, then "fixed" with an aqueous solution of potassium bromate. The commercial product consists sometimes of a ready-made solution of the acid and a package of solid potassium bromate for making fresh solutions at home. If the thioglycolic acid solution stands open, water evaporates and the acid becomes concentrated. On contact, the two chemicals ignite and can start a fire. Several such cases have actually occurred in Sweden.

Silver Nitrate, Magnesium, and Water. A mixture of silver nitrate and powdered magnesium is immediately ignited with a blinding flash by a single drop of water. The probability of this reaction's occurrence is of course slight, but in a chemical or photographic laboratory it can still conceivably happen.

Electrical Causes

The following electrical phenomena, of interest to the fire examiner, differ greatly with respect to their duration, the amount of heat developed, and the temperatures reached.

TABLE 21–9. QUANTITIES, SYMBOLS, AND UNITS USED IN THE DISCUSSION OF ELECTRICAL PHENOMENA

QUANTITY	SYMBOL	UNIT
Voltage	U	Volt (v)
Current	I	Ampere (amp)
Resistance	R	Ohm (ohm)
Effect	P	Watt (w)
Energy	E	Watt-second (ws) Joule (J) Kilogram-calorie (kcal)
Capacitance	C	Farad (f)

Prefix	pico-	nano-	micro-	milli-	kilo-	mega-
Equal to	10^{-12}	10^{-9}	10^{-6}	10^{-3}	10^{3}	10^{6}

They may be grouped into three categories: technical faults in the components of generating, distributing, or using electrical energy; atmospheric electricity; and other static electricity generated in solid, liquid, or gaseous media. The quantities, symbols, and units used are listed in Table 21–9.

Technical Faults in Electric Installations and Components

In spite of considerable improvement in the quality of and standards for electrical components, technical faults still cause numerous fires. Some of these faults are: overloading of wiring or apparatus, loose contacts, inadequate insulation that allows sparking or arcing between lines, and faulty safety devices (relays, fuses). Mishaps can also be due to the human factor (careless handling of electrical components, covering of hot apparatus with inflammable material, overheating of toasters, irons, cooking plates, heating baths).

Overloading of Electric Wiring. When an electric current flows through an insulated wire, some of its energy is turned into heat. As a rule this leads to a negligible rise in temperature since the resistance of the wire is less than the resistance of the appliance connected to it. The increase in temperature is proportional to the square of the current and to the time. It is further a function of the material through which the current flows.

$$\Delta T = \frac{kI^2t}{A^2} \qquad \text{(Eq. 3)}$$

in which ΔT = increase in temperature, I = current, t = time, A = cross section of wire, and k = a constant of the material.

In places where the cross section of a conductor is diminished, the temperature will rise appreciably. The better the heat insulation, the more rapid the rise in temperature. If the insulation finally melts, is pyrolyzed, or burns, an electric contact can ensue and cause further heating or arcing or both. Under normal conditions such accidents are rare nowadays, owing to strict regulations, in force in most countries, concerning the cross section of wiring, the quality of its insulation, the capacity and quality of fuses, and the quality of all the installation work.

Overloading of Electrical Equipment. The relation between cross section and rise of temperature just discussed also applies to the windings in magnets, relays, generators, motors, and transformers. In equipment with large effects, special cooling systems are often installed to lessen or hinder heat development.

The most common applications of electrical energy are the production of heat, light, and mechanical power. The essential part of a heating device is a length of resistance wire wound around a ceramic core. This wire of high resistance yields heat by radiation or convection or both. Its effect is:

$$P_n = \frac{U^2}{R} \qquad \text{(Eq. 4)}$$

The heat produced is proportional to the square of the voltage applied; if connected to too high a voltage, the heater can produce a great deal of excess heat.

Another risk is an internal short circuit in part of the resistance wire. An example of this is shown in Figure 21–2. If $R' = \frac{R}{2}$, then $P' = 2\,P_n$, i.e., the effect is doubled within about half the volume of the heating coil. Again, a considerable rise in temperature ensues. To make things worse, such overloads often are not great enough to melt the fuses.

Bad Contacts and Contact Resistance. During operation of an electrical system, increased heat resistance can occur close to a bad contact.

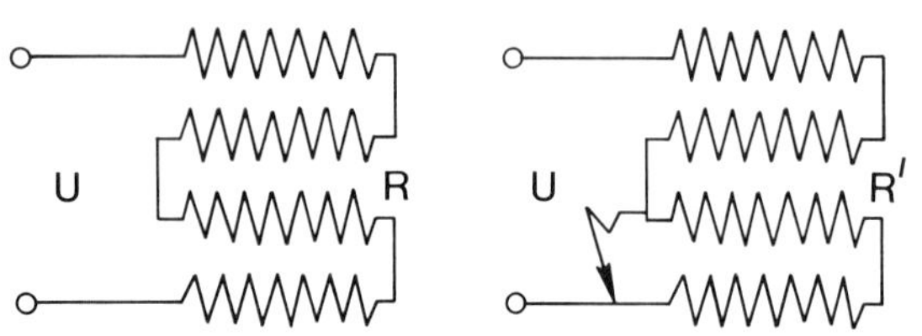

Figure 21–2. Schematic wiring diagram of a heating appliance. *Left:* Heating appliance under normal working conditions. *Right:* Conditions after internal short-circuiting of the resistance wire. U, voltage applied; R, resistance of the heating coil under normal operating conditions; R′, resistance of the heating coil after internal short circuit.

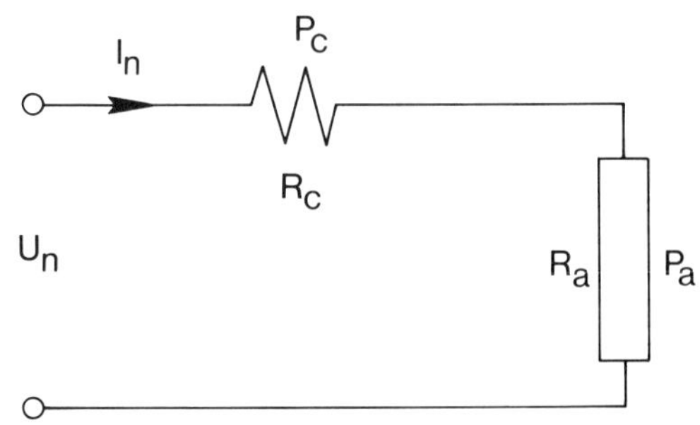

Figure 21–3. Schematic wiring diagram of an electrical appliance with a bad (loose) contact. U_n, net voltage; I_n, current; R_a, resistance of the appliance; P_a, effect of the appliance; R_c, resistance of the bad contact; P_c, effect of the bad contact.

This in turn can lead to a considerable rise in temperature. Consider the system shown in Figure 21–3 and Equations 5 and 6.

$$I_n = U_n\,(R_c + R_a)^{-1} \qquad \text{(Eq. 5)}$$

$$P_c = R_c \cdot I_n^2 = R_c \cdot U_n^2\,(R_c + R_a)^{-2} \qquad \text{(Eq. 6)}$$

Here R_a is the normal resistance of an appliance, and R_c is the extra resistance due to a bad contact. If $R_c = 0$ (proper contact), the effect is $P_n = \frac{U_n^2}{R_a}$, and if $R_c = \infty$ the current is completely interrupted. It can be shown that the effect, P_c, has a maximum value when $R_c = R_a$. Under these conditions the effect at the bad contact is 25 per cent of that of the rated effect (P_n) of the appliance:

$$P_c = R_a \cdot U_n^2\,(R_a + R_a)^{-2} = \frac{P_n}{4} \qquad \text{(Eq. 7)}$$

But even for large ratios of $\frac{R_c}{R_a}$ appreciable effects can occur at a bad contact. Calculation shows that for $0.1R_a < R_c < 10R_a$ this effect becomes greater than $0.08P_a$.

Since the current flowing through such a system actually is less than normal, the fuses are not affected. This must be kept in mind when evaluating the state of the electric system at the site of a fire.

Partial Short Circuit. A partial short circuit is the establishment of an electric current between conductors or components that normally are insulated from each other. This type of phenomenon varies greatly in its duration and the energy (heat) developed. Such shorting is a very common electrical cause of fire. It can be brought about by a number of different physical or chemical mechanisms. One example is schematically represented in Figure 21–4.

The appliance has the resistance R_a. Nor-

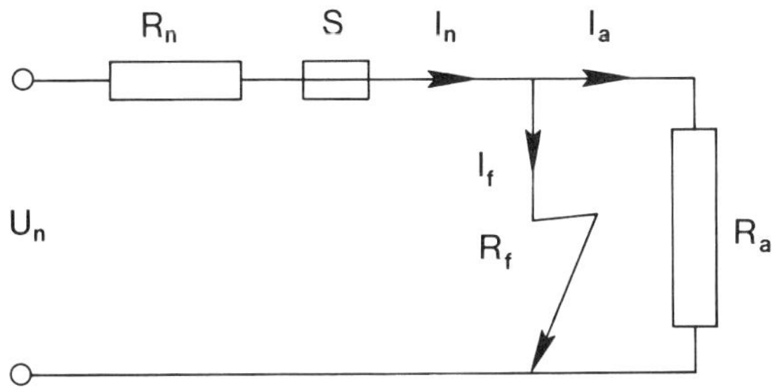

Figure 21–4. Schematic wiring diagram of an appliance in which a partial short circuit has occurred. U_n, net voltage; I_n, total current; I_a, current through the appliance alone; I_f, current through the fault; R_n, feed impedance of the net; R_a, resistance of the appliance; R_f, resistance of the fault; S, fuse.

mally, the current I_n from the net with the voltage U_n flows through the fuse S. The feed impedance of the net is symbolized by resistance R_n (neglecting its inductive and capacitance components). When a partial short circuit occurs with a resistance of R_f, a current I_f will flow through it.

From the fundamental laws of electricity the following relations between I_n, I_f, and P_f can be arrived at.

$$I_n = U_n\,[R_n + R_aR_f\,(R_a + R_f)^{-1}]^{-1} \quad \text{(Eq. 8)}$$

$$I_f = U_n\left[R_n\left(1+\frac{R_f}{R_a}\right)+R_f\right]^{-1} \quad \text{(Eq. 9)}$$

$$P_f = R_f \cdot I_f^2 = R_f \cdot U_n^2\left[R_n\left(1+\frac{R_f}{R_a}\right)+R_f\right]^{-2} \quad \text{(Eq. 10)}$$

By differentiation, it can be shown that R_f has its maximal value when

$$R_f = R_aR_n\,(R_a + R_n)^{-1} \quad \text{(Eq. 11)}$$

In this case the values for I_n, I_f, and P_f are:

$$I_n = U_n\,(R_a + 2\,R_n)\,[2\,R_n\,(R_a + R_n)]^{-1} \quad \text{(Eq. 12)}$$

$$I_f = \frac{U_n}{2\,R_n} \quad \text{(Eq. 13)}$$

$$P_f = R_a \cdot U_n^2\,[4\,R_n\,(R_a + R_n)]^{-2} \quad \text{(Eq. 14)}$$

Let us assume, for example, that in a given circuit $R_n = 2.3$ ohms, $R_a = 26$ ohms and $U_n =$ 230 v or 115 v respectively. A maximal effect at the short circuit will occur when $R_f = 2.11$ ohms. The resulting currents and effects will become:

for $U_n = 230$ v:	for $U_n = 115$ v:
$I_n = 54.1$ amp	$I_n = 27$ amp
$I_f = 50$ amp	$I_f = 25$ amp
$P_f = 5{,}280$ w	$P_f = 1{,}320$ w

The potential danger of the situation depends largely on the functioning of the fuses. Normally, these are so constructed that the melting time is a function of the magnitude of the current, i.e., the excess energy developed. Characteristic curves for regular fuses with rated currents from 2 to 60 amp are shown in Figure 21–5.

On the basis of Equations 8 through 10 and Figure 21–5, the magnitudes of I_n, P_f, the time period t, and the energy developed E_f can be determined as functions of the resistance R_f at the point of the partial short circuit. These relationships are plotted in Figure 21–6 for a range of R_f between 10^{-3} through 10^4 ohms.

At very small values of R_f, the effect P_f and the energy E_f are small, but I_n is large (short circuit) and the fuse is activated. At somewhat higher values of R_f, the current I_n is no longer sufficient to activate the fuse, and P_f is still large but has passed its maximal value. As time goes on, the value of E_f rises and can lead to appreciable production of heat. This region of the diagram is of special interest to the fire examiner, since fires can occur under these conditions.

At even higher values of R_f, the effect P_f becomes so slight that even prolonged operation does not lead to an appreciable rise in temperature: a new steady state is established in

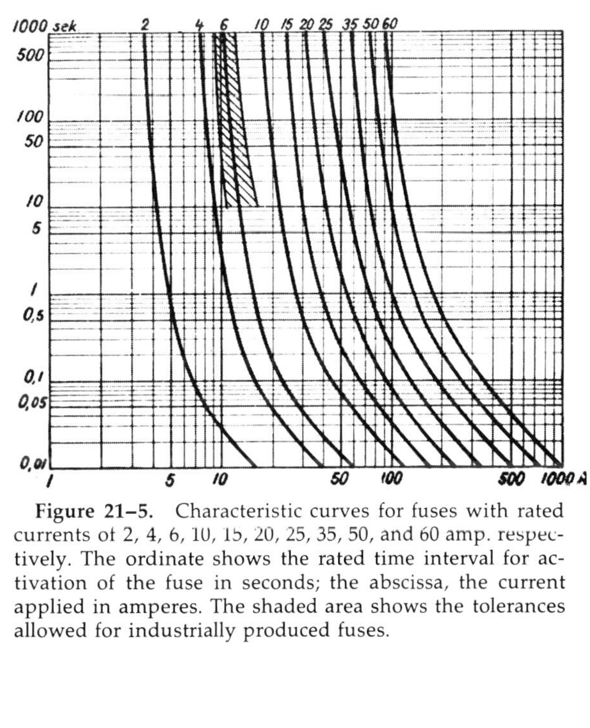

Figure 21–5. Characteristic curves for fuses with rated currents of 2, 4, 6, 10, 15, 20, 25, 35, 50, and 60 amp. respectively. The ordinate shows the rated time interval for activation of the fuse in seconds; the abscissa, the current applied in amperes. The shaded area shows the tolerances allowed for industrially produced fuses.

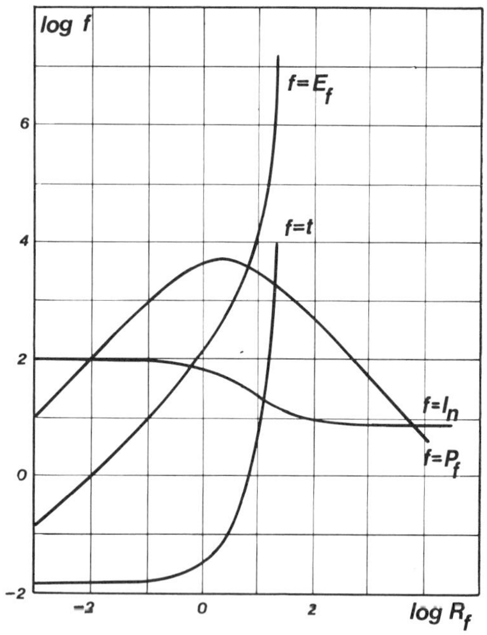

Figure 21–6. A logarithmic (log/log) plot of the energy (E_f), the period of time (t), the current (I_n), and the effect (P_f) as functions of the resistance of a fault (R_f) in a circuit with a partial short circuit shown in Figure 21–4. The magnitudes are the same as in Figure 21–4, and their relationships are discussed in the text.

which the heat generated becomes equal to the heat lost from the region of the fault.

A partial short circuit can occur in any circuit to which a voltage is applied—even when no current is flowing through the system. By contrast, a fault due to a bad contact can only occur when the current is "switched on." Partial short circuits are very unstable phenomena. Sometimes they "correct themselves," e.g., when the heat developed evaporates water from humid insulating material. More frequently, however, the situation deteriorates; the material keeps getting hotter all the time, and finally ionization sets in. This in turn can lead to arcing and a drastic decrease of resistance.

Electric Arcs. Electric arcs consist of jets of charged particles (electrons and ions) through a gas. Prerequisites for the formation of arcs are the presence of an ionizable gas and a sufficient potential difference in electrical field strength between two nearby points. Several other factors are of importance: the material, the shape and surface condition of the conductors, the composition and pressure of the gas (atmosphere), and of course the distance between the ends of the arc. The temperature in an electric arc can reach thousands of degrees, and intense heat and light are produced within a relatively small and concentrated area. Hot spots of this kind can obviously cause fires if inflammable material is nearby.

Electric arcs can originate from bad contacts or from partial short circuits. Also, breaking of the current in circuits with high inductivity—leading to pulses of high voltage—can cause arcs.

Faulty Function of Safety Devices. The simplest type of electrical heating devices are intended for continuous, or at least prolonged, operation: radiators, heating plates, toasters, soldering irons, and the like. These do not usually require any safety devices except regular fuses.

Other apparatus are built for intermittent operation, and their safety depends on properly working thermostats. Examples of this kind of equipment are stoves and especially laundry irons.

Finally, some types of appliances require special wiring or active safeguards. Among these are heating fans, including hair dryers, in which the heat must be interrupted when the fan is switched off. Other examples are boilers or electrically heated baths (water, oil), in which the current has to be cut off when either the liquid drops below a safe level or the temperature rises above a certain value.

Human Error. Numerous fires are caused by electrical components that work properly but are—by carelessness, negligence, or intention—so placed that excessive heat is transferred to inflammable material. Frequently, electric heaters or stoves are covered with clothes (for drying), with shawls, or with curtains. Such heating appliances are constructed for safe continuous operation provided that air can freely circulate through and around them. A thermal equilibrium is then reached at around 70° to 125°C. If the circulation of air is impeded, a new equilibrium is reached—often at a temperature sufficient to ignite the cover. In such cases, traces of fabric can frequently be found within or close to the appliance.

Another hazard is the ordinary light bulb. If such bulbs are covered, the temperature can rise until a glowing fire is started in the surrounding materials. Cases have been known in which even Christmas tree lights (3- to 4-watt effect) have caused fires in this fashion.

On electric stoves or heating plates, pans containing fat or oil can get so hot that the liquid is ignited. Many fires in restaurants and hotels have started this way. Under certain circumstances, negligence can be proved and legal action be taken against the responsible parties.

Atmospheric Electricity

Lightning was, no doubt, a blessing for early man, who learned how to maintain a fire before learning how to start one at will. Nowadays, thunderstorms are a potential threat to human dwellings and agricultural and industrial installations.

The theory of the formation of lightning bolts is not complete. It seems probable that small droplets of water become ionized by particle bombardment in the upper atmosphere. By several stepwise processes of charge separation, the strength of the electrical field is increased to about 400 kv per meter. The lower part of a thundercloud carries a negative charge. When finally a discharge takes place, currents of 10^5 amp can occur—but the duration of the discharge is only on the order of a few microseconds.

The electric charge hits the earth's surface at places where conductivity is high and follows regions or paths of low resistance. The amount of energy in a single lightning bolt is relatively small, since its large effect is offset by its short duration. At a voltage of 100 Mv, a current of 50 kamp, and a duration of 10 μsec the energy is:

$$E = U \times I \times t = 10^8 \cdot 5 \cdot 10^4 \cdot 10^{-5} \cdot 10^{-3} \cdot 3600^{-1} = 14 \text{ kwh} \simeq 12{,}000 \text{ kcal} \quad \text{(Eq. 15)}$$

Most of this energy is converted into heat and light during the passage through the atmosphere, but the remaining energy is quite sufficient to produce serious damage. This damage can be thermal, setting buildings on fire, or electrical, causing large oscillations of the voltage in electrical distribution networks (by direct hits, or by induction caused by near hits). These voltage shock waves can then in turn cause damage to insulation and thereby initiate short circuits. Protection is afforded by lightning rods on buildings, oil tanks, masts, and the like, and by nonlinear resistance arresters in major electrical installations.

Static Electricity Other Than Atmospheric

An electrostatic charge can accumulate in solid, liquid, or gaseous materials through external or internal friction and by induction (influence). In solid bodies with little conductivity (especially insulators), the charge tends to remain concentrated on the surface, whereas in conducting bodies the charge becomes distributed throughout. When two relatively nonconductive materials are rubbed against each other, an exchange of their charges can take place (triboelectric phenomenon). A so-called triboelectric series begins with the most strongly positively charged material and ends with the most negatively charged, as for example: glass—hair—nylon—wool—cotton—paper—steel—hard rubber—polyethylene.

Liquids such as oil or gasoline can become charged by friction against the walls of pipes or orifices as they flow through them. Clouds of vapor or small solid particles (dust) can become charged by friction of the particles against each other as well as when streaming through pipes. Such a system of particles with separated charges is in a metastable electrical state. A local increase of the ionization in the atmosphere can lead to a discharge (spark). Although the volume of these sparks is small, temperatures of up to 10,000°C have been reported. This is sufficient to ignite inflammable gases, vapors, mist, or dust particles. In normal air, solid materials are—as a rule—not ignited, but in atmospheres enriched with oxygen even those can catch fire. The rapid ignition of solid materials in an oxygen atmosphere was tragically demonstrated in the lethal fire in an Apollo capsule at Cape Kennedy in 1967.

The accumulation of an electric charge by human beings constitutes a special problem. An adult has a capacitance of around 200 pf and can under certain conditions (low atmospheric humidity, rubber soled shoes, nylon clothing) become electrostatically charged with voltages on the order of 15 kv. This corresponds to a static energy of about 0.02 ws (J). This voltage is sufficient to generate sparks 4 to 13 mm in length, depending on the geometry of the end points. An energy of 0.02 ws, suddenly released, suffices to ignite gas and air or vapor and air mixtures as well as mixtures of air and dust of, e.g., wood, sulfur, and shellac (Table 21–10).

TABLE 21–10. IGNITION ENERGY FOR EXPLOSIVE MIXTURES OF AIR WITH SOME GASES, VAPORS, AND DUSTS

COMPOUND	LOWER LIMIT OF IGNITION ENERGY (mws = mJ)
Acetylene	0.019
Ethyl ether	0.19
Propane	0.25
Methane	0.30
Sulfur	15
Cellulose acetate	30
Sucrose (sugar)	30
Polystyrene	40
Urea	80

THE SEARCH FOR THE ORIGIN OF A FIRE

Procedures While the Fire Is Raging

The first pertinent facts related to a fire are the time and nature of the alarm. Major fire companies register all alarms on tape recorders and also automatically record the time and number of each alarm. In smaller communities these facts must be manually recorded immediately. It is essential to make notes of the identity (true or assumed) of the caller and his or her location. After the first alarm has been sounded, further alarms may be necessary, depending on the nature and size of the blaze. These concern the police, ambulance services, hospitals, and doctors. The police see to it that their own technical groups and, if needed, also the district attorney, fire specialists, and the medical examiner are called in as soon as feasible.

The police should have immediate access to at least the following equipment:

- Automobiles with two-way radio
- Protective clothing (overalls, boots, gloves, goggles, helmets, smoke masks if possible)
- Portable searchlights with at least 25 m of cable
- Cameras (black and white, color, in certain cases movie camera) and flash equipment
- Tape recorder
- Material for access control (ropes, barriers, signs)
- Shovels, spades, crowbars
- First aid kit
- Fire trunks, which should contain: (1) handtools (hammer, pliers, monkey wrenches, several screwdrivers, small crowbar, hacksaws for wood and metal, small rakes and shovels); (2) brushes and trowel; (3) knives; (4) nails, screws, and thumbtacks; (5) flashlights; (6) magnet; (7) measuring tape; (8) magnifying glass; (9) gloves; (10) simple test equipment for checking electric wiring; (11) sensing device for organic vapors; (12) notebook and sketch pad; (13) pens, pencils, marking pencils, chalk; and (14) material for packing physical evidence (glass and metal containers, nylon bags, test tubes with corks, string, tape, soft wire, cardboard, wrapping paper, labels, envelopes).

Even during phase 1, facts can emerge that point to a particular cause of the fire, and in this case, effort can be directed toward proving or disproving this cause. For instance, there may have been a thunderstorm, and it may be possible that lightning started the fire. In such a case great caution is required, however, since an arsonist often chooses such a time in order to mislead the investigators. Witnesses may have noticed negligence with fire, electric installations, or industrial processes. There may be circumstantial evidence suggesting arson, such as the presence of suspiciously acting individuals, knowledge or rumors about financial difficulties of the owner (inviting insurance fraud), a series of fires in the same area or neighborhood, or multiple starting points for the fire. In general, arsonists avoid starting fires in daylight and in areas with considerable pedestrian traffic.

In most cases, however, a systematic search is required, either because circumstantial evidence is weak or because nothing is known about the cause of the fire. Under such circumstances, one cause after another has to be meticulously excluded until only one or, at worst, a few possible explanations for the fire remain.

It might be well to note at this point that small fires, threatening (but not materialized) fires, and narrow escapes all constitute excellent occasions for studying possible mechanisms and conditions for starting damaging fires. Especially should younger, less experienced investigators be encouraged to study such events, since the physical evidence generally is not damaged or is damaged only slightly.

When an actual fire is out of control, one must try to locate its starting point as soon as possible, preferably during phase 1. If several starting points are found, the probability of arson increases considerably. The location of the start of a fire can be deduced from photographs or sketches, from direct visual observation, through statements of witnesses, and especially by listening to the firemen fighting the blaze. The experience and practical knowledge of firemen is of great value during the whole investigation, and the investigator is well advised to respect their opinions. In this way, smooth teamwork between police and firemen and technical investigator can be established.

Obviously, the firemen's first tasks are the saving of life and the protection of valuable property, and they must not be hindered in carrying out these tasks. Whenever possible, especially after the fire has been brought under control, their aid may be enlisted in efforts to preserve valuable evidence by avoiding unnecessary demolition of walls or ceilings, or excessive damage by water. The use of smaller amounts of water (dousing) and the drying of larger puddles with sawdust or the like are recommended. At the later stages of the fire, closer questioning of firefighters also becomes possible.

During phase 1, the flow of information between the firemen and investigators must be continuous and unimpeded. If it is decided that specialists or personnel from a forensic science laboratory should be called in, these calls should be made forthwith so that their work can start early.

Investigations at the Site

Some general aspects of the search for the cause of a fire have already been mentioned. For practical reasons the operation was divided into three somewhat arbitrary steps: phase 1 (collection of facts and witness statements prior to and during the fire), phase 2 (investigations on the site after the fire has been brought under control), and phase 3 (laboratory tests on physical evidence brought from the fire, reconstruction of the initial period of the blaze, and theoretical and practical work by experts in special fields). Sharp boundaries between these phases do not and should not exist, however, and close cooperation between all individuals and organizations involved in clarifying the cause and the course of the conflagration is essential.

Phase 1

Among the frustrations of investigating a fire that is raging out of control is the unfortunate frequency with which it destroys much of the evidence one is searching for. It is therefore important to record pertinent facts as soon as possible by making notes, tape recordings, sketches, or photographs of all important events. Sometimes, press photographers, television teams, or others have taken pictures that became useful evidence. Also, informal talks with witnesses should start as early as possible while their memory is fresh and their statements not influenced by discussions with others or by exposure to mass media.

Among the facts to be noted are the weather conditions (especially the direction and strength of winds, and the presence and intensity of thunderstorms), the color and size of flames, the color and smell of smoke, the development of the fire (size, direction, special events like breaking of flames through roofs or partitions), and anything that can give an indication of where the fire started.

Firemen and police officers must speedily inquire if any persons are missing or not accounted for. Also individuals leaving the scene of the fire for no obvious reason should be questioned. The injured and homeless must be taken care of, but measures of this nature lie outside the scope of this chapter.

By direct observation and by questioning the firemen, the condition of each door, window, hatch, and the like must be checked to ascertain whether it was open, closed, locked, bolted, or even nailed shut. These observations can be essential for discovering if any crime was committed prior to (or even during) the fire, and for excluding certain theories about how the fire started. For the same reason the condition of all electric fuses must be noted.

Additionally, it is valuable to know the manner of fighting the fire (with hoses, sprinklers, spray, water mist, foam, or carbon dioxide) and the timing of these measures. Have other people than the fire brigade attempted to extinguish the blaze?

The firemen and persons familiar with the premises may supply information about the nature, the amount, and the location of any inflammable materials present at the site. The firemen also usually notice if it was especially hard to put out the fire in some particular spot.

Phase 2

While the fire is being brought under control, measures can be initiated that lead into phase 2. It is often quite possible to enter part of the fire area while the rest of the blaze is still being actively fought.

If any persons have been reported missing, the search for them must have been started at an early period. When a victim is found—and it has been ascertained that death has occurred—the medical examiner (and the district attorney if not previously alerted) must be called to the scene. The body should not be touched until it has been photographed. One's mind should be open to the possibility that the victim was killed or injured prior to or during the fire, accidentally or intentionally.

The search proper generally begins at those places where, according to preliminary evidence, the fire probably had its start. If no such evidence is available, a systematic search must be carried out. The areas close to the start of a fire are often revealed by the greatest fire damage (evidence of high temperatures and signs of deep carbonization). Soot is generally formed more abundantly near the origin of the fire, since the surrounding surfaces were then still relatively cool. All these indications must be evaluated with care because exceptions occur; for instance, frequently a fire can be locally intensified by the presence of particularly inflammable material or by strong drafts. Here again, talks with the persons fighting the fire are very useful and important.

The site of an extinguished fire is usually a dangerous, messy, and dirty scene. Far from getting discouraged, however, the investigator starts his task by clearing away large debris such as wooden beams, iron girders, and brick or concrete walls. Care must be exercised in two respects: the persons involved must be protected from injury, and valuable evidence should not be destroyed.

The next step consists of a finer clearing of the area, which includes making careful notes and sketches and taking photographs. It is not possible to pinpoint just what the investigator should look for, since the variations from fire to fire are obviously enormous. Anything unusual must be noted, however, such as strange locations of electrical equipment, furniture, containers, residues of inflammable material (paper baskets, crates), and the like.

Finally a patient, detailed search will usually have to be made. In some textbooks, this activity has been compared to archeologic "combing" of a site. With a brush and a dustpan, a mason's trowel, and possibly a sieve, the debris is sifted to bring to light items of interest such as matches, lighters, candle wax, fuses, textiles, parts of electric wiring, switches, bits from lamps, molten glass, plastic, metals, debris with an unusual smell or "wet" appearance. If such items are found, their location is noted on grids laid over sketches, plans, or photographs. If necessary, they are photographed before being removed. The depth of the find may be of importance for reconstruction of the event. Special attention should be paid to evidence suggesting arson, such as timing mechanisms (mechanical or chemical), fuses, containers for inflammable liquids, batteries, explosive devices, especially in places where these items should not normally be found. If clocks or watches are found, the position of the hands should be noted. Other objects of interest are all kinds of equipment and installations for heating—fireplaces, stoves, ovens, electric heaters, laundry irons, hair dryers, toasters, grills, immersion heaters, water boilers, heating pads.

It is advisable to rope off and protect the fire area for several days after the search has been finished. Often, the examiner has to return to the site for further investigation or a search for missing details. Also, it can very well happen that specialists are called in later who should have a chance to visit the site. The same can apply to the district attorney, the counsel for the defense, and possibly the court or the jury.

Investigation of Fires Caused by Chemicals. Rapid spreading of the fire, small or large explosions, and the presence of unusual smells are strong indications that inflammable liquids or gases were involved. The experienced investigator will further be suspicious of stains and discolorations on furniture or floors, and of the presence of containers for liquids or gases.

Whenever a fire has multiple starting points, arson can be suspected, and a search for inflammable liquids, candles, and the like is indicated. The fire may, however, have flared up at more than one place for quite different reasons. Sparks, trapped fire gases (especially carbon monoxide), or radiating heat can spread a fire to other locations at the same site. In order to localize and secure inflammable liquids, the sense of smell is of great help. But the nose is not the only and often not the best sensor. It can and should be supplemented by chemical sensing devices such as the commercially available vapor sensing tubes (e.g., by Draeger). The technical squads of the Swedish police are equipped with such apparatus, which consist of bellows to which short glass tubes filled with silica can be attached (Fig. 21–7). The vapors are sucked through the filling, which contains chemicals that give a color reaction with the vapor in question. For the purpose of fire investigation tubes that will indicate aliphatic hydrocarbons, aromatic hydrocarbons, alcohols, and ketones are of special value. Irrespective of the type of sensor used (nose or instrument), experience, imagination, perseverance, stubbornness, and a little luck are the prerequisites for a fire investigator looking for remaining traces of inflammable liquids.

It must also be stressed that a positive result of a vapor test may only be taken as a preliminary indication of the presence of a vapor: false positive results are frequent at the site of a fire. For obvious reasons, tubes with little specificity of response are not recommended for this purpose. The used tubes should be sealed and sent to the laboratory with the other physical evidence.

When securing and packing physical evidence suspected of containing inflammable liquids from a fire, one should observe the following points.

1. The time element is of great importance; samples should be collected and packed promptly.

2. Proper labeling is essential. The location of the sample must be carefully noted, as must the time of the collection, and a note should be

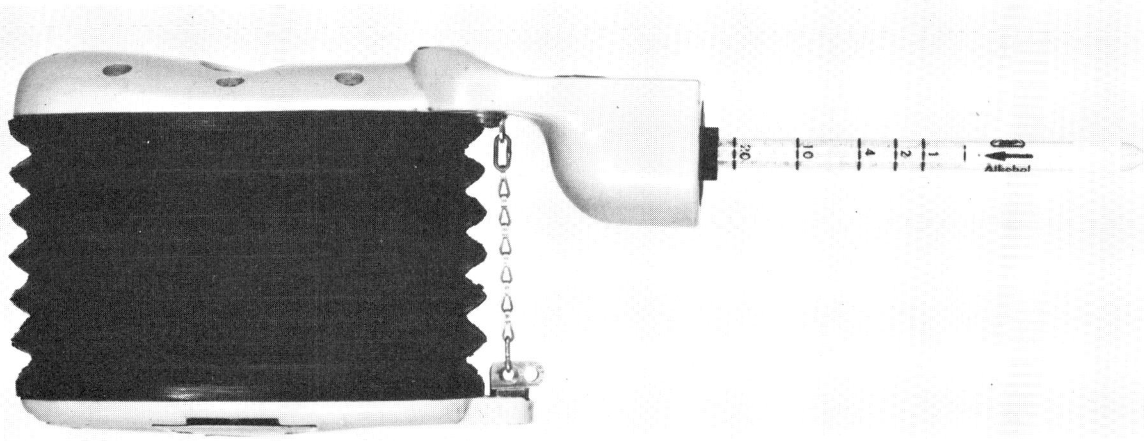

Figure 21–7. A gas and vapor sensing device (Draegerwer, Lübeck). Sensing tubes of different kinds are attached to bellows with a calibrated volume. Sampling is carried out by breaking the tip off the glass tube and sucking the gas sample through it by activating the bellows once or several times.

included stating whether the evidence has been placed in one or in several containers.

3. The packing material should be tight and inert. Glass containers that seal tightly, or tightly closed (taped) metal containers are best. Bags of nylon can be used, but plastic bags are not suitable since they may absorb solvents. The containers can be cleaned and tested for leaks by filling them with clean tap water.

4. For each type of sample secured, a reference sample should be collected from a place nearby.

5. If possible, the material secured should come from locations with relatively little fire damage (e.g., under floor boards, between partitions, under rugs or furniture, or from the soil close to the building). Thoroughly carbonized material is usually not suitable for the isolation of inflammable liquids.

6. Containers for liquids or gases must be securely closed immediately and should be checked for fingerprints before they are sent for analysis.

Spontaneous Combustion and Dangerous Chemicals. If the fire investigator finds clues or evidence pointing to spontaneous combustion as the cause of the fire, he must not be led to believe that arson can be excluded. The investigation has to continue with the same thoroughness as otherwise, as the spontaneous combustion (if proved) can be produced by any of the three processes that cause fires in general: accident, negligence, or intent. Many a skillful arsonist has arranged conditions for "spontaneous" ignition.

Clues pointing to spontaneous ignition of oils can originate from the owner or user of the premises in question, from statements of witnesses (firemen, primarily), or from a careful investigation of the site. If any material or its residue is found that by its smell or appearance suggests that oils have ignited spontaneously, a police investigation must be carried out. It should be aimed at finding out (1) the kind and amount of any unsaturated oils, paint pigments, or solvents present on the premises; (2) the kind and amount of the porous material that contained the oil; (3) when the oil was spilled or soaked up; (4) the temperature, air currents, and similar characteristics of the location in question during the interval between spilling of the oil and the start of the fire; and (5) the presence of witnesses and the time and nature of their activities and observations. Physical evidence from the primary site of the fire, and—whenever possible—comparison (reference) samples of the oil as well as the porous carrier material must be secured and sent to the laboratory for further tests.

The products formed by the reaction of dangerous chemicals with air, with other chemicals, or with ignitable material are usually heat resistant and can, therefore, be expected to survive a fire. Many of these products, however, are more or less water soluble and are apt to be washed away by the fire fighters. Where this has taken place, it is nevertheless usually possible to find local remains of powders, crusts of salts, or lumps of inorganic materials. If these are found near locations with severe fire damage (deep charring, holes burned through flooring or walls) the suspicion that a "chemical fire" caused the conflagration is strengthened. Witnesses should be heard, as mentioned earlier in the case of suspected spontaneous combustion, in order to find out—if possible—what kind of chemicals one should look for. If such chemicals were present, reference samples should be sent to the laboratory together with the samples found at the site of the fire.

INVESTIGATIONS AT THE LABORATORY

Facilities and Equipment

A practical fire laboratory can consist of a row of offices (allowing for undisturbed reading, report writing, and telephone conversations with local investigators and specialists) and four laboratory units (a mechanical unit, an electrical unit, a chemical unit, and a fire reconstruction room). All units must have appropriate hoods and ventilation equipment, and the laboratories for electrical work need to have access to a variety of power outlets for both direct and alternating current and a large choice of voltages.

Generally, the physical evidence arriving at the laboratory is unpacked and examined at the mechanical unit. Investigations carried out there can comprise checking pipes and tubing, testing valves and regulators and stopcocks, measuring flows and pressures of liquids or gases, and assessing the damage caused by heat or mechanical stress to metals, plastics, glass, wood, and the like.

The electrical unit is concerned with the investigation of fuses, wiring, relays, contacts, switches, motors, and heating coils. In addition to various kinds of microscopes, a variety of instruments for measuring electricity are used.

Work at the chemical unit is mainly focused on two areas: the analysis of inflammable liquids isolated from material sent in by local fire investigators, and the testing of such material with respect to its spontaneous combustion properties. Other experimental work includes the determination of melting and boiling points, ignition temperatures, and flash points, as is described later. The equipment consists mainly of chemical and physical instruments and the usual chemical glassware.

Reconstruction of the event is an essential part of many fire investigations since it frequently allows one to confirm a theory of how a fire started or to decide between several such theories. The reconstruction room must of course be fireproof within certain, but rather wide, limits. It should be large enough for car-

TABLE 21–11. SUGGESTED EQUIPMENT FOR MECHANICAL UNIT OF FIRE INVESTIGATION LABORATORY

Basic Equipment
- Hand tools
- Sinks with hot and cold water
- Hood with compressed air and gas
- Balances
- Areometers and specific weight balance
- Measuring tape, calipers, micrometers
- Manometers, anemometers, flowmeters
- Macroscope (about ×5), microscope, stereomicroscope (about ×5 to ×50)
- Thermometers, thermocouples, pyrometer
- Water bath and electrical furnace
- Piping, tubing, valves, stopcocks for gases and liquids
- Cleaning equipment: solvent bath, ultrasonic bath
- Reference collection of diverse material

Optional Equipment
- Stroboscope, high pressure test bath, access to comparison microscope and scanning electron microscope

TABLE 21–12. SUGGESTED EQUIPMENT FOR CHEMICAL UNIT OF FIRE INVESTIGATION LABORATORY

Basic Equipment
- Sinks with hot and cold water
- Hood with gas and compressed air
- Safety equipment: fire extinguishers, goggles, gas mask, gloves, shower, eye washing shower, fire blanket
- Glassware for chemical laboratory
- Chemicals, including comprehensive collection of solvents
- Balances, pycnometers, aerometers
- Microrefractometer
- Melting and boiling point apparatus
- Flash point meters (Abel-Pensky, Pensky-Martens)
- ASTM apparatus for following distillation processes
- Gas testing device (e.g., Draeger) employing color reactions on small silica tubes
- Gas chromatograph
- Apparatus for measuring spontaneous combustion (Mackey)
- Stopwatches
- Steam distillation unit, adaptable to various sample sizes
- Water bath, heating cabinet, furnace, refrigerator

Optional Equipment
- Infrared spectrophotometer and high-pressure liquid chromatograph or access to these

TABLE 21–13. SUGGESTED EQUIPMENT FOR ELECTRICAL UNIT OF FIRE INVESTIGATION LABORATORY

Basic Equipment
- Compressed air and gas
- Electrical outlets for direct and alternating current of various voltages
- Hand tools
- Macroscopes and microscopes as for mechanical unit
- Length measuring equipment as for mechanical unit
- Thermometers, thermocouples, resistor elements
- Stopwatches
- Electrical instruments: meters for current, voltage, resistance, capacitance, inductance
- Electrical components: resistors, rheostats, transformers, capacitors, induction coils, fuses, switches, contacts of all sorts, wiring, insulating material

Optional Equipment
- Multichannel oscilloscope, instruments for measuring phase angle and phase sequence and frequency, recorders for various instruments

TABLE 21–14. SUGGESTED EQUIPMENT FOR RECONSTRUCTION ROOM

BASIC EQUIPMENT
A good ventilation system of sufficient capacity and versatility
Fire fighting equipment: hose, fire extinguishers of various types
Observation windows
Fireproof doors (large)
Appropriate lighting for photographic work under adverse conditions
Heating and cooling equipment for experiments at high or low temperatures
Outlets for electric power, compressed air, and gas
Provisions for wiring connections to an adjacent observation room
Recording equipment in observation room
Cleaning tools: brushes, shovels etc.
Access to still and movie cameras
OPTIONAL EQUIPMENT
Cameras with remote controls, closed-circuit TV equipment

rying out major operations such as a fire in a car, a bed, or part of a furnished room, and should be so constructed that the experimental fires can be observed, photographed, and measured from an adjacent room and in safety.

The kind and amount of equipment needed in the fire investigation laboratory depends, of course, on the workload, the level of ambition, and the funds available. Some practical suggestions are summarized in Tables 21–11, 21–12, 21–13, and 21–14. In addition to this equipment, the necessary technical literature should be available at any time and within easy reach. A good drawing board and the usual office equipment are also necessary.

Investigation of Electrical Phenomena

The aim of the laboratory investigation is to ascertain whether electrical phenomena could have caused development of local heat sufficient to cause a fire. Such development of heat can be brought about when electrically charged particles (electrons or ions) pass through solid, liquid, or gaseous media under special conditions. The locally developed heat can be transported (by conduction, convection, or radiation) to areas susceptible to exothermic oxidative reactions, causing a fire. The examination is thus concerned with two separate sets of phenomena: the production of excessive heat by electrical processes and the action of this heat on inflammable material in the presence of oxygen.

Outline of Procedures

Before a fire investigation is started at the laboratory all available information (police reports, witnesses' statements, photographs, specialists' reports) should be taken into account. The physical evidence delivered to the laboratory is then described, is photographed if necessary, and its condition is noted. With the reports as a first lead, the material is checked for any signs of electrical phenomena that might have caused excessive heat, sparks, or electric arcs. Frequently, indications of such phenomena are quickly detected and can be shown to be responsible for the fire. Even if no clear-cut evidence is found, it is still often possible to arrive at one or several hypotheses for an electrical cause of the fire. These hypotheses are then subjected to experiments or to reconstruction of the initial phase of the fire.

The state of the material sent in, the outcome of reconstruction experiments, and the reports received together form the base for a graded statement concerning the start and the initial course of the fire in question.

If the physical evidence collected at the site of the fire is not seriously damaged, the components' electrical properties can be checked. For example, measurements of resistance at various applied voltages can give an indication of technical faults. It is obviously a great help if the laboratory has a collection of standard electrical components, so that comparative measurements can be carried out. In certain cases it is imperative to buy (or borrow) equipment of the same type and model as that from the site of the fire in order to make adequate comparisons.

If the evidence is seriously damaged (insulation burned or components melted), it has to be checked millimeter by millimeter under a large properly lighted magnifying glass or a stereomicroscope at moderate magnification. When damage is found, its position must be noted and its physical appearance described or photographed. The form, color, and surface texture of the damaged area can give important leads to its formation.

It is usually possible to determine in this way if the damage was caused by heat (from the fire) or by electrical phenomena (bad contact, partial short circuit, arc, spark formation). It is, on the other hand, rarely possible to discriminate between "primary" and "secondary" electrical damage. "Primary" damage is caused by electrical phenomena that lead to a fire, whereas "secondary" damage, while also electrical in nature, is a consequence of a fire (Figs. 21–8 and 21–9). Various procedures have been

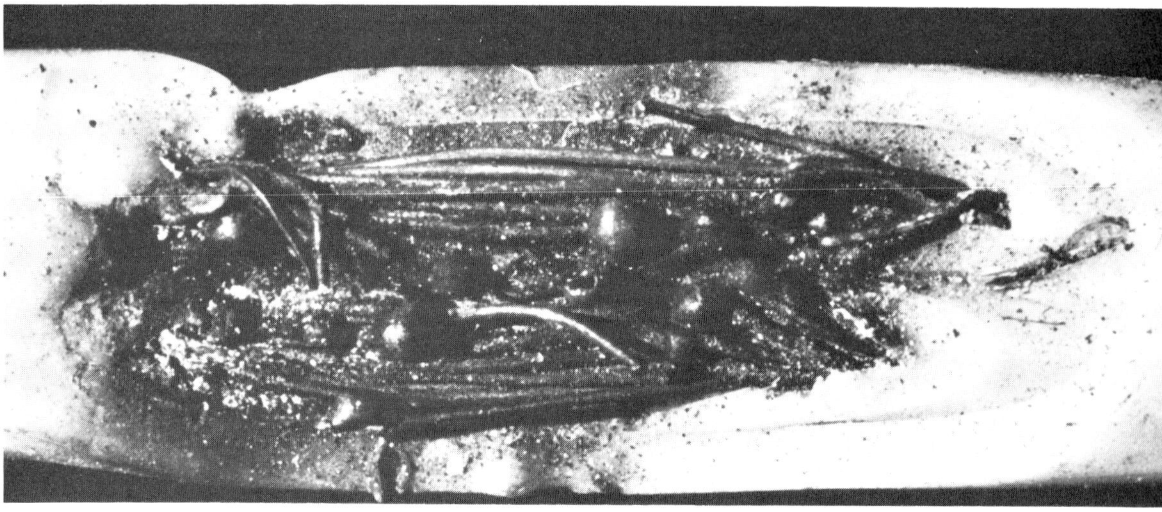

Figure 21–8. Laboratory demonstration of primary electrical damage. A piece of insulated two-pole conducting wire shows damage typical of a partial short circuit. The insulation was cut away in order to show the details of the phenomenon. Scale: 8:1.

proposed by which such discrimination can supposedly be made, but these procedures have, at least in our hands, not given clear-cut results in actual cases.

The condition of the fuses is of great importance. It is usually possible to decide if a fuse has melted because of heat or because of electrical overloading. In many cases the appearance of the fuse can tell if the melting was due to a strong current (short circuit) or to prolonged moderate overloading (Figs. 21–10 and 21–11). It is also necessary to ascertain if any fuses were short-circuited on purpose.

In many fire investigations it is desirable to

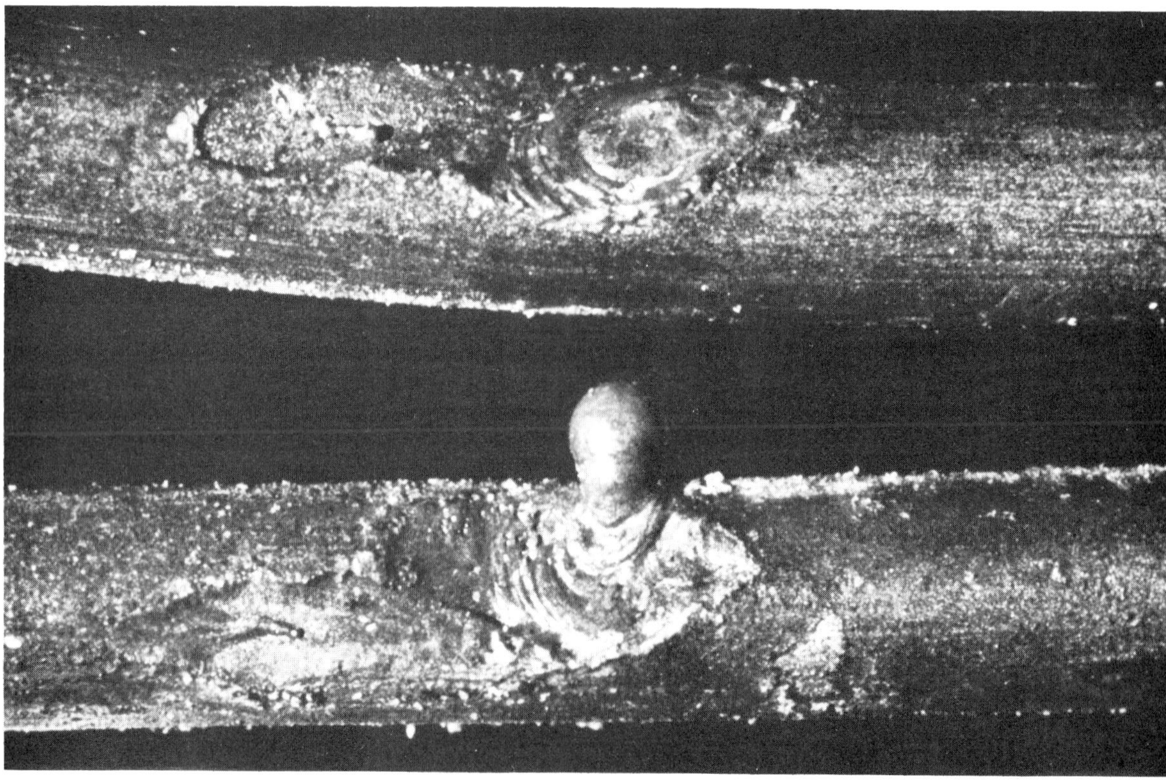

Figure 21–9. Laboratory demonstration of secondary electrical damage. The hot zone is sharply localized to a small drop. This drop is surrounded by circular "waves" of a cooler melt. Scale: about 8:1.

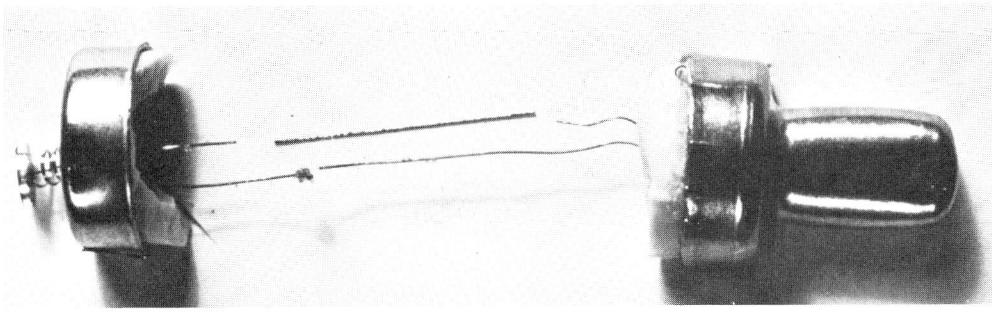

Figure 21–10. A fuse that was melted by overloading it for a period of time (on the order of 20 minutes). Note the localized oxidation and melting of the resistance wire.

check whether a proposed hypothesis for the start or spreading or both of a fire is reasonable and can explain all observations. To this end, experiments and reconstruction of pertinent phases in the development of a fire are needed. Such tests, in contrast to the complexity of a theoretical evaluation, can often give clear-cut and decisive results on which an opinion and graded statement can be based.

Case 1. Death Due to Inappropriate Construction of Electrical Apparatus

At a hospital an 18-month-old infant was treated for severe burns. As part of the therapy a stream of dry warm air from an electric hair dryer was directed upon the burned area during five days. The hair dryer was fixed to the head of the metal bedstead by strips of tape.

On the day of the accident, the patient had been left unattended for about 30 minutes when smoke was observed coming from the room (as in most European hospitals, the double doors to the room were closed). On entering the room, the nurse discovered that the bed was on fire and the child was dead.

Badly damaged pieces of the dryer were found on top of the bed and on the floor beneath it. The mattress (made of plastic foam with a plastic cover and covered by a bed sheet) was badly burned.

At the laboratory, the electrical connections of the hair dryer were checked; no malfunction was found except in the fan motor. One of the graphite brushes was completely used up and had apparently ceased to function. Presumably, the motor had then stopped, but the heating coil had continued to glow, owing to the method of wiring used (Fig. 21–12). This in turn raised the temperature until the plastic parts melted and caught fire. As the figure shows, although the heater could not be turned on without starting the fan motor, no provision was made for a malfunction of the motor; when it stopped, the current through the heater was not interrupted.

In order to determine whether the fire really started in the way just described, the situation was reconstructed in the laboratory. First the function of the fan motor was tested separately. Another hairdryer of the same kind, also used in the children's ward, was left running while the heating coil was disconnected. After 13.5 hours the motor stopped running. It was disassembled, and it was found that the brushes were used up.

In a second experiment, a "bed" was prepared by placing a mattress of the same kind as the one used in the hospital room on a plywood board. At the correct position, a "bed end" was constructed, and a new, duplicate hair dryer (same make, same model) was fixed to it with the same kind of tape as in the actual case. One of the leads to the fan motor was disconnected, simulating motor failure. The events were observed and photographs taken. Figure 21–13 shows the most significant phases of the reconstruction experiments.

Case 2. The Danger of Faulty Manufacture

A newly bought electric laundry iron was tested by the owner. She placed the iron, according to the

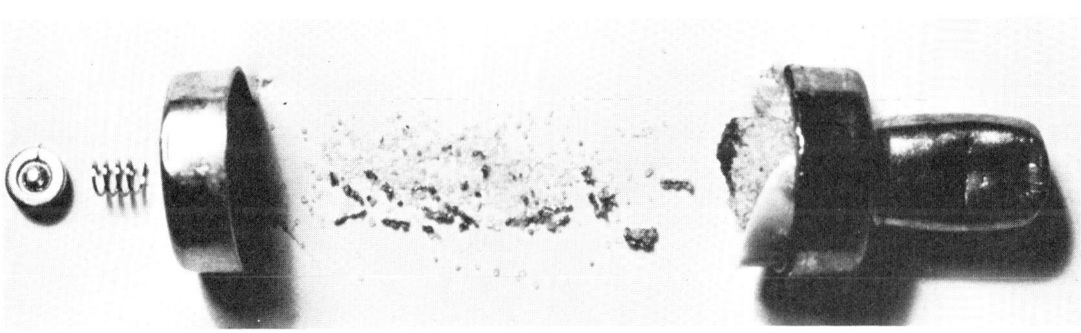

Figure 21–11. A fuse that was subjected to a short circuit. The wires partly melted and partly evaporated. Some of the melted drops are fused to the ceramic insulating material.

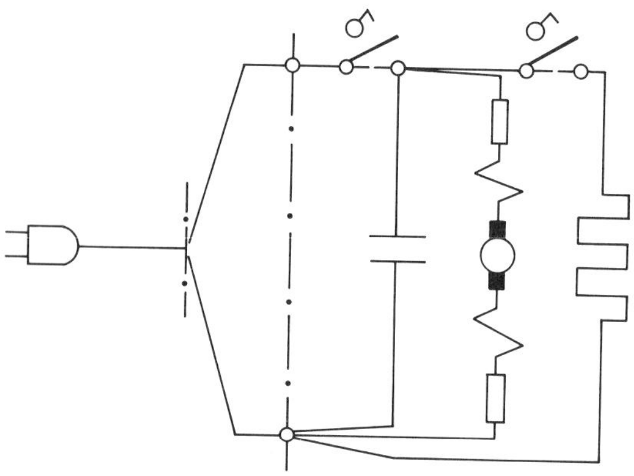

Figure 21–12. The wiring diagram of the hair dryer. The two switches are arranged in such a way that the heating coil cannot be switched on unless the fan motor also is on. No provision is made, however, to interrupt the current flowing through the heating coil when the motor ceases to function.

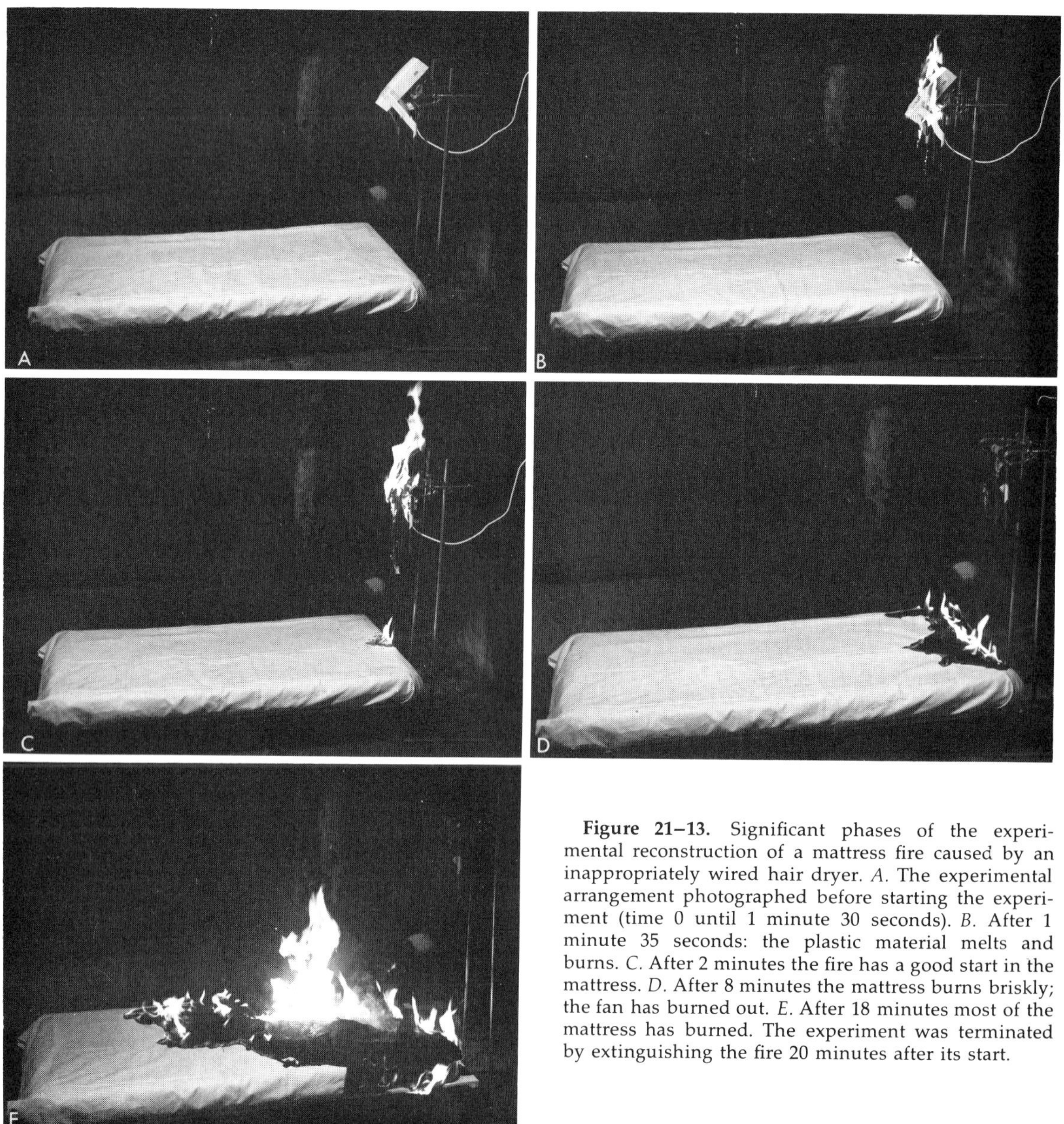

Figure 21–13. Significant phases of the experimental reconstruction of a mattress fire caused by an inappropriately wired hair dryer. *A*. The experimental arrangement photographed before starting the experiment (time 0 until 1 minute 30 seconds). *B*. After 1 minute 35 seconds: the plastic material melts and burns. *C*. After 2 minutes the fire has a good start in the mattress. *D*. After 8 minutes the mattress burns briskly; the fan has burned out. *E*. After 18 minutes most of the mattress has burned. The experiment was terminated by extinguishing the fire 20 minutes after its start.

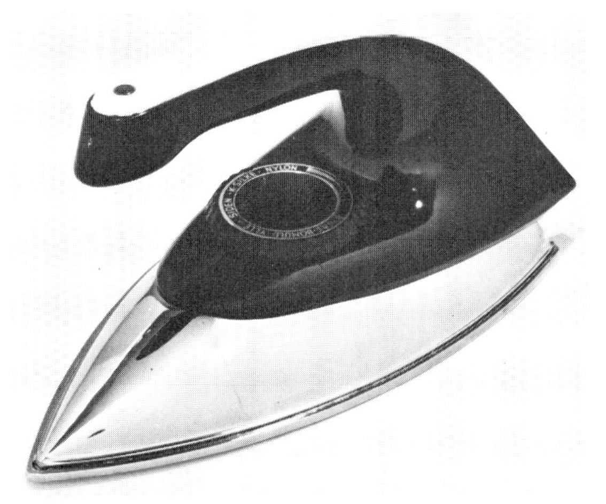

Figure 21–14. A newly purchased iron of the same type and model as the iron received from the site of the fire.

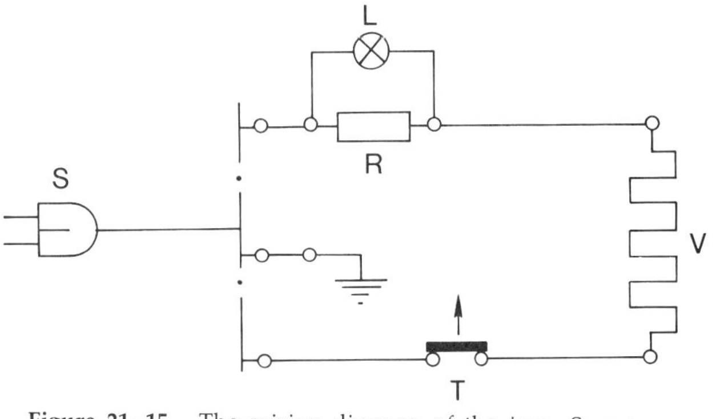

Figure 21–15. The wiring diagram of the iron. S, net plug; L, indicator lamp; R, resistor; V, heating element; T, thermostat.

written instructions on its end, on an ironing board, set the thermostat for "wool," and connected the iron. When she returned after 10 minutes she found the iron on fire. The bottom plate (of light metal) had melted, and the melt had dropped onto a chair and the floor, igniting them. The fire was rapidly put out.

The iron, or what was left of it, was sent to the laboratory for a thorough examination. Figure 21–14 shows an overall view of a new iron of the same make and model; Figure 21–15, a diagram of the wiring scheme.

It was soon discovered that the thermostat of the burned iron lacked two important parts that were present in the thermostat of the newly purchased iron, as shown in Figure 21–16. A careful search for these parts (a kind of ceramic spacer to keep the mechanism stable and aligned) was unsuccessful. It seemed, therefore, that the fire had been caused by faulty assembly of the thermostat. In order to try this theory, a number of tests were carried out.

Test No. 1. Purpose: to measure the working temperature of correctly assembled irons. Three new irons were purchased. They were placed on an ironing board, and their temperature was measured by means of a thermal element. The thermostats were set at the "wool" position, and the irons were switched on. It was found that the working temperatures varied between a low of 135° ± 18°C and a high of 171° ± 27°C for the three irons.

Test No. 2. Purpose: to test the thermostat of the burned iron after insertion of two new spacers. The burned iron's thermostat was built into a new iron and two new spacers were inserted into their proper positions as shown in Figure 21–16. The temperature (measured as in Test No. 1) fluctuated between 161° and 175°C.

Test No. 3. Purpose: to reconstruct the probable chain of events leading to the outbreak of the fire. In two of the new irons, the thermostat spacers were removed. The irons were set on end and switched

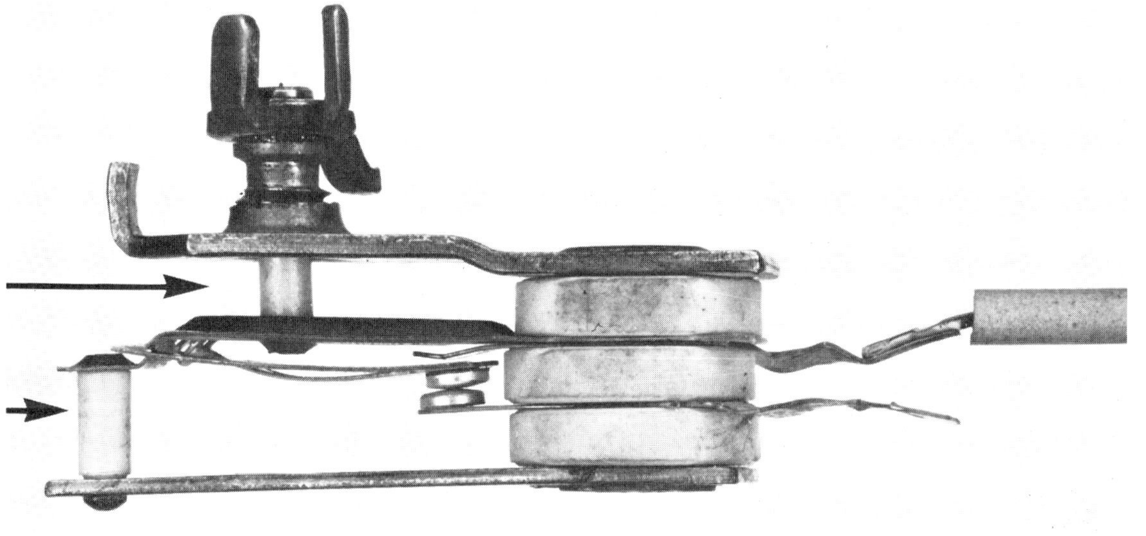

Figure 21–16. A properly constructed thermostat (from a newly purchased iron). The two ceramic spacers are indicated by arrows.

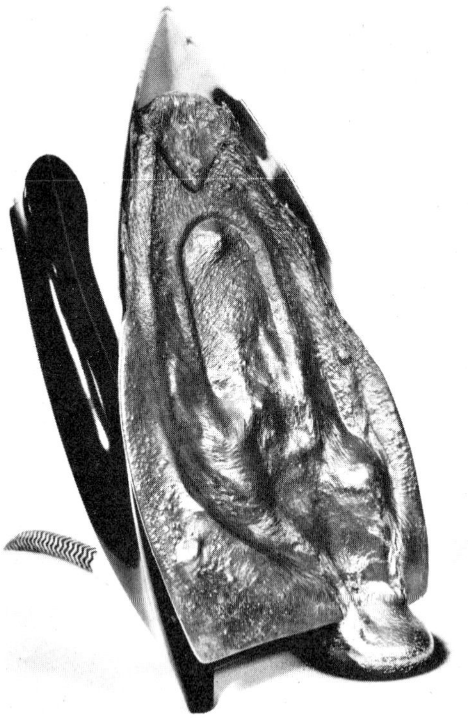

Figure 21–17. A purchased iron after carrying out Test No. 3. The bottom plate has melted.

on, the thermostats set at the "wool" position. After five minutes, the bottom plate had melted and started a fire in the ironing board (Fig. 21–17). The built-in fuse interrupted the current one half to one minute later.

Test No. 4. Purpose: to test whether the thermostat spacers, properly installed, could be dislodged by dropping the iron. A new iron was dropped from a height of over 1 m onto a plywood board lying on a concrete floor. This was repeated over and over with the iron held in different positions. A check showed that the spacers were not displaced by this rough treatment.

It was concluded that the iron had caused the actual fire because of a defect in its manufacture: the spacers were missing, the thermostat did not function, and the temperature rose unchecked to melt the bottom plate (of an aluminum alloy). The hot melt had then set the chair and the floor on fire.

Investigations of Chemical Processes

Upon arrival at the laboratory, the physical evidence is properly registered and identified. All measures taken are carefully noted, and a written report is prepared. The investigation usually starts with analysis of smell and head space, usually with a vapor testing instrument or gas chromatograph. Such tests are much easier to perform at a laboratory than at the site of the fire where smoke, fumes, and smells abound.

Before suspected liquids can be analyzed, they must be isolated from the evidence sent in. Only in this way is it possible to test for volatile compounds, and only isolated substances can be subjected to discriminating analytical methods such as infrared spectrophotometry, mass spectrometry, or fluorometry. For organometallic compounds, emission spectroscopy or atomic absorption can come into play. Various methods are available for isolating inflammable liquids from the debris of a fire. The most useful technique for volatile compounds is steam distillation; for less volatile substances extraction with ether or similar solvents is satisfactory.

Steam distillation is superior to dry distillation because the relatively low temperature required does not char or pyrolyze the majority of materials found at a fire (wood, plastic, fabrics). When two liquids (an azeotropic mixture) are heated, each exerts its own vapor pressure irrespective of the other, the two distill over together at a constant temperature, and the composition of the distillate, a function of the vapor pressure and the molecular weight of the components, remains constant.

$$\frac{m_A}{m_B} = \frac{p_A \cdot MV_A}{p_B \cdot MV_B} \qquad \text{(Eq. 16)}$$

in which m_A and m_B = amounts of components A and B, p_A and p_B = vapor pressures of A and B, and MV_A and MV_B = molecular weights of A and B. Any basic chemistry text can be consulted for further discussion of azeotropy, or constant-boiling mixtures.

Water has a low molecular weight and a relatively low vapor pressure, and this explains why compounds with higher molecular weight and intermediate vapor pressure can be distilled at relatively low temperatures. The efficiency of the process increases when superheated steam is used. An additional advantage is that the samples heated do not contain much moisture after the process is finished. For example, at 150°C, the vapor pressure is 4.70 atm for water, 9.70 atm for ethanol, and 5.70 atm for benzene. The composition of the distillates becomes therefore 5.27:1 for ethanol and water and 5.26:1 for benzene and water at 150°C. In actual practice, temperatures above 120°C are usually avoided.

Various kinds of distillation apparatus can be used. It should, however, be constructed with the following points in mind: (1) Superheated steam should preferably be used. (2) The sample compartment should be adaptable for various sizes of samples. (3) The samples must not clog the steam intake. (4) Condensation traps should be so constructed that small amounts of immiscible compounds (lighter than water) can accumulate in a narrow tube and be collected easily, and it should be possible to collect the first drops (up to several milliliters) of a mixture of water and a miscible solvent.

After distillation, the residue can still contain relatively nonvolatile organic liquids (e.g., lubricating oils, paraffins, vegetable oils, candle stearin, waxes, and resins). These can often be isolated by extraction with ethyl ether or chloroform and careful evaporation or distillation of the volatile solvent.

The identification of the isolated liquids can be carried out in a number of ways. The choice of the methods depends on the equipment available at the laboratory or at other laboratories in the region, the amount of liquid available, the nature of the case, the ambition of the investigator, and the time available for his experiments.

Color reactions such as those observed in the vapor testing tubes have very limited value for identification purposes.

In order to test a liquid for flammability, a small amount is drawn up into a glass capillary tube and then blown into the edge of a (blue) gas flame. Gas chromatography can be considered a good tool for investigating the presence of certain compounds that are volatile. The larger the number of peaks obtained in a gas chromatogram, the more powerful this tool becomes; the use of capillary columns has therefore proved extremely useful for discriminating between even closely similar mixtures of hydrocarbons. Less volatile compounds can also be subjected to gas chromatography, but only after increasing their volatility by attachment of nonpolar substituents. Pyrolysis gas chromatography is another method of analyzing these substances.

Positive identification can be achieved by the use of mass spectrometry, infrared spectrophotometry, and microchemical tests, with or without a preliminary fractionation by distillation, gas chromatography, or high-pressure liquid chromatography. If the amount of an isolated liquid is sufficient, its density, refractive index, and distillation properties can be measured. It is not, however, always necessary to identify the liquid; on the contrary, it is often quite sufficient to compare it with samples found at the site of the fire (in bottles, cans, drums) or in the possession of a suspect. In making such a comparison, it is essential to evaluate the relative abundance of the product in question and to relate this fact to the circumstances of the fire and its investigation. An important point to remember is that the composition of many solvents such as petroleum products varies greatly according to their exposure to heat, drafts, water, and air. The more volatile fractions will, of course, evaporate first and change the appearance of a chromatogram. Automobile gasoline after having lost some of its more volatile components can thus resemble white spirit.

Gasoline represents a special case because of its content of tetraethyllead. This additive is found in the steam distillate in spite of its high boiling point of about 200°C. The organic layer of the distillate can then be analyzed for lead by atomic absorption spectroscopy or emission spectrography. A direct analysis of the fire debris is not conclusive, since lead is commonly found in paint and other building materials.

Ethyl alcohol in more or less pure form is frequently used by arsonists. Since it is miscible with water, it cannot be physically separated from the distillate. It is concentrated, however, in the first fraction or fractions and can, if necessary, be further enriched by repeated redistillation of the original distillate. There are, of course, a large number of analytical methods available for the determination of ethanol in aqueous solutions. An elegant and specific method is its enzymatic assay with alcohol dehydrogenase. This method is widely used for blood alcohol determinations and is therefore available in many forensic laboratories. Gas chromatography is, in this case, of great value since the retention times for ethanol on several column materials are rather specific and matched only by very unusual organic compounds. A simple test for ethanol can be carried out as follows: One of the first drops of a steam distillate suspected of containing ethanol is diluted and placed in a small beaker or crucible. A few drops of a saturated solution of potassium dichromate and one or two drops of concentrated sulfuric acid are added. Immediately afterward, a microscope slide with a hanging drop of *p*-nitrophenylhydrazine in 15 per cent acetic acid is placed on the slide. The ethanol is oxidized to gaseous acetaldehyde, which forms crystals of acetaldehydenitrophenylhydrazone. The crystals are washed with small portions of acetic acid and dried on the coverglass. Their melting point is then determined on a Kofler block, Mettler hot-stage, or the like (it should be 128°C).

Case 3. Ignition of a Finely Divided Spray of Paint by an Electrical Discharge

For spraying anticorrosive paint in a confined space in a freighter lying in dock, a painter employed at a wharf used a spray muzzle attached to a pressure hose under pressure of about 80 psi (5.5 atm). During the operation, the room suddenly burst into flame and the man was burned to death.

The police investigation showed that the pressure hose used for spraying was entwined with electrical cables carrying a voltage of 110 v.

Laboratory investigation showed mechanical damage to one of the electrical cables. The copper wires were exposed and showed beads of molten metal, apparently the result of a short circuit. In the pressure hose for the paint sprayer a burned hole was found that extended through both the steel mesh and the plastic inner hose. By emission spectroscopy, the presence of copper was demonstrated in the burned area, indicating that electric wiring had been involved in the burning of the hole.

The spraying liquid consisted of aluminum powder and an anticorrosive agent suspended in ligroin. The liquid's flash point was found to be 41°C; normally this material should not constitute a great fire hazard.

In a reconstruction, the liquid was sprayed at the pressure of 88 psi (6 atm), and a spark plug (0.5-mm gap) was placed in the resulting cloud of finely divided paint. When the circuit was closed, sudden and violent combustion took place. The experiment was repeated under varied conditions, but always with the same result.

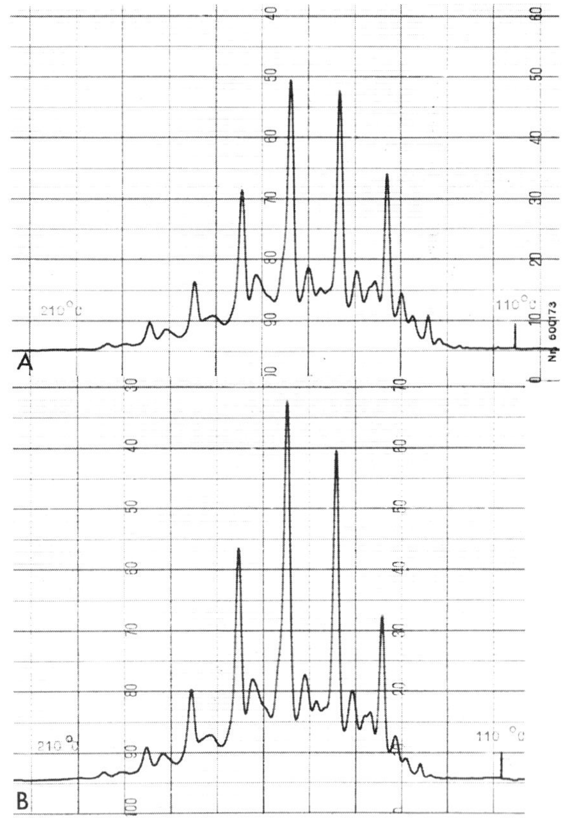

Figure 21–18. The gas chromatograms of the sample isolated from the burned cabin, *A*, and of the contents of the plastic container, *B*. Experimental conditions: gas chromatograph; Perkin-Elmer 800; column, 6 f × 1/8" o.d. with DC-710 on Chromosorb W; Temperature programming, 110° to 210° with an increase of 13.3° per minute; FID detector; injection temperature, 150°; injected volume, 1.2 μl.

Case 4. Isolation and Identification of an Inflammable Liquid from Fire Debris

A small, home-built cabin in the country caught fire, and the only inhabitant barely escaped before the place burned down. Near the entrance to the dwelling, the fire damage was especially intense.

Wooden planks and parts of the door threshold as well as pieces of wood and burned paper were secured in tightly closed glass jars and sent to the laboratory. Also sent in was a partially melted 5-liter plastic container with a few drops of a liquid. The questions to be answered were: Can inflammable liquids be isolated from the burned material? If so, can the liquids be identified? Are any of the liquids isolated identical with the liquid in the plastic container?

The contents of the plastic container had a smell similar to that of kerosene. No smell could be noticed on the other material. When tested with the Draeger gas-sensing device, most of the material sent in yielded positive reactions. Steam distillation yielded 2.5 ml of a clear, water-insoluble liquid from one of the objects sent in, but no measurable amounts of such a liquid could be isolated from the other samples.

The plastic container was emptied, and 0.5 ml of a clear liquid was collected.

Both liquid samples were inflammable. Their gas chromatograms were recorded and showed identical patterns (Fig. 21–18). These patterns were checked against a reference collection of gas chromatograms and found to resemble closely those of kerosene.

The investigation showed that the area around the entrance to the house contained an inflammable liquid, that this liquid could not be distinguished from the sample found in the plastic container, and that it closely resembled a make of kerosene available at the laboratory as a reference sample.

A suspected arsonist was consequently apprehended. He pleaded guilty and was sentenced in court to six months in prison for arson and for driving under the influence of alcohol.

Spontaneous Combustion

The laboratory experiments in cases of suspected spontaneous combustion can be divided into two groups: chemical analysis of the samples sent in and practical tests with the same materials in order to reconstruct the events.

TABLE 21–15. IODINE NUMBERS OF SOME FATS AND OILS

Coconut oil	8–10
Cocoa butter	34–43
Palm oil	52–57
Olive oil	80–88
Cottonseed oil	103–113
Whale oil	110–135
Herring oil	131–147
Cod-liver oil	136–180
Linseed oil	174–200
Perilla oil	202–208

The chemical tests often include a determination of an oil's acid and iodine numbers as a measure of its degree of unsaturation. Table 21–15 shows the iodine numbers for some unsaturated oils. Identification can be carried out by such methods as infrared spectrophotometry and gas chromatography (with or without pyrolysis). If siccatives are present in the samples, emission spectrography and atomic absorption are additional methods of value. Many siccatives contain salts of lead, cobalt, manganese, or zirconium.

In reconstruction experiments, a lead may be provided by determining the ability of an oil to react with oxygen and the amount of the temperature increase during spontaneous oxidation. The oxygen uptake can be measured gravimetrically (by repeatedly weighing a sample of oil smeared on a glass plate) or volumetrically (by enclosing a sample of the oil, soaked into a porous material, and measuring the decrease of volume of the air isobarically).

A classic way to measure the rise in temperature during spontaneous oxidation is the method of Mackey, in which the suspected oil is soaked into cheesecloth (proportion 1:1 by weight). The oily cloth is tightly rolled and placed in an air bath kept at 100°. The rise in temperature is read off at known intervals. This test can give useful results, but they must be evaluated with care because of the temperature difference between experimental and actual conditions.

Case 5. Spontaneous Combustion

Some boys had polished a wooden wagon with so-called teak oil, a blend of turpentine and a self-drying oil. When they had finished they threw the oil-soaked rags on a workbench, close to a window facing south. A fire started in the room; the fire damage was concentrated on the workbench.

The technical squad of the police sent rags of the same type and a sample of the teak oil the boys used to the laboratory. The questions asked were: What kind of oil does the sample consist of? Can the rags soaked with this oil undergo spontaneous combustion?

The first question could not be answered precisely, since all kinds of mixtures of oils are sold under the name of teak oil. One such product was purchased, and it was found that its distillation properties and its infrared spectrum were closely similar to those of the oil sent in.

In order to answer the second question a sample of the oil sent in was tested in a Mackey apparatus at 100°C. A temperature rise of 19°C was registered after 30 minutes. Fifty grams of rags sent in were soaked with 50 g of the oil, and the sample was rolled together. After lying at room temperature for two hours, the temperature began to rise, and after three and a half hours a fire started.

The investigation showed that the fire might well have started from spontaneously ignited oil-soaked rags.

Dangerous Chemicals

While it is usually not very difficult to analyze the products of a chemical reaction, reconstructing the events—and thereby arriving at an identification of the starting materials—can present a major problem. For instance, if a lump of sodium chloride has been found at the site of a fire, it is not obvious whether this represents the end product of a reaction of sodium chlorate with organic materials or whether it is simply some unchanged table salt. A careful quantitative assay, however, might show the presence of traces of sodium chlorate, which would decide the question in most cases.

REFERENCE

1. Tryon, G. H. (Ed.): *Fire Protection Handbook.* 13th Ed. Boston, National Fire Protection Association, 1969.

SELECTED READINGS

2. Frei-Sulzer, M., and Suter, A.: *Leitfaden zur Bearbeitung von Brandursachen und Explosionen.* Hamburg, Kriminalistik Verlag, 1971.
3. Fitch, R. D., and Porter, E. A.: *Accidental or Incendiary.* Springfield, Ill., Charles C Thomas, 1968.
4. Freytag, H. H.: *Handbuch der Raumexplosionen.* Weinheim, Verlag-Chemie GmbH., 1965.
5. Kirk, P. L.: *Fire Investigation.* New York, John Wiley's Sons, 1969.
6. Lewis, B., and Von Elbe, G.: *Combustion, Flames and Explosions of Gases.* 2nd Ed. New York and London, Academic Press, 1961.
7. Nabert, K., and Schön, G.: *Sicherheitstechnische Kennzahlen brennbarer Gase und Dämpfe.* 3rd Ed. Berlin, Deutscher Eichverlag, 1968.
8. National Fire Protection Association. *National Fire Codes.* Vol. 1. Flammable Liquids; Vol. 2. Gases; Vol. 3. Combustible Solids, Dusts, Chemicals and Explosives. Boston, 1973.
9. Von Schwartz, E.: *Handbuch der Feuer- und Explosionsgefahr.* München, Feuerschutzverlag, Ph. L. Jung, 1964.

SECTION 6. THERMAL INJURY

chapter 22

SYSTEMIC AND LOCAL EFFECTS OF HYPOTHERMIA

by Jorma Hirvonen

SYSTEMIC HYPOTHERMIA

The term "systemic hypothermia" is used to indicate cooling of the human body below 35° C (95° F). This occurs when loss of body heat exceeds heat production. The most common cause of accidental hypothermia is exposure to environmental low temperature. Taking into account the absence or the presence of additional circumstances, four major situations can be envisioned: (1) hypothermia caused by exposure to severe cold alone or possibly in conjunction with exhaustion (this type can be called environmental hypothermia because it is mostly dependent on climatic factors); (2) hypothermia caused by environmental conditions under the concurrent influence of alcohol or drugs affecting the generation or conservation of body heat; (3) hypothermia caused by climatic conditions with disease of some sort as an additional factor, expectedly lowering the resistance of the organism to cold exposure; and (4) hypothermia ending fatally in connection with therapeutic procedures (a rare occurrence but the most likely to lead to medicolegal controversy).

Accidental hypothermia can occur during hiking or skiing expeditions, in shipwrecks, from a fall into icy water, or in connection with insufficient heating in the home during a cold winter.[1,2] According to circumstances, two major types are usually recognized: *dry cold hypothermia* and *immersion hypothermia*. The effects of the latter are more disastrous because of the more rapid loss of heat in water than in air. Wetting of clothing is sufficient to increase the risk of ill effects.[3]

Immersion hypothermia causes loss of body heat about three times as fast as does exposure to the same temperature in dry cold air.[4] This is because water conducts heat 25 times faster than dry air; furthermore the insulating layer between skin and water is only about one tenth of that between skin and air. Because of their thicker layer of subcutaneous fat, women endure cold water better than men do.[5,6] Humans are able to retain body heat balance in water at 22° C, but below this temperature loss of heat gradually occurs. According to Molnar's calculations, survival time decreases sharply in water below 16° C (60° F).[4]

With respect to age, victims of hypothermia can be divided into three distinct categories: infants, young adults, and elderly people.

It is typical of the infant that he is unable to regulate body temperature and thus can be affected by hypothermia even in a tropical climate.[7] Hypothermia in the infant most frequently occurs in the home or at the time of delivery.[8] The most dangerous period is the first two weeks of life, and the mortality rate is quite high, varying between 26 per cent and 50 per cent.[9]

The most frequent cause of hypothermia among young adults is exposure to low ambient temperature (around or below 0° C) in sports, under conditions of physical exhaustion, or under the influence of alcohol or drugs.

Underlying the hypothermia of the elderly, there are often a debilitating disease, impaired ability to maintain body temperature, and inadequate nutrition.[10] The death rate is high, varying from 30 to 80 per cent.[11, 12] After the original hypothermic episode, thermic regulation can remain impaired for as long as three years.[13]

Pathophysiologic Effects of Cold

The critical level of ambient air temperature for a naked man is about 27° C. At this temperature he is able to retain constant body temperature in the absence of physical activity.[14] Races differ in their tolerance to cold exposure. Australian aborigines are able to reduce their rectal temperature to 35° C during sleep on cold nights, thus saving metabolic energy. Negroes have a somewhat weaker response to cold stress than do Caucasians.[15] The responses to cold of Arctic Indians and Eskimos do not seem to differ from that of the white man.[16-19]

Conservation, dispersion, and production of heat are under the control of the thermoregulatory center that in mammals, including humans, is located in the anterior hypothalamus. Any lesion in this area can lead to hypothermic crisis. This is well illustrated by the case of a young man who suffered repeated attacks of spontaneous hypothermia; at postmortem examination, this condition was explained by a degenerative lesion associated with scarring in the anterior portion of the third ventricle.[20]

The function of maintaining body temperature is mediated by the sympathetic system. Vasoconstriction in skin and skeletal muscles is the most important mechanism of heat conservation. This mechanism can be abolished by toxic levels of alcohol.

The phenomenon of shivering that is triggered both from deep temperature-sensitive structures and from reflexes elicited by lowered skin temperature is the most important source of heat. Common in conjunction with infectious states, it has been described as well in paraplegic or curarized men.[21, 22] The peak of shivering occurs about three hours after the start of severe cold exposure (−29° C, −20° F).[23] The response to cold depends to a considerable extent on the thickness of the subcutaneous insulating fat layer: fat men tolerate both dry cold and immersion hypothermia much better than thin ones do.[15, 18] The compensatory increase of heat production is maintained at a body temperature of about 32° C (90° F), but below this level rapid decrease of temperature occurs and the metabolic processes fail. Shivering stops at about 30° C (86° F).[19]

Nervous System

At about 32° C (90° F) impairment of cerebral functions is manifest in analgesia, clouding of consciousness, hallucinations, and slowing of reflexes. Cold narcosis appears at 30° C (86° F), and reflexes are abolished at 27° C (81° F). Pupillar reaction disappears at 26° C (79° F).[24] At 26° to 27° C the victim of hypothermia fails to understand when spoken to, and retrograde amnesia has been recorded in patients cooled to or below 34° C (93° F). This disorder, as a rule, is reversible, as are local paresthesias.[25]

Manifestations of permanent brain lesions, however, including epilepsia and dysphasia, have been reported following exposure to cold for a considerable time, and they have been attributed to diminished blood flow.[26] A general view derived from animal experiments is that hypothermia does not cause permanent lesions in the central nervous system as long as blood flow is maintained.[27] Cerebral blood flow is decreased and oxygen consumption is sharply reduced at body temperature of 28° to 29° C (83° to 85° F).[28, 29] Shivering can increase cerebral metabolism more than 100 per cent even at a low body temperature (28° C, 82° to 83° F).

Conduction velocity in peripheral nerves in man (peroneal nerve) decreases in proportion to the lowering of the nerve temperature; within the temperature range from 35.5° C to 23.5° C (96° to 74° F) the velocity can drop from 49.6 m per second to 25.9 m per second, i.e., to one half; at 21.5° F (71° F) the velocity is only 12.1 m per second, i.e., one fourth of normal. Paralysis of peripheral nerves occurs at a temperature below 20° C (68° F).[30] Diminished hand dexterity and clumsiness in walking are clear indications of impaired nervous transmission.

Heart and Circulatory System

Decrease in pulse rate is the most prominent change taking place in the heart in conjunction with lowering of body temperature. The relation is quite linear, except for spasmodic elevations associated with shivering.[31] The change depends on slowing of depolarization, which is recorded on the electrocardiograph with prolongation of the P-QRS wave. Repolarization is also disturbed, as indicated by inverted T waves. Around 30° C (86° F) an extra wave position after the P-QRS complex makes its appearance—the so-called J-wave.[32]

Just below 30° C (86° F) atrial fibrillation

often occurs. The most dangerous condition is ventricular fibrillation, which appears at about 25° to 28° C (77° to 82° F). The cause is not known; one possibility is the impairment of the sodium-potassium pump below 28° C (82° F), and another is the development of ectopic foci of excitation in the ventricular wall. The latter possibility is supported by experiments on dogs that indicate the occurrence of microscopic lesions in myofibers and platelet thrombi in the myocardial capillaries.[33] Similar microthrombi can be seen in other organs. Below 20° C (68° F), the heart, if it escapes fibrillation, continues to beat very slowly. For instance, the pulse rate of a woman was four beats per minute at 11° C (52° F), and the heart action finally ceased entirely at 10.5° C (51° F); however, normal rhythm was reestablished when the patient was rewarmed.[34] During the first or excitation phase of hypothermia—between 37° to 34° C (98° to 93° F)—the blood pressure becomes elevated, but with progressive hypothermia blood pressure gradually decreases until hypotension develops. At 25° C (77° F) blood pressure as low as 30 mm of mercury has been measured, and usually blood pressure is unrecordable below 29° C (84° F).[35, 36] Lowering of pulse rate and blood pressure is followed by sludging of red cells in postcapillary venules.[33]

Respiratory System

Respiratory frequency and tidal volume decline in hypothermia. Airway dead space is increased by 50 per cent at 25° C (77° F) owing to blockage of the vagus nerve. Physiologic dead space is also increased, but alveolar dead space is unchanged.[37] Pulmonary circulation time is reduced toward 29° C (84° F) because of diminished output of the right side of the heart.[38] Respiratory regulation seems to remain effective even at 25° C (77° F) although respiratory rhythm can be reduced to a few excursions per minute.[39] Cases of accidental hypothermia have been recorded in which the respiratory excursions were reduced to 7 to 15 per minute at a body temperature of 30° C (86° F).

It has been stated that cold may cause mild lesions in the bronchiolar and alveolar epithelium that open the way to bacterial invasion; this is well substantiated by the frequent occurrence of respiratory complications (bronchitis, bronchopneumonia) following exposure to environmental cold.[40] Against the assumption of a relation between cold and respiratory disease, however, is the lack of evidence that controlled surgical hypothermia affects the lungs adversely.

Respiratory acidosis is commonly found in hypothermia if respiration is not aided artifically.[37]

Gastrointestinal Tract

Hypothermia causes paralysis of the intestines, as is well documented by roentgenologic observations showing air-fluid levels indicative of stasis.[41] This explains why victims rescued from cold exposure frequently complain of abdominal pains.[42] The gastric mucosa is a well-known target of cold stress, as indicated by the far from uncommon occurrence of hemorrhages and erosions, sometimes called Wischnevsky ulcers, following accidental hypothermia.[42–44] The pathogenesis of these ulcerations is not clear, but animal experiments point to changes in mucosal microcirculation and to liberation of the vasoactive amines, histamine and serotonin, as the most likely underlying factors.[45] Ulcers of the same nature can also be found in the ileum and colon.

Pancreas and Liver

A peculiar finding in accidental hypothermia is pancreatitis. Elevated amylase values have been recorded in many cases, and hemorrhagic pancreatitis has been found at necropsies. Pancreatitis is possibly linked to paralytic ileus and to the reflux of enteric contents into the pancreatic ducts.[46–48]

Liver cells are quite resistant to hypothermia; however, nonspecific changes, such as vacuolization of hepatic cells and intracellular neutral lipid deposits have been found in fatal cases of hypothermia.[49] In dogs exposed to systemic hypothermia, glycogen depletion has been observed to take place within four hours of the exposure.[50] Experience drawn from therapeutic hypothermia indicates that when changes do occur in the liver they are of a reversible nature.

Kidneys

The kidneys react to cold exposure with diuresis that affects loss of both water and nitrates. This type of response has been seen both in adults and in newborn infants.[52] Exposure to an environmental temperature of 15° C (59° F) is sufficient to trigger diuresis. Two major factors have been advanced in explanation of the phenomenon: (1) impeded reabsorption due to impairment of enzymatic activity that in general occurs when the body temperature is 2° to 3° C below normal; and (2) peripheral vasoconstriction leading to increased blood flow to the internal viscera and therefore to increased diuresis. The opposite condition, namely oliguria and associated azotemia, takes place on longer exposure to low temperatures (around 30° C, 86° F), particularly in older persons, and the characteristic changes of acute tubular necrosis have been recorded in fatal cases.[49, 53]

Endocrine Glands

Decrease in body temperature activates the function of most of the endocrine glands. Plasma cortisol levels are higher in a cold than in a warm environment, and urinary cortisol excretion is also increased on longer exposure.[54-56] According to the results of some experiments in adult humans, thyroid stimulating hormone (TSH) and thyroxine values remain unchanged upon exposure to a cold environment, but elevated concentrations have also been noted under similar experimental conditions.[54, 57, 58] Growth hormone levels in plasma remain stable.[58, 59] In infants cooled to 18° C (64° F) during surgery, elevated plasma concentrations of thyroid stimulating hormone have been noted; this in contrast to the values in other infants submitted to comparable surgical procedures without induced hypothermia, which did not seem to be affected. These findings point to a rather specific effect of hypothermia on infants' thyroid function, an effect that is not seen in adults.[60] Adrenal medulla is rapidly activated in a cold environment, and excretion of both epinephrine and norepinephrine in the urine is increased. Catecholamines are very potent calorigenic hormones because they enhance lipolysis. The rate of excretion is roughly dependent on the degree of exposure. Exposure for one hour at 15° C (60° F) causes a slight, insignificant increase, whereas in subjects exposed to −5° to +2° C (23° to 26° F) temperatures for three hours, the excretion of epinephrine can increase as much as 83 per cent, and that of norepinephrine as much as 54 per cent.[54, 55] In another experiment, the epinephrine excretion increased to 0.93 ng per minute at the second day and was as much as 5.00 ng per minute on the fourth day; likewise, norepinephrine excretion rose from 22.00 to 58.10 ng per minute during the same time (72 hours) at 15° C (59° F). Rectal temperature fell by 0.5° C, and skin temperature from 34.1° C (93.4° F) to 30.0° C (86° F).[61] The conclusion can perhaps be drawn from these experiments that under exposure to cold, epinephrine secretion has greater importance for survival than does norepinephrine secretion.

Two other biogenic amines, histamine and serotonin are also affected by cold. Experiments on rats indicate that both are excreted into the urine in manifold amounts during cold exposure.[62] Whether this occurs in man is uncertain, because the average concentration of these amines in the urine of men who died from cold did not vary significantly from that of victims of rapid violent death.[63] The significance of histamine and serotonin release for cold survival is not known.

Blood

Hemoconcentration is likely to occur in profound hypothermia. It is caused by two mechanisms: cold diuresis and leaking of plasma into the extracellular spaces, known as *cold edema.* Hemoconcentration in man is about 12 per cent in moderate exposure (from −5° to +10° C, 23° to 50° F).[54] Hemoconcentration is mirrored by high hematocrit values that further increase circulatory resistance.

In a cold environment the dissociation curve of hemoglobin is shifted to the left, causing a tighter binding between oxygen and red blood cells. Some investigators favor the theory that under these conditions oxygen is not available to the tissues and a condition of systemic anoxia results.[17] This is partly compensated for by acidosis; the blood pH can be lowered to 7.2, which tends to loosen oxygen from hemoglobin, thus attenuating the anoxic state.[18, 64, 65]

Hyperglycemia occurs quite often in the early phase of hypothermia.[36, 53] It is caused by the action of glucocorticoids and epinephrine on the liver, followed by glycogen depletion. Free fatty acids and glycerol concentrations rise in cold exposure, both in adults and in infants.[66-69] This is caused by the lipolytic effect of epinephrine and norepinephrine on the adipose tissue; mild ketosis tends to follow.[66] Connected with the liberation of corticosteroids is the decrease in the number of blood eosinophils that has been noticed in swimmers in ice water.[70] In deep hypothermia the electrolyte balance is disturbed. Water and sodium are driven into the cells, and potassium is eliminated, causing an elevation of the serum potassium level.[71, 72] The resulting imbalance does not seem to affect the electrocardiographic pattern, however. Reports on plasma magnesium levels are controversial; an elevation has been noted, but this has not been confirmed.[71] Normal values have been found in the vitreous in fatal cases of hypothermia.[47]

Hypothermia, Alcohol, and Drugs

The effects of alcohol in cold exposure are somewhat controversial. It has been said that alcohol contributes to the fatal outcome by causing cutaneous vasodilatation and thus loss of heat. Some results, however, show that modest amounts of alcohol do not significantly increase vasodilatation and loss of heat in mild cold exposure at rest (15° C, 59° F). This applies both to dry and to wet exposure.[18, 73] Conversely, if small amounts of alcohol are ingested after strenuous exercise, loss of heat may take place.

Hypothermia is then partly due to the hypoglycemia caused by both exercise and alcohol.[74] Present experience of fatal cases is that the blood alcohol concentration has been around 0.16 per cent (0.13 to 0.25 per cent). This figure might represent the average alcohol concentration that dangerously affects the thermoregulation of man.

Observations on surviving victims of deep hypothermia after prior alcohol intake have lead to the assumption that alcohol may have a protective effect.[75] An apparent protection by alcohol administration against cardiac fibrillation has been described in hypothermic rats and dogs. This observation has been duplicated in humans during operations at body temperature of 25° to 26° C in which alcohol was administered concurrently to maintain a blood concentration of 0.4 g per 100 ml.[76, 77] Increased in circulation and reduction of oxygen consumption in the brain might explain, at least in part, the protective effects, if any, of alcohol.[78]

The intake of two other depressing drugs, namely barbiturates and promazine, is not infrequently found in the history of victims of cold exposure. Barbiturate intoxication has been recorded in association with body temperatures as low as 21° to 26° C (70° to 79° F).[79–82] It is also well known that hypothermia is one of the manifestations of barbiturate poisoning.

Hypothermia victims under promazine medication show impairment of thermoregulation, and hypothermic episodes are usually abolished when chlorpromazine is discontinued.[83–85] According to the results of animal experiments, chlorpromazine affects the hypothalamic thermoregulatory center.[86]

Survival Time in Cold

According to the results of the infamous experiments in Dachau concentration camp, it takes about one hour for a man to die when immersed in water at 4° (39° F).[87] The subjects used in these experiments were poorly nourished, and the survival time of one hour represents half of that calculated by Molnar for shipwreck victims.[4] Data from civil accidents give about the same survival time.[88]

The water temperature in the northern Atlantic is about 0° C (32° F) in winter. Fatal cooling can occur within half an hour at this temperature.[89] The experiments of Keatinge show that swimming in cold water is dangerous because muscular activity increases heat loss owing to blood flow to the body surface. This explains some surprisingly rapid accidental "drownings" occurring in young athletes following immersion in cold water. On the other hand, long-distance swimmers can endure water temperatures as low as 15° to 16° C (59° to 61° F) for several hours without developing marked hypothermia. If the water is 20° C (68° F) or more, a fit man can swim almost indefinitely without manifestations of hypothermia.[18]

Survival time in dry cold is much longer than in cold water. No exact data are available, however, primarily because factors such as wind velocity and the degree of dryness or humidity of the air play a role in determining environmental conditions.

The physical condition of the individual plays an equally important role in establishing his degree of resistance—whether he is young or old, well or sick, thin or fat, under the influence of drugs or sober, or protected or not by adequate clothing. A young woman died within about half an hour of exposure to a temperature of −30° C (−20° F). She had no overcoat and was inebriated, with a blood alcohol level of 0.15 per cent (a case from northern Finland).

Cause of Death and Temperature Levels

The mechanism of death in hypothermia is cessation of circulation, usually preceded by ventricular fibrillation.[90] The dangerous body temperature for ventricular fibrillation is 26° to 30° C (79° to 86° F). The case of a Negro woman surviving a body temperature of 18° C (64° F) is on record, however.[75] Similar cases have been reported.[91] Most unusual is that of a man with a body temperature of 0° C (32° F) who was revived although the body felt frozen and there were no apparent signs of life.[81] Also on record is the case of a three-year-old boy exposed for about 15 hours to a temperature of 0° C (32° F). Rectal temperature was 17° C (63° F). The boy survived and no permanent lesions occurred.[92] In the report of the Committee on Accidental Hypothermia of the Royal College of Physicians it is stated that none of

136 individuals survived with a body temperature below 26° C (80° F). The mortality rate was 30 per cent 34° C (93° F) and 35° C (95° F). The death rate for the whole group was 37 per cent.[93]

Diagnosis of Hypothermia

Clinical Signs and Symptoms

Body temperature must be measured with a low-reading thermometer. Esophageal registration is preferable, but deep rectal reading is also satisfactory. Clinically hypothermia can be divided into three phases: (1) from 37° to 32° C (99° to 90° F), shivering and vasoconstriction are present; (2) from 32° C to 24° C (90° to 74° F), the body responses and production of heat gradually disappear; and (3) below 24° C (75° F), the body is no longer able to withstand the loss of heat, and general paralysis takes place.[94] Clinical findings in infants include cold skin, redness of face (45 per cent), subcutaneous edema (77 to 89 per cent), sclerema (40 per cent), and muscular stiffness. The cry is feeble, and the infant is reluctant to suck. Cutaneous and mucosal lesions are uncommon; conversely convulsions, bradycardia, bradypnea, oliguria, and bowel paralysis are frequent manifestations.[41, 72, 95-97]

Similar signs and symptoms are shown in adults; red patches are often present on the skin, or the skin can be pale, with subcutaneous edema, particularly in the face, and the neck muscles are stiff (Fig. 22–1). Mental disorders are common. Frequently the victim of the exposure is unconscious. Blood pressure is low or unrecordable, pulse is slow and often irregular, and respiration is equally shallow and slow.[36, 98-101] The signs of life at body temperatures of 18° C to 27° C (64° to 81° F) are hardly observable, and one should be extremely careful before declaring dead the victim of the exposure.[102]

Laboratory Findings

Electrocardiography is mandatory. The most conspicuous change in hypothermia is the occurrence of the J wave. Other changes are widening of the QRS complex, prolongation of the PQ interval, flattening or even inversion of the T wave, and atrial or ventricular fibrillation.[32, 36, 99, 103] Laboratory tests may reveal hyperglycemia, hemoconcentration, increase of serum urea, high serum lactic acid level, and elevated pH.[36, 100, 101] Of 11 patients exposed to systemic hypothermia, 9 showed an elevation of

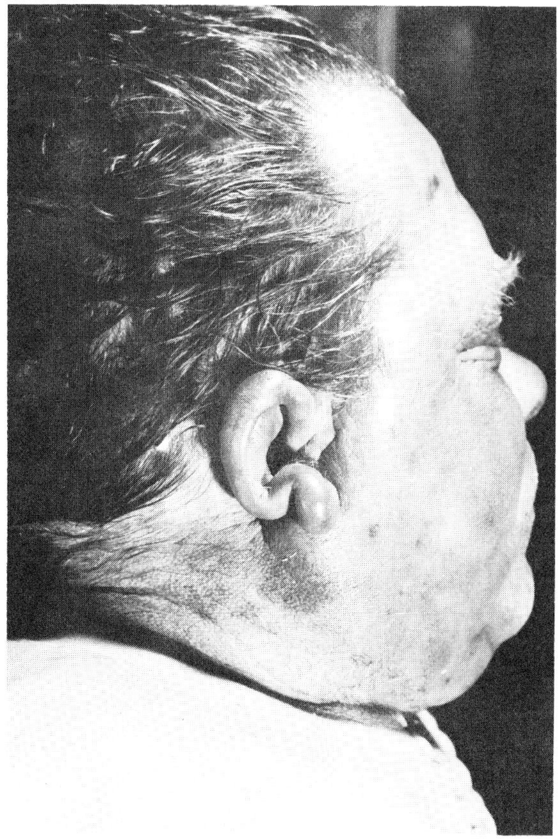

Figure 22–1. Swelling of the face and ears in a case of suicidal hypothermic death. The skin was pinky-red and the conjunctivae very hyperemic. Time of exposure was unknown.

serum amylase values that could be interpreted as an indication of pancreatic damage.[46, 48, 99]

Autopsy Findings

The inspection of the body usually reveals widespread red livor, reddish-pink discoloration of the skin, particularly in the extremities. The characteristic red livor of the skin is due to antemortem binding of oxygen to hemoglobin and its postmortem diffusion through the skin.[47, 98] Cases have been reported, however, in which the body was totally whitish—the so-called "white death."[18] Spots of bluish discoloration are also usually seen on the hands, elbows, knees, and feet, probably representing minor frostbite lesions (Fig. 22–2).[104] Histologically, they are characterized by edema and hyperemia of the dermis with occasional foci of inflammatory cell infiltration. Dilatation of the right atrium and ventricle, congestion of the vena cava, frothy sanguinous fluid in trachea and bronchi, edema and congestion and hemorrhages in the lungs, and congestion of

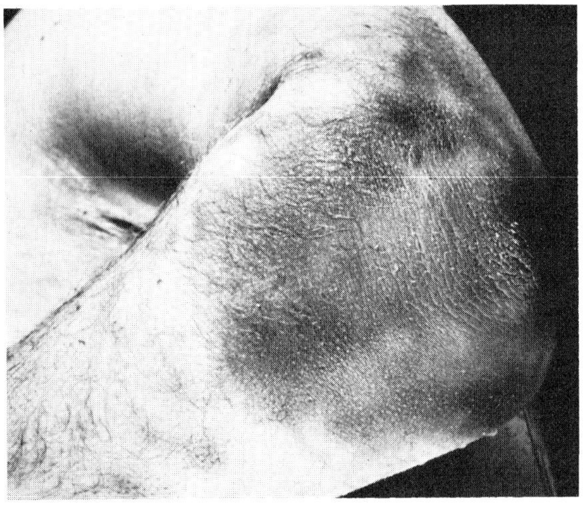

Figure 22–2. Purple-red patches of discoloration in the skin and engorgement of vessels in the elbow following suicidal cold exposure. Same case as Figure 22–1.

liver and spleen, in brief, the usual manifestations associated with acute heart failure, are the most consistent findings in both infants and adults.[9, 105–107] Bronchopneumonia is a frequent complication that develops in approximately 50 per cent of cases.[40, 108]

The incidence of gastric erosions is variable (Fig. 22–3). According to Wischnevsky, they are found in 90 per cent of cases; Krjykoff quotes an incidence of 72 per cent, and comparable data have been reported by Mant.[44, 47, 49] Pugh, however, does not mention their occurrence in three young men who died of cold exposure and exhaustion.[109] Possibly, those series that indicate a high incidence rate for this condition include mostly elderly people exposed to stress for a long period. Equally controversial is the incidence rate of acute pancreatitis—high in some series and low in some others.[40, 46–48]

Acute tubular necrosis, lipid deposition in glomeruli, in cardiac and skeletal muscle, and in liver, and brain edema have been equally reported.[40, 49] Cardiac muscle degeneration has been described, but the focal myocardial necrosis seen in dogs submitted to experimental hypothermia has not been recorded in man.[110] Lipid depletion both in the adrenals and in brown adipose tissue in infants has been stressed.[43, 111]

Measuring the catecholamines in the urine might be of value, because they are sometimes found in ample amounts in victims of fatal hypothermia.[63]

It is apparent that the diagnosis of hypothermic death rests on the assessment of several data, none of which is pathognomic. When circumstantial evidence, clinical manifestations, and autopsy findings correlate, the diagnosis can be made with a high degree of probability. Blood alcohol and toxicologic analyses should never be omitted.

The Manner of Death

Most deaths from hypothermia are accidental, and physical exhaustion and use of alcohol or drugs are frequently contributing factors. Exercise in a cold environment leads easily to rapid exhaustion because the demand for oxygen is increased both by generation of heat and by muscular activity. Exercise, inducing perspiration, also reduces the insulation of clothing to half its dry value.[112]

Insufficient nutrition can be a precipitating factor. Negligence or carelessness must be suspected whenever infants or children are affected, as in the case of an Eskimo family who deliberately left their weak infant unattended in cold weather. Fortunately, the infant was rescued in time.[113] Suicide by deliberate exposure to environmental cold has been seen by the author on two occasions.

Hypothermic death not infrequently can be

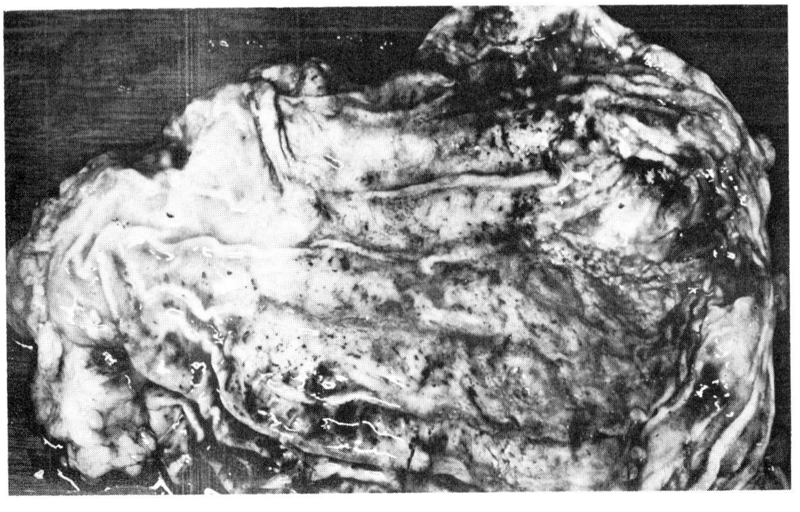

Figure 22–3. Wischnevsky ulcerations, erosions and hemorrhages in the gastric mucosa. Same case as Figures 22–1 and 22–2.

misinterpreted because of misleading circumstantial evidence. The victim of hypothermia can be found undressed, simulating a sexual attack or manslaughter.[114] Hallucinations, a feeling of warmth due to paralysis of thermoregulatory mechanisms, the effects of drugs and alcohol, and a large output of epinephrine have been suggested as explanations for this puzzling behavior.

Peculiar Adverse Effects of Cold

The adverse effects of cold are not restricted to lowering of body temperature. Aside from hypothermia, cold urticaria, cold syncope, and the effects of cold on the coronary and cerebral circulation deserve consideration.

Cold Urticaria. Cold urticaria is a hypersensitivity reaction of the skin that can be associated with cardiovascular collapse. This condition, when occurring at work, in conjunction with the individual's occupation, may lead to litigation on matters of compensation. Cold urticaria is hereditary. Cases are on record in which half the members of a family were affected by cold.[115] A serum factor, with characteristics similar to those of IgE skin-sensitizing antibodies, has been identified in the cold-sensitive patient.[116] Circulating basophilic leukocytes and skin mast cells of patients with this condition lose their granules when exposed to low temperature. Both systemic and local effects of cold urticaria have been attributed to liberation of histamine, but this was not confirmed by measurements of histamine of urticarial wheal contents.[117, 118]

Other allergic conditions resembling cold urticaria are cold erythema and cold vasculitis. The former is thought to be mediated by local release of 5-hydroxytryptamine; the latter affects mainly fingers, toes, and face, and probably represents a type of necrotizing angiitis.[119, 120]

Cold Syncope. It is known that certain individuals exhibit abnormal central nervous system responses to cold stimuli. These individuals can faint after ingesting a cold drink; the phenomenon has been attributed to cardiospasm followed by esophageal dilatation, vagal stimulation, and slowing of heart rate.[121]

Cold syncope can also be caused by vasocutaneous reflexes following sudden immersion in cold water or exposure to a cold shower.[122, 123] The term "hydrocution" has been introduced in the French literature to indicate the suddenness of the event.[124] The danger of syncope is greater after a warm bath or sauna. Cold showers (0° to 2.5° C, 32° to 36° F) over the chest cause increase of arterial pressure, pulse rate, and cardiac output; hyperventilation also occurs. The chest and abdomen are the two body areas most sensitive to cold, and electrocardiographic changes have been demonstrated following cooling of the chest wall, especially in thin subjects.[125, 126] It has been shown that even the immersion of one foot in cold water can elevate blood pressure and increase the cardiac output.[127] Both hyperactivity of sympathetic vasoreflexes and histamine sensitivity have accounted for the occasional syncope of participants in swimming contests.[128]

Cold and Coronary and Cerebral Circulation. The death rate for coronary disease and the outdoor temperature are statistically correlated: the lower the temperature, the greater is the risk of a coronary attack.[129-131] Patients suffering from angina pectoris almost invariably experience anginal pain on exposure to air temperature of less than −10° C (+15° F). The pain is caused by coronary spasm or increased stroke volume induced by breathing cold air.[132, 133] Exposure to intense cold also results in slight airway obstruction.[134] Each of these factors or their combination is apt to cause myocardial hypoxemia, infarction, or irreversible arrhythmia and sudden death. The same risk exists for cerebral hemorrhage. Data have been presented to the effect that the hospital admission rate for cerebral hemorrhages is higher on cold days (below −10° C) and that 90 per cent of the patients have been outdoors at the onset of the attack.[135] Environmental cold can be regarded as a serious hazard to the patient with preexisting vascular disease.

Other Diseases and Cold. Other diseases that can be aggravated by exposure to cold are cold hemoglobinuria and hemolysis. Both conditions are based on immunologic abnormalities.

LOCAL COLD INJURY

A profuse literature is available on localized cold injury in experimental animals; however, results of observations on rabbits, dogs, and other animal species hardly apply to man. In this review, consideration of localized cold injury is limited to those conditions that are most likely to reach the courts of law. These include chilblains, pernios, cold panniculitis, immersion foot, trench foot, and frostbite.

Chilblain can be categorized as a first-degree frostbite; it is also called *acute pernio*.[136] The skin is red or bluish, owing to capillary congestion associated with mild inflammation. As a rule the lesion recovers completely without residual deficit of the affected part.

Pernio, in its chronic form, is characterized by a reddish flat nodule in the skin, is more prevalent in women, and is inclined to affect the lower limbs. Ulceration, hemorrhage, and ultimately, scarring may occur, and frequently the lesion becomes activated in cold weather. The microscopic counterpart of the lesion consists of atrophy of the skin, dermic fibrosis, chronic panniculitis, mild angiitis and periangiitis, and sclerosis of arterial walls.[137]

Cold panniculitis is underlain by necrosis and inflammation of the subcutaneous adipose tissue. The etiology of this condition was first associated with cold injury by Haxthausen. Children are most frequently affected, and the relation of the lesion to exposure to cold air and wind is well established.[138, 139] The lesion has been reproduced by topical application of ice.[140] The susceptibility of children is probably explained by the fact that their fat contains saturated fatty acids in greater proportion than does the fat of adults.[141] Cold panniculitis may be mimicked by sclerema neonatorum, but the relation of the latter to local or systemic cold exposure is doubtful.[137] In the case of a young woman with cold panniculitis localized on cheek and chin, the condition was assumed to be linked to the presence of cryofibrinogens as well as to excessive fibrinolytic activity and platelet abnormalities.[142] Legal interest in cold panniculitis is evoked by a case of attempted infanticide in which the condition developed as a consequence of deliberate exposure to cold; the mother threw the child in snow for two hours after delivery. The baby was rescued and brought to the hospital, but developed panniculitis, broncopneumonia, and atrophy of the subcutis.[143]

Immersion foot and *trench foot* are similar types of cold injury occurring at temperatures above 0° C (32° F). Wetness is an important contributing factor in both. The injury can occur following exposure to sea water, which has a freezing point below 0° C (32° F), and may result in severe gangrene and loss of tissue, which is caused by obliterating angiitis.

Frostbite occurs on exposure to dry cold as well as following immersion at temperatures below 0° C (32° F). The distinction between superficial and deep frostbite is generally accepted. In the superficial type, only the skin is affected. In the deep type, subcutaneous fat, muscles, nerves, and bone may be involved, and massive gangrene may result. A more complicated and older classification of frostbite parallels the categories of burn injury. First-degree frostbite is characterized by redness and edema of the skin; as a rule the lesion heals promptly without permanent damage. In second-degree frostbite, the epidermis is affected and there is blister formation, but the underlying tissues are not involved. In third-degree frostbite, skin and subcutaneous tissue are necrotized. In fourth-degree injury there is total loss of tissues in the exposed area, including muscle and eventually bone.

Pathogenetic Considerations

Extremities

When a limb is immersed in ice water or exposed to cold air, arterial constriction occurs and is then followed after 10 to 15 minutes by vasodilatation.[19] With continued exposure to cold the temperature of the limb fluctuates because of intermittent vasoconstriction and dilatation (the so-called hunting phenomenon). The vascular reaction is probably elicited by cutaneous axon reflexes, and during vasodilatation, the blood flows into the cutaneous arteriovenous shunts; the blood vessels of the unexposed limb also undergo alternate constriction and dilatation.[144] Sludging of red blood cells, stasis, and edema develop in the affected part, the end result being tissue ischemia. Vascular insufficiency is thus one of the prominent factors in the development of cold injury.[145] Whereas the effects of arterial spasm and arteriovenous shunting are reversible, arterial occlusion, unless promptly compensated for by a valid collateral circulation, unavoidably leads to irreversible injury. This is primarily the case in deep (fourth-degree) frostbite.[146] Impairment of circulation from cold angiitis plays an equally important role in the pathogenesis of trench and immersion foot.[147]

The muscular and neural lesions seen in immersion foot can be caused by vascular impairment, but some evidence has been presented that lowering of temperature (10° C, 50° F) per se can be responsible for structural alterations in muscle fibers and peripheral nerves.[148–150] Bone changes may become manifest from 4 to 10 weeks later, and alterations in bone density can be the first revealing sign of this occurrence.[151] A widely accepted view is that cell death following exposure to severe cold is caused by hyperosmosis. Intercellular water freezes, and intracellular water flows out into the interstitial spaces.[152] The longer the involved tissue remains in the frozen state, the greater the tissular damage; the same is true for repeated alternating episodes of thawing and freezing.[153, 154] The freezing point of human skin is between −0.53° C and −0.65° C.[154] Thus human tissue can freeze in sea water, the freezing point of which is −1.9° C (+29° F).

In order to minimize the loss of tissue, the frozen limb must be thawed rapidly by immersing it in water heated to 40° to 42° C (104° to 108° F). In deep (fourth-degree) frostbite, a demarcation line develops just below the point of active circulation. The gangrenous distal part dries out and must be amputated. Early sympathectomy has been recommended to improve local circulation and reduce loss of tissue.[146, 155]

Moisture and lack of motion in a cold environment predispose to immersion and trench foot. Poor foot hygiene increases local moisture and therefore the risk of cold injury. Lack of mental alertness is another distinct contributory factor. Wind as well as contact with metals or plastic material increases the heat loss and likewise promotes frostbite; this is just what not infrequently happens to snowmobile drivers.[156] If the limb has suffered a previous frostbite, the danger of incurring a subsequent one is far greater, because of impaired circulation. Similarly, elderly people with poor peripheral circulation are more susceptible to frostbite.[157] Observations on Army personnel during the Korean war indicated that Negroes are more prone to frostbite than Caucasions or Eskimos. This seems to be based on different physiologic reactions to cold exposure.[158]

Acclimation to cold environment and repeated exposure to mild cold improve the ability to withstand severe cold. Fishermen and construction workers are able to keep up the dexterity of their hands and to escape cold injury even at subzero temperatures.[159]

Frostbite is nowadays mainly the concern of military personnel; cases among the civilian population are mostly limited to alcoholics and to inhabitants of extreme northern climates.[160] On the other hand, moderate concentrations of alcohol (0.06 to 0.15 per cent in blood) may have a protective effect against frostbite because alcohol tends to inhibit cold vasoconstriction in the exposed limb.[161] The risk of frostbite is greater in some occupations than in others; in the food industry, for example, the workers handle goods in a cold environment. In one case of occupational frostbite, a farmer's wife dipped her hand into a vat of brine to take out preserved meat. It was a cold day and the solution was below 0° C. Within a few minutes of exposure she developed second-degree frostbite of the hand.[162]

Ear, Nose, and Eyes

Frostbite of the ears, nose, and eyes not infrequently occurs in arctic and subarctic regions, mostly in children. Alcoholics are also inclined to develop frostbite in this pattern. The ears first become pale and hard, and then lose sensation. When thawed, they swell, become red or cyanotic, and may develop blisters; mummification follows in 7 to 10 days. Loss of the ear cartilage is quite infrequent, however. Rapid rewarming is the best treatment. Hyperhidrosis and extreme sensitivity to temperature changes are among the sequelae.[163] Frostbite of the nose is the ailment of children, but permanent defects are not seen; the same is true of snowmobile drivers.

Cold injury of the eye caused by snow and frost has been known to occur from the times of ancient military campaigns.[164] The target structures are the corneal and conjunctival epithelia. The lesion, quite common among Eskimos, is seen with increasing frequency among snowmobile drivers and occasionally among skiers.[165, 166] As a rule, mild lesions heal within 24 hours and no persistent changes arise. Permanent damage, however, such as corneal scarring and blurring of vision has been recorded.[165]

Sequelae and Complications of Frostbite

Fat embolism can be an early complication of severe frostbite. It can even represent the immediate cause of death.[167]

Late sequelae may have legal implications when the question of compensation arises. Comprehensive information on this subject is to be found in excellent review articles.[168, 169] Sequelae of frostbite in armed forces personnel in World War II included discoloration of the skin (73 per cent), hyperhidrosis (59 per cent), hyperkeratosis (1.6 per cent), skin ulceration (16 per cent), transitory edema (5 per cent), blistering (1 per cent), cold sensitivity (82 per cent), pain (39 per cent), hypesthesia (24 per cent), and phantom pains (10 per cent). Atrophy and keratinization of skin, neurologic abnormalities, and muscular atrophy were also mentioned.[168] Bone and joint changes associated with previous frostbite have also been described and attributed either to direct cold injury of the structures involved or to impaired blood supply due to arterial occlusion.[170] Cases have been reported of retarded growth of fingers in children, attributed to damage of epiphyseal cartilage at the site of previous frostbite.[171-173] Osteoarthritis of the hand 20 years after frostbite injury has also been recorded.[174]

There are reports of carcinomas arising at the site of frostbite sustained as much as 20 years earlier.[175, 176] As in the analogous situation of cancer arising at the site of injury from other causes, it is difficult to prove the relation between localized cold injury and tumor development.

COMPLICATIONS OF THERAPEUTIC HYPOTHERMIA

General Hypothermia

A comprehensive review of the use of this technique and its complications appeared in a medicolegal journal in 1969.[177] The complications of therapeutic hypothermia, including death, are difficult to evaluate accurately, primarily because morphologic changes are scarce. They are, however, prone to cause legal suits and insurance claims.

Effects on Organ Systems

General hypothermia frequently affects the *heart.* Complications may range from the rather harmless atrial fibrillation and block of the conduction system to the life-threatening ventricular fibrillation. For these reasons, deep hypothermia (28° to 30° C) (82° to 86° F) is rarely used nowadays.[178] The incidence of complications related to this procedure ranges from 1.8 to 5.2 per cent, depending on the experience of the surgical team, the nature of the operation, and the age of the patient and his general physical condition.[179-184]

Hypothermia also affects the *coagulation system.* According to Blair, disorders in coagulation become apparent only at temperatures below 25° C (77° F) and thus nowadays are rarely seen.[178] On the other hand, hypothermia seems to increase the tendency to intravascular clotting; the circulation is slowed down, and blood viscosity is greater. A case of mesenteric thrombosis during hypothermia has been reported, and the incidence of pulmonary embolism is said to be greater after hypothermic operations; thus the warning that hypothermia should not be used in patients with a tendency to red cell agglutination.[179, 185]

Brain damage after hypothermic operations has seldom been reported; however, it is not uncommon in children after cardiac operations. The lesions consist mainly of neuron and myelin loss; the globus pallidus and the Sommer's sector of the hippocampus are the areas most prone to be affected.[186] Temperatures as low as 6° to 15° C (43° to 59° F) should not be used in infants. Some investigators have attributed these cerebral changes to increased viscosity of blood, which results in the formation of microthrombi in the small vessels.[187] Since infants have recovered from exposure to 17° C (63° F) hypothermia without permanent neurologic deficit, other factors, such as the effects of anesthesia and surgery, have been taken into account to explain these changes.[188] The occurrence of subdural and subarachnoidal bleeding, possibly related to hypothermia thrombocytopenia and artificial circulation have been recorded.[189]

Among the complications affecting the *gastrointestinal tract,* a fatal gastric hemorrhage from an erosion in the stomach extending into the pancreatic duodenal artery on the tenth day after hypothermia has been reported.[190] Milder gastrointestinal bleeding occurs twice as often after hypothermic operations as after normothermic operations.[179] Intestinal peristalsis is reduced at 34° C (93° F) and ceases at 28° C (82° F) after which paralytic ileus, severe meteroism, and abdominal pain ensue.[178, 179]

Centrilobular fatty degeneration of the *liver* has been found in infants who died after surgery; conversely pancreatic damage, as found in cases of accidental hypothermia, has not been registered as a complication of hypothermic operations.[186]

Impairment of *renal function,* with increased urine flow and potassium loss, has been described.[191] Alkalosis is inclined to develop during hypothermia, and acidosis during the rewarming period, owing to respiratory and renal depression and other metabolic factors. Shivering, peripheral vasoconstriction, and alkalosis during cooling aggravate the development of acidosis during rewarming. Hence the warning that the blood pH should be kept normal or slightly below normal during hypothermia, because the acidity promotes the transfer of oxygen from the blood into the tissues.[192, 193]

Hypoglycemia is worth mentioning as one possible complication, although nowadays its underlying mechanisms are well understood and it can be prevented.[178]

The role of metabolic disorders as the cause of death is difficult to assess in postmortem material, and the pathologist, evaluating the immediate cause of death, has to rely mostly on the information obtained from hospital records. Serum and vitreous electrolyte assays can be valuable, however, if done less than one day after death.

Frostbite of the skin is a rare occurrence but has been reported.[177] Precipitation of cryofibrinogen resulting in local skin necrosis has been regarded as the cause of the frostbite that developed in one case in which a hypothermia blanket was used, but the low temperature per se was not considered the primary etiologic factor.[194]

Reports of *subcutaneous fat necrosis* come mainly from the early days of surgical hypothermia. This lesion has been described in infants undergoing surgical hypothermia, but not in adults. Its major manifestations can become apparent immediately after surgery or after a delay of two to five weeks.[195-197] They consist mainly of diffuse hardness of the subcutaneous tissue, followed within two weeks by a purplish discoloration, later on by calcification, and eventually by loss of the subcutaneous fat. The occurrence of this complication in infants only is explained by the higher melting point of the infant fat.

Rewarming shock can develop if profound (below 28° C) and extended hypothermia is used and the rewarming is done rapidly. The mechanism of the shock is probably a failure of the peripheral vessels to retain their tonus.[178]

Cryotherapy and Cryosurgery

Complications of *local freezing* from application of icebags are mainly of historical interest.[199] Cases are still being reported however.[178]

Application of liquid nitrogen (cryotherapy) to remove cutaneous *warts* may be followed by hypoesthesia and hypalgesia, pointing to a sensory nerve lesion.[200] An unexpected complication is the transmission of the wart papovavirus to other patients; the virus may withstand chilling in the −170° C liquid nitrogen in which the probe is stored.[201]

Cryosurgery is widely used in ophthalmology, mainly in cases of retinal detachment and cataract extractions. Among the complications of cryoextraction of cataracts, the following have been listed: (1) failure of freezing; (2) capsule rupture; (3) vitreous loss; and (4) accidental freezing of cornea, sclera, iris, and vitreous.[202] Complications of retinal cryotherapy include: (1) scleral edema, glazing, and rupture; (2) choroidal effusion, hemorrhage, and atrophy; (3) retinal pigment dispersal and uveitis; and (4) retinal atrophy.[203] Faulty retrobulbar positioning of the cryoprobe may cause injuries to the optic nerve, resulting in blindness.[204]

Freezing of bleeding *gastric ulcer* is a treatment still favored by some gastroenterologists. It has produced some good results, but the complications that have arisen have given reason to warnings. Complications can be caused either by faulty techniques or by unfavorable conditions. Freezing and rupture of the esophagus have occurred as a result of faulty placement of the cold balloon. Freezing of an ulcer that was adherent to the diaphragm has produced pleurisy and pneumonitis.[205] Acute ethanol intoxication developed when a patient managed to loosen the tube and the cold absolute ethanol escaped into the stomach; in this case blood alcohol climbed to 0.1 per cent, but the patient recovered.[206] Acute necrosis of the stomach wall with accompanying massive hemorrhage, formation of ulcers, and mucosal edema resulting in gastric obstruction have also been reported.[207-209]

Freezing of the prostate has been applied in the treatment of both prostatic hypertrophy and cancer. In a series including 37 patients, fatal complications occurred in four cases. In one case the orifice of the ureter was accidentally frozen, causing fatal ascending pyelonephritis. In another, the patient died of perineal abscess caused by faulty positioning of the cryoprobe. In the two remaining cases the causal relationship to the cryotherapy was less obvious; one patient died of apoplexy and the other of pulmonary embolism.[210]

Complications have also been described in coincidence with *cold conization of the uterine cervix* (in about 12 per cent of the cases), among which the most common were pyometritis, exacerbation of pelvic infection, hemorrhage, and cystitis.

Acknowledgment: This survey of the literature was supported by a grant from the Scientific Committee of National Defence of Finland.

REFERENCES

1. Pugh, L. G. C. E.: Accidental hypothermia in walkers, climbers and campers. Br. Med. J., *1*:123, 1966.
2. Keatinge, W. R.: Death after shipwreck. Br. Med. J., 2:1537, 1965.
3. Pugh, L. G. C. E.: Clothing insulation and accidental hypothermia in youth. Nature, *209*:1281, 1966.
4. Molnar, G. W.: Survival of hypothermia by men immersed in the ocean. J.A.M.A., *131*:1046, 1946.
5. Keatinge, W. R.: The effects of subcutaneous fat and of previous exposure to cold on the body temperature, peripheral blood flow and metabolic rate of men in cold water. J. Physiol. (Lond.), *153*:166, 1960.
6. Pirlet, K.: Experimentelle Studien des menschlichen Wärmehaushaltes beim kalten Seebad. Arch. Phys. Ther. (Leipz.), *21*:41, 1969.
7. Morley, D. C.: Cold injury among children severely ill in the tropics. Lancet, *2*:1170, 1960.
8. Haupt, H. C., and Mersmann, B.: Gefährdung

Frühgeborenen durch Frühauskühlung im Kreissaal. Geburtshilfe Frauenheilkd., *31*:931, 1971.
9. Mann, T. P., and Elliott, R. I.: Neonatal cold injury due to accidental exposure to cold. Lancet, *272*:229, 1957.
10. Wollner, L.: Accidental hypothermia and temperature regulation in the elderly. Gerontol. Clin. (Basel), *9*:347, 1967.
11. Exton-Smith, A. M.: Accidental hypothermia in the elderly. Practitioner, *200*:804, 1968.
12. Anderson, W. F.: Hypothermia in geriatrics. Med. Sci. Law, *9*:228, 1969.
13. Macmillan, A. L., Corbett, J. L., Johnson, R. H., Smith, A. C., Spalding, J. M. K., and Wollner, L.: Temperature regulation in survivors of accidental hypothermia of the elderly. Lancet, *2*:165, 1967.
14. Wilkerson, J. E., Raven, P. B., and Horvath, S. M.: Critical temperature of unacclimatized male Caucasians. J. Appl. Physiol., *33*:451, 1972.
15. Wyndham, C. H., Morrison, J. H., Ward, J. S., Bredell, G. A. G., von Rahden, M. J. E., Holdsworth, L. D., Wenzel, H. G., and Munro, A.: Physiological reactions to cold of Bushmen, Banta and Caucasian males. J. Appl. Physiol., *19*:868, 1964.
16. Hammel, H. T.: Effect of race on responses to cold. Fed. Proc., *22*:795, 1963.
17. Killian, H.: *Der Kälte-Unfall. Allgemeine Unterkühlung.* München, Dustin-Verlag, 1966.
18. Keatinge, W. R.: *Survival in Cold Water.* Edinburgh and Oxford, Blackwell Scientific Publications Ltd., 1969.
19. Burton, A. C., and Edholm, O. G.: *Man in a Cold Environment. Physiological and Pathological Effects of Exposure to Low Temperatures.* New York, Hafner Press, 1969.
20. Fox, R. H., Davies, T. W., Marsh, F. P., and Urich, H.: Hypothermia in a young man with an anterior hypothalamic lesion. Lancet, *2*:185, 1970.
21. Downey, J. A., Darling, R. C., and Chiodi, H. P.: The response of tetraplegia patients to cold. Arch. Phys. Med., *48*:645, 1967.
22. Johnson, R. H., Smith, A. C., and Spalding, J. M. K.: Oxygen consumption of paralysed men exposed to cold. J. Physiol. (Lond.) *169*:584, 1963.
23. Glickman, N., Mitchell, H. H., Keeton, R. W., and Lambut, E. H.: Shivering and heat production in men exposed to intense cold. J. Appl. Physiol., *22*:1, 1967.
24. Fay, T., and Smith, G. W.: Observation on reflex responses during prolonged periods of human refrigeration. Arch. Neurol. Psychiatry, *45*:215, 1941.
25. Courville, C. B.: Forensic neuropathology. VII. Changes in the brain incident to extreme variations in temperature, barometric pressure, electrical current, and x-radiation. J. Forensic Sci., *8*:82, 1963.
26. Rewerts, G.: Uber kältebedingte Schäden der Zentralnerven-System. Dtsch. Med. Wochenschr., *74*:1365, 1964.
27. Callaghan, J. C., Mcqueen, D. A., Scott, J. W., and Bigelow, W. G.: Cerebral effects of experimental hypothermia. A.M.A. Arch. Surg., *68*:208, 1954.
28. Stone, H. H., Mackrell, T. N., Fruter, M. R., Donnelly, C., and Frobese, A. S.: Effects of lowered body temperature on cerebral hemodynamics and metabolism of man. Surg. Forum, *6*:129, 1956.
29. Ehrmantraut, W. R., Ticktin, H. E., and Fazekas, J. F.: Cerebral hemodynamics and metabolism in accidental hypothermia. Arch. Int. Med., *99*:57, 1957.
30. De Jong, R. H., Hershey, W. N., and Wagman, J. H.: Nerve conduction velocity during hypothermia in man. Anesthesiology, *27*:805, 1966.
31. Barcroft, J., and Verzar, F.: Effect of exposure to cold on pulse rate and respiration of man. J. Physiol. (Lond.), *71*:373, 1931.
32. Trevino, A., Razi, B. R., and Beller, B. M.: The characteristic electrocardiogram of accidental hypothermia. Arch. Intern. Med., *127*:470, 1971.
33. Sarajas, H. S. S.: Heart damage in dogs subjected to hypothermia, with or without complicating cardiac operations. Ann. Acad. Sci. Fenn. (Med.), *86*:1, 1961.
34. Niazi, S. A., and Lewis, F. J.: Profound hypothermia in man, report of a case. Ann. Surg., *147*:264, 1958.
35. Phillipson, E. A., and Herbert, F. A.: Accidental exposure to freezing: clinical and laboratory observations during convalescence from near-fatal hypothermia. Can. Med. Assoc. J., *97*:786, 1967.
36. Prescott, L. F., Peard, M. C., and Wallace, J. R.: Accidental hypothermia, a common condition. Br. Med. J., *2*:1367, 1962.
37. Severinghaus, J. W.: Respiration and hypothermia. Ann. N.Y. Acad. Sci., *80*:384, 1959.
38. Oppenheimer, M. J., and McCravey, A.: Pulmonary circulation time in man at low body temperatures. Proc. Soc. Exp. Biol. Med., *46*:513, 1941.
39. Dill, D. B., and Forbes, W. H.: Respiratory and metabolic effects of hypothermia. Am. J. Physiol., *132*:685, 1941.
40. McNicol, M. W., and Smith, R.: Accidental hypothermia. Br. Med. J., *1*:19, 1964.
41. Arneil, G. C., and Kerr, M. M.: Severe hypothermia in Glasgow infants in winter. Lancet, *2*:756, 1963.
42. Tidow, R.: Kälteschäden der Magendarmkanals unter besonderer Berücksichtigung der Auskühlung. Münch. Med. Wochenschr., *90*:597, 1943.
43. Müller, E.: Pathology of general hypothermia in man. Acta Neuroveg., *11*:146, 1955.
44. Mant, A. K.: Some postmortem observations in accidental hypothermia. Med. Sci. Law, *4*:44, 1964.
45. Hirvonen, J., and Elfving, R.: Histamine and serotonin in the gastric erosions of rats dead from exposure to cold. A histochemical and quantitative study. Z. Rechtsmed., *74*:273, 1974.
46. Read, A. E., Emslie-Smith, D., Gough, K. R., and Holmes, R.: Pancreatitis and accidental hypothermia. Lancet, *2*:1219, 1961.
47. Mant, A. K.: Autopsy diagnosis of accidental hypothermia. J. Forensic Med., *16*:126, 1969.
48. Coopwood, T. B., and Kennedy, J. H.: Accidental hypothermia. Cryobiology, *7*:243, 1970.
49. Büchner, F.: Die Pathologie der Unterkühlung. Klin. Wochenschr., *22*:89, 1943.
50. Fisher, E. R., Fedar, E. J., and Fisher, B.: Pathologic and histochemical observations in experimental hypothermia. Arch. Surg., *75*:817, 1957.
51. Hillier, R.: The effects of dehydration on cold diuresis in recumbent man. J. Physiol. (Lond.), *206*:18P, 1970.
52. Fisher, D. A.: Cold diuresis in the newborn. Pediatrics, *40*:636, 1967.
53. Meriwether, W. D., and Goodman, R. M.: Severe accidental hypothermia with survival after rapid rewarming. Case report, pathophysiology and review of the literature. Am. J. Med., *53*:505, 1972.
54. Wilson, O., Hedner, P., Laurell, S., Norrlin, B., Rerup, C., and Rosengren, E.: Thyroid and adrenal response to acute cold exposure in man. J. Appl. Physiol., *28*:543, 1970.
55. LeBlanc, J., Pouliot, M., and Rheaume, S.: Thermal balance and biogenic amine excretion in Gaspe fishermen exposed to cold. J. Appl. Physiol., *19*:9, 1964.

56. Budd, G. M., and Warhaft, N.: Urinary excretion of adrenal steroids, catecholamines and electrolytes in man, before and after acclimatization to cold in Antarctica. J. Physiol. (Lond.), *210*:799, 1970.
57. Hershman, J. M., Read, D. G., Bailey, A. L., Norman, V. D., and Gibson, T. B.: Effect of cold exposure on serum thyrotropin. J. Clin. Endocrinol., *30*:430, 1970.
58. Golstein-Golaire, J., Vanhaelst, L., Bruno, O. D., Leclercq, R., and Copinschi, G.: Acute effects of cold on blood levels of growth hormone, cortisol, and thyrotropin in man. J. Appl. Physiol., *29*:622, 1970.
59. Okada, Y., Miyai, K., Iwatsubo, H., and Kumakara, Y.: Human growth hormone secretion in normal adult subjects during and after exposure to cold. J. Clin. Endocrinol., *30*:393, 1970.
60. Wilber, J. F., and Baum, D.: Elevation of plasma TSH during surgical hypothermia. J. Clin. Endocrinol., *31*:372, 1970.
61. Lamke, L. O., Lennquista, S., Liljedahl, S. O., and Wedin, B.: The influence of cold stress on catecholamine excretion and oxygen uptake of normal persons. Scand. J. Clin. Lab. Invest., *30*:57, 1972.
62. LeBlanc, J.: Secretion and activity of histamine and serotonin during cold adaptation. Am. J. Physiol., *204*:520, 1963.
63. Hirvonen, J.: Unpublished observations.
64. Kayser, C.: Physiological aspects of hypothermia. Ann. Rev. Physiol., *19*:83, 1957.
65. Seelye, E. R., Harris, E. A., Squire, A. W., and Barratt-Boyes, B. G.: Metabolic effects of deep hypothermia and circulatory arrest in infants during cardiac surgery. Br. J. Anaesth., *43*:449, 1971.
66. Hanson, P. G., and Johnson, R. E.: Variation of plasma ketones and free fatty acids during acute cold exposure in man. J. Appl. Physiol., *20*:56, 1965.
67. Wilson, O., Laurell, S., and Tibbling, G.: Effect of acute cold exposure on blood lipids in man. Fed. Proc., *28*:1209, 1969.
68. Nesbakken, R.: Aspects of free fatty acid metabolism during induced hypothermia. Scand. J. Clin. Lab Invest., *31*:1, 1973.
69. Schiff, D., Stern, L., and Leduc, J.: Chemical thermogenesis in newborn infants: catecholamine excretion and the plasma nonesterified fatty acid response to cold exposure. Pediatrics, *37*:577, 1966.
70. Miettinen, M.: Effect of swimming in ice cold water on blood picture. Ann. Med. Int. Fenn., *43*:298, 1954.
71. Quinn, M., Bass, D. E., and Kleeman, C. R.: Effects of acute cold exposure on serum potassium and magnesium and electrocardiogram in man. Proc. Soc. Exp. Biol. Med., *83*:560, 1953.
72. Müller, H.: Klinik und Pathologie des Unterkühlungschadens jünger Säuglinge. Münch. Med. Wochenschr., *113*:1678, 1971.
73. Anderson, K. L., Hellström, B., and Lorentzen, F. V.: Combined effects of cold and alcohol on heat balance in man. J. Appl. Physiol., *18*:975, 1973.
74. Haight, J. S. J., and Keatinge, W. R.: Human temperature regulation after severe exercise and ethanol. J. Physiol. (Lond.), *208*:22P, 1970.
75. Laufman, H.: Profound accidental hypothermia. J.A.M.A., *147*:1201, 1951.
76. White, D. C., and Nowell, N. W.: The effects of alcohol on the cardiac arrest temperature in hypothermic rats. Clin. Sci., *28*:395, 1965.
77. MacGregor, D. C., Armour, J. A., Goldman, B. S., and Bigelow, W. G.: The effects of ether, ethanol, propanol and butanol on tolerance to deep hypothermia. Experimental and clinical observations. Dis. Chest., *50*:523, 1966.
78. Battey, L. L., Heyman, A., and Pattersson, J. L.: Effects of ethyl alcohol on blood flow and metabolism. J.A.M.A., *152*:6, 1953.
79. Linton, A. L., and Ledingham, I. M.: Severe hypothermia with barbiturate intoxication. Lancet, *1*:24, 1966.
80. Lash, R. F., Burdette, J. A., and Ozdil, T.: Accidental profound hypothermia and barbiturate intoxication. A report of rapid "core" rewarming by peritoneal dialysis. J.A.M.A., *201*:269, 1967.
81. Grinsted, P.: Combined accidental hypothermia and barbiturate poisoning. Ugeskr. Laeger, *132*:933, 1970.
82. Martin, W.: Tiefe Hypothermie bei Barbituratintoxikation. Med. Klin., *65*:24, 1970.
83. Hangan, S.: Accidental hypothermia during treatment with a neuroleptic agent. Nord. Med., *75*:377, 1966.
84. Sharma, N. G., and Tihare, S. K.: Accidental hypothermia following chlorpromazine administration. J. Assoc. Physicians. India, *19*:879, 1971.
85. Laughnasse, T.: Hypothermia in a young adult. Lancet, *2*:455, 1968.
86. Gordon, M.: Phenothiazines. In *Medicinal Chemistry*. Edited by M. Gordon: New York and London, Academic Press, 1967.
87. Alexander, L.: *The Treatment of Shock From Prolonged Exposure to Cold, Especially in Water*. Combined Intelligence Objectives Sub-committee. Report No. 250. Washington D.C., United States Department of Commerce, 1946.
88. Horn, G.: Tod durch Unterkühlung. Ärztl. Wochenschr., *6*:376, 1951.
89. Cooper, K. E., Hunter, A. R., and Keatinge, W. R.: Accidental hypothermia. Int. Anesthesiol. Clin., *2*:999, 1964.
90. Hegnauer, A. H.: Lethal hypothermic temperatures for dog and man. Ann. N.Y. Acad. Sci., *80*:315, 1959.
91. Justin-Besançon, L., Péquignot, H., and Etienne, J. P.: Un cas de réfrigération à 23° 5 suivi de guérsison. Sem. Hôp. Paris, *34*:63, 1958.
92. Anderson, S., Herbring, B. G., and Widman, B.: Accidental profound hypothermia. Case report. Br. J. Anaesth., *42*:653, 1970.
93. Leading Article: Accidental hypothermia. Br. Med. J., *2*:1471, 1966.
94. Mathews, J. A.: Accidental hypothermia. Postgrad. Med. J., *43*:662, 1967.
95. Bower, B. D., Jones, L. F., and Weeks, M. M.: Cold injury in the newborn. A study of 70 cases. Br. Med. J., *1*:303, 1960.
96. Leonidas, J. C., and Golematis, T.: Primary cold injury in the newborn. Acta Paediatr. Scand., *55*:350, 1966.
97. Hutchison, J. H.: Hypothermia in infancy. Med. Sci. Law, *9*:224, 1969.
98. Trube-Becker, E.: On expert opinion in death by hypothermia. Deutsch. Z. Gerichtl. Med., *59*:211, 1967.
99. Rosin, A. J., and Exton-Smith, A. N.: Clinical features of accidental hypothermia, with some observations on thyroid function. Br. Med. J., *1*:16, 1964.
100. Kugelberg, J., Schuller, H., Berg, B., and Kallum, B.: Treatment of accidental hypothermia. Scand. J. Thorac. Cardiovasc. Surg., *1*:142, 1967.
101. Tolman, K. G., and Cohen, A.: Accidental hypothermia. Can. Med. Assoc. J., *103*:1357, 1970.
102. Edwars, H. A., Benstead, J. G., Brown, K., Makary, A.

Z., and Menon, N. K.: Apparent death with accidental hypothermia. A case report. Br. J. Anaesth., *42*:906, 1970.

103. Tomaszewski, W.: Changements électrocardiographique, observés chez un homme mort de froid. Arch. Mal. Coeur, *31*:525, 1938.

104. Prokop, O.: *Forensische Medizin.* Berlin, Volk und Gesundheit, 1966.

105. Lloyd, O. C.: Cavers dying of cold. Bristol Medico-chir. J., *79*:1, 1964.

106. Hunter, W. C.: Accidental hypothermia I. Northwest. Med., *67*:569, 1968.

107. Hunter, W. C.: Accidental hypothermia II. Northwest. Med., *67*:735, 1968.

108. Fruehan, A. E.: Accidental hypothermia. Arch. Int. Med., *106*:218, 1960.

109. Pugh, L. G. L. E.: Deaths from exposure on Four Inns walking competition. Lancet, *1*:1210, 1964.

110. Sano, M. E., and Smith, L. W.: A critical histopathologic study: fifty postmortem patients with cancer subjected to local or generalized refrigeration compared to similar control group of 37 nonrefrigerated patients. J. Lab. Clin. Med., *26*:443, 1940.

111. Aherne, W., and Hull, D.: Brown adipose tissue and heat production in the newborn infant. J. Pathol. Bacteriol., *91*:223, 1966.

112. Pugh, L. G. C. E.: Cold stress and muscular exercise, with special reference to accidental hypothermia. Br. Med. J., *2*:333, 1967.

113. Maxwell, B. E.: Neonatal cold injury in the Northwest Territories. Can. Med. Assoc. J., *97*:970, 1967.

114. Gormsen, H.: Why have some victims of death from cold undressed? Med. Sci. Law, *12*:200, 1972.

115. Witherspoon, F. G., White, C. B., Bazemore, J. M., and Hailey, H.: Familial urticaria due to cold. Arch. Dermatol. (Chicago), Syph., *58*:52, 1948.

116. Hauser, D. D., Arbesman, C. E., Ito, K., and Wicher, K.: Cold urticaria. Immunologic studies. Am. J. Med., *49*:23, 1970.

117. Juhlin, L., and Shelley, W. B.: Role of mast cell and basophil in cold urticaria with associated systemic reactions. J.A.M.A., *177*:371, 1961.

118. DeLaus, F. V., and Winkelmann, R. K.: Kinins in cold urticaria. Arch. Dermatol. (Chicago), *98*:67, 1968.

119. Shelley, W. B., and Caro, W. A.: Cold erythema. A new hypersensitivity syndrome. J.A.M.A., *180*:639, 1962.

120. Sarkany, I., and McMillan, A. L.: Cold vasculitis. Proc. R. Soc. Med., *62*:1278, 1969.

121. Rainord, D. J.: Cold drink and syncope. Br. Med. J., *3*:475, 1972.

122. Busch, J. P.: Hypersensitivity to cold as cause of sudden death while bathing. Dtsch. Med. Wochenschr., *59*:15, 1933.

123. Horton, B. T., Brown, G. E., and Roth, G. M.: Hypersensitiveness to cold, with local and systemic manifestations of histamine-like character: its amenability to treatment. J.A.M.A., *107*:1263, 1936.

124. Lartigue, G.: Allergy to cold. Hydroallergy and hydrocution. Rev. Fr. Allergol., *5*:257, 1965.

125. Keatinge, W. R., McIlory, M. B., and Goldfien, A.: Cardiovascular responses to ice-cold showers. J. Appl. Physiol., *19*:1145, 1964.

126. Rahman, S. A., Abhyankar, R. N., and Ali, T.: Effect of cooling anterior chest wall on T wave of electrocardiogram. Am. Heart. J., *47*:394, 1954.

127. Boyer, J. T., Fraser, J. R., and Doyle, A. E.: The haemodynamic effects of cold immersion. Clin. Sci., *19*:539, 1960.

128. Klaus, E. J.: Allergy to combination of cold and physical exertion as obstacle to sport; prevention of sudden death while swimming. Dtsch. Med. Wochenschr., *67*:845, 1941.

129. Rose, G.: Cold weather and ischemic heart disease. Br. J. Prev. Soc. Med., *20*:97, 1966.

130. Hall, P., Mosesson, E., Selander, H., and Selander, K.: The outdoor temperature and the mortality from cardiovascular diseases. Lakartidningen, *67*:2141, 1970.

131. Sotaniemi, E., Vuopala, U., Huhti, E., and Takkunen, J.: Effect of temperature on hospital admissions for myocardial infarction in a subarctic area. Br. Med. J., *4*:140, 1970.

132. Kavanagh, T.: A cold-weather "jogging mask" for angina patients. Can. Med. Assoc. J., *103*:1290, 1970.

133. Leon, D. F., Amidi, M., and Leonard, J. J.: Left heart work and temperature responses to cold exposure in man. Am. J. Cardiol., *26*:38, 1970.

134. Guenter, C. A., Joern, A. T., Shurley, J. T., and Pierce, C. M.: Cardiorespiratory and metabolic effects in men on the South Polar Plateau. Arch. Intern. Med., *125*:630, 1970.

135. Sotaniemi, E., Palva, I. P., and Hakkarainen, H.: Effect of environmental temperature on hospital admissions for cerebrovascular accidents. Ann. Clin. Res., *4*:233, 1972.

136. Kavanaugh, G. J.: Cold injuries in civilian practice. Heart Bull., *13*:16, 1964.

137. Montgomery, H.: *Dermatopathology.* New York, Harper and Row, 1967.

138. Lowe, L. B., Jr.: Cold panniculitis in children. Am. J. Dis. Child., *115*:709, 1968.

139. Whitwell, G.: Snowburn. Lancet, *1*:142, 1968.

140. Duncan, W. C., Freeman, R. G., and Heaton, C. L.: Cold panniculitis. Arch. Dermatol., *94*:722, 1966.

141. Tedeschi, C. G.: Pathological anatomy of adipose tissue. In Handbook of Physiology. Section 5. Adipose Tissue. Edited by A. E. Renold and G. F. Cahill. Baltimore, Williams & Wilkins Co., 1965.

142. Solmon, L. M., and Beerman, H.: Cold panniculitis. Arch. Dermatol., *88*:897, 1963.

143. McCandles, A. E.: Calcification and loss of subcutaneous tissue following trauma and hypothermia. Arch. Dis. Child., *46*:557, 1971.

144. Folkow, B., Fox, R. H., Krog, J., Oddram, H., and Thoren, O.: Studies on the reactions of the cutaneous vessels to cold exposure. Acta Physiol. Scand., *58*:342, 1963.

145. Kulka, J. P.: Cold injury of the skin. The pathogenic role of microcirculatory impairment. Arch. Environ. Health, *11*:484, 1965.

146. Martinez, A., Golding, M., Sawyer, P. N., and Wesolowski, S. A.: The specific arterial lesions in mild and severe frostbite: effect of sympathectomy. J. Cardiovasc. Surg., *7*:495, 1966.

147. Killian, H.: Kälte-Endangitis und invisible Erfrierungen. Langenbecks Arch. Klin. Chir., *292*:272, 1959.

148. Lewis, R. B., and Moen, P. W.: Further studies on pathogenesis of cold-induced muscle necrosis. Surg. Gynecol. Obstet., *95*:543, 1952.

149. Sayon, A., Meloche, B. R., Tedeschi, C. G., and Montgomery, H.: Experimental immersion foot: observations in the chilled leg of the rabbit. Clin. Sci., *19*:243, 1960.

150. Schamburg, H., Bryck, R., Herman, R., and Rosengart, C.: Peripheral nerve damage by cold. Arch. Neurol. (Chicago), *16*:103, 1967.

151. Tishler, J. M.: The soft-tissue and bone changes in frostbite injuries. Radiology, *102*:511, 1972.

152. Meryman, H.: *Cryobiology*. London, New York, Academic Press, 1966.
153. Adams-Ray, J., Eriksson, E., and Granberg, P. O.: The danger of delayed thawing in frostbite. Lakartidningen, *62*:1769, 1965 (Sw).
154. Keatinge, W. R., and Cannon, P.: Freezing-point of human skin. Lancet, *1*:11, 1960.
155. Schumacker, H. B.: Management of frostbite, Abstracts of papers: The Second International Symposium on Circumpolar Health. Oulu, Finland, 1971.
156. Erskine, L. A.: The epidemiology of snowmobiling injuries. J. Trauma, *10*:804, 1970.
157. LeRoy, N., and Juergens, J. L.: Frostbite. Mayo Clin. Proc., *40*:932, 1965.
158. Rennie, D. N., and Adams, T.: Comparative thermoregulatory responses of Negroes and white persons to acute cold stress. J. Appl. Physiol., *11*:201, 1957.
159. Rodahl, K.: *Human Acclimatization to Cold. Cold Injury.* Transactions of the Fifth Conference. Edited by J. M. Ferrer. New York, Josiah Macy, Jr., Foundation, 1958.
160. Cohen, N. M.: Severe cold injury in London. Practitioner, *200*:403, 1968.
161. Downey, J. A., and Frewin, D. B.: The effect of ethyl alcohol and chlorpromazine on the response of the hand blood vessels to cold. Br. J. Pharmacol., *40*:396, 1970.
162. Ringleb, D.: Ein eigentümlicher Erfrierungs-modus. (Odd way of freezing.) Münch. Med. Wochenschr., *98*:1778, 1957.
163. Sessions, D. G., Stallings, J. O., Mills, W. J., and Beal, D. D.: Frostbite of the ear. Laryngoscope, *81*:1223, 1971.
164. Esser, A. A. M.: Das Auge in Schnee und Frost der Antike. Klin. Monatsbl. Augenheilkd., *100*:100, 1938.
165. Forsius, H.: Climatic changes in the eyes of Eskimos, Lapps and Cheremisses. Acta Ophthalmol. (Kbh.), *50*:532, 1972.
166. Kolstad, A., and Opsahl, R., Jr.,: Cold injury to corneal epithelium. A cause of blurred vision in cross-country skiers. Acta Ophthalmol. (Kbh.), *47*:656, 1969.
167. Hardmeier, T.: Severe fat embolism in frostbite of both lower extremities. Schweiz. Med. Wochenschr., *93*:465, 1963.
168. Shafer, J. C., and Thompson, A. W.: Local cold injury sequels. A.M.A. Arch. Dermatol., *72*:335, 1955.
169. Ervasti, E.: Frostbites of the extremities and their sequelae. A clinical study. Acta Chir. Scand. (Suppl.), *229*:1, 1962.
170. Vinson, H. A., and Schatzki, R.: Roentgenologic bone changes encountered in frostbite. Radiology, *63*:685, 1954.
171. Dreyfuss, J. R., and Glimcher, M. J.: Complications and sequels of epiphysial injury following frostbite of fingers. N. Engl. J. Med., *253*:1065, 1955.
172. Selke, A. C., Jr.: Destruction of phalangeal epiphyses by frostbite. Radiology, *93*:859, 1969.
173. Lindholm, A., Nilsson, O., and Svartholm, F.: Epiphyseal destruction following frostbite. Report of three cases. Acta Clin. Scand., *134*:37, 1968.
174. Schumacher, H. R., Jr.: Unilateral osteoarthritis of the hand. J.A.M.A., *191*:246, 1965.
175. DiPirro, E., and Conway, H.: Carcinoma after frostbite: a case report. Plast. Reconstr. Surg., *38*:541, 1966.
176. Baux, S., Martinaud, A., and Roland, J.: Case of cancer on frostbite with invasion of the calcaneus. Ann. Chir. Plast., *14*:359, 1969.
177. Forrester, A. C.: Hypothermia in anaesthesia. Med. Sci. Law, *9*:233, 1969.
178. Blair, E.: *Clinical Hypothermia.* New York, McGraw-Hill Book Co., 1964.
179. Zindler, M., Dudziak, R., Eunikes, S., Pulver, K. G., and Zähle, R.: Erfahrungen bei 1290 künstlichen hypothermien für Herz- und Gefässoperationen. Anaesthesist, *15*:69, 1966.
180. Badeer, H.: Ventricular fibrillation in hypothermia, review of factors favoring fibrillation in hypothermia with and without cardiac surgery. J. Thorac. Surg., *35*:265, 1958.
181. Tsifutis, A., Burton, R. M., and Goldring, D.: The effect of hypothermia and anoxia upon oxygen consumption and contractility of human and rat heart muscle. Am. Heart. J., *79*:88, 1970.
182. Martinez, J. B., Kass, I., and Hoffman, M. S.: Factors involved in the recovery of a patient after prolonged ventricular fibrillation during hypothermia. J. Thorac. Surg., *36*:749, 1958.
183. Newman, B. J.: Control of accidental hypothermia. Occurrence and prevention, of accidental hypothermia during vascular surgery. Anaesthesia, *26*:177, 1971.
184. Speicher, C. E., Ferrigan, L., Wolfson, S. K., Jr., Yalav, E. H., and Rawson, A. J.: Cold injury of myocardium and pericardium in cardiac hypothermia. Surg. Gynecol. Obstet., *114*:659, 1962.
185. Stoddart, J. C.: Mesenteric infarction during hypothermia, a case report. Br. J. Anaesth., *34*:825, 1962.
186. Björk, V. O., and Hultquist, G.: Brain damage in children after deep hypothermia for open-heart surgery. Thorax, *15*:284, 1960.
187. Björk, V. O., and Hultquist, G.: Contraindications to profound hypothermia in open heart surgery. J. Thorac. Cardiovasc. Surg., *44*:1, 1962.
188. Anderson, S., Herbring, B. G., and Widman, B.: Accidental profound hypothermia. Br. J. Anaesth., *42*:653, 1970.
189. Brierley, J. B.: Neuropathological findings in patients dying after open-heart surgery. Thorax, *18*:291, 1963.
190. Forst, H.: Fatal stomach hemorrhage during artificial hibernation. Anaesthesist, *3*:159, 1954.
191. Gil-Rodrigues, J. A., and O'Gorman, P.: Renal function during profound hypothermia. Br. J. Anaesth., *42*:557, 1970.
192. Fairley, H. B., Weddell, W. G., and Bigelow, W. G.: Hypothermia for cardiovascular surgery: acidosis in the rewarming period. Br. J. Anaesth., *29*:310, 1957.
193. Astrup, P., and Engel, K.: Acid-base problem in hypothermia. Arch. Intern. Med., *116*:739, 1965.
194. Waxman, S., and Dove, J. T.: Cryofibrinogenemia aggravated during hypothermia. N. Engl. J. Med., *281*:1291, 1969.
195. Collins, H. A., Stahlman, M., and Scott, H. W. Jr.: Occurrence of subcutaneous fat necrosis in infant following induced hypothermia used as adjuvant in cardiac surgery. Ann. Surg., *138*:880, 1953.
196. Blake, H. A., Goyette, E. M., Lytor, S. C., and Swan, H.: Subcutaneous fat necrosis complicating hypothermia. J. Pediatr., *46*:78, 1955.
197. Duhn, R., Schoen, E. J., and Siu, M.: Subcutaneous fat necrosis with extensive calcification after hypothermia in two newborn infants. Pediatrics, *41*:661, 1968.
198. Boba, A.: Hypothermia. Appraisal of risk in 110 consecutive patients. J. Neurosurg., *19*:924, 1962.
199. Bunch, G. H.: Ischemic necrosis from ice bag "burn." Am. J. Surg., *32*:519, 1936.
200. Nix, T. E., Jr.: Liquid nitrogen neuropathy. Arch. Dermatol., *92*:185, 1965.
201. Charles, C. R., and Sire, D. J.: Transmission of papovavirus by cryotherapy applicator. J.A.M.A., *218*:1435, 1971.

202. Rubinstein, K.: Complications of cryoextraction of cataracts. Br. J. Ophthalmol., *51*:178, 1967.
203. Shea, M.: Complications of cryotherapy in retinal detachment surgery. Can. J. Ophthalmol., *3*:109, 1968.
204. Banks, W. S., and Havener, W. H.: Unanticipated posterior freezing. A hazard in retinal cryosurgery. Trans. Am. Acad. Ophthalmol. Otolaryngol., *74*:80, 1970.
205. Holland, R. H., and Morkovin, D.: Complications of gastric freezing. J.A.M.A., *186*:863, 1963.
206. Perey, B. J., Helle, S. J., and McLean, L. D.: Acute alcoholic poisoning, a complication of gastric hypothermia. Can. J. Surg., *8*:194, 1965.
207. White, R. R., Hightower, N. C., and Adalid, R.: Problems and complications of gastric freezing. Ann. Surg., *159*:765, 1964.
208. Manlove, C. H., Jr.: Complications after gastric hypothermia. Am. J. Surg., *109*:185, 1965.
209. Cali, J. R., Glaubitz, J. P., and Crampton, R. S.: Gastric necrosis due to prolonged local gastric hypothermia. J.A.M.A., *191*:858, 1965.
210. Haschek, H.: Klinische Erfahrungen mit der Anwendung extremer Kälte in der Urologie. Med. Klin., *64*:1959, 1969.
211. Villasante, U., and Durkan, J. P.: Cauterization of the cervix. Observations on 200 consecutive cases. Obstet. Gynecol., *27*:717, 1966.
212. Curry, S. L., Weed, J. C., and Creasman, W. T.: Pyometra. A complication of cervical cryosurgery. Obstet. Gynecol., *40*:499, 1972.

SECTION 7. ULTRASOUND INJURY

chapter 23

APPLICATIONS OF ULTRASOUND IN MEDICINE

by Jordan B. Greenfield

The use of diagnostic ultrasonics in medicine has a relatively short history. The first successful two-dimensional sonograms were produced by Howry and Bliss in 1950.[1] The principle on which the procedure is based is similar to the principle of sonar developed during World War I for the detection of German U-boats. Since the early 1950s we have seen great advances in the field and their ever-increasing clinical application.

PHYSICAL PRINCIPLES OF ULTRASOUND

Ultrasound is defined as sound with a frequency greater than 20,000 cycles per second, which places it above the audible range for humans. Ultrasound is more useful than audible sound because it can more readily be directed as a beam and because it obeys the laws of refraction and reflection more easily. Its principal drawback is that it propagates very poorly through a gaseous medium such as air. Certain terms must be defined if one is to understand the basic principles of sound. Sound is a series of condensations and rarefactions. The combination of one condensation and one rarefaction represents one cycle, and the distance between the beginning of one cycle and the beginning of the next is the wavelength (λ). Frequency is the number of cycles per given time and is inversely related to wavelength: velocity equals frequency times the wavelength ($V = f \times \lambda$).

The velocity at which sound travels through a medium depends in part on the density of that medium; sound travels faster through a dense medium (solid) than it does through a less dense medium (liquid). Temperature also effects the velocity of sound, but since body temperature varies little, this factor can be discounted. The velocity of sound in human tissue averages 1,540 m per second.[2]

Acoustic impedance determines how sound will travel through a medium and is defined as the density of that medium times the velocity. When sound reaches an interface between two media of different density, the beam undergoes reflection and refraction. The reflected waves give us information in diagnostic ultrasound. The greater the difference in densities between the two media at the interface, the greater the reflection. The angle of incidence is also of importance, i.e., the closer to 90 degrees the angle is, the greater is the amount of sound reflected. Other factors also play a role in penetration and reflection, namely wavelength and frequency, and the thickness of the medium.

INSTRUMENTATION

Sound is formed and propagated by means of a vibrating crystal located in a transducer that acts as both sender and receiver. The crystal is of the piezoelectric (pressure electric) type, which changes shape under the influence of an electric field. Expansion and contraction of the crystal produces sound waves. The re-

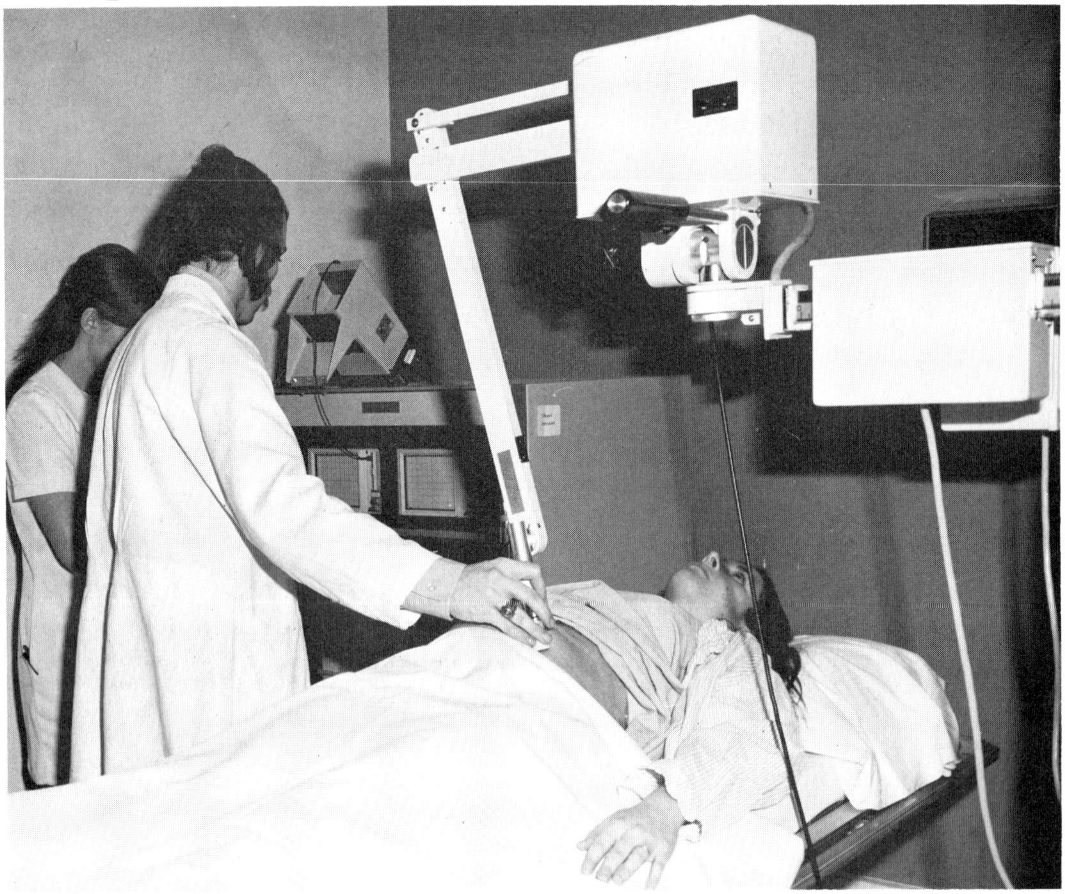

Figure 23–1. A pregnant patient is undergoing diagnostic ultrasound to determine gestational age, fetal size and location and position, and placental location. The procedure is painless, quick, and safe. See text for explanation. (Photo by Chalue.)

verse is true when the crystal is struck by sound; namely, an electric impulse is produced. This impulse is conveyed to a cathode ray tube (oscilloscope), where it is recorded and can be visualized. Figure 23–1 shows a typical ultrasound equipment display.

Sound is sent for a brief period (about 1 μsec). The transducer acts as a receiver for 99.9 per cent of the time. The repetition rate of ultrasound is, therefore, about 1,000 pulses per second. It is possible to calculate the distance from transducer to interface. Current equipment is calibrated so that conversion from part to part, of time to distance, is automatic. Thus, the oscilloscope displays actual distance between structures, and size and volume can be easily determined.

THE IMAGE

There are three major means of displaying and recording ultrasound information. They are currently referred to as A mode, B mode, and M mode.

In the A mode, each reflected impulse is recorded on the screen as a spike in "graph-like" fashion. The next interface will produce an additional spike some distance away, and the distance between spikes represents the distance between interfaces (therefore the size of the structure). If the substance between the interfaces is homogeneous (fluid, as in a cyst), the space between the major spikes will be echo-free (sonolucent); if it is nonhomogeneous (solid tissue with stroma), there will be echoes of less intensity between the major interfaces. Thus, if one finds a mass in an organ such as the kidney, he may easily distinguish between cyst and solid tumor by means of "A scanning." In A-mode scanning, the transducer and the reflecting surface are stationary and the strength of an echo is indicated by the amplitude of the spike (Figs. 23–2 and 23–3).

B-mode scanning involves recording each echo as a dot on the scope. By moving the

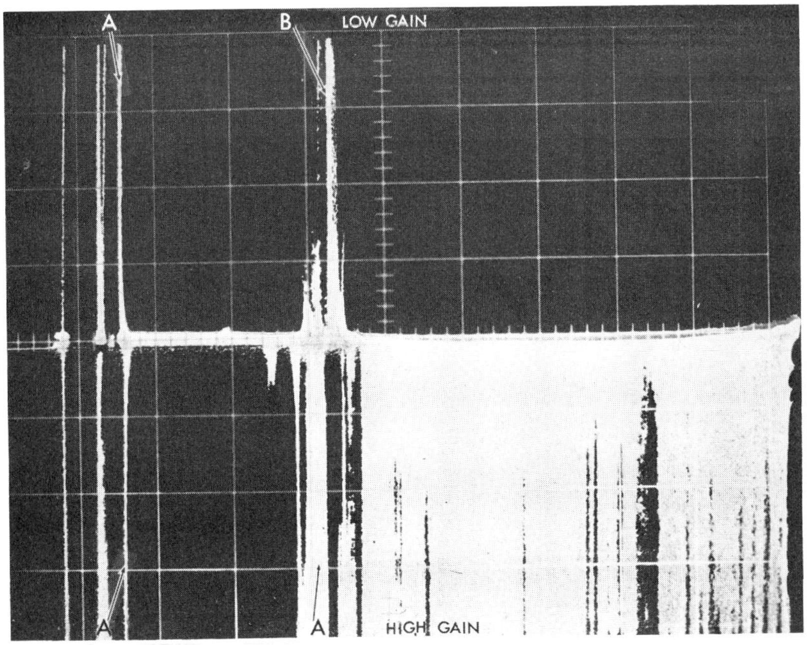

Figure 23–2. This is an A-mode scan demonstrating no echoes between the major interfaces (A and B). As the gain is increased, the space between the interfaces is still echo-free (sonolucent) indicating the homogeneous nature of the structure, which in this case was a renal cyst. Note that the image is inverted at high gain.

transducer, one can record a series of dots that form a picture. The effect is that of a tomographic "cut." Echoes are recorded in their correct spatial orientation by a system of potentiometers. In this manner, the entire outline of an organ or mass can be visualized and volumes can be calculated. Figure 23–4 shows a B-mode sonogram as a transverse cut demonstrating both kidneys in cross section.

Finally, M-mode presentation, also known as time-motion study, presents a picture as a series of dots that are in motion. The transducer is stationary, but the structure being scanned is in motion, e.g., cardiac structures in

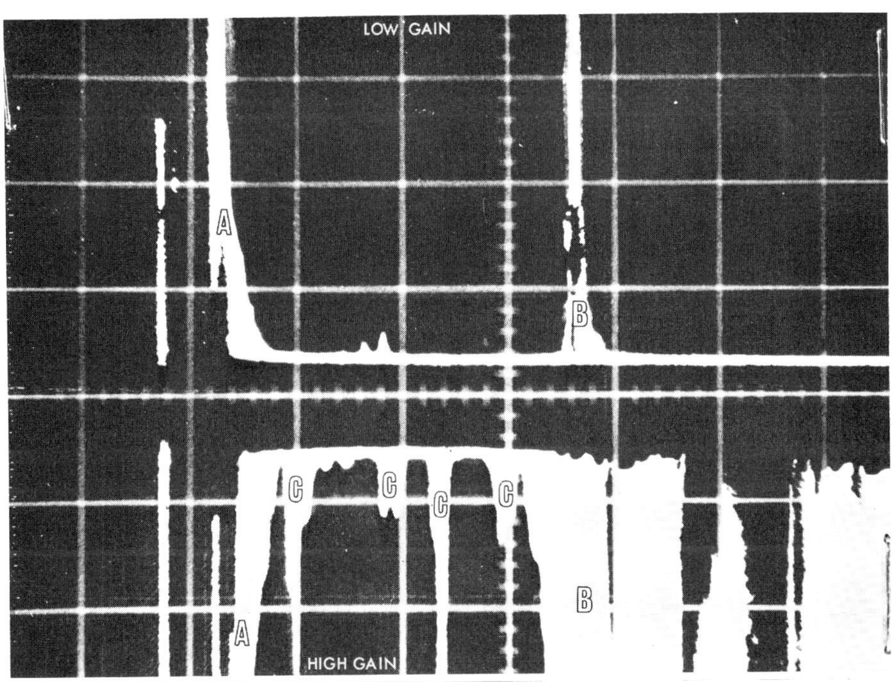

Figure 23–3. At low gain, the space between interfaces (A and B) is echo-free, but at high gain there are echoes between major interfaces (C), which indicates the solid nature of this mass, a Wilms' tumor. Image is inverted at high gain.

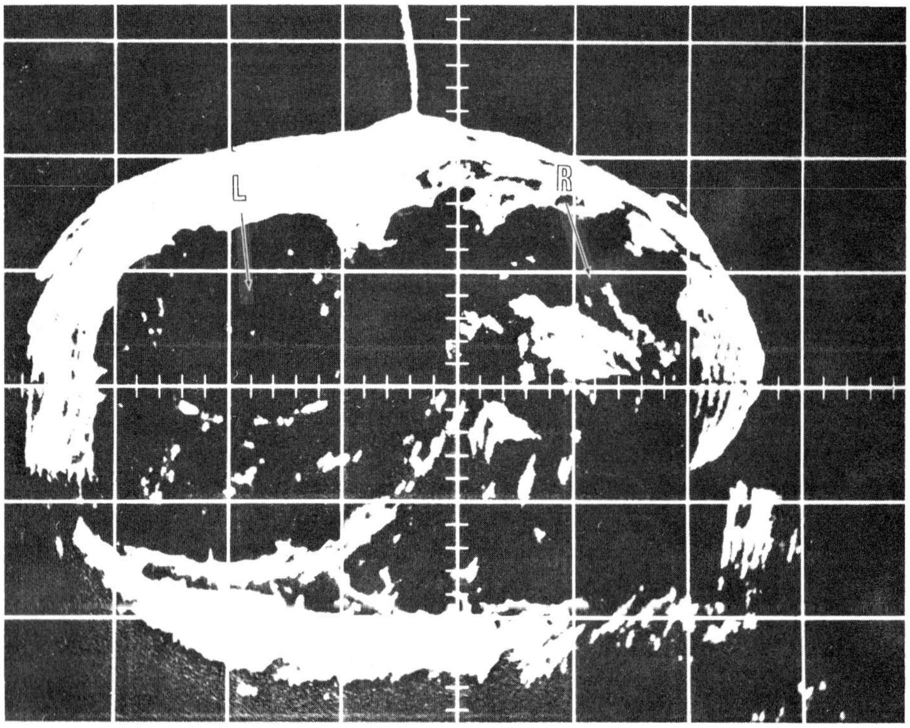

Figure 23–4. This is a B-mode transverse "tomogram" demonstrating both kidneys in cross section. The patient's right kidney (R) is of normal size while the left kidney (L) is markedly enlarged because of a tumor. This patient had a Wilms' tumor (seen on A scan in Figure 23–3).

an echocardiogram. The display is swept across the screen in a fashion similar to that seen in electrocardiography. This mode is used in studying major vessels as well as the heart itself. A typical picture of mitral valve appearance is seen in Figure 23–5.

CLINICAL APPLICATION OF ULTRASOUND

It is not pertinent to this text to discuss at length the multitude of clinical applications of diagnostic ultrasound. It is, however, of great importance to realize that ultrasound is a noninvasive technique that utilizes nonionizing energy. The equipment requires little space and can be brought to the patient's bedside if necessary. The examination is quick and painless. Following is a brief survey of the current major uses of this modality:

Echoencephalography is used in neurology to detect midline shift due to tumor, hemorrhage, edema, and the like. It is also valuable as an emergency diagnostic tool in head trauma (Fig. 23–6).[3, 4]

In *ophthalmology*, foreign bodies and tumors can be detected, and anatomy can be depicted ultrasonically.

Echocardiography applies ultrasound to the diagnosis of valvular disease, the detection of pericardial effusion, and the evaluation of cardiac motion and function (Fig. 23–7).[6, 7]

Abdominal echography can be used for detection of tumors and cysts and abscesses, evaluation of organ size and shape, and evaluation of the aorta.[8, 9]

Pelvic ultrasound and *obstetrical ultrasound* are used to evaluate pregnancy, placenta previa, twinning, breech presentation, missed abortion, moles, cysts, fetal progress, and gestational age (Fig. 23–8).[10–12]

TOXICITY OF ULTRASOUND

In Diagnostic Applications

Because of the widespread application of ultrasound in diagnostic medicine, one is justifiably required to be familiar with the potential dangers of its use, if any. A recent editorial in the *New England Journal of Medicine* cites ultrasound as being essential to good patient care.[13] If this is so, is it safe? At the levels of energy used in diagnostic work, all indications are that ultrasound is harmless. This statement

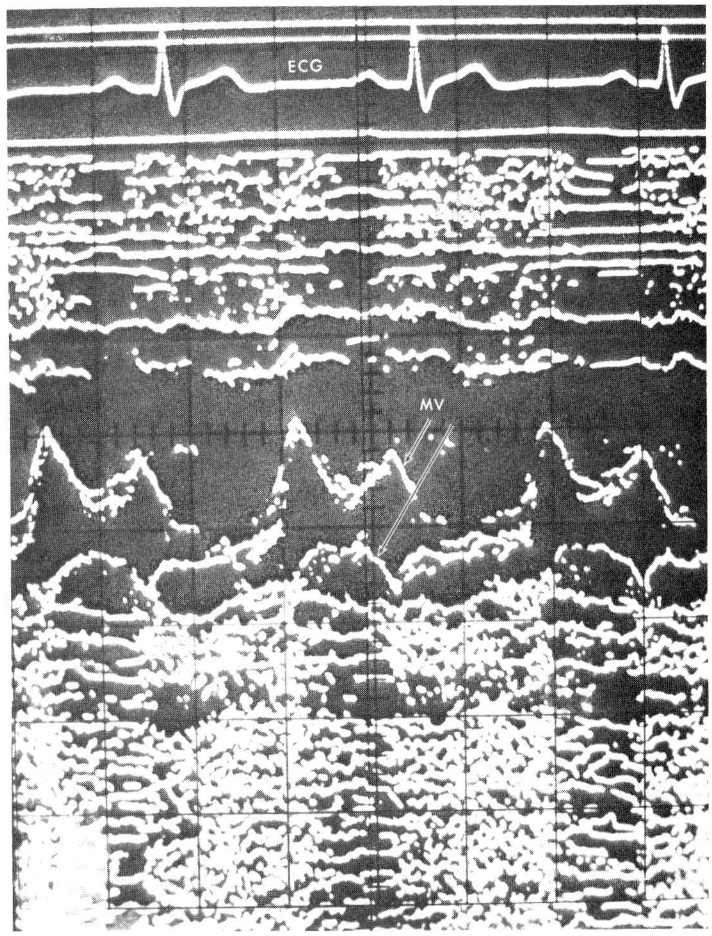

Figure 23–5. A typical "echocardiogram" with the electrocardiogram (ECG) above and the heart structures displayed by M mode. The mitral valve (MV) is displayed (anterior leaflet above and posterior leaflet below).

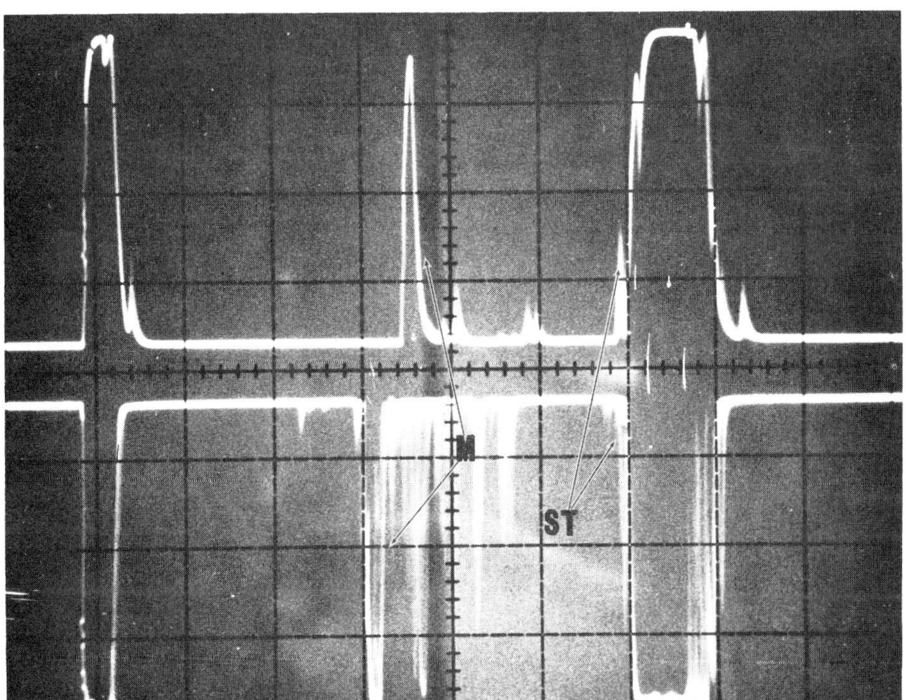

Figure 23–6. This A scan shows a midline shift in a patient with a subdural hematoma. The upper display is done from right to left and the lower display from left to right. The midline (M) is shifted from right to left because of a right-sided lesion. ST, skull table.

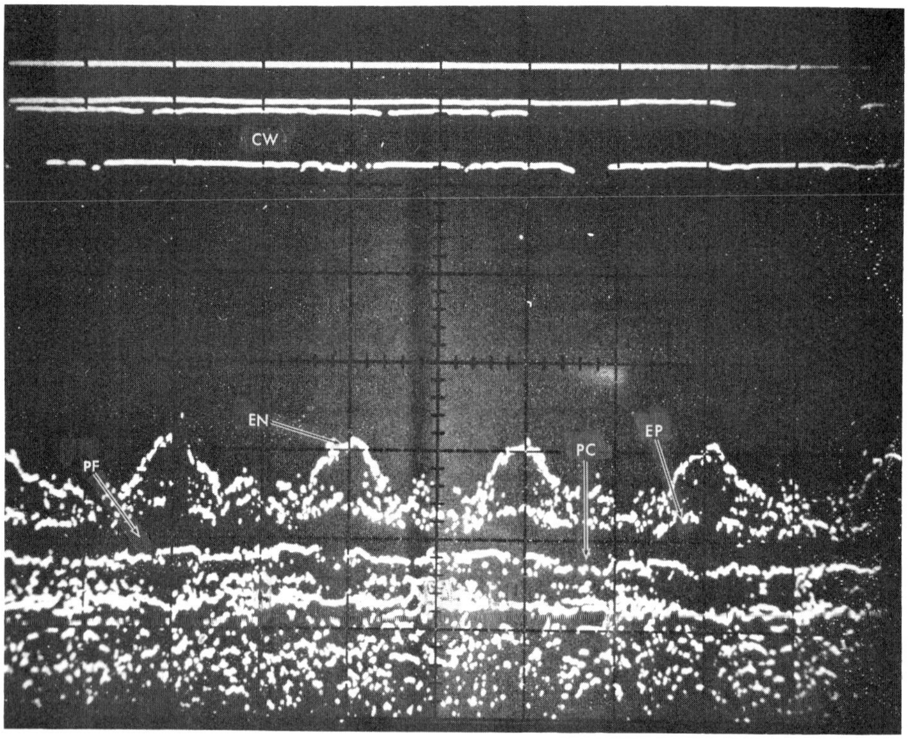

Figure 23–7. An echocardiogram in a patient with pericardial effusion. CW, chest wall; EN, endocardium; PC, pericardium; PF, pericardial fluid.

is supported by extensive research, which will be reviewed forthwith.

Ultrasonic intensity is usually measured and expressed as watts per square centimeter. Most experimental data indicate that harmful effects of ultrasound are related to the duration of exposure.[14] Since diagnostic ultrasound utilizes a pulsed system, transmission is brief (1 μsec)

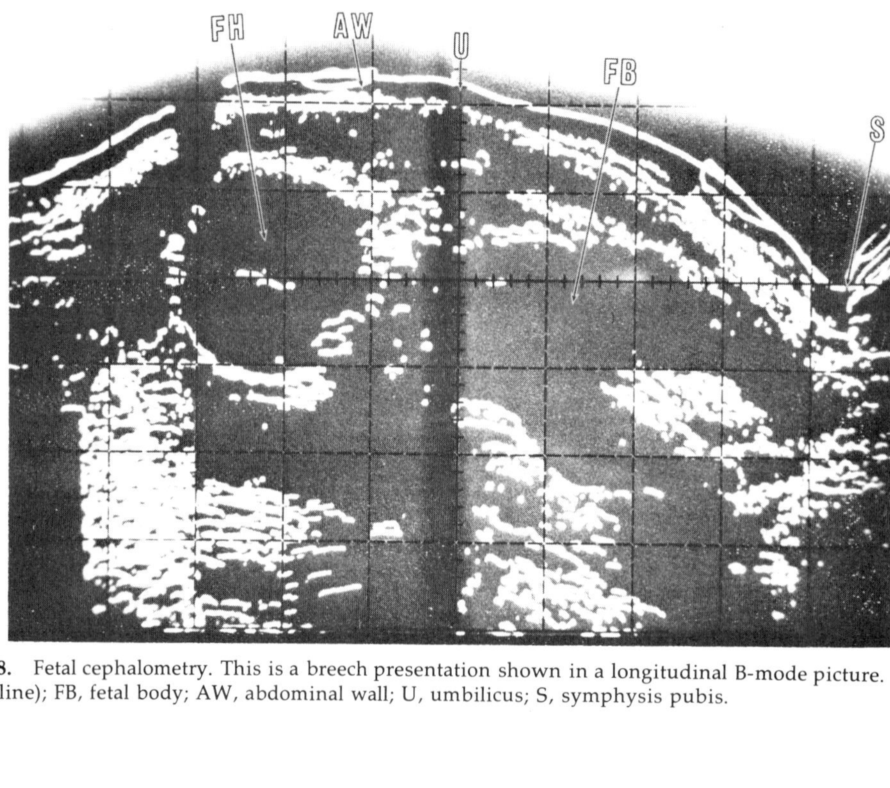

Figure 23–8. Fetal cephalometry. This is a breech presentation shown in a longitudinal B-mode picture. FH, fetal head (note the midline); FB, fetal body; AW, abdominal wall; U, umbilicus; S, symphysis pubis.

and average intensity is very low. Peak intensity may reach as high as 40 w per square centimeter, but average intensity is 1,000 times less than that, or 0.04 w per square centimeter (range 1 to 10 mw per square centimeter). Therapeutic ultrasound utilizes energies far greater than this. All available evidence indicates that 0.04 w per square centimeter is well below all known limits of safety for living tissue. Investigations of safety have focused on three areas: animal experiments, tissue culture in vitro experiments, and retrospective and prospective studies of pregnant humans.

There were early conflicting reports regarding the in vitro effect of low-energy ultrasound on human chromosomes. Recent work has shown, however, that even at a prolonged exposure time (three to four days) no chromosomal damage was detected either in fetal lymphocytes (from umbilical cord blood) or adult lymphocytes.[15] The chromosomal aberrations found in earlier studies are felt to have been due to environmental conditions rather than to ultrasonic energy.[16]

Animal experiments add additional support to our contention that diagnostic ultrasound is safe. Woodward and Warwick exposed pregnant mice to a wide range of ultrasonic energies (20 to 490 w per square centimeter) that greatly exceeded levels used in human diagnostic work. The outcome of the pregnancies were compared to control groups and no differences were seen in the two groups, even in subsequent generations.[17]

At high levels (25–50 w per square centimeter) of energy with prolonged pulses (10 msec) Taylor and Pond were able to produce cord injuries in mice. These cords, however, were surgically exposed directly to energy that greatly exceeded that used in human diagnostic work, (which operates in a range of 1 to 10 mw per square centimeter at up to 10 μsec).

Finally, our results in human studies are most conclusive. Donald and Abdulla used sonar in all stages of pregnancy and failed to demonstrate any hazard or effect on mother or fetus in hundreds of pregnancies studied.[19] Hellman and co-workers studied 1,114 normal pregnancies exposed to diagnostic sonar and found that the incidence of fetal malformation did not exceed that in the general population.[20] In a later study conducted by Abdulla and his colleagues, continuous and pulsed ultrasound was applied to pregnant women for 10 hours prior to therapeutic abortions. There was no increase in the number of chromosomal aberrations in blood cultures from fetus or mother when compared to controls.[21]

Diagnostic ultrasound has now been widely used for more than 10 years. At diagnostic levels of intensity, no harmful biologic effects have been shown. All the available evidence appears to establish the safety of diagnostic ultrasound. There exists a remote possibility that obscure or subtle damage that we cannot yet recognize may yet appear. Against this faint possibility, however, we must weigh the known positive advantages to the patient for whom diagnosis has been aided or established by this modality.

In Therapeutic Capacities

Therapeutic ultrasound presents an entirely different picture. Briefly, the energy intensity of sound used as therapy ranges up to 3 w per square centimeter. In addition, application is constant rather than pulsed, and the actual exposure of tissue to energy is considerably greater than in diagnostic work. High-energy ultrasound does cause chromosome damage in plants and animals.[22] There appears to be a linear relationship between increased dosage (intensity × time) and the degree of chromosomal damage. In the therapeutic range, ultrasound produces heat. Heat increases at interfaces between different tissues. As energy increases beyond the therapeutic range, actual cell destruction occurs. High-dosage focused ultrasound has been used to destroy lesions such as neuromas and to destroy brain tissue in patients with Parkinson's disease or intractable pain.[23–26] Patients with Meniere's disease have been treated with high-energy ultrasound.[27] This therapy abolishes the symptoms by destroying the vestibular apparatus.

There is little doubt, therefore, of the potential and real cellular effect of sound energy. Basic experiments on the effects of ultrasound on simple, unicellular organisms have opened an avenue to the understanding of the effect of ultrasound on more intricate structures, such as animal tissues and complex organs.[28,29] The most dramatic effect exhibited by unicellular organisms suspended in liquid media close to the source of ultrasound waves of intermediate strength is the so-called "cavitation phenomenon," which is characterized by the formation of gaseous bubbles in the protoplasm of the cell, resulting in the disruption of cell organelles. When exposed to greater ultrasound energy, cells actually explode. Thus, for example, red blood cells suspended in an isotonic solution become immediately hemolized.

The biologic effect of ultrasound can be classified in two major categories of phenomena: mechanical and chemical.[26,30] The mechanical effects are due to the rapid alternating compression and decompression phases of the waves. To the same order of phenomena belongs the conversion into heat of a large portion of mechanical energy. This is primarily the case for tissues with a high acoustic absorption coefficient, e.g., bone.

The chemical effects are similar to those elicited by ionizing radiation. They include oxidative phenomena, depolymerization of complex molecules, denaturation of proteins, inactivation of some enzymes, rupture of the ring of aromatic amino acids, and transition of some colloids from the state of gel to that of sol and vice versa.

The destructive effect of ultrasound on tumor cells has also been proved, but, because tumor eradication is incomplete, this method of treatment is not in use. A study done by Loch and associates compared the effect of ultrasound in diagnostic and therapeutic ranges on various types of cells (in vitro) including malignant cells. No effect on cells was observed when diagnostic levels were used for as long as 45 minutes. In the therapeutic range, however, cells were damaged and lost their ability to proliferate with increasing intensities.[31]

CONCLUSIONS

This chapter deals primarily with ultrasound safety in relation to its use in medical diagnosis. Tissue damage by heat or cavitation does occur at therapeutic levels of ultrasound, but its evolution has taken ultrasound from therapeutic application to diagnostic application. Therefore, our present concerns must be for ultrasound at diagnostic levels of intensity.

At present, we cannot state without reservation that ultrasonic intensities used in diagnosis are safe. All available evidence, however, does imply that the modality is safe, and it seems unlikely that any hazard does exist. Long-term follow-up studies may eventually turn up some genetic alteration, but the continued use of diagnostic ultrasound is justified by the existing reports of its safety and, perhaps more important, by the value of the diagnostic data that it supplies. Nevertheless, until final safety data are available, it is undesirable to exceed the intensities in current diagnostic use or to perform unnecessarily lengthy examinations.

REFERENCES

1. Howry, D. H., and Bliss, W. R.: Ultrasonic visualization of soft tissue structures of the body. J. Lab. Clin. Med., *40*:579, 1952.
2. Ludwig, G. O.: The velocity of sound through tissue and the acoustic impedance of tissues. J. Acoust. Soc. Am., *22*:862, 1950.
3. Brinker, R. A., King, D. L., and Tavera, J. M.: Echoencephalography. Am. J. Roent., *93*:781, 1965.
4. Brylski, J. R., and Izenstark, J. L.: Anatomic localization of midline echo in sonograms of the brain. Am. J. Roentgenol. Radium Ther. Nucl. Med., *93*:811, 1965.
5. Gitter, K., Keiney, A., Sarin, L., and Meyer, D.: *Ophthalmic Ultrasound: An International Symposium.* St. Louis, C. V. Mosby Co., 1969.
6. Feigenbaum, H.: Echocardiographic diagnosis of pericardial effusion. Am. J. Cardiol., *26*:475, 1970.
7. Popp, R., and Harrison, D.: Ultrasonic cardiac echography for determining stroke volume and valvular regurgitation. Circulation, *41*:493, 1969.
8. Damascelli, B., Lattuada, A., Musumeci, R., and Severini, A.: Two-dimensional ultrasonic investigations of the urinary tract. Br. J. Radiol., *41*:837, 1968.
9. Freimanis, A. K., and Asher, W. M.: Development of diagnostic criteria in echographic study of abdominal lesions. Am. J. Roentgenol. Radium Ther. Nucl. Med., *108*:747, 1970.
10. Donald, I.: Diagnostic uses of sonar in obstetrics and gynaecology. J. Obstet. Gynaecol. Br. Commonw., *72*:907, 1965.
11. Kobayashi, M.: *Atlas of Ultrasonography in Obstetrics and Gynecology.* New York, Appleton-Century-Crofts, 1972.
12. Donald, I.: On launching a new diagnostic science. Am. J. Obstet. Gynecol., *103*:609, 1969.
13. Lele, P. P.: Application of ultrasound in medicine. N. Engl. J. Med., *286*:1317, 1972.
14. Lehmann, J.: Present status of ultrasonic therapy. Arch. Phys. Med., *34*:139, 1953.
15. Mermut, S., Katayama, P., DelCastillo, R., and Jones, H. W.: The effect of ultrasound on human chromosomes in vitro. Obstet. Gynecol., *41*:4, 1973.
16. Coakley, W. T., Hughes, D. E., Slade, J. S., and Lawrence, K. M.: Chromosome aberrations after exposure to ultrasound. Br. Med. J., *1*:109, 1971.
17. Woodward, B., and Warwick, R.: How safe is diagnostic sonar? Br. J. Radiol., *43*:719, 1970.
18. Taylor, K. J. W., and Pond, J. B.: A study of the production of haemorrhagic injury and paraplegia in rat spinal cord by pulsed ultrasound of low megaHertz frequencies in the context of the safety for clinical usage. Br. J. Radiol., *45*:343, 1972.
19. Donald, I., and Abdulla, V.: Ultrasonics in obstetrics and gynecology. Br. J. Radiol., *40*:604, 1967.
20. Hellman, L. M., Duffus, G., Donald, I., and Sunden, B.: Safety of diagnostic ultrasound in obstetrics. Lancet, *1*:1133, 1970.
21. Abdulla, V., Campbell, S., Dewhurst, C. J., Talbert, D., Lucas, M., and Mullarkey, M.: Effect of diagnostic ultrasound on maternal and fetal chromosomes. Lancet, *2*:829, 1971.
22. Brown, B., and Gordon, D.: *Ultrasonic Techniques in Biology and Medicine.* Springfield, Ill., Charles C Thomas, 1967.
23. Ballentine, H. T., Jr., Bell, E., and Manlapaz, J.: Progress and problems in the neurological applications of focussed ultrasound. J. Neurosurg., *17*:858, 1960.
24. Myers, R., Fry, W. J., Fry, F., Dreyer, L. L., Schultz, D. F., and Noyes, R. F.: Early experiences with ultrasonic irradiation of the pallidofugal and nigral complexes in hyperkinetic and hypertonic disorders. J. Neurosurg., *16*:32, 1959.
25. Lindstrom, P. A.: Prefrontal ultrasonic irradiation—a substitute for lobotomy. A.M.A. Arch. Neurol. Psychiatry, *72*:399, 1954.
26. Nelson, E., Lindstrom, P. A., and Haymaker, W.:

Pathological effects of ultrasound on the human brain. A study of 25 cases in which ultrasonic irradiation was used as a lobotomy procedure. J. Neuropathol. Exp. Neurol., *18*:489, 1959.

27. McLay, K., Flinn, M., and Ormerod, F. C.: Histological changes in the inner ear resulting from application of ultrasonic energy. J. Laryngol. Otol., *75*:345, 1961.
28. Harvey, E. N., Harvey, E. B., and Loomis, A. L.: Further observations on the effect of high frequency sound waves on living matter. Biol. Bull., *55*:459, 1928.
29. Lynn, J. G., Zwemer, R. L., Chick, A. J., and Miller, A. E.: A new method for the generation and use of focused ultrasound in experimental biology. J. Gen. Physiol., *26*:179, 1942.
30. Fry, W. J., Brennan, J. F., and Barnard, J. W.: Histological study of changes produced by ultrasound in the gray and white matter of the central nervous system. In *Ultrasound in Biology and Medicine.* Edited by E. Kelly. Vol. 3. Washington, D.C., American Institute of Biological Sciences, 1957.
31. Loch, E. G., Fischer, A. B., and Kuwert, E.: Effect of diagnostic and therapeutic intensities of ultrasonics on normal and malignant human cells in vitro. Am. J. Obstet. Gynecol., *110*:457, 1971.

INDEX

Page numbers in *italics* indicate illustrations; those followed by (t) indicate tables.

Abalone, dermatitis from, 1402
Abdomen. See also *Gastrointestinal tract.*
  hemorrhage in, from explosion, 622
  injuries of, 210–215
    and cardiac injury, 204
    and kidney injury, 230, 232
    and retroperitoneal hematoma, 218–219
    and ruptured spleen, 211–212
    and traumatic retinopathy, 110, *111*
    associated injuries with, 211
    diagnosis of, 215–216
    electrical, 661
    firearm, *512*, 519–520, *520*
    in automobile accidents, 855
    in children, 216
      battered, *502*, 503, *503*, 504
    in immersion blast, 624
    in pelvic fractures, 344
    in pregnancy, 424–429
    multiple, 211
    perinatal, 439–441, *440*, *441*
    seat belt, 216, 856–857, *856*
  radiography of, 687
  surgery of, complications of, 1229–1233
    ureteral injury in, 234
  ultrasonic scanning of, 778
Abducens nerve, injury of, 62
ABH blood group, identification of, from saliva, 1144–1145
    from semen, 954–955
ABO blood groups, identification of, from bloodstains, 813–815, 813(t), 814(t)
    from semen, 954–955
Abortifacient(s), plant, 1457–1458
  potassium permanganate as, injury from, 254–255
Abortion, self-induced, injury from, 498
    potassium permanganate for, injury from, 254–255
  spontaneous, post traumatic, 428, 431–432
  therapeutic, failed, cause of action for, 492–493
    in second trimester, 483
Abortion (*Continued*)
  therapeutic, Supreme Court ruling on, and action for wrongful fetal death, 491
    uterine injury in, 255–256
Abralin, 1505
Abrasion, defined, 5
  from coral, 1389, *1389*
  from explosion missiles, 626–630, *625–630*
  marginal, in firearm entrance wound, 512, *512–514*
  of teeth, 172
Abrasion collar, in firearm entrance wound, 512, *512–514*
Abrin, 1505
Abruptio placentae, posttraumatic, 426–427, 432–433
Abrus precatorius, 1504–1508, *1506–1507*
Abscess. See also *Infection.*
  epidural, 45
  of brain, 50
    mycotic, *11*, *12*
  of hand, 368–369, *369*
  of oral structures, 164
  sterile, and fever, 712
  subdural, 45
Absolute liability, in products liability, 1657
Absorption, percutaneous, of toxins, 1274, 1572
Absorption-elution technique, for bloodstain typing, 814
Absorption-inhibition technique, for bloodstain typing, 814
Acceleration, negative, 128
  ocular effects of, 128
  positive, 128
Acceleration concussion, vs. compression concussion, 34–35
Accidents, agricultural, 1163–1166
  aircraft, 875–885. See also *Aircraft accidents.*
  alcohol and, 823, 823(t), 824
  anesthesiologic, 905–906, *905*. See also *Anesthesia; Anesthetics.*
  automobile, 853–863, *854–858*, *860–862*. See also *Automobile accidents.*
  bicycle, 858–859
Accidents (*Continued*)
  coal mining, 1182–1184
  compensation for. See *Damages.*
  cost of, 901–935
  definition of, in workmen's compensation laws, 1676
  domestic, 886–900
    asphyxiation in, 892–895, *894*
    burns in, 889–892, *889*, *891*
    drowning in, 898
    electrical, 897–898
    falls in, 886–889, *887*
    firearm, 896–897, *896*, *897*
    fires in, 889–892, *889*, *891*
    hypothermic, 899
    poisoning in, 895–896
    prevention of, 900
  drowning, 898, 1329–1330
  emergency treatment in, 865–874. See also *Emergency treatment.*
  farm, 1163–1166
  glider, 883
  helicopter, 882–883, 883(t)
  hit-and-run, 861
  hospital, 901–909. See also *Iatrogenic injuries.*
  iatrogenic, 901–909. See also *Iatrogenic injuries.*
  in fishing industry, 1167–1171
  in home. See *Accidents, domestic.*
  industrial. See *Occupational injuries.*
  liability for. See *Liability; Negligence.*
  litigation involving. See *Lawsuits.*
  motorcycle, 339, 859
  motorkart, 859
  negligence causing. See *Negligence.*
  parachute, 883–885, *884*
  pedestrian-automobile, 857–858, *857*, *858*
  pharmacologic, 906–908, *907*. See also *Drugs.*
  physical environment and, 1627–1640
  prevention of, legal-economic sanctions for, 910–935
  radiation, in hospitals, 903–904
    in laboratories, 1180
  railway, 1186–1191
    train-automobile, 858
  sailplane, 883

Accidents (*Continued*)
snowblower, 898–899
snowmobile, 859
surgical, 904–906, *905*, *906*. See also *Iatrogenic injuries; Malpractice.*
tractor, 1163–1164, *1164*
train-automobile, 857
treatment in, 865–874. See also *Emergency treatment.*
vehicular, 853–864. See also *Automobile accidents.*
Accident room, hospital, 871
Accident scene, preservation of firearm evidence at, 561–569
Accident victims, emergency care of. See *Emergency care.*
intoxicated, 873
medical records of, 867, 872–873
minors as, 873
transport of, interhospital, 871–872
to hospital, 867–869
Acclimatization, 1629
thermal, 710
Accommodation, phenomenon of, 1629
Acetabulum, fracture of, with posterior hip dislocation, 287, *287*
Acetaminophen, injury from, 1583
Acetylcholine, 1548
Acetylene, with chlorine, spontaneous combustion of, 738–739
Acids, and tooth decalcification, 193, *193*
burns from, 718, 1581, *1582*
of eye, 125–126
vs. alkali burns, 125, 127–128
effects of, on protein, 127
Acid phosphatase, in postmortem blood, 1038
Acid phosphatase test, for semen, 953–954
Ackee plant, 1530–1532, *1531*
Acokanthera spectabilis, 1477–1478
Acokanthera venenata, 1477–1478
Acokantherin, 1477
Aconite, 1525, 1526
Aconitine, 1525
Aconitum napellus, 1525
Acromioclavicular joint, injuries of, 266, *266*, *267*
Acromion, fracture of, 269
Acropora, 1389, *1389*
Actaea spicata, 1525–1526
Actinomycosis, 1337
cervicofacial, iatrogenic, 186–187
oral injury and, 164
Activation energy, for oxidizing reactions, 731–732, *731*
Addicts, narcotic. See *Drug addicts.*
Adenosine triphosphatases, activity of, in wound, *25*, *26*
Adhesions, posttraumatic, 347–348
Adhesive capsulitis, 270–271
Adipocere formation, in drowning, 1321, *1321*
Adipose tissue, injuries of, 361–364, *362*
hypothermic, 766
iatrogenic, 769
loss of, in burn injury, 722
Adipose tissue (*Continued*)
traumatic necrosis of, in female breast, 361–363, *362*
in newborn, 363–364
Adrenal glands, in burn victim, 726
infarction of, perinatal, *464*
surgery of, complications of, 1234
Adrenergic drugs, and eye injury, 129, 130, 131
Adrenocorticosteroids, and fungal infections, 11
Adult hyaline membrane disease, 392, *393*
Adult respiratory distress syndrome, 392
Aerobacter, and burn wound infection, 723
Aerocele, 45
Aerodontalgia, 637
Aeroembolism, 128, 641
Aerosinusitis, 637
Aesculin, 1504
Aesculus pavia, 1504
Aflatoxins, 791–793, 793(t)
African milk bush, 1503–1504
Afterdamp, injury from, in coal mine explosions, 631, 632
Age, determination of, from radiographs, 1157–1158
from skeletal remains, 1104–1106, 1104(t)
from teeth, 1124–1125, *1124*
meteorologic stress and, 1628, 1630
Age of consent, for statutory rape, 956
Aged persons. See *Elderly.*
Agglutination test, mixed, for bloodstain typing, 814–815
Agglutinogens, bloodstain identification by, 813–815
Aggravation, medicolegal concept of, 9, 11, 13
Agricultural chemicals, in bombs, 581, 582, 588–589, 591, 592–594
toxic, 1165
Agricultural fertilizers, spontaneous combustion of, 738
Agricultural pesticides, food contamination by, 788
Agriculture, injuries in, 1163–1166, *1164*, *1165*
electrical, 671
mortality rate in, 1163
occupational disease in, 1165, 1166
Air blast. See *Blast, air.*
Air cyst, vs. postnecrotic cyst, 45
Air embolism, 8, 208, 413–416
arterial, 414–415
in barotrauma, 637
in diving fatalities, 639
in explosion injury, 622
iatrogenic, 415–416, 905–906
postoperative, 1245
suicidal, 415
venous, 414
Air hammer, vascular injury from, 224
Air pressure. See also *Atmospheric pressure.*
in explosions, 617–618, *618*
Air rifle, injury from, *897*
Aircraft, decompression sickness in occupants of, 641–644
Aircraft accidents, 875–885
carboxyhemoglobin levels in victims of, 847
environmental causes of, 876
injuries in, 876–885, *878–882* 882(t), 883(t), *884*. See also *Crash injuries, aircraft.*
investigation of, 875–876
involving general aviation aircraft, 879–882, *880–882*, 882(t)
involving gliders, 883
involving helicopters, 882–883, 883(t)
involving high-speed aircraft, 877–879, *878*, *879*
involving jets, 877–879, *878*, *879*
involving light aircraft, 879–882, *880–882*, 882(t)
involving low-speed aircraft, 879–882, *880–882*
involving parachute descent, 883–885, *884*
pilot's preexisting disease and, 876
Aircraft seat belts, injury from, 880
Airplane accidents. See *Aircraft accidents.*
Airway obstruction. See also *Asphyxiation.*
by food, 893–894, 1614–1616
by foreign bodies, 207–208
in facial injury, 140, 143
Akee plant, 1530–1532, *1531*
Akinetic mutism, after head injury, 56
Alcohol, amyl, poisoning by, 820
beverage, and barbiturates, synergistic effect of, 823
and hypothermia, 762
as carcinogen, 191, 820
blood levels of, 1572–1577, 1576(t), 1578(t)–1579(t), 1580(t)
measurement of, 823–824
statutory limits for, 824, 863(t)
causing fire, laboratory identification of, 755
effects of, 818–825
in postmortem vitreous humor, 1051, *1052*
injury from, of gastrointestinal tract, 820
of heart, 821–822
of liver, 820–821
of musculoskeletal system, 822
of nerves, 822–823
interaction of, with drugs, 1206
intoxication by. See *Alcohol intoxication.*
metabolism of, 818–819
butyl, poisoning by, 820
ethyl. See *Alcohol, beverage.*
isopropyl, poisoning by, 820
methyl, poisoning by, 819–820
Alcohol intoxication, 818–825
acute, 819
and accidents, 823, 823(t), 824
in automobile, 823–824, *858*, 862–863, 863(t)

Alcohol intoxication (*Continued*)
and consent to emergency treatment, 873
and drowning, 638, 1329–1330
and homicide, 823, 823(t), 824
and house fires, 891–892, *891*
and suicide, 823, 823(t), 824, 1008
complicating crash injuries, 863
fatal, 819
measurement of, 823–824
medicolegal aspects of, 823–824, 823(t)
tests for, 863
Alcoholism, acute, 819
chronic, and heat cramps, 703
and heat stroke, 704
malnutrition in, 820, 821
nerve injury in, 822–823
organic injury in, 820–823
oral manifestations of, 191
symptoms of, 820
types of, 820
Aleurites fordii, 1491
Aleurites moluccana, 1491–1492
Aleurites trisperma, 1491
Algae, in drowned corpses, 1326–1327
toxic, 1429
Algolagnia, 963, *963*
Algor mortis, 34
Alkaline phosphatase, in postmortem blood, 1038
Alkali burns, 718
of eye, 125–126
vs. acid burns, 125, 127–128
Alkali grass, 1518
Alkali metals, spontaneous combustion of, 738
Alkalosis, respiratory, trauma and, 387
Allergy, anaphylaxis in, 1202–1204, 1204(t)
and sudden infant death, 1025–1026
contact, oral, 188–189, *189*
hepatitic anesthetic, 1249–1251, 1250(t)
to anesthetics, 1202–1204, 1204(t), 1247, 1249–1251, *1250*
dental, 185
to cold, 765
to drugs, 1202–1204, 1204(t)
fever in, 711–713
to dust, 1454
to foods, 793(t), 795, 1204(t)
to insect bites, 1447–1454
to insect stings, 1445–1447
to insects, ingested, 1455
inhaled, 1454–1455
to plant foodstuffs, 793(t), 795
to radiographic contrast media, 690–692
to toothpaste, 188
Allopurinol, with ethacrynic acid, effects of, 1201
with thiazide, effects of, 1201
Alpha-amanitin, 1552
Alpha rays, 680
Alternating current, injury from, 645–646
Altitude, high. See *High altitude.*
Altitude dysbarism, 641
Alveolus, dental, fracture of, 167, 168–169
Amanita muscaria, 1551
Amanita pantherina, 1551–1552
Amanita phalloides, 1552
Amblyopia, toxic, 131
Ambulance transport, interhospital, 871–872
to hospital, 867–869
Amebiasis, 1346–1347
American dog tick, 1451–1452
American Indians, racial characteristics of. See *Mongoloids.*
Amines, biogenic, extraction of, for wound timing, 26–28
Amino acids, in postmortem blood, 1036
in postmortem cerebrospinal fluid, 1044
in postmortem vitreous humor, 1048–1049
Ammonia, in postmortem blood, 1036
in postmortem cerebrospinal fluid, 1044
Ammonium, in explosives, tests for, 606
Ammonium nitrate, in bombs, 589, 591, 592–594
Ammunition. See also *Bullet(s); Cartridge(s); Shot; Shotshell.*
components of, 511
discharge residue from, 563–567
historical development of, 537–539, *538*
types of, 543–554, *545–552*, 553(t), *554*, *555*
Amnesia, in electrical injury, 659
in electroshock therapy, 662–663
indicating brain damage, 52
Amniotic fluid, postmortem analysis of, 1053
Amobarbital, injury from, 1215
Amperage, 646
Amphetamine, injection injury from, 226
poisoning by, 832
use of, 827
Amphotericin, and kidney injury, 401
Amputation, after vascular injury, 222
complications of, 1236
phantom limb sensation after, 381
traumatic, in electrical injury, *652*
of penis, 241
Amputation neuroma, 67–68
Amygdalin, 1529
Amyl alcohol, poisoning by, 820
Amylase, in postmortem blood, 1038
Amyloidosis, after spinal cord injury, 84
Anabasine, 1538
Anacardiaceae, toxic, 1470–1477, *1475*
Anacardium occidentale, 1470–1471
Analgesics, action of, smoking and, 1217
Anaphylaxis. See also *Allergy.*
drug-induced, 1202–1204, 1204(t)
Andromedotoxin, 1489, 1490
Anemia, Cooley's, oral manifestations of, 153, *153*
in burn injury, 722
Anemonin, 1527
Anesthesia, complications of, 905–906, 1239–1260
dental, and optic nerve injury, 118
oral injury in, 184–185, *184*
general, air embolism after, 1245
aspiration after, 1244
atelectasis after, 1244
bronchospasm after, 1245
complications of, from machinery malfunction and misuse, 1256–1258
hepatic, 1249–1251, 1250(t)
intraoperative, 1242
postoperative, 1243–1246
preoperative, 1241–1242
renal, 1251
flowmeters for, misuse of, 1258
hyperventilation in, 1242, 1243
hypoventilation after, 1243
hypoventilation in, 1241–1243
from mechanical failure, 1256
hypoxia in, 1241–1243
machinery for, malfunction and misuse of, 1256–1258
mechanical ventilation in, complications of, 1256
neurologic sequelae of, 1246–1249
oxygen intoxication in, 1245–1246
pneumonia after, 1244–1245
pneumothorax after, 1245
pulmonary edema after, 1245
respiratory insufficiency after, 1243–1244
toxic reactions to, 1246–1249
tracheal intubation in, complications of, 1251–1256
vaporizers for, misuse of, 1257
local, and optic nerve injury, 118
systemic toxic reaction to, 1247–1248
malpractice in, 905–906, *905*, 1239–1260
regional, cardiovascular effects of, 1247
central nervous system effects of, 1247
neurologic sequelae of, 1246–1247
systemic toxic reaction to, 1246–1248
spinal, complications of, 1248–1249
legal case involving, 1266–1267
Anesthetic(s), allergy to, 185, 1247
anaphylaxis in, 1202–1204, 1204(t)
hepatitic, 1249–1251, *1250*
and fever, 712–713
and kidney injury, 401
dental, allergy to, 185
injection of, infection from, 184–185
overinjection of, 184
gas, abuse of, 832, 832(t)
halogenated, and fever, 712–713
immunosuppression by, 389
injury from, 905–906, 1239–1260
in porphyria, 1246
legal cases involving, 1221, 1266–1267
inhalation, abuse of, 832, 832(t)

Anesthetic(s) (*Continued*)
  injection of, and chemical gangrene, 377, *378*
    and nerve injury, 373
  injury from, 905–906, 1239–1260
  local, systemic toxicity of, 1247
  overdosage of, 1247
Aneurysm, false, 225
    of forearm, *377*
    of hand, 376
  occupational, 377
  traumatic, 225
    of brain, 47
    of hand, 376–377, *377*
Angel's trumpet, 1534
Angina, Ludwig's, 187
Angina pectoris, anxiety and, 13
Angina pectoris electrica, 657
Angiocardiography, 688
Angiography, cardiac, 688
  cerebral, 688
  injury from, 903–904
  renal, 228–229, 232
Angioneurotic edema, *184*, 185
Anhydrosis, thermogenic, 704
Aniline dyes, and ear injury, 137
Animals, as infectious disease vectors, 1369–1377
  as railway hazards, 1188
  domestic, postmortem injury from, 1068–1069, *1070*, 1096–1097, *1096*
  farm, injury from, 1165, *1165*
  laboratory, injury from, 1181
  marine, injury from, 1378–1444
  wild, postmortem injury from, 1068–1069, *1068*, *1069*
Anisomorphic scar, 55
Ankle, calcification in, 320
  exostoses of, 328
  injuries of, 319–328
    dislocation, 323, 328
    eversion, 323–324
    fracture, 324–328, *326*, *327*
      bimalleolar, 325
      trimalleolar, 325, *326*, *327*
    fracture-dislocation, 325
    in explosions, 625
    inversion, 320–323, *321*, *322*
    ligamentous, 320–324, *320–322*
    soft-tissue, 319–320
    sprain, 320–324, *320–322*
Ankylosis, dental, 167–168, *168*
  in burn victims, 726–727
  of cervical spine, 63, 77
  of great toe, 337
Annelids, hazardous, 1390–1391, *1391*
Anoxia. See also *Asphyxiation.*
  injury from, in carbon monoxide poisoning, 844–845
  tissue tolerance to, 223
Ant(s), postmortem injury from, 1067, *1067*
  stinging, 1447
Antemortem wounds, adenosine triphosphatase activity in, *25*, *26*
  characteristics of, 23
  enzyme activity in, 25, *25*, *26*
  leukocytic infiltration of, 23
  timing of, 22–28
  zones of, 25, *25*
Anterior chamber, of eye, anatomy of, 99
  epithelialization of, 98
  hemorrhage in, 101, *101*
  injuries of, 99–102, *100*
Anterior tibial compartment syndrome, 314–315, *315*
Anthozoa, 1380, 1383(t), 1387
Anthracosilicosis, 1185
Anthrax, cutaneous, 9, *9*, 10
Anthropology, forensic, 1101–1115
Antibiotics, anaphylactic reaction to, 1202–1204, 1204(t)
  and fungal infections, 11
  and kidney injury, 401
  and oral injury, 188, *189*
  and postanesthetic hypoventilation, 1243
  in pregnancy, 1199–1200
  injection of, and chemical gangrene, 377
Anticholinergic drugs, and glaucoma, 131
  interaction of, with decongestants, 1205
Anticoagulant drugs, interaction of, with decongestants, 1205
Antidepressant drugs, interaction of, with estrogen, 1205–1206
Antigens, ABH, identification of, in saliva, 1144–1145
    in semen, 954–955
  ABO, identification of, in bloodstains, 813–814, 813(t), 814(t)
    in semen, 954–955
  fungal, response to, 1338–1339
  identification of, in bloodstains, 813–816
    in saliva, 1144–1145
    in semen, 954–955
Antiglobulin tests, for species identification of bloodstains, 811–812
Antihistamines, and fever, 711
Antimalarial drugs, synthetic, and eye injury, 129
Antivenin, 1442, 1443
Anuria, traumatic, 351
Anus, injuries of, 219–220
Anxiety, cardiac response to, 13
Anxiety neurosis, 17
  vs. compensation neurosis, 18
Aorta, injuries of, *13*, *14*, 205–206
  radiography of, 688
  stenosis of, calcific, *14*
Aortic arch vessels, injuries of, 206
Aortography, 688
Apallic syndrome, 56
Apgar score, 442
Aphids, 1454
Apocynaceae, toxic, 1477–1481
Appendectomy, complications of, 1231
Apple of Sodom plant, 1541
Appliances, electrical. See *Electrical appliances.*
Apricot tree, 1528
Aqueous humor, chemical injuries of, 127
  circulation of, in secondary glaucoma, 99, *100*
Araceae, toxic, 1481–1483
Arachnidism, 1454
Arachnoid cyst, 65–66
Arachnoiditis, spinal anesthesia and, 1249
Arbol del diablo plant, 1496–1497
Arc, electric, 742
Arc burns, 718
Arc current, 646
  injury from, 654–655
Arc flash, eye injury from, 662
Arm. See also names of specific parts.
  injuries of, agricultural, 1163
    fracture, 261–285
    in electrical injury, 656–657
    injection, 379
    musculoskeletal, 261–285
    vascular, acute, 222–223, 376–379, *377*, *378*
      chronic, 224–225
  paralysis of, in humeral fractures, 271
Arrhythmias, anxiety and, 13
  electrical injury and, 658
  in digitalis poisoning, 1197
  posttraumatic, 8, 13, 399–400
  vs. asphyxia, postmortem diagnosis of, 1056
Arrow grenade, 595
Arrowroot plant, 1488–1489, *1489*
Arsenic, and eye injury, 129
  as carcinogen, 20
Arsenic poisoning, toxicologic analysis in, 805
Arson, causes of, 732
  incidence of, 733(t)
  inflammable liquids used in, 737
  investigation of, 730–757
    at site, 744–747, *747*
    in laboratory, 748–757, 748(t), *751–754*
    organization of, 733–735, 734(t)
    statistical data for, 732–733, 733(t)
Arteriography, 689
  in genitourinary injuries, 228–229
  in kidney injuries, 232
  injury from, 696, 903–904
    of hand, 379
    vascular, 224
Arteriosclerosis, peripheral, trauma and, 16, *16*, *17*
Arteriovenous fistula, traumatic, 225–226
    of hand, 377
Artery(ies), air embolism in, 414–415
  catheterization of, 688–689
    injury from, 224
  foreign bodies in, 208
  injuries of, 221–227
    acute, 222–224
    chronic, 224–225
    injection, 226
      in drug abusers, illicit drug, 833
  of upper extremity, injuries of, 365, 376–379, *377*, *378*
  radiography of, 688–689
  surgery of, complications of, 1228–1229
  thromboembolism of, 408
Arthritis, degenerative, posttraumatic, 349

Arthritis (*Continued*)
degenerative, posttraumatic, in central hip dislocation, 288–289, *289*
of shoulder, 262
of temporomandibular joint, 171
drugs for, effects of, 1201
Arthrography, 688
Arthrokatadysis, 288, *288*
Arthropods, as disease vectors, 1366–1368, 1370–1371
hazardous, 1391–1393, *1392–1393*
ingestion of, injury from, 1455
succession of, in corpses, 1073–1079, 1073(t), *1074–1077*, 1076(t), *1079*
Asbestos, as carcinogen, 1278, 1279(t)–1281(t), 1284–1286, *1285*
detection of, in tissue, 1286–1290, 1286(t), *1287, 1289, 1290*
diseases caused by. See *Asbestos-related disease(s).*
exposure to, mechanisms of, 1278–1279, 1279(t)
sources of, 1277–1278, 1278(t)
Asbestos bodies, identification of, in tissue, 1286–1290, *1289*
Asbestos pneumoconiosis, 1282, *1282, 1283*
Asbestos-related disease(s), 1277–1291
asbestosis as, 1279(t)–1281(t), 1281–1282, *1282, 1283*
cancer as, 1279(t)–1281(t), 1284–1286, *1285*
incidence of, 1280(t), 1281(t)
litigation involving, 1290
lung cancer as, 1279(t)–1281(t), 1284–1285, *1285*
mesothelioma as, 1279(t)–1281(t), 1282–1284, *1283, 1284*
parenchymal asbestosis as, 1279(t), 1280(t), 1282, *1282, 1283*
pleural asbestosis as, 1279–1282, 1279(t)–1281(t), *1282*
Asbestosis, incidence of, 1280(t), 1281(t)
parenchymal, 1279(t)–1281(t), 1282, *1282, 1283*
pleural, 1279–1282, 1279(t)–1281(t), *1282*
Ascariasis, 1356
Asclepiadaceae, toxic, 1483
Ascorbic acid, in postmortem vitreous humor, 1047
Aspergillosis, 1337–1338
Aspergillus flavus, food poisoning by, 791–793, 791(t)
Aspergillus fumigatus, and brain abscess, *11, 12*
Aspergillus parasiticus, food poisoning by, 791–793, 791(t)
Asphyxia. See also *Hypoxia.*
crush, in explosion, 630–631, *631*
in carbon monoxide poisoning, 843–845
mechanisms of, 203–204
vs. cardiac arrhythmia, postmortem diagnosis of, 1056
Asphyxiation, 203–204
by carbon monoxide. See *Carbon monoxide poisoning.*
Asphyxiation (*Continued*)
by chemical inhalation, 1570
by food, 893–894, 1614–1616
by foreign body, 207–208, 893
by hanging, *6*, 203, 1006, *1006*, 1063
by plastic bags, 893
homicidal, 1010, *1011*, 1063
in chest injury, 203, *1164*
in domestic accidents, 892–895, *894*
in explosions, 630–631, *631*
in infants, vs. sudden infant death, 1018–1023, *1021, 1022, 1024*
in masturbatory acts, 894, *894*, 961–962, *962*
mechanisms of, 203–204
sexual, 894, *894*, 961–962, *962*
suicidal, 6, 1006, *1006*
simulated, 1063
Aspiration, needle, of chest, and spleen injury, 212
of chemicals, 1570
of food, 893–894, 1614–1616
of foreign bodies, 207, 893
of insects, injury from, 1454–1455
of poisons, 1570
of water, in drowning, 204, 1322, 1324
postoperative, 1244
Aspiration pneumonia, meconium, 477, *478*
Aspiration pneumonitis, postoperative, 1244
Aspirin, and ear injury, 137
and fever, 711
and oral burns, 189–190, *190*
in postmortem vitreous humor, 1052
Assassin bugs, as disease vectors, 1367
Assault, sexual, 939–964. See also *Rape.*
Asthma weed, 1483
Atelectasis, postoperative, 1244
Atlas, fracture of, 63–64, 77
fracture-dislocation of, 64–65
Atmospheric pressure, and barotrauma, 636–644
decreased, injury from, 641–644
increased, injury from, 636–640
measurement of, 641
Atomic absorption spectroscopy, of firearm discharge residue, 567
Atomic explosion, injury from, 683–684
of eye, 125
Atropa belladonna, 1532–1533
Atrophy, of bone, acute traumatic, 349, *350*
of muscle, after nerve injury, 69
of spine, after electrical injury, 659
Sudeck's, 329, 349, *350*, 387
Atropine, and glaucoma, 131
in toxic plants, 1533, 1535, 1540
Attitudinal pathosis, 17
Audiometry, 133
Auditory nerve, anatomy of, 132
injury of, 62
Autoclaves, injury from, 1178–1179
Automatic weapon(s), 542. See also *Rifled weapons.*
as rifled weapon, 510
Automatic weapon(s) (*Continued*)
barrel size of, 510–511
wounds from, *513, 517*. See also *Firearm wounds.*
Automatism, 1569
Automobile accidents, 853–863, *854–858, 860–862*
alcohol and, 823–824, *858*, 862–863, 863(t)
and abruptio placentae, 426–427, 432
and fetal injuries, 426–427, 429–433
and premature labor, 427–428, 432
and spontaneous abortion, 428, 431–432
biometeorologic study of, 1635–1637
carbon monoxide poisoning and, 846
drugs and, 862–863
hit-and-run, 861
homicidal, 861–862
in pregnancy, 424–433
injury in. See *Crash injuries, automobile.*
investigation of, 859–863
involving pedestrians, 857–858, *857, 858*, 861
involving trains, 858
physics of, 847–848, *848*
single-vehicle, 861–863, *861, 862*
suicidal, 861, *862*
weather and, 1635–1637
Automobile bomb, 589–591
Automobile drivers, carbon monoxide levels in, 846
Automobile exhaust, and carbon monoxide poisoning, *842*, 843, 846
Automobile-pedestrian accidents, 857–858, *857, 858*
Automobile seat belts. See *Seat belts, automobile.*
Autonomic nerves. See also *Nerves.*
dysreflexia of, after spinal cord injury, 82
Autonomic nervous system, trauma and, 386–387
Autopsy, bacteriologic studies in, 999
biochemical studies in, 999
clothing examination in, 997
in firearm fatalities, 523–524
findings in, as evidence, 1002
hospital, 971–972, 980
identification procedures in, 999–1000
in burn deaths, 723–727, 1000–1002
in cancer deaths, 1678–1679
in carbon monoxide poisoning, 843–845, *843–847*, 848(t)
in drowning, 639, 1323–1328
in drug abuse deaths, 835–837
in firearm deaths, 523–525
in food asphyxiation deaths, 1616
in heart disease deaths, 1679
in high altitude residents, 1295, 1302–1306, *1303–1305*
in hypothermic deaths, 763–764, *763, 764*
in workmen's compensation cases, 1675–1680
injury from, 908–909

Autopsy (*Continued*)
  medicolegal, 972, 995–1003
  nonofficial, 971–972
    statutes regulating, 980
  of exhumed corpses, 1000
  official, 972, 995–1003
  radiography in, in firearm deaths, 524
  religious attitudes toward, 975–976
  statutes regulating, 980
  toxicologic analysis in, 999
  toxicologic analysis prior to, 802
Autumn crocus, 1513–1514
Avascular necrosis, of bone, 346–347
    in talar fractures, 333–334
    in tarsal fractures, 332
Aviation accidents, 875–885. See also *Aircraft accidents.*
Aviators' aeroembolism, 128, 641
Avulsion, of ankle ligaments, *321, 322*
  of knee ligaments, 307
  of patellar tendon, 301
  of penile skin, 240
  of quadriceps muscle, 301
  of scalp, 37
  of teeth, *158*, 159, 167, *167, 168*
  of tibial tubercle, 304
Avulsion fractures. See also *Fractures.*
  of iliac spines, 338, *338*
  of ilium, in motorcycle accidents, 339
  of ischial tuberosity, 338, *338*
  of medial malleolus, *322*
  of pelvis, 338–339, *338*
  of ulnar styloid process, 284
Axillary artery, injuries of, acute, 222, 223
    chronic, 224, 225
Axonotmesis, 67
Azalea, 1490–1491
Azadarin, 1521
Azaridine, 1521
Azathioprine, injury from, 1201–1202

Bacillus anthracis, and wound infection, 10
Bacteremia, benign, 10
  tests for, at autopsy, 999
Bacteria, causing food poisoning, incubation periods for, *1589*
Bacterial endocarditis, posttraumatic, 16, *16*
Bacterial food poisoning, 1588–1612. See also *Food poisoning, bacterial.*
Bacterial infections, 1372–1375. See also *Infections.*
Bacteriophage typing, 1598, 1601, 1605, 1609
Bacteroides fragilis infection, intrauterine devices and, 256–257
Bahama tea plant, 1549–1550
Baker's cyst, 304
Balantidiasis, 1348–1349, *1349*
Ballistics, 527–569
  bullet identification in, 560–561, *561*
  cartridge identification in, 557–560, *557, 559, 560*

Ballistics (*Continued*)
  defined, 527–528
  evidence preservation in, 561–569
  exterior, defined, 527
  historical development of, 532–537
  identification methods in, 557–561, *557, 559–561*
  instrumentation in, 530–531, *531*
  interior, defined, 527
  physics of, 528
  terminal, defined, 527
  terminology of, 527–528
  tests in, for firearm discharge residue, 565–567
  wound, defined, 527
Ballistics coefficient, 529
Ballistics laboratory, 529–532
Ballistics report, 532, *533–535*
Baneberry, 1525
Barbados nut plant, 1497–1498
Barberio's test, for semen, 953
Barbiturates, and alcohol, synergistic effect of, 823
  and fever, 711
  and hypothermia, 762
  in postmortem vitreous humor, 1051
  injury from, in porphyria, 1246
  poisoning by, suicidal, 1007
  use of, 826–827
Barium carbide, spontaneous combustion of, 738
Barium enema, injury from, 695–696, 904
Barium sulfate, as contrast medium, 695–696
Barodontalgia, 637
Barometric pressure. See *Atmospheric pressure.*
Barosinusitis, 637
Barotalgia, 136, 637
Barotrauma, 636–644. See also *Dysbarism; High altitude.*
  decreased atmospheric pressure and, 641–644
  in divers, 636–640
  increased atmospheric pressure and, 636–640
  of ear, 136, 637
  of eye, 128
  of lung, 636–637
Barracuda, 1406, *1406*
Barrel, firearm, bullet markings from, 560–561, *560, 561*
    choke, 515–516
    cylinder, 515
    impression of, in self-inflicted firearm wounds, 37
    in shotguns, 515–516
    manufacture of, 554–555, *555*
    rifling of, 529, *529*, 554–555, *555*
    size of, 510–511
Barton's fracture, 283
Basal metabolism, 701
Basal skull fracture, 38
Baseball finger, 372
Baseball players, vascular injuries in, 225
Bathtub death, 1330–1332, *1331*
Battered child, 500–509, *501–505*. See also *Child abuse.*
Battery, unauthorized medical treatment as, 693

Beach apple plant, 1495–1496, *1496*
Bead tree, 1521–1522
Bear's foot plant, 1526
Beat elbow, 1184
Beat hand, 1184
Beat knee, 1184
Bedbugs, 1449
Bedsores, after spinal cord injury, 83
Behavior, effect of weather and climate on, 1627–1642
Belladonna, 1532–1533
Bellyache bush, 1498–1499
Bends, 642–643
Bennett's fracture, 374
Benzene, eye injury from, 129
Benzidine test, for bloodstains, 810
Benzodiazepines, injury from, 1581–1583
Benzoyl peroxide, spontaneous combustion of, 738
Berlandier lobelia, 1483
Berlin's edema, 109
Be-still tree, 1479–1481, *1480*
Beta burn, 634
Beta-phenylethylamine, 1520
Beta rays, 680
Biceps tendon, injuries of, 262, 272
Bicycle accidents, 858–859
Bile, toxicologic examination of, 804
Bile ducts, radiography of, 687, 688
  surgery of, complications of, 1230
Bilirubin, in postmortem blood, 1037, 1037(t)
  in postmortem cerebrospinal fluid, 1045
  in postmortem vitreous humor, 1049
Bioavailability, of drugs and chemicals, 1574–1575
Biochemical analysis, for wound timing, 26
  postmortem, 999
    in sudden infant death, 1025, 1025(t)
    of blood, 1034–1043, *1036*, 1037(t), *1038*, 1040(t), *1041*, 1042(t), 1043(t)
Bioequivalence, of drugs and chemicals, 1574–1575
Biogenic amines, extraction of, for wound timing, 26–28
Biologic rhythm, 1629
Biometeorology, pathologic, 1627–1642, 1630(t)–1632(t)
Biopsy, percutaneous pleural, injury from, 209
Birth, premature. See *Premature infants.*
  "wrongful," legal case involving, 491–493
Birth defects. See also *Fetus, injuries of.*
  and action for "wrongful birth," 491–493
  and time of conception, 634
  antibiotics and, 1199–1200
  causes of, *1620*
  hormones and, 1200
  intrauterine devices and, 1617–1626
  litigation involving, 491–493, 1617–1626
  methotrexate and, 1198–1199

Birth injuries, 436–486
breech delivery and, 439, *440, 441*, 446, *449*
causes of, 437–438
cephalic delivery and, 447–456, *448–452*, 454(t), *455*
crush, 439–441, *440*
hypoxic, 439(t), 456–484, 456(t), 466(t). See also *Hypoxic injuries.*
iatrogenic, 437–438
in premature infants, 482–483
mechanical, 439–456, 439(t), 454(t)
of abdomen, crush, 439–441, *440*
of adipose tissue, 363–364
of brain, 447–456, *452*, 454(t), *455*
of brain stem, 441–447, 441(t), *443, 445*
of central nervous system, 439(t), 456–484, 456(t), 466(t)
mechanical, 439(t), 441–456, 454(t)
of eye, 89, 93, 109
of head, 447–456, *448–452*, 454(t), *455*
of liver, 439–441, *440, 441*
of maxilla, 163
of oral structures, 163
of retina, 109
of soft tissues, *449*
of spine, 441–447, 441(t), *442–446*
Birth rate, seasonal variations in, 1634
Bismuth stomatitis, 191
Bitemark evidence,1143–1147, *1144–1147*
Bites, animal, infectious disease transmission by, 1369–1377
in battered child, 503, *503*, 1143
insect, infectious disease transmission by, 1370–1377
injury from, 1447–1454
self-inflicted, 176, 497, *497*
snake, 1437–1441
Bitter almond plant, 1528
Bittersweet, European, 1542
Bivalves. See *Mollusks.*
Black eye, 90
Black-eyed Susan plant, 1504–1508, *1506–1507*
Black flies, as disease vectors, 1367
Black hairy tongue, 188
Black locust plant, 1510–1511
Black snakeroot plant, 1518
Black widow spider, 1453–1454
Blackening, around firearm entrance wound, 514, *515*
Bladder, cancer of, after spinal cord injury, 84
injuries of, 236–238
in pelvic injury, 341
radiography of, 688
Bladder dysfunction, after spinal cord injury, 79
Bladder pod plant, 1483
Blank cartridges, injury from, 525
Blast. See also *Explosion(s).*
air, 616–622
biophysics of, 619
immersion, 622–624, *623, 624*
in nuclear explosion, 633
injury from, 619–622, *620, 621.* See also *Explosion, injuries from.*
Blast (*Continued*)
immersion, physics of, 617–618, *617, 618*
solid, 624–625
underwater, 622–624, *623, 624*
Blasting devices, in mining, injury from, 1183–1184
Blasting gelatin, 581
Blastomycosis, North American, 1336
South American, 1338
Bleeding. See *Hemorrhage.*
Bleeding disorders, in therapeutic hypothermia, 768
posttraumatic, 390
Blighia sapida, 1530–1532, *1531*
Blindness. See *Visual loss.*
Blisters, in second-degree burns, 720, *721*
Blood, agglutination of, by plant toxins, 793(t), 794
alcohol levels in, measurement of, 823–824
statutory limits for, 824, 863(t)
altitude and, 1296
antemortem, vs. postmortem, 1034–1043, 1037(t), *1038*, 1040(t), *1041*
bacteria in, 10
postmortem tests for, 999
blood group antigens in. See *Blood group.*
carboxyhemoglobin levels in, in carbon monoxide poisoning, 804–805, 840, 841(t)
in fire victims, 847, 848(t)
chemical levels in, 1572–1577, 1576(t), 1578(t)–1579(t), 1580(t)
circulating volume of, posttraumatic reduction in, 8
clotting of, in disseminated intravascular coagulation, 390
in therapeutic hypothermia, 768
mechanism of, 406–407
posttraumatic, 13, 390, 407
collection of, for postmortem toxicologic examination, 999
drug levels in, 1572–1577, 1576(t), 1578(t)–1580(t)
foreign bodies in, 8, 208, 418
hypothermia and, 761
in carbon monoxide poisoning, 804–805, 840, 841(t), 847, 848(t)
in drowning, 1322–1323
in electrial injury, 660
infections of, helminthic, 1364–1366
protozoan, 1350–1354
lead levels in, 806
menstrual, identification of, 812
of fish toxic, 1420
oxygen content of, in trauma, 8, 391–392, *392*
postmortem, analysis of, 1034–1043, *1036*, 1037(t), *1038*, 1040(t), *1041*, 1042(t), 1043(t)
for timing of death, 1056(t), 1057
bilirubin in, 1037, 1037(t)
carbohydrates in, 1034–1035
cholesterol in, 1036–1037
collection of, 1052
electrolytes in, 1040–1042, *1041*
enzymes in, 1038–1039
Blood (*Continued*)
postmortem, gases in, 1042–1043, 1042(t), 1043(t)
glucose in, diagnosis of diabetes from, 1053
hormones in, 1039–1040, 1040(t)
lipids in, 1036–1037
nitrogenous compounds in, 1036–1037, *1036*
oxygen tension of, in diagnosis of asphyxia, 1056
pH of, 1043
protein in, 1037–1038, *1038*
vitamin E in, 1039
production of, trauma and, 389–390
proteins in, after spinal cord injury, 82
radiation and, 683
Blood-brain barrier, in cerebral concussion, 53–54
Blood clot. See also *Embolism; Hematoma; Thromboembolism.*
and exophthalmos, 117
and superior orbital fissure syndrome, 118
posttraumatic, 8
Blood dyscrasias, oral injury in, 154
Blood flow, impairment of. See *Ischemia.*
Blood group, ABH, identification of, from saliva, 1144–1145
from semen, 954–955
ABO, identification of, from bloodstains, 813–815. 813(t), 814(t)
from semen, 954–955
MNS, identification of, from bloodstains, 815
rhesus, identification of, from bloodstains, 815
Blood pressure, altitude and, 1298(t)
posttraumatic, 8
Blood samples, as evidence, 603
Blood transfusion, acute respiratory failure, 393
air embolization in, 416
and fever, 712
injury from 905–907
Blood types. See *Blood group.*
Blood vessels. See also *Arteries; Veins.*
aortic arch, injuries of, 206
foreign bodies in, 208
great, injuries of, 205–206
injuries of, 221–227. See also *Vascular injuries.*
intrathoracic, injuries of, 208
of brain, injuries of, 42–45, *42–44*
electrical, 659
of hand, 365
injuries of, 225, 376–379, *377, 378*
iatrogenic, 379
radiography of. See *Angiography; Arteriography.*
surgery of, complications of, 1228–1229
Bloodstains, agglutinogens in, 813–815
chromosomes in, 812
enzymes in, 816
gender origin of, 812
haptoglobins in, 815–816

Bloodstains (*Continued*)
 identification of, 810–817
 individual source of, 813–816
 proteins in, 816
 racial origin of, 812–813
 species origin of, 811–812
 typing of, 813–816, 813(t), 814(t)
Blow out fracture, 146
Blowflies. See *Fly(ies), sarcosaprophagous.*
Blowguns, injury from, 1172
Blue cardinal flower plant, 1484
Blue lobelia plant, 1484
Blunt injuries, of abdomen, and cardiac injury, 204
  and ruptured spleen, 211–212
  diagnosis of, 216
  in children, 216
   battered, *502*, 503, *503*, 504
  in domestic accidents, 899–900
  in seat belt syndrome, 216
 of arteries, 223–224
 of bladder, 236–238
 of blood vessels, 223–224
 of chest, 202, 203
 of colon, 220
 of diaphragm, 207
 of duodenum, 216–217
 of esophagus, 206
 of fetus, in automobile accidents, 425–427
 of great vessels, 205–206
 of kidney, 230, 231
 of large intestine, 220
 of liver, 212–213
 of lung, 202
 of penis, 240–241
 of rectum, 220
 of renal pedicle, 229
 of scrotum, 241
 of small intestine, 217
 of stomach, 216
 of testis, 241
 of tracheobronchial tree, 203
 of ureter, 233
 of urethra, 238–239
 of uterus, 255
  in automobile accidents, 424–425
 of vagina, non–sex-related, 252–253
  sex-related, 248–252
 postmortem examination, 998
Body, foreign. See *Foreign body.*
 human, dead. See *Corpse.*
  elastic properties of, 4
  principal meteorologic receptors of, 1627–1633, 1628(t)–1629(t), 1630(t)–1632(t)
Body image, and organ transplantation, 990–994
Body lice, 1450–1451
 as disease vectors, 1367
Body temperature, in hypothermia, 758–763
 maintenance of, 701–702
  after spinal cord injury, 81
  in cold, 759
  in heat, 701–702, 709–710
Bojer plant, 1483
Bolt face, firearm, manufacture of, 555–557, *556*, *557*
Bomb(s). See also *Explosives; Mines.*
 atomic, injury from, 683–684
  of eye, 125
 automobile, 589–591
 booby trap, 586, *586*, 594–595, *594*
 car, 589–591
 classification of, 571–572
 explosive, 581–594
  from commercial explosives, 581–588, *581–583*, *585*, *586*
  from improvised explosives, 588–594, *589*
 fragments of, as evidence, 602
 incendiary, 572–578, *573–577*
  investigation of, 575–578
 investigation of, 570–611
 letter, 587
 mortar, 596–598, *597*, *598*
 nail, 581–582, *581*
 nuclear, 633–634
 pipe, 588
 rocket, 595–596, *595*
 time, 584–587, *585*, *586*
 types of, 571–572
Bombing(s). See also *Blast; Explosion(s).*
 explosive, 578–611
  air blast in, 616–622
  biologic evidence in, 603, 603(t)
  burns in, 615–616, *616*, 634
  deafness after, 620
  debris from, examination of, 601–603
  investigation of, 600–608, 603(t), *608*
  injuries from, 612–635
   abrasion, 626–630, *625–630*
   contusion, 626–630, *625–630*
   crush, 630–631, *631*
   fracture, 325, 625
   laceration, 626–630, *625–630*
   musculoskeletal, 625
   of ear, 619–620
   of eye, 630
   of leg, 625
   of lung, 620–621, *620*, *621*
   of skin, 626–630, *625–630*
  scene of, examination of, for evidence, 600–603
    for human remains, 612–614, *613*, *614*
  tissue disruption from, 612–615, *613–615*
  victims of, determining number of, 603, 612–614, *613*, *614*
   identification of, 614–615, *614*, *615*
 incendiary, 572–578, *573–577*
  investigation of, 575–578, *575–577*
Bone(s). See also names of specific bones.
 atrophy of, acute, traumatic, 349, *350*
 avascular necrosis of, posttraumatic, 332, 333–334, 346–347
 changes in, dating of skeletal remains from, 1102, 1104–1106
 cysts of, oral injury and, 149–150, *150*
Bone(s) (*Continued*)
 demineralization of, after spinal cord injury, 81–82
 density of, in Negro vs. Caucasian, 154
  oral injury and, 154
 ectopic, formation of, after spinal cord injury, 83–84
 epiphyses of, dating of skeletal remains from, 1105
 facial, racial differences in, 1108–1111, 1108(t), *1109*, *1110*
 fissuring of, in electrical injury, 657
 fractures of. See *Fracture(s).*
 infection of. See *Osteomyelitis.*
 inflammation of. See *Osteitis; Osteomyelitis.*
 injuries of, 259–361
  and fat embolism, 409
  electrical, 656–657
  frostbite, 767–768
  radiation, 682
 long, dating of skeletal remains from, 1104–1105
 marble, and oral injury, 153
 "melting" of, in electrical injury, 657
 necrosis of, avascular, 332, 333–334, 346–347
  radiation therapy and, 196, *196*
 ossification of, dating of skeletal remains from, 1105
 radiography of, 687
 systemic diseases affecting, 150–154, *151–153*
Booby trap, bombs, 586, *586*, 594–595, *594*
Bore, of firearm, 510–511
Botulism, 1589–1596, *1591–1593*
Bougienage, injury from, 209
Bowel. See *Intestine.*
Bowel dysfunction, after spinal cord injury, 79
Boyd and Griffin's classification, of hip fractures, *293*
Brachial artery, injuries of, acute, 222, 223
  chronic, 224–225
Brachial plexus, injuries of, 261, *261*
Bracken, 1550–1551
Brain. See also *Cerebral.*
 abscess of, 45, 50
  mycotic, *11*, *12*
 accessory elements of, injury of, 42–45, *42–44*
 aneurysm in, traumatic, 47
 angiography of, 688
 atrophy of, in chronic alcoholism, 822–823
 concussion of, 53–55
  acceleration vs. compression, 34–35
  vascular changes after, 42
 disease of, head injury and, 56–58, *57*
 edema of, 48–50
 fat embolism in, 411
 hemorrhage in, 45–47, *46–49*.
   See also *Hemorrhage, intracranial; Subdural hematoma.*
  cold and, 765

Brain (*Continued*)
hemorrhage, in carbon monoxide poisoning, *844*, 845
perinatal, hypoxic injury in, 462–477, *466–476*, 466(t)
herniation of, 49–50, *49*
perinatal, 445
in hypothermia, 759
infarction of, as indication of death, 23
perinatal, 462–477, *466–476*, 466(t)
in premature infants, 466–473, *466–473*, 466(t)
patterns of, 464–466, 466(t)
injuries of, 45–60
after whiplash injury, 63
alcoholic, 822–823
concussion, 34, 51–53, *51*, *52*
acceleration vs. compression, 34–35
blood-brain barrier in, 53–54
vascular changes after, 42
contusion, 46–47, *47–49*
electrical, 659
healing of, 55–56
in carbon monoxide poisoning, 843–844, *843–846*
in children, 59–60
in heat stroke, 707–709, *707–709*
in infants, 59–60
microscopic, 51–53
neuronal, 50–51
of accessory elements, 42–45, *42–44*
perinatal, 447–456, *452*, 454(t), *455*, 462–477, *466–476*, 466(t)
hypoxic, 462–477, *466–476*, 466(t)
scar formation in, 55
thermal, 726
timing of, 55–56
vascular, 42–45, *42–44*
electrical, 659
ischemia of, 8, 47–48, *53*, *54*. See also *Brain, infarction of*.
postmortem findings in, in burn victim, 726
thrombosis in, in children, 59
tissue of, embolization of, 416–417
Brain damage, assessment of, 52
in premature infants, 472–473, *472*, *473*, 482–483
ischemic, 8, 47–49, *53*, *54*
minimal, 481–482
perinatal, 462–484, 466(t)
latent, 481–482
sequelae of, 472–473, *472*, *473*, 475–476, *476*, 479–484
prenatal, 480–481
therapeutic hypothermia and, 768
Brain mushroom, 1553–1554
Brain stem, hemorrhage in, 466(t)
herniation of, perinatal, 445, *445*
in loss of consciousness, 52
injury of, compression, perinatal, 443–445, *444*, *445*
electrical, 649
perinatal, 441–447, 441(t), *443*, *445*
Brain stem (*Continued*)
perinatal, traction, 443–446, *443–445*
Brake fern, 1550–1551
Breach of contract, by physician, 1653–1654
damages for, vs. tort damages, 1665
Breach of duty, in negligence, 1645–1646
Breach of warranty, treatment failure as, 693
Bread poisoning, 1486, 1487
Breast, female, injuries of, 361–363, *362*
steatonecrosis in, 361–363, *362*
radiography of, 688
surgery of, complications of, 1233
male, enlargement of, after spinal cord injury, 82
Breech delivery, liver rupture in, 439, *440*, *441*
soft tissue injury in, *449*
spinal injury in, 446
Breech face, firearm, manufacture of, 555–557, *556*, *557*
Bromate, in explosives, test for, 605
Bronchography, 688
Bronchopneumonia, after hip fracture, 888
Bronchoscopy, complications of, 1238
Bronchospasm, in tracheal intubation, 1254
postoperative, 1245
Bronchus(i), foreign bodies in, 207–208
injuries of, 202–204
thermal, 724
postmortem findings in, in burn victims, 724
radiography of, 688
Brown recluse spider, 1452–1453
Brucellosis, 1373–1374
Brucine, 1519
Bruise. See *Contusion*.
Bruxism, 148, 175, 497
in narcotic addicts, 148, *1136*, 1137
Bucket handle injury, of pelvis, 343, *343*
Bullet(s). See also *Cartridge(s)*.
accidental characteristics of, 560–561, *560*, *561*
as cardiovascular foreign body, 208, 418
as evidence, 562–563, *562*
ballistics coefficient for, 529
characteristics of, 560–561, *560*, *561*
class characteristics of, 560–561, *560*
examination of, 560–561, *560*, *561*. See also *Ballistics*.
gravitational forces on, 528, *528*
gross characteristics of, 560–561, *560*
identification of, 560–561, *560*, *561*
individual characteristics of, 560–561, *561*
kinetic energy of, 528
Bullet(s) (*Continued*)
markings on, 560–561, *560*, *561*
primary characteristics of, 560–561, *560*
radiography of, 1156–1157
secondary characteristics of, 560–561, *560*, *561*
tail-wag of, 515
track of, 525
trajectory of, 528, *528*
tumbling of, 515
types of, 543–550, *545–550*, *554*
velocity of, 528, *546*
Bullet track, 525
Bullet wound. See *Firearm wound(s)*.
Bullous keratopathy, 98, *98*
in chemical burns, 126
Bur plant, 1541
in malpractice cases, 1653
Burden of proof, in products liability cases, 1263–1264, 1656–1657
Burial, statutes regulating, 971
testamentary instructions for, 979–980
Burn(s), 715–727, 716(t), *718*, 720(t), *721*
acids, 718, 1581, *1582*
of eye, 125–126
vs. alkali burn, 125, 127–128
alkali, 718, 1581
vs. acid burn, 125, 127–128
antemortem, vs. postmortem, 1069–1070
arc, 718
around firearm entrance wound, 513–514
beta, 634
brain in, 726
causes of, 717–719
central nervous system in, 726
chemical, 1175–1176, 1176–1177, 1581, *1582*
acid, vs. alkali, 125, 127–128
of esophagus, 206–207
of eye, 125–128, *126*, *127*
of oral cavity, 189–192, *190*, *191*, 1177, 1581, *1582*
of stomach, 1581, *1582*
of vagina, 253–255
physiologic effects of, 722
postmortem, 1070
classification of, 719–721, *721*
complications of, 722–723
death from, autopsy in, 723–727, 1000–1002
diathermic, of eye, 121
effects of, local, 719–722, 720(t), *721*
systemic, 722–723
electrical, 205, 651–655, *651–654*
of eye, 120, 661
of hand, 380–381
of muscle, 656
of oral cavity, 193–194, *194*
types of, 718–719, *718*
electrothermal, 718
endocrine system in, 726
extent of, estimation of, 719
first-degree, 719, 720(t), *721*
flash, electrical, 718
explosion, 615–616, *616*, 634

Burn(s) (*Continued*)
flash, of eye, 123
from clothing, 892
from hot pavement, 719
full-thickness, 721
gastrointestinal system in, 726
heart in, 722, 725
iatrogenic, diathermic, 121
laser, 122
radiation, 123–125, 695
in aircraft accidents, 882(t)
in battered child syndrome, 504–505, *505*
in domestic accidents, 889–892, *889*, *891*
in laboratories, 1175–1176
in warfare, 718
incidence of, 717–718, 717(t)
infection of, 723
postmortem examination for, 724
infrared, of eye, 121
kidneys in, 725–726
laser, of eye, 122
lightning, 669, *669*
liver in, 725
lymphatic system in, 725
metabolic response to, 722–723
microwave, of eye, 121
musculoskeletal system in, 726–727
occupational, 717–718, 1175–1176
of esophagus, chemical, 206–207
of eye, chemical, 125–128, *126*, *127*
diathermic, 121
electrical, 120, 661
flame, 119
iatrogenic, 121, 122, 123–125
laser, 122
microwave, 121
radiation, 123–125
solar, 123
of hand, 380
electrical, 380–381
of muscle, electrical, 656
of oral cavity, 193–194, *194*
chemical, 189–192, *190*, *191*
electrical, 193–194, *194*
of vagina, chemical, 253–255
partial-thickness, 721
pathophysiology of, 719–723
physiologic effects of, 719–723
postmortem, accidental infliction of, 1066, *1066*, 1069–1070
deliberate infliction of, 1062
for concealment of homicide, 1063
radiation, 682–683
in fluoroscopy, 695
in nuclear explosion, 634
of eye, 121–125
respiratory system in, 724–725
rule of nines for, 719, *891*
sadistic, 963
second-degree, 719–720, 720(t), *721*
self-inflicted, 497
shock in, 722
solar, of eye, 123
spleen in, 725
suicidal, 1006
third-degree, 720–721, 720(t), *721*

Burn(s) (*Continued*)
treatment of, complications of, 1235–1236
history of, 715–716
ulcer formation after, 396, *398*
Burn toxin, 722
Burning bush, 1530
Burrow weed, 1485
Bursitis, of elbow, 272
of foot, 329
of hip, 285
of knee, 304–306, *305*
olecranon, 272
Burst pelvis, 342–343
Bursting fracture, of skull, 40, *41*
Bushman's poison plant, 1477–1478
Busulfan, injury from, 1198
Buttercup, celery-leaved, 1527
Butyl alcohol, poisoning by, 820

Cadaver. See also *Corpse*.
infection from, 908–909
radiation injury from, 909
statutes concerning, 980
Caddisflies, 1454
Cadmium poisoning, food-borne, 788
Café coronary, 1614–1616
Caisson disease, 637, 641–644
eye injury in, 128
Calcaneus, fractures of, 334–336, *334*
Calcific aortic stenosis, *14*
Calcific tendinitis, 285
of hand, 372
Calcification, in ankle, 320
in hip, 285
in knee, 304
in shoulder, 262
in wrist, 279
periarticular, in burn victims, 727
posttraumatic, 348–349
Calcium, in explosives, tests for, 606
in postmortem blood, 1041
in postmortem vitreous humor, 1050
metabolism of, disorders of, postmortem diagnosis of, 1054–1055
Calcium carbide, spontaneous combustion of, 738
Calcium oxide, spontaneous combustion of, 738
Calculus formation, after spinal cord injury, 82–83
Calf muscle, rupture of, 315–316
Caliber, of firearm, 510–511, 529, *529*
Caliche, spontaneous combustion of, 738
Calico bush, 1489
Calliphoridae. See *Fly(ies), sarcosaprophagous*.
Camas plant, 1518
Campanulaceae, toxic, 1483–1484
Cancer. See also *Carcinoma*.
after spinal cord injury, 84
agents causing. See *Carcinogen(s)*.
asbestos-related, 1278, 1279(t)–1281(t), 1284–1286, *1285*
death from, autopsy in, 1678–1679
frostbite and, 768
hormone treatment for, 1200

Cancer (*Continued*)
in high altitude residents, 1306
in scars, 371
metastasis of, trauma and, 417–418
occupational-environmental, causes of, 20, 1273(t)–1274(t)
signal tumors in, 1275–1276
of brain, head trauma and, 58
of gastrointestinal tract, asbestos-related, 1279(t)–1281(t), 1286
of lung, asbestos-related, 1279(t)–1281(t), 1284–1285, *1285*
of oral structures, 178, *178*
alcohol and, 191
iatrogenic injuries and, 188
nicotine and, 191–192, *192*
of skin, radiation and, 682
of testis, posttraumatic, 241
osteomyelitis and, 19, *19*
preexisting, trauma and, 18–19, 417–418
pyretotherapy for, 713
radiation and, 682, 684
radiation therapy for. See *Radiation, therapeutic*.
trauma and, 18–20
Cancer cells, embolization of, 417–418, *417*
Candelabra cactus, 1493
Candida, burn wound infection from, 723
Candidiasis, 1337
oral, antibiotics and, 188, *189*
Candlenut plant, 1491–1492
Cannabinoids, effects of, 830
Cannabis. See *Marihuana*.
Caper spurge plant, 1494
Capsaicin, 1533
Capsicum frutescens, 1533
Capsulitis, adhesive, 270–271
Caput succedaneum, 448, *448*
Car. See *Automobile*.
Car bomb, 589–591
Carbamates, as food contaminants, 788
Carbides, spontaneous combustion of, 738
Carbohydrates, in postmortem blood, 1034–1035
in postmortem cerebrospinal fluid, 1043–1044
in postmortem vitreous humor, 1046–1047, *1047*
metabolism of, disorders of, postmortem diagnosis of, 1053
trauma and, 390–391
Carbon, activation of combustion of, 731–732
Carbon dioxide, in postmortem blood, 1042
in postmortem vitreous humor, 1049–1050
solid, injury from, 1177
Carbon monoxide, absorption of, 840
ear injury from, 137
exposure to, 840–849
permissible, levels of, 840
sources of, 842–843, *842*
inhalation of. See *Carbon monoxide poisoning*.
levels of, in automobile exhaust, *842*, 843

Carbon monoxide (*Continued*)
levels of, in cigarette smokers, 842–843
in fires, 841–842
in spaceship cabins, 842
permissible, 840
metabolism of, 840
occupational exposure levels for, 840
sources of, 842–843, *842*
Carbon monoxide poisoning, and automobile accidents, 846
and sudden infant death, 1026
as cause of death in fire, postmortem examination for, 1069–1070
autopsy in, 843–845, *843–847*, 848(t)
brain in, 843–844, *843–846*
carboxyhemoglobin levels in, 804–805, 840, 841(t)
in fire victims, 1069–1070
central nervous system in, 843–845, *843–846*
death from, 843–845
investigation of, 845–846
in coal mine explosions, 632
in domestic accidents, 895
in domestic gas explosions, *632*, 633
in fires, 202–203, 841–842, 889, 890–891, 1069–1070
pallidal necrosis in, 843–844, *843*, *846*
sequelae of, 841
symptoms of, 841–842, 841(t)
suicidal, 1007
toxicologic analysis in, 804–805, 846–848, *847*, 848(t)
Carbonization, of tissue, in third-degree burns, 720–721, *721*
Carbonyl hemoglobin. See *Carboxyhemoglobin.*
in carbon monoxide poisoning, 804–805, 840, 841(t)
in fire victims, 847, 848(t)
postmortem analysis of, 1069–1070
Carcinogen(s), aflatoxins as, 792
alcohol as, 191, 820
asbestos as, 1278, 1279(t)-1281(t), 1284–1286, *1285*
in food, cycasin as, 793(t), 795
diethylstilbestrol as, 788
from wood smoke, 789
nitrosamines as, 797
pesticides as, 788
in laboratories, 1179
introduction of, through wound, 20
nicotine as, 191–192, *192*
occupational exposure to, 20, 1179, 1278–1279, 1279(t)
pesticides as, 788
Carcinoma. See also *Cancer.*
asbestos-related, 1279(t)–1281(t), 1284–1286, *1285*
epidermoid, of oral structures, 178, *178*
alcohol and, 191
iatrogenic injuries and, 188
nicotine and, 191–192, *192*
Carcinoma (*Continued*)
epidermoid, osteomyelitis and, 19, *19*
trauma and, 20
radiation therapy for. See *Radiation, therapeutic.*
Cardiac arrhythmias. See *Arrhythmias.*
Cardiac catheterization, altitude and, 1299, 1300(t)
injury from, 209, 672, 906, *906*
Cardiac disorders, after head injury, 13
treatment of, electrical injury in, 672
Cardiac massage, complications of, 1238
Cardiac neurosis, intracardiac foreign bodies and, 418
Cardiac pacemaker, implantation of, complications of, 209, 1228
malfunction of, 672
Cardiac tamponade, *13*, *14*, 204
Cardinal flower, 1483
Cardiomyopathy, alcoholic, 821–822
Cardiopulmonary dysfunction, in chest injuries, 200, 201
Cardiopulmonary resuscitation, injury from, 209
Cardiovascular collapse, head injury in, 36–37
Cardiovascular system. See also *Blood vessels; Heart.*
altitude and, 1296
foreign bodies in, 208, 408
in heatstroke, 707
injuries of, 204–206
in aircraft accidents, 880, *881*, 882(t), 883(t)
regional anesthesia and, 1247
Cardol, 1471
Carotid artery, angiography of, injury from, 903–904
Carpal tunnel syndrome, 279, 373
Carpometacarpal joint, of thumb, dislocations of, 376
Carpus. See *Wrist.*
Carrageenan, as food preservative, toxicity of, 797
Carrion, arthropod succession in, 1073–1079, 1073(t), *1074–1077*, 1076(t), *1079*
Cartilage, in osteochondritis dissecans, 311–312, *311*, 347, *347*
of femoral condyle, fracture of, 310–311
of knee, degeneration of, 303
in osteochondritis dissecans, 311–312, *311*
injuries of, 303, 308–309
of patella, fractures of, 303
of wrist, injuries of, 279
Cartridge(s), firearm. See also *Bullet(s).*
accidental characteristics of, 558
as evidence, 563
blank, injury from, 525
centerfire, 543, *546–549*, *554*
reloaded, identification of, 560
reloading of, 553–554
characteristics of, 557–558
class characteristics of, 557–558
ejector markings on, 558
Cartridge(s) (*Continued*)
firearm, examination of, 557–560, *559*
extractor markings on, 558
firing pin markings on, *557*, 558
gross characteristics of, 557–558, *557*
hand loading of, 553–554
identification of, 557–560, *559*
ignition of, 550–551
historically, 538–539, *538*
impression-type markings on, 558–559
individual characteristics of, 558
manufacturers' markings on, 552–553, *554*
markings on, 557–561, *557*, *559*
powders for, 550–551
primary characteristics of, 557–558, *557*
primers for, 550–551
propellants for, 550–551
reloaded, identification of, 560
reloading of, 553–554
rimfire, 543, *545*, *546*
secondary characteristics of, 558
stampings on, 558–559
striations on, 558–559
types of, 543, *545–549*
for power tools, 542, *544–545*
Cashew nut plant, 1470–1471
Cassava plant, 1500–1501
Casteroil fishes, 1419, *1419*
Casting, of fractures, injury from, 908
Castor bean plant, 1501–1503, *1503*
Castor oil plant, 1501–1503, *1503*
Castration, self-inflicted, 498
Cat, postmortem injury by, 1097
Cat's milk plant, 1494–1495
Cat scratch disease, 1376–1377
oral manifestations of, 173, *174*
Cataract(s), cryosurgery for, injury from, 769
drugs and, 130
electrical burns and, 120–121, 661
in welders, 662
infrared radiation and, 121, 662
intraocular foreign bodies and, 113, *113*
microwaves and, 121
traumatic, 105–106, *105*
ultrasound and, 120
Caterpillars, 1449
Catfishes, 1411, *1411*
Catheterization, arterial, 688–689
injury from, 224
cardiac, injury from, 209, 672, 906, *906*
injury from, 696
percutaneous subclavian vein, injury from, 209
ureteral, in ureteral surgery, 235
urethral, injury from, 239
Caucasians, bone density in, 154
facial bones in, 1108–1111, 1108(t), *1109*, *1110*
identification of, from skeletal remains, 1108–1111, 1108(t), *1109*, *1110*
from teeth, 1119–1122, *1120*, *1121*

Cauliflower ear, 135
Causalgia, 329, 349, 382, 387
of hand, 382
Causation, legal, "but-for," 1661
in fetal injury, 429–433
in negligence, 1649, 1661–1664
in occupational-environmental diseases, 1271
in pregnancy complications, 429–433
Cause of action. See *Lawsuits; Liability.*
Caustics, injury from. See *Burns, chemical.*
Cavitation phenomenon, in therapeutic ultrasound, 781
Celandine, 1522–1523
Celery-leaved buttercup, 1527
Cells, hypoxia of, hypovolemia and, 8
injury of, radiation, 680–681, 683
ultrasound, 781–782
nerve. See *Neurons.*
response of, to trauma, 391–392, *392*
Cellulitis, oral, 164
Cementum, of tooth, fracture of, 165, *165*
Central nervous system. See also *Brain; Nerves.*
in decompression sickness, 643
in drug abuse, 831
injuries of, alcoholic, 822–823
hypoxic, in carbon monoxide poisoning, 843–845, *843–846*
perinatal, 439(t), 456–484, 456(t), 466(t)
of accessory elements of, 42–45, *42–44*
perinatal, hypoxic, 439(t), 456–484, 456(t), 466(t)
mechanical, 439(t), 441–456, 454(t)
thermal, 726
postmortem findings in, 726
regional anesthesia and, 1247
spinal anesthesia and, 1248–1249
Central zone, of antemortem wound, 25, *25*
Centrifuge, injury from, 1178, 1181
Cephalhematoma, perinatal, 448–450, *449*
Cephalic delivery, head injury in, 447–456, *448–452*, 454(t), *455*
Cephalopods. See *Mollusks.*
Cerbera thevetia, 1479–1481, *1480*
Cerebellar pressure cone of Cushing, 49
Cerebellum, atrophy of, in chronic alcoholism, 822
herniation of, perinatal, 445, *445*
Cerebral cortex. See *Cortex, cerebral.*
Cerebral hemorrhage, 45–47, *46–49*
cold and, 765
in infant, 59
perinatal, hypoxic injury in, 462–477, *466–477*, 466(t)
Cerebral herniation, 49–50, *49*
Cerebral infarction, as indication of death, 23
perinatal, 462–476, *466–476*, 466(t)
in premature infants, 466–473, *466–473*, 466(t)
patterns of, 464–466, 466(t)
Cerebral ischemia, 8, 47–49, *53*, *54*
Cerebral palsy, in premature infants, 472–473, *472*, *473*, 482–483
Cerebral thrombosis, in children, 59
perinatal hypoxia and, 472–473, *472*, *473*, 475–476, *476*, 479–481
Cerebrospinal fluid, analysis of, for timing of brain injury, 55
antemortem vs. postmortem, 1043–1046, 1045(t)
collection of, for postmortem toxicologic analysis, 999
enzyme levels in, in head injury, 54–55
in hydrocephalus, 50
postmortem, analysis of, 1033, 1043–1046, 1045(t)
for timing of death, 1056(t), 1057
bilirubin in, 1045
carbohydrates in, 1043–1044
electrolytes in, 1045–1046, 1045(t)
enzymes in, 1045
nitrogenous compounds in, 1044–1045
urobilinogen in, 1045
toxicologic analysis of, 804, 999
Cerebrospinal fluid otorrhea, 45, 62
Cerebrospinal fluid rhinorrhea, 45
in maxillary fracture, 145
Cerebrum, cortex of. See *Cortex, cerebral.*
hemorrhage in, 45–47, *46–49*
cold and, 765
perinatal, hypoxic injury in, 462–477, *466–477*, 466(t)
infarction of, perinatal, 462–476, *466–476*, 466(t)
in premature infants, 466–473, *466–473*, 466(t)
Cervical spine, ankylosis of, 63, 77
injuries of, 63–64
parturitional, *444*
tracheal intubation and, 1253
Cervical spondylosis, 63, 77
Cervix, uterine, anatomy and physiology of, 248
cryotherapy and, 769
injuries of, iatrogenic, 255–256
Cesium, spontaneous combustion of, 738
Cesium-137, levels of, in humans, 680
Cestrum diurnum, 1534
Cestrum nocturnum, 1534
Chagas' disease, 1352–1353, *1353*, 1367, 1376
Chain of evidence, 561
Chalcosis, 114
Chalice vine, 1539
Chanterelle, false, 1553
Chauffeur's fracture, 283–284
Cheek biting, 176
Cheek bone, fractures of, 146
racial differences in, 1108(t) 1109–1110, *1110*
Cheilosis, solar, of lips, 194
Chelidonine, 1522–1523
Chelidonium majus, 1522–1523
Chemicals, agricultural, in bombs, 581, 582, 588–589, 591, 592–594
Chemicals *(Continued)*
agricultural, injury from, 1165
asphyxiation by, 1570, 1571. See also *Carbon monoxide poisoning.*
aspiration of, 1570
bioavailability of, 1574–1575
bioequivalence of, 1574–1575
blood levels of, 1572–1577, 1576(t), 1578(t)–1579(t), 1580(t)
burns from. See *Burns, chemical.*
contaminating food, 787–799
corrosive, injury from. See *Burns, chemical.*
hazardous mixtures of, 738–739
in explosives, 581, 582, 588–594
inhalation of. See *Asphyxiation; Inhalation injury.*
injury from. See *Chemical injury.*
pharmaceutical. See *Drugs.*
poisoning by. See *Poisoning.*
spontaneous combustion of, 737–739
Chemical additives, to food, 796–797
Chemical analysis, for timing of wound, 24–28
postmortem, 999
for diagnosis of antemortem disease, 1033–1060
in sudden infant death, 1025, 1025(t)
of blood, 1034–1043, *1036*, 1037(t), *1038*, 1040(t), *1041*, 1042(t), 1043(t)
of cerebrospinal fluid, 1033, 1043–1046, 1045(t)
of vitreous humor, 1033, 1046–1052, *1047*, *1048*, *1051*
Chemical burns. See *Burns, chemical.*
Chemical elements, ignition temperature for, 730(t)
Chemical explosions, 578–579
Chemical fires, 735(t), 736–739, 737(t)
investigation of, at site, 746–747, *747*
in laboratory, 748(t), 754–757, *756*, 757(t)
Chemical gangrene, of hand, 377, *378*
Chemical injury, 787–850, 1568–1586. See also *Poisoning.*
blood levels in, 1572–1577, 1576(t), *1577*, 1578(t)–1579(t)
by ingestion, 1569–1570, 1570(t)
by inhalation, 1570, *1571*
by injection, 1572
by percutaneous absorption, 1572
by rectal administration, 1572
chronic. See *Occupational environmental diseases.*
defined, 1568
from abused drugs, 826–839
from alcohol, 818–825
from carbon monoxide, 840–849
from caustics. See *Burns, chemical.*
from food contaminants, 787–799
from therapeutic drugs. See *Drugs, therapeutic.*
gangrenous, 377, *378*
homicidal, 1569–1572, 1569(t)
in agricultural accidents, 1165
in domestic accidents, 895–896
in laboratory, 1176–1177

Chemical injury (*Continued*)
mortality rate in, 1568–1569, 1568(t), 1569(t)
of ear, 137
of esophagus, 206–207
of eye, 125–128, *126*, *127*
of hand, 377, *378*
occupational, 379
of lungs, 203, 713–714. See also *Inhalation injury*.
of nerves, 373
of stomach, 1581, *1582*
of vagina, 253–255
postmortem, 1070
routes of entry in, 1569–1572
suicidal, 1007, 1569–1572, 1569(t)
toxicologic analysis in, 804–807
Chemical neuritis, 373
Chemical preservatives, in food, toxicity of, 796–797
Chemical reactions, oxidizing. See *Oxidation reactions*.
Chemoreceptors, at high altitudes, 1297–1298
Chemosis, 92
Chenodeoxycholic acid, as experimental drug, 1211
Cherry laurel, 1528
Cherry plant, 1543
Cherry trees, 1528, 1529
Chest, flail, 200
foreign bodies in, 207–208
injuries of, 199–209
asphyxiating, 203
blunt, 200, 202, 203
cardiopulmonary dysfunction in, 200, 201
crash, *13–15*, 200, *854*, 855
crush, 7, 200
and traumatic retinopathy, 110, *111*
in explosions, 630–631, *631*
firearm, 200, *513*, *514*, 519
hemothorax in, 201
iatrogenic, 208–209
in automobile accidents, *13–15*, *854*, 855
in pedestrians, 857, *858*
mechanisms of, 199–200
penetrating, 200, 202, 203
pneumothorax in, 201–202
steering wheel, *854*, 855
types of, 200–209
with abdominal injuries, 211
with kidney injuries, 232
needle aspiration of, and spleen injury, 212
radiography of, 687
surgery of, complications of, 1227–1228
wounds of, firearm, 200, *513*, *514*, 519
stab, 200
sucking, 201
Chest tube, injury from, 209
Chest wall, injuries of, 200
Chigger mites, 1451
Chilblain, 765–766
Child abuse, 501–509, *501–505*
bites in, 503, *503*, 1143
evidence of, dental, 1137–1138, *1138*
Child abuse (*Continued*)
evidence of, radiographic, 1156
eye injuries in, 111
reporting of, 1138–1140
Children. See also *Fetus; Infant; Newborn*.
abdominal injuries in, 216
asphyxiation in, 892–895
battered, 500–509, *501–505*. See also *Child abuse*.
brain damage in, perinatal hypoxia and, 479–484
brain lesions in, 59–60
burns in, 889–892
cold panniculitis in, 766
congenital defects in, intrauterine devices and, 1617–1626
litigation involving, 433, 487–488, 491–493, 1617–1626
methotrexate and, 1198–1199
domestic accidents involving, 886–900
drowning in, 898
electrical injuries in, of oral cavity, 194, *194*
emergency treatment of, consent to, 873
firearm injuries in, 896–897, *896*, *897*
food poisoning in, 792
head banging in, 60
head injuries in, 59–60
kidney injuries in, 230
oral injuries in, 147–148
electrical, 194, *194*
poisoning in, 895–896
psychologic disorders in, after head trauma, 59–60
radiation injuries in, 682, 683
rape of, physical examination in, 955
consent to, 943
statutory, 956
restlessness of, weather and, 1634–1635
skeletal remains of, identification of, 1104–1106, 1104(t)
skull in, 38
spinal injuries in, 65
teeth in. See *Tooth, deciduous*.
unwanted, birth of, cause of action for, 491–493
ureteral injuries in, 233
vulvovaginal injuries in, 252
Chile saltpeter, spontaneous combustion of, 738
Chinaberry, 1521–1522
Chinese wisteria, 1512
Chinese wood-oil tree, 1491
Chinkerinchee plant, 1516
Chironex, 1381, *1381*, 1382, 1383(t), 1384, 1385
Chloramphenicol, injury from, of ear, 137
litigation involving, 1214
interaction of, with diphenylhydantoin, 1206
Chlorates, in explosives, tests for, 604
spontaneous combustion of, 738
Chloride, in postmortem blood, 1040, *1041*
Chloride (*Continued*)
in postmortem vitreous humor, 1049
Chlorinated hydrocarbons, as food contaminants, 788
Chlorinated naphthalenes, poisoning by, 789
Chlorite, in explosives, tests for, 604
Chloroacetophenone, burns from, 718
Chloroacetophenothane, food contamination by, 788
Chloroquine, and cataract, 130
and eye injuries, 129
Chlorpromazine, and impotence, 1198
in treatment of schizophrenia, 1207
injury from, of eye, 129
package insert warning of, 1219
Choanal atresia, in newborn, 38
Choke barrel, of shotgun, 515–516
Chokecherry plant, 1528, 1529
"Chokes," 643
Choking, on food, 1614–1616
Cholangiography, intravenous, injury from, 695
surgical use of, 1230
Cholecystectomy, complications of, 1230
Cholecystography, oral, 687
injury from, 695
Cholesterol, in postmortem blood, 1036
postmortem analysis of, for diagnosis of antemortem disease, 1055
Cholinesterase, in postmortem blood, 1039
Cholinesterase inhibitors, and cataract, 130
Chondromalacia, of patella, 303
Chordates, injury from, 1406–1429
Choriomeningitis, lymphocytic, 1369
Chorionic embolism, 416
Chorionic gonadotropin, in postmortem blood, 1040
Choroid, detachment of, 108
hemorrhage in, 108
injuries of, electrical, 120
mechanical, 108, *109*, 111
radiation, 122
Christmas flower plant, 1493–1494
Christmas rose plant, 1526–1527
Chromatolysis, in neurons, 52, 53
Chromosomes, abnormalities of, and sexual identity, 958
identification of, in bloodstains, 812
radiation injury of, 681
Chronic mountain sickness, 1308–1314, 1309(t), 1310(t), *1311–1313*
Cicuta, 1546–1547
Cicutoxin, 1546
Cigar smoking, and oral injuries, 191–192, *192*
Cigarette smokers, carbon monoxide levels in, 842–843
Cigarette smoking, and asbestos-related lung cancer, 1285, *1285*
and drug utilization, 1217
and oral injuries, 191–192, *192*

Ciguatera, 1496
Ciguatera disease, 796, 1402, 1420, 1421–1426, *1422–1424*
Ciguatoxin, *1408*
  chemistry of, 1425
Ciliary body, anatomy of, 103
  injuries of, 104–105, *104*
Cinderella syndrome, 501
Circuit, electrical, short in, 740, *740*
    partial, 740–742, *741*, *742*
Circular enamel hypoplasia, 160, *160*
Circulation, coronary, high altitude and, 1300–1302, *1304–1305*
  enteric, 1569
Circulatory failure, after trauma, 8
  in perinatal hypoxia, 458
Circulatory system, at high altitude, 1298–1302, *1298*, 1298(t), *1299*, 1300(t), *1302–1305*
  foreign bodies in, 208
  hypothermia and, 759
  injuries of, 204–206. See also *Heart, injuries of; Vascular injuries.*
Circumcision, injuries from, 240
Clams, hazardous, 1394, *1394*, 1402
Claviceps purpurea, 1552–1553
Clavicle, fracture of, 268
Claymore mine, 582, *582*, *583*
Climate. See *Weather.*
Clitocybe illudens, 1553
Clonorchiasis, 1363
Clostridium botulinum, 1588, 1589, 1590–1591, *1591*
Clostridium perfringens, 1596–1598, *1596*
Clostridium tetani, 10
Clothing, burns from, 892
  postmortem examination of, at autopsy, 997
    in firearm fatalities, 523–524
Clupeoid poisoning, 796, 1426
Coagulation, blood, disseminated intravascular, 390
      causes of, 407
      kidney failure in, 402
    in therapeutic hypothermia, 768
    mechanism of, 406–407
    posttraumatic, 13, 390, 407
Coal miners' cramps, 703
Coal miners' nystagmus, 1184
Coal miners' pneumoconiosis, 1185
Coal mining, explosions in, 632, 1183–1184
  injuries in, 1182–1184
  mortality rate in, 1182
  nontraumatic disorders in, 1184–1185
Cocaine, and fever, 711
  overdose of, 832
  use of, historically, 827
Coccidioidomycosis, 1335–1336
Coccyx, fractures of, 345
Cochlear hearing loss, 134
Cochlear-vestibular system. See also *Ear, inner.*
  anatomy of, 132–133
  measurements of hearing in, 133–134
Cockroaches, ingestion of, injury from, 1455
Coelenterates, hazardous, 1380–1389, *1380–1381*, 1383(t), *1384–1389*
Coffee bean plant, 1511–1512
Cohosh plant, 1525
Coitus. See *Sexual intercourse.*
Colchicine, 1513, 1515
Colchicum autumnale, 1513–1514
Cold, and cerebral hemorrhage, 765
  and heart disease, 765
  hypersensitivity to, 765
  injuries from, 758–774. See also *Hypothermia.*
  survival time in, 762
Cold erythema, 765
Cold panniculitis, 766
Cold syncope, 765
Cold urticaria, 765
Cold vasculitis, 765
Colistin, and kidney injuries, 401
Colitis, ulcerative, effects of drugs for, 1201–1202
Collateral ligaments, injuries of, 307
Colles' fracture, 281–283, *282*
  reverse, 283, *283*
Collisions. See also *Automobile accidents.*
  elastic, 4
  injuries in. See *Crash injuries.*
  nonelastic, 4
Colon, injuries of, 219–220. See also *Intestine(s).*
    seat belt, 856, *856*
  surgery of, complications of, 1231–1232
Colorado tick fever, 1371
Coma, drug-induced, 835
    ischemic muscular injuries in, 379
Coma vigile, 56
Combustion. See also *Fire(s).*
  activation energy for, 731–732
  as source of carbon monoxide, 842–843
  heat of, for chemical elements, 730(t)
  spontaneous, fires started by, evidence of, 747
      investigation of, 756–757
    substances capable of, 737–739
Combustion residues, from firearms, 563–567, *564–566*
Commensalism, 1343
Commotio retinae, 109
Comparison microscope, in forensic ballistics, 530–531, *531*
    bullet identification with, 561, *561*
    cartridge identification, with, 559, *559*
Compensated shock, 8
Compensation, for injuries. See *Damages.*
Compensation neurosis, 17
  vs. anxiety neurosis, 18
Complex fracture, of skull, 40
Complicated injury, defined, 19
Complications, of anesthesia, 1239–1260
  of surgery, 1226–1238
  of trauma, 8–20
Compositae, poisonous, 1484–1487
Compound fractures, 259–261
Compressed air, injury from, 1172
Compression concussion, vs. acceleration concussion, 34–35
Compression fractures, of os calcis, 335
  of pelvis, *342*
  of talus, 331–332
  of tibia, 325–328
  of wrist, 284–285
Compression injury, and traumatic retinopathy, 110, *111*
  of brain stem, perinatal, 443–446, *444*, *445*
Comptie plant, 1488–1489, *1489*
Concentrated explosion, chemical, 578
  evidence of, 600–601
  vs. dispersed explosion, 600–601
Concussion, brain, 51–53
    acceleration vs. compression, 34–35
    vascular changes after, 42
  spinal, 64–65
Condensed explosion, chemical, 579
  evidence of, 600–601
  vs. dispersed explosion, 600–601
Conductive hearing loss, 134
Cone shells, hazardous, 1394–1396, *1395–1396*
Conflagration. See *Fire(s).*
Congenital malformations. See *Birth defects.*
Congestive heart failure. See *Heart failure.*
Coniine, 1547
Conjum maculatum, 1547
Conjunctiva, anatomy of, 89, 91
  edema of, 92
  emphysema of, 92
  hemorrhage in, 91
  injuries of, chemical, 126, *127*
    drug-induced, 129
    mechanical, 91–92
    radiation, 123, 124
    thermal, 119
Consciousness, loss of. See also *Syncope.*
    in electrical injury, 658–659
    indicating brain damage, 52
Consent, age of, for statutory rape, 956
  informed, doctrine of, 693, 1669–1674
    of child, 873, 943
    to medical treatment, 1669–1674
      and disclosure of risk, 1669–1674
      and malpractice, 1654–1655
      in emergency, 873–874, 1670
      involving experimental drugs, 1211–1212
      requirements for, 1671–1673
      written form for, 697
    to radiography, 696–697
  to making of forensic dental impressions, 1140–1141
  to postmortem odontologic examination, 1130–1132
  to sexual intercourse, age and, 956
  validity of, 941
Conservation of energy, 4

Conservation of momentum, 4
Contact firearm wounds, 7–8, *47*, 520–521
  contact ring of, 37, *41*
Conti plant, 1488–1489, *1489*
Contraceptive, intrauterine. See *Intrauterine devices.*
  oral, and toxic optic neuropathy, 131
    injury from, legal case involving, 1214
  postcoital, for rape victim, 955–956
Contract, breach of, by physician, 1653–1654
    damages for, vs. tort damages, 1665
  law of, and products liability, 1656
Contracture, Dupuytren's, 330, 382–383
    muscular, after nerve injury, 69
      ischemic, 377–378, *378*
    Volkmann's, 69, 349, 377–378, *378*
Contralateral injury, defined, 7
  of head, 35, 46
Contrast media, radiographic, injury from, 186, *187*, 690–692, 695–696, 904
Contrast studies, radiographic, 687
Contrecoup fracture, of skull, 40
Contrecoup injury, 7
Controlled Substances Act of 1970, drug classification in, 828–829
Contusion(s), around firearm entrance wound, 512–513
  defined, 5, *5*, *6*, *7*
  in battered child syndrome, 501–503, *501*, *502*
  in rape victim, 946–947
  of bladder, 237
  of brain, 46–47, *47–49*
  of choroid, 108
  of heart, 204–205
    in steering wheel injury, 12
  of kidney, 231
    radiographic appearance of, 232
  of lung, 7, 202
  of skin, from explosion missiles, 626–630, *625–630*
  of spine, 64–65
  retroperitoneal, *6*
  timing of, 22
  vs. postmortem hypostasis, 5, 36
Contusion compression, of spinal cord, 65
Convalla toxin, 1514
Convallaria majalis, 1514–1515
Convulsions, drug-induced, 1200–1201
"Cook-off," 578
Cooley's anemia, oral manifestations of, 153, *153*
Cooling, atmospheric, and physiologic processes, 1630, 1630(t)–1632(t)
  rate of, in submerged body, 1319
Coontie plant, 1488–1489, *1489*
Co-op sugar, 589
Coracoid process, fracture of, 269
Coral, poisonous, 1386
  abrasions from, 1389, *1389*
Coral plant, 1499
Coral sumac, 1473–1474
Corn lily, 1517–1518
Corn picker, hand injuries from, 380
Cornea, 92–98
  anatomy of, 92–93, *93*
  edema of, 93
    intraocular foreign body and, 112, *113*
  infection of. See *Keratitis.*
  injuries of, chemical, 126–127, *126*, *127*
    drug-induced, 129
    electrical, 120–121
    mechanical, 92–98, *94–98*
    radiation, 122, 123, 124
    thermal, 119
Cornucopia plant, 1534
Coronary artery thrombosis, trauma and, 13, *15*
Coronary circulation, at high altitude, 1300–1302, *1304–1305*
Coronary tree, *1304*, *1305*
Corpse, age of, dental evidence of, 1124–1125, *1124*
    radiographic evidence of, 1157–1158
    skeletal evidence of, 1104–1106, 1104(t), 1157–1158
  arthropod succession in, 1073–1079, 1073(t), *1074–1077*, 1076(t), *1079*
  autopsied, infection from, 908–909
    radiation injury from, 909
    statutes concerning, 980
  autopsy of. See *Autopsy.*
  burial of, statutes regulating, 971
    testamentary instructions for, 979–980
  buried, arthropod succession in, 1078–1079, *1079*
  burned, identification of, 1000–1002
  clothing of, examination of, 997, 523–524
  drowned, algae in, 1326–1327
    decomposition of, 1319–1321, *1319–1321*
    diatoms in, *1321*, 1326–1328
    identification of, 1317–1319, *1318*
    injuries of, 1068, *1068*, 1097–1098, 1328, *1329*
      from recovery of, 1065–1066
    postmortem findings in, 1323–1328
    water in, 1324–1325
  effects of sarcosaprophagous flies on, 1079–1081, *1083*, *1085*
  English civil law concerning, 970–971
  examination of. See *Autopsy.*
    odontologic, 999–1000, 1115–1153
  exhumation of, injury in, 1064–1065, *1065*
  exhumed, autopsy of, 1000
  exposed, arthropod succession in, 1073–1078, 1073(t), *1074–1076*, 1076(t), *1077*
  gender of, dental evidence of, 1123–1124
    radiographic evidence of, 1157
Corpse (*Continued*)
  gender of, skeletal evidence of, 1102, 1106–1108, 1106(t), 1157
  identification of, 995–996, *996*
    fingerprinting for, 33
    from dental photographs, 1134–1136, *1135*, *1136*
    from dental radiographs, 1134–1136, *1135*, *1136*
    from oral structures, 999–1000, 1115–1153
    from radiographs, 1157–1158
    from skeletal remains, 1101–1115. See also *Skeletal remains.*
    from teeth, 999–1000, 1115–1153
    in explosions, 614–615, *614*, *615*
    odontologic, methods of, 1128–1130, *1130–1132*
  illegal disposal of, 1063–1064
  injury of. See *Postmortem injuries.*
  livor mortis in, 34, 997
    in carbon monoxide poisoning, 843, 847, *847*
  mutilation of, 1064. See also *Postmortem injuries.*
  odontologic examination of, 999–1000, 1115–1153
  organ transplants from. See *Transplants, organ.*
  oviposition in, by sarcosaprophagous flies, 1080–1084, *1083*
  postmortem injuries of. See *Postmortem injuries.*
  property of, 967–977
    religious attitudes concerning, 975–976
  race of, dental evidence of, 1119–1122, *1119–1122*
    radiographic evidence of, 1158
    skeletal evidence of, 1102–1103, 1108–1111, 1108(t), *1109*, *1110*, 1158
  rigor mortis in, 34, 997
    in drowning, 1319–1320
  skeletal remains of. See *Skeletal remains.*
  stature of, skeletal evidence of, 1103, 1111–1115, 1158
  unidentified, dental examination of, 999–1000
    disposition of, statutes regulating, 980
  United States law concerning, 971–975, 974(t)
  weathering of, 1070–1071
Corrosive, injury from. See *Burns, chemical.*
Corrosive esophagitis, 206–207
Corrosive vaginitis, potassium permanganate and, 254–255
Cortex, cerebral, atrophy of, in chronic alcoholism, 822
    contusions of, 46
    gutter hemorrhage, in, 46
    infarction in, perinatal, *466*, 466(t), 473–477, *474–476*
Corticosteroids, and cataract, 130
  and glaucoma, 130
Corticotropin, and fungal infections, 11

Cortisol, in postmortem blood, 1039
Cosmic rays, 680
Cotton fracture, 325, *327*
Cotton-leaved physic nut, 1498–1499
Courville's classification, of skull fractures, 39–40
Crab lice, 1451
Crabs, hazardous, 1391–1392, *1392*
 horseshoe, hazardous, 1392–1393, *1393*
Crab's eyes plant, 1504–1508, *1506–1507*
Crafton weed, 1485
Cramps, heat, 703
Cranial nerves, injuries of, 62–63
Cranial sutures, closure of, dating of skeletal remains from, 1106
Craniocervical junction, injuries of, 63
Crash injuries. See also *Blunt injuries.*
 aircraft, 875–885, *879–882*, 882(t), 883(t), *884*
  in glider accidents, 883
  in helicopter accidents, 882–883, 883(t)
  in jet accidents, 876–879, *878*, *879*
  in light plane accidents, 879–882, *890–882*, 882(t)
  in parachute descents, 883–885, *884*
  in sailplane accidents, 883
 automobile, *5*, *7*, *13–15*, 853–864, *854*, *856*, *858*, *860*
  alcohol complicating, 863
  ejection, 855–856
  from seat belt, 216, 856–857, *857*
  from steering wheel, 204, 216, 217
  in pedestrians, 857–858, *857*, *858*
  in pregnancy, of fetus, 425–433
   maternal, of mother, 424–425
  nonejection, 854–855, *854*, *855*
  of abdomen, 216, 217
  of chest, *13–15*, 200, 216, 217, *854*, 855
  of heart, 12, 204
  of spinal cord, 77
  physics of, 847–848, *848*
Creatine, in postmortem cerebrospinal fluid, 1045
Creatine kinase, levels of, in head trauma, 55–56
Creatine phosphokinase test, for semen, 954
Creatinine, in postmortem blood, 1035–1036
 in postmortem cerebrospinal fluid, 1044
 in postmortem vitreous humor, 1048
Crepitine, 1497
Crepitus, defined, 118
Crib death. See *Sudden infant death.*
Crime(s), homicidal. See *Homicide.*
 involving explosives. See *Bombings.*
 involving fire. See *Arson; Bombings.*
 physical environment and, 1627–1640
Crime(s) (*Continued*)
 sadistic, *961*, 962–963, *963*
 sexual, 939–964. See also *Rape.*
  bitemarks in, 1143
  homicidal, 1010
   postmortem injury in, 1061–1062
Crime scene, investigation of, in arson, 744–747, *747*
  in bombings, 600–603, 612–614, *613*, *614*
 preservation of firearm evidence at, 561–569
Criminalist, in automobile accident investigations, 862
Crocus, autumn, 1513–1514
Crotalaria sericea, 1508–1509
Crotalaria spectabilis, 1508–1509
Crowfoot plant, 1527
Cruciate ligaments, rupture of, 307–308
Crush asphyxia, in explosions, 630–631, *631*
Crush injuries, 7, *7*. See also *Blunt injuries.*
 in explosions, 630–631, *631*
 of abdomen, perinatal, 439–441, *440*
 of chest, *7*, 200
 of forearm, 277–278
 of spinal cord, 65
Crush syndrome, 351
 in drug-induced coma, 8, 35
 kidney failure in, 400
Crustaceans, injury from, 1391–1392, *1392*
  postmortem, 1068, 1097–1098
Crutches, vascular injuries from, 224
Cryosurgery, injury from, 769
Cryotherapy, in ear disorders, 137
 injury from, 769
Cryptic hamartomas, 47
Cryptococcosis, 1337
Cryptograndioside A and B, 1483
Cryptostegia grandiflora, 1483
Cryptostegia madagascariensis, 1483
Cuboid, fractures of, 336
Cuneiform, fractures of, 336
Cup of gold plant, 1539
Curare, injection of, and chemical gangrene, 377
Curcin, 1499
Curling's ulcer, 396, *398*, 726
Current, electrical. See *Electrical current.*
Current marks, in electrical injury, 648, 651–655, *651–654*
Cushing's ulcer, 396–397
Cyanea, 1385, *1385*
Cyanide gas, inhalation of, 203
Cyanide poisoning, 793(t), 794, 1581
Cycadaceae, poisonous, 1487–1489
Cycas circinalis, 1487–1488
Cycas revoluta, 1487–1488
Cycas siamensis, 1487–1488
Cycasin, 1487, 1488
 as carcinogen, 793(t), 795
Cylinder shotgun barrel, 515
Cypress spurge plant, 1494
Cyst, air, vs. postnecrotic cyst, 45
 arachnoid, 65–66
Cyst (*Continued*)
 Baker's, 304
 bone, oral injuries and, 149–150, *150*, 168, *169*
 hydatid, 1365–1366
 macular, 110
 mandibular, 168, *169*
 meniscial, 309
 oral, 149–150, *150*, 176, *176*
 popliteal, 304
 postnecrotic, vs. air cyst, 45
Cyst stage, of parasite, 1345
Cystogram, in bladder injuries, 236–237
Cystography, 688
 in genitourinary injuries, 228
Cytisine, 1509
Cytisus laburnym, 1509

Dacryocystography, 688
Damages, assessment of, in negligence, 1665–1668
  fault system for, 910–935
 for breach of contract, 1665
 for emotional injuries, 1666–1668
 for fetal injuries, 429–433
 punitive, 1666
Daphne laureola, 1546
Daphne mezereum, 1546
Daphne plant, 1546
Daphnin, 1546
Darvon, injury from, 1583
Datura candida, 1534
Datura innoxia, 1535
Datura metel, 1535, *1536*
Datura meteloides, 1535
Datura stramonium, 1535
Datura suaveolens, 1534
Datura tatula, 1535
Daubentonia cavanillesii, 1511–1512
Daubentonia drummondii, 1511–1512
Daubentonia longifolia, 1511–1512
Daubentonia punicea, 1511
Daubentonia texana, 1511–1512
DDT, food contamination by, 788
Dead body. See *Corpse.*
Deadly nightshade, 1532–1533
Deafness. See *Hearing loss.*
Death, accidental, alcohol and, 823, 823(t), 824
  domestic, 886–900
 alcoholic, 819
 autopsy in. See *Autopsy.*
 biological, defined, 974
 carbon monoxide, 843–846, *843–846*
 cause of, determination of, 996–997
  blood levels and, 1576–1577
  chemical analysis for, 1033–1060
  from skeletal remains, 1113, *1113*
  in workmen's compensation cases, 1677–1680
 homicidal, attempted concealment of, 1062–1063
 cerebral, defined, 974
 clinical, defined, 974

Death (*Continued*)
  drowning, 1321, 1326
  drug, 831–832
    investigation of, 835–837
  electrical, 648–651, 648(t). See also *Electrocution.*
  fetal, amniotic fluid analysis in, 1053
    in automobile accidents, 425–428
    wrongful death statutes and, 430, 488–491
  from falls, 886–889
  from head injury, investigation of, 33–35
  from sexual practices, 961–962, *962, 963*
  homicidal. See *Homicide.*
  hypothermic, 764–765
  injuries inflicted after, 1061–1064. See also *Postmortem injuries.*
  Judeo-Christian attitudes toward, 968–970
  legal definition of, 973–974
  medical definition of, 973–974
  moment of, definition of, 23
  radiation, 683
  sudden, in infant, 1015–1032. See also *Sudden infant death.*
  suicidal. See *Suicide.*
  time of, determination of, 996–997, 1056, 1057(t)
    by sarcosaprophagous insect invasion, 1073–1095
Death certificate, in sudden infant death, 1029–1030, 1030(t)
  wrongful, 430, 488–491
    from skeletal remains, 1113–1114
Death cup fungus, 1552
Deceleration, ocular effects of, 128
Deceleration injuries. See also *Blunt injuries.*
  in aircraft accidents, 876–885
  in automobile accidents, 853–855
  of great vessels, 205
  of renal pedicle, 229
Decibel, defined, 134
Deciduous dentition. See *Tooth, deciduous.*
Deck feet, 330
Decompression, explosive, injury from, 643
  rapid, injury from, 643
Decompression sickness, 637, 641–644
  eye injury in, 128
Decongestants, interaction of, with anticholinergics, 1205
    with anticoagulants, 1205
Decubitus ulcers, after spinal cord injury, 83
Defecation, after spinal cord injury, 79
Deflagrating explosives, 580
Delayed union, of fractures, 345
  radiographic evidence of, 699–700
Delirium tremens, 823
Delivery. See also *Labor.*
  breech, liver rupture in, 439, *440, 441*
Delivery (*Continued*)
  breech, spinal injury in, 446
    soft tissue injury in, *449*
  cephalic, head injury in, 447–456, *448–452*, 454(t), *455*
  precipitous, fetal injury in, 446, 454
  prolonged, fetal injury in, 446, 454
Delphinium, 1526
Dementia praecox, trauma and, 17
Dementia pugilistica, 56–57, *57, 58*
Dental anesthesia, and optic nerve injuries, 118
  and oral injuries, 184–185, *184*
Dental appliances, geographical origin of, 1121–1122, *1121, 1122*
  injury from, 183, 187–188, *188*
Dental caries, radiation therapy and, 196, *196*
Dental charting, systems of, 1133–1134, *1133–1135*
Dental examination, forensic. See *Odontology, forensic.*
Dental impressions, as evidence, 1140–1141
  for bitemark comparison, 1146–1147, *1146*
Dental radiography, postmortem, 1134–1136, *1135, 1136*
Dental injuries. See *Oral injuries; Tooth.*
Dental instruments, injury from, 181, *181*, 185, *185*
Dental procedures, injury from, 178–188, *179–188*
Dental prostheses, injury from, 179, *180*, 182, 187–188, *188*
Dental radiography, postmortem, 1134–1136, *1135, 1136*. See also *Odontology, forensic.*
Dental restorations, determination of race from, 1121–1122, *1121, 1122*
  determination of socioeconomic status from, 1122–1123, *1123*
Dentin, of tooth, fracture of, 157, *157*, 165, *165*
Dentistry, forensic, vs. forensic odontology, 1118–1119
Dentists, legal responsibilities of, 1140–1143
  reporting of child abuse by, 1138–1140
Dentition. See *Tooth.*
Denture sores, 182
Dentures, injury from, 182, 187, *187*
Dependence, drug, 827–829
Depressant drugs, effects of, 829
  use of, historically, 826–827
  withdrawal from, 829
Depressed skull fracture, 40, *41*
  and scalp laceration, 6
  in newborns, 450, *450*
DeQuervain's disease, 349, 367, 383–384
Dermal nitrate test, for firearm discharge residue, 565–566
Dermatitis, abalone and, 1402
  factitial, 496
  fish processing and, 1169
  friction, 1170
  of eyelids, metallic salts and, 129
Dermatitis (*Continued*)
  of mouth, 188–189, *189*
  radiation, 682
Dermatomes, 78, *78*
Dermatomycosis, 1376
Desert syndrome, 704
Destroying angel fungus, 1552
Detonating explosives, 580–581
Devices, medical, injury from, legal case involving, 1261–1262, 1617–1626
Devil tree, 1496–1497
Devil's tobacco plant, 1484
Devil's trumpet, 1535, *1536*
Dextro propoxyphene hydrochloride, injury from, 1583
Diabetes, burn injury and, 723
  electrical injury and, 660–661
  head injury and, 61
  postmortem diagnosis of, 1053
Diagnostic procedures, air embolization in, 415–416
  injury from, electrical, 672
    of spleen, 212
    vascular, 224
      of hand, 379
  radiologic. See *Radiography.*
  ultrasonic. See *Ultrasound.*
Diaphragm, injuries of, 207
    in seat belt syndrome, 216
Diathermy, short-wave, injury from, of eye, 121
Diatoms, in drowned corpses, *1321*, 1326–1328
Diatrizoates, injury from, 690–692
Dichromate, in explosives, tests for, 605
Dictamnine, 1530
Dictamnolacton, 1530
Dictamnus albus, 1530
Dieffenbachia, 1481–1483
Diethylene glycol, poisoning by, 820
Diethylstilbestrol, food contamination by, 788
  for prevention of pregnancy, in rape victim, 955–956
Digestive tract. See *Gastrointestinal tract.*
Digit(s). See *Finger(s); Toe(s).*
Digital arteries, laceration of, 376
  thromboses of, from chronic injury, 224–225
Digital nerve block, and chemical gangrene, 377, *378*
Digitalis, injury from, 1197, 1532
Digitoxin, 1532
Digoxin, in postmortem vitreous humor, 1052
Dihydrostreptomycin, and ear injury, 137
Dihydroxycoumarin, 1546
Dilantin. See *Diphenylhydantoin.*
Dinitrophenol, and cataract, 130
Dinoflagellates, poisonous, 1398–1400, *1398–1399*, 1403, 1429
Diphenylamine test, for firearm discharge residue, 565–566
Diphenylhydantoin, and gingival hyperplasia, 189, *189*
  injury from, 1198
  interaction of, with chloramphenicol, 1206

Diphyllobothriasis, 1360–1361, *1361*
Diplopia, in orbital fractures, 117, 146
  in orbital hemorrhage, 116
Dipylidiasis, 1362
Direct current, 645–646
Disability, compensation for. See *Damages.*
  defined, 354
  evaluation of, for workmen's compensation, 354–355
Discharge residue, from firearms, 563–567, *564–566*
Disease(s), infectious, animal-transmitted, 1369–1377
  influence of physical environment on, 1627–1640, 1630(t)–1632(t)
  noninfectious, agents of, in laboratories, 1179–1180
  occupational. See *Occupational-environmental diseases.*
  parasitic, 1343–1368
  postmortem diagnosis, 1033–1060
  simulation of, 498
Disk, intervertebral, radiography of, 688
    surgery of, complications of, 66
Dislocation(s), aggravating preexisting conditions, 353–354
  complications of, 345–352
  defined, 259
  disability evaluation in, 354–355
  in electrical injury, 656–657
    in electroshock therapy, 662
  Monteggia, 276–277, *277*
  nerve injury in, 68, 276–277, 285–287
  of acromioclavicular joint, 266, *266, 267*
  of ankle, 323, 328
  of atlas, 63–64
  of biceps tendon, 262
  of elbow, 272–273, *273*
  of femoral head, 285–289, *286–289*
  of fibula, from tibia, 313
  of fingers, 375
  of foot, 330–331
  of glenohumeral joint, 266–268, *267–269*
  of hand, 375
  of hip, 285–289, *286–289*
  of ilium, 342
  of knee, 308
  of lacrimal gland, 91
  of lens of eye, 106, *106, 107*
  of lunate, 280, *281*
  of metatarsal joints, 331
  of midtarsal joint, 331
  of navicular, 280–281, *281*
  of patella, 303–304
  of pelvis, 341–343, *341–343*
  of peroneal tendons, 319–320
  of radioulnar joint, 281
  of radius, in Monteggia fracture-dislocation, 276–277, *277*
  of sacroiliac joint, *219*
  of scaphoid, 280–281, *281*
  of shoulder, 265–268, *265–269*
  of spine, parturitional, *444*
  of sternoclavicular joint, 265–266, *265*
Dislocation(s) (*Continued*)
  of talus, 330–331
  of tarsal joint, 331
  of teeth, *155*, 157, *157, 158*, 159, 166–167, *166, 167*
  of testis, 241
  of thumb, 375–376, *375*
  of toes, 331
  of wrist, 280–281, *281*
  psychologic sequelae of, 354
  sciatic, 285–288, *286, 287*
  vascular injury in, 223–224
  with fracture. See *Fracture-dislocation(s).*
Dispersed explosion, chemical, 578–579
  evidence of, 600–601
  secondary, 601
  vs. concentrated explosion, 600–601
Disseminated intravascular coagulation, 390
  causes of, 407
  kidney failure in, 402
Dittany plant, 1530
Divers, barotrauma in, 636–640
  drowning in, 1330
  eye injuries in, 128
  nitrogen narcosis in, 637–638
  oxygen poisoning in, 638
Dizziness. See also *Equilibrium.*
  after head injury, 136
DNA, radiation injury of, 681
Doctor. See *Physician.*
Doctor gum plant, 1473–1474
Dogger Bank itch, 1170, 1393
Dogs, postmortem injury by, 1068–1069, *1070*, 1096–1097
Doll's eyes plant, 1525
Domestic accidents. See *Accidents, domestic.*
Domestic animals, postmortem injury by, 1068–1069, *1070*, 1096–1097, *1096*
Domestic fires, 889–892, *889, 891*
Dopamine, 1488
Double vision, in orbital fractures, 117, 146
  in orbital hemorrhage, 116
Douching, vulvovaginal injury from, 254–255
Doxorubicin, as experimental drug, 1210–1211
Drivers, automobile, carbon monoxide levels in, 846
    injuries of. See *Crash injuries, automobile.*
Drowning, 203–204, 1317–1332
  accidental, 1329–1330
    domestic, 898
  alcohol and, 638, 1329–1330
  as agricultural hazard, 1165
  bathtub, 1330–1332, *1331*
  cardiovascular disease and, 638
  defined, 1317
  diagnosis of, 1323–1328, *1324*
    from magnesium levels, 1055
    tests for, 1325–1326
  homicidal, 1331–1332
  in scuba diving, 638–639, 1330
  incidence of, 1317
Drowning (*Continued*)
  investigation of, 638–639, 1328–1332, *1329–1331*
  length of submersion in, 1319–1321, *1319–1321*
  mechanism of, 203–204, 1321–1322
  pathophysiology of, 1322–1323
  reaction phenomena in, 1323–1324, *1324*
  salt water vs. fresh water, 203–204
  signs of, external, 1323–1324, *1324*
    internal, 1324–1325
  suicidal, 1006, 1330–1331, *1330*
  swimming pool, 1329
  victims of. See *Corpses, drowned.*
Drug(s). See also generic names of specific drugs.
  abuse potential of, 828–829
  abused, absorption of, 831
    action of, factors affecting, 830–831
      on central nervous system, 831
    and impotence, 1198
    cross tolerance to, 828
    dependence on, causes of, 828–829
      defined, 827–828
    diluting agents in, injury from, 834–835, *834*
    excretion of, 831
    habituation to, defined, 828
    huffing of, 832
    idiosyncratic reaction to, 832
    ingestion of, 830
    inhalation of, 830, 832(t)
      injury from, 832
    injection of, 830
      injury from, 226, 372, 830, 832–835
    injury from, 831–835, 833(t), *834*
    metabolism of, 831
    overdose of, 831–832
      home remedies for, 835
      homicidal, 1011
      investigation of, 835–837
    recycling of, 831
    routes of administration for, 830
    sniffing of, injury from, 832
    snorting of, 832
    synergistic effects of, 831–832
      with alcohol, 823
    tolerance to, defined, 828
  action of, altitude and, 1639–1640
    smoking and, 1217
    thermal stress and, 1639–1640
  adrenergic, and eye injury, 129, 130, 131
  allergic reaction to, 185, 1247
    anaphylactic, 1202–1204, 1204(t)
  and automobile accidents, 862–863
  and cataract, 130
  and convulsions, 1200–1201
  and ear injury, 137, 1199
  and eye injury, 129–131
  and fever, 711–713
  and fungal infection, 11, *11, 12*
  and gingival hyperplasia, 189, *189*
  and glaucoma, 130–131
  and hearing loss, 1199

Drug(s) (*Continued*)
- and hypothermia, 762
- and impotence, 1198
- and infertility, 1198
- and kidney injury, 401
- and optic nerve injury, 131
- anesthetic. See *Anesthetics.*
- antiarthritic, effects of, 1201
- anticholinergic, and glaucoma, 131
  - interaction of, with decongestants, 1205
- anticoagulant, interaction of, with decongestants, 1205
- anticonvulsant, and gingival hyperplasia, 189, *189*
  - injury from, 1198
  - interaction of, with chloramphenicol, 1206
- antidepressant, interaction of, with estrogen, 1205–1206
- antihistamine, and fever, 711
- antileukemic, injury from, 1198–1199
- antischizophrenic, 1206–1207
- benefit-to risk ratio for, 1201–1202
- bioavailability of, 1574–1575
- bioequivalence of, 1574–1575
- blood levels of, 1572–1577, 1576(t), 1578(t)–1580(t)
- cannabinoid, effects of, 830
- classification of, in Federal Controlled Substances Act of 1970, 828–829
- contraceptive, injury from, legal case involving, 1214
  - of eye, 131
- decongestant, interaction of, with anticholinergics, 1205
  - with anticoagulants, 1205
- defined, 827
- depressant, and alcohol, synergistic effects of, 823
  - effects of, 829
  - injury from, 832
  - use of, historically, 826
  - withdrawal from, 829
- dosage of, and blood levels, 1575
- experimental, use of, consent for, 1211–1212
  - liability for, 1209–1211
- for ulcerative colitis, injury from, 1201–1202
- hallucinogenic, effects of, 830
  - overdose of, 832
  - use of, historically, 827
- homicide by, 837, 1011
- hypnotic, effects of, 829
- illicit. See *Drugs, abused.*
- immunosuppressive effects of, 389
- in postmortem vitreous humor, 1051–1052
- in pregnancy, effects of, 1198–1200
- inhalant, effects of, 829
- injection of, and chemical gangrene, 377, 378
  - and nerve injury, 373
  - in drug abusers, injury from, 832–835
  - intraarterial, injury from, 226
  - intracardiac injury from, 209
- injury from, 906–908, *907*, 1195–1225, 1581–1583

Drug(s) (*Continued*)
- injury from, legal cases involving, 1212–1216, 1262–1267. See also *Products liability.*
  - manufacturer's liability for, 1207–1208
    - legal cases involving, 1212–1216, 1262–1267
  - of ear, 137, 1199
  - of eye, 129–131
  - of kidney, 401
  - of optic nerve, 131
  - pharmacist's liability for, 1222–1223
  - physician's liability for, 1208–1212
    - legal cases involving, 1212–1216
    - overdosage and, 1217–1219
    - package inserts and, 1219–1222
    - prescriptions and, 1217, 1219
  - prevention of, 1216–1222
  - products liability litigation ininvolving, 1207–1209, 1262–1267
- interactions of, 1204–1206
  - with alcohol, 1206
- legal cases involving, 1212–1216, 1262–1267
- manufacturers of, liability of, for drug-induced injury, 1207–1208
    - legal cases involving, 1212–1216
  - for package inserts, 1219–1222
- metabolites of, blood levels of, 1576
- narcotic, injection of, injury from, 832–835
  - withdrawal from, 829
- nephrotoxic, 401
- opiate, effects of, 829, 831
  - use of, historically, 826
- overdosage of, 1217–1219
- package insert with, 1219–1222
- poisoning by, 1217–1219
  - accidental, 895–896
  - homicidal, 837, 1011
  - in drug abusers, 831–832
  - investigation of, 835–837
  - suicidal, 1007
- prescription of, liability for mistakes in, 1217, 1219
  - telephonic, 1219
- products liability and, 1207–1209
  - legal cases involving, 1262–1267
- psychiatric, 1206–1207
- psychic effects of, 1206–1207
- response to, variability of, 1196–1201
- sedative, effects of, 829
- side effects of, 1196–1201. See also *Drugs, injury from.*
  - failure to test for, liability for, 1263
  - failure to warn of, liability for, 1263–1264
  - injury from, 832
  - multiple, 1199
  - use of, historically, 827
  - withdrawal from, 830
- stimulant, effects of, 829

Drug(s) (*Continued*)
- suicide by, 1007
- teratogenic, methotrexate as, 1198–1199
- tranquilizing, and impotence, 1198
  - effects of, 829
- utilization of, smoking and, 1217
- vasodilating, effects of, 1202

Drug abuse, 826–837. See also *Drugs, abused.*
- defined, 827
- dental evidence of, 1136–1137, *1136*
- injury in, 832–835, 833(t), *834*

Drug addicts, and homicide, 1011
- comatose, muscular ischemia in, 379
- dental lesions in, 148, 1136–1137, *1136*
- injection injuries in, 226, 379, 830, 832–835

Drug jaundice, general anesthetics and, 1249–1251, 1250(t)

Druggist. See *Pharmacist.*

Drumstick fingers, 1294

Drunk driving, 823–824, *858*, 862–863, 863(t)

Drunkeness. See *Alcohol intoxication.*

Dumb cane plant, 1481–1483

Duodenum, injuries of, 216–217
- stress ulcers of, 395–397, *398*
- surgery of, complications of, 1229–1230

Dupuytren's contracture, 330, 382–383

Dupuytren's fracture-dislocation, 325, *326*

Dural-venous laceration, perinatal, 452–456, *452*, 454(t), *455*

Dust allergy, 1454

Dust explosions, 579, *580*
- ignition energy for, 743(t)

Dust tattooing, from explosion missiles, 627, *628*

Duty, breach of, in negligence, 1645–1646

Dyes, analine, and ear injury, 137

Dysbarism, 636–644. See also *High altitude.*
- altitude, 641
- evolved-gas, 641–642
- hyperbaric, 636–640
- hypobaric, 641–644
- injury from. See *Barotrauma.*
- post-descent shock in, 643–644
- trapped-gas, 641–642

Dysproteinemias, postmortem diagnosis of, 1055

Dystrophic ulcer, 16

Dystrophy, of disuse, of hand, 381
- reflex sympathetic, of hand, 382, *382*

Ear, amputation of, traumatic, 135
- anatomy of, 132–133
- bleeding from, in skull fracture, 38, 40
- cauliflower, 135
- cerebrospinal fluid discharge from, 45, 62
- external, anatomy of, 132

Ear (*Continued*)
  injuries of, abrasion, 134
    and hearing loss. See *Hearing loss.*
    barotrauma and, 136, 637
    blast, 619–620, 637
    blunt, 135–136
    chemical, 137
    contusion, 135
    drug-induced, 137, 1199
    electrical, 661
    explosion, 619–620
    frostbite, 137, 767
    in head injury, 135–136
    in temporal bone fracture, 62, 136–137
    laceration, 135
    mechanical, 134–135
    noise-induced, 138–139
    radiation, 137–138
    thermal, 137
    whiplash and, 136
  inner, anatomy of, 132–133
    fistula in membranes of, 136
  innervation of, 132, 133
  middle, anatomy of, 132
Eardrum, rupture of, 135
    barotrauma and, 637
    explosions and, 619
Echinococciasis, 1365–1366
Echinoderms, hazardous, 1402–1406, *1403–1405*
Echocardiography, 778, *780*. See also *Ultrasound, diagnostic.*
Echoencephalography, 778, *779*. See also *Ultrasound, diagnostic.*
Echography, abdominal, 778. See also *Ultrasound, diagnostic.*
Ectoparasite, 1343
Ectoplasm, 1344
Ectromelia, causes of, legal case involving, 1617–1626
Edema, angioneurotic, of hip, *184*, 185
  Berlin's, 109
  of brain, 48–50.
  of conjunctiva, 92
  of cornea, 93, 94
  of glottis from tracheal intubation, 1254–1255
  of lung. See *Pulmonary edema.*
  of scalp, perinatal, 448, *448*
  of skin, in radiation therapy, 123
  posttraumatic, 391
Edema electricum, 657
Eels, Moray, 1407–1408, *1408*
Eight-ball hemorrhage, of eye, 101, *101*
Ejaculation, after spinal cord injury, 80
Ejector, of firearm, manufacture of, 555–557, *556*
    markings from, on cartridge, 558
Elastic collision, 4
Elastic energy, 4
Elastic properties, of human body, 4
Elasticity, law of, 4–5
Elbow, beat, 1184
  bursitis of, 272
  dislocation of, 272–273, *273*
  fractures of, 274–275
Elbow (*Continued*)
  injuries of, 271–277, *272–274*, *277*
    soft-tissue, 271–272, *272*
  osteochondritis dissecans of, *347*
  strain of, 272
  tennis, 271–272
Elderly, asphyxiation in, from aspirated food, 893–894
  falls in, 886–889, *887*
  fractures in, of hip, 887–889, *887*
    treatment of, 260
  heart failure in, 888
  heat stroke in, 704–705
  hypothermia in, 758–759, 889, *889*
  postmortem injuries in, 1066
  thermal injuries in, 889–892, *889*, *891*
Electric fishes, hazardous, 1409
Electrical appliances, causing fire,
    faulty contacts in, 740, *740*
    faulty safety devices in, 742
    internal short circuit in, 740, *740*
    laboratory examination of, 748(t), 749–754, *750–754*
    partial short circuit in, 740–742, *741*, *742*
Electrical arcs, 742
Electrical burns. See *Burns, electrical.*
Electrical circuit, short in, 740, *740*
    partial, 740–742, *741*, *742*
Electrical contacts, faulty, causing fire, 740, *740*
Electrical current, alternating, 645–646
  amperage of, 647, 647(t)
  arc, 646
    injury from, 654–655
  density of, 647
  direct, 645–646
  duration of contact with, 647–648
  path of, 647, *648*
  resistance of, 646–647
  voltage of, 646
Electrical damage, primary, 749, *750*
  secondary, 749, *750*
Electrical death. See *Electrocution.*
Electrical equipment, faulty, causing fire, 739–742
    laboratory examination of, 748(t), 749–754, *750–754*
  laboratory, injury from, 1176
  overloading of, causing fire, 740
Electrical fires, causes of, 735(t), 739–743
  investigation of, at site, 746–747, *747*
    in laboratory, 748(t), 749–754, *750–754*
Electrical fuses, laboratory examination of, 750, *751*
  tolerance of, *741*
Electrical injuries, 205
  blood in, 660
  current marks in, 651–655, *651–654*
  from arc flash, 662
  from electromagnetic waves, 663–664
  from lightning, 666–670, *668–670*
  from static electricity, 664–665
  homicidal, 665–666
Electrical injuries (*Continued*)
  iatrogenic, 662–663
  in agricultural accidents, 671, 1164–1165
  in cardiac procedures, 672
  in domestic accidents, 671, 897–898
  in hospital, 671–672, 904
  in laboratory, 1176
  in operating room, 671–672
  in pregnancy, 663
    lightning and, 670
  incidence of, 648(t)
  investigation of, 672–673
  occupational, 662, 663–664, 664–665
    causes of, 670–671
  of abdomen, 661
  of bone, 656–657
  of brain, 659
  of brain stem, 649
  of central nervous system, 649, 658–660
  of ear, 661
  of endocrine system, 660
  of eye, 120–121, 661–662
  of gastrointestinal tract, 661
  of hand, 380–381
  of joint, 656–657
  of kidney, 661
  of liver, 660
  of lung, 660
  of muscle, 655–656
  of nerve, 660
  of oral structures, 193–194, *194*, 655
  of pancreas, 660–661
  of renal pedicle, 229
  of skin, 651–655, *651–654*. See also *Burns, electrical.*
  of spinal cord, 650
  of tendon, 655–656
  suicidal, 665, *666*, *667*, 1006
Electrical wiring, overloaded, causing fires, 739–740
    laboratory examination of, 748(t), 749–754, *750–754*
Electricity, and fires, 739–743
  atmospheric. See *Lightning.*
  injury from. See *Electrical injuries.*
  physics of, 645–648
  quantities of, 739(t)
  static, causing fire, 743
    injury from, 664–665
  units of, 739(t)
Electrocardiograph, injury from, 672
Electrocution, 205, 649–650
  accidental, 650, 897–898, 1176
  apparent, 649
  defined, 648
  experimental findings in, 649
  homicidal, 665–666
  incidence of, 649(t)
  judicial, 650
  railway, 1190, 1191
  suicidal, 665, *666*, *667*, 1006
  types of, 649
  ventricular fibrillation in, 649–650, 649(t)
Electrolytes, in postmortem blood, 1040–1042, *1041*
  in postmortem cerebrospinal fluid, 1045–1046, 1045(t)

Electrolytes *(Continued)*
in postmortem vitreous humor, 1049–1050, *1051*
Electrolyte imbalance, decomposition pattern in, 1054
dehydration pattern in, 1054
in burn injury, 722–723
in sudden infant death, 1025 1025(t)
low-salt pattern in, 1054
postmortem diagnosis of, 1054–1055
uremia pattern in, 1054
Electrolyte therapy, injury from, 907
Electromagnetic waves, injury from, 663–664
of eye, 121–125
Electron radiography, 687
Electronic gears, injury from, 1170
Electroshock therapy, injury from, 662–663
Electrothermal burns, 718
Elephantiasis, 1364–1365
Embolism. See also *Thromboembolism.*
air. See *Air embolism.*
cancer cell, 417–418, *417*
catheter, 208–209
chorionic, 416
fat. See *Fat embolism.*
foreign body, 208–209, 418
nitrogen bubble, 641
oxygen. See *Air embolism.*
posttraumatic, 8, 351–352, 406–422
saddle, 408
tissue, 416–418, *417*
Embolus, defined, 407
Emergency Medical Service Systems Act, 873–874
Emergency treatment, consent to, 873–874, 1670
for snake venom poisoning, 1442
Good Samaritan laws and, 1670
hospital, 870–874
complications of, 1236–1237
liability for, 873–874
of intoxicated persons, 873
of minors, 873
refusal of, 873
standard of care for, 873–874
malpractice in, 908
pre-hospital, 866–869
liability for, 869
medical records of, 867
Emotional disorders. See *Psychologic disorders.*
Emphysema, defined, 118
of conjunctiva, 92
of eyelid, 92
of face, 183–184
of lung, from barotrauma, 637
postnatal, 478–479, *478*
of orbit, 118
subcutaneous, posttraumatic, *860*
Emphysema aquosum, 204, 1324
Empyema, 45
Emulsin, 1529
Enamel, dental, circular hypoplasia of, 160, *160*
decalcification of, in orthodontic treatment, 180–181, *180*
Enamel (*Continued*)
dental, mottled, in fluorosis, 192–193, *193*
Encephalitis hemorrhagica superior, 822
Encephalopathy, protracted, posttraumatic, 56–57, *57*
End bulbs, in neurons, 55–56
Endocarditis, bacterial, posttraumatic, 16, *16*
Endocrine glands, altitude and, 1296–1297
head injury and, 61
hypothermia, 761
in burn victims, 726
injury of, electrical, 600
thermal, 726
Endodontics, and oral injury, 149
Endoparasite, 1343
Endophthalmitis, 102, *102*, 107
Endoplasm, 1344
Enema, barium, injury from, 695–696, 904
Energy, activation, for oxidizing reactions, 731–732, *731*
conservation of, 4
elastic, 4
ignition, for gases, vapors, and dusts, 743(t)
in ballistics, 528
kinetic, 4
potential, 4
Energy wall, for oxidation reactions, 731, *731*
Engine room, of ship, accidents in, 1170
Enophthalmos, 117
Enteric circulation, 1569
Enterobiasis, 1355
Entomology, forensic, 1072–1095
Entrance wound, firearm, 7
abrasion collar of, 512, *512*
characteristics of, 511–516, *512–515*
from rifled weapon, 515
from shotgun, *512–515*, 515–516
Envenomation, by insects, 1441–1444
by marine animals, 1378–1436
medical aspects of, 1383–1385
by snakes, 1437–1444
Environment, physical. See *Weather.*
Environmental pollution, and disease. See *Occupational-environmental diseases.*
Enzymes, defined, 24
histochemical analysis of, for timing of wound, 24, *25*, *26*
in blood, postmortem, 1038–1039
in cerebrospinal fluid, in head injury, 54–55
postmortem, 1045
in vitreous humor, postmortem, 1048
polymorphic, identification of, in bloodstains, 816
postmortem levels of, 1055
Eosinophilic granuloma, oral injury and, 151–152, *152*
Ephedrine, 1544
Epicondyle, humeral, fractures of, 275
Epicondylitis, lateral, 271–272
medial, 272
Epidermoid carcinoma, of oral structures, 178, *178*
alcohol and, 191
iatrogenic injuries and, 191–192, *192*
nicotine and, 191–192, *192*
osteomyelitis and, 19, *19*
radiation therapy for. See *Radiation therapy.*
trauma and, 20
Epidural abscess, 45
Epidural hematoma, 42
in fire victims, 715
Epidural hemorrhage, 39, 42
spinal, perinatal, 442, *442*, 466(t)
Epiglottis, edema of, in tracheal intubation, 1254–1255
Epilepsy, drugs for, injury from, 1198
oral injuries in, 150, *150*
perinatal hypoxia and, 472–473, *472*, *473*, 475–476, *476*, 479–481
Epinephrine, in postmortem blood, 1039
injury from, legal case involving, 1221
of eye, 129, 130, 131
Epithelium, oral. See *Oral injuries*
Epoxides, food contamination by, 789
Epulis fissuratum, 187, *187*
Equilibrium, measurement of, 134
vestibular system for, 131
Erection, penile, after spinal cord injury, 80
Ergot, fungal, 1552–1553
Ergot alkaloids, 1552–1553
Ergot preparations, and chemical gangrene, 377
Ergotamine, 1552
Ericaceae, poisonous, 1489–1491
Escherichia coli, burn wound infection from, 10, 723
Esophagus, injuries of, 206–207
iatrogenic, 209, 1227–1228
in cervical disk surgery, 66
in tracheal intubation, 1253–1254
obstruction of, 206
surgery of, complications of, 1227–1228
Esterases, in postmortem blood, 1039
Estrogen, administration of, in pregnancy, 1200
interaction of, with antidepressants, 1205–1206
Ethacrynic acid, and ear injury, 137
interaction of, with allopurinol, 1201
Ethanol. See *Alcohol.*
Ethchlorvynol, in postmortem vitreous humor, 1052
Ether peroxides, spontaneous combustion of, 738
Ethyl alcohol. See *Alcohol, beverage.*
Ethylene chlorhydrin, food contamination by, 789
Ethylene glycol, poisoning by, 820, 1581
Ethylene glycol dinitrate, in explosives, tests for, 606–607
Ethylene oxide, food contamination by, 789

Eupatorium adenophorum, 1485
Eupatorium ageratoides, 1484–1485
Eupatorium glandulosum, 1485
Eupatorium rugosum, 1484–1485
Eupatorium urticaefolium, 1484–1485
Eupatorium wrightii, 1485
Euphorbia, 1492–1495
Euphorbia antiquorum, 1493
Euphorbia continifolia, 1493
Euphorbia cyparissias, 1494
Euphorbia helioscopia, 1494–1495
Euphorbia lactea, 1493
Euphorbia lathyrus, 1494
Euphorbia marginata, 1494
Euphorbia pulcherrima, 1493–1494
Euphorbia royleana, 1493
Euphorbia tirucalli, 1493
Euphorbiaceae, poisonous, 1491–1504, *1496*, *1503*
Euphorbon, 1492
European bittersweet, 1542
Euthanasia, 1010
Evan's classification, of hip fractures, *294*
Evidence, autopsy findings as, 1002
  ballistic, preservation of, 561–569
  bitemark, 1143–1147, *1144–1147*
  blood samples as, 603
  bomb fragments as, 602
  bullets as, 562–563, *562*
  chain of, 561
  dental, 1116–1153
    and preserving chain of evidence, 1141–1142
    bitemark, 1143–1147, *1144–1147*
    collection of, 1140–1141
    of child abuse, 1137–1140, *1138*
    of drug addiction, 1136–1137, *1136*
  in explosions and bombings, 600–603
  in fires, 735
    collection of, 744–747, *747*
    packing of, for transport to laboratory, 746–747
  of child abuse, dental, 1137–1140, *1138*
    radiographic, 1156
  of smuggling, radiographic, 1158
  of time of death, sarcosaprophagous insects as, 1072–1095
  radiographic, in tort cases, 699–700
    of child abuse, 1156
    of smuggling, 1158
    presentation of, in court, 1154–1155
  shot as, 563
  toxicologic, preparation of, 808–809
Excoriation, neurotic, 496, *496*
Exhaust, automobile, and carbon monoxide poisoning, *842*, 843, 846
Exhibitionism, 958
Exit wound, firearm, 7, 516–518, *516*, *517*
Exophthalmos, in orbital emphysema, 118
  in orbital fracture, 117
  in orbital hemorrhage, 116
Exostoses, traumatic, of ankle, 328
  of tibia, 319
Experimental drugs, use of, consent for, 1211–1212
  liability for, 1209–1212
Expert witness, fire investigator as, 734
  in products liability cases, 1621
  medical, 697–699
  pathologist as, 1002
  radiologist as, 1154–1155
  toxicologist as, 808–809
Explosion fracture, of distal tibia, 326
Explosions. See also *Blast; Bombings.*
  accidental vs. deliberate, 601
  air blast in, 616–622
  atomic, 683–684
  biologic evidence in, 603, 603(t)
  chemical, 578–579
  classification of, 578–579
  coal mine, 632, 1183–1184
  concentrated, chemical, 578
    evidence of, 600–601
    vs. dispersed explosion, 600–601
  condensed, chemical, 579
    evidence of, 601
    vs. dispersed explosion, 600–601
  deafness after, 620
  debris from, examination of, 601–603
  dispersed, chemical, 578–579
    evidence of, 600–601
    secondary, 601
    vs. condensed explosion, 600–601
  dust, 579, *580*
  effects of, on tissue, 612–615, *613–615*
  from lightning, 666–667
  from static electricity, 664–665
  gas, 578–579, 579(t), 632–633, *632*
    evidence of, 600–601
    in laboratories, 1177–1178
  immersion blast in, 622–624, *623*, *624*
  injuries from, 612–635
    abrasion, 626–630, *625–630*
    burn, 615–616, *616*, 634
    contusion, 626–630, *625–630*
    crush, 630–631, *631*
    fracture, 625
    from missiles, 625–630, *625–630*
    in air blast, 619–622, *620*, *621*
    in atomic explosions, 125, 683–684
    in coal mine explosions, 632
    in gas explosions, 632–633, *632*
    in immersion blast, 623–624
    in nuclear explosions, 633–634
    in solid blast, 624–625
    laceration, 626–630, *625–630*
    of ear, 619–620
    of eye, 125, 630
    of leg, 625
    of lung, 620–621, *620*, *621*
    of musculoskeletal system, 625
    of penis, 239
    of skin, 615–616, *616*, 626–630, *625–630*, 634
  investigation of, 600–608, 603(t), *608*
  mechanical, 578
    dispersed, evidence of, 601
  mine, 632, 1183–1184
  nuclear, 633–634
Explosions (*Continued*)
  physicis of, 616–618, *617*, *618*
  scene of, examination of, for evidence, 600–603
    for human remains, 612–614, *613*, *614*
  solid blast in,
  underground, 1184
  underwater, 622–624, *623*, *624*
  victims of, determining number of, 603, 612–614, *613*, *614*
    identification of, 614–615, *614*, *615*
Explosive(s), classification of, 580–581
  commercial, identification of components of, 606–607
    illegal use of, 581–588
  deflagrating, 580
  detonating, 580–581
  fireworks, injury from, 892
  high, 580–581
  identification of, 603–608, *608*
  improvised, 588–594, *589*
    identification of components of, 606
  investigation of, 570–611
  low, 580
  mining, 1183–1184
  vapor analysis of, 607–608, *608*
Explosive bombs. See *Bombs, explosive.*
Explosive limits, of gases, 579(t)
Explosive range, of inflammable substances, 736–737, 737(t)
Exposure, injury from, antemortem. See *Hyperthermia; Hypothermia.*
  postmortem, 1070–1071
  suicidal, *763*, 764, *764*
Exsanguination, in abdominal injuries, 211
  in heart injuries, 204
  in liver injuries, 212–213
  in pancreatic injuries, 214
Exterior ballistics, defined, 527
Extractor, firearm, manufacture of, 555–557, *556*
    markings from, on cartridge, 558
Extradural hemorrhage, 40
  in infants, 59
Extraocular muscles, anatomy of, 115
  injuries of, 116
Extremities. See names of specific parts.
Eye. See also names of specific parts.
  anatomy of, 88, *88*
  aqueous humor of, 99
  black, 90
  effects of meteorologic stimuli on, 1628(t)–1629(t)
  flash, 123
  fluid in, toxicologic examination of, 804
  foreign bodies in, 112–114, *113*
    ultrasonic diagnosis of, 778
  infection in, 102, *102*, 107
  injuries of, 88–131
    acceleration, 128
    burn. See *Burns, of eye.*
    chemical, 125–128, *126*, *127*, 129–131, *130*
    concussion, 107

Eye (*Continued*)
injuries of, contusion, 99, 101
drug-induced, 129–131
electrical, 120–121, 661–662
from arc flash, 662
from barotrauma, 128
from cryotherapy, 769
from diathermy, 121
from explosion missiles, 630
from swarf particles, 1172
from ultrasound, 120
hypothermic, 119–120, 767
iatrogenic, 120, 121–125, 129–131, 769
in battered child, 111, 503
in miners, 1184
in welders, 123, 662
mechanical, 89–119
nonmechanical, 119–131
of anterior chamber, 99–102
of choroid, 108–109, *109*, 111
of ciliary body, 104–105, *104*
of conjunctiva, 91–92
of cornea, 93–98, *94–98*
of extraocular muscles, 116
of iris, 104–105, *104*
of lacrimal glands, 90–91, *91*
of lens, 105–107, *105–107*
of orbit, 116–119, *117*, 146–147
of retina, 109–114, *109–111*, *113*
of sclera, 98–99
of vitreous humor, 107–108, *108*
penetrating, 99, 102, 105, 107
radiation, 121–125
rupture, 98
stress, 128–129
thermal, 119–120
toxicologic, 129–131, *130*
protrusion of, in orbital emphysema, 116
in orbital fracture, 117
in orbital hemorrhage, 116
recession of, in orbital fracture, 117
ultrasonic scanning of, 778
Eyelid, anatomy of, *88*, 89
arsenic dermatitis of, 129
emphysema of, 92
hemorrhage in, 90
injuries of, blunt, 89–90, 143
burn, 119–121
electrical, 120–121
frostbite, 119–120
in orbital fractures, 117
laceration, 90, 143
ligamentous, 90
penetrating, 90, *91*
radiation, 123, 124
scarring of, 119

Fabella, fractures of, 313
Face, bones of. See *Facial bones.*
injuries of, 37–38, 140–147
abrasion, 141
accidental vs. nonaccidental, 38
contusion, 141
emergency treatment of, 140–141
fracture, 37–38, 143–147
laceration, 38, 141–143
soft-tissue, 141–143
Facial asymmetry, posttraumatic, 162, *162*
Facial bones. See also *Mandible; Maxilla; Orbit.*
fractures of, 38, 143–147
racial characteristics of, 1108–1111, 1108(t), *1109*, *1110*
Facial nerve, injuries of, 142–143
paralysis from, 174
ear injuries and, 135
head injuries and, 62
iatrogenic dental injuries and, 188
in infants, 135
temporal bone fracture and, 136
pathway of, 133
Factitial dermatitis, 496
Facultative parasite, 1343
Fainting. See *Syncope.*
Fallout, nuclear, 679
Falls, in fishing industry, 1168
in home, 886–889, *887*
in hospital, by employees, 901–902
by patients, 902–903
on farm, 1163, 1165
suicidal, 1006
False acacia plant, 1510–1511
False aneurysm, 225
of forearm, *377*
of hand, 376
False blusher fungus, 1551–1552
False labor, posttraumatic, 427
False parasol mushroom, 1555
False poinciana, 1511
False sago palm, 1487–1488
Farmers, occupational diseases of, 1166
occupational injuries of, 1163–1166
Farmer's lung, 1166
Fascia, herniation of, 316
in foot, 329
in thigh, 297, 316
of foot, injuries of, 329, 330
of hand, 366–367
Dupuytren's contracture of, 382–383
of knee, injuries of, 304
Fasciitis, plantar, 330
Fascioliasis, 1362–1363
Fasciolopsiasis, 1362
Fat cells. See *Adipose tissue.*
Fat embolism, 8, 409–413, *411*, *412*
and acute respiratory failure, 393, *394*
and air embolism, 413–414
fractures and, 351
Fat metabolism, trauma and, 390–391
Fat necrosis, traumatic, of female breast, 361–363, *362*
of newborn, 363–364
Fatigue fractures, 336, 352–353, *353*
Fault, as legal concept, 910–911
Fault system, in negligence law, damages and, 910–935
Favism, 793, 795(t)
F. D. I. system, for dental charting, 1133–1134, *1134*, *1135*
Federal Controlled Substances Act of 1970, drug classification in, 828–829
Federation Dentaire Internationale, dental charting system of, 1133–1134, *1134*, *1135*
Felons, 368
Female. See *Women.*
Femoral cutaneous nerve, lateral, entrapment of, 297
Femur, fractures of, condylar, 310–311
in elderly, complications of, 887–889
in falls, 887–889, *887*
in pedestrians, 857
intercondylar, 310
of distal end of, 310–312, *311*
of head of. See *Femur, head of, fractures of.*
of shaft of, 297–299, *299*
of single condyle of, 310
osteochondral, 310–311
supracondylar, 299–300, *300*
head of, avascular necrosis of, *286*
in elderly, 889
determination of gender from, 1106(t), 1107–1108
dislocations of, 285–289, *286–289*
fractures of, 289–296, *290–296*
in elderly, 887–889, *887*
with posterior hip dislocation, 287
Fern, poisonous, 1469(t), 1550–1551
Fern palm, 1487
Fertility, altitude and, 1294–1295
drugs and, 1198
Fertilizers, agricultural, spontaneous combustion of, 738
Fetishism, 958–959
Fetus, abortion of. See *Abortion.*
as legal person, 430
and wrongful death statutes, 489, 490
bloodstains from, identification of, 812
brain damage in, 462–484, 466(t). See also *Brain damage.*
caput succedaneum in, 448, *448*
cephalohematoma in, 448–450, *449*
circulatory failure in, 458
death of, amniotic fluid analysis in, 1053
in automobile accidents, 425–428
wrongful death statutes and, 488–491
delivery of, breech, liver rupture in, 439, *440*, *441*
soft tissue injury in, *449*
spinal injury in, 446
cephalic, cranial injury in, 447–456, *448–452*, 454(t), *455*
head molding in, 450–452, *451*
hemorrhage in, 458–460
subdural, 452–456, *452*, 454(t), *455*
injuries of, blunt, 425–427
causation in, 429–433
cause of action for, 488–499, 1617–1626
crush, 439–441, *440*
drug-induced, 1198–1199, 1199–1200
during birth. See *Birth injuries.*

Fetus (*Continued*)
injuries of, electrical, 663
firearm, 429
fracture, 427, 450, *450*
hypoxic, 439(t), 454–484, 456(t), 466(t)
causes of, 457–458
of adrenal, *464*
of brain, 462–484, 466(t)
of heart, *462*
of intestines, *462*
of kidney, 461–462, *463*
of lung, *465*
of placenta, *459*, *460*, *463*
of testis, *464*
of thymus, *461*
of viscera, 461–462, *461–465*
placental disorders and, *458–460*
sequelae of, 472–473, *472*, *473*, 477–484
stages of, 457–460
umbilical cord and, *457*
iatrogenic, legal case involving, 1617–1626
in automobile accidents, 425–433
in maternal shock, 427
intrauterine devices and, 1617–1626
mechanical, 439–456, 439(t), 454(t)
medicolegal considerations in, 429–433
methotrexate and, 1198–1199
of abdomen, 439–441, *440*
of brain stem, 441–447, 441(t), *443*, *445*
of central nervous system, 436–486
hypoxic, 439(t), 456–484, 456(t), 466(t)
mechanical, 439(t), 441–456, 454(t)
of head, 447–456, *448–452*, 454(t), *455*
of liver, 439–441, *440*, *441*
of spine, 441–447, 441(t), *442–446*
parturitional. See *Birth injuries.*
penetrating, 429
perinatal, 436–484. See also *Birth injuries.*
stabbing, 429
malposition of, and spinal injury, 446, *446*
premature, mechanical injury in, *442*, 446–447
radiography of, 688
subdural hemorrhage in, 452–456, *452*, 454(t), *455*
ultrasonic scanning of, 776, 778, *780*
safety of, 781
venous infarction in, 458–460
viability of, as precondition to injury compensation, 488
gestational age and, 488
in second trimester, 483
legal definition of, 430
medical definition of, 488
Fetus-in-coma, 438, 476–477
Fever, 710–711
drug-induced, 711–713
hemorrhagic, 1371
Fibrillation, defined, 69
ventricular, in drowning, 1322
in electrical injury, 649–650, 649(t)
in hypothermia, 760
Fibroma, irritation, oral, 176, *177*
ossifying, 296
Fibromatosis, of plantar fascia, 330
Fibroses, posttraumatic, of hand, 382–384
Fibula, dislocation of, from tibia, 313, *314*
fractures of, of head of, 313
of shaft of, 316–319, *317*
Field machines, agricultural, injury from, 1164
Filefish poisoning, 1426–1427
Finger(s), anatomy of, 366
baseball, 372
chemical gangrene of, 377, *378*
clawing of, in Dupuytren's contracture, 382–383
in Volkmann's contracture, 377–378, *378*
drumstick, 1294
injuries of, chemical, 377, *378*
dislocation, 375
fracture, 374
from narcotic injections, 379
occupational, 379–380
in fishing industry, 1169, 1170
vascular, 376
mallet, 372
muscular ischemia of, 377–378, *378*
trigger, 366
Fingernails, analysis of, in arsenic poisoning, 805
beds of, infections of, 368
biting of, 497
Fingerprinting, of unidentified corpse, 33
Fire(s), alcohol and, 891–892, *891*
carbon monoxide in, 842–843
levels of, 841–842
carbon monoxide poisoning in, 202–203, 841–842, 889, 890–891, 1069–1070
caused by incendiary bombs, investigation of, 575–578
caused by negligence, 732, 742
caused by spontaneous combustion, investigation of, 756–757
caused by static electricity, 664–665
causes of, 735–743, 735(t)
determination of, 744–747
technical, 735–743, 735(t)
thermal, 735(t)
chemical, causes of, 735(t), 736–739, 737(t)
investigation of, at site, 746–747, *747*
in laboratory, 748(t), 754–757, *756*, 757(t)
deliberate. See *Arson.*
domestic, 889–892, *889*, *891*
electrical, causes of, 735(t), 739–743
investigation of, at site, 744–746
Fire(s) (*Continued*)
electrical, investigation of, in laboratory, 748(t), 749–754, *750–754*
farm, 1163
ignition phase of, 736
in coal mines, 1184
in laboratories, 1175–1176
incendiary. See *Arson.*
injuries in, burn. See *Burns.*
inhalation, chemical vs. thermal, 713–714
non-burn, 713–715
investigation of, 730–757
at site, 744–747, *747*
in bombings, 575–578
in laboratory, 748–757, 748(t)
organization of, 733–735, 734(t)
phases of, 734
reasons for, 732
statistical data for, 732–733, *733*
while fire is raging, 744–745
railway, 1188, 1189
reconstruction of, in laboratory, 748–749, 749(t), 751–754, *752–754*
suicide by, 1006
victims of, autopsy of, 1000–1002, 1069–1070
carbon monoxide poisoning in, 1069–1070
carboxyhemoglobin levels in, 847, 848(t)
toxicologic examination in, 805
Fire ants, 1447
Fire bombs, 572–578, *573–577*
Fire coral, 1386, *1386*
Fire investigation laboratory, 748–757, 748(t), *751–754*
Fire worm, 1390–1391, *1391*
Firearm(s). See also *Ballistics;* and names of specific types.
accidents involving, *517*, 522, 896–897, *896*, 897
in men vs. women, 897
ammunition for, 511
identification of, 557–561, *557*, *559–561*
types of, 543–554, *545–552*, 553(t), *554*, *555*
as evidence, 561–562
automatic, 542
barrel of. See *Barrel.*
bolt face of, 555–557, *556*, *557*
breech face of, 555–557, *556*, *557*
bullets for. See *Bullets.*
caliber of, 510–511, 529, *529*
cartridges for. See *Cartridges.*
discharge residues from, 563–567, *564–566*
ejector of, cartridge markings from, 558
manufacture of, 555–557, *556*
evidence involving, preservation of, 561–569
extractor of, cartridge markings from, 558
manufacture of, 555–557, *556*
firing pins of, cartridge markings from, *557*, 558

Firearm(s) (*Continued*)
firing pins of, characteristics of, 556, *556*, *557*, 558
manufacture of, 556, *556*, 557
for animal slaughter, injury from, 525–526
gauge of, 510–511, 529
historical development of, 537–539, *538*
homicide by, 522–523, 1012
identification of, 527–528. See also *Ballistics*.
ignition systems for, 538–539, *538*
injuries from. See *Firearm wounds*.
manufacture of, 554–557, *555–557*
primers for, 550–551
suicide by, 521–522, 1004–1005, *1004*, *1005*
types of, 510–511, 540–542, *540–542*
veterinary slaughtering, injury from, 525–526
Firearm wounds, 5, 511–526
accidental, *517*, 522, 896–897, *896*, *897*
bullet track in, 525
categorization of, 7–8
contact, 7–8, *47*, 520–521
contact ring of, 37, *41*
discharge residue around, 563–567, *564–566*
entrance, 7, 511–516, *512–515*
exit, 7, 516–518, *516*, *517*
from blank cartridges, 525
homicidal, *512–514*, *516*, 522–523, 1012
in children, 896–897, *896*, *897*
of abdomen, *512*, 519–520, *520*
of artery, 222
of chest, 200, *513*, *514*, 519
of fetus, 429
of head, 518–519, *515–519*
of liver, 212
of mouth, 174–175, *175*
of penis, 239
of scalp, 37
postmortem examination of, 523–525
range of, estimation of, 520–521
sites of election in, in homicide, 523
in suicide, 521
suicidal, *41*, *515*, 521–522, 1004–1005, *1004*, *1005*
barrel impression in, 37
survival time in, 523
Firedamp, poisoning by, in coal mine explosions, 1184
Fireworks, injury from, 892
Firing pins, cartridge markings from, *557*, 558
characteristics of, 556, *556*, *557*, 558
manufacture of, 556, *556*, *557*
First aid. See *Emergency treatment*.
Fish, electric, hazardous, 1409
poisonous, 795–796, 1417–1426
postmortem injury from, 1068, *1068*, 1097–1098, 1328, *1329*
stinging, 1409–1417, *1410–1413*, *1416*
Fish (*Continued*)
with endogenous toxins, 1417–1420, *1417*, *1419*
with exogenous toxins, 1420–1426, *1421–1424*
Fish liver, excessive vitamin A in, 1428–1429
Fish processing, injuries in, 1169
Fishing industry, injuries in, 1167–1171
incidence of, 1167–1168
mortality rate in, 1168
Fistula, in inner ear membranes, 136
traumatic arteriovenous, of hand, 225–226, 377
traumatic urethrovaginal, 238
Flail chest, 200
Flammable. See *Inflammable*.
Flash burns, electrical, 718
in explosion, 615–616, *616*, 634
Flash eye, 123
Flash point, 736–737, 737(t)
Fleas, as disease vectors, 1367
biting, 1450
Fleshflies. See *Flies, sarcosaprophagous*.
Flight response, 386
Florence test, for semen, 953
Florida arrowroot plant, 1488–1489, *1489*
Floripondio plant, 1534
Flukes, intestinal, 1362–1364
liver, 1362–1364
lung, 1362–1364
Fluoroscopy, 687
injury from, 695
Fluorosis, 192–193, *193*
Fly(ies), as disease vectors, 1367
biting, 1448–1449
postmortem injury from, 1067–1068. See also *Flies, sarcosaprophagous*.
sarcosaprophagous, adult, on corpse, 1090–1091
as forensic indicators, 1079–1091
biology of, 1079–1080, *1080*, 1080(t)
development of, 1079–1080, *1080*, 1080(t), 1081(t)
environmental conditions affecting, 1079–1080, *1080*, 1080(t), 1081–1082
larvae of, in corpse, 1084–1089, *1086*, 1086(t), *1088*, *1089*
age of, 1084–1087, *1086*, 1086(t), *1087*
migration of, 1087–1089, *1088*
oviposition by, in corpse, 1080–1084
puparia of, in corpse, 1089–1090, *1090*
Fly agaric fungus, 1551
Foehn weather, 1634
Food(s), allergens in, 793(t), 795
and anaphylaxis, 1204(t)
asphyxiation by, 893–894, 1614–1616
aspiration of, 893–894, 1614–1616
bitemarks on, as evidence, 1144, *1144*
Food(s) (*Continued*)
carcinogens in, cycasin as, 795
from wood smoke, 789
nitrosamines as, 797
residues as, pesticide, 788
contamination of, by aflatoxins, 791–793, 791(t)
by bacteria, 1588–1612
by cadmium, 788
by chemicals, 787–790
by *Clostridium botulinum*, 1589–1596, *1591–1593*
by *Clostridium perfringens*, 1596–1598, *1596*
by diethylstilbestrol, 788
by extraction solvents, 789–790
by food additives, 796–797
by fumigants, 789
by mercury, 787–788
by mycotoxins, 790–793, 791(t)
by nitrosamines, 797
by PCB, 789
by pesticide residues, 788
by preservatives, 796–797
by processing agents, 789–790
by *Salmonella*, 1598–1606, *1600*
by *Shigella*, 1610–1611
by *Staphylococcus*, 1606–1610, *1607*
by *Streptococcus*, 1610
by trichloroethylene, 789–790
by unknown agents, 1611–1612
by *Vibrio parahaemolyticus*, 1611
by weeds, 1457
by wood smoke, 789
in processing, 789–790
cyanide poisoning by, 793(t), 794
goitrogenic, 793(t), 794
hemagglutinins in, 793–794, 793(t)
lipid oxidation in, 789
protease inhibitors in, 793–794, 793(t)
saponins in, 793–794, 793(t)
smoked, carcinogens in, 789
solvent extraction in, toxins generated by, 789–790
toxins in, injury from, 787–799, 793(t), 1459–1461
Food additives, toxicity of, 796–797
Food plants, poisonous, 793–795, 793(t), 1459–1461
Food poisoning, bacterial, 1588–1612
agents of, 1588–1599, *1588*
incubation periods for, 1589(t)
incidence of, 1588–1589, *1588*, *1589*
legal cases involving, 1588, 1603–1604, 1611–1612
by marine animals, 795–796, 1388–1389, 1417–1426, 1427–1428, *1428*
by plants, 793–795, 793(t), 1459–1461
by shellfish, 795
by unidentified agents, 1611–1612
chemical, 787–790
microbial, 790–793, 791(t)
mycotoxic, 790–793, 791(t)
prevention of, 1612
Food preservatives, toxicity of, 796–797

Food processing, toxins generated by, 789
Food-borne disease, streptococcal, 1610
Food-borne shigellosis, 1610–1611
Food-borne typhoid fever, 1604–1605
Foot, bursitis of, 329
  fascial hernia of, 329
  ganglion of, 329
  immersion, 766–767
  injuries of, 328–337
    burn, from hot pavement, 719
    dislocation, 330–331
    explosion, 625
    fracture, 331–337, *332*, *334*, *337*
    hypothermic, 766–767
    ligamentous, 330
    soft tissue, 328–329
    sprain, 328–329, 330
  neuralgia of, 329
  trench, 766–767
Foramen magnum, herniation through, 50
Force, concept of, 3–5
Forceps, obstetrical, injury from, 439–456
Forearm, injuries of, 277–278. See also *Radius; Ulna.*
Foreign body, air embolus as, 414
  asbestos fibers as, 1286–1290
  aspiration of, 207–208
    in children, 893
  embolic, 418
  illicit drug contaminants as, 834, *834*
  in artery, 208
  in cardiovascular system, 8, 208, 408, 418
  in chest, 207–208, 418
  in esophagus, 206
  in eye, 112–114, *113*
    from explosion, 630
    ultrasonic diagnosis of, 778
  in heart, 418
  in orbit, 118–119
    and orbital fracture, 117
  in vagina, 252–253
  left in surgical wounds, 66
  radiography of, 1154, 1156–1157
Forensic anthropology, 1101–1115
Forensic ballistics, 527–569,
Forensic dentistry, vs. forensic odontology, 1118–1119
Forensic entomology, 1072–1098. See also *Flies, sarcosaprophagous.*
Forensic odontology, 1116–1153. See also *Odontology, forensic.*
Forensic toxicology, 800–809, 1568–1586
Foreseeability of harm, in negligence, 1645–1646
Formaldehyde, with permanganate, spontaneous combustion of, 739
Fouling, around firearm entrance wound, 514, *515*
Foxglove, 1532
Fracture(s), age of, radiographic evidence of, 699
  aggravating preexisting conditions, 353–354
  and genitourinary injury, 228
Fracture(s) (*Continued*)
  and nerve injury, 68
  and traumatic retinopathy, 110
  and vascular injury, 223–224
  avulsion. See *Avulsion fractures.*
  Barton's, 283
  Bennett's, 374
  blow out, 146
  bumper, 857
  casting of, injury from, 908
  chauffeur's, 283–284
  chondral, of femoral condyle, 310–311
  Colles', 281–283, *282*
    reverse, 283, *283*
  complications of, 345–352
    in elderly, 887–889
    in treatment, 908, 1234–1235
    radiographic evidence of, 699–700
  compound, 259–261
  compression. See *Compression fractures.*
  contrecoup, 46
  Cotton, 325, *327*
  defined, 259
  delayed union of, 345
    radiographic evidence of, 699–700
  depressed, 40, *41*, 59
    and scalp laceration, 6
    in newborns, 450, *450*
  disability evaluation in, 354–355
  diseases predisposing to, 150–154, *151–153*
  dislocations with. See *Fracture-dislocations.*
  Dupuytren's, 325
  evidence of, in skeletal remains, 1113
  fatigue, 336, 352–353, *353*
  gutter, 40–41
  in aircraft accidents, 875–885, *879*, *880*, *882*, 882(t), 883(t), *884*
    incidence of, 882(t)
  in automobile accidents, 855
  in battered child, 504, *504*
  in elderly, 887–889, *887*
    treatment of, 260
  in electrical injury, 656–657
  in electroshock therapy, 662
  in explosions, 325, 625
  in falls, 887–889, *887*
  in fetus, 427
  in motorcycle accidents, 339
  in pedestrians, 857
  intrauterine, 427
  LeFort, of maxilla, 144, 170
  malunion of, 345–346
    radiographic evidence of, 699–700
  march, 336, 352–353, *353*
  Monteggia, 276–277, *277*
  nonunion of, 346
    radiographic evidence of, 699–700
  of acetabulum, with posterior hip dislocation, 287, *287*
  of acromion, 269
  of alveolus, dental, 167, 168–169
  of ankle, 324–328, *326*, *327*
    in explosions, 625
Fracture(s) (*Continued*)
  of arm, 261–285
  of atlas, 63–64
  of calcaneus, 334–336, *334*
  of cartilage, of femoral condyl, 310–311
  of cervical spine, 63–64, 77
  of clavicle, 268
  of coccyx, 345
  of cranial fossa, anterior, 37–38
  of cuboid, 336
  of cuneiform, 336
  of elbow, 274–275
  of fabella, 313
  of facial bones, 38, 143–147
  of femur. See *Femur, fractures of.*
  of fibula, 313, 316–319, *317*
  of fingers, 374
  of foot, 331–337, *332*, *334*, *337*
  of forearm, 278. See also *Radius; Ulna.*
  of glenoid cavity, 269
  of hand, 374
  of heel, 334–336, *334*
  of hip, 289–296, *290–296*
    in elderly, 887–889, *887*
  of humerus. See *Humerus, fractures of.*
  of ilium, 338–339, *338*
  of ischium, 338, *338*, 339, *339*
  of leg, 285–337
    in aircraft accidents, *880*, 882(t), *884*
    in pedestrians, 857
  of malleoli, of ankle, 324–325, *321*, *322*, *326*, *327*
  of mandible. See *Mandible, fractures of.*
  of maxilla. See *Maxilla, fractures of.*
  of metatarsus, 336–337
  of navicular, of foot, 336
    of wrist, 284, *284*
  of nose, 38
  of olecranon, 275
  of orbit, 116–118, *117*, 146–147
    hemorrhage in, vs. subconjunctival hemorrhage, 91
  of patella, 301–303, *302*
  of pelvis. See *Pelvis, fractures of.*
  of penis, 240
  of phalanges, of fingers, 374
    of toes, 337
  of pisiform, 285
  of radius. See *Radius, fractures of.*
  of ribs, 200
    in battered child, 504
  of sacrum, 344
  of scaphoid, 284, *284*
  of scapula, 269–270
  of sesamoid bones, of foot, 337, *337*
  of shoulder, 268–270, *270*
  of skull. See *Skull, fractures of.*
  of spine, 63–64, 77
    parturitional, *444*
  of sustentaculum tali, 335
  of talus, of dome of, 328
    of posterior process of, 331–332
  of temporal bone, 62, 136–137
    signs of, 38
  of tibia. See *Tibia, fractures of.*
  of toes, 337

Fracture(s) (*Continued*)
of tooth. See *Tooth, fractures of.*
of ulna. See *Ulna, fractures of.*
of wrist, 281–285, *282–284*
osteochondral, of femoral condyl, 310–311
of patella, 303
parry, 276–277, *277*
pathologic, 352
in burn victims, 726
radiation therapy and, 196, *196*
systemic disease and, 150–154, *151–153*
ping pong, 59
Pott's, 325
psychologic response to, 354
pyramidal, 144
radiography of, 143–144, 687
in tort cases, 699–700
Smith's, 283, *283*
stress, 352–353, *353*
of fibula, 318–319
treatment of, 260–261
complications of, 908, 1234–1235
tripod, 146
union of, complications of, 345–346
radiographic evidence of, 669–700
Fracture-dislocation, Dupuytren's, 325, *326*
Monteggia, 276–277, *277*
of ankle, 325
of mandibular condyle, 41
of pelvis, *219*, 343–344, *343*
of spine, 63–64, 77
parturitional, *444*
Fraxin, 1504
Fraxinella plant, 1530
Free balls, in neurons, 55–56
Friar's cap plant, 1525
Friedelin, 1477
Fright response, 386
Frostbite, 766–768
complications of, 767–768
in therapeutic hypothermia, 769
of ear, 137, 767
of eye, 119–120, 767
of eyelid, 119–120
sequelae of, 767–768
Froth of drowning, 1323, 1324, *1324*
Frozen shoulder, 270–271
Fuchsinophilic degeneration, of heart, head injury and, 400
Fulvine, 1508
Fumes, poisonous. See also *Carbon monoxide poisoning.*
inhalation of, in explosions, 631
in coal mines, 632, 1184
in fires, 713–714
and pulmonary injury, 724–725
toxicologic analysis for, 806
Fumigants, food contamination by, 789
Functional overlay, in musculoskeletal injuries, 354
Fungal antigens, response to, 1338–1339
Fungal infections, 1334–1342
drug-induced, 11, *11*
Fungal infections (*Continued*)
of burns, 723
of cornea, 96, *96*
of skin, in agricultures, 1166
opportunistic, 1337–1338
secondary, 11, *11*
Fungi, food contamination by, 790–793, 791(t)
infections from. See *Fungal infections.*
injury from, 1464, 1456–1557, 1469(t)–1470(t), 1551–1557
Furosemide, and ear injury, 137
Fuses, electrical, laboratory examination of, 750, *751*
tolerances of, *741*

Gallbladder, injuries of, 213
radiography of, 687
surgery of, complications of, 1230
toxicologic examination of, 804
Galley, of ship, accidents in, 1170
Gamma rays, 680
in radiation therapy, 690
injury from, in nuclear explosions, 634
of eye, 123–125
Ganglion, of ankle, 320
of foot, 329
of wrist, 279
Gangrene, chemical, of hand, 377, *378*
in peripheral arteriosclerosis, 16, *16*, *17*
thrombotic occlusion and, 16
Garden's classification, of hip fractures, 289–290, *291*
Gas(es), anesthetic, abuse of, 832, 832(t). See also *Anesthetics.*
explosion of. See *Gas explosions.*
from shotgun discharge, 511
in postmortem blood, 1042–1043, 1042(t), 1043(t)
inflammable, 736–739
causing fire, identification of, in laboratory, 754–757
on-site, 746–747, *747*
explosive limits of, 579(t)
explosive range of, 736–737
flash point of, 736–737, 737(t)
ignition of, by static electricity, 743, 743(t)
ignition temperature of, 736–737
inhaled as drugs, 832(t)
abuse of, 832, 832(t)
effects of, 829
injury from, 832
injection of, diagnostic, 688
injury from, in dysbarism, 636–644
in laboratories, 1177–1178
natural, explosion of, 632–633, *632*
poisonous. See *Fumes, poisonous.*
radioactive, 679
Gas chromatography, in carbon monoxide poisoning, 846
in explosion investigations, 606–607
in fire investigations, 755, *756*
Gas explosions, 578–579, 579(t)
evidence of, 600–601
Gas explosions (*Continued*)
in coal mines, 632, 1184
in homes, 632–633, *632*
in laboratories, 1177–1178
Gas plant, 1530
Gasoline, causing fire, laboratory identification of, 755
Gastrectomy, complications of, 1229–1230
Gastrocnemius muscle, rupture of, 315–316
Gastrointestinal function, after spinal cord injury, 84
Gastrointestinal tract. See also *Abdomen;* and names of specific organs.
carcinoma of, asbestos-related, 1279(t)–1281(t), 1286
injuries of, 215–220
alcoholic, 820
blunt, 215–216
chemical, 189–192, *190*, *191*, 206–207, 1177, *1581*, *1582*
diagnosis of, 215–216
electrical, 661
explosion, 621–622, 624
firearm, 215
hypothermic on, 760, 768
iatrogenic, 768
in children, 216
in dysbarism, 637
in immersion blast, 624
radiation, 683
seat belt, 216
thermal, 726
postmortem findings in, in burn victims, 726
radiography of, 687
surgery of, complications of, 1229–1233
ulceration of, in burn victims, 726
Gastropods. See *Mollusks.*
Gaucher's disease, and oral injury, 152, *152*
Gauge, of firearm, 510–511, 529
Gaze nystagmus, 134
Gc protein groups, identification of, in bloodstains, 816
Gelatin, blasting, 581
Gelignite, in explosives, 581, 582
tests for, 606
Gelsemine, 1518
Gelsemium sempervirens, 1518–1519
Gender, chromosomal abnormalities and, 958
determination of, from bloodstains, 812
from radiographs, 1157
from skeletal remains, 1106–1108, 1106(t)
from teeth, 1123–1124
meteorologic stress and, 1628, 1630
Genes, radiation injury of, 681
Genitals, female, 243–258, *246*
anatomy and physiology of, 243–248, *244*, *245*
injury of, in rape, 947–951
postmortem, 1061–1062
self-inflicted, 498
sex-related, 248–252
male, injuries of, 239–241
self-inflicted, 498

Genitourinary tract, injuries of, 227–243
associated injuries with, 228
diagnosis of, 228–229
pelvic injuries and, 341, 344
postmortem, 1061–1062
symptoms of, 227–229
Gentamicin, and ear injury, 137
and kidney injury, 401
Germidine, 1517
Gettler test, 1325
Giardiasis, 1347–1348, *1348*
Gingiva. See also *Oral injuries.*
abscess of, 164
abrasion of, *156*, 157
contusion of, *156*, 157
dental cement in, 183, *184*
hyperplasia of, drug-induced, 189, *189*
laceration of, 157, *157*
normal appearance of, 148, *148*
pregnancy tumor of, 176, *177*
recession of, 175, *175*
toothbrush trauma of, 173
Gingivitis, 175, *175*
Gingivostomatitis, primary herpetic, 182–183, *183*
Glancing wounds, of scalp, 37
Glands, endocrine. See *Endocrine glands.*
Glaucoma, anticholinergic drugs and, 131
secondary, traumatic, 99–101, 102, 106
Glenohumeral dislocations, 266–268, *267*, *268*
Glenoid cavity, fracture of, 269
Glider accidents, 883
Globe, of eye, injuries of, concussion, 107
contusion of, 99, 101
penetrating, 99, 102, 105, 107
rupture, 98
Gloriosa rothschildiana, 1515–1516
Gloriosa simplex, 1515–1516
Gloriosa superba, 1515–1516
Gloriosine, 1515
Glossitis, antibiotics and, 188, *189*
Glossopharyngeal nerve, injury of, 63
Glucose, in postmortem blood, 1034–1035
in postmortem cerebrospinal fluid, 1043
in postmortem vitreous humor, 1046, *1047*
Glutamic oxaloacetic transaminase, levels of, in head injury, 54
Glutamine, in postmortem cerebrospinal fluid, 1045
Glycerol, with permanganate, spontaneous combustion of, 739
Glycogen, accumulation of, in neurons, 53
Glycol, with permanganate, spontaneous combustion of, 739
Gm protein, identification of, in bloodstains, 816
Goitrogens, in plants, 793(t), 794
Gold, injury from, 1584–1585
of eye, 129
Gold dermatitis, of eyelid, 129
Goldbricking, 497
Golden bough plant, 1520–1521
Golden chain plant, 1509
Golden rain plant, 1509
Goldenrod, 1485
Gokart accidents, 859
Gonadotropin, chorionic, in postmortem blood, 1040
Gonzalez test, for firearm discharge residue, 565–566
Good Samaritan statutes, 869, 1670
Granuloma, dental, 163–164
eosinophilic, oral injury and, 151–152, *152*
milker's, 368
of lip, 173, *173*
of tongue, 173, *174*
pyogenic, of oral soft tissues, 173, *174*
iatrogenic, 185
Graveyard weed, 1494
Gravitational forces, effects of, on eye, 128
on projectile, 528
Grazing wounds, of scalp, 37
Grease ring, around firearm entrance wound, 513
Greasing equipment, injury from, 379, 1174
Great vessels, injuries of, 205–206. See also *Blood vessels.*
Green gill fungus, 1555
Grenade, arrow-launched, 595
improvised, 588, *589*
spigot, 595
Groin strains, 285
Groundsel plant, 1485–1487
Groupers, hazardous, 1407, *1408*
Growth hormone, in postmortem blood, 1040
Gun. See *Firearm(s).*
Gunpowder, as low explosive, 580
historical development of, 537–538
Gunshot wounds. See *Firearm wounds.*
Gutter cortical hemorrhage, 46
Gynecologic examination, of rape victim, 947–951
Gynecologic procedures, air embolization in, 416
bladder injury in, 237–238
complications of, 1233–1234
ureteral injury in, 233–234
uterine injury in, 255–257
Gynecomastia, after spinal cord injury, 82
Gyri, contusion of, 46
Gyromitra esculenta, 1553–1554

Habituation, to abused drugs, 828
to meteorologic stress, 1629
Hair, analysis of, in arsenic poisoning, 805
head, racial differences in, 1108(t), 1111
pubic, as evidence in rape, 947
Hallucinatory mullet poisoning, 1427, *1427*
Hallucinogens, effects of, 830
overdose of, 832
plant sources of, 1556–1557
D. stramonium as, 1537
use of, historically, 827
Hallux rigidus, 337
Halogens, with acetylene, spontaneous combustion of, 738–739
Haloperidol, side effects of, 1206–1207
Halothane, and liver injury, 1249–1251, 1250(t)
Hamartomas, cryptic, 47
Hand, abscess of, 368–369, *369*
anatomy of, 365–368, *366*, *367*
arteriovenous fistula of, 377
beat, 1184
causalgia of, 382
chemical gangrene of, 377, *378*
Dupuytren's contracture of, 330, 382–383
fibroses of, posttraumatic, 382–384
in shoulder-hand syndrome, 264–265
infections of, posttraumatic, 368–370, *369*
injuries of, 365–385
burn, 380–381
dislocation, 375–376, *375*
electrical, 380–381
fracture, 374
from narcotic injections, 379
from spraying equipment, 1173
iatrogenic, 379
occupational, 379–380, 1173
of joints of, 374–376
of nerves of, 372–374
of skin of, 370–371, *370*
of tendons of, 371–372, *371*
sprain, 374–375
treatment of, complications of, 1235
vascular, 225, 376–379, *377*, *378*
ischemic local contracture of, 378
pain in, posttraumatic, 381–382, *382*
reflex sympathetic dystrophy of, 382, *382*
stiffness in, posttraumatic, 381
Volkmann's contracture of, 69, 349, 377–378, *378*
Handball players, vascular injuries in, 225
Hand grenade, improvised, 588, *589*
Handgun. See also *Firearm(s); Rifled weapons.*
as rifled weapon, 510
barrel of, bullet markings from, 560–561, *560*, *561*
manufacture of, 554–555, *555*
sizes of, 510–511
breech face of, manufacture of, 555–557, *556*, *557*
bullets for. See *Bullets.*
cartridges for. See *Cartridges.*
ejector of, cartridge markings from, 558
manufacture of, 555–557, *556*
extractor of, cartridge markings from, 558
manufacture of, 555–557, *556*
firing pin of, cartridge markings from, *557*, 558
manufacture of, 555–557, *556*, *557*
injury from. See *Firearm wounds.*
manufacture of, 554–557, *555–557*

Handgun (*Continued*)
types of, 540–541, *540*
Hand-Schüller-Christian disease, and oral injury, 152–153, *152*
Hanging, 203
suicidal, *6*, 1006, *1006*
simulated, 1063
Haplopappus fruticosus, 1485
Haplopappus heterophyllus, 1485
Haptoglobins, identification of, in bloodstains, 815–816
Hard palate. See *Palate.*
Harrison and Gilroy test, for firearm discharge residue, 566–567
Head. See also *Skull.*
examination of, posttraumatic, 35–38
hair of, racial differences in, 1108(t), 1111
injuries of. See *Head injuries.*
molding of, during birth, 450–452, *451*
and dural venous laceration, 452–453, *452*, 454, 454(t)
radiography of, 688
surgery of, complications of, 1226–1227
Head banging, in children, 60, 497
Head injuries, 29–63
and acute respiratory failure, 394
and akinetic mutism, 56
and brain lesions, 41–60
and brain tumors, 58
and diabetes insipidus, 61
and ear injury, 135–136
and hearing loss, 136
and heart disorders, 13, 400
and intracranial nerve injury, 62–63
and kidney dysfunction, 401
and life expectancy, 58–59
and myocardial lesions, 400
and olfactory disorders, 62
and pituitary gland injury, *57*, 60–61
and traumatic retinopathy, 110
and ulcer formation, 396–397
and vertigo, 136
contralateral, 35
contrecoup, 35
defined, 29
during birth, 447–456, *448–452*, 454(t), *455*
examination in, 35–38
from acceleration concussion, 34–35
from compression concussion, 34–35
from firearms, 518–519, *515–519*
history-taking in, 33
in aircraft accidents, 877, *879*, *882*, 882(t), 883(t), *884*
in automobile accidents, 855
in battered child, 503–504, *504*
in cardiovascular collapse, 36–37
in children, 59–60, 503–504, *504*
in infants, 59–60
in newborns, 447–456, *448–452*, 454(t), *455*
investigation of, 33–35
mechanisms of, 34–35
misdiagnosis in, 908

Head injuries (*Continued*)
perinatal, 447–456, *448–452*, 454(t), *455*
psychoneurologic sequelae of, 57–58
in infants and children, 59–60
ultrasonic diagnosis of, 778, *779*
with facial injury, 141
Head lice, 1451
Headstamps, 552–553, *554*
Hearing, anatomical system for, 132
tests of, 133
Hearing loss, after explosion, 620
after head injury, 136
cochlear, 134
conductive, 134
drug-induced, 1199
noise-induced, 138–139
temporal bone fracture and, 136–137
types of, 134
Heart, angiography of, 688
anxiety and, 13
arrhythmias of. See *Arrhythmias.*
catheterization of, injury from, 209, 672, 906, *906*
circulation in, altitude and, 1300–1302, *1304–1305*
foreign bodies in, 418
fuchsinophilic degeneration of, head injury and, 400
hemorrhagic shock and, 8
hypothermia and, 759, 763–764
in burn injury, 722, 725
infection of, posttraumatic, 16, *16*
injuries of, 12–17, 204–205
alcoholic, 821–822
cardiac tamponade in, *13*, *14*, 204
contusion, 12, 204–205
electrical, 205, 657–658, *658*
from catheterization, 209, 262, 906, *906*
heart failure in, 204, 205
hypothermic, 768
hypoxic, perinatal, *462*
iatrogenic, 208–209, 768
in aircraft accidents, 880, *881*, 882(t)
laceration, *13*
penetrating, 209
rupture, 205, 880, *881*, 882(t), 883
steering wheel, 12
thermal, 722, 725
local anesthetics and, 1247
massage of, complications of, 1238
myocardium of. See *Myocardium.*
myocytolysis, of, head injury and, 400
paper bag rupture of, 883
postmortem findings in, in burn victims, 725
radiography of, 687, 688
surgery of, complications of, 1228–1229
transplantation of, 986
trauma and, 8, 12–17, *13–16*, 398–400, *399*
ultrasonic scanning of, 778, *780*
valves of, infection of, post-traumatic, 16, *16*

Heart (*Continued*)
ventricular fibrillation in, in drowning, 1322
in electrical injury, 649–650, 649(t), 650
in hypothermia, 760
Heart disease, cold and, 765
death from, autopsy in, 1679
postmortem diagnosis of, 1055
trauma and, 12–17, *13–16*
Heart failure, after femoral fracture, in elderly, 888
anxiety and, 13
cardiac massage in, complications of, 1238
concurrent with trauma, causation in, 15–16
in drug anaphylaxis, 1202–1203
in heart injury, 204, 205
in heatstroke, 707
in hypothermia, 763–764
perinatal, and hypoxic injury, 456–486, 456(t)
senile, 888
subclinical, posttraumatic, 398, *399*
vs. food aspiration, 1614
Heat, body, elevated. See *Fever; Hyperpyrexia; Hyperthermia.*
regulation of, 701–702
environmental, 701
acclimatization to, 710
injury from, 701–729. See also *Hyperthermia.*
physiologic response to, 709–710
in prevention of food poisoning, 1612
inhaled, injury from, 714
Heat cramps, 703
Heat exhaustion, 703–704
anhydrotic, 704
Heat hyperpyrexia, 704–710, *706–709*
Heat load, 701
Heat of combustion, for chemical elements, 730(t)
Heatstroke, 704–710, *706–709*
Heavy metals, and ear injury, 137
contaminating food, 787–788
injection of, and chemical gangrene, 377
toxicologic examination for, 806
Heel, fractures of, 334–336, *334*
lover's, 335
policeman's, 330
Helicopter accidents, 882–883, 883(t)
Hellaborus foetidus, 1526
Hellaborus niger, 1526–1527
Hellaborus orientalis, 1526
Hellaborus viridis, 1526
Hellebore, 1526–1527
Hellebore plant, 1516
Helleborein, 1527
Helminthic infections, 1355–1366, *1359–1361*
Helvella esculenta, 1553
Helvellic acid, 1553–1554
Hemagglutinins, in plants, 793–794, 793(t)
Hemarthrosis, traumatic, of knee, 309–310
Hematoma, cerebral, 46
duodenal, 216, *218*

Hematoma *(Continued)*
  epidural, 42
  intracranial, vs. cerebral fat embolism, 411
  of fetal pericranium, 448–450, *449*
  ossifying, 296, 348
  retroperitoneal, 218–219, *219*
  retroplacental, *460*
  subdural. See *Subdural hematoma.*
  subpleural, *7*
Hematomyelia, 65
Hematorrhachis, 65
Hematuria, in genitourinary injury, 227
  in kidney injury, 231
Hemianopia, bitemporal, 62
Hemlock, 1546, 1547
Hemodynamic alterations, in shock, 13
Hemodynamic parameters, 8
Hemoglobin, carbonyl. See *Carboxyhemoglobin.*
Hemoglobin tests, for racial origin of bloodstains, 812
Hemoglutinin, 1505
Hemopericardium, *13, 14*
Hemorrhage, alveolar, from air blast, 620–621, *620, 621*
  and shock, 387–388
  and venous infarction, 458–460
  cerebral, 45–47, *46–49*
    cold and, 765
    in infant, 59
    perinatal, hypoxic injury in, 462–477, *466–477*, 466(t)
  choroidal, 108
  conjunctival, 91
  epidural, 39, 42
    spinal, perinatal, 442, *442*, 466(t)
  extradural, 40
    in infants, 59
  gastrointestinal, from air blast, 622
    from immersion blast, 624
    from stress ulcers, 395
  gutter cortical, 46
  in abdominal injuries, 211, 622, 624
  in facial injuries, 140–141
  in fetus, 460. See also *Subdural hemorrhage, perinatal.*
  in great vessel injuries, 205, 206
  in heart injuries, 204
  in liver injuries, 212–213
  in newborn, 460. See also *Subdural hemorrhage, perinatal.*
  in pancreatic injuries, 214
  into pleural cavity, 201
  intracranial, death from, autopsy in, 1680
    delayed, 46–47
    perinatal, 462–466, 466(t)
      of brain stem, 442–443, *443*, 466(t)
  intraocular, 101–102, *101*, 109
    in battered child, 111
  intraorbital, 116
  perinatal, 458–460
    spinal epidural, 442, *442*
    subdural. See *Subdural hemorrhage, perinatal.*
  petechial, in sudden infant death, 1028
Hemorrhage *(Continued)*
  pulmonary, from air blast, 620–621, *620, 621*
  retinal, 109
  retroperitoneal, traumatic, in pregnancy, 425
  spinal epidural, perinatal, 442, *442*
  subarachnoid, 44–45
  subconjunctival, 91
  subdural, 42–44, *42–44*
    in infants, 59
    perinatal. See *Subdural hemorrhage, perinatal.*
    timing of, 43
  traumatic, 387–388
    coagulopathy and, 390
    in pregnancy, 425
Hemorrhagic fever, 1371
Hemorrhagic shock, 8, 387–388
  in facial injuries, 140, 143
  in heart injuries, 204
  organ failure in, 8
Hemothorax, 201
  iatrogenic, 209
Henbane, 1537
Henschel test, 1633
Hepatitis, alcoholic, 821
  halothane, 1249–1251, 1250(t)
  viral, from cadavers, 909
    vs. halothane hepatitis, 1249–1251
    vs. hepatitic drug jaundice, 1249–1251
Herb Christopher plant, 1525
Herbicides, as food contaminants, 788
Hernia, abdominal, surgery of, complications of, 1232–1233
  diaphragmatic, 207
  fascial, 316
    of foot, 329
    of thigh, 297, 329
  synovial, of ankle, 320
    of foot, 329
    of wrist, 279
Herniation, of brain parts, 49–50, *49*
  of brain stem, perinatal, 445, *445*
  of mesencephalon, 50
Heroin, injection of, injury from, 832–835. See also *Drugs, abused.*
Hesitation wounds, 1005
High altitude, biologic effects of, 1293–1294
    on newborns, 1295–1296, 1296(t)
  chemoreceptors at, 1297–1298
  circulatory system at, 1298–1302, *1298*, 1298(t), *1299*, 1300(t), *1302–1305*
  coronary circulation at, 1300–1302, *1304–1305*
  defined, 1293
  drug action at, 1639–1640
  endocrine system at, 1296–1297
  hematologic system at, 1296
  homeostatic balance at, 1293, 1294
  injury from, 641–644
  mortality at, 1302–1306
  pathologic conditions at, 1306–1314
    nonspecific, 1306
  placenta at, 1295, *1295*, 1296(t)
High altitude *(Continued)*
  physiopathologic aspects of, 1293–1314
  population density at, 1293–1294, 1294(t)
  respiratory system at, 1297
  tumors at, 1306
High altitude acute pulmonary edema, 1306–1308, *1307–1308*
High altitude disease, 1308–1314, 1309(t), 1310(t), *1311–1313*
High altitude residents, characteristics of, 1294
  reproduction in, 1294–1295
High explosives, 580–581
High pressure equipment injury from, 1172–1174
Hip, bursitis of, 285
  calcification in, 285
  dislocations of, 285–289, *286–289*
    posterior, 285–288, *286, 287*
      recurrent, 287–288
  fractures of, 289–296, *290–296*
    extracapsular, 292–296, *293–296*
    in elderly, complications of, 887–889, *887*
    intertrochanteric, 292–293
    intracapsular, 289–292, *290–292*
    subtrochanteric, 293–296, *293, 299*
  injuries of, 285–296, *285–296*
    posttraumatic disability from, 296
    soft tissue, 285
  snapping, 285
Hippocastanaceae, poisonous, 1504
Hippomane mancinella, 1495–1496, *1496*
Histamine, 1548
  in wound timing, analysis of, 1096
    extraction of, 26–28
Histochemical examination, for wound timing, 24, *25*, 26
Histologic examination, for wound timing, 23–24
Histoplasmosis, 1334–1335
History taking, in head injury, 33
  in occupational-environmental disease, 1276
Hit-and-run accident, investigation of, 861
Hitrine, 1497
Home, accidents in, 886–900
  asphyxiation in, 892–895, *894*
  burns in, 717, 889–892, *889, 891*
  cuts and lacerations in, 899–900
  drowning in, 898
  electrical injury in, 671, 897–898
  falls in, 886–889, *887*
  firearm accidents in, 896–897, *896*
  fires in, 889–892, *889. 891*
  gas explosions in, 632–633, *632*
  hypothermia in, 899
  poisoning in, 895–896
  snowblower accidents at, 898–899
Home permanents, causing fires, 739
Homeostasis, at high altitude, 1293, 1294
  thermal, 701–702
    in sauna bath, 709–710
Homicidal wounds, 6, 7
  firearm, *512–514*, *516*, 522–523

Homicide, alcohol and, 823, 823(t), 824
  attempted concealment of, 1062–1963
  by automobile, 861–862
  by drowning, 1317, 1331–1332
  by electrocution, 665–666
  by poisoning, incidence of, 1569, 1569(t)
    with drugs, 837, 1011
    with plants, 1456
  by shooting, *512–514*, *516*, 522–523, 1012
  by strangulation, 1010, *1011*, 1063
  crime-related, 1010–1013, *1012*
  gangland, 1011–1012, *1012*
  homosexual, 962, *962*, 1010, *1011*
  methods of, 1008–1014, *1008–1113*
  postmortem injury in, 1013, *1013*, 1061–1064, *1064*
  premeditated, injuries in, 1009–1013
  sexual, 962, *962*, 1010, *1011*
    bitemarks in, 1143
    terroristic, 1012–1013
  unpremeditated, injuries in, 1009
Homicide victims, radiography of, 1157
Homosexuality, 959
  and homicide, 962, *962*, 1010, *1011*
  and suicide, 962
Homotransplantation. See *Transplants, organ.*
Hooke's law of elasticity, 4–5
Hookworm infections, 1357–1358
Hormones, administration of, during pregnancy, 1200
  in burn injury, 722
  in cancer treatment, 1200
  in hypothermia, 761
  in postmortem blood, 1039–1040, 1040(t)
  postmortem levels of, 1055
  response of, to trauma, 386–387
Hospital, accidents in, 901–909
  electrical injury in, 671–672
  emergency treatment in. See *Emergency treatment, hospital.*
Hospital accident room, 871
Hospital autopsy, 971–972, 980
Hospital emergency department, 871–874
Hospital employees, occupational injuries in, 901–903, 908–909
Host, to parasite, 1343
    definitive, 1345
  intermediate, 1345
Hottentot's poison bush, 1477
Houseflies. See *Fly(ies), sarcosaprophagous.*
Housemaid's knee, 304
Human body, dead. See *Corpse.*
  elastic properties of, 4
Human growth hormone, in postmortem blood, 1040
Humerus, fractures of, of condyl of, 275
    of distal end of, 273–274, *274*
    of epicondyl of, 275
    of proximal end of, 270, *270*
Humerus *(Continued)*
  fractures of, of shaft of, 271
    of trochlea of, 275
Hura crepitans, 1496
Hura polyandra, 1496–1497
Hurin, 1497
Hurtado's disease, 1306–1308, *1307–1308*
Hyaline membrane disease, 479, *479*
  adult, 392, *393*
Hydatid cyst disease, 1365–1366
Hydrocephalus, 50
Hydrogen ion concentration, in postmortem blood, 1043
Hydrogen peroxide, spontaneous combustion of, 738
Hydroma, 44
Hydromedusae, 1385, *1386*
Hydrostatic lung, 1325
Hydroxycorticosteroids, in postmortem blood, 1039
Hydroxytryptamine, 1548
Hydrozoa, 1380, 1383(t), 1385–1387, *1386–1387*
Hygroma, 44
Hymen, examination of, in rape victim, 947–950, *949*
  lacerations of, 249–250
Hymenolepiasis, 1361–1362
Hyoscine, 1540
Hyoscyamine, 1533, 1535–1536, 1537
Hyoscyamus muticus, 1537
Hyoscyamus niger, 1537
Hyperbarism, injury from, 636–640
Hypercalcemia, antemortem, postmortem diagnosis of, 1054–1055
Hyperdynamic state, in trauma, 388–389
Hyperemia, of skin, in radiation therapy, 124
  of tooth pulp, 163
Hyperextension-hyperflexion injury, of spine, 63, 64. 77
    perinatal, 446, *446*
Hyperglycemia, postmortem diagnosis of, 1053
  posttraumatic, 391
Hyperkeratosis, oral, 176–177, *177*
    nicotine and, 191–192, *192*
Hyperoxia, in divers, 638
Hyperparathyroidism, and oral injury, 150, *151*
Hyperplasia, chronic inflammatory papillary, 187, *187*
  gingival, drug-induced, 189, *189*
Hyperpyrexia. See also *Hyperthermia.*
  conflagration, 713–715
  drug-induced, 710–711
  febrile, 710–711
  heat, 704–710, *706–709*
  malignant, 712–713
Hypersensitivity. See *Allergy.*
Hypertension, after spinal cord injury, 84
  at high altitude, 1298–1300, 1306
  pulmonary arterial, 1306
Hyperthermia, local. See *Burns.*
  systemic, 702–715
    causes of, 703
    conflagration, 713–715
    drug-induced, 711–713
Hyperthermia *(Continued)*
  systemic, effects of, 701–715
    endogenous, 710–711
    exogenous, 703–710
  febrile, 710–711
    malignant, 712
    nonfebrile, 703–710
    therapeutic, 713
Hyperventilation, in anesthesia, 1242, 1243
  trauma and, 387
Hypervitaminosis A poisoning, 1428–1429
Hyphema, 101, *101*
Hypnotic, drugs, effects of, 829
Hypobarism, injury from, 641–644
Hypocalcemia, antemortem, postmortem diagnosis of, 1054–1055
Hypoglossal nerve, 63
Hypoglycemia, postmortem diagnosis of, 1053
Hypoglycine, 1531
Hypoplasia, of dental enamel, 160, *160*, 180–181, *180*
Hypoproteinemia, in burn injury, 722
Hypopyon, 102, *102*
Hypostasis, postmortem, 34, 997
    in carbon monoxide poisoning, 843, 847, *847*
    in drowning, 1320
    vs. contusion, 5, 36
Hypotension, orthostatic, after spinal cord injury, 81
Hypothalamus, as thermoregulatory center, 1627
  in schizophrenia, 1633–1634
Hypothermia, local, 765–768. See also *Frostbite.*
  systemic, 758–765, *763*, *764*
    alcohol and, 762
    barbiturates and, 762
    coagulation disorders in, 768
    death from, 764–765
      at home, 899, *899*
      cause of, 762
    diagnosis of, 763–765
    drugs and, 762
    environmental, 758
    immersion, 758
    laboratory findings in, 763
    postmortem findings in, 763–764, *763*, *764*
    promazine and, 762
    rewarming shock in, 769
    signs and symptoms of, 763
    survival time in, 762
  therapeutic, injury from, 768–769
Hypotropia, 117
Hypoventilation, after anesthesia, 1243
  in anesthesia, 1241–1243, 1256
Hypovolemic shock, 8, 351, 388
Hypoxia, in anesthesia, 1241–1243
  in drowning, 1322
  in hemorrhagic shock, 8
  injury from, in carbon monoxide poisoning, 843–845, *843–846*
    of eye, 128
    perinatal, 439(t), 456–484, 456(t), 466(t)
      causes of, 457–458

Hypoxia *(Continued)*
  injury from, perinatal, in placental disorders, *458–460, 463*
    in premature infants, 472–473, *472, 473*, 482–483
    of adrenal, *464*
    of brain, 462–484, 466(t)
    of central nervous system, 439(t), 456–484, 456(t), 466(t)
    of intestines, *462*
    of kidney, 461–462, *463*
    of lung, *465*
    of testis, *464*
    of thymus, *461*
    of thyroid, *465*
    of viscera, 461–462, *461–465*
    sequelae of, 472–473, *472, 473*, 475–476, *476*, 477–484
    stages of, 457–460
Hysterectomy, complications of, 1233
Hysterosalpingography, 688

Iatrogenic injuries, and arteriovenous fistula, 226
  and pneumothorax, 201
  electrical, in cardiologic procedures, 672
  from air embolism, 415–416, 905–906
  from anesthesia, 905–906, *905*
  from dental procedures, 178–188
  from cryosurgery, 769
  from cryotherapy, 769
  from diathermy, 121
  from drugs, 906–908, *907*, 1195–1225. See also generic names of specific drugs.
    experimental, 1209–1212
    legal cases involving, 1212–1216
  from electroshock therapy, 662–663
  from fluoroscopy, 695
  from intraarterial injections, 226
  from laser therapy, 123
  from radiation therapy, 694–695, 908
  from radiographic contrast media, 186, *187*, 690–692, 695–696, 904
  from radiography, 186, *187*, 690–692, 694, 695–696, 902, 903–904
  from surgical procedures, 904–906, *905, 906*, 1226–1260. See also *Anesthesia; Surgery.*
  from therapeutic hypothermia, 768–769
  from ultrasound, 778–782
  in hospital, 901–909
  of bladder, 237–238
  of blood vessels, 224, 377, *378*, 905, *905*
  of chest, 208–209
  of esophagus, 206, 1227–1228
  of eye, 123–125
  of fetus, legal case involving, 1623–1625
  of hand, 379
  of kidney, 230–231, 401
  of musculoskeletal system, 908
  of nerves, anesthetic, 1246, 1248–1249

Iatrogenic injuries *(Continued)*
  of nerves, injection, 373
    surgical, 66, 68, 280
  of newborn, 437–438
  of oral structures, 178–188
  of penis, 240
  of renal pedicle, 229
  of spine, perinatal, 443, *444*
  of spleen, 212
  of teeth, 178–188, 1252–1253
  of trachea, 203
  of ureter, 233–236
  of urethra, 239
  of uterine cervix, 255–256
  of uterus, 255–257
  of vagina, 253
  perinatal, 437–438
Ibotenic acid, 1551
Ichthyotoxism, 795–796, 1417–1426
Ignition, of fires, causes of, 735–743, 735(t)
Ignition energy, for gases, vapors, and dusts, 743(t)
Ignition temperature, for chemical elements, 730(t)
  for inflammable substances, 736–737, 737(t)
Ileum. See *Small intestine.*
Iliopsoas tendon, strain of, 285
Ilium, dislocation of, 342
  fractures of, 338, *338*, 339
Illegitimacy, cause of action for, 492
Immersion blast, 622–624, *623, 624*
Immersion foot, 766–767
Immunologic tests for bloodstain identification, 816
Immunosuppression, in shock, 390–391
Impact, primary, 4
  secondary, 4
Impotence, drug-induced, 1198
  posttraumatic, 238
Incendiarism, 959. See also *Arson.*
Incendiary bombs, 572–578, *573–577.* See also *Bomb(s); Bombing(s).*
Incendiary fires. See *Arson.*
Incised wounds, defined, 6
Incontinence, posttraumatic, 238, 239
Incubation period, defined, 10
  in food poisoning, 1589(t)
  in wound infection, 10
India rubber vine, 1483
Indian licorice plant, 1504–1508, *1506–1507*
Indian lobelia plant, 1484
Indian pink plant, 1483
Indian poke plant, 1516
Indian tobacco plant, 1483
Indians, American, racial characteristics of. See *Mongoloids.*
Indomethacin, injury from, of eye, 129
    products liability case involving, 1264–1266
Industrial chemicals, use of, in bombs, 588–589, 592–594
Industrial diseases. See *Occupational-environmental diseases.*
Industrial injuries. See *Occupational injuries.*
Inertia, principle of, 3
  in ballistics, 528

Infant. See also *Newborn.*
  asphyxiation in, vs. sudden infant death syndrome, 1018–1023, *1021, 1022, 1024*
  birth defects in. See *Birth defects.*
  birth injuries in, 436–486. See also *Birth injuries.*
  bloodstains from, identification of, 812
  brain lesions in, 59–60
  death in, unexplained, 1015–1032. See also *Sudden infant death.*
  facial paralysis in, 135
  hypothermia in, 758
    diagnosis of, 763
  injuries of, from radiographic contrast media, 904
    of head, 59–60
    of spine, 65
  intestinal surgery in, complications of, 1232
  premature. See *Premature infant.*
  skull of, 38
Infanticide, 1010
  skull fractures in, 450
Infarct, septic, 16, 408–409
Infarction, defined, 23
  in brain, as indication of death, 23
    perinatal, 462–476, *466–476*, 466(t)
      in premature infants, 466–473, *466–473*, 466(t)
      patterns of, 464–466, 466(t)
  in kidney, perinatal, 461–462, *463*
  in placenta, 426, *459, 460, 463*
  in thymus, perinatal, *461*
  perinatal, 458–484
  venous, 458–460
Infection(s). See also names of specific organs and body parts.
  as fracture complication, 349–350, *351*
  as surgical complication, 1237
  as trauma complication, 389–390
  bacterial, 1372–1375
  drug therapy and, 11
  from autopsy cadavers, 908–909
  from illicit drug injections, 833–834
  fungal, 1334–1342
    secondary, 11
  helminthic, 1355–1366, *1359–1361*
  mycobacterial, 1334–1342
  of burns, 723
    postmortem examination for, 724
  of thrombus, 16, 408–409
  of wounds, 9–11. See also *Wound infection.*
  pelvic, intrauterine devices and, 256–257
  preexisting, trauma aggravating, 11
  protozoan, 1346–1354, *1348–1349, 1353–1354*, 1375–1376
  psychosomatic approach to, 11–12
  respiratory, and sudden infant death, 1023–1025, *1024*
  rickettsial, 1371–1372
  stress and, 11–12
  trauma and, 9–12, *9*
  viral, 1369–1370
    arthropod-borne, 1370–1371
Infectious diseases, animal-transmitted, 1369–1377
  insect-transmitted, 1370–1377

Inferior oblique muscle, anatomy of, 115, *115*
Inferior rectus muscle, anatomy of, 115, *115*
  entrapment of, in orbital fracture, 117, 147
Infertility, altitude and, 1294–1295
  drug-induced, 1198
Inflammable substance(s), explosive range of, 736–737, 737(t)
  flash point of, 736–737, 737(t)
  identification of, in fire investigation, 745–757
  ignition temperature of, 736–737, 737(t)
  spontaneous combustion of, 737–739
Informed consent. See *Consent, informed.*
Infrared radiation, eye injury from, 121–122
Ingestion, of insects, 1455
  of toxins, 1569, 1570, 1570(t)
Inhalant, drugs, abuse of, 832
  effects of, 829
Inhalation, of solids and liquids. See *Aspiration.*
Inhalation anesthetics, abuse of, 832, 832(t)
Inhalation injury, from carbon monoxide. See *Carbon monoxide poisoning.*
  from chemicals, 203, 1570, *1571.* See also *Fumes, poisonous.*
    in fires, 713–714, 724–725
  from drugs, 832
  from heat, 713–714, 724–725
  from smoke, 202–203, 713–714, 724–725
  in explosions, 631, 632, 1184
  in fires, 202–203, 713–714
    postmortem findings in, 724–725
  occupational, 632, 1184, 1274–1275
  suicidal, 1007
  toxicologic analysis in, 806
Injection injury, chemical, 1572
  chemical gangrene in, 377, *378*
  from intraarterial injection, 226
  in drug addicts, 379
Injury. See also *Wound*; and name of specific organ or body part.
  definition of, in workmen's compensation laws, 1676
  evidence of, in skeletal remains, 1113, *1113*
  postmortem examination of, 997–998
  radiography of, 1155–1157
  response to, patterns of, 1155–1156
  timing of, at autopsy, 998
  treatment of. See *Emergency treatment.*
Inkberry, 1523–1524, *1524*
Inner ear, anatomy of, 132–133. See also *Ear.*
Innervation. See *Nerves.*
Inocybe geophylla, 1554
Inocybe infida, 1554
Inocybe patouillardi, 1554
Inorganic compounds, identification of, in commercial explosives, 606–607
Inorganic compounds *(Continued)*
  identification of, in improvised explosives, 604–606
Inositol, in postmortem cerebrospinal fluid, 1044
Insects, as infectious diseases vectors, 1370–1377
  as parasitic disease vectors, 1366–1368
  bites of, injury from, 1447–1454
  ingestion of, 1455
  inhalation of, 1454–1455
  postmortem injury from, 1067–1069, *1067–1069.* See also *Fly(ies), sarcosaprophagous.*
  sarcosaprophagous, as forensic indicators, 1072–1095. See also *Fly(ies), sarcosaprophagous.*
  stings of, hypersensitivity to, 1445–1447
Insensible perspiration, 701
In-shot wounds. See *Entrance wounds.*
Insulin, and convulsions, 1200–1201
  in postmortem blood, 1039–1040
Intercourse, sexual. See *Sexual intercourse.*
Interior ballistics, defined, 527
Interment, statutes regulating, 971
  testamentary instructions for, 979–980
Interphalangeal joints, of hand, dislocations of, 375
Intersexuality, 959
Interstitial emphysema, from barotrauma, 637
  postnatal, 478–479, *478*
Intervertebral disk, radiography of, 66
  surgery of, complications of, 66
Intestinal flukes, 1362–1364
Intestinal infections, protozoan, 1346–1349, *1348–1349*
  round worm, 1355–1359, *1359*
  tapeworm, 1359–1362, *1360–1361*
Intestines, injury of, from barotrauma, 637
    hypoxic, perinatal, *462*
    in battered child, *502*, 504
    in immersion blast, 624
  large, injuries of, 219–220
    seat belt, 856, *856*
    surgery of, complications of, 1231–1232
  parasitic infestation of, 1346–1349, *1348–1349*, 1355–1359, *1359*, 1359–1362, *1360–1361*
  small, injuries of, 217–218
    surgery of, complications of, 1230
Intoxicant drugs. See *Drugs, abused.*
Intoxicant plants, 1457
Intoxication, alcoholic. See *Alcohol intoxication.*
  chemical. See *Poisoning.*
Intracranial hematoma, vs. cerebral fat embolism, 411
Intracranial hemorrhage, death from, autopsy in, 1680
  delayed, 46–47
Intracranial hemorrhage *(Continued)*
  perinatal, 462–466, 466(t)
    of brain stem, 442–443, *443*, 466(t)
Intracranial injuries. See *Head injuries.*
Intraocular foreign bodies, 112–114, *113*
Intraocular infection, 102, *102*, 107
Intraocular pressure, elevated. See *Glaucoma.*
Intrapelvic dislocation, 288–289, *288*
Intrauterine device, and birth defects, legal case involving, 1617–1626
  injury from, 256–257
Intrauterine transfusion syndrome, *458*
Intravenous feeding, complications of, 1237
Intravenous fluid, administration of, injury from, 907
Intubation, tracheal. See *Tracheal intubation.*
Iodide fever, 712
Iodine, in postmortem vitreous humor, 1050
  radioactive, as contrast medium, injury from, 690–692
Ion trapping, 1569
Ionizing radiation. See *Radiation, ionizing.*
Iothalamates, injury from, 690–692
Iris, anatomy of, 103
  injuries of, blunt, 104, *104*
    chemical, 127, *127*
    electrical, 120
    from laser therapy, 122
    iatrogenic, 122
    penetrating, 104–105
  prolapse of, 97–98, *97*, *127*
Irradiation, therapeutic. See *Radiology, therapeutic.*
  ultrasonic. See *Ultrasound.*
Ischemia, cerebral, 8, 47–49, 53, *54*
  in arterial injuries, 222, 223
  in hemorrhagic shock, 8
  in spinal cord injury, 65, 77, 83
  muscular, 69, 349, 377–378, *378*
    in drug-induced coma, 379
  neural, 373
  tissue tolerance to, 223
Ischemic contracture, local, of hand, 378
Ischemic ulceration, after spinal cord injury, 83
Ischium, fractures of, 338, *338*, 339, *339*
Isomorphic scar, 55
Isoniazid, injury from, 1198
Isopropyl alcohol, poisoning by, 820
Itches, in decompression sickness, 642
Itchweed, 1516
IUD. See *Intrauterine device.*
Ivory shell poisoning, 1401
Ivy-bush, 1489

Jack-o'-lantern fungus, 1553
Jacks, venomous, 1415
Japanese wisteria, 1512

Jatropha curcas, 1497–1498
Jatropha gossypifolia, 1498–1499
Jatropha multifida, 1499
Jatrophine, 1499
Jaundice, drug, general anesthetics and, 1249–1251, 1250(t)
Jaw. See *Mandible; Maxilla.*
Jejunum. See *Small intestine.*
Jellyfish, 1381–1383, *1381*, 1384
Jequirity bean, 1504–1508, *1506–1507*
Jessamine, 1518–1519, 1534
Jet aircraft accidents, 876–879, *878*, *879*
Jimmyweed, 1485
Jimsonweed, 1535
Joint(s). See also names of specific joints.
  adhesions in, posttraumatic, 347–348
  ankylosis of, in burn victims, 726–727
    in spinal cord injury, 63, 77
  arthritis of. See *Arthritis.*
  arthrography of, 688
  calcification in, posttraumatic, 348–349. See also *Calcification.*
  in decompression sickness, 642–643
  infection of, posttraumatic, 349–350
  injuries of, 259–361
    dislocation. See *Dislocations.*
    electrical, 656–657
    fracture. See *Fractures.*
  radiography of, 687, 688
  stiffness of, posttraumatic, 347–348
Joint mice, 303
Judicial electrocution, 650

Kalmia angustifolia, 1489–1490
Kalmia latifolia, 1489
Kanamycin, and ear injury, 137
  and kidney injury, 401
Kastle-Meyer test, for bloodstains, 810
Keloids, 67
Keratitis, 96, *96*
  in chemical burns, 126
  in photophthalmia, 123
  in radiation therapy and, 124
Keratopathy, bullous, 98, *98*
  in chemical burns, 126
Ketosteroid levels, after spinal cord injury, 82
Kidney. See also *Renal pedicle.*
  angiography of, 228–229, 232
  disease of, postmortem diagnosis of, 1054
  hypothermia and, 760–761
  infarction of, perinatal, 461–462, *463*
  injuries of, 230–232
    anesthetics and, 1251
    colistin and, 401
    electrical, 661
    iatrogenic, 401
      hypothermic, 768
    thermal, 725–726
  ischemia in, posttraumatic, 8
  postmortem findings in, in burn victims, 725–726
Kidney *(Continued)*
  radiography of, 231–232, 688, 689
  surgery of, complications of, 1234
  transplantation of, 985–986
Kidney failure, posttraumatic, 351, 400–402, *401*
Kinetic energy, 4
  in ballistics, 528
Kissing bugs, bites of, 1449
Knee, beat, 1184
  bursitis of, 304–306, *305*
  calcification in, 304
  cartilage of, degeneration of, 303
    in osteochondritis dissecans, 311–312, *311*
    injuries of, 308–309
  housemaid's, 304
  injuries of, 300–313, *302*, *305*, *306*, *311*, *314*
    cartilaginous, 308–309
    dislocation, 308
    fascial, 304
    ligamentous, 306–308, *306*
    extensor apparatus, 300–301, *302*
    sprain, 306–307
  instability of, posttraumatic, 308
  loose bodies in, 303
  osteochondritis dissecans of, 311–312, *311*
  radiography of, 688
  snapping, 309
Kneecap. See *Patella.*
Knife wounds. See *Stab wounds.*
Koa haole plant, 1509–1510
Koonti plant, 1488–1489, *1489*
Korsakoff's syndrome, 822–823
Kymography, 688

Labor, false, posttraumatic, 427
  fetal injuries during. See *Birth injuries.*
  precipitous, and fetal injury, 454
  premature, posttraumatic, 427–428, 432
  prolonged, and fetal injury, 446, 454
Laboratory, ballistics, 529–532
  fire investigation, 748–757, 748(t), *751–754*
  injuries in, 1175–1181
  toxicology, 800–809
Laboratory animals, injury from, 1181
Laburnum alpinum, 1509
Laburnum anagyroides, 1509
Laburnum vulgare, 1509
Labyrinth, acoustic. See *Ear, inner.*
Laceration(s). See also *Blunt injuries; Rupture.*
  defined, 6–7, *7*
  dural-venous, perinatal, 452–456, *452*, 454(t), *455*
  in aircraft accidents, 877, *879*, *881*, 882(t)
  in battered child, 501–503, *502*, *503*
  of choroid, 108, *109*, 111
  of face, 38
Laceration(s) *(Continued)*
  of hymen, 249–250
  of kidney, 231
  of lung, 202
  of nerves, 373–374
  of penis, 240
  of perineum, in aircraft accidents, 877, *879*
  of scalp, 6, 37
  of skin, in explosions, 626–630, *625–630*
  of stomach, 216
  of tendon, 371–372, *371*
  of tentorium, perinatal, *452*, 454, 454(t)
  of trachea, 203
  of vagina, coital, 249–250
    from foreign bodies, 251
    in rape victim, 950
    self-inflicted, 252
Lacrimal ducts, anatomy of, 89
  injuries of, 90–91, *91*, 143
  radiography of, 688
Lactic acid, in postmortem blood, 1035
  in postmortem cerebrospinal fluid, 1043
  in postmortem vitreous humor, 1046–1047
Lactic dehydrogenase, in postmortem blood, 1038–1039
Lady-of-the-night plant, 1534
Lambkill plant, 1489–1490
Lantadene A, 1549
Lantana camera, 1549–1550
Lap belts. See *Seat belts.*
Laportea canadensis, 1547–1548
Large intestine, injuries of, 219–220. See also *Intestine(s).*
    seat belt, 856, *856*
  surgery of, complications of, 1231–1232
Larkspur, 1526
Larva, of sarcosaprophagous flies, 1084–1090. See also *Fly(ies), sarcosaprophagous.*
Laryngography, 688
Laryngoscopy, dental injury in, 1252–1253
  injury of, in cervical disk surgery, 66
    in tracheal intubation, 1255
  radiography of, 688
Laser burns, iatrogenic, of eye, 122
Latent period, in radiation injury, 121
Lateral rectus muscle, anatomy of, 115, *115*
Latex, of *Euphorbia*, injury from, 1492, 1493, 1494, 1495, 1496
Lathyrogens, in plants, 793(t), 795
Laurel, cherry, 1528
Laurel, spurge, 1546
Laurel plant, 1489
Law, of negligence. See *Negligence.*
  of torts. See *Negligence.*
Law of elasticity, 4–5
Laws of motion, 3–5
Law of Wilder, 1628
Lawsuit, damages in. See *Damages.*
  evidence in. See *Evidence.*
  expert witness in. See *Expert witness.*

Lawsuit *(Continued)*
involving drug injury, 1212–1216, 1262–1267
involving fetal injury, 433, 487–494, 1617–1626
involving food poisoning, 1588, 1603–1604, 1611–1612
involving hazardous products, 1261–1267, 1621–1623, 1656–1660. See also *Products liability.*
involving medical device injury, 1261–1262, 1617–1626
involving occupational-environmental diseases, 1276–1277, 1290. See also *Workmen's compensation.*
malpractice, 696–700, 1212–1216, 1623–1625. See also *Malpractice.*
burden of proof in, 1653, 1656–1657
statute of limitations for, 1652–1653
Lead, eye injury from, 129
poisoning by, 1584(t), 1585
and sudden infant death, 1026
toxicologic analysis in, 805–806
radioactive, average levels of, in humans, 680
Lead tree, 1509–1510
Lectins, food poisoning from, 793–794, 793(t)
LeFort fractures, of maxilla, 144, 170
Left ventricular failure, posttraumatic, 398–400
Leg. See also names of component parts.
anterior tibial compartment syndrome in, 314–315, *315*
injuries of, 285–337
agricultural, 1163
bicycle spoke, 859
in aircraft accidents, *880*, 882(t), *884*
in explosions, 625
soft tissue, 313–316, *315*
Legal cases. See *Lawsuits.*
Leguminosae, poisonous, 1504–1513, *1506–1507*
Leishmaniasis, 1350–1352, 1375
Lemons, and tooth decalcification, 193
Lens, of eye, anatomy of, 105
in pupillary block, 100, *100*
injuries of, blunt, 105–107, *106*, *107*
drug-induced, 130
electrical, 120
iatrogenic, 124–125
penetrating, 105, *105*
radiation, 121
opacities of. See *Cataract.*
Lenten rose plant, 1526
Lepiota morgani, 1555
Leptomeningitis, traumatic, 45
Leptospirosis, 1185, 1374
agricultural, 1166
Letter bombs, 587
incendiary, 574–575
Letterer-Siwe disease, and oral injury, *152*, 153
Leucaena glauca, 1509
Leucaena leucocephala, 1509–1510
Leukemia, and oral injury, 154
drugs for, injury from, 1198–1199
Leukocytic infiltration, of wound, 23
Leukoplakia, 177–178, *177*
alcohol and, 191
nicotine and, 191–192, *192*
Liability. See also *Malpractice; Negligence; Products liability.*
absolute, in products liability, 1657
causation and, 1661–1664
fault system for, 910–935
for birth injuries, 437–438
for drug-induced injury, 1207–1216
involving overdosage, 1217–1219
involving package insert, 1219–1222
involving prescriptions, 1217, 1219
legal cases, involving, 1212–1216, 1262–1267
for emergency treatment, 869, 873–874, 1670
for emotional injuries, 1666–1668
for fetal injury, 433, 437–438, 487–494, 1617–1626
for food poisoning, 1588, 1603–1604, 1611–1612
for hazardous products. See *Products liability.*
for malpractice, 696–700, 1212–1216, 1623–1625
for medical device injury, 1261–1262, 1621–1623
for occupational-environmental disease, 1276–1277
for wrongful death, 430, 488–491
for "wrongful life," 491–493
in products liability, 1656–1660
risk theory of, 1662
standards for, 1645–1649. See also *Negligence.*
statute of limitations for, 1652–1653
strict, in products liability, 1656
vicarious, in malpractice, 1653
in medical partnerships, 1653
Lice, as disease vectors, 1367
biting, 1450–1451
plant, 1454
Lidocaine, and convulsions, 1200–1201
Ligaments, injuries of. See also *Sprains.*
of ankle, 320–324, *320–322*
of elbow, in Monteggia fracture-dislocation, *277*
of foot, 330
of knee, 306–308, *306*
Ligature strangulation, 203
Light aircraft accidents, 879–882, *880–882*
Lightning, causing fire, 743
injury from, 666–670, *668–670*
Lightning marks, 669, *669*, *670*
Lightning syndrome, 667
Lilac, persian, 1521–1522
Liliaceae, poisonous, 1513–1518
Lily of the valley plant, 1514–1515
Lily plant, 1515–1516
Limb. See also names of specific components of.
phantom, 381
Limb deformities, causes of, litigation involving, 1617–1626
Limber neck disease, of poultry, 1457
Limulus, 1392–1393, *1393*
Linamarin, 1500
Linase, 1500
Linear skull fracture, 6, 40, *41*
Linseed oil, spontaneous combustion of, 737–738
Lip, angioneurotic edema of, *183*, 184
granuloma of, 173, *173*
injuries of, iatrogenic, 185
in anesthesia, 184, *184*
in battered child, 502
laceration, 142
self-inflicted, 497, *497*
solar cheilosis of, 194
Lip prints, identification from, 1117–1118
Lipids, in postmortem blood, 1036–1037
postmortem analysis of, for diagnosis of antemortem disease, 1055
Lipiodol, in sialography, injury from, 186, *187*
Liquids, inflammable, 736–737
causing fire, identification of, in laboratory, 754–757, *756*
on-site, 746–747, *747*
explosive range of, 736–737, 737(t)
flash point of, 736–737, 737(t)
ignition temperature of, 736–737, 737(t)
used in arson, 736
Lithium, poisoning by, 1585–1586
spontaneous combustion of, 738
Litigation. See *Lawsuits.*
Liver, aflatoxins and, 792
cirrhosis of, alcoholic, 821
disease of, postmortem diagnosis of, 1055
hypothermia and, 760
injuries of, 212–213
alcoholic, 820–821
anesthetics and, 1249–1251, 1250(t)
electrical, 660
hypothermic, iatrogenic, 768
in battered child, *503*, 504
perinatal, 439–441, *440*, *441*
thermal, 725
metabolism in, of alcohol, 819
posttraumatic, 390–391
of fish, excessive vitamin A in, 1428–1429
postmortem findings in, in burn victims, 725
Liver flukes, 1362–1364
Livestock feed, contamination of, by chlorinated naphthalenes, 789
by diethylstilbestrol, 788
by mycotoxins, 790
Livor mortis, 34, 997
in carbon monoxide poisoning, 843, 847, *847*
in drowning, 1320
vs. contusion, 5, 35
Loaiasis, 1365
Lobelanidine, 1484
Lobelia berlandierei, 1483

Lobelia cardinalis, 1483
Lobelia inflata, 1483
Lobelia nicotianaefolia, 1484
Lobelia siphilitica, 1484
Lobelia tupa, 1484
"Lobelia" plant, 1518
Lobeline, 1484
Lobinaline, 1484
Local anesthetics, systemic toxicity of, 1247
"Locust" plant, 1511
Loganiaceae, poisonous, 1518–1520
Loose bodies, in knee, 303
Loranthaceae, poisonous, 1520–1521
Lorchel fungus, 1553
Lorel fungus, 1553
Loss of consciousness. See also *Syncope.*
  in electrical injury, 658–659
  indicating brain damage, 52
Lover's heels, 335
Low explosives, 580
Lower extremity. See *Leg;* and names of specific parts.
Lower worms, parasitic, marine, 1389–1390
LSD, 827, 830
Lucky nut plant, 1479–1481, *1480*
Ludwig's angina, 187, *187*
Lumbang nut plant, 1491
Lunate, dislocation of, 280, *281*
Lung. See also *Tracheobronchial tree.*
  biopsy of, percutaneous, injury from, 209
  carcinoma of, asbestos-related, 1279(t)–1281(t), 1284–1285, *1285*
  collapse of, postoperative, 1244
  edema of. See *Pulmonary edema.*
  fat embolism in, 410–411
  fluid in, posttraumatic, 8
  hemorrhage in, from air blast, 620–621, *620, 621*
  honeycomb, in asbestosis, 1282, *1283*
  hydrostatic, 1325
  in drowning, 204, 1324–1325, 1326
  in sudden infant death syndrome, 1020, *1021,* 1023, *1024*
  infarction of, perinatal, *465*
  injuries of, blunt, 202
    chemical, 203, 713–714
    contusion, 7, 202
    electrical, 660
    from asbestos, 1277–1291. See also *Asbestos-related diseases.*
    from barotrauma, 636–637
    from explosions, 202, 620–621, *620, 621*
    from oxygen intoxication, 1245–1246
    iatrogenic, 209
    inhalation. See *Inhalation injuries.*
    laceration, 202
    thermal, 714, 724–725
  meteorologic stimuli and, 1628(t)–1629(t)
  postmortem findings in, in burn victims, 724–725
  shock, 392, *393*
  stiff, 392
  surgery of, complications of, 1227
Lung *(Continued)*
  trauma and, 392–395, *393–396*
  wet, 392
Lung flukes, 1362–1364
Luxation. See *Dislocation.*
Lymph system, in sudden infant death syndrome, 1028
  postmortem findings in, in burn victims, 725
  radiography of, 689
  thermal injury of, 725
Lymphadenitis, regional, 10
Lymphangiography, 689
Lymphocytic choriomeningitis, 1369
D-Lysergic acid diethylamine, 827, 830

Mace, chemical, burns from, 718
Maceration of skin, in drowning, 1319
Machinery, anesthetic, misuse and malfunction of, 1256–1258
  injury from, in agriculture, 1164
    in coal mining, 1183
    in fishing industry, 1169–1171
    of hand, 380
Macula, radiation, injury of, 122
Macular cyst, 110
Macular hole, 110, *111*
Madagascar rubber vine, 1483
Madura foot, 1338
Maduromycosis, 1338
Maggots, in corpses, 1080–1084, *1081, 1083*
Magnesium, burns from, 722
  in postmortem blood, 1042
  in postmortem vitreous humor, 1050
  with silver nitrate and water, spontaneous combustion of, 739
Malabar tree, 1493
Malar. See *Zygoma.*
Malaria, 1353–1354, *1354*
Malignant disease. See *Cancer; Carcinoma.*
Malleoli, of ankle, fractures of, 324–325, *321, 322, 326, 327*
Mallet finger, 372
Malnutrition, in chronic alcoholics, 820, 821
  nerve injury from, 823
Malocclusion, in facial fractures, 143
  in untreated jaw fracture, 171, *171*
Malpractice, 692–693. See also *Iatrogenic injuries.*
  anesthesiologic, 905–906, *905,* 1239–1260
  causation in, 1649
  defined, 692
  elements of, 692
  in drug administration, 1208–1212
    legal cases involving, 1212–1216
    of experimental drugs, 1209–1212
  in emergency treatment, 870, 873, 908, 1670
    of snake bite, 1437–1438
  in hospital, 901–909
  informed consent and, 1654–1655
  legal concepts of, 1651–1655
Malpractice *(Continued)*
  obstetrical, 437–438, 491–493, 1617–1626
  orthopedic, 908
  pharmacologic, 906–908, 907, 1195–1225. See also *Drugs, injury from.*
  proximate cause in, 1649, 1663–1664
  radiologic, 694–696
  reasonably prudent man standard for, 1646–1649, 1651–1652
  res ipsa loquitor doctrine in, 1653
  standard of care in, 1646–1649, 1651–1652
  surgical, 904–906, *905, 906,* 1226–1260
  vicarious liability for, 1653
Malpractice lawsuits, 696–700, 1212–1216, 1623–1625
  burden of proof in, 1653
  damages in, computation of, 1665–1668
  evidence in, 699–700. See also *Evidence.*
  expert witness in, 697–699. See also *Expert witness.*
  statute of limitations for, 1652–1653
Mammals, marine, hazardous, 1408–1409
Mammography, 688
Manchineel plant, 1495–1496, *1496*
Mandible, fracture-dislocation of, 41
  fractures of, 169–172, *170, 171*
    classification of, 159, *159, 160,* 170–171
    faulty treatment of, 181, *182*
    systemic diseases predisposing to, 150–154, *151–153*
  racial differences in, 108(t), 1110, *1110,* 1111
  underdevelopment of, 162, *162*
Mangifera indica, 1471–1473
Mango plant, 1471–1473
Mangrovin, 1521
Manic-depressive states, trauma and, 17
Manihot esculenta, 1500–1501
Manihot utilissima, 1500–1501
Manioc plant, 1500–1501
Manzanilla plant, 1495–1496, *1496*
Marble bones, and oral injury, 153
March fractures, 336, *353*
Marchiafava-Bignami syndrome, 822
Marginal abrasion, in firearm entrance wound, 512, *512–514*
Margosine, 1521
Marihuana, 827, 830
Marine algae, toxic, 1429
Marine animals, injury from, 1378–1444
    by food poisoning, 795–796, 1388–1389, 1417–1426, 1427–1428, *1428*
Marine parasitic worms, 1389–1390
Marine turtles, poisonous, 1427–1428, *1428*
Marine venomous snakes, 1437–1444
Marjolin's ulcer, 371
Mark II mortar bomb, 596
Mark III mortar bomb, 596–597

Mark IV mortar bomb, 597, *597*
Mark VI mortar bomb, 598, *598*
Masochism, 959
Masochistic injuries, 963, *963*. See also *Self-inflicted injuries*.
Mastectomy, complications of, 1233
Mastoid air system, anatomy of, 132
Mastoid process, anatomy of, 132
Masturbatory practices, asphyxiation in, 894, *894*, 961–962, *962*, *963*
  penile injuries from, 239–240
  vulvovaginal injuries from, 251–252
Maxilla, birth, injury of, 163
  cyst of, *176*
  fractures of, 144–146, 169–172
    classification of, 159, *159*, *160*, 170
  underdevelopment of, 162
Maxillofacial injuries. See *Face, injuries of*.
Mayfly, inhalation of, injury from, 1454
McLaughlin's classification, of hip fractures, *290*
Meadow saffron plant, 1513–1514
Mechanical explosions, 578
  accidental vs. deliberate, 601
  dispersed, evidence of, 601
Mechanical injury, 3–509
Meconium aspiration pneumonia, 477, *478*
Medial rectus muscle, anatomy of, 115, *115*
Median nerve, of hand, anatomy of, 367
    entrapment of, in carpal tunnel syndrome, 279, 373
Medical devices, litigation involving, 1261–1262, 1617–1626
Medical records, of hospital emergency care, 872–873
  of prehospital emergency care, 867
Medications. See *Drugs*.
Medicinal plants, 1456–1457
Melia azedarach, 1521–1522
Meliaceae, toxic, 1521–1522
Men, bones of, vs. female bones, 1106–1108, 1106(t)
  breast enlargement in, after spinal cord injury, 82
  dental characteristics of, 1123–1124
  firearm injury in, 897
  genital injuries in, 239–241
    self-inflicted, 239–241
  identification of bloodstains from, 812
  identification of skeletal remains of, 1106–1108, 1106(t)
  meteorologic stress and, 1628, 1630
  rape of, 940
  sexual dysfunction in, after spinal cord injury, 80
  urethral injuries in, 238–239
Meningioma, and head trauma, 58
Meningitis, posttraumatic, 45
  rhizopus, 1338
  spinal anesthesia and, 1248–1249
Menisci, of knee, injuries of, 308–309
Menstrual bloodstains, identification of, 812
Mental anguish, damages for, 1666–1668
Mental disorders. See *Psychologic disorders*.
Mental processes, weather and, 1633–1637
Mental retardation, and self-mutilation, 497, *497*
  and time of conception, 1634
  in premature infants, 472–473, *472*, *473*, 482–483
  perinatal hypoxia and, 472–473, *472*, *473*, 475–476, *476*, 479–481
Mentation, changes in, in decompensated shock, 8
Meperidine, and smoking, 1216
Meprobamate, in postmortem vitreous humor, 1051–1052
Mercurialentis, 129
Mercury, as laboratory hazard, 1179
  eye injury from, 129
  poisoning by, 1583–1584
    chronic, and oral injury, 190–191, *191*
    from food, 787–788
Meridional skull fracture, 40
Mesencephalon, herniation of, 50
Mesothelioma, 1279(t)–1281(t), 1282–1284, *1283*, *1284*
Metabolism, alterations in, after spinal cord injury, 81–82
  basal, 701
  disorders of, in therapeutic hypothermia, 768–769
  of alcohol, 818–819
  of calcium, disorders of, postmortem diagnosis of, 1054–1055
  of carbohydrates, trauma and, 390–391
  of carbon monoxide, 840
  of drugs, 1576
  in burn injury, 722–723
  in shock, 390–391
  trauma and, 390–391
Metabolites, drug, and drug blood levels, 1576
Metacarpophalangeal joints, of hand, dislocations of, 375–376, *375*
Metal(s), alkali, spontaneous combustion of, 738
  blood levels of, 1578(t)–1579(t)
  contaminating food, 787–788
  injury from, 1583–1586, 1584(t)
    of ear, 137
  toxicologic examination for, 806
Metallic salts, and eye injury, 129
Metallization of skin, in electrical injury, 654
Metaraminol, and kidney injury, 401
Metastability, of earth's biosphere, 731–732, *731*
Metastases, trauma and, 19, 417–418
Metatarsal bones, dislocations of, 331
  fractures of, 336–337
Metatarsalgia, 330
  Morton's, 329
Metel plant, 1535, *1536*
Meteorologic phenomena, and human behavior, 1627–1642
Meteorotropic typology, 1628, 1630
Methane poisoning, in coal mine explosions, 1184
Methanol poisoning, 819–820
Methohexital, injury from, legal case involving, 1215
Methotrexate, injury from, 1198–1199
    legal case involving, 1213–1214
Methoxyflurane, and kidney injury, 401
Methyl alcohol poisoning, 819–820
Methyl mercury poisoning, from food, 787–788
Methysergide, and chemical gangrene, 377
Metopium toxiferum, 1473–1474
Mezereon plant, 1546
Microangiomas, 47
Micrognathism, 162, *162*
Micromandible, 162, *162*
Micromaxilla, 162, *162*
Microorganisms, as laboratory hazard, 1180–1181
Microscope, comparison, in forensic ballistics, 530–531, *531*
    bullet identification, with, 561, *561*
    cartridge identification with, 559, *559*
Microwaves, injury from, 121, 663–664
Micturition, after spinal cord injury, 79
Middle ear. See *Ear, middle*.
Military injuries, burns as, 718
Milk bush, 1493
Milker's granuloma, 368
Milkstripe euphorbia plant, 1493
Mill-wheel murmur, of air embolism, 414
Mimosine, 1510
Mine, claymore, 582, *582*, *583*
  nail, 582, *582*
Miners' cramps, 703
Miners' nystagmus, 1184
Miners' pneumoconiosis, 1185
Mining, coal. See *Coal mining*.
Minors, and statutory rape, 956
  consent of, validity of, 873, 943
Miosis, defined, 123
Miscarriage, posttraumatic, 428, 431–432
Missiles, as foreign bodies, in cardiovascular system, 208
  explosive, injury from, 625–630, *625–630*
Missile wounds. See *Firearm wounds*.
Mistletoe, 1520–1521
Mites, as disease vectors, 1367
  biting, 1451
MNS blood group, identification of, from bloodstains, 815
Mold toxins, 790–793, 791(t)
Mole plant, 1494
Mollusks, hazardous, 1393–1402, *1394–1399*, *1401–1402*
  poisonous, 1397–1402, *1398–1399*, *1401–1402*
  venomous, 1394–1397, *1395–1397*
Moment of death, definition of, 23
Momentum, principle of conservation of, 4
Monge's disease, 1308–1314, 1309(t), 1310(t), *1311–1313*
Mongoloids, facial bones of, 1108–1111, 1108(t), *1109*, *1110*
  identification of, from teeth, 1119–1122, *1119*

Mongoloids *(Continued)*
identification of, from skeletal remains, 1108–1111, 1108(t), *1109, 1110*
Moniliasis, 1337
oral, antibiotics and, 188, *189*
Monkey fiddle plant, 1493
Monkey pistol tree, 1496
Monkshood plant, 1525
Monocrotaline, 1508
Monteggia fracture-dislocation, 276–277, *277*
Moonshine, toxic ingredients of, 818
Morel, false, 1553
Morphine, and cataract, 130
smoking and, 1216
Mortar bombs, 596–598, *597, 598*
Morton's toe, 329
Mosquitoes, as disease vectors, 1366
bites of, 1447–1448
Moss animals, 1393
Mother-in-law plant, 1481–1483
Motion, laws of, 3–5
Motor nerves. See *Nerves.*
Motor paralysis, defined, 69. See also *Paralysis.*
Motorcycle accidents, 859
Motorcycle injury, of pelvis, 339, *340*
Motorkart accidents, 859
Mottled candlestick plant, 1493
Mountain ivy, 1489
Mountain laurel, 1489
Mountain sickness, chronic, 1308–1314, 1309(t)–1310(t), *1311–1313*
Mouth. See *Oral structures; Tooth.*
Mucocele, oral, 176, *176*
Mucor, burn wound infection from, 723
Mucormycosis, 1338
Mucous membranes, oral, injuries of, *156,* 157, *157*
electrical, 655
radiation, 682
normal appearance of, 148–149
Multinucleation, of nerve cells, 52
Münchausen syndrome, 498
Murine typhus, 1372
Muscarine, 1553, 1554
Muscazone, 1551
Muscidae. See *Flies, sarcosaprophagous.*
Muscimole, 1551
Muscle, atrophy of, after nerve injury, 69
contractures of, after nerve injury, 69
Dupuytren's, 330, 382–383
ischemic, 377–378, *378*
Volkmann's, 69, 349, 377–378, *378*
heat cramps of, 703
herniation of, 316
injury of, alcoholic, 822
electrical, 655–656
in anterior tibial compartment syndrome, 314–315, *315*
ischemic, 69, 349, 377–378, *378*
in drug-induced coma, 379
of calf, 315–316
of eye, 116
of hip, 285
of knee, 301
of shoulder, 261–265, *263, 264*
Muscle *(Continued)*
injury of, of thigh, 297
radiographic evidence of, 700
innervation of, 78, *78*
loss of, in burn injury, 722
paralysis of. See *Paralysis.*
Musculoskeletal injuries, 259–361. See also *Dislocations; Fractures.*
aggravating preexisting conditions, 353–354
alcoholic, 822
by hospital employees, 901–902
complications of, 345–352
disability evaluation in, 354–355
fat embolism in, 409, 351
hypothermic, 766–767
iatrogenic, 908
in aircraft accidents, 875–885, *879, 880, 882,* 882(t), 883(t), *884*
in automobile accidents, 855
in battered child, 504
in explosions, 625
infection in, 349–350
kidney failure in, 351
psychiatric aspects of, 354
soft-tissue, radiographic evidence of, 700
systemic effects of, 351–352
thermal, 726–727
treatment of, 259–261
urinary complications of, 351
vascular complications of, 351–352
Musculoskeletal system, postmortem findings in, in burn victims, 726–727
radiography of, 687
trauma and, 259
Mushrooms, canned, botulism from, 1589–1590
poisonous, 1464, 1551–1557
Mutilation, self-inflicted, 496–497, *496, 497*
of female genitals, 252
of male genitals, 241
sexual, of females, 251
Mutualism, 1343
Mycobacteria, atypical, 1340–1342
infection by, 1334–1342
cerebral, *11, 12*
drug therapy and, 11
nonphotochromogenic, 1342
photochromogenic, 1340–1341
rapid grower, 1342
scotochromogenic, 1341–1342
Mycotoxins, 1456–1557, 1469(t)–1470(t), 1551–1557
food poisoning by, 790–793, 791(t)
Myelography, 688
complications of, 67
Myelopathy, from spinal anesthesia, 1248–1249
Myiasis, in corpses, 1080–1084, *1081, 1083*
Myocardial depression, posttraumatic, 398–400, *399*
Myocardial failure, senile, 888
Myocardium. See also *Heart.*
injury of, alcoholic, 821–822
blunt, 204–205
contusion, 204–205
electrical, 658, *658*
Myocardium *(Continued)*
injury of, head injury and, 400
perinatal hypoxic, *462*
rupture, 204–205
thermal, 725
Myocytolysis, cardiac, head injury and, 400
Myomectomy, complications of, 1233
Myopathy, alcoholic, 822
Myositis ossificans, 296, 348, *348*
Myrtle spurge plant, 1494
Mytilotoxism, 795

Nail bomb, 581–582, *581*
Nail guns, hand injury from, 380
Nail mine, 582, *582*
Nails, of fingers. See *Fingernails.*
Naked ladies plant, 1513–1514
Naphthalene(s), and cataract, 130
chlorinated, poisoning by, 789
Narcosis, nitrogen, in divers, 637–638
Narcotics, effects of, 829, 831
injection of, injury from, 832–835
of hand, 379
use of, historically, 826
withdrawal from, 829
Narcotics addicts. See *Drug addicts.*
Nasal aperture, racial differences in, 1108–1109, 1108(t), *1109*
Natural gas explosions, 632–633, *632*
Navicular, carpal, dislocation of, 280–281, *281*
fractures of, 284, *284*
tarsal, fractures of, 336
Neck. See also *Cervical spine.*
injuries of, 63–64
surgery of, complications of, 1226–1227
Necklace weed, 1525
Necrosis, avascular traumatic, of bone, 332, 333–334, 346–347
pallidal, in carbon monoxide poisoning, 843–844, *843, 846*
Needle aspiration, of chest, and spleen injury, 212
Needle biopsy, pleural, injury from, 209
Negative vital reactions, 25
Negligence, as legal concept, 1645–1650
by physician. See *Malpractice.*
causation in, 1649, 1661–1664
compensation for, costs of, 910–935
computation of, 1665–1668. See also *Damages.*
deterrence of, collective system for, 913–914
fault system for, 910–935
legal-economic sanctions for, 910–935
market system for, 914–915
due care and, 1646
elements of, 1645
fault system for, 910–935
foreseeability of harm and, 1645–1646
hazardous products and. See *Products liability.*

Negligence *(Continued)*
in drug and device manufacture and distribution, 1207–1208, 1262–1267, 1621–1623
intervening acts and, 1662–1663
legal definition of, 1645
liability for. See *Liability.*
litigation involving. See *Lawsuits.*
medical. See *Malpractice.*
products liability and. See *Products liability.*
proximate cause and, 1649, 1661–1662
reasonably prudent man standard and, 1646–1649, 1651–1652
res ipsa loquitor doctrine and, 1653
respondeat superior doctrine and, 1651
risk theory of, 1662
statute of limitation for, 1652–1653
Negroes, blood stains from, identification of, 812
bone density in, 154
facial bones in, 1108–1111, 1108(t), *1109, 1110*
identification of, from skeletal remains, 1108–1111, 1108(t), *1109, 1110*
from teeth, 1119–1122, *1120, 1122*
Nematocysts, 1380–1385, *1380–1381*
Neomycin, injury from, legal case involving, 1213
of ear, 137
Neonate. See *Newborn.*
Neoplastic disease. See *Cancer; Carcinoma.*
Neoplastic embolus, 417–418
Neovascularization, in corneal injury, 126–127, *126*
in scleral injury, 99
Nephrectomy, complications of, 1234
Nerioside, 1478
Nerium indicum, 1478–1479, *1478*
Nerium odorum, 1478–1479, *1478*
Nerium oleander, 1478–1479, *1478*
Nerve(s). See also names of specific nerves.
dysreflexia of, after spinal cord injury, 82
entrapment of, in foot, 329–330
in hand, 279, 373
in thigh, 297
injuries of, 67–70
alcoholic, 822–823
and causalgia, 329, 349, 382, 387
and muscular contractures, 69
and vascular injury, 69
assessment of, 69–70
chemical, 373
electrical, 660
from lightning, 670
iatrogenic, anesthetic, 1246, 1248–1249
injection, 373
surgical, 66, 68, 280
in carbon monoxide poisoning, 844
in drug injection, 373
Nerve(s) *(Continued)*
injuries of, in heatstroke, 707–709, *707–709*
in Monteggia fracture-dislocation, 276–277
in pelvic fractures, 344
in posterior hip dislocations, 285–287
ischemic, 373
laceration, 373–374
of eye, 118
of foot, 329–330
of hand, 280, 372–374
and causalgia, 382
of spine, 66, 1248–1249. See also *Spinal cord injury.*
recovery from, grading of, 70, 70(t)
rupture, loads required for, 68(t)
of hand, anatomy of, 367–368
of spine, anatomy of, 78, *78*
paralysis of. See *Paralysis.*
regeneration of, 68, 373–374
Nerve cells. See *Neurons.*
Nervous system, effects of hypothermia on, 759
effects of meteorologic stimuli on, 1628–1629(t)
injury of, electrical, 658–660
from anesthesia, 1246–1249
Nettle, 1541
Nettle plants, 1547–1549
Neuralgia, plantar digital, 329
traumatic prepatellar, 304
Neurapraxia, 67
Neurinoma, Morton's, 329
Neuritis, chemical, 373
Neurofibroma, Morton's, 329
Neurohormonal disorders, trauma and, 8
Neuroma, amputation, 67–68
of oral soft tissues, 173, *173*
iatrogenic dental injuries and, 188
pain from, 381–382
posttraumatic, 381–382
Neurons, balls of retraction in, 53
chromatolysis in, 52, 53
end bulbs in, 55–56
ferrugination in, 53
free balls in, 55–56
glycogen accumulation in, 53
injury of, assessment of, by silver impregnation method, 53
in cerebral concussion, 51, *51, 52*
nonstructural, 50–51
pigmentary infiltration of, 53
Neuropsychiatric disorders, and perinatal hypoxia, 472–473, *472, 473,* 475–476, *476,* 479–484
and prematurity, 472–473, *472, 473,* 482–483
Neurosis, anxiety, 17
vs. compensation neurosis, 17
cardiac, intracardiac foreign body and, 418
compensation, 17
vs. anxiety neurosis, 18
war, 17
Neurosurgery, ureteral injury in, 234
Neurotic excoriation, 496, *496*
Neurotmesis, 67
Neutron, 680
Neutron activation analysis, for firearm discharge residue, 567
Newborns. See also *Infants.*
birth defects in. See *Birth defects.*
brain damage in, 462–484, 466(t)
breech delivery of, liver rupture in, 439, *440, 441*
soft tissue injury in, *449*
spinal injury in, 446
caput succedaneum in, 448, *448*
cephalhematoma in, 448–450, *449*
cephalic delivery of, head injury in, 447–456, *448–452,* 454(t), *455*
circulatory failure in, 458
death in, unexplained, 1015–1032. See also *Sudden infant death.*
effects of high altitude on, 1295–1296, 1296(t)
head molding in, 450–452, *451*
hemorrhage in, 458–460
injuries of, hypoxic. See *Hypoxic injuries, perinatal.*
perinatal. See *Birth injuries.*
intestinal surgery in, complications of, 1232
iris color in, 103
premature. See *Premature infants.*
subdural hematoma in, 452–456, *452,* 454(t), *455*
traumatic fat necrosis of, 363–364
venous infarction in, 458–460
Newton's Laws of Motion, 4
Nicotiana glauca, 1537–1538
Nicotiana rustica, 1538
Nicotiana tabacum, 1538
Nicotine, 1538
as carcinogen, 191–192
oral injury from, 191–192, *192*
Nightshade plants, 1542–1543, 1544
Nitrates in explosives, tests for, 605
spontaneous combustion of, 738
Nitre, spontaneous combustion of, 738
Nitric acid, spontaneous combustion of, 738
Nitrites, as food preservatives, toxicity of, 796–797
Nitrobenzene, in improvised explosives, 588–589, 593–594
tests for, 607
Nitrogen, amino acid, in postmortem blood, 1036
in postmortem cerebrospinal fluid, 1044
nonprotein, in postmortem blood, 1036
in postmortem cerebrospinal fluid, 1044
in postmortem vitreous humor, 1048
Nitrogen narcosis, in divers, 637–638
Nitrogen poisoning, in coal mine explosions, 632
Nitrogenous compounds, in postmortem blood, 1035–1036, *1036*
in postmortem cerebrospinal fluid, 1044–1045

Nitrogenous compounds *(Continued)*
in postmortem vitreous humor, 1047–1048, *1048*
Nitroglycerin, as secondary high explosive, 581
in explosives, tests for, 606–607
Nitrosamines, in foods, toxicity of, 796–797
Nocardiosis, 1336–1337
Noise-induced hearing loss, 138–139
Nonelastic collision, 4
Nonphotochromogenic mycobacteria, 1342
Nonstructural neuronal injury, 50–51
Nonunion, of fractures, 346
radiographic evidence of, 699–700
Noratropine, 1540
Norepinephrine, and kidney injury, 401
in postmortem blood, 1039
Norscopolamine, 1535
North American blastomycosis, 1336
Nose, cerebrospinal fluid discharge from, 45
effect of meteorologic stimuli on, 1629(t)
fracture of, 38
frostbite of, 767
racial differences in, 1108–1109, 1108(t), *1109*
Nuclear explosions, 633–634
Nuclear fallout, 679
Nudibranchs, 1394, *1395*
Numbness, facial, 174
Nurses, occupational injuries in, 901–903
Nutritional paralysis, after nerve injury, 69
Nux-vomica plant, 1519–1520
Nymphomania, 959
Nystagmus, gaze, 134
in measurement of equilibrium, 134
miners', 1184
positional, 134
spontaneous, 134

Obesity, and heatstroke, 705
Obligate parasite, 1343
Obstetric procedures, air embolization in, 416
injuring fetus and newborn, 436–486. See also *Birth injuries; Hypoxic injuries, perinatal.*
ureteral injury in, 234
Obstetrical ultrasound, safety of, 781
Obstetrician, liability of, for birth injuries, 437–438
Obturator dislocation, 288
Occupational aneurysm, 377
Occupational diseases. See *Occupational-environmental diseases.*
Occupational injuries, burn, 662, 717–718, 1175–1176
chemical, 190–191, 1176
death from, autopsy in, 1675–1680
electrical, 670–671, 1164, 1176
Occupational injuries *(Continued)*
electrical, from arc flash, 662
from electromagnetic waves, 663–664
from static electricity, 664–665
from high pressure equipment, 1172–1175
from plants, 1458–1459, *1460*
hypothermic, 767
in agriculture, 1163–1166
in autopsy workers, 908–909
in coal mining, 1182
in fishing industry, 1167–1171
in hospitals, 901–902, 903
in laboratories, 1175–1181
of eye, 662, 1172
of forearm, 277–278
of hand, 368, 379–380
Dupuytren's contracture as, 383
stenosing tenovaginitis as, 383
vascular, 224–225, 376
of shoulder, 262
of teeth, 172
radiation, 677, 684, 903, 909, 1180
railway, 1186–1191
thermal, 717–718, 1175–1176
vascular, 376
weather and, 1635–1637
workmen's compensation for. See *Workmen's compensation.*
Occupational-environmental diseases, 1271–1292. See also *Occupational injuries.*
agents causing, 1271–1274, 1273(t)–1274(t)
multiple, 1274
multiple effects of, 1274
routes of entry for, 1274–1275
types of exposure to, 1275
asbestos-related, 1277–1291. See also *Asbestos-related diseases.*
cancer as, 20. See also *Cancer.*
history taking in, 1276
in agricultural workers, 1165, 1166
in coal miners, 1184–1185
in laboratory workers, 1179–1181
latent period in, 1275
litigation involving, 1276–1277, 1290
medicolegal investigation of, 1276, 1277
proof of causation in, 1271
signal tumors in, 1275–1276
Octopi, hazardous, 1396–1397, *1397*
Oculomotor nerve, injury of, 62
Odontogenic tumors, malformations resembling, 160–161, *161*
Odontologic examination, at autopsy, 999–1000
forensic, bitemark evidence in, 1143–1147, *1144–1147*
equipment for, 1133
in child abuse cases, 1137–1140
in narcotic addiction cases, 1136–1137, *1136*
in sex crimes, 960–961
of unidentified corpses, 1128–1136
in drownings, 1318–1319
photography in, 1136
preserving chain of evidence, in, 1141–1142
Odontologic examination *(Continued)*
forensic, radiography in, 1134–1136, *1135, 1136*
teeth charting in, 1133–1134, *1133–1135*
Odontology, forensic, 1115–1153
identification methods in, 1128–1136
legal aspects of, 1130–1132, 1140–1143
Oils, causing spontaneous combustion, iodine numbers of, 757, 757(t)
unsaturated, spontaneous combustion of, 737–738
Old age. See *Elderly.*
Oleander plant, 1478–1479, *1478*
Oleandroside, 1478
Olecranon, fracture of, 275
Olecranon bursitis, 272
Oleoma, 379
Olfactory nerve, injury of, in head injury, 62
Oliguria, in genitourinary injury, 227–228
in hemorrhagic shock, 8
posttraumatic, 400
Ontoid process, displacement of, 63
Onychophagia, 497
Open fractures, 259–261
Operating room, electrical injury in, 671–672
Ophthalmology, ultrasound in, 778
Opiates, idiosyncratic reaction to, 832
use of, 826
Opium, use of, 826
Optic nerve, anatomy of, 114–115
injuries of, 118
drug-induced, 131
in head injury, 62
Oral contraceptives, and toxic optic neuropathy, 131
injury from, legal case involving, 1214
Oral injuries, 147–199
abrasion, *156*, 157
alcoholic, 191
and cerebral abscess, 50
burn, 193–194, *194*
causes of, 147–148
chemical, 188–193, *188–193*
classification of, 156–159
complications of, 163, *163*
contusion, *156*, 157
drug-induced, 189–190, *189, 190*
electrical, 193–194, *194*, 655
firearm, 174–175, *175*
from abnormal habits, 188
from food, 175–176
from nicotine, 191–192, *192*
from toothpaste, 188
iatrogenic, 178–188, *178–188*
in children, 147–148
battered, 1137–1138, *1138*
in dental anesthesia, 184–185, *184*
in narcotics addicts, 1136–1137, *1137*
incidence of, 147–148
laceration, 142
mechanical, 172–178, *172–178*
morphologic variations and, 154, *154*

Oral injuries *(Continued)*
of developing hard tissues, 159–162, *160*
of jaw. See *Mandible; Maxilla.*
of teeth. See *Tooth.*
perinatal, 163
principles of, 154–156
radiation, 194–196, *195, 196*, 682
self-inflicted, 173, 188, 497
sequelae of, 159–169, *159–169*
smoking and, 191–192, *192*
systemic diseases predisposing to, 150–154, *151–153*
thermal, 193–194, *194*
Oral route, for chemical injury, 1569–1570, 1570(t)
Oral structures. See also *Mandible; Maxilla; Palate; Tongue; Tooth.*
abscess of, 164
carcinoma of, 177, *177*, 188, 191–192, *192*
cellulitis of, 164
development of, and trauma, 162–163, *162*
granuloma of, 173, *173, 174*
hyperkeratosis of, 176–177, *177*
identification from. See *Odontologic examination.*
in cat scratch disease, 173–174, *174*
inflammation of, 182, *183*. See also *Stomatitis.*
injuries of. See *Oral injuries.*
irritation fibroma of, 176, *177*
leukoplakia of, 177–178, *177*
alcohol and, 191
malignant tumors of, 178, *178*
mucocele of, 176, *176*
necrosis of, 164
neuroma of, 173, *173*
normal appearance of, 148–149, *148*
papilloma of, 176, *176*
pregnancy tumors of, 176
racial differences in, 1108–1111
traumatic vesicle of, 181–182
ulceration of, 183, *183*
Oral surgery. See *Dental procedures.*
Orbicular ligament, injury of, in Monteggia fracture-dislocation, *277*
Orbit, anatomy of, 115–116
emphysema of, 118
foreign body in, 118–119
fractures of, 116–118, *117*, 146–147
and orbital emphysema, 118
and superior orbital fissure syndrome, 118
hemorrhage in, vs. subconjunctival hemorrhage, 91
with zygomatic fracture, 146
hemorrhage in, 91, 116
infection of, 119
injuries of, 116–119, 146–147
racial differences in, 1108(t), 1109–1110, *1109*
Orbital apex syndrome, 118
Orbital syndromes, 118
Organ failure, in hemorrhagic shock, 8
Organ of Corti, anatomy of, 132
noise-induced injury of, 138
Organ transplants. See *Transplants, organ.*
Organic compounds, identification of, in commercial explosives, 606
in improvised explosives, 606
Organophosphates, as food contaminants, 788
Orgasm, female, after spinal cord injury, 81
male, after spinal cord injury, 80
Orientals, racial characteristics of. See *Mongoloids.*
Ornithogalum thyrsoides, 1516
Ornithogalum umbellatum, 1516
Orthodontic appliances, injury from, 179, *180*, 183, *183*, 185–186, *186*
Orthopedic injuries. See *Dislocations; Fractures; Musculoskeletal system, injuries of.*
Orthopedic procedures, malpractice in, 908
ureteral injury in, 234
Orthostatic hypotension, after spinal cord injury, 81
Orthotolidine test, for blood stains, 810
Os calcis, fractures of, 334–336, *334*
Osmolality, of postmortem vitreous humor, 1050
Osseous schisis, 657
Ossicles, auditory, anatomy of, 132
Ossification, heterotopic, in burn victim, 727
posttraumatic, 348, *348*
Ossifying fibroma, 296
Ossifying hematoma, 296
Osteitis, radiographic evidence of, 700
Osteitis deformans, and oral injury, 150, *151*
Osteochondral fractures, of femoral condyle, 310–311
Osteochondritis dissecans, 347, *347*
of elbow, *347*
of knee, 311–312, *311*
Osteogenesis imperfecta, and oral injury, 153
Osteomyelitis, and oral injury, 153–154, *153*
chronic, and cancer, 19, *19*
posttraumatic, 164, 349–350, *351*
radiographic evidence of, 700
Osteopetrosis, and oral injury, 153
Osteophyte, marginal, 328
Osteoporosis, posttraumatic, 387
in spinal cord injury, 81–82
radiographic evidence of, 700
systemic diseases causing, 150–154, *151–153*
Osteoradionecrosis, 196, *196*
Otaheite walnut plant, 1491–1492
Otorrhea, cerebrospinal fluid, 45, 62
Otto pelvis, 288, *288*
Otto's disease, 288, *288*
Ouabain, 1477, 1534
Out-shoot wound. See *Exit wound.*
Oxidation reaction, energy threshold for, 731, *731*
temperature coefficients for, 730(t), 731
Oxygen, retinal injury from, 130
spontaneous combustion in, 737–739
Oxygen deprivation. See *Hypoxia.*
Oxygen embolism. See *Air embolism.*
Oxygen poisoning, in anesthesia, 1245–1246
in divers, 638
Oxygen tension, in postmortem blood, 1042–1043, 1042(t), 1043(t)
Oxytocin, and precipitous obstetric delivery, 453

Pacemaker, cardiac, implantation of, complications of, 209, 1228
malfunction of, 672
Pachymeningitis hemorrhagica, 44, *44*
Pachymeningitis interna chronica, 44, *44*
Paget's disease, and oral injury, 150–151, *151*
Pain, chronic, after disk surgery, 67
after spinal cord injury, 84
phantom limb, 381
posttraumatic, in hand, 381–382, *382*
in nerve injury. See *Causalgia; Neuralgia.*
Paint guns, hand injury from, 379
Palate, burns of, 193, 194
epidermoid carcinoma of, *178*
leukoplakia of, *177*
normal appearance of, 148
racial differences in, 1110–1111
Palay rubber vine, 1483
Pallidal necrosis, in carbon monoxide poisoning, 843–844, *843, 846*
Palma christi plant, 1501–1503, *1503*
Palmar fascia, anatomy of, 367
Dupuytren's contracture of, 382–383
Palmer's notation, for dental charting, 1133, *1134*
Pancreas, in hypothermia, 760
injuries of, 213–214
alcoholic, 820
chemical, from plants, 793–794, 793(t)
electrical, 660–661
surgery of, complications of, 1231
Pancreatitis, in hypothermia, 760
Panniculitis, cold, 766
Panther cap fungus, 1551–1552
Papaveraceae, poisonous, 1522–1523
Papillary hyperplasia, chronic inflammatory, 187, *187*
Papilloma, oral, 176, *176*
Paracentesis, abdominal, complications of, 1238
Parachute accidents, 883–885, *884*
Paraffin test, for firearm discharge residue, 565–566
Paragonimiasis, 1363–1364
Paralysis, 69, 77. See also *Spinal cord injury.*
after cervical disk surgery, 67
after polio vaccination, legal case involving, 1213
after spinal anesthesia, 1248–1249

Paralysis *(Continued)*
  divers', eye injury in, 128
  facial. See *Facial nerve, injury of.*
  motor, defined, 69
  of arm, in humeral fractures, 271
  sensory, defined, 69
  sudomotor, defined, 69
  temporary, in lightning injury, 670
  tick, 1452
  vasomotor, defined, 69
Paralytic shellfish poisoning, 795, 1398–1400, *1398–1399*
Paramedics, emergency care by, 866–869
Paraosteoarthropathy, 83
Paraplegia, defined, 77. See also *Spinal cord injury.*
Parasite, adult phase of, 1345
  asexual phase of, 1345
  cyst stage of, 1345
  facultative, 1343
  injury from, modes of, 1345
  obligate, 1343
  pathogenic, 1343
  sexual phase of, 1345
  spurious, 1343
Parasitic diseases, 1343–1368
Parasitic worms, marine, 1389–1390
Parasitism, 1343–1346, *1344*
  climate and, 1344–1345
  limiting factors in, 1344–1345
  vector control in, 1345–1346
Parasitosis, delusional, 496
Parenteral route, of chemical injury, 1572
Parenteral therapy, complications of, 1237
Paronychia, 368
Parotid duct, laceration of, 142
Parotid gland, radiography of, 688
   injury from, 186, *187*
Parquine, 1534
Parrotfish, ciguateric, *1424*
Parry fracture, 276–277, *277*
Partnership, medical, vicarious tort liability in, 1653
Parturition, injuries during. See *Birth injuries; Hypoxic injuries, perinatal.*
Pasteurella tularensis, wound infection from, 10
Patella, avulsion of quadriceps muscle from, 301
  avulsion of tendon from, 301
  chondromalacia of, 303
  dislocation of, 303–304
  fractures of, 301–303, *302*
Patent ductus arteriosus, altitude and, 1306
Pathogenic parasite, 1343
Pathologic fractures, 352
  in burn victims, 726
  radiation therapy and, 196, *196*
  systemic diseases causing, 150–154, *151–153*
Pathologist, as expert witness, 1002
  autopsy by. See *Autopsy.*
  occupational injuries in, 908–909
Patient, consent of. See *Consent, informed.*
Patterned wound, *6*, 7
Pauwels' classification, of intracapsular hip fractures, 289, *290*
PCB. See *Polychlorinated biphenyls.*
Peach tree, 1529
Pectoralis major muscle, rupture of, 261–262
Pedestrians, injury of, 857–858, *857, 858*
Pedicellariae, venomous, 1405, *1405*
Pellegrini-Stieda disease, 306, 307, 349
Pelography, retrograde, in genitourinary injury, 228
Pelvis. See also *Hip.*
  bucket-handle, injury of, 343, *343*
  burst, 342
  dating of skeletal remains from, 1105
  determination of gender of skeletal remains from, 1106–1107, 1106(t), *1107*
  dislocations of, 341–343, *341–343*
  female, *246*
  fracture-dislocations of, 343–344, *343*
  fractures of, *219*, 337–341, *338–341*
   associated injuries in, 344
   bladder injuries in, 236, 237
   compression, *342*
   in pedestrians, 857
   in pregnancy, 425
    and fetal skull fractures, 427
   rectal injuries in, 220
   shear, 341, *341*
   stable, 339, *339*
   unstable, 339–341, *340, 341*
   urethral injuries in, 238
   vertical shear, 341, *341*
   visceral injuries in, 344
  motorcycle injury of, 339, *340*
  Otto, 288, *288*
Pencil tree, 1493
Penetrating injuries, autopsy examination of, 998
  defined, 7
  from explosion missiles, 626–630, *625–630*
  from firearms. See *Firearm wounds.*
  from knives. See *Stab wounds.*
  introduction of carcinogenic substances through, 20
  of artery, 222–223
  of bladder, 236
  of blood vessels, 206, 222–223
  of chest, 200, 202
  of choroid, 111
  of ciliary body, 105
  of colon, 219–220
  of diaphragm, 207
  of esophagus, 206
  of fetus, 429
  of great vessels, 206
  of kidney, 230
  of large intestine, 219–220
  of lung, 202
  of penis, 239
  of rectum, 219–220
  of renal pedicle, 229
  of scrotum, 241
  of testis, 241
  of tracheobronchial tree, 203
  of vagina, non-sex-related, 252–253
   sex-related, 248–252
Penetrating injuries *(Continued)*
  of ureter, 233
  of uterus, 255–257
   pregnant, 429
  suicidal, 1005–1006, *1006*
Penicillin, and convulsions, 1200–1201
  and fever, 711
  as anaphylactic agent, 1202–1204, 1204(t)
Penis, injuries of, 239–241
Pennaria, 1383, *1384,* 1385
Pentobarbital injection, injury from, 905, *905*
Pepper plant, 1533
Peppering, around firearm entrance wound, 514
Peptic ulcer, after spinal cord injury, 84
Perborate, in explosives, tests for, 605
Perchlorate, in explosives, test for, 604
Percutaneous route, of chemical injury, 1274, 1572
Perforation. See also *Penetrating injuries.*
  of esophagus, 206
   iatrogenic, 209, 1227–1228
    in tracheal intubation, 1253–1254
  of heart, iatrogenic, 209
  of intestines, in immersion blast, 624
  of stomach, 216
  of trachea, in tracheal intubation, 1254
  of uterus, 255–257
Pericardiocentesis, injury from, 209
Pericoronitis, 176
Perinatal injuries. See *Birth injuries; Hypoxic injuries, perinatal.*
Perineum, laceration of, in aircraft accidents, 877–879
  straddle injury of, 238–239
Peripheral arteriosclerosis, trauma and, 16, *16, 17*
Peripheral nerves. See also *Nerves.*
  injuries of, and causalgia, 329, 349, 382, 387
   electrical, 660
   in cervical disk surgery, 66
  regeneration of, 68
Peripheral vascular disease, trauma aggravating, 16, 17, *16, 17*
Peripheral zone, of antemortem wound, 25, *25*
Peritoneal lavage, in abdominal injury, 216
Permanents, for hair, causing fires, 739
Permanganate, in explosives, tests for, 605
Pernio, acute, 765–766
  chronic, 766
Peroneal nerve, entrapment of, 329–330
  injuries of, in fibular dislocation, 313
   in ligament rupture, 307
Peroneal tendons, injuries of, 319–320

Peroxide, in explosives, test for, 605
  spontaneous combustion of, 738
Perphenazine, and impotence, 1198
Persian lilac, 1521–1522
Perspiration, absence of, after nerve injury, 69
  in sauna bath, 709
  insensible, 701
  mechanism of, 703
Persulfate, in explosives, tests for, 605
Peruvoside, 1479, 1481
Pesticides, as carcinogens, 788
  as food contaminants, 788
  poisoning by, toxicologic analysis in, 806–807
pH, of postmortem blood, 1043
Phage typing, 1598, 1601, 1605, 1609
Phalanges, of fingers, dislocations of, 375
    fractures of, 374
  of toes, dislocations of, 331
    fractures of, 337
Phalloidin, 1552
Phantom limb, 381
Pharmaceuticals. See *Drugs.*
Pharmacist, liability of, for drug injury, 1222–1223
Pharmacokinetics, 830
Pharmacology, biometeorologic, 1639–1640
  of marine animal toxins, 1385
  of snake venoms, 1439–1441, 1440(t)
Phenelzine sulfate, and impotence, 1198
Phenol, causing oral burns, 190, *190*
Phenolphthalein, eye injury from, 129
Phenolphthalein test, for bloodstain, 810
Phenothiazines, and cataract, 130
  and convulsions, 1200
  and eye injury, 129
  in treatment of schizophrenia, 1207
Phenylephrine, and glaucoma, 131
Phenylephrine hydrochloride, and kidney injury, 401
Phlebothrombosis, after spinal cord injury, 83
Phocomelia, causes of, litigation involving, 1617–1626
Phoradendron flavescens, 1520–1521
Phoradendron serotinum, 1520–1521
Phosphorus, in postmortem blood, 1041
  in postmortem vitreous humor, 1050
  injury from, 1580–1581
  spontaneous combustion of, 738
Photochemical activation, of oxidizing reactions, 731
Photochromogenic mycobacteria, 1340–1341
Photocoagulation, ophthalmologic, 122
Photography, in autopsy, 997–998
  in forensic odontology, 1136, 1141
  of unidentified corpses, 33
Photophthalmia, 123
Physalia, 1381, 1382, 1383(t), 1384, 1385, 1386
Physic nut plant, 1497–1498
Physical environment. See *Weather.*
Physician, as expert witness, 697–699
  as reasonably prudent man, 1647–1649, 1651–1652
  contractual obligations of, to patients, 1653–1654
  drug prescription by, telephonic, 1219
    written, 1217
  duty of, to obtain informed consent, 1669–1674. See also *Consent, informed.*
  to warn of risks, 1654–1655, 1669–1674
  injuries by. See *Iatrogenic injuries; Malpractice.*
  liability of, for drug-induced injury, 1208–1212
    legal cases involving, 1212–1216
  vicarious, 1653
  negligence of. See *Malpractice.*
  standards of care for, 692, 1647–1649, 1651–1652
    in drug administration, 1195, 1207–1212
Phytolacca americana, 1523–1524, *1524*
Phytolacca decandra, 1523–1524, *1524*
Phytolaccaceae, poisonous, 1523–1524
Phytolaccine, 1523
Pieplant, 1524–1525
Pilot, aircraft, preexisting disease of, and accidents, 876
Ping-pong skull fracture, 59
Pinna. See *Ear, external.*
Pinworm infection, 1355
Pipe bomb, 588
Pipe smoking, and oral injury, 191–192, *192*
Piperocaine, injury from, products liability case involving, 1266–1267
Pisiform, fracture of, 285
Pisiform-triquetral joint, sprain of, 279
Pistol. See also *Firearm(s); Handguns.*
  semiautomatic, 540–541, *541*
  single-shot, 540
Pituitary gland, injury of, in head injury, 57, 60–61
Pizza palate, 193, *194*
Placenta, altitudes and, 1295, *1295,* 1296(t)
  disorders of, fetal hypoxia in, *458–460*
  infarction of, 426, *459, 460, 463*
  pathologic examination of, 483–484
  premature separation of, post-traumatic, 426–427, 432–433
Placental cerebral syndrome, *459,* 484
Placental transfusion syndrome, *458*
Plague, 1373
Plankton blooms, 1398–1399, 1400
Planography, 688
Plantar digital neuralgia, 329
Plantar fascia, injuries of, 330
Plantar fasciitis, 330
Plantaris muscle, rupture of, 315
Plants, injurious, 793–795, 793(t), 1456–1557, 1465(t)–1470(t)
  abortifacient, 1457–1458
Plants *(Continued)*
  injurious, edible, 793–795, 793(t), 1459–1461
    flowering, 1465(t)–1469(t), 1470–1550
    homicidal use of, 1456
    intoxicant, 1457
    legal aspects of, 1462–1470, 1465(t)–1470(t)
    nonpoisonous, 1461–1462, *1461–1462*
    occupational injury from, 1458–1459, *1460*
    protection of, 1463–1464
    regulation of, 1463–1464
  medicinal, 1456–1457
Plastics, molten, hand injury from, 379
Pleura, perforation of, in cervical disk surgery, 67
Pneumatic tools, and vascular hand injury, 376
Pneumocele, 45
Pneumoconiosis, asbestos, 1282, *1282, 1283*
  coal miners', 1185
  collagenous, 1282, *1282, 1283*
Pneumoencephalography, 688
Pneumography, presacral, 688
Pneumonectomy, complications of, 1227
Pneumonia, meconium aspiration, 477, *478*
  postoperative, 1244–1245
Pneumonitis, aspiration, postoperative, 1244
Pneumoperitoneum, diagnostic, 688
Pneumothorax, 201–202
  iatrogenic, 209
  in dysbarism, 637
  postnatal, 477–479, *478*
  postoperative, 1245
Poinsettia, 1493–1494
Poison(s). See also *Toxin(s).*
  analysis of. See *Toxicologic analysis.*
  blood levels of, 1572–1577, 1576(t), *1577,* 1578(t)–1580(t)
  carbon monoxide as, 840–849. See also *Carbon monoxide poisoning.*
  drugs as, 831. See also *Drugs;* and generic names of specific drugs.
  inorganic, eye injury from, 129
  organic eye injury from, 129–131
Poison bean plant, 1511–1512
Poison bush, 1477
Poison control center, 801
Poison hemlock, 1547
Poison ivy, 1474–1477, *1475*
Poison nut plant, 1519–1520
Poison oak, 1474–1477, *1475*
Poison parsley, 1547
Poison sego plant, 1518
Poison sumac, 1477
Poison tobacco, 1537
Poisoning. See also *Chemical injuries.*
  accidental, incidence of, 1568(t), 1569(t)
    domestic, 895–896
  acetaminophen, 1583
  alcohol, 819–820
  and sudden infant death, 1026
  animal, 1378–1455

Poisoning *(Continued)*
arsenic, 805
benzodiazeoine, 1581–1583
bread, 1486, 1487
butyl alcohol, 820
by aspiration, 1570
by ingestion, 1569–1570, 1570(t)
by inhalation, 1570
by injection, 1572
by percutaneous absorption, 1274, 1572
by rectal administration, 1572
cadmium, food-borne, 788
carbon monoxide, 840–849, 895. See also *Carbon monoxide poisoning.*
chlorinated napthalene, 789
chronic. See *Occupational-environmental diseases.*
ciguatera, 796, 1420, 1421–1426, *1422–1424*
clupeoid, 796, 1426
coelenterate, 1388–1389
cyanide, 1581
by plants, 793(t), 794
DDT, food-borne, 788
drug, 831–835, 1196–1201, 1217–1219, 1581–1583
metabolism in, 1576
ethyl alcohol, 819–820
ethylene glycol, 1581
filefish, 1426–1427
fish, 795–796, 1417–1426
food. See *Food poisoning.*
fungal, 1551–1557
gaseous, in explosions, 631, 632, 1184
gold, 1584–1585, 1584(t)
heavy metal, 1583–1586, 1584(t)
food-borne, 787–788
toxicologic analysis in, 806
homicidal, 1456, 1569, 1569(t)
incidence of, 1568(t), 1569(t)
isopropyl alcohol, 820
ivory shell, 1401
lead, 1584(t), 1585
and sudden infant death, 1026
toxicologic analysis in, 805–806
lithium, 1584(t), 1585–1586
marine algae, 1429
marine animal, 795–796
marine turtle, 1427–1428, *1428*
mercury, 1583–1584, 1584(t)
food-borne, 787–788
in laboratories, 1179
methane, 1184
methanol, 819–820
methyl alcohol, 819–820
mullet, hallucinatory, 1427, *1427*
mushroom, 1464, 1551–1557
occupational, acute, 190–191, 1176, 1458–1459, *1460*
chronic. See *Occupational-environmental diseases.*
oxygen, in anesthesia, 1245–1246
in divers, 638
paralytic shellfish, 795, 1398–1400, *1398–1399*
PCB, food-borne, 788–789
pesticide, food-borne, 788
toxicologic analysis in, 806–807
phosphorus, 1580–1581

Poisoning *(Continued)*
plant, 793–795, 795(t), 1456–1568
indirect, 1461
legal aspects of, 1462–1470, 1465(t)–1470(t)
symptoms of, 1464
propoxyphene, 1583
pufferfish, 796
routes of entry in, 1569–1572, *1571, 1572*
scombroid, 1420–1421, *1421*
shellfish, 795, 1398–1400, *1398–1399*
snake venom, 1437–1441
suicidal, 1007
tetraodon, 796
toxicologic analysis in. See *Toxicologic analysis.*
venom, 1437–1441
vitamin A, 1428–1429
vitamin C, 1197
vitamin D, 1197–1198
whelk, 1401
Poison-tree, 1473–1474
Poisonwood tree, 1473–1474
Pokeberry, 1523–1524, *1524*
Pokeweed, 1523–1524, *1524*
Pokeweed mitogen, 1523
Polar bears, excessive vitamin A in, 1428–1429
Policeman's heel, 330
Polio vaccine, oral, injury from, legal case involving, 1213
Pollution, environmental, and disease. See *Occupational-environmental disease.*
Polychlorinated biphenyls, contaminating food, 788–789
Polygonaceae, toxic, 1524–1525
Polymyxin B, and ear injury, 137
and kidney injury, 401
Polynesians, identification of skeletal remains of, 1111
Polyneuritis, alcoholic, 823
Polyp, of tooth pulp, 163, *163*
Pompano, ciguateric, *1422*
Popliteal cyst, 304
Porphyria, anesthetic injury in, 1246
Positional nystagmus, 134
Positive vital reaction, 25
Possum bug, 1449–1450
Posterior fossa subdural hemorrhage, perinatal, 455, *455*, 466(t)
Postmenopausal women, vulvovaginal injuries in, 250
Postmortem chemical analysis. See *Chemical analysis, postmortem.*
Postmortem examination, of body. See *Autopsy.*
toxicologic, 802
Postmortem findings. See *Autopsy, findings in.*
Postmortem hypostasis. See *Hypostasis.*
Postmortem injuries, 1061–1071, *1064–1071*
accidental, 1066–1071, *1064–1071*
burn, 1062, 1066, *1066*, 1069–1070
chemical, 1070
crime-related, 1061–1064
deliberate, 1061–1064, *1064*
from ants, 1067, *1067*

Postmortem injuries *(Continued)*
from crustaceans, 1068, 1097–1098, *1097*
from domestic animals, 1068–1069, *1070*, 1096–1097, *1096*
from exposure, 1070–1071, *1071*
from fish, 1068, *1068*, 1097–1098, 1328, *1329*
from flies, 1067–1068, 1079–1081, *1083, 1085*. See also *Fly(ies), sarcosaprophagous.*
from rodents, 1068–1069, *1068, 1069*
from wild animals, 1068–1069, *1068, 1069*
in disposal of body, 1063–1064
in drowning, 1065–1066, 1068, *1068*, 1097–1098, 1328, *1329*
sexual, 1061–1062
thermal, 1062, 1066, *1066*, 1069–1070
vs. antemortem injuries, 22
Postmortem interval, determination of, 1056(t), 1057
Posttraumatic syndrome, 57–58
Potassium, average levels of, in humans, 680
in explosives, tests for, 605–606
in postmortem blood, 1040–1041
in postmortem cerebrospinal fluid, 1045(t), 1046
in postmortem vitreous humor, 1050, *1051*
spontaneous combustion of, 738
Potassium bromate, with thioglycolic acid, spontaneous combustion of, 739
Potassium nitrate, in bombs, 593
spontaneous combustion of, 738
Potassium permanganate, as abortifacient, 254–255
Potential energy, 4
Pott's fracture, 325
Poultry, *Salmonella* food poisoning from, 1602–1603
Powder, for firearm cartridges, 550–551
Powder blackening, around firearm entrance wound, 514, *515*
Powder residue, firearm, 563–567, *564–566*
Powder tattooing, around firearm entrance wound, 514
Powder-actuated tools, 542, *544–545*
Power take-off injuries, of penis, 240
Power tools, cartridge-firing, 542, *544–545*
Precipitin test, for semen, 954
for species origin of bloodstains, 811
Pregnancy, abnormal, and time of conception, 1634
abortion in. See *Abortion.*
after spinal cord injury, 81
automobile accidents in, 424–433
breech delivery in, liver rupture in, 439, *440, 441*
soft tissue injury in, *449*
spinal injury in, 446
cephalic delivery in, head injury in, 447–456, *448–452*, 454(t), *455*

Pregnancy *(Continued)*
complications of, causation in, 429–433
drugs in, 1199–1200
injuries in, cause of action for, 487–493
electrical, 663
from lightning, 670
fetal. See *Fetus, injuries of.*
in automobile accidents, 424–433
miscarriage in, posttraumatic, 428, 431–432
prevention of, in rape victim, 955–956
seat belt use during, 428–429
shock in, 427
trauma in, 423–435
and fetal injury, 436–486
and maternal injury, 424–425
medicolegal considerations in, 429–433
travel during, 423–424
ultrasound in, *776*, 778, *780*
safety of, 781
uterus in. See *Uterus, pregnant.*
with intact intrauterine device, 257
and birth defects, litigation involving, 1617–1626
Pregnancy tumor, 176, *177*
Pregnant women. See *Women, pregnant.*
Premature infants, birth injuries in, *442*, 446–447
brain damage in, 472–473, *472*, *473*, 482–483
cerebral infarction in, 466–473, *466–473*, 466(t)
hyaline membrane disease in, 479, *479*
neuropsychiatric disorders in, 472–473, *472*, *473*, 482–483
respiratory distress syndrome in, 479, *479*
Premature labor, posttraumatic, 427–428
Prenatal injuries. See *Fetus, injuries of.*
Prescriptions, drug, liability for mistakes in, 1217, 1219
telephonic, 1219
Preservation necrosis, in cerebral concussion, 52
Preservatives, food, toxicity of, 796–797
Pressure, air, in explosions, 617–618, *618*
atmospheric. See *Atmospheric pressure.*
gas, and dysbarism, 636–644
in mechanical explosions, 578
subatmospheric, death from, 643
Pressure cone, cerebellar, of Cushing, 49
tentorial, of Jefferson, 49
Pride of India plant, 1521–1522
Primary dentition. See *Tooth, deciduous.*
Primary impact, 4
Primary wound infection, 11
Primer, for firearm cartridges, 550–551
for shotgun shells, 550
residue from, 563–567, *564–566*
Prochlorperazine, and impotence, 1198
Products liability, absolute liability in, 1657
breach of warranty in, 1659–1660
drug injury and, 1207–1209, 1262–1267
law of, 1656–1660
manufacturer's warning in, 1659
medical device injury and, 1261–1262, 1621–1623
strict liability in, 1657
unreasonable danger requirement in, 1657–1658
warranty in, 1621–1623
Products liability litigation, burden of proof in, 1263–1264, 1657–1658
defendants in, 1660
involving drugs, 1207–1209, 1262–1267
involving medical devices, 1261–1262, 1621–1623
proceedings in, 1621–1623
proof of negligence in, 1263–1264, 1657–1658
Projectiles. See *Missiles.*
firearm. See *Bullets; Cartridges; Shot; Shotgun shells.*
Prolapse, of iris, 97–98, *97*, *127*
Promazine, and hypothermia, 762
and impotence, 1198
injury from, legal case involving, 1221–1222
Promethazine, and impotence, 1198
Proof, burden of, in malpractice cases, 1653
in products liability cases, 1263–1264, 1656–1657
Propellants, for firearm cartridges, 550–551
for shotgun shells, 511
Propoxyphene, injury from, 1583
Proptosis, in orbital emphysema, 118
in orbital fractures, 117
in orbital hemorrhage, 116
Prostate, cryotherapeutic injury of, 769
Prostatovesiculitis, 1349–1350
Prostheses, dental, and oral injury, 179, *180*
Protease inhibitors, in plants, 793–794, 793(t)
Protective scar, 55
Protein(s), blood, identification of in bloodstains, 816
effects of acids on, 127
Gc, identification of, in bloodstains, 816
Gm, identification of, in bloodstains, 816
in postmortem blood, 1037, *1038*
in postmortem vitreous humor, 1048–1049
metabolism of, after spinal cord injury, 82, 84
postmortem analysis of, for diagnosis of dysproteinemias, 1055
Proteus, burn wound infection from, 723
Proteus vulgaris, wound infection from, 10
Protoanemonin, 1526, 1527
Protopine, 1523
Protoveratrine A and B, 1517
Protozoa, disease-causing, 1343–1344, *1344*
injury causing, 1378
Protozoan infections, 1346–1354, *1347–1349*, *1353–1354*
Protrusio acetabuli, 288, *288*
Proximate cause, 1661–1662. See also *Causation.*
in malpractice, 1663–1664
in negligence, 1649
in prenatal injury cases, 488
Prudent man standard, in negligence, 1646–1649, 1651–1652
Prunus armeniaca, 1528
Prunus avium, 1528
Prunus caroliniana, 1528
Prunus cerasus, 1528
Prunus demissa, 1528
Prunus laurocerasus, 1528
Prunus padus, 1528
Prunus pennsylvanica, 1528
Prunus persica, 1529
Prunus serotina, 1529
Prunus virginia, 1529
Prussian disease, 348
Pseudoarthrosis, 346
Pseudomonas aeruginosa, in burn wounds, 723
Pseudomonas mallei, wound infection from, 10
Psilocin, 1556
Psilocybe, 1556–1557
Psilocybe cubensis, 1556–1557
Psilocybin, 1556
Psittacosis, 1376
Psychiatric disorders, after electrical injury, 659
after head injury, 57–60
in children, 59–60
after perinatal hypoxia, 472–473, *472*, *473*, 475–476, 476, 479–484
after premature birth, 482
and death from exposure, 899, *899*
drugs for, 1206–1207
self-mutilation in, 497
trauma aggravating, 17–18
Psychologic injuries, damages for, 1666
tort liability for, 1666
Psychologic reaction, to insect stings, 1446
to intracardiac foreign body, 418
to musculoskeletal injury, 354
to organ transplant, 990–994
to penile injury, 241
to trauma, 17–18
Pteridium aquilinum, 1550–1551
Ptomaine poisoning, 1607
Ptosis, traumatic, 90
in orbital fractures, 117
Pubic hair, as rape evidence, 947
Pubic lice, 1451
Pubic symphysis, dating of skeletal remains from, 1105
determination of gender from, 1106–1107, 1106(t), *1107*
diastasis of, 342–343
Pubis, fractures of, stable, 339, *339*
unstable, 339–341, *340*
straddle injury of, 339–341, *340*

Puerperal women, vulvovaginal injuries in, 250
Pufferfish poisoning, 796, 1417–1419, *1417*
Pulmonary arterial hypertension, 1306
Pulmonary artery, altitude and, 1299–1300
Pulmonary edema, acute, high-altitude, 1306–1308, *1307–1308*
  in acute respiratory failure, 394
  in idiosyncratic drug reaction, 832
Pulmonary embolism, after hip fracture, 888
  after spinal cord injury, 83
  fat, 410–411
  postoperative, 1245
  posttraumatic, 8, 407, *408*
  tissue, 416–418, *417*
Pulmonary hypertension, altitude and, 1298–1300, 1306
Pulmonary route, of chemical injury, 1570, *1571*
Pulmonary thromboembolism, posttraumatic, 407, *408*
Pulp, of tooth. See *Tooth, pulp of.*
Pulpitis, 163, *163*
Punch-drunk syndrome, 56–57, *57*, *58*
Puncture wound, 7
  from illicit drug injection, age of, 835
  of scalp, 37
Punitive damages, for negligence, 1666
Punkies, as disease vectors, 1367
Puparia, of sarcosaprophagous flies, 1089–1090. See also *Flies, sarcosaprophagous.*
Pupil, dilation of, 103
  in uveal tract injury, 104, 105
Pupillary block, 104
  and secondary glaucoma, 100, *100*
  in traumatic cataract, 106
Purging nut plant, 1497–1498
Purple allamanda, 1483
Purple rattlebox plant, 1511
Purtscher's retinopathy, 111, *111*
Pyelography, intravenous, in genitourinary injury, 228
  in kidney injury, 231
  preoperative, for prevention of ureteral injury, 235
Pyramidal fracture, 144
Pyretotherapy, 713
Pyruvic acid, in postmortem vitreous humor, 1047

Q fever, 1372
Quadriceps extensor mechanism, injuries of, 300–304, *302*
Quadriceps muscle, avulsion of, from patella, 301
  injuries of, 301
Quadriceps tendons, rupture of, 301
Quadriplegia, 77. See also *Spinal cord injury.*
Queiloscopy, 1117, 1118
Quicklime, spontaneous combustion of, 738
Quinacrine, and eye injury, 129
Quinine, and ear injury, 137
  injection of, and chemical gangrene, 377

Rabbitfish, venomous, 1416
Rabies, 1369–1370
Race(s), ABO blood group distribution in, 813, 814(t)
  determination of, from bloodstains, 812–813
    from radiographs, 1158
    from skeletal remains, 1102–1103, 1108–1111, 1108(t), *1109*, *1110*, 1158
    from teeth, 1119–1122, *1119–1122*
Radial artery, injury of, 365
Radial nerve, anatomy of, 367
  injury of, in humeral fractures, 271
Radiation, infrared, eye injury from, 121–122
  ionizing, and cancer, 682, 684
    average dose rates for, 680, 680(t)
    dental dose rates for, 680(t)
    diagnostic. See *Radiography.*
    exposure to, average, 680, 680(t)
    in nuclear explosions, 634
    injury from. See *Radiation injuries.*
    medical dose rates for, 680(t)
    occupational dose rates for, average, 680, 680(t)
      permissible, 680
    sources of, 678–680
    therapeutic. See *Radiation therapy.*
    types of, 680
  laser, eye injury from, 122–123
  microwave, injury from, 121, 664
  short wave, injury from, 121, 663–664
  solar, injury from, of eye, 122, 123
    of lip, 194–195
  thermal, in explosions, 615–616
    injury from, 615–616
      in nuclear explosions, 634
  ultraviolet, non-solar, eye injury from, 123
Radiation cataract, 124
Radiation dermatitis, 682
  from fluoroscopy, 695
Radiation injury, 677–700
  and cancer, 682, 684
  burn, 682–683, 695
  criteria for identifying, 682–684
  from cadavers, 909
  from whole-body exposure, 683–684
  generalized, 683–684
  historically, 677–678
  iatrogenic, 686–700, 903, 908
  in nuclear explosions, 634
  localized, 682–683
  occupational, 677, 684, 903, 909, 1180
  of bone, 196, *196*, 682
  of cells, 680–681, 683
  of chromosomes, 681
  of ear, 137–138
  of eye, 123–125
  of genes, 681
Radiation injury *(Continued)*
  of oral cavity, 194–196, *195*, *196*
  of skin, 682–683, 695
  signs and symptoms of, 682–684
  somatic, 681–682
  types of, 680–682
Radiation therapy, 689–690
  injury from. See *Radiation injury.*
  malpractice in, 694–695, 908
  non-ionizing, eye injury from, 121–123
  occupational injury in, 908
Radiocarpal joint, dislocation of, 280
Radiograph, as evidence, 1154–1155
Radiography, 686–689
  body-section, 688
  consent for, 696–697
  contrast media for, injury from, 186, *187*, 690–692, 695–696, 902
  contrast studies in, 687
  dental, in forensic odontology, 1134–1136, *1135*, *1136*
  electron, 687
  fluoroscopic, 687
    injury from, 695
  forensic, 1154–1159
  iatrogenic injuries in, 186, *187*, 690–692, 694–696, 902, 903–904. See also *Radiation injuries.*
  in autopsy, 997–998
  in battered child, 504, 1156
  in forensic anthropology, 1157–1158
  in negligence cases, 699–700
  in nuclear medicine, 689
  malpractice in, 695–696, 903–904
  of abdomen, 688
  of arteries, See *Arteriography.*
  of bile ducts, 687, 688
  of blood vessels. See *Angiography; Arteriography.*
  of breast, 688
  of bullets, 1156–1157
  of chest, 687
  of cranium, 688
  of fetus, 688
  of fractures, 144–145, 687
  of gallbladder, 687
  of gastrointestinal tract, 687
  of genitourinary injuries, 228
  of heart, 687, 688
  of injuries, 1155–1157
  of joints, 687, 688
  of kidney, 231–232, 688, 689
  of lacrimal duct, 688
  of lymphatic system, 689
  of salivary glands, 688
    injury from, 186, *187*
  of skull, 687
  of spine, 687, 688
  of temporal bone, 134
  of tracheobronchial tree, 688
  of uterus, pregnant, 688
  personal identification by, 1157–1158
  postmortem, 1157–1158
    dental, 1134–1136, *1135*, *1136*
    in firearm fatalities, 524
  procedures for, 686–689, *686*
  xonics, 687
Radioisotopes, average levels of, in humans, 680

Radioisotopes *(Continued)*
in radiation therapy, 689
injury from, 690–692
Radioisotope scanning, 689
Radiologist, malpractice by, 694–695
occupational injuries in, 903, 908
Radiology, diagnostic. See *Radiography.*
therapeutic. See *Radiation therapy.*
Radionuclide scanning, 689
Radionuclides, as contrast media, injury from, 690–692
Radioulnar joint, dislocation of, 281
Radium-226, average levels of, in humans, 680
Radius, dislocation of, in Monteggia fracture-dislocation, 276–277, *277*
of head of, 273
fracture of, 278, *281*
Barton's, 283
Colles', 281–283, *282*
reverse, 283, *283*
of head and neck of, 275–276
of styloid process of, 283–284
Smith's, 283, *283*
Ragwort plant, 1485–1487
Railroad injuries, 858, 1186–1191, *1190*
electrical, 671
Ranunculaceae, toxic, 1525–1528
Ranunculus soeleratus, 1527–1528
Rape, elements of, 939–943
incidence of, 939, *940, 941*
investigation of, 959–961, *960*
legal definitions of, 939–943
postmortem, 1061–1062
pubic hair as evidence in, 947
statutory, 956
time of, sperm motility tests for, 951–952
Rape victim, clothing of, examination of, 945
injuries of, contusions, 946–947
genital, 249, 947–951
non-genital, 945–947
photographing of, 945–946
interview of, by physician, 943–945
laboratory examination of, 951–955
physical examination of, 250, 251, 945–951
consent to, 943
report of, 955
pregnancy prevention in, 955–956
resistance by, 941–942
treatment of, 955–956
Rattlebox plant, 1511
Rattlebush, 1511–1512
Ray, alpha, 680
beta, 680
cosmic, 680
gamma, 680
x, 680, 690
Reaction phenomena, in drowning, 1323–1324, *1324*
Reaction time, weather and, 1635
Reasonably prudent man, in negligence, 1646–1649
medical professional as, 1647–1649, 1651–1652
Rectal route, of chemical injury, 1572, *1572*
Rectum, injuries of, in pelvic injury, 220
surgery of, complications of, 1231–1232
Rectus femoris, rupture of, 301
Red buckeye plant, 1504
Red snapper, ciguateric, *1423*
Red spurge plant, 1493
Red tide, 1398, 1403
Reflex sympathetic dystrophy, 349, *350*
of hand, 382, *382*
Regional lymphadenitis, 10
Relapsing fever, 1374
Relapsing juvenile chronic subdural hematoma, 44
Renal arteries, injuries of, 229–230
Renal failure, posttraumatic, 351, 400–402, *401*
Renal pedicle, injury of, 229–230
Renal scanning, 232
in genitourinary injuries, 229
Renal veins, injuries of, 229–230
thrombosis of, perinatal, 462
Report deafness, 620
Reproduction, human, altitude and, 1294–1295
weather and, 1637
Res ipsa loquitur, 693, 1653
Resistance, to electrical current, 646
Respiration, trauma and, 8, 387
Respiratory alkalosis, trauma and, 387
Respiratory distress, in decompression sickness, 643
Respiratory distress syndrome, adult, 392
of newborn, 479, *479*
Respiratory failure, acute, 392–395, *393–396*
Respiratory insufficiency, after spinal cord injury, 79–80
in anesthesia, 1241–1243
in flail chest, 200
in pulmonary injuries, 202
in rib fractures, 200
in tracheal intubation, 1254
in tracheobronchial injuries, 203
intraoperative, 1241–1242
postoperative, 1243–1244
Respiratory system, at high altitudes, 1297
foreign bodies in, 207–208
in burn victim, 724–725
in hypothermia, 760
in sudden infant death, 1020, *1021*, 1023, *1024*
injuries of, inhalation. See *Inhalation injuries.*
mechanical, 202–204
Respondeat superior, doctrine of, 1651
Restlessness, weather and, 1634–1635
Resuscitation, cardiopulmonary, injury from, 209
Reticuloendothelial system, trauma and, 389–390
Retina, anatomy of, 108
detachment of, 110, *110*
scleral injury, 99
in vitreous infection, 107
foreign body in, 113, *113*
hemorrhage in, 109, *109*
Retina *(Continued)*
injuries of, 109–114, *109–111, 113*
concussion, 109
contusion, 109, *109*
drug-induced, 129
electrical, 120
iatrogenic, in cryosurgery, 769
lacerating, 109–110, 111
oxygen and, 130
perforating, 111–112
perinatal, 109
radiation, 122
Retinopathy, Purtscher's 111, *111*
traumatic, 111, *111*
Retrocochlear hearing loss, defined, 134
Retrograde amnesia, indicating brain damage, 52
Retrograde pyelography, 228
Retrolental fibroplasia, 130, *130*
Retroperitoneal contusion, *6*
Retroperitoneal hematoma, 218–219, *219*
Retroplacental hematoma, *460*
Retrosine, 1486, 1508
Retrosternoclavicular dislocation, 265–266
Revolvers. See *Handguns.*
Rhesus blood groups, identification of, from bloodstains, 815
Rheum rhaponticum, 1524–1525
Rhinorrhea, cerebrospinal fluid, 45
in maxillary fracture, 145
Rhinosporidiosis, 1338
Rhizopus meningitis, 1338
Rhododendron, 1490–1491
Rhubarb, 1524
Rhus toxicodendron, 1474–1477, *1475*
Rhus vernix, 1477
Rib fractures, 200
and abdominal injury, 211
in battered child, 504
Richweed plant, 1484–1485
Ricin, 1501
Ricinoleic acid, 1501
Ricinus communis, 1501–1503, *1503*
Rickettsial infections, 1371–1372
Rickettsialpox, 1372
Rifle. See also *Firearm(s); Rifled weapons.*
air, injury from, *897*
as rifled weapon, 510
bolt-action, 541, *541*
lever-action, 541, *541*
semiautomatic, 541–542, *541*
slide-action, 541, *541*
Rifled slugs, shotgun, 550
Rifled weapons, ammunition for, 511, 543–550, *545–550, 554*
barrel of, bullet markings from, 560–561, *560, 561*
manufacture of, 554–555, *555*
rifling in, 529, *529*
size of, 510–511
bullets for, See *Bullets.*
caliber of, 529
cartridges for. See *Cartridges.*
characteristics of, 510
ejector of, cartridge markings from, 558
manufacture of, 555–557, *556*
entrance wounds from, 515

Rifled weapons (*Continued*)
  exit wounds from, 516–518, *516*, *517*
  extractor of, cartridge markings from, 558
    manufacture of, 555–557, *556*
  firing pin of, cartridge markings from, *557*, 558
    manufacture of, 555–557, *556*, *557*
  manufacture of, 554–557, *555–557*
  types of, 540–542, *540*, *541*
  wounds from, *516*, *517*, *519*. See also *Firearm wounds.*
    contact, 520–521
    estimation of range of, 520–521
Rifling of gun barrel, 529, *529*
    historical development of, 539
    process of, 554–555, *555*
Rigor mortis, 34, 997
  in drowning, 1319–1320
Rimfire cartridge, 543, *545*, *546*
Risk, warning of, by manufacturer, 1659
    by physician, 1654–1655, 1669–1674
Risk theory, in negligence, 1662
Ristocetin, and ear injury, 137
Road crashes. See *Automobile accidents.*
Robin, 1510
Robinia pseudoacacia, 1510–1511
Robinin, 1510
Robitin, 1510
Rocket bombs, 595–596, *595*
Rocky Mountain spotted fever, 1372
Rocky Mountain wood tick, 1451, 1452
Rodents, postmortem injury from, 1068–1069, *1068*, *1069*
Roe, toxic, 1420
Roentgen rays, 680, 690
Roentgenography. See *Radiography.*
Rosaceae, toxic, 1528–1530
Rosary pea, 1504–1508, *1506–1507*
Rose bay plant, 1478–1479, *1478*, 1490–1491
Rose laurel plant, 1478–1479, *1478*
Rotator cuff, injuries of, 262–264, *263*, *264*
Round worm infections, 1355–1359, *1359*
Rubidium, spontaneous combustion of, 738
Rule of nines, for burn estimation, 719, *891*
Rupture. See also *Blunt injuries; Lacerations.*
  of biceps tendon, 262, 272
  of bladder, 237–238
  of calf muscle, 315–316
  of choroid, 108, *109*
  of diaphragm, 207
  of duodenum, 216
  of heart, 205
    in aircraft accidents, 880, *881*, 882(t)
    paper bag, 883
  of kidney, 231
  of knee ligaments, 307–308
  of liver, perinatal, 439–441, *440*, *441*
  of pancreas, 214
Rupture (*Continued*)
  of plantaris muscle, 315
  of quadriceps muscle, 300–301
  of quadriceps tendons, 301
  of spleen, 211–212
    in pregnancy, 425
  of stomach, 216
  of testis, 241
  of thigh muscles, 297
  of thoracic aorta, 205
  of trachea, 203
  of tympanic membrane, in dysbarism, 637
    in explosions, 619
  of uterus, 255
    pregnant, in automobile accidents, 424–425
  of vagina, 253
Rutaceae, toxic, 1530
Rye fungus, 1552–1553

Sacroiliac joints, diastasis of, 342
  dislocations of, *219*, 339
Sacrum, fractures of, 339, *339*, 344
Saddle embolism, 408
Sadism, 959
  sexual, injury from, 252. See also *Rape.*
Sadistic crimes, *961*, 962–963, *962*
Sage plants, 1549–1550
Sailplane accidents, 883
Salicylates, and ear injury, 137
  and fever, 711
  and oral burns, 189–190, *190*
  in postmortem vitreous humor, 1052
Saliva, blood group antigens in, 814–815, 1144–1145
Saliva washings, of bitemarks, 1144–1145
Salivary duct, laceration of, 142
Salivary glands, radiography of, 688
  injury from, 186, *187*
Salmonella food poisoning, 1598–1606, *1600*. See also *Salmonellosis.*
Salmonellae, carriers of, 1601–1602, 1604–1605
  identification of, 1600–1601, *1600*
Salmonellosis, 1374–1375
  causes of, identification of, 1605
  control of, 1605–1606
  death from, 1599
  foods causing, 1602–1605
  incidence of, 1599–1600, *1600*
  symptoms of, 1599, *1600*
Saltpeter, in bombs, 593
  spontaneous combustion of, 738
Salts, metallic, and eye injury, 129
Sandbox tree, 1496
Sandflies, as disease vectors, 1367
Sapindaceae, toxic, 1530–1532
Saponin, 793–794, 793(t), 1491, 1499, 1511, 1523, 1534
Sarcophagidae. See *Fly(ies), sarcosaprophagous.*
Satyriasis, 959
Saurine toxin, 1421
Saxitoxin, 1399–1400
Scalp, edema of, perinatal, 448, *448*
  injuries of, 36–37
Scalp (*Continued*)
  injuries of, in skull fracture, 6
    perinatal, 449–450
  tissues of, 35
Scanning, radioisotope, 689
  ultrasonic. See *Ultrasound.*
Scaphoid, dislocation of, 280–281, *281*
  fracture of, 284, *284*
Scapula, fracture of, 269–270
Scapulocostal syndrome, 264
Scar, anisomorphic, 55
  isomorphic, 55
  keloid formation in, 67
  malignant changes in, 371
  of eyelid, 119
  protective, 55
Scatophogid fishes, venomous, 1415
Schistosomiasis, 1364
Schizophrenia, drugs for, side effects of, 1206–1207
  time of birth and, 1634
  trauma aggravating, 17
  weather and, 1633–1634
Sciatic dislocation, 285–288, *286*, *287*
Sclera, injuries of, 98–99
Scombroid poisoning, 1420–1421, *1421*
Scopolamine, 1533, 1535, 1537
  and glaucoma, 131
Scorpionfish, 1412–1415, *1412–1413*
Scotch laburnum, 1509
Scotochromogens, 1341–1342
Scotoma, defined, 131
Scrophulariaceae, toxic, 1532
Scrotum, injuries of, 241
Scrub typhus, 1372
Scuba diving. See also *Divers.*
  and high-altitude flying, 642
  barotrauma in, 638–639
  drowning in, 1330
Scyphozoa, 1380, 1383(t), 1387
Sea anemones, 1387, 1388–1389, 1402
Sea cucumbers, hazardous, 1403, 1406
Sea hares, toxic, 1401–1402, *1402*
Sea urchins, toxic, 1403, 1404–1406, *1404–1405*
Sea water boils, 1170
Seat belts, aircraft, injury from, 880
  automobile, in pregnancy, 428–429
      injury from, 424
        fetal, 427
    injury from, 216, 856–857, *856*
Secondary glaucoma, and chemical burns, 127
  and drugs, 130–131
Secondary impact, 4
Secondary infection, 11
Secretions, human, personal identification from, 814–815, 954–955, 1144–1145
  marine animal, toxic, 1388–1390
Secretors, 814–815, 954–955, 1144–1145
Sedatives, effects of, 829
Selenium, in postmortem blood, 1042
Self-inflicted injuries, 496–499, *496*, *497*
  "benign," 497
  firearm, *515*, 521–522

Self-inflicted injuries *(Continued)*
of female genitals, 252
of male genitals, 241
of oral structures, 173, 188
suicidal. See *Suicide.*
Semen, blood group antigens in, 814–815, 954–955
tests for, in rape victim, 952–955
Sempervirine, 1518
Senecio, 1485–1487
Senecionine, 1486
Sensorineural hearing loss, 134
Sensory nerves. See *Nerves.*
Sensory paralysis, 69
Sepsis. See *Infections.*
Septic infarcts, 16
Septic shock, 389
Septic thrombosis, 16, 408–409
Septicemia, defined, 723
in burn injury, 723
postmortem examination for, 999
in burn injury, 724
Serotonin, in wound timing, analysis of, 1096
extraction of, 26, 28
technique for, 27
Serum protein, after spinal cord injury, 82
Serum sickness, 712
Sesamoid bones, of foot, fractures of, 337, *337*
Sesbania drummondii, 1511–1512
Sesbania punicea, 1511
Sex, of person. See *Gender.*
Sexual asphyxia, 894, *894*, 961–962, *962*
Sexual brutality, injury from, 252. See also *Rape.*
Sexual crimes. 939–964. See also *Rape.*
bitemarks in, 1143
homicidal, 962, *962*, 1010, *1011*
postmortem injury in, 1061–1062
Sexual identity, chromosomal abnormalities and, 958
deviations in, 959
Sexual intercourse, after spinal cord injury, 80–81
consent to, validity of, 941
age and, 956
involuntary. See *Rape.*
legal vs. medical definition of, 941
penile fracture in, 240
physiologic response to, in female, 247–248, *247*
tests for, in rape victim, 951–955
vulvovaginal injury in, 248–251, 249(t)
Sexual practices, deviant, 958–964, *960–964*
death from, 961–962, *962*, *963*
Sharks, 1406–1407
Shear fracture, pelvis, 341, *341*
Sheep laurel, 1489–1490
Sheepkill plant, 1489–1490
Shells, marine, hazardous, 1394–1396, *1395–1396*, 1401, *1401*
shotgun. See *Shotshell.*
Shellfish poisoning, paralytic, 795, 1398–1400, *1398–1399*
Shigellosis, food-borne, 1610–1611
Shin splints, 313–314
Shock, anaphylactic, 1202–1203
and fat embolism, 410
and thrombosis, 13
biochemical response to, 391–392, *392*
cardiac arrhythmias in, 399–400
cellular response to, 391–392
coagulopathy in, 390
compensated, 8
from explosion, 622
hemodynamic alterations in, 13
hemorrhagic, 8, 387–388
hyperdynamic state in, 388–389
hypovolemic, 8, 351, 388
immunosuppression in, 390–391
in burn injury, 722
in facial injury, 143
in heart injury, 204
in pregnancy, and fetal death, 427
kidney failure in, 400–402, *401*
metabolic response to, 390–391
myocardial depression in, 398–400, *399*
postdescent, 643–644
respiratory failure in, 392–395, *393–396*
rewarming, 769
septic, 389
traumatic, 387–388
Shock lung, 392, *393*
Shock wave, effects of, on tissue, 619
in air, 617, *617*
in water, 623, *623*, *624*
Short circuit, causing fire, 740, *740*
partial, causing fire, 740–742, *741*, *742*
Short-wave diathermy, and eye injury, 121
Short waves, injury from, 663–664
Shot, shotgun, 544–550, 550–552, 553(t)
discharged, 511
as evidence, 563
patterns of, 567–569, 567(t), *568*
radiography of, 1157
Shotgun. See also *Firearm(s).*
as smooth-bore weapon, 510
barrel of, manufacture of, 554
size of, 510–511
types of, 515–516, 542
bolt face of, manufacture of, 555–557, *556*, *557*
breech face of, manufacture of, 555–557, *556*, *557*
characteristics of, 510
choke barrel, 542
cylinder bore, 542
double-barreled, 542, *542*
ejector of, cartridge markings from, 558
manufacture of, 555–557, *556*
extractor of, cartridge markings from, 558
manufacture of, 555–557, *556*
firing pin of, cartridge markings from, *557*, 558
manufacture of, 555–557, *556*, *557*
gauge of, 529
manufacture of, 554–557, *555–557*
pellets for. See *Shot.*
Shotgun *(Continued)*
rifled slugs for, 550
semiautomatic, *542*
shells for. See *Shotshell.*
shot for. See *Shot.*
slide-action, *542*
types of, 542, *542*
Shotgun wounds, *512–515*, *517*, *520*, *896*. See also *Firearm wounds.*
contact, 520
entrance, *512–515*, 515–516
exit, *517*
range of, estimation of, 520
Shotshells, components of, 511, 551–552, *552*, *553*
loads of, 553(t)
manufacturers' markings on, 552–553, *554*
primer for, 550
velocities of, 553(t)
wad for, patterns made by, 568
types of, 551, 568–569, *569*
Shoulder, calcification in, 262
dislocation of, anterior, 266, *267*
inferior, 268
posterior, 268, *268*, *269*
recurrent, 267
superior, 268
fractures of, 268–270, *270*
frozen, 270–271
musculotendinous injuries of, 261–265, *262–264*
soft-tissue injuries of, 261–265, *261–264*
Shoulder-hand syndrome, 264–265
Shoulder harnesses, automobile, injury from, 856
Showy rattlepod, 1508–1509
Shredding machines, hand injury from, 379
Sialography, 688
injury from, 186, *187*
Siderosis, 114
Siganid fish, venomous, 1416
Silver, and eye injury, 129
Silver impregnation method, for detecting neuronal injury, 53
Silver nitrate, and oral injury, 190, *190*
with magnesium and water, spontaneous combustion of, 739
Silverleaf nightshade, 1541
Siphonophores, 1386–1387, *1387*
Skeletal remains, determination of gender from, 1106–1108, 1106(t)
determination of origin of, 1101–1102, 1101(t), 1102(t)
determination of race from, 1102–1103, 1108–1111, 1108(t), *1109*, *1110*, 1158
determination of stature from, 1103, 1111–1112, 1158
determination of time of death from, 1103–1104, 1113–1114
evidence of injury in, 1103
human vs. nonhuman, 1101–1102, 1101(t), 1102(t)
personal identification from, 1101–1115
Skimmianine, 1530
Skin, bitemarks on, as evidence, 1143–1147, *1144–1147*

Skin *(Continued)*
blistering of, in second degree burns, 720, *721*
cancer of, radiation and, 682
trauma and, 20
chemical absorption through, 1572
current marks on, 651–655, *651–654*
frostbite of. See *Frostbite.*
hypersensitivity of. See *Allergy.*
in carbon monoxide poisoning, 843, 847, *847*
in decompression sickness, 643
in drowning, 319, *1319*, *1320*, 1323
in firearm entrance wounds, 512–514, *512–516*
in hypothermia fatalities, 763, *763*, *764*
injuries of. See also names of specific types of injuries, e.g., *Contusions.*
burn. See *Burns.*
electrical, 651–655, *651–654*
hypothermic, 765–768, 769
iatrogenic, 695, 769
in drug abuse, 833
in explosions, 626–630, *625–630*
in fish processing, 1169
of hand, 370–371, *370*
radiation, 123–124, 682–683
self-inflicted, 496–497, *496*, *497*
irritation of. See *Dermatitis.*
maceration of, in drowning, 1319, *1319*
metallization of, in electrical injury, 654
meteorologic stimuli and, 1628–1629(t)
of hand, 365
physiologic effects of burns on, 719–722, 720(t), *721*
resistance of, to electrical current, 646
scarring of. See *Scars.*
ulceration of, after spinal cord injury, 83
vesication of, in second degree burns, 720, *721*
washerwoman's 1319, *1319*
Skin anthrax, 9, *9*, 10
Skull, anatomy of, 38–39
development of, 38–39
electrical injuries of, 657
firearm injuries of, 518–519, *515–519*
fractures of, 39–41, *40*, *41*, 59
basal, 38
bursting, 40, *41*
by diastasis, 40
complex, 40
contrecoup, 40
Courville's classification for, 39–40
depressed, 40, *41*
in newborns, 450, *450*
with scalp laceration, 6
gutter, 40–41
healing of, 41
in aircraft accidents, *879*, *882*, 882(t), *884*
in battered child, 503–504, *504*
in fetus, 427
Skull *(Continued)*
fractures of, in infanticide, 450, *450*
intrauterine, 427
linear, 40, *41*
with scalp laceration, 6
meridional, 40
perinatal, 450, *450*
ping-pong, 59
simple, 40
symptoms, 38
gender differences in, 1106(t), 1108
in adults, 39
in infants, 38
indentation of, 40
molding of, during birth, 450–452, *451*
penetration of, by explosion missiles, 627–628, *628*
racial differences in, 1108–1111, 1108(t), *1109*, *1110*
radiography of, 687
venation in, 39
Skunk cabbage, 1517
Skydiving accidents, 883–885, *884*
Slaughtering guns, animal injury from, 525 526
Sleeping sickness, 1352–1353, 1375–1376
Slugs, rifled, shotgun, 550
Small intestine. See also *Duodenum; Ileum; Jejunum.*
injuries of, 217–218. See also *Intestine(s).*
surgery of, complications of, 1230
Smell, disorders of, after head injury, 62
Smith's fracture, 283, *283*
Smoke blackening, around firearm entrance wound, 514, *515*
Smoke inhalation, injury from, 202–203, 713–714
Smokers, cigarette, carbon monoxide levels in, 842–843
Smoking, and asbestos-related lung cancer, 1285, *1285*
and drug utilization, 1217
and oral injury, 191–192, *192*
Smooth-bore weapons. See *Shotguns.*
Smudging, around firearm entrance wound, 514, *515*
Snake bite, 1437–1441
Snake venoms, chemistry of, 1438–1439
pharmacology of, 1439–1441, 1440(t)
Snake venom poisoning, 1437–1441
Snakeberry, 1525
Snakes, venomous, 1437–1444
Snapping hip, 285
Snapping knee, 309
"Sniffer," for vapor analysis of explosives, 60
Snow blindness, 123
Snow-on-the-mountain plant, 1494
Snowblowers, injury from, 898–899
Snowmobile accidents, 859
Snuff, and oral injury, 191–192, *192*
Soap plant, 1518
Sodium, in explosives, tests for, 605
in postmortem blood, 1040, *1041*
in postmortem vitreous humor, 1049
Sodium *(Continued)*
spontaneous combustion of, 738
Sodium chlorate, in bombs, 574, 582, 588–589, 591, 592–594
Sodium chlorite, in bombs, 593
Sodium dichloroisocyanurate, in bombs, 592–593
tests for, 606
Sodium nitrate, in bombs, 593
spontaneous combustion of, 738
Sodium nitrite, as food preservative, toxicity of, 796–797
in bombs, 593, *593*
Sodium pentobarbital, injection injury from, 226
Soft tissue injuries. See also names of specific body parts.
in breech delivery, *449*
radiography of, 700
Soil, as wound contaminant, 10
Soiling, around firearm entrance wound, 512–514, *512–515*
Solanaceae, 1532–1544
Solandra hartwegii, 1539
Solandra maxima, 1539
Solandra mitida, 1539–1541
Solandrine, 1540
Solanidine, 1543, 1544
Solanine, 1541, 1542, 1543, 1544
Solanocapsidine, 1543
Solanocapsine, 1543
Solanum, 1541–1544
Solar burns, of eye, 123
Solar cheilosis, of lips, 194–195
Solenopsis geminata, postmortem injury from, 1067, *1067*
Solid blast, 624–625
Solids, inflammable, ignition temperature of, 737(t)
Soroche, chronic, 1308–1314, 1309(t), *1311–1313*
Sound waves, injury from. See *Ultrasound.*
South American blastomycosis, 1338
Spanish physic nut, 1499
Spasticity, after spinal cord injury, 84
Spectabilin, 1477
Spectabiline, 1508
Spectroscopy, for firearm discharge residue, 567
Sperm, test for, in rape victims, 951–955
Spiders, biting, 1452–1454
Spigot grenade, 595
Spinal accessory nerve, injury of, 63
Spinal anesthesia, complications of, 1248–1249
legal case involving, 1266–1267
Spinal cord, segmental nerve distribution in, 78, *78*
Spinal cord function, critical levels of, 79, *79*
Spinal cord injury, 64
amyloidosis after, 84
bladder cancer after, 84
bladder dysfunction after, 79
body temperature regulation after, 81
bowel dysfunction after, 79
calculus formation after, 82–83
cancer after, 84
cervical spondylosis after, 63, 77

Spinal cord injury *(Continued)*
complications of, 82–84
contusion-compression, 65
crush, 65
ectopic bone formation after, 83–84
electrical, 659
gastrointestinal function after, 84
homeostasis after, 81
hypertension after, 83
hypotension after, 81
in cervical disk surgery, 67
in spinal anesthesia, 1248–1249
legal case involving, 1266–1267
incidence of, 76–77
ischemia in, 65, 77, 83
ischemic ulceration after, 83
long-term disability from, 76–87
mechanisms of, 77–78
metabolic alterations after, 81–82
mortality rates in, 76
pain after, 84
paralysis after, 78–79, 79(t)
penetrating, 65
perinatal, 441–447, 441(t), *442–446*
phlebothrombosis after, 83
rehabilitation after, 85
respiratory dysfunction after, 79–80
sequelae of, 77
long-term, 80–82
sexual dysfunction after, 80–81
spasticity after, 84
thrombophlebitis after, 83
treatment of, historically, 76–77
hospital units for, 85
urinary tract infections after, 82–83
vascular impairment after, 77
Spinal nerve dermatome, 78, *78*
Spinal nerves, segmental distribution of, 78, *78*
Spine, atrophy of, after electrical injury, 659
cervical. See *Cervical spine.*
epidural hemorrhage in, perinatal, 442, *442*
injuries of, 63–65. See also *Spinal cord injuries.*
compression, 64
concussion, 64–65
contusion, 64–65
electrical, 659
fracture, 63–64, 77
fracture-dislocation, 77
perinatal, *444*
hyperextension-hyperflexion, 63, 64, 77
in breech delivery, 446
in children, 65
perinatal, 441–447, 441(t), *442–446*
traction, perinatal, 443–446, *443–445*
vascular complications of, 64
radiography of, 687
surgery of, complications of, 65–67
Spines, iliac, avulsion fractures of, 338
sea urchin, venomous, 1404–1405, *1404–1405*
Spleen, injuries of, 211–212, 213
rupture, in pregnancy, 425
Spleen *(Continued)*
injuries of, thermal, 725
postmortem findings in, in burn victims, 725
surgery of, complications of, 1231
Splenoportogram, injury from, 212
Spondylosis, cervical, 63, 77
Sponge fisherman's disease, 1379, 1387
Sponge toxins, 1379–1380
Sponges, marine, toxic, 1378–1380, *1379*
Spontaneous abortion, posttraumatic, 428, 431–432
Spontaneous combustion, fires due to, investigation of, 747, 756–757
substances capable of, 737–739
Spontaneous nystagmus, 134
Sporotrichosis, 1338
Sports injuries, musculoskeletal. See *Musculoskeletal system, injuries of.*
vascular, 225
vulvovaginal, 253
Sprain(s), defined, 259, 328
of ankle, 320–324
of elbow, 272
of foot, 328–329, 330
of knee, 306–307
of pisiform-triquetral joint, 279
of wrist, 278–279
fractures misdiagnosed as, 284–285
static, 328
Spraying equipment, industrial, injury from, 1172–1173
Spurge olive plant, 1546
Spurge plant, 1492–1495
Spurious parasite, 1343
Stab wound(s), 7. See also *Penetrating injuries.*
categorization of, 8
of chest, 200
of fetus, 429
of gastrointestinal tract, 216
of liver, 212
of pregnant uterus, 429
of scalp, 37
sadistic, *962*, 963
suicidal, 1005–1006, *1006*
Standard of care, for hospital emergency treatment, 873–874
in malpractice, 1651–1652
Staphylococci, burn wound infection from, 723
food poisoning from, 1606–1610
wound infection from, 10
Staphyloma, corneal, 98
Star-of-Bethlehem plant, 1516
Starfish, hazardous, 1403, *1403*
Stargazer fish, poisonous, 1415–1416
Static electricity, causing fire, 743
injury from, 664–665
Stature, radiographic evidence of, 1158
Statute of limitations, in malpractice, 1652–1653
Statutory rape, 956
Stavesacre plant, 1526
Steatonecrosis, traumatic, 361–364, *362*
of newborn, 363–364
Steering wheel injury, *15*, *854*, 855
of abdomen, 216, 217
of heart, 204
Stenosis, aortic calcific, *14*
colonic, posttraumatic, 220
Stensen's duct, laceration of, 142
Stereomicroscope, in forensic ballistics, 530, *531*
Sterilization, failure of, cause of action for, 491–493
Sternoclavicular joint, injuries of, 265–266, *265*
Steroids, and fungal infections, 11, *11*, *12*
Sticky agrimony plant, 1485
Stiff lung syndrome, 392
Stimulants, effects of, 829–830
injury from, 832
use of, 827
withdrawal from, 830
Stinging coelenterates, 1380–1387, *1380–1381*, *1386–1387*
Stinging fish, 1409–1417, *1410–1413*, *1416*
Stinging insects, 1445–1447
Stingrays, 1409–1410, *1410*
Stinking amanita fungus, 1552
Stinkweed, 1535
Stippling, around firearm entrance wound, 514
Stoker's cramps, 703
Stomach, contents of, toxicologic examination of, 804, 999, 1569, 1570
injuries of, 216
alcoholic, 820
chemical, 1581, *1582*
iatrogenic, 769
surgery of, complications of, 1229–1230
ulceration of, posttraumatic. See *Ulcer(s).*
Stomatitis, bismuth, 191
iatrogenic, 186–187, *187*
nicotine, 191–192, *192*
Straddle injury, defined, 238–239
pelvic, 339–341, *340*
Strain, of elbow, 272
of foot, 328
of iliopsoas tendon, 285
of muscle, 259
Strangulation, 203
homicidal, 1010, *1011*, 1063
penile, 239–240
suicidal, *6*, 1006, *1006*
simulated, 1063
Streptococci, burn wound infection from, 723
food poisoning from, 1610
wound infection from, 10
Streptomycin, and ear injury, 137
Stress, and infections, 11–12
and pseudodiabetes, 723
neurohormonal response to, 386–387
Stress fractures, 352–353, *353*
of fibula, 318–319
of metatarsus, 336–337
of tibia, 318–319
Stress injuries, of eye, 128–129
Stress ulcers, 395–397, *397*, *398*
in hypothermia, 760, 764, *764*

Stretch injury. See Traction injury.
Strict liability, in products liability, 1656
Strictures, posttraumatic, esophageal, 207
urethral, 238
Strongyloidiasis, 1358–1359, *1359*
Strontium-90, levels of, in humans, 680
Stropharia cubensis, 1556–1557
Strychnine, 1519
Strychnine tree, 1519–1520
Strychnos nux-vomica, 1519–1520
Stud guns, injury from, 542, *544–545*
Styloid process, of radius, fractures of, 283–284
of ulna, fractures of, 284
Subarachnoid hemorrhage, 44–45
Subarachnoid-pleural fistula, 64
Subclavian vein catheterization, percutaneous, injury from, 209
Subdural abscess, 45
Subdural hematoma, 42–44, *42–44*, *48*, *49*
chronic, 44, *44*
in battered child, 503–504
organization of, 43, *43*
relapsing juvenile chronic, 44
timing of, 43–44
ultrasonic imaging of, *779*
Subdural hemorrhage, 42–44, *42–44*
in infants, 59
perinatal, 447–456, *448–452*, 454(t), *455*, 466(t)
dural venous laceration and, 452–456, 454(t), *455*, 466(t)
hypoxic injury in, 462–477, *466–476*, 466(t)
injuries associated with, 447–452, *448–451*, 466(t)
timing of, 43
Subluxation, defined, 259
of peroneal tendons, 319–320
of sacroiliac joints, 339
Submaxillary duct, laceration of, 142
Submersion, diagnosis of drowning after, 1326–1328
estimating length of, 1319–1321, *1319–1321*
in grain, 1165–1166
Subpleural hematoma, *7*
Sudden infant death, autopsy in, 1018–1026, *1021*, *1022*, *1024*, 1025(t)
causes of, 1026–1029
chemical analysis in, 1025, 1025(t)
choanal atresia and, 38
death certificate in, 1029–1030, 1030(t)
definition of, 1015–1016
evidence of organic disease in, 1020–1026
family counseling in, 1030–1031
immunohematologic studies in, 1025–1026
incidence of, 1016–1017, 1017(t)
infection and, 1023–1025, *1024*
interstitial pneumonitis and, 1023, *1024*
investigation of, 1017–1018
mechanisms of, 1026–1029
Sudden infant death *(Continued)*
microbiologic studies in, 1023–1025, *1024*
research in, 1028–1029, 1031
respiratory infection and, 1020–1023, *1021*, *1022*
toxicologic studies in, 1026
Sudeck's atrophy, 329, 349, *350*, 387
Sudomotor paralysis, 69
Suffocation. See *Asphyxiation.*
Sugar, in bombs, 574, 582, 588–589, 591, 592–594
tests for, 606
with chlorates, spontaneous combustion of, 739
with potassium bromate, spontaneous combustion of, 739
Suicide, after organ transplant, 990
alcohol and, 823, 823(t), 824, 1008
by air embolization, 415
by asphyxiation, 1006, *1006*
by automobile, 861, *862*
by burning, 1006
by carbon monoxide poisoning, 1007
by drowning, 1006, 1330–1331, *1330*
by drug administration, 1007
by electrocution, 665, *666*, *667*, 1006
by exposure, *763*, 764, *764*
by falls, 1006
by hanging, *6*, 1006, *1006*
simulated, 1063
by homosexuals, 962
by poisoning, 1007, 1569–1572, 1569(t)
by railway accident, 1190, *1190*
by shooting, *41*, *515*, 521–522, 1004–1005, *1004*, *1005*
by stabbing, 1005–1006, *1006*
by strangulation, *6*, 1006, *1006*
methods, of, 1004–1008, *1004–1006*
physical environment and, 1627–1640
Sulfadiazine, and eye injury, 129
and fever, 711
Sulfathiazole, and fever, 711–712
Sulfonamides, and cataract, 130
and fever, 711–712
Sulfur, in postmortem blood, 1041–1042
in postmortem cerebrospinal fluid, 1046
Sumac plant, 1477
Sun, injury from, of eye, 123
of lip, 194–195
Sun spurge plant, 1494–1495
Superior oblique muscle, anatomy of, 115, *115*
paralysis of, 116
Superior orbital fissure syndrome, 118
Superior rectus muscle, anatomy of, 115, *115*
injury of, in orbital fracture, 117
Surgeonfish, venomous, 1416, *1416*
Surgery, air embolism after, 1245
aspiration after, 1244
atelectasis after, 1244
bladder injury in, 237–238
Surgery *(Continued)*
bronchospasm after, 1245
complications of, postoperative, 1243–1246
consent to, 1669–1674. See also *Consent, informed.*
gastrointestinal, in infants, 1232
gynecologic, complications of, 1233
hypoventilation in, 1242–1243
infection after, 1237
intravenous feeding in, complications of, 1237
malpractice in, 904–906, *905*, *906*, 1226–1260
of abdomen, complications of, 1229–1233
of adrenal glands, complications of, 1234
of appendix, complications of, 1231
of arteries, complications of, 1228–1229
of bile ducts, complications of, 1230
of blood vessels, complications of, 1228–1229
of breast, complications of, 1233
of chest, complications of, 1227–1228
of colon, complications of, 1231–1232
in infants, 1232
of duodenum, complications of, 1229–1230
of esophagus, complications of, 1227–1228
of gallbladder, complications of, 1230
of great vessels, complications of, 1228–1229
of head, complications of, 1226–1227
of heart, complications of, 1228–1229
of hernia, complications of, 1232–1233
of intervertebral disk, complications of, 66
of intestines, complications of, 1230, 1231–1232
in infants, 1232
of large intestine, complications of, 1231–1232
of lungs, complications of, 1227
of neck, complications of, 1227–1228
of pancreas, complications of, 1231
of rectum, complications of, 1231–1232
of small intestine, complications of, 1230
of spleen, complications of, 1231
of ureter, complications of, 1234
of urinary tract, complications of, 1234
of veins, complications of, 1229
oxygen intoxication in, 1245–1246
parenteral feeding in, complications of, 1237
pneumonia after, 1244–1245
pneumothorax after, 1245
pulmonary edema after, 1245

Surgery *(Continued)*
respiratory complications of, 1243–1246
respiratory insufficiency after, 1243–1244
ureteral injury in, 233–235
urologic, urethral injury in, 239
vascular, complications of, 1228–1229
Sustentaculum tali, fractures of, 335
Swamp sumac, 1477
Sweating, absence of, after nerve injury, 69
in sauna bath, 709
insensible, 701
mechanism of, 703
Swimming pool drowning, 1329
Symbiosis, 1343
Symblepharon, defined, 126
Sympathetic dystrophy, reflex, of hand, 382, *382*
Sympathetic nervous system, electrical injury of, 660. See also *Nerve(s).*
Sympathetic ophthalmitis, 111
Symphysis pubis, dating of skeletal remains from, 1105
determination of gender from, 1106–1107, 1106(t), 1107
diastasis of, 342–343
Synadenium grantii, 1503–1504
Syncope, cold, 765
trauma and, 386
Synovia, of hands, anatomy of, 367
Synovial hernia, of ankle, 320
of foot, 329
of wrist, 279
Synovitis, acute traumatic, 309–310. See also *Bursitis.*

T fracture, of proximal end of tibia, 313
Taeniasis, 1359
Tail-wag, of bullet, 515
Takayama test, for blood stains, 811
Talus, dislocations of, 330–331
fractures of, compression, 331–332
of body of, 331–332
of dome of, 328
of head of, 333
of neck of, 332–333, *332*
of posterior process of, 331–332
Tangential wound, 37
Tapeworm infections, 1359–1362, *1360–1361*
Tapioca plant, 1500–1501
Tarsal joint, dislocations of, 331
Tarsal tunnel syndrome, 329
Tarsus, navicular of, fractures of, 336
Tattooing, around firearm entrance wound, 514
Taxaceae, toxic, 1544–1546
Taxine, 1544
Taxus baccata, 1544–1545
Tazetine, 1521
Teeth, abscesses of, 164
alveoli of, fractures of, 167, 168–169

Teeth *(Continued)*
ankylosis of, 167–168, *168*
attrition of, dating of skeletal remains from, 1105
bitemarks from, as evidence, 1143–1147, *1144–1147*
calcification defects of, 159, 160, *160*
calculus build-up on, and soft tissue injury, 176
caries of, radiation therapy and, 196, *196*
cementum of, fractures of, 165, *165*
charting of, systems of, 1133–1134, *1133–1135*
crowns of, dilaceration of, 161
fractures of, 157, *158,* 164–165, *165*
dating of skeletal remains from, 1104, 1104(t), 1105
decalcification of, from acids, 193, *193*
in orthodontic treatment, 180–181, *180*
deciduous, avulsion of, 167, *167*
characteristics of, 1124–1125, *1124*
dislocations of, 166–167, *166–167*
fractures of, 164–166, *165*
mechanical injuries of, 159–163, *160, 161*
sequelae of, 159–163, *160, 161*
reimplantation of, 181, *183*
root resorption in, 168
dentin of, fractures of, 157, *157,* 165, *165*
determination of age from, 1124–1125, *1124*
determination of gender from, 1123–1124
determination of geographical origin from, 1121, *1121, 1122*
determination of race from, 1119–1122, *1119–1122*
determination of socioeconomic status from, 1122–1123, *1123*
discoloration of, 159–160, *160,* 168
in fluorosis, 192–193, *193*
tetracycline and, 193, *193*
enamel of, fractures of, 157, *157,* 165, *165,*
hypoplasia of, 160, *160,* 180–181, *180*
mottled, in fluorosis, 192–193, *193*
endodontically treated, and oral injury, 149
eruption of, abnormal, trauma and, 162
age at, 1104(t)
ethnic characteristics of, 1125
evidence of oral habits from, 1125, *1125*
examination of, 38
for identification of corpses, 999–1000. See also *Odontology, forensic.*
extrusion of, *158,* 159, 166, *166*
fluorosis of, 192–193, *193*
granulomas of, 163–164, *163*

Teeth *(Continued)*
grinding of, 148, 175, 497
in narcotics addicts, 148, *1136,* 1137
hypersensitivity of, 175
impressions of, as evidence, 1140–1141
for bitemark comparison, 1146–1147, *1146*
in narcotics addicts, 1136–1137, *1136*
injuries of, abrasion, 172
acute, 163–168, *163, 165–168,* 175
as evidence. See *Evidence, dental.*
avulsion, *158,* 159, 167, *167, 168*
chemical, 192–193, *193*
chronic, 175
deciduous teeth injury and, 159–163, *160, 161*
dislocation, *155,* 157, *157, 158,* 159
fracture, *149, 155, 157, 158,* 175
classification of, 157, *157, 158*
factors influencing, 154–156, *154, 156*
with pulpal exposure, 157, *157*
from abnormal habits, 188
from barotrauma, 637
from child abuse, 1137–1138, *1138*
from tracheal intubation, 1252–1253
iatrogenic, 168, 178–181, *178, 180–183*
radiation, 196
without fracture, 163, *163,*
intrusion of, 157, *158,* 166–167, *166*
loss of, and cerebral abscess, 50
malformations of, resembling odontomas, 160–161, *161*
morphologic variations in, and oral injury, 154, *154*
postmortem examination of. See *Odontology, forensic.*
protrusion of, and oral injury, 149, *149*
pulp of, abscess of, 164
calcific degeneration of, 163, *163*
denticles of, 163, *163*
hyperemia of, 163
inflammation of, 163, *163*
necrosis of, 164
polyps of, 163, *163*
stones of, 163, *163*
racial characteristics of, 1119–1122, *1119–1122*
radiography of, postmortem, 1134–1136, *1135, 1136.* See also *Odontology, forensic.*
reimplantation of, 167, *168*
restorations in, and oral injury, 149
faulty, 178, *179*
roots of, arrested formation of, 161–162, *161*
dilaceration of, 161, *161*
fractures of, 157, *158,* 165–166, *165,* 175
iatrogenic, 181
resorption of, 168, 175
and oral injury, 149, *149*

Teeth *(Continued)*
roots of, resorption of, orthodontic treatment and, 179, *180*
sockets of, fractures of, 167, 168–169
supporting bone of, fractures of, 159, *159*
Teichmann's test, for blood stains, 811
Temperature, ambient, and behavior, 1627–1642
and sarcosaprophagous fly development, 1080, *1080*, 1081(t)
body. See *Body temperature.*
ignition, for chemical elements, 730(t)
for inflammable substances, 736–737, 737(t)
Temperature coefficient, of oxidation reaction, 730(t), 731
Temporal bone, fractures of, 62, 136–137
longitudinal, 62
signs of, 38
transverse, 136
mastoid process of, 132
petrous portion of, 132
radiography of, 134
Temporal lobe, herniation of, 49–50, *49*
Temporomandibular joint, injuries of, 171–172
Tendinitis, bicipital, 262
cacareous, of shoulder, 262, *262*
calcific, 285
of hand, 372
of wrist, 279
Tendon(s), electrical injuries of, 655–656
iliopsoas, strain of, 285
inflammation of. See *Tendinitis; Tenosynovitis.*
of ankle, calcification of, 320
injuries of, 319–320
of hand, anatomy of, 365–366, *366*
injuries of, 371–372, *371*
stenosing tenovaginitis of, 383–384
of shoulder, injuries of, 261–265, *262*, *263*
patellar, avulsion of, 301
peroneal, injuries of, 319–320
quadriceps, rupture of, 301
tibial, anterior, rupture of, 320
posterior, dislocation of, 320
Tennis elbow, 271–272
Tenosynovitis, bicipital, 262
of ankle, 319
of foot, 329
of hand, 369
of wrist, 279
Tenovaginitis, stenosing, 383–384
Tension pneumothorax, 201–202
Tentorial pressure cone of Jefferson, 49
Tentorium, laceration of, perinatal, *452*, 454, 454(t)
Teratogen(s), litigation involving, 1617–1626
methotrexate as, 1198–1199
Terminal ballistics, defined, 527
Termites, ingestion of, 1455
Terrestrial venomous snakes, 1437–1444
Test(s). See also names of specific tests.
bacteriologic, at autopsy, 999
biochemical, at autopsy, 999
for bloodstain identification, 810–817
for drowning, 1325–1328
for explosives components, 604–607
for skin metallization, 654
immunologic, for bloodstain identification, 816
in fire investigation, 748–757
in rape victim, 951–955
of sperm motility, in rape victim, 951–952
toxicologic, at autopsy, 999
Testis, infarction of, perinatal, *464*
injuries of, 241
Tetanus, agricultural, 1166
prophylaxis for, malpractice in, 907, 908
Tetracycline, and tooth discoloration, 193, *193*
injury from, injection, 226
legal case involving, 1215
Tetraodon poisoning, 796
Tetraodotoxin, 1418
Thalassemia, and oral injury, 153, *153*
Thermal activation, of oxidizing reactions, 731–732
Thermal burns. See *Burns.*
Thermal homeostasis, 701–702
Thermal injuries. See also *Burns; Hyperthermia; Hypothermia.*
domestic, 889–892, *889*, *891*
of brain, 726
of central nervous system, 726
of endocrine glands, 726
of eye, 119–120
of gastrointestinal tract, 726
of heart, 725
of kidney, 725–726
of liver, 725
of lung, 202, 724–725
of lymphatic system, 725
of musculoskeletal system, 726–727
of spleen, 725
postmortem, 1069–1070
Thermal radiation, injuries from, in bombings, 615–616
in nuclear explosion, 634
Thermal stress, and drug action, 1639–1640
Thermogenic anhydrosis, 704
Thermography, 688
Thermophilia, 497
Thevetia peruviana, 1479–1481, *1480*
Thevotoxin, 1479
Thiaminase, 1550
Thiazide, with allopurinol, effects of, 1201
Thigh, injuries of, 296–300, *299*, *300*
Thiobarbiturates, injury from, in porphyria, 1246
Thioglycolic acid, with potassium permanganate, spontaneous combustion of, 739
Thiopental sodium, injection injury from, 226
and chemical gangrene, 377
Thioridazine, and impotence, 1198
injury from, 1199
of eye, 130
Third ventricle downward shift, 50
Thoracentesis, complications of, 209, 1238
Thoracic aorta, disruption of, 205–206
Thoracic spine, injuries of, 64
fracture-dislocation, 77
Thorax. See *Chest.*
Thorium-228, levels of, in humans, 680
Thorn apple, 1535
Throat, effect of meteorologic stimuli on, 1628–1629(t)
Throatwort, 1532
Thromboembolism. See also *Embolism.*
arterial, 408
posttraumatic, 351–352, 406–409, *408*
pulmonary, 407, *408*
after hip fracture, 888
after spinal cord injury, 83
septic, 16
systemic, 408
Thrombophlebitis, after spinal cord injury, 83
posttraumatic, 351–352
Thrombosis, arterial, arteriography and, 224
from acute injury, 222
from chronic injury, 224–225
cerebral, in children, 59
of coronary artery, trauma and, 13, *15*
of renal vein, perinatal, 462
postoperative, 1229
posttraumatic, 351–352
septic, 408–409
shock and, 13
vascular injury and, 222, 224–225
venous, of hand, 376
perinatal, 458–460
Thrush, 1337
antibiotics and, 188, *189*
Thumb, anatomy of, 366
chemical gangrene of, 377, *378*
dislocations of, 375–376, *375*
fractures of, 374
occupational injuries of, 379–380
trigger, 366
Thunderwood plant, 1477
Thymelaeaceae, toxic, 1546
Thymus, in burn victims, 726
perinatal infarction of, *461*
Thyroid, in burn victims, 726
perinatal infarction of, *465*
plants toxic to, 793(t), 794
surgery of, complications of, 1227
Thyroid stimulating hormone, in postmortem blood, 1039, 1040(t)
Thyroxine, in postmortem blood, 1039, 1040(t)

Tibia, anterior tibial compartment syndrome, in, 314–315, *315*
dislocation of fibula from, 313
fractures of, avulsion, 304
compression, 325–328
in pedestrians, 857
of condyls of, 312–313
of distal end of, *353*
of proximal end of, 312–313
of shaft of, 316–319, *317*
stress, 318–319
traumatic exostoses of, 319
Tibial nerve entrapment, 329
Tibial tendon, anterior, rupture of, 320
posterior, dislocation of, 320
Tick(s), as disease vectors, 1368
bites of, 1451–1452
Tick paralysis, 1452
Tick-borne togavirus infection, 1370
Time bomb, 584–587, *585*, *586*
Tirucallol, 1492
Tissue, cherry-red color of, in carbon monoxide poisoning, 843, *847*
effects of acids on, 127
effects of alkalis on, 127
effects of explosives on, 612–615, *613–615*
effects of radiation on, 681–682
resistance of, to electrical current, 646
Tissue embolism, 416–418, *417*
Titanium tetrachloride, and oral injury, 191, *191*
Toadfish, hazardous, 1415
Tobacco, and oral injury, 191–192, *192*
Tobacco plant, 1538
Toe(s), dislocations of, 331
fractures of, 337
great, fixed ankylosis of, 337
Morton's, 329
neuralgia of, 329
Togavirus infections, tick-borne, 1370
Tomography, 688
Tongue, bites of, 173, *173*
in anesthesia, 184, *184*
in epileptics, 150, *150*
black, hairy, 188
chronic injuries of, 176
hyperkeratosis of, *177*
normal, 148
radiation injury of, *195*
Tongue thrusting, 175
Tools, powder-actuated, 542, *544–545*
power, cartridge-firing, injury from, 552, *554–555*
Toothbrush trauma, 173
Toothpaste, allergy to, 188
Tort. See also *Negligence.*
defined, 692
Torulosis, 1337
Tourniquets, and nerve injury, 373
Toxic amblyopia, 131
Toxic optic neuropathy, 131
Toxicodendron diversilobum, 1474–1477, *1475*
Toxicodendron quercifolium, 1474–1477, *1475*
Toxicodendron radicans, 1474–1477, *1475*
Toxicodendron vernix, 1477
Toxin(s). See also Poison(s); *Poisoning.*
analysis of. See *Toxicologic analysis.*
aspiration of, 1570
autopsy, 999
blood levels of, 1572–1577, 1576(t), *1577*, 1578(t)–1580(t)
burn, 722
chemistry of, 1382–1383, 1384, 1395
fish, endogenous, 1417–1420, *1417*, *1419*
exogenous, 1420–1426, *1421–1424*
food poisoning from, 795–796
stinging, 1409, 1410, 1411, 1412, 1414–1415
food-borne, 787–799, 1588–1613. See also *Food poisoning.*
fungal, 1456–1557, 1469(t)–1470(t)
food poisoning by, 790–793, 791(t)
ingestion of, 1569–1570, 1570(t)
inhalation of, 1570
injection of, 1572
injury from. See *Poisoning.*
marine animal, 1388–1389
food poisoning from, 795–796
mold, 791–793, 791(t)
percutaneous absorption of, 1572
pharmacology of, 1385
plant, 1456–1557, 1465(t)–1470(t)
food poisoning by, 793–795, 793(t), 1459–1461
rectal administration of, 1572
sea urchin, 1404–1406, *1404–1405*
shellfish, 795, 1398–1400, *1398–1399*
Toxicologic analysis, 800–809
in carbon monoxide poisoning, 804–805, 846–848, *847*, 848(t)
in chemical poisoning, 804–807, 1572–1577, 1576(t)
in drug death, 836–837
in sudden infant death, 1026
interpretation of results of, 808
of postmortem blood, 999
of postmortem cerebrospinal fluid, 999
of postmortem vitreous humor, 1056
postmortem, 999
preautopsy, 802
report of, as evidence, 808–809
specimens for, collection of, 802–807, *803*
information to accompany, 807–808
marking of, 807
submission of, to laboratory, 808
Toxicology, forensic, 800–809, 999, 1568–1586
Toxicology laboratory, 800–809
Toxoplasmosis, 1350, 1376
Trachea, foreign bodies in, 207
injuries of, 203
iatrogenic, 1254
thermal, 724
postmortem findings in, in burn victims, 724
radiography of, 688
Tracheal intubation, in anesthesia, complications of, 1251–1256
sequelae of, 1254–1255
in facial injury, 140, 143
Tracheobronchial tree. See also *Lung.*
disruption of, 203
foreign bodies in, 207–208
inhalation injuries of. See *Inhalation injuries.*
thermal injuries of, 202, 724–725
Tracheostomy, in facial injury, 140, 143
Traction injury, of brachial plexus, 261, *261*
of nerves, 68, 261, *261*
of spine, perinatal, 443–446, *443–445*
Tractor accidents, 1163–1164, *1164*
Traffic accidents. See *Automobile accidents.*
Trains, injury from, 1186–1191
in train-automobile accidents, 858
Trajectory, of projectile, 528, *528*
Tranquilizers, and impotence, 1198
effects of, 829
injury from, 1581–1583
of eye, 129
Transaminase, in postmortem blood, 1038
Transfusion. See *Blood transfusion.*
Transient traumatic occipital blindness, 62
Transitional resistance, to electrical current, 646
Transplants, organ, 978–994
and body image, 990–994
donation for, compulsory, 982–985
definition of death for, 23
determination of death for, 973–974
legal alternatives for, 980–985
statutes for, 972–973, 974(t), 978–980
reform of, 980–985
voluntary, proposals for, 981–982
emotional sequelae of, 990–994
experimental, 1236
tissue, 986
Uniform Anatomical Gift Act for, 972–973, 974(t), 987
Transsexualism, 969
Transvestism, 959, *962*
Trauma, aggravating preexisting conditions, 9–20
and cancer, 18–20, 417–418
of brain, 58
and coagulopathy, 13
and heart disease, 12–17
and infection, 9–12, *9*

Trauma *(Continued)*
and fetal injuries, 429–433
and peripheral vascular disease, 16, 17, *16, 17*
and pregnancy complications, 429–433
and spontaneous abortion, 430–433
and thrombosis, 13, *15*
biochemical response to, 391–392, *392*
cellular response to, 391–392, *392*
complications of, 8–20
defined, 3
evolutionary history of, 3
hyperdynamic state in, 388–389
in pregnancy, 423–495
mortality in, 8
neurohormonal response to, 386–387
perinatal, 436–486
prevention of, 20–21
psychologic response to, 17–18. See also *Psychologic reaction.*
systemic response to, 386–405
treatment of, 21. See also *Emergency treatment.*
Traumatic aneurysms, 225
of brain, 47
of hand, 376–377, *377*
Traumatic arteriovenous fistulae, 225–226
Traumatic asphyxia, 203
Traumatic shock, hemorrhage and, 387–388
hyperdynamic state in, 388–389
Travel, during pregnancy, 423–424
Treatment, of injuries. See *Emergency treatment.*
Tree tobacco, 1537–1538
Tremetol, 1484
Trench foot, 766–767
Treponema pallidum, 10
Triamcinolone, injury from, legal case involving, 1212–1213
Trichinosis, 1356–1357
Trichloroethylene, food contamination by, 789–790
Trichomonad vaginitis, 1349–1350
Trichotillomania, 497
Trichuriasis, 1355–1356
Trifluoperazine, injury from, legal case involving, 1213
Trigeminal nerve injury, in head injury, 62
Trigger finger, 366
Trigonelline, 1530
Triparanol, injury from, legal case involving, 1216
Tripod fracture, 146
Trismus, defined, 143
Trochanter, fractures of, 296
Trochlea, humeral, fracture of, 275
ocular, anatomy of, 115, *115*
detachment of, 116
Trochlear nerve, injury of, 62
Trockenes Ödem, 1324
Tromp's waterbath test, 1633
Tropical anhydrotic asthenia, 704
Trumpet flower, 1539
Trypanosomiasis, 1352–1353, *1353*, 1375
Tryptophan, 1550
Tsetse flies, 1367
Tubercle bacilli, 1339–1340
and wound infection, 10
Tuberculoma, local, 10
Tuberculosis, altitude and, 1306
drugs for, injury from, 1199
from cadavers, 908–909
Tularemia, 1373
Tumbling, of bullet, 515
Tumor, benign, traumatic conversion of, to malignant tumor, 19
malignant. See also *Cancer; Carcinoma.*
altitude and, 1306
metastasis of, trauma and, 417–418
of brain, head injury and, 58
radiation and, 684
odontogenic, malformations resembling, 160–161, *161*
pregnancy, 176, *177*
signal, in occupational-environmental disease, 1275–1276
Tumor cell embolus, 417–418, *417*
Tung nut plant, 1491
Tung oil tree, 1491
Turban shells, toxic, 1401, *1401*
Turbojet accidents, 876–879, *878, 879*
Turtles, marine, poisonous, 1427–1428, *1428*
Tuw-tua, 1498–1499
Tympanic membrane, rupture of, 135
in dysbarism, 637
in explosions, 619
Typhoid carriers, 1601–1602, 1604–1605
Typhoid fever, 1601, 1604–1605
Typhus, murine, 1372
scrub, 1372
Tyramine, 1488, 1520

Ulcer(s), corneal, 96, 124
Curling's, 396, *398*, 726
Cushing's, 396–397
decubitus, after spinal cord injury, 83
dystrophic, 16
gastric, cryotherapy for, injury from, 769
gastroduodenal, posttraumatic, 395–397, *397, 398*
in burn injury, 396, *398*, 726
Marjolin's, 371
neurogenic, 396–397
peptic, after spinal cord injury, 84
radiation and, 682, 683
stress, 8, 395–397, *397*, 398
hypothermia and, 760, 764, *764*
Wischnevsky, 760, 764, *764*
Ulcerative colitis, drugs for, side effects of, 1201–1202
Ulna, fractures of, 278
in Monteggia fracture-dislocation, 276–277, *277*
Ulna *(Continued)*
fractures of, of coronoid process of, 276
of olecranon of, 275
of proximal end of, 276–277, *277*
of styloid process of, 284
Ulnar artery, injury of, 385
thrombosis of, in hand injury, 376
Ulnar nerve, anatomy of, in hand, 367–368
entrapment of, 280, 373
Ultrasonography, 688
Ultrasound, diagnostic, A-mode scan in, 776, *777, 779*
B-mode scan in, 776–777, *778*
imaging in, 776–778, *777–780*
instrumentation in, 775–776, *776*
M-scan in, 777–778, *779*
obstetrical, *776*, 778, *780*
safety of, 781
pelvic, *776*, 778, *780*
safety of, 779–781, 782
time-motion study in, 777–778, *779*
types of, *776–780*, 778
medical applications of, 775–783
physics of, 775
therapeutic, and cataract, 120
injury from, 781–782
of eye, 120
Ultraviolet radiation, non-solar, eye injury from, 123
Umbelliferae, toxic, 1546–1547
Umbilical cord, and fetal injury, *457*
Unconsciousness. See *Loss of consciousness.*
Uniform Anatomical Gift Act, 972–973, 974(t), 987
Universal system, of dental charting, 1133, *1133*
Upper extremity. See *Arm;* and names of specific parts.
Urea, in postmortem blood, 1035, *1036*
in postmortem cerebrospinal fluid, 1044
in postmortem vitreous humor, 1047–1048, *1048*
Uremia, posttraumatic, 400
Ureter, catheterization of, in ureteral surgery, 235
injuries of, 232–236
radiography of, 688
surgery of, complications of, 1234
Urethra, injury from, in catheterization, 239
in pelvic injury, 341
strictures of, posttraumatic, 238
Urethritis, 1349–1350
Urethrography, retrograde, in genitourinary injuries, 228
Urethrovaginal fistula, posttraumatic, 238
Uric acid, in postmortem blood, 1036
in postmortem cerebrospinal fluid, 1044
in postmortem vitreous humor, 1048
Urinary bladder. See *Bladder.*

Urinary tract, cancer of, after spinal cord injury, 84
in musculoskeletal injuries, 351
injuries of, in pelvic injury, 341, 344
radiography of, 687, 688
surgery of, complications of, 1234
Urinary tract infections, after spinal cord injury, 82–83
protozoan, 1349–1350
Urination, after spinal cord injury, 79
Urine, absence of, posttraumatic, 351
collection of, for postmortem toxicologic examination, 999
decreased, posttraumatic, 8
in genitourinary injuries, 227–228
postmortem, analysis of, 1053
toxicologic examination of, 804
Urobilinogen, in postmortem cerebrospinal fluid, 1045
Urography, 687, 688
Urologic surgery, ureteral injury in, 234
urethral injury in, 239
Urtica dioica, 1548
Urtica gracilis, 1548–1549
Urticaceae, toxic, 1547–1549
Urticaria, cold, 765
Urticin, 1548
Uterus, anatomy and physiology of, 248
cervix of. See *Cervix, uterine.*
injuries of, 255–257
in abortion, 255–256
pregnant, firearm wounds of, 429
radiography of, 688
rupture of, in automobile accidents, 424–425
stab wounds of, 429
ultrasonic scanning of, *776*, 778, *780*, 781
surgery of, complications of, 1233
Uveal tract. See also *Choroid; Ciliary body; Iris.*
anatomy of, 103
injuries of, 104–105, *104*, 108–109
drug-induced, 129
Uveitis, chronic, 105, 111
in sympathetic ophthalmitis, 111–112
posttraumatic, 104

Vaccine, oral polio, injury from, legal case involving, 1213
Vacuum equipment, laboratory, injury from, 1178
Vagina, anatomy and physiology of, 246–248, *246–248*
examination of, in rape victim, 947–951
injuries of, 248–255, 249(t)
chemical, 253–255
in rape victim, 950
non-sex-related, 252–255
sex-related, 248–252
surgery of, complications of, 1233–1234
Vaginismus, 946
Vaginitis, trichomonad, 1349–1350
Vagus nerve, injury of, 63
Valves, of heart, posttraumatic infection of, 16, *16*
Vancomycin, and ear injury, 137
Vapors. See *Gas(es).*
Vapor sensing tubes, for fire investigation, 746, *747*
Vapor analysis, of explosives, 607–608, *608*
Varicose veins, stripping of, complications of, 1229
Vascular complications, of musculoskeletal injuries, 351–352
Vascular disease, peripheral, trauma aggravating, 16, *16*, 17, *17*
Vascular injuries, 221–227
acute, 222–224
amputation rates in, 222
and nerve injury, 69
chemical gangrene in, 377, *378*
chronic, 224–226
electrical, 639, 657
from anesthetic injection, 905, *905*
from arteriography, 224
from axillary crutches, 224
from illicit drug injection, 833
from physical exertion, 17
hypothermic, 765, 766
iatrogenic, 224, 377, *378*, 379, 905, *905*
in brain concussion, 42
in fractures and dislocations, 233–234
in pelvic fractures, 344
in renal pedicle injuries, 229–230
of brain, 42–45, *42–44*
electrical, 659
of hand, 225, 376–379, *377*, *378*
perinatal, 456–484, 465(t)
radiation, 682, 683
Vascular surgery, ureteral injury in, 234
Vascularization, posttraumatic. See *Neovascularization.*
Vasculitis, cold, 765
Vasoactive amines, extraction of, for wound timing, 26, 28
techniques for, 27
Vasodilators, effects of, 1202
Vasomotor paralysis, after nerve injury, 69
Vasopressor amines, and kidney injury, 401
Vastus intermedius, injuries of, 301
Vastus lateralis, injuries of, 301
Vastus medialis, injuries of, 301
Vehicular accidents, 853–864. See also *Automobile accidents.*
Veins, foreign bodies in, 208
injuries of. See *Vascular injuries.*
radiography of, 688–689
surgery of, complications of, 1229
varicose, stripping of, complications of, 1229
Venereal disease, prophylaxis for, in rape victim, 956
Venerupin toxin, 1400
Venography, iatrogenic hand injuries in, 379
Venom poisoning, 1437–1441
Venous infarction, in perinatal hypoxia, 458–459
Ventilation, mechanical, in anesthesia, complications of, 1256
Ventricle thickness, altitude and, 1298–1299, *1299*
Ventricular failure, posttraumatic, 398–400
Ventricular fibrillation in drowning, 1322
in electrical injury, 649–650, 649(t)
in hypothermia, 760
Ventriculography, 688
Veratrum album, 1516
Veratrum californicum, 1517–1518
Veratrum viride, 1516
Verbenaceae, toxic, 1549–1550
Vertebrae. See *Spine.*
Vertebral artery, puncture of, in cervical disk surgery, 67
rupture of, in spinal injury, 64
Vertical compression, of spine, 64
Vertigo. See also *Equilibrium.*
after head injury, 136
Vesication, in second-degree burns, 720, *721*
Vessels, blood. See *Blood vessels.*
Vestibular system. See *Ear, inner.*
Vestibulocochlear nerve, auditory portion of, 132
injury of, 62
Veterinary slaughtering guns, injuries from, 525–526
Viability, of fetus. See *Fetus, viability of.*
Vibrational stress, ocular effects of, 128
Vibrio parahaemolyticus food poisoning, 1611
Vicarious liability, in malpractice, 1653
in medical partnership, 1653
Viomycin, and ear injury, 137
Viral hepatitis, from cadavers, 909
Viral infections, 1369–1370
arthropod borne, 1370–1371
Virginity and vulvovaginal injuries, 249–250
Viscum album, 1521
Vision, double, in orbital fractures, 117, 146
in orbital hemorrhage, 116
Visual disorders, after head injury, 62
Visual loss, acceleration and, 128
corneal edema and, 93
drug-induced, 130
head injury and, 62
in intraorbital hemorrhage, 116
in optic nerve injury, 118
in oxygen deprivation, 128
in toxic amblyopia, 131
in toxic optic neuropathy, 131
vibrational stress and, 128
Vital injury. See *Antemortem wound.*
Vital reaction, defined, 23
negative, 25

Vital reaction *(Continued)*
positive, 25
systemic, 23
Vital wound. See *Antemortem wound.*
Vitamin A, injury from, 1428–1429
Vitamin C, injury from, 1197
Vitamin D, injury from, 1197–1198
Vitamin E, in postmortem blood, 1039
Vitreous humor, anatomy of, 107
detachment of, 107
fibrosis in, 107, *108*
hemorrhage in, 107
infection in, 107
injuries of, 107–108, *108*
postmortem, alcohol in, 1051, *1052*
amino acids in, 1048–1049
analysis of, 1033, 1046–1052, *1047, 1048, 1051*
barbiturates in, 1051
bilirubin in, 1049
carbohydrates in, 1046–1047, *1047*
collection of, 1052–1053
drugs in, 1051–1052
electrolytes in, 1049–1050, *1051*
enzymes in, 1048
nitrogenous compounds in, 1047–1048, *1048*
osmolality of, 1050
proteins in, 1048–1049
toxicologic analysis of, 1051–1052, *1052*, 1056
syneresis of, 107
Volkmann's contracture, 69, 349, 377–378, *378*
Voltage, electrical, 646
Volvulus, altitude and, 1306
Vomitwort plant, 1483
Voyeurism, 959
Vulva, anatomy of, 244–245, *244, 245*
injuries of, 248–255, 249(t)
chemical, 253–255
non-sex-related, 252–255
sex-related, 248–252

Wad, shotshell, 511, 551
as evidence, 563
patterns made by, 568
types of, 568–569, *569*
War injuries, burns as, 718
War neurosis, 17
Warning of risk, by manufacturer, 1659
by physician, 1654–1655, 1669–1674
Warranty, breach of, in products liability, 1659–1660
treatment failure as, 693
in products liability, 1621–1623
Wartweed, 1494–1495, 1522–1523
Washerwoman's skin, 1319, *1319*
Water, with silver nitrate and magnesium, spontaneous combustion of, 739
Water Accident Investigation Team, 638–639
Water celery, 1527
Water jet equipment, injury from, 1172–1173
Water skiing, vulvovaginal injuries in, 253
Waterbath test of Tromp, 1633
Waves, injury from. See *Radiation, injuries from.*
shock. See *Shock wave.*
Weapons, automatic, 542
projectile. See *Firearms.*
Weather, effect of, on accidents, 1635–1637
on behavior, 1627–1642
on body, 1627–1633, 1628–1629(t), 1630–1632(t). See also *Hyperthermia; Hypothermia.*
on diseases, 1639
on mental processes, 1633–1637
on suicide, 1637–1639
foehn, 1634
Weathering, of corpse, 1070–1071, *1071*
Weaver's bottom, 285, 349
Weeds, contaminating foods, 1457
Weeverfish, 1411
Weil's disease, 1185
Welders, cataract in, 662
eye injury in, 662
photophthalmia in, 123
Wet lung, 392
Whelk poisoning, 1401
Whiplash injury, 63
temporomandibular joint symptoms in, 171–172
Whipworm infection, 1355–1356
White cedar, 1521–1522
White sanicle plant, 1484–1485
White snakeroot plant, 1484–1485
White thoroughwort plant, 1485
Wilder's law of initial value, 1628
Wild potato plant, 1544
Wild tobacco plant, 1484
Wine plant, 1524–1525
Winter sweet plant, 1477–1478
Wiring, electrical, overloading of, causing fires, 739–740
Wischnevsky ulcers, 760, 764, *764*
Wistarin, 1512
Wisteria, 1457, 1512
Wisteria chinensis, 1512
Wisteria floribunda, 1512
Wisteria sinensis, 1512
Wistin, 1512
Witness, expert. See *Expert witness.*
Wolf's milk plant, 1494–1495
Wolfsbane, 1525
Women, firearm injury in, 897
genital tract of. See *Genitals, female.*
identification of blood stains from, 812
identification of skeletal remains of, 1106–1108, 1106(t)
meteorologic stress and, 1628, 1630
orgasm in, after spinal cord injury, 81
postmenopausal vaginal injuries in, 250
Women *(Continued)*
pregnant, drug administration in, 1199–1200
injuries in, electrical, 663, 670
in automobile accidents, 424–425
medicolegal considerations in, 429–433
shock in, and fetal death, 427
ultrasonic scanning in, *776*, 778, *780*
safety of, 781
uterus in. See *Uterus, pregnant.*
rape of. See *Rape.*
skeletal characteristics of, 1106–1108, 1106(t)
ureteral injuries in, 233–234
urethral injuries in, 239
virginal, vulvovaginal injuries in, 249–250
Woolly worm, toxic, 1449
Workmen's compensation, autopsy requirement for, 1675–1680
disability evaluation for, 354–355
Worms, parasitic, infection from, 1355–1366, *1359–1361*
marine, 1389–1390
Wounds, 3–22. See also *Injury;* and names of specific organs or body parts.
age of. See *Wound, timing of.*
antemortem. See *Antemortem wound.*
deep, 5, *5*
firearm. See *Firearms wounds.*
hesitation, 1005
identification of, in skeletal remains, 1113, *1113*
incised, 6
infection of. See *Wound infection.*
laceration, 6–7. See also *Lacerations.*
leukocytic infiltration of, 23
patterned, *6*, 7
penetrating, 5, *5*, 7. See also *Penetrating injuries.*
postmortem vs. antemortem, 22
puncture, 7
stab, 7. See also *Stab wounds.*
stages of healing in, 24
superficial, 5
timing of, 22–28
antemortem, 22
at autopsy, 998
by biochemical examination, 26
by clinical examination, 22
by histochemical examination, 24, *25*
by histologic examination, 23
clinical signs for, 22
histamine analysis for, 1096
in brain, 55–56
serotonin analysis for, 1096
types of, 5–9
vital. See *Antemortem wounds.*
Wound ballistics, defined, 527
Wound formation, and Hooke's law of elasticity, 5
Wound infection, 9–12
after spinal surgery, 66
and timing of wound, 22, 24

Wound infection *(Continued)*
causes of, 10
soil as, 10
incubation period for, 10
occupational hazards of, 10
primary, 11
secondary, 11
systemic infection from, 10–11
Wound man, 30, *31*
Wrasse, ciguateric, *1423*
Wringer injuries, of forearm, 277–278
Wrist, calcification in, 279
injuries of, 278–285, *281–284*
cartilaginous, 279
dislocation, 280–281, *281*
fracture, 281–285, *282–284*
iatrogenic, 280
soft-tissue, 278–280
sprain, 278–279
fractures misdiagnosed as, 284–285
Wrongful death statutes, and fetal death, 430, 488–491
Wrongful life, cause of action for, 491–493
Wuchereriasis, 1364–1365

Xanthine, in postmortem cerebrospinal fluid, 1044
Xeroradiography, 688
Xonics radiography, 687
X-rays, 680
diagnostic, use of, 686–687, *686*. See also *Radiography*.
in radiation therapy, 690. See also *Radiation therapy*.
injuries from. See *Radiation injuries*.

Y fracture, of proximal end of tibia, 313
Yellow fever, 1371
Yellow oleander plant, 1479–1481, *1480*
Yellow rattlebox plant, 1511–1512
Yew, 1544–1545
Yuca plant, 1500–1501

Zamia floridana, 1488–1489, *1489*
Zamia integrifolia, 1488–1489, *1489*
Zigadenus, 1518
Zoanthus, 1388, *1388*
Zones, of antemortem wound, 25, *25*
Zoonoses, 1369–1377
Zygadenine, 1518
Zygadenus, 1518
Zygoma, fractures of, 146
racial differences in, 1108(t), 1109–1110, *1110*